AF771528

Clinical Geropsychology

Clinical Geropsychology

Editor
Barry Edelstein
West Virginia University, Morgantown, WV, USA

Comprehensive Clinical Psychology Editors-in-Chief
Alan S. Bellack
The University of Maryland at Baltimore, MD, USA
Michel Hersen
Pacific University, Forest Grove, OR, USA

Comprehensive Clinical Psychology
Volume 7

2001

AN IMPRINT OF ELSEVIER SCIENCE

AMSTERDAM—LONDON—NEW YORK—OXFORD—PARIS—SHANNON—TOKYO

Elsevier Science Ltd., The Boulevard, Langford Lane, Kidlington, Oxford, OX5 1GB, UK

First edition 1998
Paperback edition 2001

Library of Congress Cataloging in Publication Data
Comprehensive clinical psychology / editors-in-chief. Alan S. Bellack, Michel Hersen. —1st ed.
p. cm.
Includes indexes.
Contents: v. 1. Foundations / volume editor, C. Eugene Walker — v. 2. Professional issues / volume editor, Arthur N. Wiens — v. 3. Research and Methods / volume editor, Nina R. Schooler — v. 4. Assessment / volume editor, Cecil R. Reynolds — v. 5. Children & adolescents / volume editor, Thomas Ollendick — v. 6. Adults / volume editor, Paul Salkovskis — v. 7. Clinical geropsychology / volume editor, Barry Edelstein — v. 8. Health psychology / volume editors, Derek W. Johnston and Marie Jonhston — v. 9. Applications in diverse populations / volume editor, Nirbhay N. Singh — v. 10. Sociocultural and individual differences / volume editor, Cynthia D. Belar — v. 11. Indexes.
1. Clinical psychology. I. Bellack, Alan S. II. Hersen, Michel.
[DNLM: 1. Psychology, Clinical. WM 105 C737 1998]
RC467.C597 1998
616.89--dc21
DNLM/DLC
for Library of Congress 97-50185
CIP

British Library Cataloguing in Publication Data
Comprehensive clinical psychology
1. Clinical psychology
II. Bellack, Alan S. (Alan Scott), 1944- II. Hersen, Michel
616.8 ' 9

ISBN 0-08-042707-3 (set : alk. paper)
ISBN 0-08-043146-1 (Volume 7)
ISBN 0-08-044069-X (Volume 7 paperback)

∞™ The paper used in this publication meets the minimum requirements of the American National Standard for Information Sciences—Permanence of Paper for Printed Library Materials, ANSI Z39.48–1984.

Typeset by Bibliocraft, Dundee, UK.
Printed and bound in The Netherlands by Giethoorn Media Group.

Contents

Introduction to *Comprehensive Clinical Psychology*

Co-Editors-in-Chief

Alan S. Bellack and Michel Hersen

Background

Clinical psychology is a relatively new field. While its roots can be traced back to at least the late nineteenth century, its evolution as a distinct academic discipline and profession dates only to the Second World War. The first 20 years of this postwar period saw steady, albeit nonspectacular, growth. Based substantially in the United States and Europe during this period, the study of clinical psychology developed as an alternative to medical school and psychiatry for many students interested in clinical service careers or the scientific study of human behavior. Postgraduate training was conducted exclusively in large university psychology departments within a strict scientist–practitioner model. The total number of Ph.D. candidates admitted to graduate school programs each year was relatively small; there were fewer than 50 accredited programs in the United States during much of this period, each admitting only 5–10 students. The number of new Ph.D.'s produced each year was substantially less, as many students failed to complete the rigorous scientific requirements of these elite programs. Career opportunities were similarly delimited, due in no small part to restraints on clinical practice imposed by psychiatrists and other physicians. The dominant form of psychotherapy was psychoanalysis, and psychologists were either excluded from psychoanalytic institutes or trained only as lay analysts who were proscribed from clinical practice. Few jurisdictions awarded licenses for independent practice, and psychologists generally were not reimbursed for their activities unless they worked under the direction of a physician. A sizable minority of clinical psychologists followed their mentors into university positions, teaching and conducting research. The majority, who were more interested in clinical service, opted for work in large psychiatric or Veterans Administration hospitals, where the modal activity was psychological testing; verbal psychotherapy was provided at the discretion of medical supervisors. A gradually increasing number of psychologists elected to be in private practice, where there was a greater professional autonomy. Medical hegemony over services for psychiatric disorders was even greater in Europe and Latin America.

The last 30 years has witnessed a massive change in the profession, stimulated by a number of scientific, clinical, and economic factors. Psychoanalysis gradually fell out of favor due to a dearth of data on its effectiveness and a desire for shorter term treatments that were not the primary purview of psychiatrists. First, client-centered therapy and then behavior therapy emerged as brief, highly effective alternatives. The former was entirely a product of clinical psychology, and was the intellectual and technical forebear of the current mandate for empirical evaluation of psychotherapies.

Carl Rogers, his colleagues, and students were the first to demonstrate the feasibility of careful, objective evaluation of the therapy process as well as outcome. While behavior therapy owes much of its legacy to psychiatrists such as Joseph Wolpe, it was substantially a product of academic psychologists searching for an approach with a strong scientific underpinning (in this case learning theory) that could be subjected to rigorous scientific scrutiny. Early behavior therapy emerged simultaneously in the UK and the US: in the UK psychologists such as Hans Eysenck based their work on Pavlov and classical conditioning, while in the US researchers were following Skinner and operant conditioning theories. The two schools merged with cognitive therapy, developed largely by Beck and Ellis through the 1960s, when the limitations of behavior therapy in isolation became apparent, particulary with depressed patients, and cognitive-behavior therapy is now widely practised.

Behavior therapy and cognitive-behavior therapy have not only proven themselves to be effective with a broad array of disorders, they have since been shown to be very successful alternatives to pharmacotherapy as well. Notably, behavior therapy was able to produce significant changes in populations that had previously been warehoused as untreatable, including people with physical and developmental disabilities and schizophrenia. Many of the most important contributions to the behavior therapies came from the UK, The Netherlands, South Africa, Australia, and Scandinavia, providing a tremendous stimulus for the development of clinical psychology globally. The availability of cost-effective, scientifically sound nonmedical treatments has decreased the medical monopoly of psychiatric/mental health services around the world and fostered the evolution of clinical psychology as a legally sanctioned helping profession, as well as a prestigious scientific discipline.

Scientific advances in our understanding of the brain and the role of psychosocial factors in physical health and illness have led to the development of two other rapidly growing subspecialties of clinical psychology: neuropsychology and health psychology. Novel assessment and treatment technologies in these two areas have created professional opportunities for clinical psychologists in medical schools, general medical hospitals, and other nonpsychiatric settings. Clinical psychologists can now be found conducting research and providing services in departments of neurology and neurosurgery, medicine, cardiac surgery, pediatrics, anesthesiology, oncology, and other medical specialty areas, as well as in the traditional psychiatric settings. They increasingly serve as directors of governmental agencies and service facilities. They comprise a large percentage of research grant recipients in the US, Canada, and the UK, and sit on prestigious government and foundation review boards. In fact the field has earned sufficient public recognition that it now has the somewhat dubious distinction of having clinical psychologists as lead characters on television shows and in cinema.

Stimulated, in part, by these exciting developments in scientific progress and clinical creativity, the field has grown geometrically in the past two decades. Psychology is now the second leading undergraduate major in the US and is increasingly popular elsewhere in the world as well. There are now more than 175 doctoral programs in the United States, each admitting many more students per annum than the 5–10 that has been typical of traditional scientist–practitioner Ph.D. programs over the past 25 years. Some of these schools have entering classes as large as 200 per year. Moreover, along with the professional school movement, which began in the 1970s, a new degree, the Psy.D. (or Doctorate in Psychology), is regularly being offered as an alternative to the Ph.D. Basically a professional rather than an academic degree, the Psy.D. is reflective of the local practitioner–scientist model rather than the scientist–practitioner.

Yet another trend in the field is the proliferation of master's level psychologists, specifically trained to carry out some of the more mundane functions formerly implemented by doctoral level psychologists. Indeed, each year in the United States alone 10 000 new master's level psychologists graduate from university programs. The financial and programmatic implication of such large numbers is obvious.

Statistics are not readily available about the size of the profession in all regions of the globe, but anecdotal evidence supports the hypothesis that the field is growing worldwide. As previously indicated, behavioral and cognitive-behavioral therapies owe a substantial debt to scientists and clinicians from Europe, Australia, and South Africa. There are now enough cognitive-behavior therapists to support national societies in most Western European countries, as well as Asia, Australia, and Latin America. Many of the most important developments in the psychosocial treatment of severe and persistent mental illness in the last decade have come from the United Kingdom, Australia, Switzerland, and Germany. Psychologists in Scandinavia, the United Kingdom, and the Netherlands have played a central role in the development of cognitive-behavioral treatments for anxiety and depression, and there have also been notable contributions from these regions to health psychology. As the hold of psychoanalytic therapies on psychiatric treatment in Europe continues its inevitable decline, there will be increasing opportunities for clinical psychologists to provide shorter term behavioral and cognitive-behavioral treatments. In addition, exciting developments are also emerging from Japan, China, and other countries in the Pacific rim. It seems likely that the global influence of regional approaches and thinking will lead to a more multicultural and universal psychology than has been the case in the past.

The scientific and clinical literatures have burgeoned along with the number of clinical psychologists in the world. This has been an era of rapid growth of knowledge and increasing specialization. General topics, such as psychological assessment, clinical child psychology, and psychotherapy, that used to merit only one or two graduate courses to establish expertise, have expanded and are subdivided to the extent that circumscribed specialty areas, such as neuropsychology, geropsychology, behavioral pediatrics, or cognitive-behavior therapy for depression can each require postdoctoral training. Consequently, hundreds of undergraduate, graduate, and professional level texts are published each year. Specialty journals abound. Where a few key generalist journals such as the *Journal of Consulting and Clinical Psychology* used to represent the entire field, each subdiscipline now has multiple journals, and there are both national journals (e.g., the *British Journal of Clinical Psychology*, the *British Journal of Health Psychology*, the *Australian Journal of Cognitive and Behavioral Therapy*) and journals representing specific populations or disorders (e.g., *Addictive Behaviors*, *Journal of Family Violence*, *Journal of Clinical Geropsychology*), or domains of practice (e.g., *Journal of Clinical Psychology in Medical Setting*). Specialization has made it difficult for professionals to keep abreast of developments within their immediate areas of expertise, and impossible for them to be conversant with the literature in other areas. Moreover, given the plethora of choices, it is also virtually impossible for either students or professionals to know where to find the most accurate, up-to-date information in most areas.

The combination of a large and increasing number of students and professionals, and rapidly growing scientific and clinical literature, makes this a particularly appropriate time for *Comprehensive Clinical Psychology*. This multivolume work encompasses the entire field, and represents a single source of information on the scientific status of clinical psychology and its subspecialties, on theory, and on clinical techniques. The work covers the history of the field, and current thinking about training, professional standards and practices, and sociocultural factors in mental health and illness.

Genesis of Comprehensive Clinical Psychology

Following preliminary conceptual discussions between Elsevier Science and Alan S. Bellack at several international conferences in 1994, Michel Hersen was asked to join as Co-Editor-in-Chief. The first official planning meeting for the project took place in June 1995. In addition to Elsevier Science staff, Alan S. Bellack and Michel Hersen invited Tom Ollendick, Nina Schooler, and Warren Tryon to serve as consultants. At that meeting, the philosophical and international scope of the project was agreed upon and established, with the scientific underpinnings of the field identified as the model. The objective here was to ensure that chapters reflect our core knowledge and that the material stand the test of time.

At that meeting, we also underscored that since clinical psychology was now an international discipline, the work should reflect contributions at the cross-cultural level, with chapters solicited from eminent psychologists worldwide. Although it was acknowledged that the United States was in the forefront of the field, the work could not simply represent the American perspective but to the extent possible would represent diversity at its best. Consistent with the international perspective, at the initial planning meeting, the importance of having an Honorary International Editorial Advisory Board comprised of international representatives was acknowledged, and the 10 specific volumes to comprise *Comprehensive Clinical Psychology* were identified. Preliminary outlines for each volume were developed and volumes editors were considered.

The international perspective was to be reflected at a tripartite level. First, diversity among editors and contributors for their respective volumes was selected as a goal. Second, chapters in each volume were designed to reflect diversity by providing the reader with worldwide examples, not simply the Anglo-Saxon view. Of course, where basic facts and principles were the same, there was no need to present regional diversity. Third, and related to the first two parts, the Honorary International Editorial Advisory Board provided us with an international perspective on overall organization and specifics for the individual volumes.

Between June and October 1995, Alan S. Bellack and Michel Hersen, in consultation with Elsevier Science, invited the ten volume editors to assume their positions, and a meeting of the Editors-in-Chief, the ten volume editors (C. Eugene Walker, Arthur N. Wiens, Nina R. Schooler, Cecil R. Reynolds, Thomas Ollendick, Paul Salkovskis, Barry Edelstein, Marie Johnston and Derek W. Johnston, Nirbhay N. Singh, and Cynthia D. Belar), and Elsevier Science staff was convened in October of that year. At that meeting, each of the volume editors presented his or her conception of the relevant volume, and the nature of coverage and particular contributors was discussed at length. Most of all the philosophical underpinnings of the work were stressed so as to insure intervolume consistency.

Subsequent to the October 1995 meeting, the enormous work to bring this project to fruition began, with potential authors invited to contribute, manuscripts reviewed, and then edited. Were it not for the wonders of electronic communication, a project of this scope would not have been possible, especially given the international aspects involved. A lengthy series of checks and balances was instituted to guarantee the quality and excellence of each contribution. The volume editor first approved each contributor's chapter outline, followed by editing and approval of the text. This process frequently required several revisions. The Co-Editor-in-Chief then reviewed each chapter for scope, level, and overlap, but only after the volume editor had first verified the accuracy of references cited. After the Co-Editor-in-Chief's labors, the manuscript was reviewed by Elsevier staff for format, writing style, reference checking, and other technical issues.

Aims and Scope

The final organization and contents of the work evolved over a series of discussions between the Editors-in-Chief, the volume editors, and Elsevier Science. It was comparatively easy to select the primary domains that needed to be covered: history, treatment, assessment, research, training, and professional issues. It was also comparatively easy to identify the first two-thirds, or so, of specific topics that required chapter-length coverage: treatment of the primary *DSM/ICD* disorders, basic research strategies, standard assessment techniques, etc. However, organizing the vast set of requisite topics into coherent volumes, determining which topics warranted independent chapters, and assigning page limits to individual chapters proved to be daunting. Two broad organizational themes immediately suggested themselves: a focus on core themes or techniques across populations vs. integrated coverage of populations. For example, the former would have entailed volumes on treatment modalities, such as behavior therapy, as they are applied to children and adults, while the latter would call for separate volumes on children and adults that covered diverse approaches. To complicate matters, some topics, such as Research Methods and Professional Issues, do not lend themselves to breakdown by population, and others, such as Behavioral Medicine, do not lend themselves to a breakdown by themes or techniques. Volume length was also an important factor, making some content-based solutions less practical than others. For example, we determined that treatment should receive more attention than assessment; a strict population-based solution would have led to separate short volumes on assessment of adults and children. Ultimately, we opted for an organizational structure that balanced practical considerations with our collective prediction about how the individual volumes would be used. While it was different earlier in the development of the field, we believe that the current trend is for people to be more organized around populations than techniques. Hence, more people are likely to pick up and cross-reference a single volume on children or the elderly than a volume on Behavior Therapy. Our strategy for identifying chapter length topics and associated page limits is more difficult to explain. Once again, we relied on our collective judgement, honed by negotiation. In rough order, priority was given to topics that had established empirical literatures, that were deemed to be "important," that had broad interest, and that were likely to be at least as important in the next decade. Page limits were determined substantially by estimates of the first two criteria. We began with an overall target for the entire work and minimums and maximums for volumes, and then worked backwards to divide up the allotted pages among the chapters designated for each volume. Given that no scheme will please everyone, we are confident that the organization of the work adequately reflects the field now and in the foreseeable future.

Under the careful aegis of the outstanding group of experts comprising the Honorary International Editorial Advisory Board, 10 leading international scholars were selected to edit the 10 specific volumes.

Volume 1 (*Foundations*), edited by C. Eugene Walker, provides a complete overview of the basic foundations of clinical psychology, with special emphasis on the relationship between clinical psychology and other fields of science. Beginning with a brief history of clinical psychology, as well as a look at its current scientific status, this informative volume covers such topics as the biological bases of clinical psychology, elucidating research in genetics, psychobiology, psychopharmacology, and the use of animal models in human mental health problems; clinical psychology in the behavioral sciences, including anthropology, epidemiology, sociology, and research psychology; and the major systems and theories that are used in clinical psychology. The volume also describes various techniques for library research and information retrieval in psychology.

Volume 2 (*Professional Issues*), edited by Arthur W. Wiens, focuses on the professional, legal, and ethical issues that are relevant to clinical psychology. The volume addresses the various educational and training programs available, such as doctoral study, internship training, and postdoctoral residency programs, and reviews the accreditation of these programs. Also highlighted are the various international government guidelines for registration, certification, and licensing, including a discussion of the advantages of specialty recognition and practice certificates. The volume concludes with a look at ethical and legal guidelines in the management of clinical psychology practices, national healthcare policies, and advocacy efforts for government support for practitioners.

Volume 3 (*Research and Methods*), edited by Nina R. Schooler, explores the function of research in clinical psychology. The volume begins with an in-depth look at research approaches, including the use of descriptive studies, single case designs, observational methods, and other methods of analysis. The volume goes on to explore a broad range of topics that have been the focus of research, such as test development and validation, personality assessment, clinical interventions, and service evaluations and outcomes. Finally, various statistical techniques are reviewed, including descriptive and inferential statistics, factor analysis, and sampling and generalizability.

Volume 4 (*Assessment*), edited by Cecil R. Reynolds, provides valuable information on the development and role of assessment in clinical practice, analyzing such topics as psychometrics; taxonomic, functional, and actuarial approaches to diagnosis; and specific instruments, techniques, and procedures. Chapters also review the range of assessment techniques and procedures used in clinical practice, with emphasis on intelligence, neuropsychological, personality, projective, computer-assisted, therapeutic, and forensic assessment. The volume concludes with a review of legal guidelines and regulations in the use of psychological testing.

Volume 5 (*Children & Adolescents: Clinical Formulation & Treatment*), edited by Thomas Ollendick, draws on the experience and research of leading scientists and clinicians from Australia, Canada, Israel, the United Kingdom, and the United States to present state-of-the-art information on all aspects of child psychology and psychiatry, with special attention given to the psychopathology, assessment, treatment, and prevention of childhood behavioral disorders. The volume highlights the developmental-contextual framework used in the clinical formulation of these disorders, as well as process and outcome issues in treatment. Various theoretical perspectives are also reviewed, including applied behavior analysis, family systems therapy, play therapy, and pharmacologic therapy. In the final section, all of the major childhood disorders found in the *DSM* and *ICD* are described, with information on their prevalence, etiology, assessment, and treatment. This section also analyzes the empirical status of the various therapies used for treatment of childhood disorders.

Volume 6 (*Adults: Clinical Formulation & Treatment*), edited by Paul Salkovskis, provides valuable insights into the basis of the psychological theories and interventions used for behavioral and emotional problems and reviews how to integrate clinical skills with these theories. Various treatment approaches are addressed, such as cognitive therapy, family therapy, and Humanistic/Rogerian/Gestalt approaches, as well as the issues related to treatments, including stress management, arousal reduction methods, suicidal behavior, and specific issues in working with groups. The final section details specific problem areas and disorders, ranging from such universally recognized problems as gambling and substance abuse to more specific disorders such as post-traumatic stress, depression, obsessive-compulsive, and the various phobias. Each chapter in the volume emphasizes approaches that have an empirical basis.

Volume 7 (*Clinical Geropsychology*), edited by Barry Edelstein, addresses the emerging field of clinical psychology in the aging population. The volume begins with a review of this area of research, presenting important epidemiological information. The volume then offers a detailed look at issues that range from analyzing physiological and cognitive aspects to cognitive changes and specific neurological disorders common among older adults. Specific topics covered include sexuality, bereavement, anxiety, substance abuse, and schizophrenia. Each chapter presents a summary of clinical research and its practical application. Voids in the knowledge base are also noted, along with recommendations for the direction of future investigations. The volume also addresses management problems, such as incontinence, wandering, and aggressive behavior, and reviews the various mental healthcare systems available in different countries.

Volume 8 (*Health Psychology*), edited by Derek W. Johnston and Marie Johnston, provides a comprehensive overview of the development and application of clinical health psychology. Beginning with a discussion of training, assessment, and measurement issues, this volume analyzes the key behaviors that either affect or are related to health. Topics covered include stress and disease, the experience of illness, and behavior that can affect the neuroendocrine, cardiovascular, and immune systems. The volume also provides a detailed analysis of specific clinical problems and their psychological aspects and interventions. These include cancer, diabetes, epilepsy, disfigurement, and smoking.

Volume 9 (*Applications in Diverse Populations*), edited by Nirbhay N. Singh, covers the broad spectrum of diverse issues that clinical psychologists typically face in their work. Four sections outline the various psychological aspects found in different populations, as well as methods for assessment, diagnostic information, and interventions useful with these different groups. Section I focuses on select child, adolescent, and adult populations, including those with developmental disorders, learning disabilities, and mental retardation. Section II is devoted to various types of families and their issues, including families of individuals with HIV or AIDS, families of alcoholics, and families of children with serious emotional disturbances. Section III covers victims of violence and abuse, including child sexual abuse. Section IV examines perpetrators of violence and abuse, including sex offenders and issues of domestic violence.

Volume 10 (*Sociocultural and Individual Differences*), edited by Cynthia D. Belar, covers cross-cultural psychopathology and interventions. Chapters examine such select topics as gender, sexual orientation, socioeconomic status, religions, and training for clinical psychologists. The volume also provides valuable insights into the use of clinical psychology in different parts of the world, as well as personality assessment across international settings.

Given the scope and detail of *Comprehensive Clinical Psychology*, Volume 11 is devoted to: (i) a Name Index, (ii) a Subject Index, (iii) a List of Contributors, and (iv) a list of the Contents of All Volumes. The Name Index is an accumulation of all the authors who are cited in text in the reference sections throughout the entire work. The Subject Index, consisting of more than 40 000 entries, is a consolidation of all the individual volume subject indexes. It is presented in word-by-word alphabetical sequence with a maximum of three levels of heading. Terminology in the index is based on standard internationally recognized sources. Cross-references are provided to assist the user to locate preferred terms and terms of related interest.

Acknowledgments

To produce a tome of this magnitude requires an enormous number of individuals with unique talents working in concert. To begin with, we applaud the herculean efforts of our driving force and friend at Elsevier Science, Barbara Barrett. We also gratefully acknowledge the efforts of two other publishing editors at Elsevier Science, Susan Hanscom and David Hoole, who provided guidance and encouragement along the way. We are particularly thankful for the exceptionally hard work of Angela Greenwell and her staff in Oxford, who made sure that all tasks were implemented reasonably on time and who orchestrated the day-to-day management of this huge undertaking. Next, we thank our eminent volume editors, who had the difficult job of soliciting, tracking, and editing manuscripts for their respective volumes. Similarly, we thank the Honorary International Editorial Advisory Board for their excellent input in developing the outline for the work and suggestions as to potential international contributors. Of course, we owe a great deal to the individual contributors who agreed to share their expertise with us in a timely fashion. Finally, we are most appreciative of our own editorial assistants, Sonia McQuarters and Burt G. Bolton, who repeatedly have provided us with the kind of support that makes all of this a possibility.

HONORARY INTERNATIONAL EDITORIAL ADVISORY BOARD

Preface

In 1900 the average life expectancy in the USA was 49 years. There was relatively little need at that time for a psychology of aging, much less a clinical psychology of aging. That situation has dramatically changed over the past century and will continue to do so for many years. Today, adults 65 years of age and older comprise approximately 12.7% of the US population. In 1994 there were 33.2 million individuals in this age group and this number is expected to increase to 35.3 million by the year 2000 (Association for the Advancement of Retired Persons [AARP], 1995). Though the growth in number of older adults is expected to slow somewhat during the 1990s due to the decrease in births during the Great Depression of the 1930s, a rapid increase is expected as baby boomers reach the age of 65. According to estimates by the AARP (1995), there will be approximately twice as many older adults in 2030 as there were in 1990, representing approximately 20% of the total population.

With increasing age comes increased risks of physical health problems. In 1993, 8% of the US population under the age of 65 years rated their health as fair or poor, in contrast to 28% of adults 65 years and older. Approximately 80% of older adults suffer from at least one chronic health problem (Knight, Santos, Teri, & Lawton, 1995), with arthritis, hypertension, and heart disease being among the most prevalent (AARP, 1995). Mental health problems continue to be experienced as we age. Older adults suffer from the same psychological problems as younger adults, although the prevalence of the various disorders varies somewhat across the lifespan. Gatz, Kasl-Godley, and Karel (1996) have estimated that approximately 23% of adults 65 years of age and older meet diagnostic criteria for some mental disorder. The authors note that this proportion is approximately the same for younger adults (National Advisory Mental Health Council, 1993) and individuals under the age of 18 (Kazdin & Kagan, 1994). Many older adults are also potentially more vulnerable than younger adults to develop psychological problems resulting from factors associated with increasing age, such as retirement, loss of friends and family members, diminishing cognitive skills, and changes in living situations. The psychological and physical health problems of older adults have significant implications beyond the individuals experiencing the problems, as their caregivers often experience significant mental health problems arising from the stress of caregiving (Stone, Cafferata, & Sangl, 1987; see also Chapters 15 and 22, this volume).

Knight, Santos, Teri, and Lawton (1995) have identified several factors that collectively reveal the urgency and importance of addressing the mental health needs of older adults. "These include the numbers of elderly adults involved, the growing proportion of individuals and families affected the emotional, functional, and social disabilities related to these problems, and their overwhelming impact on our social service and health care delivery systems" (p. 2).

Clinical psychologists have met the challenge presented by older adults through the years, often without the benefit of specialized knowledge and skills. Ample evidence of these contributions are well documented at least back to the early 1900s (see Knight, Kelly, & Gatz, 1992, for a historical account). In more recent years the relatively new field of clinical geropsychology has emerged, with the clear understanding that to be most effective in dealing with the mental health problems of older adults, one must have "special knowledge of the aging process and the unique characteristics and situations of older adults," coupled with "additional training, the degree of which will depend on the types of clinical issues with which the practitioner will be dealing" (Niederehe, 1995, p. 3). By 1981 the training of psychologists to work with older adults was viewed as sufficiently important and pressing to warrant a training conference in Boulder, Colorado devoted to the topic (known as the Older Boulder Conference). A second training conference, co-sponsored by the National Institute of Mental Health and the American Psychological Association and chaired by Linda Teri, was held in 1992 and entitled "The 1992 National Conference on Clinical Training in Psychology: Improving Psychological Services for Older Adults." 1993 saw the initiation of a Section on Clinical Geropsychology within the Clinical Division (12) of the American Psychological Association. Most recently, in 1997, the new section and Division 20 submitted an application to the American Psychological Association for the recognition of clinical geropsychology as a proficiency within clinical psychology.

Clinical geropsychology has come to be defined as "the growing area of practice that applies the knowledge and techniques of clinical psychology to help older persons and their families maintain well-being, overcome problems, and achieve maximum potential during later life" (Petition for the Recognition of a Proficiency in Psychology, 1997, p. 1). The field of clinical geropsychology continues to evolve as more researchers and clinicians begin to address the mental health needs of our increasing older adult population.

The Current Volume

The principal goal of this volume was to assemble the contributions of a group of international experts whose work has focused on the psychology of aging and the field of clinical geropsychology. The chapters in this volume survey many of the significant contributions to our knowledge of the mental health problems of older adults, their clinical assessment, and the empirical support for our clinical interventions.

Chapter 1 is a very thoughtful consideration of the many physiological changes that occur with aging. In this chapter Whitbourne emphasizes the importance of considering a variety of psychological disorders (e.g., depression, anxiety) in light of the changes occurring within the body as one ages. Moreover, she emphasizes the distinction between chronic diseases often associated with aging and normal age-related changes in the body. A person's identity, sense of self over time, is discussed with the aging process conceptualized as a constant challenge to the maintenance of a stable identity. Whitbourne then introduces a multiple threshold model of aging that comprises physical changes to identity, coping processes, adaptational outcomes, and age-related control behaviors. Whitbourne ends with a discussion of changes in the major systems of the body and the clinical implications of changes in each.

In Chapter 2, Johansson and Wahlin offer the reader an understanding of age-related changes in memory and cognition, two extremely important domains of functioning that are often assessed by clinical geropsychologists. Aging is conceptualized as an interaction between biological, psychological, and social processes. The authors take an idiographic approach, emphasizing the patterns of aging that are unique to each individual. Learning, memory, and intellectual functioning are discussed, followed by a consideration of how older adults cope with cognitive change. Finally, the authors address the transition from the basic research laboratory to the "real world," followed by a brief discussion of what is known about cognition in everyday life. Overall, the authors do a stunning job of reviewing relevant research with an eye to bridging the more basic experimental literature and the questions that might be faced by the clinical geropsychologist.

In Chapter 3, Lang and Carstensen address the role of social relationships in late-life adaptation. Normative changes in the characteristics of social relationships and social networks across adulthood are discussed with a focus on friendships and family relationships. The authors review the health-related functions of social relationships, including the negative outcomes of negative social interactions. Finally, the findings regarding social relationships, age, and health are considered in light of recent theoretical perspectives on adaptive social behaviors.

Zank explores issues of older adult sexuality in Chapter 4, beginning with an enlightening discussion of the previous reviews of sexual behavior among older adults. The results of various epidemiological studies of sexual behavior are discussed followed by a very thoughtful critique addressing methodological and theoretical problems. Zank then reviews the physiological changes related to sexual functioning that are associated with aging in females and males. Age-related diseases and psychological disorders that can affect sexual functioning are also addressed. Finally, Zank reviews the literature on the treatment of sexual disorders.

In Chapter 5, Lund examines the complexities of the bereavement process, beginning with a discussion of bereavement experiences, with particular emphasis on bereavement in later life. He emphasizes the multidimensional context of bereavement, which can impact family life, social interactions, life satisfaction, and even the financial stability of the bereaved. Theories and models of bereavement are briefly discussed, ranging from psychoanalytic to stress, appraisal, and coping theories. Of particular importance is the discussion of predictors of bereavement adjustment in which the author, dispelling the myth that time heals the wound of grief, addresses the importance of active coping. This chapter ends with a review of promising methods for working with the bereaved.

In Chapter 6, Frank and Smyer explore psychological and legal issues associated with the decisional capacity of older adults. The doctrine of informed consent is briefly reviewed, followed by a discussion of issues surrounding competence to provide informed consent and its psychological assessment. A particularly important element of this chapter is the contrasting of forensic and cognitive psychological views of competence. Advance directives are discussed in light of the Patient Self-determination Act, which has reinforced older adults' rights to self-determination and substantially influenced the relationship between caregivers and those for whom care is being provided. This chapter is the most thorough and thoughtful presentation of issues surrounding decision-making capacity to date.

In Chapter 7, Crawford, Venneri, and O'Carroll offer an unusually thorough consideration of the many issues associated with the neuropsychological assessment of older adults. For many clinical geropsychologists, neuropsychological assessment represents the most substantial element of their practices. For others, it is an essential first step in the broader assessment of individuals whose problems range from depression to difficulties accomplishing activities of daily living. The authors of this chapter begin by noting the changes in neuropsychological assessment over the past two decades from a focus on differential diagnosis and lesion localization to the identification of cognitive and behavioral consequences of cerebral dysfunction. The authors go on to a consideration of specific assessment issues, the neuropsychological interview, and basic psychometric issues. This latter consideration is particularly important in light of the potential consequences of neuropsychological assessment, which can range from rehabilitation recommendations to legal determinations ranging from competence to the settlement of civil disputes. From the perspective of the average clinical geropsychologist, the section on screening tests for mental status is particularly important, as this is a key ingredient in the assessment of older adults by non-neuropsychologists. Finally, very specific recommendations are made regarding the interpretation of various psychological tests and their use in differential diagnosis.

In Chapter 8, Stanley and Beck explore the relatively under-researched area of anxiety disorders among older adults. Anxiety disorders are the most prevalent of the many psychiatric disorders among older adults, even more prevalent than clinical depression, which is often mistakenly thought to be particularly prevalent among older adults. The authors appropriately qualify their discussion by noting the lack of well-established measures of anxiety for older adults and the limitations of studies due to the failure to use strict diagnostic criteria. The prevalence of anxiety disorders among older adults, their onset and associated risk factors are initially discussed, with particular attention to gender and ethnicity. The psychopathology of anxiety disorders and their differential diagnosis follows, with appropriate attention to problems of many older adults that complicate the diagnostic picture (e.g., medical problems, sleep disturbances, depression, and cognitive impairment). The paucity of support for measures of anxiety and the attendant psychometric limitations of most measures is well documented. Finally, the authors discuss the general issue of older adults' utilization of mental health services followed by a discussion of pharmacological and psychosocial interventions. The authors end with an appeal for more research addressing the durability of treatment response.

In Chapter 9, Gatz, Fiske, and Kasl-Godley provide an overview of mood disorders in late life. The authors initially address diagnostic issues with particular attention to the adequacy of our current diagnostic system for the affective disorders of older adults. Prevalence rates are then discussed with appropriate caveats regarding the definitional problems that cloud our understanding of the prevalence and etiology of affective disorders. Different diagnostic classification systems are discussed as an illustration of this problem. One of the more interesting and important topics addressed is the difference in symptom presentation between younger and older adults. The authors provide an excellent review of factors associated with depression among older adults. They have also done a marvelous job of addressing the assessment of affective disorders with careful attention to the psychometric properties of current measurement instruments. Finally, the course, treatment, and prevention of depression are addressed.

Small, Herlitz, and Bäckman examine dementia in Chapter 10, with particular emphasis on Alzheimer's disease, its development and cognitive course. The authors begin with an interesting discussion of preclinical cognitive markers of dementia, proceeding through the detection of dementia, its staging, and the progression of decline in cognitive functioning. The authors make a compelling case for the predictability of changes accompanying dementia, specifically addressing predictors of dementia-related differences and changes.

Pearson provides an exceptionally thorough review of the literature on suicide among older adults in Chapter 11. This is a particularly important topic for clinical geropsychologists, as the suicide rate among older adults, particularly those aged 85 years and older, surpasses that of all other age groups. Pearson begins with the epidemiology of suicidal behavior in late life and then examines the correlates of suicide completions among older adults. She also reviews studies of suicide attempters, followed by an exploration of older adult subgroups who are at increased risk for suicide. Pearson then addresses some of the more difficult bioethical issues associated with suicide, including physician-assisted suicide, competency assessment of depressed older adults, and the need for bioethical research. This section of the chapter is particularly timely in light of the increasing publicity and public concern regarding passive and active euthanasia, advance directives, and physician-assisted suicide. Finally, she explores a variety of clinical resources for the suicidal older adult, followed by a brief discussion of psychotherapeutic approaches for suicidal older adults.

Segal and Coolidge explore the literature on personality disorders among older adults in Chapter 12. The authors very thoughtfully place their initial discussion of personality disorders in the historical context of personality disorders as they evolved through the various versions of the *Diagnostic and statistical manual of mental disorders (DSM)*. Interestingly, the *DSM-IV* was the first of these to specifically consider the developmental issues of aging with regard to personality disorders. The authors briefly present various theories regarding the etiologies of personality disorders and the relevance of these theories for older adults. Segal and Coolidge have worked at a considerable disadvantage in preparing this chapter in light of the paucity of literature on personality disorders among older adults, and the inconsistencies of epidemiological information regarding incidence and prevalence. The more prominent personality assessment measures are discussed followed by discussions of their applications to older adults. Finally, the treatment of personality disorders is addressed, again with the disadvantage of the lack of relevant literature for older adults. Overall, the authors have done a noteworthy job of addressing this topic in spite of the paucity of literature and theoretical considerations of this age group.

Schizophrenia, which was once thought to be a disorder arising only among younger adults, is competently discussed by Harvey in Chapter 13. The author approaches the diagnosis of schizophrenia and related conditions in late life with the goals of informing the reader regarding the impact of these disorders on older adults, and encouraging the development of new treatments specifically targeting older adults. He does a particularly good job of explaining the differences between individuals with early- and late-onset schizophrenia. Harvey offers an in-depth discussion of cognitive functioning in late-life schizophrenia and the resulting impairment in adaptive behavior. Finally, he notes the lack of any specialized literature on the treatment of late-life schizophrenia, noting that we have no evidence that our current therapeutic practices would be ineffective with late-onset schizophrenia.

In Chapter 14, Ancoli-Israel, Martin, and Pat-Horencyzk discuss sleep and its disorders among older adults. Older adults spend more time in bed than younger individuals but sleep less. Moreover, they are more easily aroused from sleep and experience decreases in slow wave sleep. The authors address these points and review what constitutes sleep, how it is measured, the major theories of sleep, and then the changes that occur in sleep as one ages. Sleep disorders (e.g., sleep-disordered breathing, periodic limb movements in sleep, and insomnia) are reviewed in considerable depth, followed by a discussion of dementia and sleep. For each of the disorders, the authors describe prevalence, symptoms, evaluation, and treatment of the disorder. This is not only a useful guide for clinicians, but also a very thorough and up-to-date review of the state of our knowledge regarding the assessment and treatment of sleep disorders among older adults. Finally, the authors dispel two common myths of sleep among older adults, noting that aging does not cause sleep problems and older adults do not need less sleep than younger individuals.

In Chapter 15, Heller addresses the very complication issue of later life caregiving for intellectually disabled individuals. Many of us do not stop to think that intellectually disabled individuals require care throughout their lifespan and the families of these individuals are the caregivers for almost 80% of these individuals. Heller examines caregiving of intellectually disabled individuals from a life-course perspective that takes into account social trends and changes in service patterns. As the number of older adults with intellectual disabilities increases, so do the demands on the social system in general and their caregivers in particular. Heller addresses the reasons for increased life expectancy of intellectually disabled individuals, age- related changes, and trends in services and supports. She also reviews theories of family caregiving over the lifespan and discusses the empirical support for these theories. The roles of mothers, fathers, and siblings are addressed along with the need for future planning and possible placement of the intellectually disabled individuals who have or will lose their caregivers to poor health, death, or other factors that preclude continued care. Heller ends with several excellent recommendations for future research.

Edelstein and Drozdick address falls among older adults in Chapter 16, initially noting that a significant percentage of older adults fall each day, with approximately 50% of long-term residents falling every year. The authors begin with a discussion of the conceptual and methodological issues that have plagued this area of research, followed by a discussion of the physical, psychological, and economic consequences of falls. Internal and external risk factors for falls are discussed in depth, with particular attention to the variability in findings across studies. Finally, the authors describe approaches to the prevention of falls, including medical, rehabilitative, and environmental strategies. The authors end on an optimistic note, indicating that numerous risk factors have been identified that can be changed through a variety of interventions.

In Chapter 17, Algase offers an extraordinarily comprehensive review of the literature on wandering among older adults, a very significant problem for cognitively-impaired individuals and their caregivers. The author begins with a discussion of various conceptual schemes and typologies of wandering, noting that few empirical descriptions or characterizations exist. Epidemiological data are presented, including potential contributors to and consequences of wandering behavior. Perhaps the most interesting element of this chapter is the very thoughtful discussion of etiologic theories and factors, culminating in a multifactorial explanation for wandering. Extraordinarily detailed reviews and discussions of assessment methods, assessment instruments, and interventions fill the remainder of the chapter. Algase ends with an extensive set of important research questions.

Chapter 18 is a very thorough review of the assessment and treatment of agitated and aggressive behavior among older adults. Fisher, Swingen, and Harsin address the rather frequent and quite significant problems among cognitively impaired older adults. These behaviors increase the likelihood of one being institutionalized and experiencing physical and/or pharmacological restraint. They are the bane of psychologists consulting in long-term care facilities and the source of considerable suffering among caregivers. The authors initially address definitional issues, prevalence, and etiological factors associated with aggressive and agitated behavior. Assessment of these behaviors is thoughtfully considered, including discussions of the psychometric properties of various assessment instruments. Finally, a broad array of interventions are critically evaluated. This chapter is an excellent critical review of the literature and an excellent resource for the practicing clinical geropsychologist.

In Chapter 19, Schnelle offers an exceptionally thorough treatment of incontinence among older adults, a problem that affects 30% of individuals over the age of 60 years and over 50% of residents of nursing facilities. The author also discusses how and why psychologists should be involved in the management of incontinence among older adults. Schnelle begins with an overview of the prevalence, morbidity, and consequences of incontinence. This is followed by in-depth discussions of the various types of urinary incontinence, the assessment of incontinence, and treatment options. Interventions include the use of drugs, surgery, and a variety of behavioral interventions. Of substantial utility is a very thoughtful and thorough discussion of how to implement an incontinence management program in a nursing home, including methods of assessment, determination of candidates for various interventions, and staff management issues that can influence the effectiveness of continence programs. Finally, future directions are addressed with respect to both community-dwelling and nursing home populations.

Knight, Kaskie, Woods, and Phibbs offer an interesting and unique comparison between US and UK systems of mental health for older adults in Chapter 20. The authors highlight the similarities and differences in community mental health services for older adults and explore the development of these systems. The authors initially explore the many systems in which older adults with mental health problems are embedded and explain how such systems are confusing and characterized by numerous gaps in service because of the conditions under which each of the services developed. A broad array of community-based services are described, beginning with long-term institutional psychiatric care. Community-based care in the UK and USA are described and contrasted. Finally, the histories of development of clinical geropsychology in the UK and USA are contrasted, ending with an appeal to training programs to rethink their training goals for the twenty-first century.

In Chapter 21, Lomranz and Bar-Tur address the topic of mental health care in the nursing home. The authors describe the effects of institutionalization and the mental health of residents in light of their transition and adaptation to a nursing home. Mental disorders common among nursing home residents are discussed, followed by a discussion of a proposed model of clinical geropsychological services. The model proposed, which is quite impressive for its innovativeness and comprehensiveness, is currently operative in Israel.

In Chapter 22, Zarit, Davey, Edwards, Femia, and Jarrott inform us that families are caring for disabled older adults more often and for longer periods of time than ever before. It is clear from their presentation that we must be as concerned about the mental health and well- being of the caregivers as we have been with the recipient of the care. These authors review the research findings on family caregiving and discuss the clinical implications. They begin with a very lucid presentation of several basic issues in family caregiving, followed by a presentation of the various stages of caregiving or careers assumed by caregivers as those under their care progressively change. What follows are discussions of a variety of caregiving topics including caregiving stress, the family context of caregiving, the perspective of the care recipient, normative family relationships in later life, health and mental health outcomes of caregiving, current clinical research and services, and the consequences of institutionalization.

In Chapter 23, Tesch-Römer and Wahl provide a very broad and comprehensive survey of the rehabilitation of older adults with particular attention to the psychosocial issues involved. The authors discuss issues of assessment, restoration of functional independence, and a variety of strategies for accomplishing this. Motivation and compliance are addressed as key factors in the success of any rehabilitation program. Rehabilitation of specific client groups (e.g., stroke patients, arthritis patients, sensory impaired patients) is discussed from a multidisciplinary perspective. Finally, the authors address various practical issues and ethical problems associated with rehabilitation efforts. This chapter is an excellent overview of the many problem areas in which geropsychological knowledge and skills can play significant roles in the rehabilitation of older adults.

In the last chapter Zeiss and Steffen advocate an interdisciplinary health care team approach to the assessment and treatment of older adults residing in medical facilities. The authors build a strong case for the use of such teams, with much of their rationale based upon two characteristics of geriatric patients: their problems are complex and chronic. The heterogeneity of capacities and problems of older adults argue for interdisciplinary teams, which the authors distinguish from unidisciplinary, intradisciplinary, and multidisciplinary teams. Because the interdisciplinary team as a whole takes responsibility for team effectiveness and function, it functions quite differently from teams that are hierarchically organized. Advantages and disadvantages of such teams are considered, followed by a discussion of the natural history of team development.

In closing I would like to take this opportunity to thank George Niederehe for his many thoughtful suggestions for chapter topics and potential authors. Margy Gatz was also very helpful with this project, particularly through her suggestions for international authors. Finally, I wish to thank Angela Greenwell at Elsevier, who consistently provided answers to all of my often odd questions and who repeatedly offered assistance in motivating chapter authors.

References

Association for the Advancement of Retired Persons (1995). *A profile of older Americans*. Washington, DC: Author.

Gatz, M., Kasl-Godley, J. E., & Karel, M. J. (1996). Aging and mental disorders. In J. E. Birren & K. W. Schaie (Eds.), *Handbook of the psychology of aging* (4th ed., pp. 365–382). New York: Academic Press.

Kazdin, A. E., & Kagan, J. (1994). Models of dysfunction in developmental psychopathology. *Clinical Psychology: Science and Practice, 1,* 35–52.

Knight, B. G., Santos, J., Teri, L., & Lawton, M. P. (1995). The development of training in clinical geropsychology. In B. G. Knight, L. Teri, P. Wohlford, & J. Santos (Eds.), *Mental health services for older adults* (pp. 1–8). Washington, DC: American Psychological Association.

Knight, B., Kelly, M., & Gatz, M. (1992). Psychotherapy with the elderly. In D. K. Freedheim (Ed.), *The history of psychotherapy*. Washington, DC: American Psychological Association.

National Advisory Mental Council (1993). Health care reform for Americans with severe mental illnesses. Report of the National Advisory Mental Health Council. *American Journal of Psychiatry, 150,* 1447–1465.

Niederehe, G. (1995). Progress and prospects in clinical geropsychology. *The Clinical Psychologist, 48,* 3–4.

Petition for the Recognition of a Proficiency in Psychology (1997). Unpublished manuscript.

Stone, R., Cafferata, G. L., & Sangl, J. (1987). Caregivers of the frail elderly: A national profile. *The Gerontologist, 27,* 616–626.

Contributors

Dr. D. L. Algase
School of Nursing, University of Michigan, 400 North Ingalls, Room 2306, Ann Arbor, MI 48109-0482, USA

Dr. S. Ancoli-Israel
Department of Psychiatry (116A), Veterans Affairs Medical Center, 3350 La Jolla Village Drive, San Diego, CA 92161, USA

Dr. L. Bäckman
Stockholm Gerontology Research Center, Box 6401, Stockholm S-113 82, Sweden
Department of Psychology, Göteborg University, Göteborg, Sweden

Dr. L. Bar-Tur
The Herczeg Institute on Aging, Tel Aviv University, PO Box 39040, Ramat Aviv, 69978 Tel Aviv, Israel

Dr. J. G. Beck
Department of Psychology, State University of New York at Buffalo, 230 Park Hall, Buffalo, NY 14260, USA

Dr. L. L. Carstensen
Department of Psychology, Stanford University, Jordan Hall, Building 420, Stanford, CA 94305-2130, USA

Dr. F. L. Coolidge
Department of Psychology, University of Colorado, PO Box 7150, Colorado Springs, CO 80933-7150, USA

Dr. J. R. Crawford
Department of Psychology, King's College, University of Aberdeen, Aberdeen, AB9 2UB, UK

Dr. A. Davey
Department of Human Development and Family Studies, Pennsylvania State University, 110 Henderson Building South, University Park, PA 16802-6504, USA

Dr. L. W. Drozdick
Department of Psychology, West Virginia University, PO Box 6040, Morgantown, WV 26506-6040, USA

Professor B. A. Edelstein
Department of Psychology, West Virginia University, PO Box 6040, Morgantown, WV 26506-6040, USA

Ms. A. B. Edwards
Department of Human Development and Family Studies, Pennsylvania State University, 110 Henderson Building South, University Park, PA 16802-6504, USA

Ms. E. E. Femia
Department of Human Development and Family Studies, Pennsylvania State University, 110 Henderson Building South, University Park, PA 16802-6504, USA

Dr. J. E. Fisher
Department of Psychology/298, University of Nevada at Reno, Reno, NV 89557-0062, USA

Ms. A. Fiske
Department of Psychology, University of Southern California, 3620 McClintock, Los Angeles, CA 90089-1061, USA

Dr. L. Frank
MEDTAP International, 7101 Wisconsin Avenue, Suite 600, Bethesda, MD 20814, USA

Dr. M. Gatz
Department of Psychology, University of Southern California, 3620 McClintock, Los Angeles, CA 90089-1061, USA

Ms. C. M. Harsin
Department of Psychology/298, University of Nevada at Reno, Reno, NV 89557-0062, USA

Dr. P. D. Harvey
Department of Psychiatry, Box 1229, Mount Sinai School of Medicine, New York, NY 10029, USA

Dr. T. Heller
Institute on Disability and Human Development, University of Illinois at Chicago, 1640 West Roosevelt Road, Chicago, IL 60608, USA

Dr. A. Herlitz
Stockholm Gerontology Research Center, Box 6401, Stockholm S-113 82, Sweden
Department of Psychology, Stockholm University, Stockholm, Sweden

Mr. S. E. Jarrot
Department of Human Development and Family Studies, Pennsylvania State University, 110 Henderson Building South, University Park, PA 16802-6504, USA

Dr. B. Johansson
Institute of Gerontology and Centre for Psychology, University College of Health Sciences, Box 1038, S-551 11 Jönköping, Sweden

Mr. B. Kaskie
Andrus Gerontology Center, University of Southern California, Los Angeles, CA 90089-0191, USA

Ms. J. E. Kasl-Godley
Department of Psychology, University of Southern California, 3620 McClintock, Los Angeles, CA 90089-1061, USA

Dr. R. G. Knight
Andrus Gerontology Center, University of Southern California, Los Angeles, CA 90089-0191, USA

Dr. F. R. Lang
Department of Gerontopsychiatry, Freie Universität Berlin, Nussbaumallee 38, 14050 Berlin, Germany

Dr. J. Lomranz
The Herczeg Institute on Aging, Tel Aviv University, PO Box 39040, Ramat Aviv, 69978 Tel Aviv, Israel

Dr. D. A. Lund
Gerontology Center, 25 South Medical Drive, 311 College of Nursing, University of Utah, Salt Lake City, UT 84112, USA

Ms. J. Martin
Department of Psychiatry (116A), Veterans Affairs Medical Center, 3350 La Jolla Village Drive, San Diego, CA 92161, USA

Dr. R. E. O'Carroll
Department of Psychology, University of Stirling, Stirling, FK9 ULA, UK

Dr. R. Pat-Horenczyk
Sleep Medicine Center, 24 Strauss Street, Jerusalem, Israel 95142

Dr. J. L. Pearson
National Institute of Mental Health, Room 18-101, 5600 Fishers Lane, Rockville, MD 20857, USA

Ms. E. Phibbs
Department of Clinical Health Psychology, University College London, Gower Street, London, WC1E 6BT, UK

Dr. J. F. Schnelle
Borun Center, University of California, Los Angeles, 7150 Tampa Avenue, Los Angeles, CA 91335, USA

Dr. D. L. Segal
Department of Psychology, University of Colorado, PO Box 7150, Colorado Springs, CO 80933-7150, USA

Dr. B. J. Small
Department of Gerontology, SOC 107, University of South Florida, 4202 East Fowler Avenue, Tampa, FL 33620-8100, USA

Dr. M. Smyer
Graduate School of Arts and Sciences, McGuinn 221, Boston College, Chestnut Hill, MA 02167, USA

Dr. M. A. Stanley
Department of Psychiatry and Behavioral Sciences, University of Texas Medical School, 1300 Moursund Avenue, Msl, Houston, TX 77030-3497, USA

Dr. A. Steffen
Department of Psychology, University of Missouri at St. Louis, 8001 Natural Bridge Road, St. Louis, MO 63121-4499, USA

Ms. D. N. Swingen
Department of Psychology/298, University of Nevada at Reno, Reno, NV 89557-0062, USA

Dr. C. Tesch-Römer
Ernst Moritz Arndt University, Greifswald, Franz Mehring Strasse 47, D-17487 Greifswald, Germany

Dr. A. Venneri
Department of Psychology, King's College, University of Aberdeen, Aberdeen, AB9 2UB, Scotland, UK

Professor H.-W. Wahl
German Center for Research on Aging at the University of Heidelberg, Bergheimer Strasse 20, D-69115 Heidelberg, Germany

Dr. Å. Wahlin
Stockholm Gerontology Research Center, Karolinska Institute, Box 6401, S-113 82 Stockholm, Sweden

Professor S. K. Whitbourne
Department of Psychology, University of Massachusetts–Amherst, Amherst, MA 01003-7710, USA

Professor R. Woods
School of Psychology, University of Wales, Bangor, Gwynedd, LL57 2DG, UK

Dr. S. Zank
Department of Gerontopsychiatry, Freie Universität Berlin, Nussbaumallee 38, 14050 Berlin, Germany

Dr. S. H. Zarit
Department of Human Development and Family Studies, Pennsylvania State University, 110 Henderson Building South, University Park, PA 16802-6504, USA

Dr. A. M. Zeiss
VA Palo Alto Health Care System, 3801 Miranda Avenue, Palo Alto, CA 94303, USA

Comprehensive Clinical Psychology

This volume was previously published as part of the eleven-volume work *Comprehensive Clinical Psychology*, the contents of which are outlined here.

Volume 1: Foundations
Professor C. Eugene Walker, *University of Oklahoma Health Sciences Center, Oklahoma City, OK, USA*

Volume 2: Professional Issues
Professor Arthur N. Wiens, *Oregon Health Sciences University, Portland, OR, USA*

Volume 3: Research and Methods
Professor Nina R. Schooler, *University of Pittsburgh, PA, USA*

Volume 4: Assessment
Professor Cecil R. Reynolds, *Texas A&M University, College Station, TX, USA*

Volume 5: Children & Adolescents: Clinical Formulation & Treatment
Professor Thomas Ollendick, *Virginia Tech, Blacksburg, VA, USA*

Volume 6: Adults: Clinical Formulation & Treatment
Professor Paul Salkovskis, *University of Oxford, Warneford Hospital, UK*

Volume 7: Clinical Geropsychology
Professor Barry Edelstein, *West Virginia University, Morgantown, WV, USA*

Volume 8: Health Psychology
Professor Derek W. Johnston and Professor Marie Johnston, *University of St. Andrews, UK*

Volume 9: Applications in Diverse Populations
Dr Nirbhay N. Singh, *Virginia Commonwealth University, Richmond, VA, USA*

Volume 10: Sociocultural and Individual Differences
Professor Cynthia D. Belar, *University of Florida Health Sciences Center, Gainesville, FL, USA*

Volume 11: Indexes

7.01
Physiological Aspects of Aging: Relation to Identity and Clinical Implications

SUSAN K. WHITBOURNE
University of Massachusetts–Amherst, MA, USA

7.01.1 INTRODUCTION

Understanding the normal physiological changes associated with aging is of essential importance to clinical psychologists who work with the elderly. Issues related to depression, anxiety, and other psychological disorders are seen from new perspectives when interpreted in terms of the changes within the body that older clients are likely to experience. Of particular importance is the necessity of distinguishing between the processes of normal aging and alterations in functioning that are the result of specific diseases. Although it is true that older individuals are at heightened risk of developing chronic health problems such as arthritis, cardiovascular disease, cancer, and diabetes, these are diseases rather than normal age-related changes. Clinicians should be aware that they need to persist in the treatment of an elderly client rather than assume that the symptoms of chronic disease represent inevitable losses due to aging.

After reading this chapter, it should be clear that the physical changes associated with the aging process are complex, multifaceted, and multidirectional. Individuals age in their own unique ways, due to their genetic inheritance and lifestyle choices. Clinicians can be of tremendous help to an older person by being aware of expectable age-related changes that affect the aging population as a whole but also by planning interventions that take into account the individual's unique characteristics, life history, and resources.

In general, with regard to physical functioning, it is beneficial to advocate the "use it or lose it" principle; that is, the individual maximizes functioning by maintaining maximum levels of activity. This philosophy gives the clinician concrete tools to design treatment plans and helps to communicate a sense of optimism rather than hopelessness about aging. Furthermore, this approach often results in demonstrable gains in the older individual's daily functioning. However, the clinician is best advised to tailor the application of this principle to the client's preferences, lifestyle, and resources. It is of little help to prescribe an exercise regimen for an individual who has no access to supervised exercise facilities, has never had an interest in exercise, and who cannot afford even the proper pair of sneakers. Apart from such restrictions, however, clinicians may expect to encounter resistance of a different nature when proposing lifestyle changes to older clients. Those who have incorporated into their own identities the belief that there is in fact nothing they can do to alter their own aging will not be led by even the most effective clinician down the activity path unless this resistance can be approached and sensitively overcome. Therefore, in this chapter, a perspective incorporating the notion of identity will be discussed in regard to physical changes. With this perspective, clinicians can target interventions that take into account the ways that older individuals incorporate views about aging into their identities.

7.01.2 IDENTITY AND PHYSICAL CHANGES IN LATER LIFE

7.01.2.1 Identity Processes

The construct of identity has been used in the area of adult development to refer to the individual's sense of self over time. It is conceptualized as incorporating various content areas, including physical functioning, cognition, social relationships, and experiences in the world. In this model (Whitbourne, 1986, 1996a), identity is theorized to form an organizing schema through which the individual's experiences are interpreted. The affective content of identity, for psychologically healthy adults, takes the positive self-referential form encapsulated in the expression "I am a competent, loving, and good person;" that is, competent at work, loving in family life, and good in the sense of being morally and ethically righteous. In this model, such self-attributions are seen as contributing to the individual's emotional well-being. The developmental imperative for normal, nondepressed adults to regard themselves as having these qualities may be seen as providing a driving force in development in the adult years.

The individual's experiences, both past and present, are postulated to relate to identity through processes of assimilation and accommodation. Identity assimilation is defined as the interpretation of life events relevant to the self in terms of the cognitive and affective schemas that are incorporated in identity. The events and experiences to which the assimilation function applies can include major life events, cumulative interactions with the environment over time, or minor incidents that can have a potential impact on identity. Each type of experience can have different meanings depending on the nature of the individual's current self-conceptualizations in identity. The process of identity accommodation, by contrast, involves changing identity in response to identity-relevant experiences. An event that reflects unfavorably on identity is likely to be processed first through assimilation and, only after such efforts prove unsatisfactory, will identity accommodation follow (Brandtstadter & Renner, 1990). As a general principle, it is theorized that a healthy state of emotional adaptation involves a balance or equilibrium between the two identity processes so that the individual maintains a sense of consistency over time but is able to change when there are large discrepancies between the self and experiences (Kiecolt, 1994).

The aging process is a constant challenge to the maintenance of a stable sense of identity over time. Events caused by physical aging are qualitatively different from other experiences that are of a more transitory or fleeting nature. An unpleasant encounter in a chance meeting with a stranger that reflects unfavorably upon one's social identity will fade through time as it is dismissed through identity assimilation as lacking direct personal relevance. Aging, however, is a process that does not fade with time but may in fact grow with importance as the individual must find ways to integrate age-related changes into identity throughout adulthood.

7.01.2.2 A Multiple Threshold Model

Integrating these factors into a comprehensive framework is a "multiple threshold model" of aging (Whitbourne, 1996a, 1996b), that relates age changes to identity, coping processes, adaptational outcomes, and age-related control behaviors. The term "threshold" in this model refers to the point at which an age-related change is recognized by the individual. Before this threshold is reached, the individual does not think of the self as "aging" or "old," or even perhaps as having the real potential to be "aging" or "old." After crossing the threshold, the individual recognizes the possibility that functions may be lost through aging (or disease), and begins to accommodate to this possibility by changing identity accordingly.

The term "multiple" in this model refers to the fact that the aging process involves potentially every system in the body, so that there is in actuality no single threshold leading to the view of the self as aging. The individual may feel "old" in one domain of functioning, such as in the area of mobility, but feel "not old," "middle-aged," or possibly "young" in other domains, such as in the area of sensory acuity or intellectual functioning. Whether a threshold is crossed depends in part on the actual nature of the aging process and whether it has affected a particular area of functioning. However, it is also the case that individuals vary widely in the areas of functioning that they value. Mobility may not be as important to an individual whose major source of pleasure is derived from sedentary reading activities. Changes in the area of mobility will not have as much relevance to the individual's direct adaptation to the environment or to identity as would be the case for losses in vision or memory. In the multiple threshold model, it is assumed that changes in areas important to adaptation and competence have the greatest potential for affecting identity.

Not only are changes in central functions likely to have a greater impact on adaptation and identity, but it is possible to assume further that changes in these functions are watched for most carefully by the individual and early signs of age-related changes will be noticed in these areas. For example, the individual who takes great pride in a full and vibrant head of hair will be on the lookout for gray hairs and thinning, and the individual who values intellectual skills will scrutinize performance on activities involving memory for signs of deterioration. The increased vigilance for areas of functioning central to identity will theoretically heighten the impact of age changes.

On the other hand, with increased vigilance may come increased motivation to take advantage of control activities that reduce the impact of aging. The adult who values being in peak physical shape will work devotedly each day to avoid loss of muscle strength and aerobic capacity. Having valued these qualities, he or she will be more likely to hold onto them into old age. This situation presents a double-edged sword, in which heightened vigilance leads to behavior that offsets the aging process, thus reducing the dreaded outcomes, but also leads the individual to become acutely sensitive to signs that loss has occurred. It may be in this situation, then, that identity accommodation becomes important. The individual who recognizes that he or she is aging is less likely to become discouraged and frustrated at evidence that certain age-related changes cannot be completely reversed. The assimilative individual who desperately attempts to hang onto a youthful identity has the potential to be demolished when an event occurs that makes it abundantly clear that the aging process has taken its inevitable toll.

The multiple threshold concept is most easily viewed as a set of linear processes, with the outcome of passing through a threshold an alteration in the individual's level of well-being. The process is, however, cyclical. Each time a threshold is passed, the individual's identity has the potential to be altered through identity accommodation. When this happens, the crossing of the threshold serves as an event relevant to the self that becomes integrated into identity. The resulting change in identity then alters the individual's subsequent vigilance regarding future age-related in changes in other areas of functioning and the behaviors relevant to the threshold just crossed.

7.01.2.3 Physical Identity and Aging

The substantive content of identity incorporates the domains of physical, psychological, and social functioning. Within the domain of physical functioning are the attributes of appearance, competence, and health (Whitbourne & Primus, 1996). Physical identity may be regarded as one of the fundamental, yet overlooked, areas within psychological gerontology. For example, in a preliminary test of the multiple threshold model, it was found that the aspect of physical functioning in particular that seems to trigger the crossing of a threshold with regard to aging is the recognition of loss of physical competence, an area that is generally not given a great deal of attention by clinicians (Whitbourne, 1996b).

Individuals who use identity assimilation tend to deny as much as possible the importance of age-related changes in valued aspects of physical functioning. For these individuals, it might be speculated that changes in functioning that are related to age are not acknowledged as a result of the aging process, but instead are attributed to transitory states of health or health-related behaviors. This type of denial may be seen as an effort to preserve and protect the individual's sense of the self as competent and consistent over time.

Those older adults who rely more or less exclusively on identity accommodation overreact to small events or experiences and draw overly broad and sweeping conclusions from one instance or situation. With regard to aging, they may conclude prematurely that they are "over the hill" and fail to take preventative actions (Woodward & Wallston, 1987) because they adopt the self-image of being too weak or feeble to continue to maintain their participation in activities that were formerly rewarding to them (Janelli, 1993). As a result, they can become unduly depressed and hopeless (Parmalee, Katz, & Lawton, 1991). In a test of the multiple threshold model (Whitbourne, 1996b), identity accommodation was found to predict awareness of age-related physical changes. Thus, individuals who are highly responsive to their experiences and do not have a firm sense of self are more likely to be sensitive to the effects of normal aging on their bodies. Greater sensitivity to age-related changes, in turn, appears to be predictive of lower self-esteem.

A balanced approach to adapting to age-related changes in valued aspects of physical functioning involves taking precautions and attempting to preserve functions for as long as possible, and adapting to them when they occur by finding ways to compensate for losses. The individual may find a compromise between assimilation and accommodation by recognizing the reailty of aging, but not letting this knowledge interfere with daily functioning or future plans. There may be emotional costs involved in the recognition of impending losses, but individuals who maintain a balanced approach rebound from setbacks with renewed vigor and optimism (Labouvie-Vief, Hakim-Lawson, & Hobart, 1987; Ryff, 1989).

With this model as a backdrop, research on the physical aspects of aging will now be summarized. The concepts of the multiple threshold model and the identity processes of assimilation and accommodation will be used as the basis for suggesting clinical implications. The underlying assumption is not that the aging process must or should be slowed, but that the individual's adaptation to the aging process can be maximized by working with the assimilative or accommodative functions of identity. Ultimately, the value of these interventions can be measured in terms of improved physical health and in terms of an improved or perhaps more realistic outlook on the part of the individual toward the aging process.

7.01.3 THE EFFECTS OF AGE ON APPEARANCE AND MOBILITY

7.01.3.1 Skin

7.01.3.1.1 Age changes

A variety of changes contribute to the phenomena of wrinkling and sagging, the most apparent age-related effects on the skin. The epidermis, the outer layer of the skin, becomes flattened (Kligman, Grove, & Bolin, 1985), and as cells in the epidermis are replaced through cell renewal processes, their patterns become less organized and their arrangment less regular. These changes at the microscopic level are reflected in visible changes of the geometric furrows visible on the surface of exposed areas of the skin (Lavker, Kwong, & Kligman, 1980). Wrinkling and sagging can be explained in large part by changes in the middle, dermal layer of the skin, notably a decrease in the connective tissue collagen (Kligman et al., 1985). Elastin fibers become more brittle so that the ability of the skin to conform to movement of the bones is compromised. The subcutaneous fat on the limbs decreases and instead collects in areas of fatty deposits, such as around the waist and hips. A decrease in muscle mass, as will be discussed later, further adds to the loss of firmness in the skin's appearance.

There are also significant changes in the sweat and oil-producing glands within the dermis that maintain body temperature and lubricate the skin surface (Bolin & Pratt, 1989; Kurban & Bhawan, 1990). In areas such as the palms and underarms, the sweat glands become less active. The sebaceous glands that lubricate the skin with their secretions diminish in activity, and consequently the skin becomes rougher, dryer, and more vulnerable to surface damage. These changes lead to heightened risk of medical problems such as dermatitis (Grove, 1989) and pruritis (excessive itching), as well as to general discomfort (Kligman, 1989).

Age-related alterations also occur in the coloring of the skin. There are fewer melanocytes, and those that remain develop irregular areas of dark pigmentation. Under the skin surface, capillaries and small arteries become dilated, creating small irregular colored lines. Varicose veins may also form, creating an uneven surface of knotty, bluish, and cordlike irregularities. The loss of capillaries means that fair-skinned people look paler, and in general the blood vessels and bones can be seen more easily under what is a more transparent skin surface.

7.01.3.1.2 Clinical implications

Age-related changes in the skin and skin-related structures alter the skin's protective functions as well as its appearance. There is less insulation provided against extremes of temperature, and less of a barrier against environmental agents that can irritate the skin and cause dermatitis (Grove, 1989). Even if the individual is not particularly concerned about the effects of age on appearance, these changes in comfort level can trigger the crossing of an aging threshold. However, for many individuals, particularly in middle age (Whitbourne, 1996a, 1996b), age changes in the skin that lead to wrinkling are very noticeable and can have an impact on the individual's identity. In particular, comparisons of present appearance with pictures or memories of early adulthood can trigger identity accommodation in a negative way to older people who valued their youthful image (Fenske & Albers, 1990; Kleinsmith & Perricone, 1989)

Having crossed this threshold in terms of appearance, there are many steps that older individuals can take to slow, compensate for, or correct the changes in appearance caused by aging of the skin. The primary method of prevention is for fair-skinned people to avoid direct exposure to the sun and to use sunblocks when exposure cannot be avoided (Gilchrest, 1989). There are also many ways for the individual to compensate for age-related changes in the skin once they have become manifest. To counteract the fragility, sensitivity, and dryness of the skin, the individual can use sunscreens, emollients, and fragrance-free cosmetics (O'Donoghue, 1991). If a client raises concerns about these aspects of appearance, interventions here, as with hair color (see below), must attempt to strike a judicious balance between intrusiveness into matters of personal taste and the concerns of preventive practice.

7.01.3.2 Hair

7.01.3.2.1 Age changes

With increasing age in adulthood, for men and women, the hair on the head and body loses pigmentation and takes on a white appearance due to a decrease in melanin production in the hair follicles. The rate at which hair color changes varies from person to person due to variations in the timing of onset and rate of melanin production decrease across the surface of the scalp. Interestingly, although gray hair is thought to be a universal feature of aging, the degree of hair grayness is not as reliable an indicator of a person's age as is the extent to which hair on the body (axillary and pubic) has turned gray (Kenney, 1989).

Gradual and general thinning of scalp hair occurs in both sexes over the years of adulthood, although loss of hair is popularly regarded as a concern of men. Hair loss results from destruction or regression of the germ centers that produce the hair follicles underneath the skin surface. However, in men with pattern baldness, the hair follicles do not actually die but change the type of hair they produce from coarse terminal hair to fine translucent vellus hair. Men may also experience thinning of the hairs in their whiskers, and a growth of coarse hair on the eyebrows and inside the ear. Patches of coarse terminal hair may develop on the face of women, particularly around the chin.

7.01.3.2.2 Clinical implications

As is true for wrinkles, the threshold for age-related changes in the hair, at least for graying, appears to be crossed at some point in the 30s or 40s (Whitbourne, 1996b). Compared to wrinkles, gray hairs are relatively easy to detect; however, unlike wrinkles, gray hairs can be returned to virtually their original state through the use of hair dye. Changes in hair thickness, however, are not so easily reversed. The desire to disguise or stop the apparent signs of aging through surgery or the wearing of hairpieces is widespread, as is evident in the many advertisements for hair loss replacement processes.

There are many ways in which clinical intervention can be of use when changes in hair amount and color becomes a concern. Apart from providing information about commercial products that can be used if the individual chooses to try to combat the aging process, interventions can focus on ways the individual can learn to reframe age changes in the hair's appearance, particularly with regard to hair thinning, in a manner that allows for a balance between identity assimilation and accommodation. Since there are no practical implications of hair loss or hair graying, interventions in this area can be entirely at the discretion of the client and clinician. Unlike cardiovascular functioning, in which denial of age-related changes can prove fatal, the denial of changes in the hair does not have severe health consequences. The only exception is when the individual is at risk of ostracism or ridicule by others due to inappropriate attempts to maintain what he or she thinks is a youthful head of hair. In these cases, the accommodation process may need to be brought to bear on the situation so that the individual can accept that patch of skin on the top of the head or can find a hair dye that does not attempt to recreate the look of a 20-year-old. Of course, these issues quickly become matters of taste and preference, and short of major concerns or problems, should ultimately be left to the individual's discretion.

7.01.3.3 Body Build

7.01.3.3.1 Age changes

It is a well-established fact that over the course of adulthood there is a consistent pattern of a reduction in standing height, occurring at a greater rate after the 50s and particularly pronounced in women (Shephard, 1978). The major cause is loss of bone mineral content in the vertebrae, which leads them to collapse and cause compression in the length of the spine (Garn, 1975). Changes in the joints and flattening of the arches of the feet can further contribute to height loss (Kenney, 1989).

Total body weight increases from the 20s until the mid-50s, after which total body weight declines. Most of the weight gain in middle adulthood is due to an accumulation of body fat, particularly around the waist and hips. The weight loss that occurs in the later years of adulthood is not due to a slimming of the torso but to a loss of lean body mass consisting of muscle and bone (Chien et al., 1975; Ellis, Shukla, Cohn, & Pierson, 1974). Consequently, very old adults may have very thin extremities but fatty areas in the chin, waist, and hips. Middle-aged and older women are particularly likely to experience this accumulation of body fat around the torso, with a gain of abdominal girth amounting to 25–35% across the adult years compared to 6–16% for men over a comparable time period (Shephard, 1978). However, contemporary changes in lifestyle and improved nutrition may be altering this trend, with current cohorts of older women showing a decrease rather than an increase in body fat (Rico, Revilla, Hernandez, Gonzalez-Riola, & Villa, 1993).

7.01.3.3.2 Clinical implications

Changes in body fat that lead to the appearance of a sagging or heavier body shape can result in increased identification of the self as moving away from the figure of youth. The development of "middle-aged spread" is one of the first occurrences to trigger identity accommodation of the self as aging, perhaps even before the first gray hairs have sprouted. Indeed, awareness of changes in body composition can occur surprisingly early in adulthood, perhaps by the 30s (Whitbourne, 1996b).

Fortunately, the crossing of the body fat threshold may be readily compensated, and before the individual gives up on trying to slow down this particular process, there are many activities that the clinician can promote if this is an area of concern for the individual. It is well established that participation in active sports and exercise activity can offset the deleterious effects of aging on body fat accumulation. For instance, endurance athletes do not gain weight and they maintain their muscular physiques throughout adulthood for as long as they continue to train (Suominen, Heikkinen, Parkatti, Forsberg, & Kiiskinen, 1977). Participation in exercise training programs can even be of value for middle-aged and elderly adults who were sedentary throughout their lives. By engaging in vigorous walking, jogging, or cycling for 30–60 minutes a day for 3–4 days a week, the sedentary adult can expect to achieve positive results in a period as short as 10–20 weeks (Whitbourne, 1996a). Furthermore, the same activities that a middle-aged person might engage in to combat body fat changes can also have very positive cardiovascular and general health benefits. Thus, vanity might actually serve a protective function in this area.

Changes in body height are less easily compensated, but identity processes are also less likely to be engaged in this area unless the individual has had concerns about height from the early years and on. Clinical interventions here may focus on the maintenance of bone strength through weight resistance training and although these activities might not have an enhancing effect on height, they can be very important in promoting mobility (see below), another major concern for many older adults.

7.01.3.4 Mobility

7.01.3.4.1 Age changes

The individual's ability to move around in the physical environment is a function of the integrity of the muscles, bones, joints between the bones, tendons and ligaments that connect muscle to bone, and contractility of flexor and extensor muscles. Mobility changes in important ways over the course of the adult years such that movement becomes more difficult, more painful, and often less effective for the older adult.

Between ages 40–70 years, the loss of muscle strength amounts to approximately 10–20% with more severe losses of 30–40% after ages 70 to 80 years; losses that are more pronounced in the muscles of the lower extremities (McArdle, Katch, & Katch, 1991). This pattern of diminishing muscle strength appears to be due to atrophy of muscle fibers, particularly the "fast twitch" fibers important in developing the rapidly accelerating powerful contractions normally associated with strength. The "slow twitch" fibers involved in maintaining posture and muscular contractions over protacted periods of exertion remain constant over the adult years. The atrophy of fast-twitch fibers is thought to result from the loss of the motoneurons that activate the muscles. After the muscle fiber dies, it is replaced initially by connective tissue and in its final stages, by fat (Fiatrone & Evans, 1993). However, declines in muscle strength are not completely accounted for by loss of muscle mass, and there are other influences on age effects on muscle strength as yet to be determined (Kallman, Plato, & Tobin, 1990; Overend, Cunningham, Kramer, Lefeve, & Paterson, 1992).

There are individual variations that can lead to important deviations from such a general pattern of decline. The extent to which aging affects loss of muscle strength depends in part on which gender is being tested, the general level of activity in which the individual has typically engaged, the particular muscle group being tested, and whether the type of muscle strength being assessed is static (isometric) or dynamic.

Although the process of bone growth and remodeling continues, the overall course of bone development in adulthood is toward loss of bone strength, resulting in diminished ability of the bones to withstand mechanical pressure and to show greater vulnerability to fracture. The decrease in various measures of bone strength ranges from 5 to 12% per decade from the 20s through the 90s (McCalden, McGeough, Barker, & Court-Brown, 1993). Loss of bone strength is generally explained as a function of the loss of bone mineral content, meaning that the bone becomes increasingly porous and unable to support the loads it must bear. The extent to which bone mass decreases over the years of adulthood amounts to approximately 20–30% of total bone mineral content in women, and approximately half that amount in men (Mazess, 1982; Riggs et al., 1981). The period of maximum bone loss is between the 50s and the 70s (Sparrow, Beausoleil, Garvey, Rozner, & Silbert, 1982). The explanation of the underlying process that causes loss of bone mineral content is that the rate of resorption exceeds that of new bone growth in later adulthood, giving a net result of a reduction in bone mass (Sherman et al., 1992). In part, bone density and the loss of bone mass in the later years of adulthood may be a function of genetic factors (Dargent & Breart, 1993; Kelly et al., 1993). Lifestyle also seems to play a role, however, including factors such as physical activity, smoking, alcohol use, and diet which can account for 50–60% of the variation in bone density (Krall & Dawson-Hughes, 1993). There are also hormonal influences on bone mass, as indicated by the observation that bone mineral loss in women proceeds at a higher rate in postmenopausal women who are no longer producing estrogen in monthly cycles (Nuti & Martini, 1993).

Although the aging of joints is most commonly associated with the later years of life, degenerative processes that reduce the functional efficiency of the joints begin even before the individual reaches skeletal maturity. Restrictions of movement and discomfort are therefore a potential problem for adults of any age, but they occur with increasing frequency as age progresses. The decline in joint functioning can be accounted for by age losses in virtually every structural component of the joint. Starting in the 20s and 30s, the arterial cartilage begins to thin, fray, shred, and crack (Adrian, 1981). Unprotected by cartilage, the underlying bone eventually begins to wear away. At the same time, outgrowths of cartilage develop and these interfere with the smooth movement of the joint. Age-related weakening of the muscles further contributes to restrictions in range of movement due to changes in the joints themselves (Vandervoort et al., 1992). Changes at the cellular level in the structure of collagen and elastin comparable to those that occur in the dermis are thought to contribute to loss of flexibility, strength, and resiliency of connective tissue. Diminished efficiency of circulation may contribute further to deteriorative changes. Since the cartilage receives little vascular supply to begin with, any reductions in adulthood due to aging or arterial disease will further reduce its reparative ability. Furthermore, the joints are subjected to an extreme amount of trauma throughout life, including the strains and sprains encountered during everyday activities and strenuous exercise, activities that further contribute to their deterioration.

7.01.3.4.2 Clinical implications

For many individuals, thresholds of aging become painfully crossed with each newly-discovered joint ache or mobility restriction, sometimes beginning in the 40s (Whitbourne, 1996b). Changes in the structures that support movement have many pervasive effects on the individual's life, resulting in restrictions in activity and pain which can interfere with the individual's psychological adaptation and sense of well-being (Hughes, Edelman, Singer, & Chang, 1993). In part, the effects of mobility loss can be attributed to the enforced reliance on others that is created, leading to other deleterious processes such as being treated like a dependent child (Whitbourne & Wills, 1993).

One of the most serious outcomes of reduced muscle strength, bone strength, and joint mobility is the heightened susceptibility of older individuals, particularly women, to falls (Dargent & Breart, 1993; Lord, Clark, & Webster, 1991). If a broken hip results, the individual is more likely to suffer long-term disability and dependency (Roberto, 1992). Unfortunately, individuals might overreact to falls by developing a "fear of falling" (Downton & Andrews, 1990) or lowered sense of self-efficacy regarding the ability to avoid a fall (Tinetti & Powell, 1993). As a result, they become less stable on their feet and avoid physical activities that might benefit their strength and stability. Understandably, these individuals are vulnerable to feelings of depression and anxiety. Other adults may react to falls through identity assimilation, by repressing their occurrence (Wright, Aizenstein, Vogler, Rowe, & Miller, 1990), which might maintain their sense of self-efficacy but place them at risk of further serious injury.

This summary of age-related changes in mobility describes a fairly downhill process, but there are many interventions clinicians can pursue that will have practical advantages. As has been mentioned already, it is important to structure an intervention around the nature of the individual's identity processes, particularly as balanced against the individual's actual age-related losses and possiblities for compensation. Given such an assessment, older individuals can be encouraged to participate in a variety of physical exercises that can prove to be extremely helpful in maintaining or restoring mobility. A regular program of exercise can help the middle-aged and older adult compensate substantially for the loss of muscle fibers. Although there is nothing that can be done to stop the loss of muscle cells, the remaining fibers can be strengthened and work efficiency increased through exercise training even in persons as old as 90 years (Fiatrone et al., 1990). Inactivity can accelerate the loss of muscle strength, and the same is true of bone loss. Older individuals can also benefit from resistance training exercises that, within limits, increase the stress placed upon the bone (Dalsky et al. 1988; Rikli & McManis, 1990; Smith, 1981). Although degenerative changes in the joints are not reversible, it is possible for older individuals to benefit from exercise training, particularly if it is oriented toward promoting flexibility (Jirovec, 1991), strengthening the muscles that support the joints, increasing the circulation of blood to the joints thereby promoting the repair of injured tissues (Brooks & Fahey, 1984), and decreasing the risk of injury (Stamford, 1988).

7.01.4 THE EFFECTS OF AGE ON VITAL FUNCTIONS

7.01.4.1 Cardiovascular System

7.01.4.1.1 Age changes

The aging process results in serious limitations of the heart's functional requirement to pump blood continuously through the circulatory system at a rate that adequately perfuses the body's cells. Although a distinct entity in terms of underlying processes, fatal cardiovascular diseases do become more probable with advancing age in adulthood. These diseases can have widespread effects on daily life in addition to providing constant sources of reminders of the individual's mortality. For example, the chest pains associated with angina, a chronic cardiac illness, are not only uncomfortable but provide clear warning signals of the heart's impending failure.

The reduction in the heart's pumping capacity is due to a variety of changes affecting the structure and function of the heart muscle walls, particularly the left ventricle which becomes progressively thicker with each decade in adulthood and less elastic (Kitzman, Scholz, Hagen, Ilstrup, & Edwards 1988; Kitzman & Edwards, 1990) as the number of myocardial cells decreases and the remaining cells become hypertrophied (Olivetti, Melissari, Capasso, & Anversa, 1991). The decreased capacity of the ventricle walls to expand results in a reduced and delayed filling of the left ventricle and the ejection of less blood into the aorta. The cardiac muscle also becomes less responsive to the neural stimulation of the "pacemaker" cells in the heart that initiate each contraction (Montamat & Davies 1989; Schulman & Gerstenblith, 1989).

Effects of aging on the arteries further compromise the system's ability to distribute blood to the body's cells. Although it is difficult to separate the effects of aging from those of atherosclerosis (a disease in which the arteries become rigid and narrowed by fatty accumulation), the aging process itself appears to cause changes in the aorta and arteries (Shimojo, Tsuda, Iwasaka, & Inada, 1991). The wall of the aorta becomes less flexible, so that the blood leaving the left ventricle of the heart is faced by more resistance and cannot travel as far. The walls of the arteries throughout the body become thicker and less flexible. Impedence of blood flow through the arteries is further augmented by the accumulation of lipids in the blood (Heiss et al., 1980).

Although age-related changes in the heart and arteries reduce the amount of blood available to the cells of the body, under normal conditions these changes are not particularly pronounced or noticable. The effects of aging of the circulatory system are most apparent while the individual is engaging in aerobic exercise, when there is a reduction both in maximum oxygen consumption (aerobic capacity) and the maximum attainable heart rate (Lakatta, 1987; Morley & Reese, 1989). Aerobic capacity decreases in a linear fashion throughout the adult years, so that the average 65-year-old individual has 30–40% of the aerobic capacity of the young adult (McArdle et al., 1991). Other functional variables decrease to a commensurate degree, such as the amount of blood pumped at each beat of the heart (Weisfeldt & Gerstenblith, 1986), and the cardiac output per minute. These decreases in the functional capacity of the heart mean that less oxygen reaches the muscles during exercise. Changes in the heart and arteries can also account, in part, for the observation that older individuals have higher levels of systolic and diastolic blood pressure, both at rest and during exercise.

7.01.4.1.2 Clinical implications

Although not as apparent in its effects on identity as appearance, the functioning of the cardiovascular system is an important influence on the individual's feelings of well-being and identity. The efficiency of the cardiovascular system is essential to life so that threats to the integrity of this system are perceived as highly dangerous. Awareness of reduced cardiovascular efficiency can therefore serve as reminders of one's own personal mortality.

In working with middle-aged and older adults, clinicians can turn to the wealth of research pointing to the effectiveness of exercise in slowing or reversing the effects of the aging process. The results of research on the effectiveness of exercise training have consistently revealed improved functioning in long-term endurance athletes, master athletes, exercisers, and previously sedentary adults (Whitbourne 1996a; McArdle et al., 1991). Previously sedentary adults can improve to levels that approximate the improvements achieved by younger adults (Govindasamy, Paterson, Poulin, & Cunningham 1988; Hagberg et al., 1989). Even moderate or low-intensity exercise can have beneficial effects on healthy sedentary elderly (Foster, Hume, Byrnes, Dickinson, & Chatfield 1989; Hamdorf, Withers, Penhall, & Haslam, 1992). Further, aerobic exercise training has the positive effect of lowering the heart rate and improving work load intensity and duration in submaximal exercise, (Morey et al., 1991; Poulin, Paterson, Govindasamy, & Cunningham, 1988), ultimately placing less stress upon the heart during exertion. Other benefits of exercise training are improvements in the peripheral vasculature (Blumenthal et al., 1989), lipid metabolism (Tamai et al., 1988), and blood pressure during or immediately after exertion (Webb, Poehlman, & Tonino, 1993). That exercise can have such positive effects on physical functioning in old age, even if it is begun after a lifetime of sedentary patterns, provides strong evidence in favor of the view that the rate of the aging process can be altered significantly through active lifestyle choices made by the individual.

The main advantage that exercise seems to hold as a means of retaining a higher level of cardiovascular functioning is that it provides a continued potent stimulus for the muscle cells of the heart to undergo strong contractions so that they retain or gain contractile power. The greater strength of the myocardial muscle improves the functioning of the left ventricle and as a result, more blood can be ejected from the left ventricle (Ehsani, Ogawa, Miller, Spina, & Jilka, 1991). The other advantage of exercise training is that it makes it possible for the individual to "save" energy during aerobic work that is less than maximal by fulfilling the demands of the work load but placing less stress on the heart. Because more blood is ejected with each cardiac muscle contraction, the same output of blood can be pumped per minute but at a lower heart rate. The effects of training on cardiac functioning under submaximal conditions are of interest in that these performance situations are closer to the conditions under which people exert themselves in their daily lives. Exercise training also has favorable effects on the body's performance by increasing the efficiency of metabolism in the working muscles (Meredith et al., 1989).

In addition to the advantages of exercise training for the cardiovascular system, it is well established that adults who become involved in aerobic activities experience a variety of positive effects on mood, anxiety levels, and particularly feelings of mastery and control, leading to enhanced feelings of self-esteem (Hill, Storandt, & Malley 1993; McAuley, Lox, & Duncan, 1993). Although some researchers have demonstrated there to be positive effects of exercise on cognitive functioning (Chodzko-Zajko, Schuler, Solomon, Heiul, & Ellis, 1992; Stevenson & Topp, 1990), this effect is not observed consistently (Hill et al., 1993). Nevertheless, it appears clear that older adults who enter exercise training programs "feel better," and this improvement in mood can be clinically useful for many aging clients.

A great deal has been written in the area of behavioral medicine on strategies for increasing the compliance of cardiac patients with dietary and exercise controls over the progress of their disease. In terms of the normal aging process, similar interventions might be suggested. Those individuals who deny the effects of aging through identity assimilation must be brought to recognize that they will run real risks to their lives if they either fail to engage in preventative behaviors or engage in strenuous activities without proper supervision or training. In contrast, middle-aged and older individuals who overreact to age changes in what they have heard about cardiovascular functioning, or perhaps to the appearance of slight symptoms, need to be given assurance that they can nevertheless continue to engage in exercise activities and that, indeed, such activities are necessary for the prevention of further and more serious health limitations.

7.01.4.2 Respiratory System

7.01.4.2.1 Age changes

The airways in the respiratory system permit gas exchange between the blood and air, making it possible for the body's cells to receive support for their metabolic activities. Aging's primary effect is to reduce the quality of gas exchange in the lungs so that less oxygen from the outside air reaches the blood (Kenney, 1989). Aging also reduces vital capacity, the amount of air that is moved into and out of the lungs at maximal levels of exertion (Reddon, 1981), and forced expiratory volume, the amount of air that can be breathed out during a short amount of time (Smith, Cunningham, Patterson, Rechnitzer, & Koval, 1992). These reductions in respiratory functioning result from changes in pulmonary structures such that the airways, and particularly lung tissue, lose the elastic ability to resist expansion as they fill with air. The changes in lung structures that account for decreased elastic recoil and increased compliance are alterations in the composition and structure of the elastin and collagen composition of lung tissue (Brandstetter & Kazemi, 1983; D'Errico et al., 1989). Increased rigidity of the chest wall further lower the lung's ability to be fully compressed during expiration and expanded during inspiration (Mahler, Rossiello, & Lohe, 1986). These changes mean that less than the maximal amount of air can be brought into and out of the lungs, particularly under conditions of exertion (Teramoto, Fukuchi, Nagase, Matsuse, & Orimo, 1995). The greater rigidity of the chest wall also increases the amount of work that must be performed by the respiratory muscles during the inspiratory and expiratory phases of the ventilation cycle.

7.01.4.2.2 Clinical implications

Age changes in respiration can lead to feelings of dyspnea and fatigue associated with exertion, sensations that can approach the intensity of a panic attack. Adding to age effects on cardiovascular functioning, changes in the respiratory system can lead the aging individual to avoid strenuous activities, a consequence that further impairs the individual's cardiovascular and respiratory efficiency. Because both of these functions are so crucial to life, and because shortness of breath is so frightening, the individual might conclude prematurely that death is around the corner.

The effects of exercise training on respiratory functioning are encouraging (Blumenthal et al., 1989) but the specific effects of exercise on respiratory functioning are not as dramatic as the effects on the cardiovascular system. Equally, if not more, beneficial to the respiratory function is the avoidance of cigarette smoking (Hermanson, Omenn, & Kronmal, 1988).

Taking these factors into account, clinicians may wish to treat instances of dyspnea leading to panic as instances of overaccommodation, in which the individual may be brought to a more balanced state through recognizing the fact that some age-related changes in breathing capacity are in fact inevitable. On the other hand, for individuals who are using identity assimilation to deny the importance of factors that impede respiratory efficiency, notably cigarette smoking, steps need to be taken to increase identity accommodation and the recognition that this behavior can accelerate the deleterious effects of aging on respiratory efficiency and feelings of comfort during exercise.

7.01.5 THE EFFECTS OF AGE ON REGULATORY SYSTEMS

7.01.5.1 Excretory System

7.01.5.1.1 Age changes

It has been known for years that there are significant and widespread changes in the structure of the kidneys, changes that are reflected in cross-sectional studies in impaired efficiency across adulthood on every measure of renal functioning studied. (Rowe, Shock, & DeFronzo, 1976). An early estimate of the loss of renal functions over the adult years was a figure of 6% per decade from age 20 and continuing into the 90s, a loss that exists in longitudinal studies as well (Shock, Andres, Norris, & Tobin, 1978). The cause of aging of the kidney is loss of structure and function of the basic cell of the kidney, the nephron (McLacklan, Guthrie, Anderson, & Fulker, 1977). There are also independent losses in mechanism within the kidney responsible for concentrating urine (Rowe, 1982).

Particularly challenging to the aging kidney is aerobic exercise because it diverts blood to the working skeletal muscles, and thereby causes a further reduction in the blood flow through the kidneys. Equally important, the urine concentrating mechanism begins to fail during exercise or under extreme conditions of heat when the individual begins to perspire. Fatigue, changes in body chemistry, and potentially harmful changes in bodily fluid levels occur more rapidly in the older adult who cannot conserve sodium and water adequately under these conditions.

The effects of aging on the bladder are of great importance to the individual's conscious experience of aging. Adults past the age of 65 years experience a reduction in the total amount of urine they can store before feeling a need to void, and more urine is retained in the bladder after the individual has attempted to empty it. These phenomena appear to be related to age changes in the connective tissue of the bladder causing the organ to lose its expandability and contractility somewhat like that which is seen in the lung. Furthermore, recognition of the need to void may not occur until the bladder is almost or even completely filled. This means that the individual has less or perhaps no time to reach a lavatory before leakage or spillage occurs.

The most significant effect of changes with age in the bladder is on patterns of urinary incontinence. The prevalence of incontinence among the population 60 years and older is estimated to be 19% for women and 8% for men (Herzog, Diokno, Brown, Normolle, & Brock, 1990) but can reach as high as 36% among community-dwelling elderly with dementia

(Ouslander, Zarit, Orr, & Muira, 1990). Women are more likely to suffer from stress incontinence, which refers to loss of urine at times of exertion such as when one is laughing, sneezing, lifting, or bending and is the result of weakness of the pelvic muscles. Urge incontinence, which is more prevalent in men, involves urine loss following an urge to void or lack of control over voiding with little or no warning (Diokno, Brock, Brown, & Herzog, 1986); it is related to prostatic disease or incomplete emptying of the bladder. Among the community-dwelling elderly, each of these conditions, particularly urge incontinence, is reversible and may disappear within a year or two of its initial development (Herzog et al., 1990)

7.01.5.1.2 Clinical implications

Although not insignificant in terms of the body's physiological efficiency, the aging of the kidney is unlikely to have a discernible impact on everyday functioning. However, age-related changes in the bladder are another matter, and can be important threshold phenomena (Whitbourne, 1996b). Incontinence can be highly disruptive to the older individual's everyday life, causing distress and embarrassment (Hunskaar & Vinsnes, 1991; Ouslander & Abelson 1990; Wyman, Hawkins, & Fantl, 1990). Not only do such occasions involve shame, but they feed into the association in many people's minds between "senility" and urinary incontinence. Other horrors of incontinence may also trigger overaccommodation, such as loss of independence and respect. Given the many associations to urinary continence, it would not be unreasonable to suppose that even a single episode of stress incontinence could create a threshold experience and overaccommodation. Unfortunately, advertisers prey on this vulnerability of older adults in commercials for adult diapers that suggest these changes to be expectable and unpreventable. Clinicians needs to work with older adult clients to dispel these myths.

On the positive side, once identified, incontinence is a condition that in many cases can be managed if the individual is able to learn new behavioral strategies. Through behavioral techniques, sometimes involving only very simple exercises, the problem can be held in check if not reversed (Burgio & Engel, 1990; Burns et al., 1993).

Age effects on renal functioning significantly affect the older person's ability to excrete medications, a fact that can be of great importance in a therapeutic context. When an older person is given the the same dosage of medication appropriate for a younger adult, more of the drug will remain in the bloodstream over the period of time between doses. With repeated dosages of the drug it is more likely that toxic levels will build up in the blood. Unless the dosage is adjusted to take into account this lower rate of tubular transport, drugs may have an adverse impact instead of their intended benefits (Lamy, 1988; Montgomery, 1990).

7.01.5.2 Digestive System

7.01.5.2.1 Age changes

The documented effects of aging on digestion in the empirical literature are remarkably minor compared to the lavish attention devoted by advertisers and the popular media to the supposed inefficiencies of digestive processes in older adults. One change with age that may have implications for digestive functioning is a reduction in the metabolism of certain nutrients in the stomach and small intestine, but other structures such as the esophagous, liver, pancreas, and large intestine appear to be relatively spared by the aging process (Whitbourne, 1996). More important than constipation, dyspepsia, and reduced sensory capacities for enjoying food are the beliefs that people hold as communicated through the media, the social context in which food is eaten, other physical and cognitive deficiencies, and the individual's lifelong patterns of nutrition (Costello & Moser-Veillon, 1992; Fischer & Iohson 1990; Ryan, Craig, & Finn, 1992; Wedman et al., 1991).

7.01.5.2.2 Clinical implications

Changes in the digestive system at the physiological level due to aging are not likely to propel the individual over an aging threshold (Whitbourne, 1996b). However, so many elders have been exposed to inaccurate conceptions in the media about the aging digestive system that clinicians have an important psychoeducational role to play. In the area of digestion and particularly elimination, embarrassment may lead the older individual to avoid discussions of anxiety-provoking issues that, if discussed and allayed, could ease these very uncomfortable feelings. Furthermore, questions about food intake are essential for clinicians to explore, as inadequate nutrition may lead to symptoms that mimic those of psychological or cognitive impairment disorders. Unchecked, a vicious cycle may be created, as depression can lead to loss of interest in food and food preparation (Rosenbloom & Whittington, 1993).

Another clinical issue related to digestion concerns fecal incontinence. Older adults, particularly those who overrely on identity accommodation, may associate irregularities in defecation with feared diseases and the prospects of institutionalization in later life (Holt, 1991; Wald, 1990). Older persons who believe that "senility" is an inevitable feature of aging may regard with alarm any indication that their patterns of elimination are changing, seeing in such changes a more ominous significance that can risk putting them over the threshold. The anxiety created by this concern may contribute further to gastrointestinal problems so that what originates as a temporary problem comes to have a more prolonged course. Clinicians can intervene in this process by sensitive discussion of this very personal and potentially frightening area of daily life.

7.01.5.3 Immune System

7.01.5.3.1 Age changes

There is substantial evidence of reduced immune system functioning across age groups of adults. T-cells, which destroy antigens (foreign substances that enter the body), lose effectiveness over the adult years (Bloom, 1994; Globerson, Eren, Abel, & Ben-Menahem, 1990), in part due to changes in the thymus gland. Autopsy studies have revealed that deterioration of the thymus gland begins shortly after sexual maturity is reached, so that by the time the individual is 45–50 years old, the thymus retains only 5–10% of its peak mass. As a result of these changes, there are more immature T-cells present both within the thymus gland and in the bloodstream. Other immune system cells, including natural killer (NK) cells, K cells, and macrophages, do appear to retain their functioning into old age (Bloom 1994; Kutza, Kaye, & Mwasko, 1995); however, another entire line of defenses is altered in the aging process through the reduced activity of helper T-cells, increased activity of suppresser T-cells, and the increasing development of certain autoimmune diseases.

7.01.5.3.2 Clinical implications

Investigations have been stimulated by progress in psychoneuroimmunology, a field in which the intricate connections are examined between affective states such as stress and depression, nervous system functioning, and operation of the immune system (O'Leary 1990; Vollardt, 1991). For example, elderly individuals with high levels of life stress have been found to experience lower T-cell functioning (McNaughton, Smith, Patterson, & Grant, 1990). Conversely, social support, at least among women, was found to be related positively to immune system competence measured in terms of lymphocyte numbers and response to mitogens (Thomas, Goodwin, & Goodwin, 1985). Older individuals are at least as susceptible to stress as younger adults in increases of T-suppressor cells and NK cell numbers, although not in terms of increased NK activity (Nabiloff et al., 1991). Stress also seems linked to the release of beta-endorphin, an opioid peptide released from the pituitary gland that has an analgesic effect. This process may play an important role in mediating the effects of emotions on the immune system (Antoni, 1987).

Apart from changes in the immune system that interact with psychological functioning, the lowered effectiveness of the immune system in older adults has important implications for health. The aging immune system has been linked to increased vulnerability to influenza, infections, cancer, and certain age-associated autoimmune disorders such as diabetes and possibly atherosclerosis and Alzheimer's disease. A less competent immune system can put the elderly individual at higher risk at least to certain forms of cancer and influenza (Ershler, 1990; Miller, 1993). Clearly, the development of severe health problems can have significant effects on the individual's psychological well-being.

There are many ways in which clinicians can take advantage of the potential interactions between identity and immune system functioning. The crossing of an aging threshold in any salient area of functioning, to the extent that it triggers a stressful reaction, can lead to deleterious effects on immune functioning. The individual then becomes more susceptible to immune-related conditions, further accentuating the effects of crossing the threshold. Overassimilation may have some beneficial aspects, in this regard, if the individual is not placed at risk by ignoring important physical changes.

7.01.6 AGE CHANGES IN THE REPRODUCTIVE SYSTEM AND SEXUALITY

7.01.6.1 Female Reproductive System

Throughout her 40s, a woman's reproductive capacity becomes gradually reduced until, by the age of 50–55 years, it ceases altogether. Associated with the ending of the monthly phases of ovulation and menstruation is a diminution of the hormones estrogen and progesterone. Other changes in sexual functioning are related to aging of the tissues in other bodily systems. For example, sagging of the breasts and torso results from decreased skin elasticity. Subcutaneous fat accumulates around the waist, leading to uneven bulges. The appearance and functioning of the genital organs also change after the menopause. The pubic hair on the mons veneris and around the vulva becomes thin and coarser. The labia majora and minora become thinner and wrinkled, the skin in the vulva atrophies, and the surface cells of the vaginal wall become thin, dry, pale, and smooth. The vagina also becomes narrower and shorter. These changes are significant not only for their effects on sexual functioning but for their effects on the woman's enjoyment of sexual intercourse. The older woman may experience discomfort during intercourse due to changes in the vagina and vulva, and the rhythmic contractions of the uterus during orgasm may become painful.

Despite changes in the reproductive system, the conclusion reached by Masters and Johnson (1966) in the mid 1960s is still generally accepted: that older women are limited in their sexual gratification more by their attitudes, values, and accessibility to partners than they are by physical changes involved in aging. The sexual response cycle might be slowed down somewhat in the older woman, but the possibility of achieving orgasm is not reduced.

7.01.6.2 Male Reproductive System

Just as women gradually lose reproductive capacity, men experience a climacteric of sorts in which there is a reduction in the number of viable sperm they produce due to degenerative changes in the seminiferous tubules of the testes (Harman, 1978). With increasing age, men may experience changes in the prostate gland that lead to a reduction of the volume and pressure of semen expelled during ejaculation. Age-related changes also include overgrowth or hypertrophy of the glandular and connective tissue in the parts of the prostate that surround the prostatic urethra. This condition, called benign prostatic hypertrophy, is increasingly prevalent in men past 50 years, rising to an estimated 50% of men 80 years and older. The adjacent penile urethra may become constricted due to this overgrowth, and urinary rentention may ensue. Discomfort and embarrassment may result from difficulties in urination and from the occurrence of involuntary penile erections (Masters & Johnson, 1966). If urinary retention becomes a chronic condition, kidney problems may develop, leading to more serious health threats.

A physiological index of reproductive function that has a decidedly noticeable effect on the older man's sense of his own sexuality is that of penile erectility. It is well documented that older men experience fewer nightly episodes of penile erections compared to younger males (Karacan, Willliam, Thornby, & Salis, 1975). By contrast, there are inconsistencies in the findings regarding increase in penile circumference during erection, with some decreases noted across age groups (Solnick & Birren, 1977), and in other research no age differences are observed (Schiavi & Schreiner-Engel, 1988).

As is true for aging women, there is a general slowing down in aging men of the progression through the human sexual response cycle. Compared to young adult men, orgasm is shorter, involving fewer contractions of the prostate, and ejection of a smaller amount of seminal fluid (Masters & Johnson, 1970). These findings may carry some negative implications for the aging male's sexual relations. However, the gains for the older man's ability to enjoy sexuality are also compelling. He may feel less driven toward the pressure to ejaculate, be able to prolong the period of sensual enjoyment prior to orgasm, and have the control to coordinate his pleasure cycle to correspond more to his female partner.

The main predictor of a man's pattern of sexuality in the earlier years of adulthood is by far the best predictor of his sexuality in old age (George & Weiler, 1985). The sexually active middle-aged man, given good health, has the potential to remain sexually active well into his later years.

7.01.6.3 Clinical Implications

The impact of the menopause depends heavily on how the woman interprets the significance of this transition, which may be met with relief or as a reminder of the inevitability of aging and mortality. Although the aging male is likely to be less preoccupied by his diminished (but not lost) reproductive capacity, he may also find age-related changes to have a negative impact on his enjoyment of sexual relations. He may overaccommodate to aging changes, believing that his masculine prowess has failed. Furthermore, the changes he perceives in his sexual functioning may be interpreted as movement toward deterioration and death. As is true for any man regardless of age, depression, heavy alcohol use, or late-life career pressures may also interfere with the aging male's ability to enjoy sexual relations. Difficulties in adjusting to age changes in the sexual response cycle may present a problem if the partners are unfamiliar with the fact that sexual responsivity naturally becomes altered in later adulthood. The woman may worry that she has lost her orgasmic capacity because it takes her longer to become aroused, excited, and stimulated. The aging male may be at high risk of developing symptoms of secondary (nonphysiological) impotence.

As is true of other sensitive areas of physical functioning, the clinician's responsibility in these areas is to explore in a patient and careful manner the level of concern the individual or couple may have about their functioning. Given cohort differences in attitudes toward sexuality, it is likely that the average older person finds it difficult to discuss specific details about problems in sexual functioning. The general level of anxiety associated with sexual matters can lead to heightened potential for either identity assimilation in the form of denial, or identity accommodation in the form of overreaction. Furthermore, in this area perhaps more so than in any other, it might be necessary for the clinician's own attitudes toward sexuality in the aged to become an area of personal focus and reflection before proceeding to the level of intervention.

7.01.7 THE NERVOUS SYSTEM

7.01.7.1 Central Nervous System

7.01.7.1.1 Age changes

In the central nervous system (CNS), as in the other major organ systems, changes that are due to aging alone are difficult to separate from changes that are the result of disease. Neurofibrillary tangles, amyloid plaques, and granulovacuolar degeneration are all deleterious changes observed in the brains of people with Alzheimer's disease, but are also thought to occur to a lesser extent in normal aging. There are thought to be decreases in acetylcholine levels in the hippocampus and a decline in the number of neurons in the hippocampus, but these are also well-known correlates of Alzheimer's disease. Similarly, decreased amounts of dopamine in the substantia nigra–basal ganglia pathway are regarded as age-related changes but are also observed in Parkinson's disease. It is not clear whether these losses occur normally in later life and are exaggerated in the case of disease, or whether they constitute discrete phenomena.

Keeping in mind the distinction between normal aging and disease processes, there is documentation that areas of the brain are differentially affected by neuronal loss in later adulthood. There appear to be signficiant losses of neurons from the hippocampus, the area affected by Alzheimer's disease and involved in short-term memory (Mouritzen Dam, 1979), and in the cerebellum (Hall, Miller, & Corsellis, 1975), the structure that regulates refined motor patterns. Age losses in these subcortical areas, however, are considered relatively minor compared to losses (as high as 50%) in the areas of the cerebral cortex responsible for processing sensory information, including the primary visual cortex (Devaney & Johnson, 1980), the primary somatosensory region (Henderson, Tomlinson, & Gibson, 1980), and the secondary auditory cortex which loses between one-third and one-half of its total number of neurons over the adult years (Brody, 1955; Henderson et al., 1980). Cells in the motor cortex show comparable losses of 20–50%, and these losses are thought to be a contributing factor to muscular stiffness, slowness, and joint pain (Scheibel, 1982). In contrast to these somewhat dramatic losses of neuron numbers is the pattern of relative stability in the prefrontal region of the cortex (Higatsberger, Budka, & Bernheimer, 1982; Huttenlocher, 1979). The stability of neurons in these regions of the cortex is important, as these are the parts of the nervous system involved in judgment, abstract thinking, and the ability to plan.

7.01.7.1.2 Clinical implications

Aging of the CNS has direct effects on a variety of sensory, motor, and cognitive capacities and behaviors including perception, short-term memory, fine motor coordination, and large muscle control. However, the view of the aging brain as a degenerating system does not take into account what is known about the compensatory processes of redundancy and plasticity (Buell & Coleman, 1979; Flood, Buell, Horowitz, & Coleman 1987; Flood & Coleman, 1988). The impact of these processes is most likely to occur in the association areas of the cerebral cortex, where higher order abstract thinking processes are mediated. In fact, these abilities may improve in the later years of adulthood as the individual stores more experiences into the long-term memory association areas on which decisions and judgment are based.

Furthermore, it is important to emphasize once again that there is tremendous variation among adults in the ways in which the aging process (apart from disease) affects CNS functions. Some of these functions in later adulthood are, in addition, affected by the extent to which the individual developed and used them during the adult years. Exposure to stimulation in the areas of perception, cognition, and motor activity through mental and physical exercise can influence, throughout old age, the degree to which the abilities that depend on these functions are maintained. The importance placed by the individual on mental and physical abilities contributes further to the personal meaning of age changes in any of these areas and whether a threshold is crossed in this domain.

Clinically, of course, it is essential that those working with the elderly are knowledgable about and sensitive to the symptoms of Alzheimer's disease, particularly as these differ from other forms of cognitive impairment or depression. Clinicians must also be aware of the extent to which elders fear the onset of Alzheimer's disease and interpret even minor changes in cognitive functions as signs that the end is in sight. Overaccommodation in the cognitive domain can prove extremely damaging to the older adult's identity as a sentient being, and vigilance in this area toward any signs of deterioration is likely to be high. This risk is perhaps greater than that of overassimilation, except when an individual who really does have early symptoms of Alzheimer's disease denies the memory or judgment problems that are interfering with daily life activities. Media attention to Alzheimer's disease, although positive in the sense of educating the public, may backfire in this domain, leaving many elders (and clinicians) with the erroneous impression that the disease is an inevitable outcome of the aging process.

7.01.7.2 Autonomic Nervous System

7.01.7.2.1 Age changes

Although in many aspects the autonomic nervous system (ANS) operates without significant age-related alterations throughout adulthood, there are important effects of aging on two functions served by the ANS that have a considerable impact on the individual's daily life: bodily temperature control and sleep patterns.

It is well established both through population health statistics and experimental studies that individuals over the age of 65 years have impaired adaptive responses to extremely hot and cold outside temperatures. The diminished response of the elderly to cold appears to be due to a diminished perception that the core body temperature is low, and to an impaired ability to raise core temperature when the body's peripheral temperature becomes lowered. Responses to extremes of heat are impaired due to decreased secretion by the sweat glands in the skin.

In the area of sleep regulation, older adults spend more time in bed relative to time spent asleep due to longer time taken to fall asleep, more periods of wakefulness during the night, and time spent lying awake before arising in the morning. The primary causes of sleep disturbance include sleep apnea (Ancoli-Israel & Kripke, 1991), periodic leg movements, heartburn, and frequent needs to urinate (Freidman, Bliwise, Tauke, & Salom, 1992). EEG sleep patterns show some corresponding age alterations, including a rise in Stage 1 sleep (drowsiness without actual sleep), and a large decrease in Stage 4 sleep (slow wave or heavy sleep). By the 60s and 70s, REM sleep starts to diminish as well, as do the observable behaviors associated with REM sleep.

7.01.7.2.2 Clinical implications

The knowledge gained from personal experience and media exposure that one's aging body is less adaptable to outside temperatures means that adults living in geographical areas with cold winters will restrict their outdoor activities and spend more time at home. They will also limit their outdoor exposure during the summer. Overaccommodation to the threshold experience of aging in this regard can reduce the well-being of the older adult who may feel forced to remain indoors unnecessarily even on days when the temperature would not pose a threat. Conversely, overassimilation can have deleterious effects when the older adult does not take precautions during physical exertion or when venturing out into a very hot or very cold day. Fortunately, the changes in the ANS described here occur gradually over a period of years. Consequently, there are many opportunities for the individual to learn to adjust to the effects of aging and find new behavioral accommodations as these become necessary. Clinicians can play an important role in this process through helping their clients establish a favorable balance between overreaction and denial of aging-related changes in temperature regulation.

Similarly, the function of sleep in everyday life is clearly crucial to the individual's sense of well-being and there is a strong relationship between quality of sleep and psychological symptoms (Bliwise, 1992). Given the sensitivity of sleep patterns to psychological distress, this is an area where identity–age change relationships might very profitably be discussed in therapy. Older adults who overreact through accommodation to slight sleep change patterns are perhaps the ones fated to experience the most significant changes in their ability to get a good night's sleep. They need to be given the information that a night's sleep need not consist of more than seven hours and that the longer the time spent in bed awake, the harder it will be for the individual to develop a normal nightly rhythm based on this more realistic sleep requirement. The clinician can also advise the client to avoid daytime naps and to follow good sleep habits.

7.01.8 AGE CHANGES IN SENSORY FUNCTIONING

7.01.8.1 Vision

7.01.8.1.1 Age changes

The optical structures in the eye focus light reflected from stimuli in the environment onto the sensory cells of the retina. Many, if not all, age effects on visual functions can be explained in terms of the effects of normal aging on these optical structures (Scheie & Albert, 1977). One effect of these changes is to reduce the clarity of the visual image reaching the retina. The image reaching the retina is clouded by increased density and opacity of the lens (Spector, 1982), and by the formation of opacities in the vitreous. Adding to these structural changes are changes in the retina itself, including declines in the number of photoreceptors (rods and cones) (Ordy, Brizzee, & Johnson, 1982), the accumulation of debris in the outermost layer of the retina (Marmor, 1980), and detachment of the vitreous from the surface of the retina (Scheie & Albert). The amount of light reaching the retina is diminished by the condition known as senile meiosis, reduction in the size of the pupil due to atrophy of the iris dilator (Carter, 1982).

In addition to these changes that reduce the quality of the visual image on the retina are changes in the lens that decrease its capacity to accommodate to necessary changes in focus as objects move closer or further away from the individual. In addition to becoming denser, the lens fibers become harder and less elastic (Paterson, 1979). The loss of accommodative power of the lens due to these changes is referred to as presbyopia, and it is a condition that typically requires correction between the ages of 40 to 50 years. By the age of 60 years, the lens is completely incapable of accommodating to focus on objects at close distance (Moses, 1981). The lens also becomes yellowed due to an accumulation of yellow pigment, and as a result the older adult is less able to discriminate colors in the green–blue–violet end of the spectrum (Mancil & Owsley, 1988).

These structural changes in the eye result in altered refractive power leading to hypermetropia (farsightedness), a condition that cannot be compensated by greater focusing of the lens due to presbyopia. There is a reduction in visual acuity which is especially severe at low levels of illumination, such as driving at night, and when tracking moving objects (Panek, Barrett, Sterns, & Alexander, 1977; Richards, 1977). Dark adaptation is reduced so that older adults have greater difficulty adjusting to movement from bright to dim lighting, and have lower absolute levels of ability to see in the dark (McFarland, Dorney, Warren, & Ward, 1960). There is also a reduction in the individual's ability to react to scotomatic glare, or sudden exposure to bright light, such as a flashbulb or the headlights of an oncoming car at night (Wolf & Gardiner, 1965). Although there are only minimal data on depth perception, there appear to be reductions in stereopsis, the perception of three-dimensional space resulting from the varying input that reaches the two eyes (Bell, Wolf, & Bernholz, 1972).

7.01.8.1.2 Clinical implications

Given the centrality of vision to many activities, changes with age in the eye's basic functions can have profound psychological effects. One set of problems relates to discomfort and frustration caused by poorer acuity and reduced focusing power. Even if visual problems can be corrected with glasses or contact lenses, there are residual symptoms that may remain in special circumstances such as when the individual overworks or is trying to read small print. Older adults report experiencing as problems sensitivity to glare, difficulty seeing in dim light, and problems focusing on near objects (Kosnik, Winslow, Kline, Rasinski, & Sekuler, 1988). When these problems become more persistent, they may propel the individual toward a threshold experience.

Presbyopia, although reached after a gradual process of changes in the lens, is often perceived with relative suddenness by the individual (Carter, 1982). The immediacy of this apparent change, given the association that many people have between presbyopia and the infirmities of age, makes it more likely that the change will be negatively interpreted. The necessity of wearing bifocals adds the complication of requiring the individual to adjust to a new and awkward way of using corrective lenses.

Difficulties in depth perception and dark adaptation can heighten the older adult's vulnerability to falls (Felson et al., 1989; McMurdo & Gaskell, 1991), adding to the tendency to overaccommodate due to concerns about bone fragility and stiffness. Visual losses can increase the individual's dependence on others (Hakkinen, 1984), interfering with the older adult's ability to complete basic tasks of living such as driving, housekeeping, grocery shopping, and food preparation (Branch, Horowitz, & Carr 1989; Rudberg, Furner,

Dunn, & Cassel, 1993). Apart from the practical implications, these changes can further erode the individual's physical identity.

Finally, age changes in vision can detract from the older adult's ability to enjoy leisure and esthetic activities, and even to choose appropriate clothes (Morgan, 1988). Although not a serious problem compared with difficulties in driving, such changes can be annoying and perhaps lead to derision by others. Other leisure activities involving the perception of color and fine detail may be interfered with, such as needlepoint, gardening, word puzzles, and painting. Loss of the ability to enjoy these activities add further to the threshold experience which may be crossed each time a new visual function is altered or affected by aging.

A number of changes in visual functioning can, fortunately, be compensated by corrective lenses, increases in the ambient lighting, and efforts to reduce glare and heighten contrast between light and dark. Corrective surgery for cataracts can have a number of widespread positive effects on daily life (Brenner, Curbow, Javitt, Legro, & Sommer, 1993). The success of these efforts depends on the individual's willingness to persist in trying new ideas when the old methods no longer work, a process that might be enhanced through clinical intervention. Nevertheless, a point may be reached within each sphere of functioning in which the individual's range of movement becomes compromised. Furthermore, the situation may not permit compensation, as is true for night driving. Again, clinical sensitivity plays an important role in helping the older person accommodate to this age-related change in a valued function.

7.01.8.2 Hearing

7.01.8.2.1 Age changes

Presbycusis, the general term used to refer to age-related hearing loss, actually includes several specific subtypes reflecting different changes in the auditory structures. The most common form of hearing loss reduces sensitivity to high-frequency tones earlier and more severely than sensitivity to low-frequency tones (Van-Rooij & Plomp, 1990). The loss of high-frequency pitch perception is particularly pronounced in men (Lebo & Reddell, 1972). Speech perception is affected both by the various forms of presbycusis operating at the sensory level and by changes in the central processing of auditory information at the level of the brain stem and above (Van-Rooij & Plomp, 1992). Translated into speech discrimination, this means that older adults suffering from presbycusis have greater dificulty perceiving sibilants, such as the "s" in plurals.

In addition to the effects of aging on speech discrimination due to the loss of high-pitched tone sensitivity are the effects of aging on the ability to hear when there is interference or distraction. Age effects begin to appear even as early as 40 years in the understanding of sentences under a variety of distorting conditions, particularly when the speech signal is interrupted (Bergman et al., 1976). Other conditions known to impair speech perception in the aged include higher rate of presentation, deletion of parts of the message, competition from background noise or competing messages, and reverberation (Neils, Newman, Hill, & Weiler, 1991).

7.01.8.2.2 Clinical implications

Hearing deficits interfere greatly with interpersonal communication, leading to strained relationships and greater caution by the elderly in an attempt to avoid making inappropriate responses to uncertain auditory signals. They also reduce the older person's ability to hear noises such as a siren or a door knock (Gatehouse, 1990). These changes are almost impossible to avoid noticing (Slawinski, Hartel, & Kline, 1993), and it is perhaps for this reason that hearing loss forms a threshold for a large percentage of individuals over the age of 70 years and particularly those in their 80s (Whitbourne, 1996b). There is evidence linking hearing loss to impaired physical functioning (Bess, Lichenstein, Logan, & Burger, 1989) and psychological difficulties including loneliness (Christian, Dluky, & O'Neill, 1989) and depression (Kalayam, Alexopoulos, Merrell, & Young, 1991).

Those who interact with hearing-impaired elders can benefit from learning ways to communicate that lessen the impact of age-related changes (Slawinski et al., 1993). Modulating one's tone of voice, particularly for women, so that it is not too high, and avoiding distractions or interference, can be important aids to communicating clearly with older adults. The clinician can also use observations of the elderly client's reaction to communication difficulties in therapy as the basis for clinical recommendations. For example, identity accommodation can be encouraged in a client who denies the existence of an obvious hearing deficit; a client who has no apparent hearing deficit but appears preoccupied with this particular threshold will need to develop a more balanced approach to this area of functioning.

7.01.8.3 Balance

7.01.8.3.1 Age changes

The effects of age on the vestibular organs involve the losses occurring in the sensory structures as well as in the pathways to the higher levels of the nervous system (Johnsson & Hawkins, 1972; Rosenhall & Rubin, 1973). There are also reductions in the numbers of Purkinje cells in the cerebellum (Hall, Miller, & Corsellis, 1975) which could result in lowering of reflexive abilities to adjust the body's posture to changes in position. The apparent results of these changes in the vestibular system are increased dizziness and vertigo in older adults (Toglia, 1975). Not only are these sensations unpleasant, but they can increase the likelihood of accidental falls.

However, structural changes in the vestibular system do not account entirely for the phenomena of dizziness and vertigo. There is considerable plasticity within the vestibular system so that loss of receptor cells may be compensated by the activity of structures in other sensory systems (Teasdale, Stelmach, & Breunig, 1991). For example, the positional receptors in the somesthetic system appear to be less vulnerable to aging effects (Babin & Harker, 1982). Conversely, the loss of information from more than one sensory system, such as the visual and the vestibular systems, can make it difficult for the older person to compensate successfully (Manchester, Woollacott, Zederbauer-Hylton, & Marin, 1989). Slowing of central integrative processes responsible for maintaining postural stability can also contribute to increased likelihood of falls. It may take longer for the older adult to integrate information from the vestibular, visual, and somesthetic systems, resulting in less efficient control of posture under changing body positions (Teasdale et al., 1991).

7.01.8.3.2 Clinical implications

Balance is an essential element of moving about effectively in the environment. Aging of the vestibular system brings with it the potential for the individual to feel insecure in moving, particularly under conditions that are less than ideal, such as sloping, steep, or uneven surfaces. Fear of falling due to other changes in mobility can increase the individual's anxiety and perhaps exacerbate any true deficits in vestibular functioning. Conversely, individuals who through identity assimilation ignore signs of dizziness and vertigo may place themselves in danger as they may not be able to avoid a fall when and if they do lose their balance.

There are social consequences of aging of the vestibular system as well. The older adult who experiences dizziness and vertigo may fear appearing disoriented in front of other people, perhaps due to concern about appearing intoxicated or mentally confused. A desire to avoid such embarrassment may lead the individual to avoid leaving the home, creating unnecessary limitations on social opportunities.

Nevertheless, it remains the case that vestibular dysfunction is not an inevitable consequence of the aging of the vestibular system. Furthermore, compensation is possible if the individual is able to adapt other sensory systems to make up for vestibular losses (Lord, Clark, & Webster, 1991). Such compensation seems to be more likely to occur if the individual is able to react in a balanced manner to the experience of dizziness or vertigo. The clinician can encourage the older client to benefit from the coping strategies that involve seeking other cues, such as those provided by the somesthetic system. During episodes of dizziness or vertigo, the individual can learn to pay attention to stance and bodily orientation, learning to judge the position of the lower body limbs to make better use of feedback in adjusting posture (Hu & Woollacott 1994a, 1994b; Meenwsen, Sawicki, & Stelmack, 1993).

7.01.9 CONCLUDING OBSERVATIONS

In this chapter, a number of age-related changes have been described that occur throughout the body's organ systems and sensory processes. The multiple threshold model postulates that an individual's reactions to these changes varies according to how central the area of functioning is to identity as well as according to whether the individual approaches the age change through identity assimilation or accommodation. The problems involved in using overaccommodation or overassimilation have also been described.

Clinicians can learn from this approach to pay greater attention to the subtle and not-so-subtle cues that elderly clients give regarding the concerns they have about the functioning of their bodies. Assessments of older adults in particular, but also adults in middle age, can benefit from detailed history-taking not only of "health" problems but also of the individual's appraisal of and reaction to normal age-related changes in physical and sensory functioning. Such questions are particularly important for the clinician to raise because older clients are likely to be reticent in raising delicate and potentially embarrassing concerns about how their bodies are aging. Clinicians should also be encouraged to narrow their questions as specifically as possible to particular areas of functioning rather than explore issues related to "aging" or "health" in general. Such general questions are easily disregarded, as most older individuals tend to report that they are in good health even if they have a number of specific age-related limitations (Heidrich & Ryff, 1993).

Authors in the field of clinical geropsychology have, for years, advised clinicians to examine their own age biases and attitudes toward elderly people. This admonition definitely applies with regard to the aging of the body, as clinicians who are a product of Western culture have undoubtedly acquired a number of negative attitudes toward the loss of functioning that is so generally associated with old age. Less well recognized, though, is the need for the clinician to examine his or her own personal aging thresholds. To the extent that the clinician harbors concern about how aging will affect his or her own appearance, physical mobility, or cognitive functioning, that clinician might approach in a defensive and unhelpful way an elderly client with apparent deficits in that area.

Finally, it is crucial for clinicians to recognize the independence, autonomy, and vitality of spirit seen in many elders, even those with severe losses or age-related limitations. The older adults seen in therapy are "survivors" who have managed to reach this point in life through resiliency and an indefatigible ability to adapt to change. They are coping daily with physical changes that would daunt individuals many years their junior. Therapists who condescend to the elderly or patronize them (perhaps as a result of their own fears of aging) are missing important treatment opportunities as well as important opportunities to learn from the wisdom of their clients.

7.01.10 REFERENCES

Adrian, M. J. (1981). Flexibility in the aging adult. In E. L. Smith & R. C. Serfass (Eds.), *Exercise and aging: The scientific basis* (pp. 45–58). Hillsdale, NJ: Enslow.

Ancoli-Israel, S., & Kripke, D. F. (1991). Prevalent sleep problems in the aged. *Biofeedback and Self Regulation, 16*, 349–359.

Antoni, M. H. (1987). Neuroendocrine influences in psychoimmunology and neoplasia: A review. *Psychology and Health, 1*, 3–24.

Babin, R. W., & Harker, L. A. (1982). The vestibular system in the elderly. *Otolaryngolic Clinics of North America, 15*, 387–393.

Balin, A. K., & Pratt, L. A. (1989). Physiological consequences of human skin aging. *Cutis, 43*, 431–436.

Bell, B., Wolf, E., & Bernholtz, C. D. (1972). Depth perception as a function of age. *Aging and Human Development, 3*, 77–81.

Bergman, M., Blumenfeld, V. G., Cascardo, D., Dash, B., Levitt, H., & Margulies, M. K. (1976). Age-related decrement in hearing for speech: Sampling and longitudinal studies. *Journal of Gerontology, 31*, 533–538.

Bess, F. H., Lichtenstein, M. J., Logan, S. A., & Burger, M. C. (1989). Hearing impairment as a determinant of function in the elderly. *Journal of the American Geriatrics Society, 37*, 123–128.

Bliwise, N. G. (1992). Factors related to sleep quality in healthy elderly women. *Psychology and Aging, 7*, 83–88.

Bloom, E. T. (1994). Natural killer cells, lymphokine-activated killer cells, and cytolytic T lymphocytes: Compartmentalization of age-related changes in cytolytic lymphocytes? *Journal of Gerontology: Biological Sciences, 49*, B85–92.

Blumenthal, J. A., Emery, G. F., Madden, D. J., George, L. K., Coleman, R. E., Riddle, M. W., McKee, D. C., Reasoner, J., & Williams, R. S. (1989). Cardiovascular and behavioral effects of aerobic exercise training in healthy older men and women. *Journal of Gerontology: Medical Sciences, 44*, M147–157.

Branch, L. G., Horowitz, A., & Carr, C. (1989). The implications for everyday life of incident self-reported visual decline among people over age 65 living in the community. *Gerontologist, 29*, 359–365.

Brandtstadter, J., & Renner, G. (1990). Tenacious goal pursuit and flexible goal adjustment: Explication and age-related analysis of assimilative and accommodative strategies in coping. *Psychology and Aging, 5*, 58–67.

Brandstetter, R. D., & Kazemi, H. (1983). Aging and the respiratory system. *Medical Clinics of North America, 67*, 419–431.

Brenner, M. H., Curbow, B., Javitt, J. C., Legro, M. W., & Sommer, A. (1993). Vision change and quality of life in the elderly: Response to cataract surgery and treatment of other chronic ocular conditions. *Archives of Ophthalmology, 5*, 680–685.

Brody, H. (1955). Organization of cerebral cortex. III. A study of aging in the human cerebral cortex. *Journal of Comparative Neurology, 102*, 511–556.

Brooks, G. A., & Fahey, T. D. (1984). *Exercise physiology: Human bioenergetics and its applications.* New York: Wiley.

Buell, S. J., & Coleman, P. D. (1979). Dendritic growth in the aged human brain and failure of growth in senile dementia. *Science, 206*, 854–856.

Burgio, K. L., & Engel, B. T. (1990). Biofeedback-assisted behavioral training for elderly men and women. *Journal of the American Geriatrics Society, 38*, 338–340.

Burns, P. A., Pranikoff, K., Nochajski, T. H., Hadley, E. C., Levy, K. J., & Ory, M. G. (1993). A comparison of effectiveness of biofeedback and pelvic muscle exercise treatment of stress incontinence in older community-dwelling women. *Journal of Gerontology: Medical Sciences, 38*, M167–174.

Carter, J. H. (1982). The effects of aging on selected visual functions: Color vision, glare sensitivity, field of vision, and accommodation. In R. Sekuler, D. Kline, & K. Dismukes (Eds.), *Aging and human visual function* . New York: Alan R. Liss.

Carter, J. H. (1982). Predicting visual responses to increasing age. *Journal of the American Optometric Association, 53*, 31–36.

Chien, S., Peng, M. T., Chen, K. P., Huang, T. F., Chang, C., & Fang, H. S. (1975). Longitudinal studies on adipose tissue and its distribution in human subjects. *Journal of Applied Physiology, 39*, 825–830.

Chodzko-Zajko, W. J., Schuler, P., Solomon, J., Heinl, B., & Ellis, N. R. (1992). The influence of physical fitness on automatic and effortful memory changes in aging. *International Journal of Aging and Human Development, 35*, 265–285.

Christian, E., Dluhy, N., & O'Neill, R. (1989). Sounds of silence: Coping with hearing loss and loneliness. *Journal of Gerontological Nursing, 15*(11), 4–9.

Costello, R. B., & Moser-Veillon, P. B. (1992). A review of magnesium intake in the elderly. A cause for concern? *Magnesium Research, 5*, 61–67.

Dalsky, G. P., Stocke, K. S., Ehsani, A. A., Slatopolsky,

E., Lee, W. C., & Birge, S. J. (1988). Weight-bearing exercise, training, and lumbar bone mineral content in post-menopausal women. *Annals of Internal Medicine, 108*, 824–828.

Dargent, P., & Breart, G. (1993). Epidemiology and risk factors of osteoporosis. *Current Opinions in Rheumatology, 5*, 339–345.

D'Errico, A., Scarani, P., Colosimo, E., Spina, M., Grigioni, W. F., & Mancini, A. M. (1989). Changes in the alveolar connective tissue of the ageing lung. An immunohistochemical study. *Archives of Pathology Anatomy and Histopathology, 415*, 137–144.

Devaney, K. O., & Johnson, H. A. (1980). Neuron loss in the aging visual cortex in man. *Journal of Gerontology, 35*, 836–841.

Diokno, A. C., Brock, B. M., Brown, M. B., & Herzog, A. R. (1986). Prevalence of urinary incontinence and other urological syptoms in the noninstitutionalized elderly. *Journal of Urology, 136*, 1022–1025.

Downton, J. H., & Andrews, K. (1990). Postural disturbance and psychological symptoms amongst elderly people living at home. *International Journal of Geriatric Psychiatry, 5*, 93–98.

Ehsani, A. A., Ogawa, T., Miller, T. R., Spina, R. J., & Jilka, S. M. (1991). Exercise training improves left ventricular systolic function in older men. *Circulation, 83*, 96–103.

Ellis, F. P., Shukla, K. K., Cohn, S. H., & Pierson, R. N. (1974). A predictor for total-body potassium in man based on height, weight, sex, and age: Application in metabolic disorders. *Journal of Laboratory and Clinical Medicine, 83*, 716–727.

Ershler, W. B. (1990). Influenza and aging. In A. L. Goldstein (Ed.), *Biomedical advances in aging* (pp. 513–521). New York: Plenum.

Felson, D. T., Anderson, J. J., Hannan, M. T., Milton, R. C., Wilson, P. W., & Kiel, D. P. (1989). Impaired vision and hip fracture: The Framingham Study. *Journal of the American Geriatrics Society, 37*, 495–500.

Fenske, N. A., & Albers, S. E. (1990). Cosmetic modalities for aging skin: what to tell patients. *Geriatrics, 45*(9), 59–67.

Fiatrone, M. A., & Evans, W. J. (1993). The etiology and reversibility of muscle dysfunction in the aged. *Journal of Gerontology, 48 (Special issue)*, 77–83.

Fiatrone, M. A., Marks, E. C., Ryan, N. D., Meredith, C. N., Lipsitz, L. A., & Evans, W. J. (1990). High-intensity strength training in nonagenarians. Effects on skeletal muscle. *Journal of the American Medical Association 263*, 3029–3034.

Fischer, J., & Johnson, M. A. (1990). Low body weight and weight loss in the aged. *Journal of the American Dietetic Association, 90*, 1697–1706.

Flood, D. G., Buell, S. J., Horwitz, G. J., & Coleman, P. D. (1987). Dendritic extent in human dentate gyrus granule cells in normal aging and senile dementia. *Brain Research, 402*, 205–216.

Flood, D. G., & Coleman, P. D. (1988). Cell type heterogeneity of changes in dendritic extent in the hippocampal region of the human brain in normal aging and in Alzheimer's disease. In T. L. Petit & G. O. Ivy (Eds.), *Neural plasticity: A lifespan approach* (pp. 265–281). New York: Alan R. Liss.

Foster, V. L., Hume, G. J. E., Byrnes, W. C., Dickinson, A. L., & Chatfield, S. J. (1989). Endurance training for elderly women: Moderate vs low intensity. *Journal of Gerontology: Medical Sciences, 44*, M184–188.

Friedman, L. F., Bliwise, D. L., Tanke, E. D., & Salom, S. R. (1992). A survey of self-reported poor sleep and associated factors in older individuals. *Behavior, Health, and Aging, 2*(1), 13–20.

Garn, S. M. (1975). Bone loss and aging. In R. Goldman & M. Rockstein (Eds.), *The physiology and pathology of aging* (pp. 39–57). New York: Academic Press.

Gatehouse, S. (1990). Determinants of self-reported disability in older subjects. *Ear and Hearing, 11* (Suppl.), 57S–65S.

George, L. K., & Weiler, S. J. (1985). Sexuality in middle and late life. In E. Palmore, J. Nowlin, E. Busse, I. Siegler & G. Maddox (Eds.), *Normal aging III*. Durham, NC: Duke University Press.

Gilchrest, B. A. (1989). Skin aging and photoaging: an overview. *Journal of the American Academy of Dermatology, 21*(3, Pt. 2), 610–613.

Globerson, A., Eren, R., Abel, L., & Ben-Menahem, D. (1990). Developmental aspects of T lymphocytes in aging. In A. L. Goldstein (Ed.), *Biomedical advances in aging* (pp. 363–373). New York: Plenum.

Govindasamy, D., Paterson, D. H., Poulin, M., & Cunningham, D. A. (1988). The time course of cardiorespiratory adaptations in elderly men. *Canadian Journal of Sport Sciences, 13*, 53–54.

Grove, G. L. (1989). Physiologic changes in older skin. *Clinics in Geriatric Medicine, 5*, 115–125.

Hagberg, J. M., Graves, J. E., Limacher, L., Woods, D. R., Leggett, S. H., Cononie, C., Gruber, J. J., & Pollock, M.L. (1989). Cardiovascular responses of 70– to 79–yr-old men and women to exercise training. *Journal of Applied Physiology, 66*, 2589–2594.

Hakkinen, L. (1984). Vision in the elderly and its use in the social environment. *Scandanavian Journal of Social Medicine, 35*, 5–60.

Hall, T. C., Miller, A. K. H., & Corsellis, J. A. N. (1975). Variations in the human Purkinje cell population according to age and sex. *Neuropathology and Applied Neurobiology, 1*, 267–292.

Hamdorf, P. A., Withers, R. T., Penhall, R. K., & Haslam, M. V. (1992). Physical training effects on the fitness and habitual activity patterns of elderly women. *Archives of Physical Medicine and Rehabilitation, 73*, 603–608.

Harman, S. M. (1978). Clinical aspects of the male reproductive system. In E. L. Schneider (Ed.), *Aging: Vol. 4. The aging reproductive system*. New York: Raven Press.

Heidrich, S. M., & Ryff, C. D. (1993). The role of social comparisons processes in the psychological adaptation of elderly adults. *Journal of Gerontology: Psychological Sciences, 48*, 127–136.

Heiss, G., Tamir, I., Davis, C. E., Tyroler, H. A., Rifkind, B. M., Schonfeld, G., Jacobs, D., & Frantz, I. D. (1980). Lipoprotein-cholesterol distributions in selected North American populations: The Lipid Research Clinics Program Prevalence Study. *Circulation, 61*, 302–315.

Henderson, G., Tomlinson, B., & Gibson, P. H. (1980). Cell counts in human cerebral cortex in normal adults throughout life using an image analysing computer. *Journal of the Neurological Sciences, 46*, 113–136.

Hermanson, B., Omenn, G. S., & Kronmal, R. A. (1988). Beneficial six-year outcome of smoking cessation in older men and women with coronary artery disease. *New England Journal of Medicine, 24*, 1365–1369.

Herzog, A. R., Diokno, A. C., Brown, M. B., Normolle, D. P., & Brock, B. M. (1990). Two-year incidence, remission, and change patterns of urinary incontinence in noninstitutionalized older adults. *Journal of Gerontology: Medical Sciences, 45*, M67–74.

Higatsberger, M. R., Budka, H., & Bernheimer, H. (1982). Neurochemical investigations of aged human brain cortex. In S. Hoyer (Ed.), *The aging brain: Physiological and pathophysiological aspects*. New York: Springer.

Hill, R. D., Storandt, M., & Malley, M. (1993). The impact of long-term exercise training on psychological function in older adults. *Journal of Gerontology: Psychological Sciences, 48*, P12–17.

Holt, P. R. (1991). General perspectives on the aged gut. *Clinics in Geriatric Medicine, 7*, 185–189.

Hu, M.-H., & Woollacott, M. H. (1994a). Multisensory training of standing balance in older adults: I. Postural stability and one-leg stance balance. *Journal of Gerontology: Medical Sciences, 49,* M52–61.

Hu, M.-H., & Woollacott, M. H. (1994b). Multisensory training of standing balance in older adults. II. Kinematic and electromyographic postural responses. *Journal of Gerontology: Medical Sciences, 49,* M62–71.

Hughes, S. L., Edelman, P. L., Singer, R. H., & Chang, R. W. (1993). Joint impairment and self-reported disability in elderly persons. *Journal of Gerontology: Social Sciences, 48,* S84–92.

Hunskaar, S., & Vinsnes, A. (1991). The quality of life in women with urinary incontinence as measured by the Sickness Impact Profile. *Journal of the American Geriatrics Society, 39,* 378–382.

Huttenlocher, P. (1979). Synaptic density in human frontal cortex—developmental changes and effects of aging. *Brain Research, 163,* 195–205.

Janelli, L. M. (1993). Are there body image differences between older men and women? *Western Journal of Nursing Research, 15,* 327–339.

Jirovec, M. M. (1991). The impact of daily exercise on the mobility, balance and urine control of cognitively impaired nursing home residents. *International Journal of Nursing Studies, 28,* 145–151.

Johnsson, L. G., & Hawkins, J. E., Jr. (1972). Sensory and neural degeneration with aging, as seen in microdissections of the human inner ear. *Annals of Otolaryngology, Rhinology, and Laryngology, 81,* 179–193.

Kalayam, B., Alexopoulos, G. S., Merrell, H. B., & Young, R. C. (1991). Patterns of hearing loss and psychiatric morbidity in elderly patients attending a hearing clinic. *International Journal of Geriatric Psychiatry, 6,* 131–136.

Kallman, D. A., Plato, C. C., & Tobin, J. D. (1990). The role of muscle loss in the age–related decline of grip strength: Cross-sectional and longitudinal perspectives. *Journal of Gerontology: Medical Sciences, 45,* M82–88.

Karacan, I., Williams, R. L., Thornby, J. I., & Salis, P. J. (1975). Sleep-related penile tumescence as a function of age. *American Journal of Psychiatry, 132,* 932–937.

Kelly, P. J., Nguyen, T., Hopper, J., Pocock, N., Sambrook, P., & Eisman, J. (1993). Changes in axial bone density with age: a twin study. *Journal of Bone Mineral Research, 8,* 11–17.

Kenney, A. R. (1989). *Physiology of aging* (2nd ed.). Chicago, IL: Yearbook Medical.

Kiecolt, K. J. (1994). Stress and the decision to change oneself: A theoretical model. *Social Psychology Quarterly, 57,* 49–63.

Kitzman, D. W., & Edwards, W. D. (1990). Age-related changes in the anatomy of the normal human heart. *Journal of Gerontology: Medical Sciences, 45,* M33–39.

Kitzman, D. W., Scholz, D. G., Hagen, P. T., Ilstrup, D. M., & Edwards, W. D. (1988). Age-related changes in normal human hearts during the first ten decades. Part II (Maturity): A quantitative anatomic study of 765 specimens from subjects 20 to 99 years old. *Mayo Clinic Proceedings, 63,* 137–146.

Kleinsmith, D. M., & Perricone, N. V. (1989). Common skin problems in the elderly. *Clinics in Geriatric Medicine, 5,* 189–211.

Kligman, A. M. (1989). Psychological aspects of skin disorders in the elderly. *Cutis, 43,* 498–501.

Kligman, A. M., Grove, G. L., & Balin, A. K. (1985). Aging of human skin. In C. E. Finch & E. L. Schneider (Eds.), *Handbook of the biology of aging* (2nd ed.). New York: Van Nostrand Reinhold.

Kosnik, W., Winslow, L., Kline, D., Rasinski, K., & Sekuler, R. (1988). Visual changes in daily life throughout adulthood. *Journal of Gerontology: Psychological Sciences, 43,* P63–70.

Krall, E. A., & Dawson-Hughes, B. (1993). Heritable and life-style determinants of bone mineral density. *Journal of Bone Mineral Research, 8,* 1–9.

Kurban, R. S., & Bhawan, J. (1990). Histologic changes in skin associated with aging. *Journal of Dermatology and Surgical Oncology, 16,* 908–914.

Kutza, J., Kaye, D., & Murasko, D. M. (1995). Basal natural killer cell activity of young versus elderly humans. *Journal of Gerontology: Biological Sciences, 50A,* B110–116.

Labouvie-Vief, G., Hakim-Larson, J., & Hobart, C. J. (1987). Age, ego level, and the life-span development of coping and defense processes. *Psychology and Aging, 2,* 286–293.

Lakatta, E. G. (1987). Why cardiovascular function may decline with age. *Geriatrics, 42,* 84–94.

Lamy, P. P. (1988). Actions of alcohol and drugs in older people. *Generations, 12*(4), 9–13.

Lavker, R. M., Kwong, F., & Kligman, A. M. (1980). Changes in skin surface patterns with age. *Journal of Gerontology, 35,* 348–354.

Lebo, C. P., & Reddell, R. C. (1972). The presbycusis component in occupational hearing loss. *Laryngoscope, 82,* 1399–1409.

Lord, S. R., Clark, R. D., & Webster, I. W. (1991). Postural stability and associated physiological factors in a population of aged persons. *Journal of Gerontology: Medical Sciences, 46,* M69–76.

Lord, S. R., Clark, R. D., & Webster, I. W. (1991). Physiological factors associated with falls in an elderly population. *Journal of the American Geriatrics Society, 39,* 1194–1200.

Mahler, D. A., Rossiello, R. A., & Loke, J. (1986). The aging lung. *Clinics in Geriatric Medicine, 2,* 215–225.

Manchester, D., Woollacott, M., Zederbauer-Hylton, N., & Marin, O. (1989). Visual, vestibular and somatosensory contributions to balance control in the older adult. *Journal of Gerontology: Medical Sciences, 44,* M118–127.

Mancil, G. L., & Owsley, C. (1988). 'Vision through my aging eyes' revisited. *Journal of the American Optometric Association, 59,* 288–294.

Marmor, M. F. (1980). Clinical physiology of the retina. In G. A. Reyman, D. R. Sanders, & M. F. Goldberg (Eds.), *Principles and practice of opthalmology* (Vol. 2, pp. 823–856). Philadelphia: Saunders.

Masters, W. H., & Johnson, V. E. (1966). *Human sexual response.* Boston, MA: Little, Brown.

Masters, W. H., & Johnson, V. E. (1970). *Human sexual inadequacy.* Boston, MA: Little, Brown.

Mazess, R. B. (1982). On aging bone loss. *Clinical Orthopaedics and Related Research, 165,* 239–252.

McArdle, W. D., Katch, F. I., & Katch, V. L. (1991). *Exercise physiology: Energy, nutrition, and human performance* (3rd ed.). Philadelphia: Lea & Febiger.

McAuley, E., Lox, C., & Duncan, T. E. (1993). Long-term maintenance of exercise, self-efficacy, and physiological change in older adults. *Journal of Gerontology: Psychological Sciences, 48,* P218–224.

McCalden, R. W., McGeough, J. A., Barker, M. B., & Court-Brown, C. M. (1993). Age-related changes in the tensile properties of cortical bone. The relative importance of changes in porosity, mineralization, and microstructure. *Journal of Bone and Joint Surgery, 75,* 1193–1205.

McFarland, R. A., Domey, R. G., Warren, A. B., & Ward, D. C. (1960). Dark adaptation as a function of age: I. A statistical analysis. *Journal of Gerontology, 15,* 149–154.

McLachlan, M. S. F., Guthrie, J. C., Anderson, C. K., & Fulker, M. J. (1977). Vascular and glomerular changes in the ageing kidney. *Journal of Pathology, 121,* 65–78.

McMurdo, M. E., & Gaskell, A. (1991). Dark adaptation and falls in the elderly. *Gerontology, 37,* 221–224.

McNaughton, M. E., Smith, L. W., Patterson, T. L., & Grant, I. (1990). Stress, social support, coping resources, and immune status in elderly women. *Journal of Nervous and Mental Disease, 178,* 460–461.

Meeuwsen, H. J., Sawicki, T. M., & Stelmach, G. E. (1993). Improved foot position sense as a result of repetitions in older adults. *Journal of Gerontology: Psychological Sciences, 48,* P137–141.

Meredith, C. N., Frontera, W. R., Fisher, E. C., Hughes, V. A., Herland, J. C., Edwards, J., & Evans, W. J. (1989). Peripheral effects of endurance training in young and old subjects. *Journal of Applied Physiology, 66,* 2844–2849.

Miller, R. A. (1993). Aging and cancer—Another perspective. *Journal of Gerontology: Biological Sciences, 48,* B8–9.

Montamat, S. C., & Davies, A. O. (1989). Physiological response to isoproterenol and coupling of beta-adrenergic receptors in young and elderly human subjects. *Journal of Gerontology: Medical Sciences, 44,* M100–105.

Montgomery, S. A. (1990). Depression in the elderly: Pharmacokinetics of antidepressants and death from overdose. *International Clinical Psychopharmacology, 5*(Suppl. 3), 67–76.

Morey, M. C., Cowper, P. A., Feussner, J. R., DiPasquale, R. C., Crowley, G. M., Kitzman, D. W., & Sullivan, R. J., Jr. (1991). Two-year trends in physical performance following supervised exercise among community-dwelling older veterans. *Journal of the American Geriatrics Society, 39,* 986–992.

Morgan, M. W. (1988). VIsion through my aging eyes. *Journal of the American Optometric Association, 59,* 278–280.

Morley, J. E., & Reese, S. S. (1989). Clinical implications of the aging heart. *The American Journal of Medicine, 86,* 77–86.

Moses, R. A. (1981). Accommodation. In R. A. Moses (Ed.), *Adler's physiology of the eye.* St. Louis, MO: Mosby.

Mouritzen Dam, A. (1979). The density of neurons in the human hippocampus. *Neuropathology and Applied Neurobiology, 5,* 249–264.

Naliboff, B. D., Benton, D., Solomon, G. F., Morley, J. E., Fahey, J. L., Bloom, E. T., Makinodan, T. et al. (1991). Immunological changes in young and old adults during brief laboratory stress. *Psychosomatic Medicine, 53,* 121–132.

Neils, J., Newman, C. W., Hill, M., & Weiler, E. (1991). The effects of rate, sequencing, and memory on auditory processing in the elderly. *Journal of Gerontology, 46*(2), 71–75.

Nuti, R., & Martini, G. (1993). Effects of age and menopause on bone density of entire skeleton in healthy and osteoporotic women. *Osteoporosis International, 3,* 59–65.

O'Donoghue, M. N. (1991). Cosmetics for the elderly. *Dermatology Clinics, 9,* 29–34.

O'Leary, A. (1990). Stress, emotion, and human immune function. *Psychological Bulletin, 108,* 363–382.

Olivetti, G., Melissari, M., Capasso, J. M., & Anversa, P. (1991). Cardiomyopathy of the aging human heart. Myocyte loss and reactive cellular hypertrophy. *Circulation Research, 68,* 1560–1568.

Ordy, J. M., Brizzee, K. R., & Johnson, H. A. (1982). Cellular alterations in visual pathways and the limbic system: Implications for vision and short-term memory. In R. Sekuler, D. Kline, & K. Dismukes (Eds.), *Aging and human visual function.* New York: Alan R. Liss.

Ouslander, J. G., & Abelson, S. (1990). Perceptions of urinary incontinence among elderly outpatients. *Gerontologist, 30*(3), 369–372.

Ouslander, J. G., Zarit, S. H., Orr, N. K., & Muira, S. A. (1990). Incontinence among elderly community-dwelling dementia patients: Characteristics, management, and impact on caregivers. *Journal of the American Geriatrics Society, 38,* 440–445.

Overend, T. J., Cunningham, D. A., Kramer, J. F., Lefcoe, M. S., & Paterson, D. H. (1992). Knee extensor and knee flexor strength: Cross-sectional areas ratio in young and elderly men. *Journal of Gerontology: Medical Sciences, 47,* M204–210.

Panek, P. E., Barrett, G. V., Sterns, H. L., & Alexander, R. A. (1977). A review of age changes in perceptual information ability with regard to driving. *Experimental Aging Research, 3,* 387–449.

Parmelee, P. A., Katz, I. R., & Lawton, M. P. (1991). The relation of pain to depression among institutionalized aged. *Journal of Gerontology: Psychological Sciences, 46,* P15–21.

Paterson, C. A. (1979). Crystalline lens. In R. E. Records (Ed.), *Physiology of the human eye and visual system.* New York: Harper & Row.

Poulin, M., Paterson, D. H., Govindasamy, D., & Cunningham, D. A. (1988). Endurance training of elderly men. Responses to submaximal exercise. *Canadian Journal of Sport Sciences, 13,* 78–79P.

Reddan, W. G. (1981). Respiratory system and aging. In E. L. Smith & R. C. Serfass (Eds.), *Exercise and aging: The scientific basis* (pp. 89–107). Hillside, NJ: Enslow.

Richards, O. W. (1977). Effects of luminance and contrast on visual acuity ages 16 to 90 years. *American Journal of Optometry and Physiological Optics, 54,* 178–184.

Rico, H., Revilla, M., Hernandez, E. R., Gonzalez-Riola, J. M., & Villa, L. F. (1993). Four-compartment model of body composition of normal elderly women. *Age and Aging, 22,* 265–268.

Riggs, B. L., Wahner, W. H., Dunn, W. L., Mazess, R. B., Offord, K. P., & Melton, L. J. (1981). Differential changes in bone mineral density of the appendicular and axial skeleton with aging. *Journal of Clinical Investigation, 67,* 328–335.

Rikli, R. E., & McManis, B. G. (1990). Effects of exercise on bone mineral content in postmenopausal women. *Research Quarterly in Exercise of Sport, 61,* 243–249.

Roberto, K. (1992). Coping strategies of older women with hip fractures: Resources and outcomes. *Journal of Gerontology: Psychological Sciences, 47,* 21–26.

Rosenbloom, C. A., & Whittington, F. J. (1993). The effects of bereavement on eating behaviors and nutrient intakes in elderly widowed persons. *Journal of Gerontology: Social Sciences, 48,* S223–229.

Rosenhall, U., & Rubin, W. (1973). Degenerative patterns in the aging human vestibular neuroepithelia. *Acta Otolaryngolica, 76,* 208–220.

Rowe, J. W. (1982). Renal function and aging. In M. E. Reff & E. L. Schneider (Eds.), *Biological markers of aging.* Bethesda, MD: National Institutes of Health, Publication No. 82-2221.

Rowe, J. W., Shock, N. W., & DeFronzo, R. A. (1976). The influence of age on the renal response to water deprivation in man. *Nephron, 17,* 270–278.

Rudberg, M. A., Furner, S. E., Dunn, J. E., & Cassel, C. K. (1993). The relationship of visual and hearing impairments to disability: An analysis using the longitudinal study of aging. *Journal of Gerontology: Medical Sciences, 48,* M261–265.

Ryan, A. S., Craig, L. D., & Finn, S. C. (1992). Nutrient intakes and dietary patterns of older Americans: A national study. *Journal of Gerontology: Medical Sciences, 47,* M145–150.

Ryff, C. D. (1989). In the eye of the beholder: Views of psychological well-being among middle-aged and older adults. *Psychology and Aging, 4,* 195–210.

Scheibel, A. B. (1982). Age-related changes in the human forebrain. *Neurosciences Research Progress Bulletin, 20,* 577–583.

Scheie, H. G., & Albert, D. M. (1977). *Textbook of opthalmology.* (9th ed.). Philadelphia: Saunders.

Schiavi, R. C., & Schreiner-Engel, P. (1988). Nocturnal penile tumescence in healthy aging men. *Journal of Gerontology: Medical Sciences, 43,* M146–150.

Schulman, S. P., & Gerstenblith, G. (1989). Cardiovascular changes with aging: The response to exercise. *Journal of Cardiopulmonary Rehabilitation, 9,* 12–16.

Shephard, R. J. (1978). *Physical activity and aging.* Chicago, IL: Yearbook Medical.

Sherman, S. S., Tobin, J. D., Hollis, B. W., Gundberg, C. M., Roy, T. A., & Plato, C. C. (1992). Biochemical parameters associated with low bone density in healthy men and women. *Journal of Bone and Mineral Research, 7,* 1123–1130.

Shimojo, M., Tsuda, N., Iwasaka, T., & Inada, M. (1991). Age-related changes in aortic elasticity determined by gated radionuclide angiography in patients with systemic hypertension or healed myocardial infarcts and in normal subjects. *American Journal of Cardiology, 68,* 950–953.

Shock, N. W., Andres, R., Norris, A. H., & Tobin, J. D. (1978). Patterns of longitudinal changes in renal function, *Proceedings XII International Congress of Gerontology, Tokyo, August 20–25* (pp. 525–527). Amsterdam: Excerpta Medica.

Slawinski, E. B., Hartel, D. M., & Kline, D. W. (1993). Self-reported hearing problems in daily life throughout adulthood. *Psychology and Aging, 8,* 552–561.

Smith, E. L. (1981). Physical activity: A preventive and maintenance modality for bone loss with age. In F. J. Nagle & H. J. Montoye (Eds.), *Exercise in health and disease* (pp. 196–202). Springfield, IL: Charles C. Thomas.

Smith, W. D. F., Cunningham, D. A., Patterson, D. H., Rechnitzer, P. A., & Koval, J. J. (1992). Forced expiratory volume, height, and demispan in Canadian men and women aged 55–86. *Journal of Gerontology: Medical Sciences, 47,* M40–44.

Solnick, R. L., & Birren, J. E. (1977). Age and male erectile responsiveness. *Archives of Sexual Behavior, 6,* 1–9.

Sparrow, D., Beausoleil, N. I., Garvey, A. J., Rosner, B., & Silbert, J. E. (1982). The influence of cigarette smoking and age on bone loss in men. *Archives of Environmental Health, 37,* 246–249.

Spector, A. (1982). Aging of the lens and cataract formation. In R. Sekuler, D. Kline, & K. Dismukes (Eds.), *Aging and human visual function.* New York: Alan R. Liss.

Stamford, B. A. (1988). Exercise in the elderly. In K. B. Pandolf (Ed.), *Exercise and Sports Sciences Reviews, 16,* 341–379.

Stevenson, J. S., & Topp, R. (1990). Effects of moderate and low intensity long-term exercise by older adults. *Research in Nursing and Health, 13,* 209–218.

Suominen, H., Heikkinen, E., Parkatti, T., Forsberg, S., & Kiiskinen, A. (1977). Effect of lifelong physical training on functional aging in men. *Scandanavian Journal of the Society of Medicine, 14* (Suppl.), 225–240.

Tamai, T., Nakai, T., Takai, H., Fujiwara, R., Miyabo, S., Higuchi, M., & Kobayashi, S. (1988). The effects of physical exercise on plasma lipoprotein and apolipoprotein metabolism in elderly men. *Journal of Gerontology: Medical Sciences, 43,* M75–79.

Teasdale, N., Stelmach, G. E., & Breunig, A. (1991). Postural sway characteristics of the elderly under normal and altered visual and support surface conditions. *Journal of Gerontology: Biological Sciences, 46,* B238–244.

Teramoto, S., Fukuchi, Y., Nagase, T., Matsuse, T., & Orimo, H. (1995). A comparison of ventilation components in young and elderly men during exercise. *Journal of Gerontology: Biological Sciences, 50A,* B34–39.

Thomas, P. D., Goodwin, J. M., & Goodwin, J. W. (1985). Effect of social support on stress-related changes in cholesterol, uric acid level, and immune function in an elderly sample. *American Journal of Psychiatry, 142,* 735–737.

Tinetti, M. E., & Powell, L. (1993). Fear of falling and low self-efficacy: A cause of dependence in elderly persons. *Journal of Gerontology, 48* (Special Issue), 35–58.

Toglia, J. U. (1975). Dizziness in the elderly. In W. Fields (Ed.), *Neurological and sensory disorders in the elderly.* New York: Grune & Stratton.

Vandervoort, A. A., Chesworth, B. M., Cunningham, D. A., Paterson, D. H., Rechnitzer, P. A., & Koval, J. J. (1992). Age and sex effects on mobility of the human ankle. *Journal of Gerontology: Medical Sciences, 47,* M17–21.

Van-Rooij, J. C., & Plomp, R. (1990). Auditive and cognitive factors in speech perception by elderly listeners: II. Multivariate analyses. *Journal of the Acoustical Society of America, 88,* 2611–2624.

Van-Rooij, J. C., & Plomp, R. (1992). How much do working memory deficits contribute to age differences in discourse memory? Special Issue: Cognitive gerontology. *Journal of the Acoustical Society of America, 91,* 1028–1033.

Vollardt, L. T. (1991). Psychoneuroimmunology: A literature review. *American Journal of Orthopsychiatry, 61,* 35–47.

Wald, A. (1990). Constipation and fecal incontinence in the elderly. *Gastroenterology Clinics of North America, 19,* 405–418.

Webb, G. D., Poehlman, E. T., & Tonino, R. P. (1993). Dissociation of changes in metabolic rate and blood pressure with erthrocyte Na-K pump activity in older men after endurance training. *Journal of Gerontology: Medical Sciences, 48,* M47–52.

Wedmann, B., Schmidt, G., Wegener, M., Coenen, C., Ricken, D., & Althoff, J. (1991). Effects of age and gender on fat-induced gallbladder contraction and gastric emptying of a caloric liquid meal: a sonographic study. *American Journal of Gastroenterology, 86,* 1765–1770.

Weisfeldt, M. L., & Gerstenblith, G. (1986). Cardiovascular aging and adaptation to disease. In J. W. Hurst (Ed.), *The heart.* New York: Macmillan.

Whitbourne, S. K. (1996a). *The aging individual: Physical and psychological perspectives.* New York: Springer.

Whitbourne, S. K. (1996b). *Identity processes and perceptions of physical functioning in adults: A test of the multiple threshold model.* American Psychological Association 104th Annual Meeting. Toronto, Ontario, Canada.

Whitbourne, S. K. (1986). *The me I know: A study of adult identity.* New York: Springer.

Whitbourne, S. K., & Primus, L. A. (1996). Physical identity in later adulthood. In J. E. Birren (Ed.), *Encyclopedia of aging.* San Diego, CA: Academic Press.

Whitbourne, S. K., & Wills, K.-J. (1993). Psychological issues in institutional care of the aged. In S. B. Goldsmith (Ed.), *Long-term care administration handbook* (pp. 19–32). Gaithersburg, MD: Aspen.

Wolf, E., & Gardiner, J. S. (1965). Studies on the scatter of light in the dioptric media of the eye as a basis of visual glare. *Archives of Opthalmology, 74,* 338–345.

Woodward, N. J., & Wallston, B. S. (1987). Age and health care beliefs: Self-efficacy as a mediator of low desire for control. *Psychology and Aging,* 3–8.

Wright, B. A., Aizenstein, S., Vogler, G., Rowe, M., & Miller, C. (1990). Frequent fallers: Leading groups to identify psychological factors. *Journal of Gerontological Nursing, 16*(4), 15–19.

Wyman, J. F., Harkins, S. W., & Fantl, J. A. (1990). Psychosocial impact of urinary incontinence in the community-dwelling population. *Journal of the American Geriatrics Society, 38*(3), 282–288.

7.02
Cognition and Geropsychological Assessment

BOO JOHANSSON
Institute of Gerontology and Centre for Psychology, University College of Health Sciences, Jönköping, Sweden
and
ÅKE WAHLIN
Stockholm Gerontology Research Center and Karolinska Institute, Stockholm, Sweden

---

7.02.1 INTRODUCTION

Understanding age-related changes, as well as stability, in highly integrated cognitive functions is of fundamental importance for the geropsychologist since memory and cognitive abilities are often focused in an assessment setting. The geropsychologist may be confronted with elderly individuals who seek help because of worries and experiences of cognitive failures, or who are referred to an assessment by family or health professionals due to impairments in memory and thinking.

A fundamental issue for an unbiased assessment of memory and other cognitive abilities is the geropsychologist's expertise in considering strengths or preserved ability as well as weaknesses or impaired ability relative to previous functioning, as well as the cognitive demands that are imposed in everyday life and how this relates to outcomes of cognitive testing. Other issues refer to the application of theoretical guidelines for analyzing performance, including the mechanisms involved, taking into account individual factors and the sociocultural context for cognitive functioning in aging.

This chapter discusses various aspects of cognitive functioning in aging in a context that is intended to correspond to that of the clinical geropsychologist, where considerations are based on detailed information about the individual in the assessment setting as well as outside the clinic. Other chapters in this volume address reasons for assessment of elderly people, including principles and methods. The present chapter provides a solid base for these more applied contributions. Given the limitation of a single chapter for discussing cognitive aspects of aging, the reader is directed to consult recent reviews for detailed information on current research on memory (e.g., Kausler, 1994), cognitive aging (e.g., Craik & Salthouse, 1992), and clinical geropsychology, including relevant chapters in the *Handbook of the psychology of aging* (Birren & Schaie, 1996 and previous editions).

This chapter is organized into subsections based on the heuristic scheme presented in Figure 1. The general idea with this scheme is that cognitive functioning must be understood and consequently analyzed within the context of noncognitive factors. The emphasis will be on aspects of memory and intellectual abilities that are likely to be addressed in an assessment setting (the term assessment is used throughout in its broadest sense and includes assessment in clinical settings as well as research approaches to various aspects of memory and cognitive aging).

The noncognitive factors depicted in Figure 1 are first discussed with reference to general aspects of memory and cognition. An overview of these domains of functioning follows, based on what is considered to be of relevance for the geropsychologist. The final section comprises an integration of cognitive aspects of aging, including messages to the geropsychologist.

7.02.2 NONCOGNITIVE INFLUENCES ON MEMORY AND COGNITION IN AGING

7.02.2.1 Types of Aging

Psychological aging is a complex interaction process involving influences from biological and social factors. In addition, the aging process is characterized by change as well as continuity and becomes manifest in a multidimensional and multidirectional manner. The former refers to the differential view on aging in which various abilities are affected differently, while the latter refers to the observation that certain abilities may deteriorate gradually, whereas still others remain stable or even improve.

The cascade metaphor of aging, proposed by Birren and Cunningham (1985), represents a heuristic simplification in the context of geropsychological assessment. The metaphor is based on the separation of primary, secondary,

A. Types of aging
- primary aging
- secondary aging
- tertiary aging

B. The individual
- demographics, skills and knowledge
- coping and self-attributions
- psychological well-being

E. Learning and memory
F. Intellectual abilities

C. Sociocultural context
- cohort and period effects
- sociocognitive development

D. Cognitive demands
- cognitive testing
- everyday life tasks

Figure 1 An analytical scheme for understanding and assessment of cognitive functioning in aging.

and tertiary aging patterns. Primary aging refers to intrinsic sources producing irreversible changes but otherwise a healthy or normal aging trajectory. Secondary aging refers to changes due to illnesses or pathology, adding to the inevitable primary aging. Tertiary aging refers to factors increasing the mortality risk and the pattern of terminal decline that becomes manifest preceding death. At the individual level this may be seen as a "curvilinear" dramatic drop while at the group level as a linear decline (cf. Berg, 1996).

It could easily be argued that it is impossible fully to separate the three theoretical aging types. However, in an assessment it is usually required that the geropsychologist concludes whether an observed impairment is to be diagnosed in terms of dysfunction or whether the impairment is to be considered within the borders of "normal aging." The phenomenon of terminal decline (e.g., Johansson & Berg, 1992) must also be taken into account, but is otherwise not an obvious diagnostic issue.

7.02.2.1.1 Primary aging

With increasing age we can expect less primary aging and more secondary and tertiary aging. Although the likelihood of sole primary aging decreases substantially with age because of increased morbidity, primary aging constitutes the bottom line for our understanding of cognitive aging.

Primary aging is, in practice, defined as the lack of illnesses that potentially could be diagnosed. In a population-based random sample of nondemented community-dwelling individuals aged 75 to 96 years, Wahlin et al. (1993) had to exclude 38% of the participants in order to meet their health criteria. Of these, 19% were excluded because of a Mini-Mental State score (MMSE) below 25 (Folstein, Folstein, & McHugh, 1975), 4% due to psychiatric disease and/or medication, and 15% due to values of serum vitamin B^{12} or thyroid-stimulating hormone indicative of disease.

Primary cognitive aging is principally characterized by a reduction in the speed at which information is processed in the cognitive system (e.g., Light, 1991; Salthouse, 1993). This slowing affects all cognitive processes where speed of behavior is an essential component, for example, in problem solving or executive functioning. In many tests, time limits are therefore more disadvantageous for an elderly person as compared to a younger individual.

A conceptual distinction within primary aging is that between usual and successful aging. According to Rowe and Kahn (1987), usual aging refers to normal aging heightened by the effects of extrinsic factors, both physical and psychosocial. In successful aging, these extrinsic influences have a neutral or positive role in maintaining functioning. As emphasized by Rowe and Kahn, the elucidation of factors that explain success is of great value for potential interventions, including preventive efforts, aiming at successful aging. Hill, Wahlin, Winblad, and Bäckman (1995) followed this route and examined the predictive strength of demographic and life-style variables for memory performance and ability to utilize cognitive support in very old age. The authors concluded that among healthy elderly persons, those who were younger, better educated, and more socially active not only improved more from cognitive support, but also demonstrated better overall performance. Further, level of exercise (in terms of walking or bicycling) was found to be a reliable predictor of episodic free recall performance. Although this was a cross-sectional study, and no conclusions can be drawn about causative relations, it was argued that the results are relevant for the selection of individuals who are likely to benefit from memory training programs. Identifying factors important for level of cognitive performance (such as level of social activity or exercise) may also have implications for other interventions.

7.02.2.1.2 Secondary aging—physical health

Secondary or disease-related aging becomes significantly more important with increasing age. It is well known that age is associated with an increased prevalence of a variety of diseases that may affect cognitive and memory functioning (e.g., Brody & Schneider, 1986; Fries & Crapo, 1981). Among persons over 65, more than 80% have at least one chronic illness, and many individuals have multiple diagnoses.

In addition to an even more pronounced slowing of speed (e.g., Salthouse, 1993), other intellectual abilites are also likely to become affected by various illnesses. A few examples are sufficient to illustrate the effects of secondary aging on cognitive abilities: the cardiovascular system is prone to age-related changes, the prevalence of heart disease among those 65 years of age and older in the Western world is estimated to be approximately 30% (Epstein et al., 1965), and the treatment of hypertension among elderly adults is considered by many geriatricians to be an almost normal and inevitable medication in aging. It has been demonstrated that cardiovascular disease has negative impacts on memory and cognition (e.g., Barclay, Weiss, Bond, & Blass, 1988; Grut, Forsell, Hill, Bäckman, & Winblad, 1995). Furthermore, the negative relation between elevated blood pressure and cognitive functioning has been documented in several longitudinal investigations (e.g, Farmer et al., 1990), and performance differences may also exist as a function of blood pressure medication (e.g., Elias, Wolf, D'Agostino, Cobb, & White, 1993). Also, older people may have health-related motor impairments that interfere with performance on psychological tests. Examples include tremor associated with Parkinson's disease, or difficulties associated with severe arthritis. Obviously, it may be necessary to modify tasks that put demands on hand motor functioning. Additional examples concern the negative relation between cognitive performance and such diverse conditions as diabetes (e.g., Bale, 1973), epilepsy (e.g., Dikman & Matthews, 1977), hyperthyroidism (Gambert, 1988), hypothyroidism (Mennemeier, Garner, & Heilman, 1993), or diseases related to vitamin deficiency (e.g., Wahlin, Hill, Winblad, & Bäckman, in press). It is well known that visual acuity (Lerman, 1983) and hearing, especially of high-frequency tones (Ordy, Brizzee, Beavers, & Medart, 1979), decline with age. In the assessment situation, it therefore becomes neccessary first to make sure that the older person has sufficient hearing or vision abilities to meet the sensory demands of the tasks at hand. It is notable that even within normal ranges, sensory functioning seems to be a strong late-life indicator of intellectual functioning (Lindenberger & Baltes, 1994).

Comprehensive health screening is rarely performed in cognitive aging studies. For the clinician, this should be kept in mind in using results from scientific reports as normative data. More recent studies of age-related effects on memory and other cognitive performance, however, have tended to screen for potentially confounded critical aspects of physical health (e.g., Bäckman & Wahlin, 1995; Hill et al., 1995; Robins Wahlin, Bäckman, Wahlin, & Winblad, 1993, 1996; Wahlin, Bäckman, & Winblad, 1995). Given the complexity of the potential impact of health-related factors, it is difficult to present clear-cut recommendations to the geropsychologist. Generally speaking, it is however important to evaluate performance, keeping in mind that influences other than what is addressed by the diagnostic question must be taken under serious consideration by the geropsychologist.

There exists at present no clear consensus about the differentiation between primary aging and pathology. This distinction becomes increasingly difficult with age, with the risk of both over- and underdiagnosis, that is, defining assessment results within the category of "normal aging" as disease/illness or ascribing an impairment to "normal aging." Also, the symptoms for many diseases change and tend to be more diffuse, in addition to prevalent comorbidity in old age (Fozard, Metter, & Brant, 1990). Furthermore, a diagnosis of disease is often accompanied by certain treatment efforts and with potential side-effects on cognitive functions. For example, Berg and Dellasega (1996), examined the relationships between cognitive function and psychotropic medication use in the H70 population-based sample in Sweden over a nine-year period (see Section 7.02.3.2.1). About one-third of the sample was on a drug regimen including anxiolytics, hypnotics, and antidepressant medications. The study showed that these psychotropics had a negative effect on most cognitive functions, although the effects generally were found to be moderate.

The dementia syndrome represents a diagnostic category of particular relevance for cognitive aging, since dementia is the single most devastating group of illnesses in which memory disturbances and cognitive impairments are cardinal outcomes. We will only address a few issues here. Dementia is extensively discussed in Chapter 10, this volume. The prevalence of dementia increases with age and the incidence rates are considerable (e.g., Fratiglioni et al., 1991; Johansson & Zarit, 1995). Dementia also demonstrates the principal difficulties in separating primary and secondary aging at an early stage, despite findings of significant impairments already present in the earliest, preclinical stage. Johansson and Zarit (1997) examined this "borderline issue" in a longitudinal study of a population-based sample of people aged 84 and older. They found that nondemented subjects who were diagnosed with "mild dysfunction" because of their performance were 11 times more likely to develop dementia within a two-year period, and seven times more likely to become demented over a four-year period. Their results also provide further evidence for terminal decline, as the likelihood for subsequent mortality was greater among individuals diagnosed with "mild dysfunction." The mortality risk was three times greater over two years and five times greater over four years compared with individuals who were rated as cognitively intact (see Figure 2).

The insidious onset of many diseases, like that of primary degenerative dementia (e.g., Alzheimer's disease) presents particular diagnostic problems. As pointed out by Sliwinski, Lipton, Buschke, and Stewart (1996), the identification of preclinical dementia is complicated by the overestimation of age effects on cognitive measures through an underestimation of the mean and an overestimation of variance. This notion becomes more important with increasing age, because of higher prevalence rates and increased likelihood of the incidence of dementia. Besides the neccessary criteria of impaired memory and other cognitive abilities, a functional criterion is generally employed for the definition of a clinically manifest dementia. This functional criterion, as in the case of the *Diagnostic and statistical manual for mental disorders* (*DSM*; American Psychiatric Association, 1987, 1994), requires that cognitive impairments need to be of sufficient severity to interfere with social or occupational functioning. A problem, however, is that cognitive demands may vary with age. The risk of underdiagnosis tends to be greater with the oldest-old due to lower cognitive demands in everyday life which makes it less likely that impairments will be uncovered. A more detailed discussion about inputs from the sociocultural context follows in Section 7.02.2.3.

7.02.2.1.3 Summary

Aging is not a unitary process but the complex outcome of numerous interactions with biological, psychological and social subprocesses. The outcome can roughly be categorized using three broad aging types: primary, secondary, and tertiary aging. The distinction between primary and secondary aging often corresponds to what is expected of the geropsychologist. A differential view of cognitive aging means that while performance in certain functions has declined and may be diagnosed as an expression of disease, for example dementia, performance in other functions may remain within the "normal aging" category or at the border of primary aging. This is especially the case when impairments are mild or changes are subtle and where there is lack of information on decline and course of change.

7.02.2.2 The Individual

Within each type of aging pattern, described above, one can discern features unique to the individual. Such individual or subject-related factors refer to exposures that have affected the individual throughout life. Whereas certain factors reflect basic demographics like age, gender, ethnicity, and socioeconomics, others refer to various aspects of personality and mental health. An understanding of the unique constellation of these influences requires the gathering of information necessary to evaluate present functioning in light of previous ability. In addition, this notion provides arguments for an interindividual difference perspective on aging.

7.02.2.2.1 Coping and self-attributions

The individual's unique repertoire of behaviors, including cognitive and emotional styles, represents another dimension to consider in an assessment. Coping and self-attributions are, in the late 1990s, more often identified as significant influences for memory and cognition. A number of coping definitions have been proposed. Most of them share the general idea

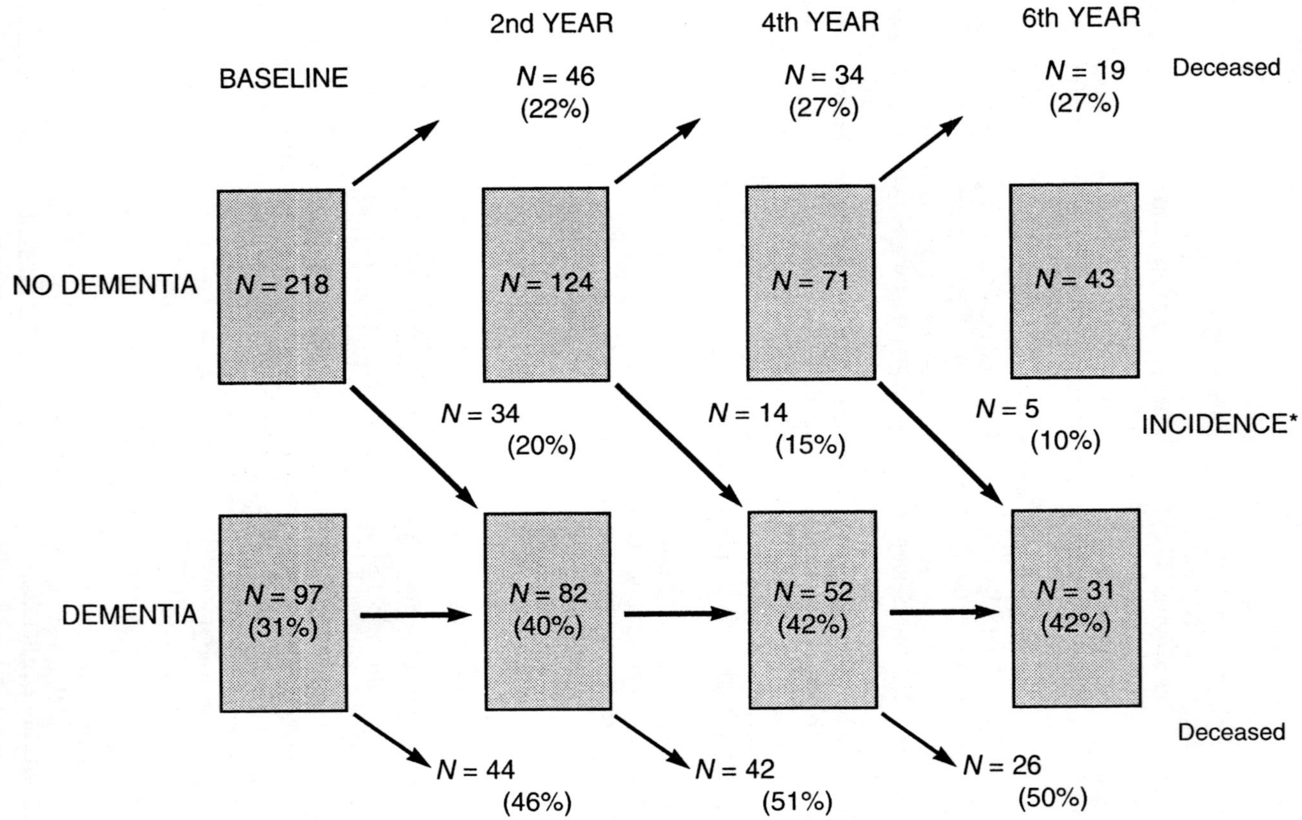

* Incidence was calculated by taking the percentage of new cases of dementia from among surviving subjects not diagnosed as demented at the previous time of assessment. (At Time 2 there was incomplete information for diagnosis in 14 cases, at Time 3 in 8 cases and at Time 4 in one case.)

Figure 2 Prevalence of dementia and incidence of demention and mortality over a six-year period in a population-based sample of 84–90 year olds ("Early cognitive markers of the incidence of dementia and mortality: A longitudinal population-based study of the oldest old" by B. Johansson and S. H. Zarit, 1997. *Journal of Geriatric Psychiatry, 12*, pp. 53–59. Copyright 1997 by John Wiley & Sons Ltd. Adapted with permission).

of Lazarus and Folkman (1984), who described coping as "constantly changing cognitive and behavioral efforts to manage specific external and/or internal demands that are appraised as taxing or exceeding the resources of the person" (p. 14). Because appraisal is a crucial component, self-attributions and personal control come into focus. Personal control, locus of control, self-efficacy, and other similar concepts all refer to the individual's feeling of being in control or lacking control over life in general or in managing certain aspects, for example intellectual tasks (see, Baltes & Baltes, 1986). In this respect, coping and dimensions of personal control are also important for daily life adjustment and performance on certain cognitive tasks.

Of particular relevance for memory and cognition in this context is metamemory and metacognition, referring to people's awareness of their own strengths and weaknesses in performing memory and other cognitive tasks. For example, less effort than necessary may be invested in performance when belief exists that one's memory and cognitive capacity is too low for a certain task, and self-attributions given to actual success or failures in performance tend to reinforce these attributions. Hayslip and Panek (1993) describe the interrelations between performance experiences, self-statements, and emotional reactions in terms of a vicious cycle (see Figure 3).

Further, the relation between conceptions or self-attributions of, for example, intelligence, may be under multifactorial influence. Much of the work on conceptions of intelligence indicates that the dimensions that make up the prototypic intelligent person may vary at different periods of development and for individuals of different ages or experiental background (e.g., Siegler & Richards, 1982; Yussen & Kane, 1983). Berg and Sternberg (1992) examined whether young, middle-aged, and older adults viewed the concept of intelligence differently depending on their own age. They found that adults perceive differences in what constitutes exceptional intelligence during young, middle, and late adulthood, but also that adults' conceptions of intelligence are characterized by multidirectionality and modifiability.

In a study of actual and perceived change in intellectual performance, Schaie, Willis, & O'Hanlon (1994) identified three groups: realists (individuals who accurately estimated actual change), optimists (those who overestimated actual change), and pessimists (those who underestimated change). This classification was based on self-reports and actual performance on several tests. Older individuals were more realistic than younger subjects on a test of number ability, while more pessimistic about verbal meaning and reasoning tests. Section 7.02.2.2.2 examines further relations between psychological well-being, self-attributions, and cognitive performance.

7.02.2.2.2 Psychological well-being

Research into the psychological well-being of elderly persons tends to emphasize prior life satisfaction and mood as important predictors. Self-attributions, in terms of subjective memory and cognition, are also concurrent markers for adjustment and well-being. Beyond normal emotional fluctuations, the interrelationships between self-reports and performance become obvious in clinical depression. An inability in the depressed person to mobilize motivation will ultimately lead to deficient performance. Depression is a prevalent and disabling mental disorder in the elderly and the symptoms tend to be more indistinguishable and often involve impairments in memory and cognition (e.g., Bäckman & Forsell, 1994), in some cases with a severity that corresponds to depressive pseudodementia (see Katona, 1994). Severity of depression seems to be correlated with the magnitude of performance deficits in tests of memory and cognition (e.g., Cipioli, Neri, Andermarcher, Pinelli, & Lalla, 1990).

Numerous studies have reported strong associations between depression and self-reports of cognitive functioning. It was, however, early recognized that complaints must be differentiated from actual performance (Kahn, Zarit, Hilbert, & Niederehe, 1979). A diagnostic scheme for different configurations of performance, complaints, and affective status was presented by Gallagher, Thompson and Levy (1980). In a meta-analysis, Burt, Zembar, and Niederehe (1995) even suggested that complaints may have a stronger association with general psychopathology than with depressive symptoms. Further studies are needed to resolve the complex interrelationships between cognitive performance, mood, and self-attributions (see Kaszniak & Ditraglia Christenson, 1995).

Zarit (1979) suggested that memory complaints also reflect "a memory and aging stereotype" that ascribes poor memory to the elderly due to their age. Such a stereotype is likely to be internalized by the elderly. Studies on self-reports show, however, a great variation, typically in the range of 40–80%, in the extent to which older people feel that their memory performance is compromised. These discrepancies may reflect sampling differences and sociocultural values. In a population-based

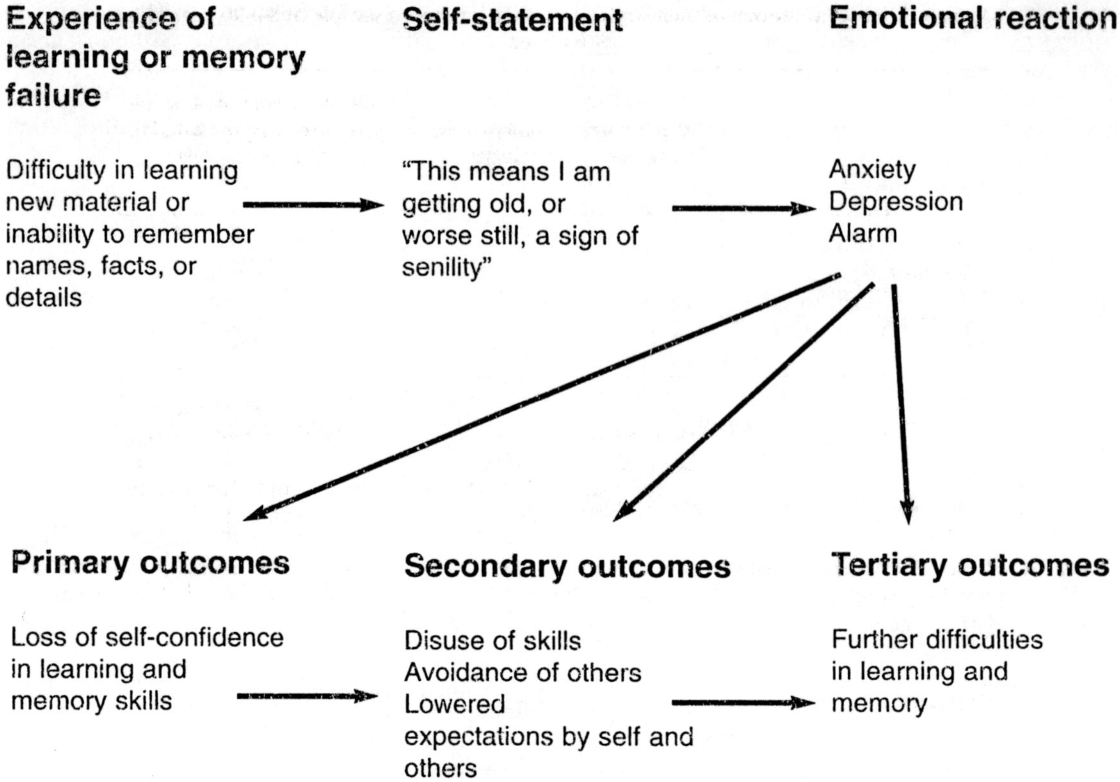

Figure 3 A vicious cycle in which memory failures, self-statements, and emotional reactions tend to compromise future performance (*Adult Development and aging* (p. 158), by B. Hayslip Jr. and P. E. Panek, 1993, New York: HarperCollins. Copyright 1993 by HarperCollins College Publishers. Adapted with permission).

sample of very old Swedish people, participants were examined four times over a six-year period, and were asked to rate their own memory and cognitive ability (Johansson, Allen-Burge, & Zarit, in press). Participants typically evaluated their abilities in a positive manner (see Table 1). A subsample of 31% were, however, excluded because of dementia, which has to be taken into account when examining the figures.

These self-evaluations were scaled and further examined in relation to concurrent, prospective, and retrospective performance on a battery of memory and cognitive tasks (Johansson et al., 1997). Individuals who evaluated their memory more positively showed significantly better concurrent test performances. In addition, they also reported less depression. The study interestingly revealed that self-evaluations predicted subsequent decline in test performance, as well as onset of dementia within the next two to four years. In the retrospective analysis, more negative self-evaluations were found in individuals who two years later reported that they had experienced declining memory. The actual strength in the associations between test scores and self-evaluations were, however, quite weak. This suggests that self-evaluations are influenced by factors not covered by performance on tests. The few existing studies on the relationships between self-rated intellectual abilities and performance on intelligence and practical problem-solving tasks also show weak associations (e.g., Cornelius, 1990).

7.02.2.2.3 Summary

Present functioning should always be related to the individual's prior level of functioning. This will obviously present difficulties as we seldom have baseline information or any other detailed information about the individual's past function at the level of various abilities in focus in an assessment. It is also necessary to consider influences from demographics and to take into account the individual's own perception of memory and cognitive functioning, as well as other expressions of psychological well-being that may exert an impact on the effort invested in a certain performance. Although self-reports are closely related to psychological well-being, self-evaluations may also be formed by experiences of success and failure in performing cognitive tasks in daily life.

Table 1 Self-evaluations of memory in a population-based sample of 84–90 year olds in Sweden.

Self-evaluation	*On the whole, how would you rate your memory? (%)*	*On the whole, how would you rate your thinking and problem solving? (%)*
Good	44%	53%
Rather good	34%	33%
Neither good nor bad	8%	7%
Rather bad	5%	6%
Bad	9%	1%
	Do you experience memory failures in everyday life that makes life more difficult? (%)	*Do you experience problems in remembering what to do and say at a later occasion (prospective memory)? (%)*
No problems	82%	66%
Minor problems	17%	32%
Major problems	1%	2%
	Have you experienced any changes with your memory in the last two years? (%)	
Better now	1%	
No change	50%	
Somewhat worse now	44%	
Worse now	5%	

Source: Johansson et al. (1997).

7.02.2.3 Sociocultural Context

Aging is certainly not a context-free process (see Blanchard-Fields & Abeles, 1996). On the contrary, health status and level of functioning in later life are dependent on cumulative outcomes from numerous sources, including influences from the sociocultural context (e.g., dietary habits, transportation, and physical mobility, or the coverage and inputs by health care institutions like dentistry or preventive pediatrics). A list of potential factors would be very extensive. The differential exposure to environmental influences generally makes people different, and it is often claimed that interindividual differences increase with age (e.g., Krauss, 1980; Nelson & Daneffer, 1992). This is still an unresolved issue, but in assessing elderly persons, attending to sociocultural influences seems as important as attending to ethnicity or social class.

7.02.2.3.1 Cohort and period effects

Cohort is a concept often used in the aging literature. Cohort generally refers to people born during a certain time and therefore exposed to similar experiences that tend to make them more alike than generations of people born earlier or later (see Rosow, 1978). Thus, age differences should be interpreted taking cohort effects into account. This was noticed early when age differences found in cross-sectional studies could be ascribed to significant cohort effects. The classical example is a study by Birren and Morrison (1961), who found higher correlations between certain tests of intelligence and years of formal schooling, than with age. The important role of education has since been identified in many studies (e.g., Inouye, Albert, Mohs, Sun, & Berkman, 1993). The educational system also represents an important social institution where different methods and content, hopefully, have long-lasting but differential effects on various cohorts. Thus, the potential impact of educational differences must be considered in evaluating cognitive performance, particularly in the presence of broad age ranges.

The importance of cohort is easily observed in the educational system. In elderly Swedish cohorts most individuals have six years of basic formal schooling only, compared to more than 12 years for persons in their twenties. Even at the level of brief cognitive screening, employing devices like the MMSE, it has been suggested that different cut-offs have to be used for elderly people at different educational levels (e.g., Crum, Anthony, Basset, & Folstein, 1993). Employing more sophisticated tests, cohort-adjusted norms have to be appropriate for accurate interpretations. Other cohort influences may be identified in the political scene, for example the 1968 movement in Europe, corresponding to the Vietnam generation in the USA, or personal experiences of the world wars that affected people differently across ages.

Period effects refer, in the context of aging, to influences that affect people throughout ages. An example is the introduction of television. Some claimed that socially and intellectually rewarding activities, such as crosswords and jigsaw puzzles, hobbies and so forth were replaced by television. The Swedish expression *dumburken* ("couch potatoes") captures these assumed negative aspects of passive television watching. At the same time no one can deny the wealth of information and general world knowledge that is easily brought to the public through television. Although period effects tend to be pervasive across ages, certain influences may affect older persons differently from younger (see Elder, 1979).

7.02.2.3.2 Sociocognitive development

Memory and other cognitive abilities develop in a sociocultural context where environmental influences tend to be normatively age-graded, that is, highly correlated with chronological age. A life-span model of intellectual development based on significant inputs from the sociocultural context was formulated by Schaie (1977–78). The model distinguishes four major developmental stages. Acquisition is the major theme in childhood and adolescence, preparing the individual with basic skills and information for later life. This basic expertise includes what society defines as essential for successful socialization and crucial for the reproduction of society. In the next stage, the young adulthood period—or the achieving stage—acquired knowledge has to be applied, whether at work, in the family, or in other social contexts. The middle age period that follows is described basically as a stage where cognitive abilities involve more social responsibilities or executive roles. The reintegrative stage in old age is a period where one's interests, attitudes, and values become the important inputs for the individual. Personal meaningfulness is ascribed a major theme in this stage. The transitions between stages proceeds from "What should I know?" through "How should I use what I know?" to "Why should I know?" In aging, the individual requires more meaning in order to be motivated to engage in a certain task.

Disuse has been identified as a main source for decline in abilities that require continuous use in order to be preserved (see Kohn & Schooler, 1983; Lee, 1991). In addition to the general slowing in primary aging, disuse is generally thought of as an important input for decline in functions not practiced. Support for this hypothesis is offered by an increased performance–capacity gap with increasing age, and interventions demonstrating considerable plasticity or modifiability in primary aging (e.g., Baltes & Kliegl, 1992). Perlmutter (1986) describes a life-span view of memory in which the individual's memory capabilities reflect past experience, and where decline in capacity can be compensated for by growth in memory contents. This leads to an increasing environmental fitness and to an increasingly adapted memory system.

7.02.2.3.3 Summary

In a sociocognitive development context, aging can be understood as a change of the behavior repertoire in accordance with the individual's own preferences, besides the influences of cohort and generation. Cohort effects refer to age differences due to influences that variously have affected different birth cohorts. Period effects, on the other hand, emphasize the need to consider certain sociocultural influences as more pervasive across ages. The actual impact of these influences may, however, vary depending on the age of the individual. The specific organization of society also imposes certain age-graded roles and tasks. Although a fixed stage model like Schaie's (1977–78) tends to neglect interindividual differences, it directs attention to the fact that certain tasks may be perceived quite differently depending on the differential use of intellect at different ages. This view emphasizes a need to consider what types of cognitive tasks could be employed in examining elderly people in an age-fair manner. The latter includes an ecological aspect of memory and cognition.

7.02.2.4 Cognitive Demands and Everyday Functioning

In cognitive aging research, age-related decline in a variety of abilities such as visuospatial functioning or episodic memory performance is well documented. In other types of task one may find that performance remains relatively stable or even improves across the adult life span. Preserved abilities are likely in tasks tapping general knowledge or language-related skills. Our knowledge is sparse on how this translates into everyday functioning (e.g., Salthouse, 1990; Searight & Goldberg, 1991). In clinical practice, the geropsychologist may have to resolve whether it is likely that impaired performance on, for example, tests of visuospatial ability is related to difficulties in everyday functioning. In other words, to what extent is it possible to infer, from certain test results, that an individual is incapable of performing adequately in everyday life? A patient with extensive prefrontal damage may be significantly impaired in everyday life, yet perform within the normal range on neuropsychological tests (e.g., Stuss & Benson, 1986). Another patient may score below cut-off for normal performance, but demonstrate adequate performance on a variety of everyday tasks, perhaps because these tasks are overlearned and because adequate performance is defined according to lower demands because of old age.

Clearly, everyday performance has to be related to the demands of daily living and available support systems, as well as baseline capacity. One can discern two major explanations for the understanding of discrepancies between elderly people's daily-life performance and scores on test of memory and cognition. The first is based on the idea that standard tests are inadequate because they simply do not measure the relevant processes underlying daily-life functioning. Thus, the assumption is that tests and everyday life differ in terms of the mechanisms involved. The other, functional, explanation, relates to age fairness emphasizing unfamiliarity and task novelty as significant inputs for lower test performance in the elderly (e.g., Bruce, 1991).

7.02.2.4.1 Cognitive mechanisms and tasks

The experimental and clinical test traditions have been criticized for their predilection for using artificial materials for remembering, or as stimuli in problem solving. The claim is that these methods have restricted relevance for the understanding of memory and cognition in everyday life (see Willis, 1996). In this vein, Neisser (1978) even suggested that naturalistic studies of memory would be more productive than their laboratory counterparts.

Some authors have argued that standard experimental tasks, in which elderly people demonstrate worse performance than younger ones, are not valid as indicators of everyday performance for older adults (e.g., Baltes & Willis, 1979; Berg & Sternberg, 1985; Labouvie-Vief, 1982, 1985). However, in spite of many efforts to develop more naturalistic measures, such as memory for texts or television programs, the results do not confirm the expected elimination of age effects or even attenuation of age differences (e.g., Denney, 1989; Hartley, 1989; Salthouse, 1983). On the contrary, performance on standard memory tasks and on more ecologically relevant tasks seem to provide similar results. It has also been claimed that certain tests may have a potential disadvantageous impact because different age groups are not equally experienced with stimulus materials or experimental and clinical tests of cognitive functions. There is, however, rather convincing evidence that differences in experience or unfamiliarity with stimulus materials cannot solely account for observed age differences (e.g., Salthouse, 1987, 1990).

The claim that standard tasks do not accurately portray everyday performance led some researchers to construct tests better suited for elderly persons, so called age-fair tasks. An example is the brief battery of tests based on ideas of ecological relevance and used by Johansson, Zarit, and Berg (1992) in studies of the oldest old. The tests, Coin Test, Clock Test, and MIR ("Memory in Reality"), were deliberately designed to minimize floor effects and to differentiate performance in cognitively impaired individuals. Age-fair testing is highly interrelated with *ecological relevance*, referring to naturalistic studies of memory and cognition. Both concepts emphasize the functional aspects, not that different mechanisms are involved in everyday performance compared to an experimental or clinical context. Ecological relevance refers to the congruence between task demands and demands imposed in everyday life. In other words, to what extent do the obtained pattern of results using psychometric or laboratory tasks generalize to situations in the everyday life of the individual? In a study by Cockburn and Smith (1991), subjects were tested with various measures of fluid and crystallized intelligence (see Section 7.02.3.2.1) in order to examine the predictive value of these tests for performances on a range of everyday memory problems, including analogs of situations met in daily life, such as remembering names or asking for the return of a hidden possession. Crystallized intelligence showed low predictive power, while fluid intelligence was a better predictor, although the authors concluded that cognitive decline in aging involves more than a simple decline in fluid intelligence. In another study on everyday memory, West, Crook, and Barron (1992) found that a measure of crystallized intelligence, vocabulary, played a significant role for almost every memory measure examined.

7.02.2.4.2 *Tests of functional abilities*

In some cases it may be preferable to perform a functional assessment of the client's abilities in parallel with cognitive testing. For this, clinicians have at their disposal several standardized methods measuring activities of daily living (ADL; e.g., Kane & Kane, 1981). These instruments assess functions that are associated with basic self-maintenance such as dressing, feeding, or hygiene. Furthermore, there are other instruments assessing a broader domain of more complex abilities such as managing transportation, communication, self-medication, or financial transactions. This domain of abilities is often called instrumental activities of daily living (IADL; e.g., Kuriansky & Gurland, 1976). One example is the Community Competence Scale (see Grisso, 1986). Using a multidimensional battery, Zarit, Johansson, and Berg (1993) found strong associations between cognitive impairment, ADL, and IADL in the oldest old. Results like this demonstrate that cognitive abilities are necessary prerequisites for adequate performance, although the sensitivity may be low within normal ranges of functioning.

7.02.2.4.3 *Summary*

Our understanding of memory and cognition are greatly determined by procedures and methods used in research. There seems to be no reason to believe that experimental and psychological tests measure functions other than those also constituting the basis for everyday functioning. The relation between test performance and level of functioning in daily life appears, however, to be influenced by numerous other factors such as social demands, support-systems, or the individual's level of experience. Everyday functioning of the client is of importance. In assessing elderly people, the degree to which test demands overlap with demands of daily life ought to be taken into consideration. Much effort has been invested in constructing tasks more suitable for the oldest people. Research suggests that results on various psychometric tests may show weak associations with everyday functioning. The inclusion of an assessment of actual performance in everyday life, such as IADL measures, can provide additional information of value to the geropsychologist.

7.02.3 MEMORY AND OTHER COGNITIVE ABILITIES

This section reviews some select research on memory and cognition in relation to current theory. Some brief outlines of models of memory, as well as processes and components involved in other cognitive abilities, will be provided. The reader is reminded of the analytical scheme (Figure 1) presented in the introductory section when critically examining reported findings and the bases for interpretations. In doing so, it is important to keep in mind the multifactorial influences on cognitive performance in old age. Furthermore, apart from noncognitive influences, it is also important to recognize that most published studies are cross-sectional and consequently demonstrate age differences only, and that the bulk of research includes convenience samples recruited for studying cognitive mechanisms or potential age-related differences in various abilities. Most studies provide no detailed information concerning physical health (relating to the distinction between primary and secondary aging). To what degree the failure to do so has influenced the typical picture of cognitive aging remains yet to be elucidated. Last, few studies of memory and cognition have included individuals beyond 80 years, which limits our understanding of the very old and oldest old.

7.02.3.1 Learning and Memory

Learning and memory represent highly interrelated processes, and the study of either requires understanding of the other. Studies of learning tend to emphasize the acquisition of new behaviors and information, while memory refers to processes involved in the retention and retrieval of what has been acquired. Learning and memory are here treated separately from other aspects of cognition because of the wealth of information available and the extensive research in the area. This subsection provides first a framework, out of several possible, for the understanding of learning and memory. In addition, there is an examination of the significance of task properties, here defined as levels of cognitive support, for variations in episodic memory performance. Finally, some relevant research is reviewed with focus on the oldest. The review is largely restricted to episodic memory, because this memory system has proved to be most affected by age, in addition to its sensitivity to depression, dementia, and other illnesses that are prevalent in aging.

7.02.3.1.1 Types of learning

Learning may mean many quite different things. It may refer to the mastering of a new skill such as learning how to ride a bicycle. The resulting procedural or motor-based memories are formed without awareness. This general area of learning and memory has been reviewed by Chiarello and Hoyer (1988) and Graf (1990). Learning may also mean acquiring and changing habits. Behavior modification is an example of this type of learning in clinical practice. Learning may further mean the acquisition of new information. This is something we all do in school. We may still remember what date World War One started, but not when that information was acquired. This is generally what we refer to as semantic memory.

This subsection restricts itself to episodic memory, and learning is concerned with the remembering of personal incidents that are, in most cases, not very distant in time. Tested persons are presupposed to remember where they picked up the requested information. The typical example is a test of memory where the psychologist reads a list of words or sentences, and the client is later asked to recall as many of the words or sentences as possible of those that were presented some minutes ago.

7.02.3.1.2 Models of memory

Many researchers classify memory phenomena in terms of memory systems, although the results are often analyzed in terms of various processes operating within these systems. For the clinician, the system model is perhaps the most intuitive, since it alludes to specific tasks. Before proceeding to some of the systems identified in modern experimental psychology, we choose as the point of departure a model that has exerted an enormous impact in the development of later theoretical accounts. This is the "Multistore" model of memory proposed by Atkinson and Shiffrin (1968). In clinical practice, their line of reasoning is perhaps still sufficient. Basically, this model of memory distinguishes between the sensory store where new information enters through sensory stimulation, the short-term store where the information is subjected to conscious mental activity, and the long-term store which is thought of as a more or less permanent store of information.

As a general guideline, it may be sufficient to distinguish between recent and remote memories, or between short- and long-term memory. These subdivisions are, however, somewhat complicated in terms of test materials. We therefore now turn to selected parts of the system model which are somewhat more clear for clinical purposes. For more detailed discussions, consult Baddeley (1990) or Parkin (1993).

Short-term memory is analogous to primary memory in that it represents the locus of conscious mental activity. Early accounts of primary memory (e.g., Waugh & Norman, 1965) stated that this system registers and retains incoming information in a highly accessible form for a short period of time after input. This conception of primary memory has been elaborated in recent years (e.g., Baddeley, 1986). It may be useful to distinguish primary memory (holding information in consciousness) from working memory (simultaneously holding information in mind and elaborating on or using that information in combination with other incoming information). Roughly, in terms of tests, this corresponds to the difference between Digit span forward and backwards (Wechsler, 1981).

The long-term store may, in terms of memory systems, be further subdivided into episodic and semantic memory. Episodic memory refers to memory of personally experienced events with a reference both in time and space, that is, we remember something we have experienced, and that memory is associated with information about when and where the information was encoded. The command "recall as many of the words as possible from the list I presented to you 10 minutes ago" evokes episodic memory. Semantic memory is memory for general knowledge (Tulving, 1983, 1985). The information task of the Wechsler Adult Intelligence Scale (WAIS) battery corresponds to a test of semantic memory.

7.02.3.1.3 Episodic memory

Most researchers agree that age differences in performance are most likely to occur in episodic memory tasks, that is, in tasks requiring conscious retrieval of information acquired in a particular place at a particular time (see Kausler, 1994; Light, 1991; Salthouse, 1991, for reviews). However, memory performance in very old age has received relatively little empirical attention. The available evidence is mixed as to whether there are differences in episodic memory functioning among different cohorts of old and very old adults. Most studies of the late adult life span indicate a gradual decline in performance with age (e.g., Bäckman, 1991; Bäckman & Larsson, 1992; Crook & Larrabee, 1992). There are, however, studies indicating no age differences (e.g., Cohen & Faulkner, 1989; Larsson & Bäckman, 1993; Olofsson & Bäckman, 1993). With reference to the previous discussion on potential impacts of health-related factors on cognitive performance, it is important to note that a careful health screening has not been performed in these memory and aging studies. This may be an essential factor underlying the contradictory findings. In studies performed by Wahlin and colleagues (e.g., Bäckman & Wahlin, 1995; Wahlin et al., 1993, 1995), careful health screening was routinely performed. The outcome of these studies showed that performance in a variety of episodic memory tasks differs reliably in comparing elderly people between 75 and 96 years of age. This was the case in tests of episodic face recognition, free recall and recognition of random word lists, and free and cued recall of organizable words. The age-related differences were, however, relatively small in raw score numbers and more pronounced in the free recall tasks as compared to the recognition tasks. In a study of 1000 healthy participants ranging in age between 35 and 80 years, a battery of episodic and semantic memory tests (Nyberg, Bäckman, Erngrund, Olofsson, & Nilsson, 1996) was employed. It was found that after controlling for differences in demographic (education, gender), cognitive (visuospatial ability), and health-related (blood pressure, serum vitamin B^{12}) factors, age did not predict performance on tests of semantic memory. The impact of age on tests of episodic memory was substantially reduced when differences in the background factors were controlled for, although still significant. These authors proposed that the failure to account for the age effects on episodic memory is because it can be attributed to age-related neuronal changes.

7.02.3.1.4 Memory tests and cognitive support

In addition to the many influences on cognitive and memory performance described in previous sections, performance may also vary depending on level of support provided. Some research indicates that age differences are large in unsupported tasks such as free recall, while relatively small in more supported tasks such as recognition (Craik & Jennings, 1992).

Before elaborating on the concept of cognitive support, this subsection will briefly describe three types of memory tests that have dominated research on episodic memory. In these tests, the retrieval conditions vary, such that free recall represents the lowest level of support, cued recall represents a more supportive test condition, and recognition of the information to-be-remembered (TBR) is the most supportive retrieval condition.

In the free recall task, subjects are presented with the items and are then asked to recall without prompting what was previously presented. In the cued recall condition, cues of some sort are provided by the examiner, and test materials are then typically organizable in some way. Questions such as "what animals do you remember?" or "what kind of furniture do you remember?" constitute the cues. Finally, in the recognition tasks, the initially presented materials are presented intermixed with a number of distractors. Subjects are asked to state whether they recognize items from the presentation.

Tasks may also vary in terms of presentation rate, where a slow presentation rate represents a more supportive condition as compared to a rapid presentation rate. Performance is also dependent upon the nature of the TBR materials. It is well known that stimulus dimensions like modality (i.e., items may be presented in a way that one or more of the sensory systems are stimulated during encoding), richness (e.g., items may be presented as objects or words), and organizability (i.e., it may or may not be possible to combine items in a meaningful fashion) are important to goodness of remembering (see Bäckman, Mäntylä, & Herlitz, 1990). Further examples include the datedness of the TBR materials (e.g., items may be faces of persons who were famous 50 years ago or faces of persons who attained their fame recently). There is a consensus that performance of older adults is facilitated by increasing the support with respect to modality, richness, organizability, and prior knowledge (Bäckman et al., 1990; Craik & Jennings, 1992) (see Figure 4).

There is converging evidence from experimental research and intervention studies that episodic memory in normal aging is modifiable (Bäckman et al., 1990; Verhaeghen, Marcoen, & Goossens, 1992). Older adults possess a substantial cognitive reserve capacity, although it seems to be less than for younger individuals (e.g., Baltes & Kliegl, 1992). However, there is no evidence for a simple relationship among cognitive support, episodic memory, and age (see Bäckman, 1995). Also, the level of support needed for the optimization of memory performance in dementia differs considerably from that required of healthy elderly people. While in dementia, support is needed at both encoding and retrieval, normally aged adults seem to require support at either encoding or retrieval only in order to enhance their performance (e.g., Herlitz, Lipinska, & Bäckman, 1992).

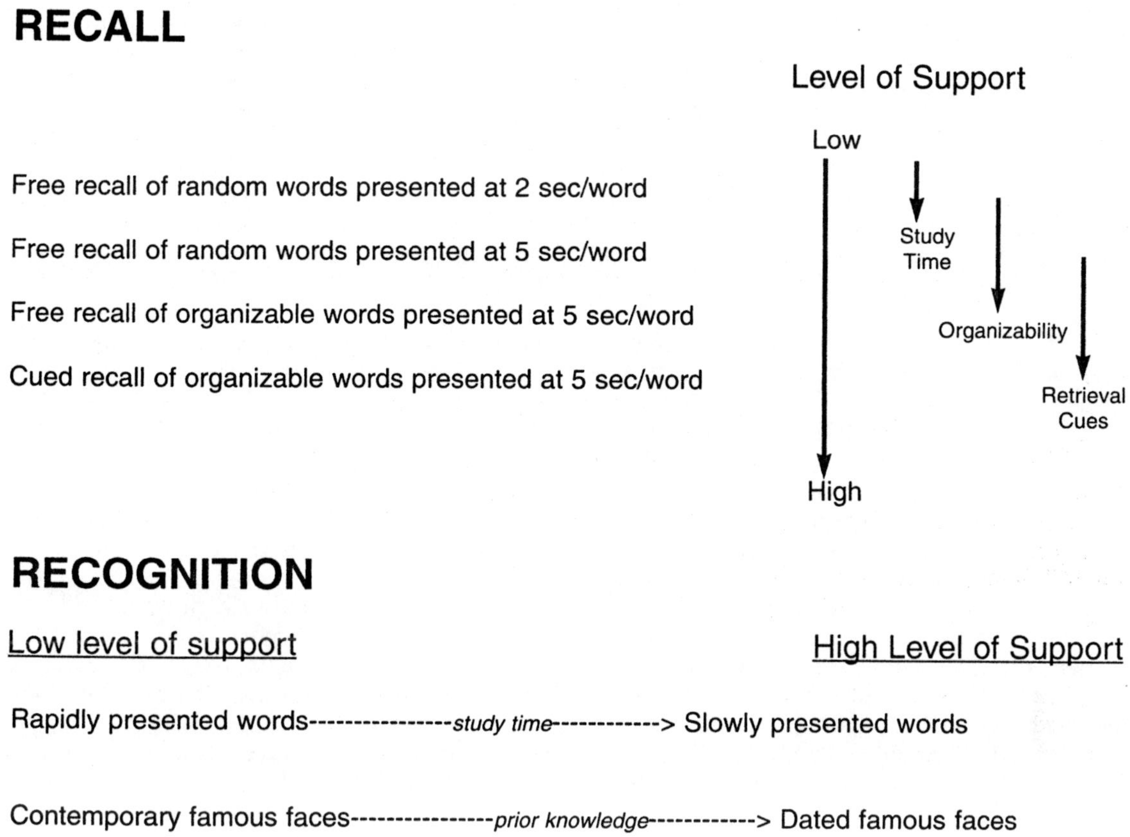

Figure 4 Memory tasks ordered along a continuum of cognitive support.

7.02.3.1.5 Summary

Learning and memory are highly interrelated and cannot be fully understood independently of each other. Most studies on memory in aging are cross-sectional and there is typically a lack of information necessary for ruling out the influence of the health status of the participants. The system model of memory employed in recent research usually distinguishes between episodic, semantic, primary, and working memory. Memory performance is seen as influenced by numerous properties acting at both encoding and retrieval stages of memory processing. Task properties may generally be recognized in terms of cognitive support (low–high), although there is no evidence of a simple relation between level of support and performance. The relatively few studies on episodic memory performance in very old age portray a gradual decline into the very late stages of the life span.

7.02.3.2 Intellectual Abilities

Learning and memory represent in a sense the input and output stages of information processing, while cognition, in a broad sense, also includes processes involved in the integration and reorganization of aquired knowledge for the sake of matching behavior in an appropriate manner, that is, intelligent behavior. Certain tasks are novel and require the execution of new behavior, while others may be practiced and require less cognitive effort. The outcome of matching task demands and cognitive resources is evaluated in the relative success, or failure, to perform a task whether measured as everyday performance or by cognitive tests. This section concentrates on abilities as expressed in aging and reported in the current literature, more than on the fundamental mechanisms involved in the mental operations necessary for intelligent behavior (see Craik & Salthouse, 1992; Rybash, Hoyer, & Roodin, 1986).

Studies on intelligence and aging have generally aimed at identifying normative patterns of age-related changes in the various ability components. The components are operationalized by the test battery. The following section describes such intelligence and aging patterns, while the next focuses on some of the specific cognitive components involved in intelligent behavior.

7.02.3.2.1 Intelligence and aging

The intelligence test tradition evolved at the beginning of the twentieth century as a differential psychology with focus on interindividual differences in intelligence. Age was recognized early as an important stratification variable in these studies. This psychometric tradition has since provided a basis for our understanding of normative aging and the typical age-related pattern. The most frequently used battery of tests in this research arena, as well as in the clinical setting, is the WAIS (Wechsler, 1955) and later modifications (WAIS-R, Wechsler, 1981) of this battery, encompassing tests of verbal ability (1, Vocabulary; 2, Information; 3, Comprehension), short-term learning and remembering (4, Digit-span forward and backwards), numerical abilities (5, Arithmetic), abstraction and generalizations (6, Similarities), and nonverbal abilities (7, Digit-symbol substitution; 8, Picture arrangement; 9, Picture completion; 10, Block design; 11, Object assembly). Wechsler divided the test battery into two broad categories: "the hold tests" (1, 2, 3, and 6) and "the don't hold tests" (7, 8, 9, 10, and 11) according to their resistance to age.

A number of cross-sectional studies over a broad age range have consistently confirmed the "classic aging pattern" (Botwinick, 1978), in which the verbal tests are identified as the hold tests and the nonverbal or performance tests as the don't hold tests. These findings were largely confirmed in later longitudinal studies, although the magnitude of age-related changes generally were found to be less than previously found by age differences. These design-related differences are intensively discussed in the gerontological literature and have supported the notion of including characteristics of the individual as well as recognizing influences from the sociocultural context when interpreting studies showing age effects.

The classical aging pattern was partly refined in a series of studies by Horn, Catell, and Donaldsson (see Horn, 1982, for an overview) who suggested a dichotomization between crystallized and fluid intelligence. This distinction was assumed to reflect different developmental trends. The label of fluid intelligence (Gf) was attached to basic processes involved in identifying complex relations among stimulus patterns and the drawing of inferences on the basis of comprehending relationships. The tests proposed to measure this broad ability component should not be greatly aided by the breadth of previous knowledge and include tests of logical reasoning and of figural and spatial relations. Crystallized intelligence (Cc) was defined as the cumulative end product of information acquired by the operation of fluid processes through interactions with the environment. The measurement of experience-based crystallized intelligence includes, for example, tests of vocabulary, information or general knowledge, comprehension, and arithmetic (Horn, 1982). The definition leads to expectations of preserved function, or even improvements with age.

The distinction between fluid and crystallized intelligence in aging differentiates intelligence components with regard to age. While development into adulthood is characterized by a differentiation of various abilities it is followed by a dedifferentiation in late adulthood and aging (e.g., Reinert, 1970). The broad categories of fluid and crystallized intelligence correspond to a dedifferentiated pattern of formerly more independent abilities. Some researchers claim that this dedifferentiation continues, and that there remains only a broad component of basic cognitive performance in the oldest old (eg., Marsiske, Lindenberger, & Baltes, 1994). The arguments for a more rudimentary intelligence system in advanced age awaits, however, further empirical support.

Although the results from some studies have been interpreted as favoring the general outcomes predicted by the fluid–crystallized dichotomy, the trend in recent research on intelligence and aging is to examine various intelligence components separately. This is consistent with the interest of a clinican when faced with separate scores for various tests. There are problems inherited in all higher-order approaches to intelligence, for example, the comparability between tests in different batteries. The greatest value, therefore, may be that higher-order approaches to intelligence can serve as heuristic frameworks for the clarification of relationships between complex abilities.

The most informative data on aging and intelligence patterns emerge from longitudinal studies using multiple measurements over longer time periods (see Berg, 1996; Schaie, 1996). In the ongoing H70 study in Gothenburg, Sweden (Rinder, Roupe, Steen, & Svanborg, 1975), a random population-based sample were included at the age of 70 and then followed over the years. Interesting patterns of age-related changes, as well as continuity, emerged. In this study, the effects of tertiary aging (terminal decline) were also examined separately for different survival intervals. That is, trends of change for individuals, for example measured at Time 1, Time 2, and Time 3, and then deceased, were compared with that of individuals who survived into the assessment at the next occasion, that is, Time 4. The main finding in the H70 study was that of a robust and pervasive terminal decline pattern in which performance levels were associated with survival. Figure 5 (a) and (b) (Berg, 1987) show this for a test of verbal meaning (Synonyms; SRB:1, Dureman & Sälde, 1959) and reasoning (Figure logic; SRB: 2, Dureman & Sälde, 1959).

The data from longitudinal studies typically show less change than is the case when examining age differences in cross-sectional studies. Although more accurate in providing a portrayal of intelligence and aging, longitudinal studies are affected by attrition and other selective influences that are likely to produce too optimistic a portrayal of aging trends.

7.02.3.2.2 *Specific cognitive abilities*

The "top-down" intelligence and aging perspective (described above) is here supplemented with a "bottom-up" approach focusing on specific cognitive abilites and some tests used for the measurement of these abilities.

(i) Speed of behavior: perceptual and psychomotor performance

Speed of behavior is a crucial ingredient in many memory and cognitive tasks because of time constraints, whether it is in everyday life, in the laboratory, or in clinical tests. While it has been argued by some that time is less important than accuracy, and that speeded tasks are unfair to elderly people, others have argued for the inclusion of speed of behavior as an important marker of intelligent behavior. The former position was supported by early assumptions that the reduced rate of processing was extrinsic or peripheral to the primary aging of the nervous system. Slowing has, however, been recognized as an intrinsic phenomenon that accompanies aging (e.g., Salthouse, 1993) caused by increased levels of noise in the nervous system (e.g., Cremer & Zeef, 1987), or broken or attenuated neural connections (MacKay & Burke, 1990). Most reseachers seem to have accepted speed as an inevitable component in various tests of intelligent behavior.

Psychomotor performance was frequently studied in the early days of gerontological inquiries. The prototype experiment compared performance of young and older people on tests of simple and complex reaction time (RT). The results of numerous RT studies consistently show that when the cognitive demands are increased by the introduction of multiple stimuli and response formats, the effects of age become more pronounced (Welford, 1977). The literature on perceptual speed also demonstrates a general agreement on age-related decline.

Attention and decision constitute two highly interwoven components in speed of behavior. Attention has been examined using experimental paradigms for divided and selective attention, vigilance, or the ability to identify less frequent signals occurring over long time periods, or in terms of concentration and search for certain signal patterns within an array of similar signals. Tests like digit-symbol in the WAIS battery represent a way to study concentration and search. The findings from this test demonstrate marked age effects. Elderly people show worse performance in terms of items accomplished per time unit, as compared to younger people. Accuracy is, however, not impaired in the elderly. The trail-making test is a frequently used clinical test for psychomotor performance and attention. Robins Wahlin et al. (1996) administered this test in a healthy sample of individuals aged 76–93. As expected, they found that the time needed to complete the test increased significantly with age. Noteworthy, however, is that they found no age differences in accuracy.

An important message is that lower speed is also related to deficient performance on a number of memory and other cognitive tasks. The pervasiveness of reduced speed of behavior in aging, thus requires that this phenomenon is taken into account in evaluating performance in tasks where speed is an ingredient (Salthouse, 1985; Stankov, 1988).

Studies in which elderly individuals' slower rate of processing is compensated for by elimination of time limits still show an overall pattern of performance decline with age, identical to that found when time constraints are present. The oldest, however, seem to benefit somewhat more from eliminated time limits (e.g., Botwinick, 1977; Robins Wahlin et al., 1993), but age and other interindividual differences remain. In everyday life, however, compensatory behaviors become essential for the functioning of the individual. Performance is better when time is less of a restriction.

(ii) Verbal abilities and language

The spontaneous use of language, as in unrestricted speech, typically reveals experience-based learning and thereby cohort differences and other sociodemographic characteristics. That is often evident in the communication across generations where younger and older persons may find themselves using different words, grammar, and syntax. In this sense, language serves as a "generation marker."

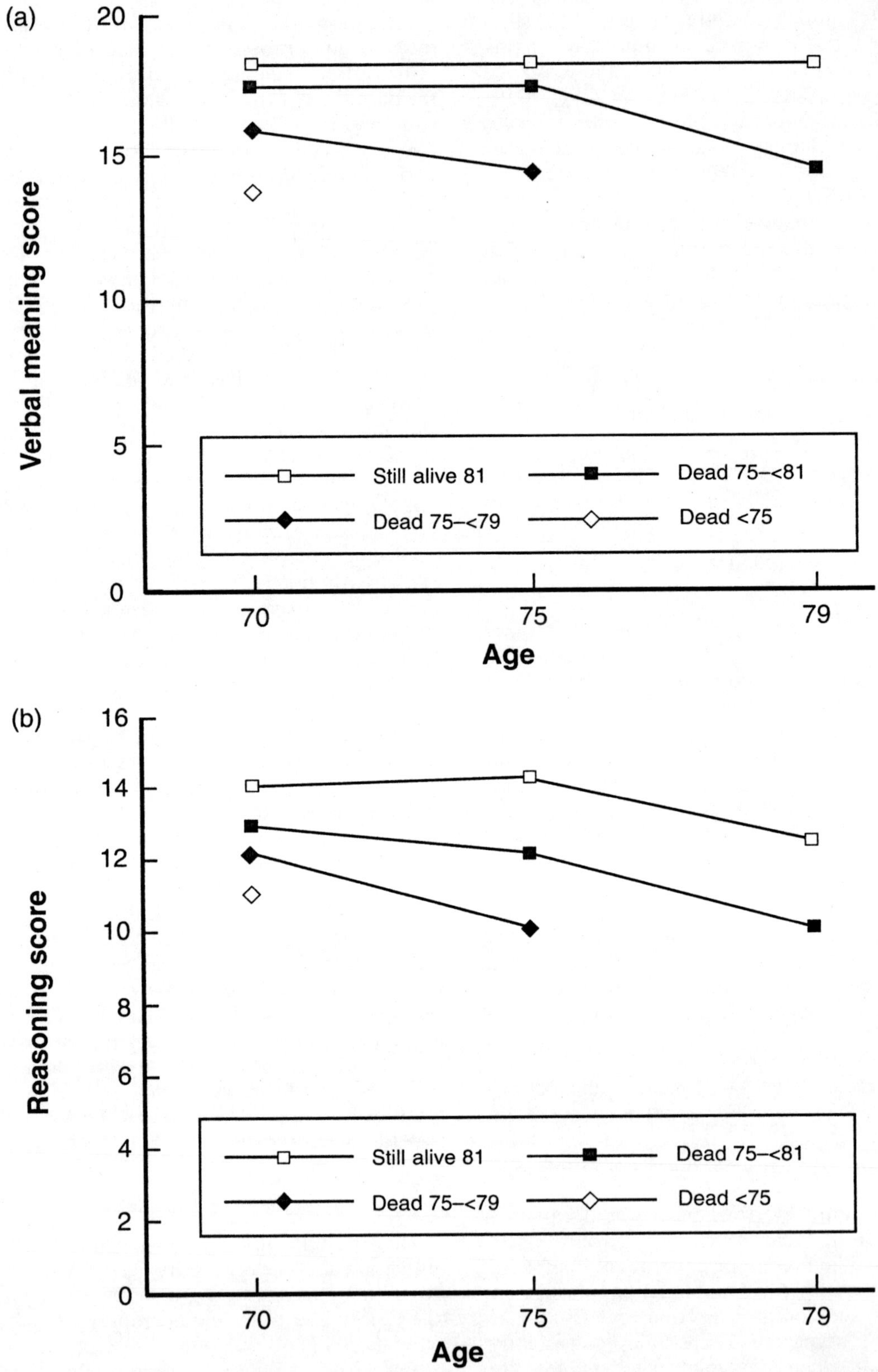

Figure 5 Longitudinal scores for a test of verbal meaning (a) and reasoning (b) showing terminal decline. ("Intelligence and terminal decline" by S. Berg, 1987. In G. L. Maddox and E. W. Busse (Eds.), *Aging: The universal experience* (pp. 414–415), New York: Springer. Copyright 1987 by Springer Publishing Company. Adapted with permission).

Besides speech comprehension, language also involves the domains of reading and writing. All these aspects of language are likely to be affected by sensory problems prevalent in the aged, including difficulties in visual acuity and hearing (presbycusis). In writing, hand motor ability also becomes important. The influences of these peripheral sources of impairment must be considered in evaluating potential cognition-related deficits in language. Despite sensory problems, language abilities are generally well preserved at the level of communication in aging (e.g., Bayles, Kaszniak, & Tomeda 1987). Furthermore, certain language difficulties may not become manifest because individuals may compensate for minor difficulties in unrestricted speech. Difficulties can be covered through the use of compensatory strategies, for example, simplifications or pauses filled with "Ums."

Language abilities require components of linguistic and lexical knowledge (vocabulary), word finding, and verbal fluency. The knowledge of linguistic structure, including syntax, seems to be a well-preserved ability in aging. In an extensive study by Emery (1985) on various aspects of language in younger individuals, normal elderly, and elderly individuals with dementia, results indicated that normal elderly people had greater difficulties with more complex syntactic structure. In the demented sample all aspects of language were affected (for details see Emery, 1985).

Vocabulary, or verbal meaning and verbal fluency have been extensively studied and tests of these aspects are often also included in comprehensive batteries. The general findings for vocabulary demonstrate continuity, whereas speeded fluency tests show lower performance in elderly individuals. In this sense, fluency becomes yet another marker of speed of behavior (Obler & Albert, 1985).

The ability of naming has been investigated using the tip-of-the-tongue (TOT) phenomenon. Studies generally show that younger individuals are more advantaged in their access to the lexical network needed for accurate naming of objects (Burke, Mackay, Worthley, & Wade, 1991). The close relationship between accuracy and speed, previously discussed, is also observed in word-finding tasks, where accurate speed tends to become a prerequsite for the primary naming. Difficulties in finding the name of objects may be described as a memory failure by subjects themselves. The literature indeed shows that memory mechanisms are involved in TOTs, although this involvement is more pronounced in the complex usage of language abilities, as for example in discourse (Burke, Worthley, & Martin, 1988).

While relatively robust in primary aging, language and verbal abilities are prone to cerebral lesions in dementia, where the "aphasia-agnosia" syndrome constitutes a diagnostic marker. Available information on various aspects of language are still relatively sparse, compared to other cognitive functions in aging (see Kemper, 1992; Light, 1988).

(iii) Visuospatial and visuoconstructive abilities

The components involved in visuospatial and visuoconstructive abilities include pattern recognition and the understanding of dimensionality. Reading a clock face, telling the time and setting the clock hands on certain times, reading maps and drawing maps represent some ecological examples of this cognitive domain.

The block design test in the WAIS battery is often thought of as a prototype test for visuospatial ability. The results from this test show worse performance in older individuls. Robins Wahlin et al. (1993) used block design and a clock test to study visuospatial functioning and spatial orientation in a healthy sample ranging from 75 to 96 years. In block design, they found significant age differences in which the youngest individuals showed superior performance. Interestingly, the test was administered both in the standard format including fixed time limits and in a format without time limits. The differences across ages remained in the no-time-limit condition, although performance levels were increased. In examining performance for each individual design, they found age effects only for the most complex designs. In the clock test, encompassing the tasks of setting hands on preprinted clock faces and time telling, they also found a slight but significant age effect in both. The oldest, aged 90 to 96 years, were less accurate than individuals in the age range of 75–89 years. It was concluded that there is an age-related deterioration in visuospatial abilities that continues into very old age.

Visuoconstructive tasks include components of perception, motor behavior, and spatial orientation. Such tasks are often included in clinical batteries, for example, in tasks where subjects are asked to copy figures at different levels of complexity. Such tests also provide qualitative information, including type of errors, that may be useful. The findings from studies on visuoconstruction generally show that the copying ability is well preserved in aging when motor and sensory difficulties are taken into account (e.g., Van Gorp, Satz, & Mirushina, 1990).

(iv) Problem solving and executive functions

A complex domain of cognitive functioning involves problem solving and logical reasoning, including inductive as well as deductive components. Problem solving encompasses all behaviors executed when facing old problems that we have learned how to solve, as well as novel problems requiring reorganization of already established modes of thinking and acting. Problem solving includes concrete as well as abstract thinking, and therefore constitutes a broad category of intelligent behavior.

Various tests of reasoning and problem solving are often included as subtests in comprehensive test batteries. For example, in Schaie's longitudinal Seattle study (Schaie, 1995), estimates of age changes in reasoning show a general decline with age. A more marked decline was found for those in their late sixties. This pattern resembles that of other abilities, suggesting that this aspect of problem solving is equally prone to aging as other cognitive abilities. In the Swedish H70 study, inductive reasoning remained remarkably stable across times of measurement in individuals with longer survival. That is, when retrospectively excluding those individuals who died after a certain occasion in the series of measurements, those who survived to the next occasion in the series showed an almost stable performance in reasoning, an ability often considered sensitive to age. This finding suggests that decline is more closely associated with subsequent mortality, rather than with age *per se* (see Berg, 1996, and Figure 5).

A well-known reasoning test is that of Raven's Progressive Matrices (Raven, 1982), including the original and the coloured matrices versions. Subjects are instructed to find a principle among certain patterns and to choose a pattern that corresponds to this principle in identifying a missing pattern. Significant age differences suggest lower performance with age in the original version of the test (see Lezak, 1983, 1995; Salthouse, 1983). This finding was also confirmed in a study by Denney and Heidrich (1990), who interestingly employed a simple training strategy before administering the test. Following training, equal improvements were found for young, middle-aged, and elderly individuals.

Another aspect of intelligent behavior is that of executive functions which refers to abilities that successfully enable a person to engage in "independent, purposive, self-serving behavior" (Lezak, 1983, p. 38). Questions about whether people will execute a certain behavior and if so, how they are doing it, capture the dimension of executive functioning. Lezak (1983) articulated four components of executive activity-related behaviors: goal formulation, planning, carrying out goal-directed plans, and effective performance. Given these components the question arises regarding how to evaluate the aspects of "whether" and "how." The interest in executive functions emerged in neuropsychology and is largely associated with interest in cerebral dysfunction, especially with dementia and frontal lobe lesions (e.g., Moss, Albert, & Kemper, 1992; Shallice & Burgess, 1991)

Symptoms like distractability, passivity and apathy, apraxia, and perseverations, affecting self-care behaviors and leading to impaired activities of daily living have often been the focus. In patients suffering from frontal lobe lesions, impairments become manifest in a more obvious manner. Executive functioning is, however, usually maintained in primary aging although affected by a slower speed of behavior. The complexity of the executive dimension requires close scrutinity of sensory and motor handicaps, and of other noncognitive factors that potentially may influence the individual's adaptation to demands in everyday life as well as performance on cognitive tests (LaRue, 1992).

The generation of alternate behaviors necessary to overcome and compensate for deficits in certain domains can be seen as an indicator of the flexibility aspect of executive functioning. Cognitive flexibility, or the ability to shift strategy in order to solve and overcome certain problems, is an essential component in many tests, as well as in real-life situations. Rigidity, the converse of flexibility, is a more visible marker for the lack of flexibility in the ecological context. Tests that require switching from one strategy to another or tasks in which overlearned responses are to be inhibited in favour of new responses generally show superior performance in younger individuals. The Wisconsin Card Sorting Test (WCST, Grant & Berg, 1948) is another test requiring cognitive flexibility. Subjects are here instructed to organize cards according to different principles, for example, color and form. Only slight age differences were found in a study of healthy, well-educated elderly individuals' performance on a modified WCST version (Haaland, Vranes, Goodwin, & Garry, 1987). The study provides support for the conclusion that executive functions in primary aging remain relatively unaffected.

Although verbal fluency and certain tests of construction and motor performance can serve as markers of executive functioning (Royall, Mahurin, & Gray, 1992; see also Lezak, 1995), noncognitive influences must be taken into account in evaluating performance. A powerful approach for examining executive functioning is the observation of naturalistic behaviors interpreted in the context of previous ability, sensory and motor functioning. An elderly person unwilling or unable to perform as before and exhibiting lower cognitive flexibility has to be assessed in a broad context, including information on coping, perceived personal control, and well-being, before any definite conclusions can be drawn about deficient executive functioning.

7.02.3.2.3 Summary

In the intelligence test tradition, the most frequently used battery is the WAIS. The subtests can be subdivided into "hold tests," assumed to measure crystallized intelligence, and "don't hold tests" measuring fluid abilities. Crystallized abilities are relatively stable across the entire adult age span, and some may improve even into old age. Fluid abilities, on the other hand, are more sensitive to age, as well as to various diseases. The findings of terminal decline (tertiary aging) in cognitive abilities demonstrate the close interrelationships between brain function and vital physiology in aging.

7.02.4 COPING WITH COGNITIVE CHANGE IN AGING: PERSPECTIVES OF THE AGING INDIVIDUAL AND THE GEROPSYCHOLOGIST

Some implications of reported findings on memory and other cognitive aspects of aging will be discussed in this section, including considerations relevant to the geropsychologist.

7.02.4.1 "From Lab to Life"

The research literature on memory and other cognitive functions conveys the general conclusion that decline and change become more likely with advancing age, although the age-related sensitivity differs for various tasks. At the same time we usually find that most elderly people maintain independence and successful functioning in everyday life even though this involves numerous tasks that require complex memory and cognitive abilities. These observations seem contradictory and address questions about the significance of reported findings on memory and cognitive changes in aging, revealed in the experimental or clinical setting. These different portrayals of aging also become evident to the geropsychologist. Salthouse (1983) suggested four explanations for the discrepancy between "lab and life": individual differences, ecological validity, cognitive demands in terms of complexity and difficulty, and everyday life experiences and learning.

7.02.4.1.1 Individual differences

The individual differences issue is a neglected aspect in the prevailing normative tradition in the gerosciences. The use of chronological age, as a proxy marker for aging, and the arithmetic mean as the typical statistic for describing performances, tends to emphasize general patterns over unique features, including that of interindividual differences.

In everyday life we may face individuals in advanced ages who show better performance than they did some years ago. The recovery from certain diseases and treatment effects are also seen in advanced ages. The normative design is, however, unlikely to show both sides of the coin, that is, while some individuals decline, others remain stable or even improve their performance over time. Besides generation and cohort differences, individuals of the same age typically manifest great differences in physical as well as psychological functioning. Elderly people are distributed between the extremes of those who experience early physical and cognitive impairments and, at the other end of the continuum, the successful agers who maintain their performance throughout life. This notion is important because it provides a basic frame of reference for assessment, as well as an accurate portrayal of aging.

An interindividual perspective is an essential element for the geropsychologist. The research literature provides the general norms for late-life functioning, and at best adequate norms for various tests. An assessment requires, however, detailed information about previous functioning of the individual. Such information, or more likely assumptions about "baseline performance" in earlier days, should provide the ultimate points of reference for the geropsychologist.

7.02.4.1.2 Ecological validity

Ecological validity refers to the congruence between laboratory and clinical tests, and everyday life tasks requiring memory and other cognitive resources. Although certain experimental tasks may be considered as esoteric, they surely activate cognitive subprocesses and components of relevance for life outside the laboratory. The overall aim in experimental aging and cognition studies is the understanding of age-related change in those subprocesses and components. In this sense, the complexity of everyday life tasks can never correspond to requirements in the laboratory setting. Although the range of available tests covers many dimensions of memory and cognitive functioning, it is important to remember that they still represent only a sample of markers for various cognitive processes.

Another aspect of ecology relates to compensatory behaviors that tend to be neglected in the laboratory. In everyday life individuals can compensate for weaknesses in certain abilities by profiting from strengths in other areas of functioning. In this sense difficulties may not become manifest in natural settings. In tests, however, individuals are usually inhibited from using compensatory strategies to overcome weaknesses. Impairments are then more likely to be evinced.

The "lab–life dimension" represents an important issue for the geropsychologist when confronted with an individual showing impaired test performance, but demonstrating relatively intact functioning in everyday life. The detection of cognitive problems on certain tests may be due to disease processes (secondary aging) and provide arguments for interventions aimed at retarding or improving performance. Low performance on tests is also indicative of the cognitive expenditure that is needed to manifest "intact" everyday functioning.

7.02.4.1.3 Complex cognitive processing

The notion that cognitive demands in everyday life are less complex and difficult than that of laboratory and clinical tests deserves attention. One might argue that the demands of the two situations are not identical (e.g., Baltes & Willis, 1979). Laboratory and clinical tests of memory and cognition are usually designed in accordance with psychometrics. This means that level of difficulty is deliberately introduced as a variable for evaluating performance. Everyday life is often highly predictable through recurrent tasks and events with which we have learned to cope. Tests of memory and cognition are also likely to introduce novel tasks, requirements, and a setting that is unfamiliar to the individual.

The familiarity with psychological testing differs across age cohorts. The oldest old tend to have fewer such experiences. Recommendations of "age-fairness" should be evaluated against this background. In addition, in real life people tend to seek those environments that fit their interests and available resources, including those that relate to cognition. This is a matching of abilities and task demands that does not occur in the laboratory or in the clinical test situation. In evaluating an individual's performance, geropsychologists have to consider how a task should be presented, how the instructions are administered, including feedback to the individual. Motivation and other noncognitive factors are also important. The importance of instructions and practice before administering a certain task is well known to the experienced clinician. Standard tests and batteries usually allow only brief instructions. Difficulties experienced by elderly people in comprehending these instructions, for example, in abstract tasks, are likely to interfere with later performance. Ensuring that the individual understands task requirements can therefore significantly improve performance (e.g. Baltes, Sowarka & Kliegl, 1989).

7.02.4.1.4 Everyday life experiences and learning

Although research on memory and cognition in aging typically confirms a deterioration view, the resources in most individuals are sufficient to cope with environmental demands of daily life. When the magnitude of decline exceeds the ecological demands it becomes a manifest deficit. For example, in the diagnosis of dementia, the impairment in memory and other cognitive abilities must interfere with daily life functioning according to diagnostic criteria (American Psychiatric Association, 1987, 1994). Many activities and tasks in everyday life are overlearned by their being practiced over and over again. As noted by Salthouse (1983), "since increased age in adulthood is generally positively correlated with experience, many highly practiced activities may be maintained at a constant level despite age-related declines in component ability because of the compensating effects of greater experience" (p. 203).

In experimental and clinical settings, memory and cognitive tasks are typically novel and the cues and instructions provided do not necessarily correspond to those available in natural, everyday life. Performance is then more unlikely to rely on previous experiences. The ability for adequate everyday functioning is also affected by more or less subtle social and cognitive support systems that constitute natural ingredients in daily-life activities (use of a calendar, reminders, and other external aids). In addition, individuals also tend to withdraw from activities that are viewed as too demanding, using excuses such as that they have lost interest (see Baltes's model below). The geropsychologist has to consider and be aware of the mechanisms of the fit between environmental demands and cognitive capabilities of the individual.

7.02.4.1.5 Current knowledge and extralaboratory cognition

As pointed out by Salthouse (1983), and by recent proponents of testing memory and cognition in daily-life contexts (e.g., Willis, 1996), "the greatest hindrance to knowledge about the relationships between laboratory performance and extralaboratory competence is simply lack of detailed information about the nature of real-world activities" (Salthouse, 1983, pp. 203–204). Clearly, more attention needs to be given to the external validity of results obtained in the laboratory or clinical setting. Improved means of evaluating everyday performances constitutes one avenue for this. Much of the literature on aging and cognitive functions can be divided into three parts on the basis of methodology. Research is conducted in the psychometric tradition, in the experimental tradition, or in the ecological tradition. It seems clear that there are possible gains by cross-fertilization between approaches. Indeed such efforts are not absent. One approach includes bringing everyday activities such as television watching into the laboratory (e.g., Stine, Wingfield, & Myers, 1990) for subsequent tests of, for example, memory. Another logical possibility is to perform clinical or laboratory-like tasks in the subject's everyday world. Weber, Brown, and Weldon (1978), conducted such a study where elderly residents in a nursing home were tested on spatial knowledge and memory for scenes and locations in their nursing home. An even broader approach may be warranted, taking into account such things as collaborative support provided by a spouse (Gould & Dixon, 1993; Gould, Trevithick, & Dixon, 1991). On the other hand, proponents of an applied approach aiming at intervention and adjustment of the environment argue that researchers have now developed sufficient understanding of older adults' cognitive systems to make it possible to improve the quality of life for older adults (see Park, 1992). The latter view relies mainly on knowledge about cognitive processes, as well as documented strengths and weaknesses of the elderly in a broader sense.

7.02.4.1.6 Cognitive aging and the individual: an integrative model

A comprehensive model for the understanding of primary cognitive aging in the real-life context that integrates much of the literature on cognitive aspects of aging was proposed by Baltes (1991). The model (see Figure 6) is based on a series of propositions. These propositions, or general statements, are to some extent already covered in previous sections of the present chapter. Briefly, it is assumed that aging is characterized by much interindividual variability; it is important to distinguish between pathological, normal, and optimal aging; there is much developmental reserve capacity in old age; aging is characterized by a loss of fluid intelligence; knowledge and crystallized abilities may compensate for the losses in fluid abilities; with aging the balance between gains and losses becomes less positive or even negative; and the self in old age continues to be a powerful system of coping and maintaining integrity.

Against the background of these general conclusions, some adaptional mechanisms were suggested for successful psychological aging. The model focuses on the dynamic interplay among selection, optimization, and compensation, all components in a general process of adaption, effective throughout life. However, because of the losses experienced in aging, whether biological, social, or mental, the model is especially applicable to elderly persons. By selection of activities from a previously more extensive repertoire of behaviours, maximizing the effort spent on maintaining certain activities by means of practice or acquisition of new knowledge, and finally fostering of compensatory behavior, performance may be maintained at high levels even in old age.

Without going into details, some conclusions apply to the present chapter. The model has obvious implications for the geropsychologist. In the clinical setting, a wide variety of functions or abilities are routinely tested. Since the purpose of an investigation is usually to arrive at a diagnosis, the focus is often on deficits and weaknesses. Planning for training or rehabilitation, on the other hand, also requires closer examination of strengths and the potential for improvements. However, with reference to the discussion about everyday cognitive performance, it may be justifiable to include a routine for evaluation of cognitive reserves and abilities to adopt compensatory behavior. The impact of interindividual variability is strongly acknowledged in Baltes's model as interindividual variability in old age applies not only to behavioral functioning, but also to indicators of biomedical functioning (Costa & Andres, 1986; Rowe & Kahn, 1987). This variability may in combination with other critical components, such as expertise in some areas, produce differential patterns in aging. Hence, both strengths and weaknesses are equally critical components in a full understanding of the individual's general level of functioning.

7.02.4.1.7 Cognitive reserves and plasticity

Some additional comments on cognitive reserve capacity may be warranted. Following the Baltes (1991) model, potential for cognitive improvement may be discussed in terms of baseline reserve capacity as well as developmental reserve capacity (see Kliegl & Baltes, 1987). Baseline reserve capacity refers to

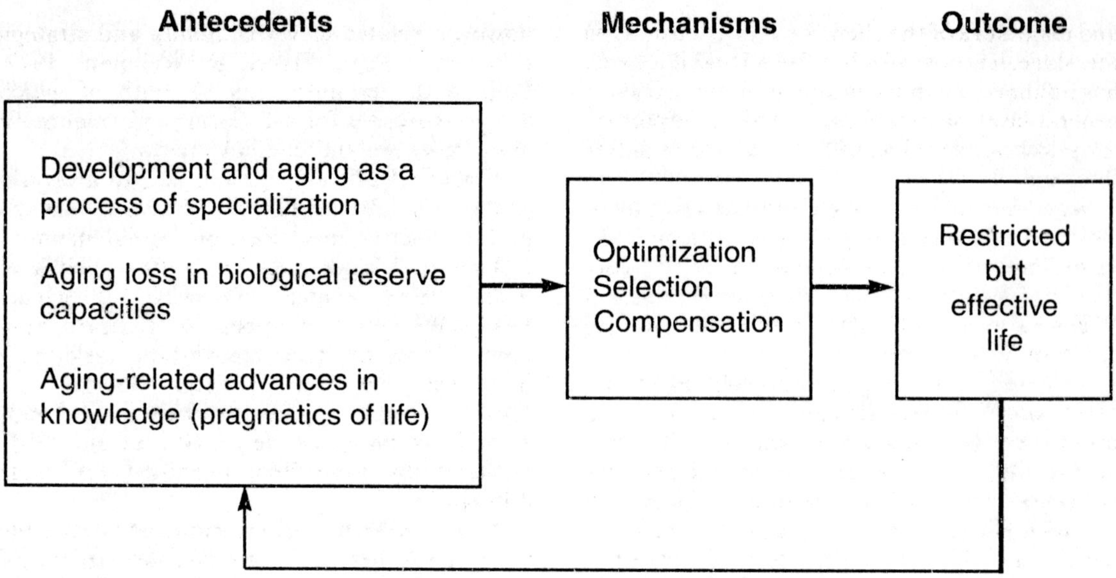

Figure 6 Baltes's selective optimization with compensation ("The many faces of human ageing: Toward a psychological culture of old age" by P. B. Baltes, 1991, *Psychological Medicine, 21,* p. 85. Copyright by Cambridge University Press. Adapted with permisssion).

variations in performance due to varying levels of task demands and support, while developmental reserve capacity denotes the range of performance under extended periods of development or practice. Reserve capacity is related to such diverse examples as the acquisition of expertise, testing the limits of an individual's capacity, and memory training.

7.02.4.2 General Assessment Guidelines

Some guidelines in the assessment of elderly persons can be extracted from previous discussions. These general guidelines by no means constitute a complete coverage of all topics. Also, advice in relation to specific diagnostic issues is not dealt with. Certain suggestions are self-evident, but nevertheless important to address explicitly.

Throughout the chapter, it has been emphasized that the level of cognitive functioning is under multifactorial influence and that interindividual variability is substantial in aging. These notions have obvious implications for the geropsychologist. Chronological age has traditionally been the sole stratification variable in the psychometric test tradition. Using test norms to aid in the interpretation of performance ought to be considered in this context. Further, the distinction between primary and secondary aging requires the integration of information from several sources, including that of physical health and social life.

Before meeting the client, we would strongly recommend the geropsychologist to review medical records. Although literature on the relation between cognition and disease is scarce for illnesses in old age other than dementia or major depression, it may be worthwhile to look for the presence of, for example, cardiovascular disease including elevated blood pressure, hyper- or hypothyroidism, diabetes, epilepsy, vitamin deficiency, previous transient ischemic attacks or stroke. The medical literature also lacks, in general, age-graded norms for the elderly, for example, age-adjusted cut-offs for laboratory tests such as the test of folic acid. (For details, see the literature listed in the previous section on secondary aging.)

In the assessment setting it is also strongly recommended to check for vision and hearing. Does the client need certain glasses or a hearing aid? Secure the use of these aids, and, when vision or hearing is poor, consider using adjusted test materials.

Testing should start with a brief interview. During this conversation, much information crucial to later interpretation of test results may be obtained. The geropsychologist should, in addition to basic information concerning education and prior work or career, also collect data about previous and present skills and interests. When necessary, a relative may provide valuable information (e.g., Jorm et al., 1996). The client's general feeling of being in control of daily life as well as beliefs about their own capacity may be informative in evaluating subsequent test performance.

Motivational factors play an important role in the assessment setting. Therefore, one should explain carefully the purpose of the assessment and make sure of the client's comprehension. At this stage, it is possible that the geropsychologist has obtained a clinical impression of the client's general level of functioning. This is important for selecting the relevant tests and for avoiding floor and ceiling effects.

When introducing tests to the client, it may be worthwile to vary task demands systematically in order to investigate reserve capacity. Also, tasks may be varied in terms of time restraints. It is generally advised that tasks be selected in terms of age-fairness.

As noted, in testing older clients, norms are often not entirely reliable. In addition to problems concerning sample selections for these norms, they seldom cover the age range above 80 years. Most studies portray, however, a continuous decline of cognitive performance in the oldest, although performance may remain at relatively high levels. In the absence of norms for the very old and the introduction of other stratification variables than age, it becomes advisable to interpret raw scores carefully.

7.02.4.3 Future Prospects and Cohorts

In the years to come, geropsychologists will meet new cohorts of elderly people who are exposed to other experiences and influences than the elderly people of today. Future clients are likely to require efforts to promote independence and growth in aging, also for aspects of life related to memory and cognition. Future cohorts may require somewhat different diagnostic considerations than today and age-fair testing may refer to something different than today. Improvements in the educational system are likely to exert an impact on performance in new cohorts of elderly people. Furthermore, it may be that successful medical treatments for conditions such as Alzheimer's disease are introduced. In that case, geropsychological expertise may require improved methods for early, preclinical, detection of the disease.

Given increasing interest in geropsychological matters, new test norms adjusted for individuals in the range 80–100 years will hopefully be available to future cohorts of clinicians. The recognition of interindividual differences may end in norms that do not apply chronological age as the sole stratification variable for differentiation within normal and pathological aging. Educational level and gender are two probable candidates among other critical variables to be considered.

The impact of education may seem somewhat far-fetched, as formal education is quite distant in time for elderly people. Education is, however, related to verbal ability and strategy knowledge (e.g., Flavell & Wellman, 1977; Gillund & Perlmutter, 1988), both of which are prerequisites for successful performance on many memory and cognitive tasks.

Norms adjusted for gender are, to a certain extent, already available. Generally, women perform better than men on verbal memory tasks (e.g., Larrabee & Crook, 1993; Schaie & Willis, 1993; Zelinski, Gilewski, & Schaie, 1993). Women also appear to perform at a higher level on face recognition tasks (see Shepherd, 1981, for review). Social (e.g., McKelvie, Standing, St. Jean, & Law, 1993) as well as biological (e.g., Gur et al., 1991) explanations have been proposed for these differences.

Aging research is being conducted around the globe and there is a continuous stream of reports and an increasing wealth of information from the psychological, medical, and social gerosciences. Many projects are designed with an interdisciplinary approach which opens potential for cross-fertilizations and analyses of complex interactions among biological, social, and psychological variables. In cognitive aging research, structural modeling techniques are now applied more often in an effort to identify critical components for successful performance (see Salthouse, 1991). Although, not theory based, the approach truly recognizes the complexity of various aging processes.

The complexity of aging processes becomes apparent for the geropsychologist in the evaluation of performance and gathering of other information in a comprehensive assessment of memory and other cognitive abilities. The challenge is to end up with appropriate conclusions for diagnosis and treatment. For this, geropsychological expertise is indispensable.

7.02.5 REFERENCES

American Psychiatric Association. (1987). *Diagnostic and statistical manual of mental disorders* (3rd ed. rev.). Washington, DC: Author.

American Psychiatric Association. (1994). *Diagnostic and statistical manual of mental disorders* (4th ed.). Washington, DC: Author.

Atkinson, R. C., & Shiffrin, R. M. (1968). Human memory: A proposed system and its control processes. In K. W. Spence (Ed.), *The psychology of learning and motivation: Advances in research and theory* (pp. 89–195). New York: Academic Press.

Bäckman, L. (1991). Recognition memory across the adult life span: The role of prior knowledge. *Memory & Cognition, 19,* 63–71.

Bäckman, L. (1995). Cognitive support and episodic memory functioning in normal aging and Alzheimer's disease: A continuity view of the modifiability of memory performance in old age. In R. Cacabelos, H. Frey, T. Nishimura, & B. Winblad (Eds.), *Neuroger-*

ontology and neurogeriatrics (pp. 85–106). Barcelona, Spain: Prous Science.

Bäckman, L., & Forsell, Y. (1994). Episodic memory functioning in a community-based sample of very old adults with major depression: Utilization of cognitive support. *Journal of Abnormal Psychology, 103,* 361–370.

Bäckman, L., & Larsson, M. (1992). Recall of organizable words and objects in adulthood: Influences of instructions, retention interval, and retrieval cues. *Journal of Gerontology: Psychological Sciences, 47,* P273–P278.

Bäckman, L., Mäntylä, T., & Herlitz, A. (1990). The optimization of episodic remembering in old age. In P. B. Baltes & M. M. Baltes (Eds.), *Successful aging: Perspectives from the behavioral sciences* (pp. 118–163). New York: Cambridge University Press.

Bäckman, L., & Wahlin, Å. (1995). Influences of item organizability and semantic retrieval cues on episodic recall in very old age. *Aging and Cognition, 2,* 312–325.

Baddeley, A. D. (1986). *Working memory.* Oxford, UK: Oxford University Press.

Baddeley, A. D. (1990). *Human memory: Theory and practice.* Boston: Allyn and Bacon.

Bale, R. N. (1973). Brain damage in diabetes mellitus. *British Journal of Psychiatry, 122,* 337–341.

Baltes, M. M., & Baltes, P. B. (Eds.) (1986). *The psychology of control and aging.* Hillsdale, NJ: Erlbaum.

Baltes, P. B. (1991). The many faces of human ageing: Toward a psychological culture of old age. *Psychological Medicine, 21,* 837–854.

Baltes, P. B., & Kliegl, R. (1992). Further testing of limits of cognitive plasticity: Negative age differences in a mnemonic skill are robust. *Developmental Psychology, 28,* 121–125.

Baltes, P. B., Sowarka, D., & Kliegl, R. (1989): Cognitive training research on fluid intelligence in old age: What can older adults achieve by themselves? *Psychology and Aging, 4,* 217–221.

Baltes, P. B., & Willis, S. L. (1979). The critical importance of appropriate methodology in the study of aging: The sample case of psychometric intelligence. In F. Hoffmeister & C. Muller: (Eds.), *Brain function in old age* (pp. 164–187). Berlin: Springer-Verlag.

Barclay, L., Weiss, E., Bond, O., & Blass, J. (1988). Unrecognized cognitive impairment in cardiac rehabilitation patients. *Journal of the American Geriatrics Society, 36,* 22–28.

Bayles, K. A., Kaszniak, A. W., & Tomeda, C. K. (1987). *Communication and cognition in normal aging and dementia.* Boston: College-Hill/Little, Brown & Co.

Berg, C. A., & Sternberg, R. J. (1985). A triarchic theory of intellectual development during adulthood. *Developmental Review, 5,* 334–370.

Berg, C. A., & Sternberg, R. J. (1992). Adults' conceptions of intelligence across the adult life span. *Psychology and Aging, 7,* 221–231.

Berg, S. (1987). Intelligence and terminal decline. In G. L. Maddox & E. W. Busse (Eds.), *Aging: The universal experience* (pp. 414–415). New York: Springer.

Berg, S. (1996). Aging, behavior, and terminal decline. In J. E. Birren & K. W. Schaie (Eds.), *Handbook of the psychology of aging* (4th ed., pp. 323–337). San Diego, CA: Academic Press.

Berg, S., & Dellasega, C. (1996). The use of psychoactive medications and cognitive function in older adults. *Journal of Aging and Health, 8,* 136–149.

Birren, J. E., & Cunningham, W. R. (1985). Research on the psychology of aging: Principles, concepts and theory. In J. E. Birren & K. W. Schaie (Eds.), *Handbook of the psychology of aging* (2nd ed., pp. 3–34). New York: Van Nostrand Reinhold.

Birren, J. E., & Morrison, D. F. (1961). Analysis of the WAIS subtests in relation to age and education. *Journal of Gerontology, 16,* 363–369.

Birren, J. E., & Schaie, K. W. (1996). *Handbook of the psychology of aging* (4th ed.). San Diego, CA: Academic Press.

Blanchard-Fields, F., & Abeles, R. P. (1996). Social cognition and aging. In J. E. Birren & K. W. Schaie (Eds.), *Handbook of the psychology of aging* (4th ed., pp. 150–161). San Diego, CA: Academic Press.

Botwinick, J. (1977). Intellectual abilities. In J. E. Birren & K. W. Schaie (Eds.), *Handbook of the psychology of aging* (pp. 580–605). New York: Van Nostrand Reinhold.

Botwinick, J. (1978). *Aging and behavior: A comprehensive integration of research findings.* New York: Springer.

Brody, J. A., & Schneider, E. L. (1986). Disease and disorders of ageing: A hypothesis. *Journal of Chronic Disorders, 39,* 871–876.

Bruce, D. (1991). Mechanistic and functional explanations of memory. *American Psychologist, 46,* 46–48.

Burke, D. M., MacKay, D. G., Worthley, J. S., & Wade, E. (1991). On the tip of the tongue: What causes word finding failures in young and older adults? *Journal of Memory and Language, 30,* 542–579.

Burke, D. M., Worthley, J., & Martin, J. (1988). I'll never forget what's-her-name: Aging and the tip of the tongue experience. In M. M. Gruneberg, P. Morris, & R. N. Sykes (Eds.), *Practical aspects of memory: Current research and issues* (Vol. 2, pp. 113–118). Chichester, UK: Wiley.

Burt, D. B., Zembar, M. J. & Niederehe, G. (1995). Depression and memory impairment: A meta-analysis of the association, its pattern, and specificity. *Psychological Bullentin, 117,* 285–305.

Chiarello, C., & Hoyer, W. J. (1988). Adult age differences in implicit and explicit memory: Time course and encoding effects. *Psychology and Aging, 3,* 358–366.

Cipioli, C., Neri, M., Andermarcher, E., Pinelli, E., & Lalla, M. (1990). Self-rating and objective memory testing of normal and depressed elderly. *Aging, 2,* 39–48.

Cockburn, J. & Smith, P. T. (1991). The relative influence of intelligence and age on everyday memory. *Journal of Gerontology: Psychological Sciences, 46,* P31–P36.

Cohen, G., & Faulkner, D. (1989). Age differences in source forgetting: Effects on reality monitoring and on eyewitness testimony. *Psychology and Aging, 4,* 10–17.

Cornelius, S. W. (1990). Aging and everyday cognitive abilities. In T. Hess (Ed.), *Aging and cognition: Knowledge, organization and utilization* (pp. 411–444). Amsterdam: North-Holland.

Costa, P. T., Jr., & Andres, R. (1986). Patterns of age changes. In I. Rossman (Ed.), *Clinical geriatrics* (pp. 23–30). Philadelphia: Lippincott.

Craik, F. I. M., & Jennings, J. M. (1992). Human memory. In F. I. M. Craik & T. A. Salthouse (Eds.), *The handbook of aging and cognition* (pp. 51–110). Hillsdale, NJ: Erlbaum.

Craik, F. I. M., & Salthouse, T. A. (Eds.) (1992). *Handbook of aging and cognition.* Hillsdale, NJ: Erlbaum.

Cremer, R., & Zeef, E. J. (1987). What kind of noise increases with age? *Journal of Gerontology, 42,* 515–518.

Crook, T. H., & Larrabee, G. J. (1992). Changes in facial recognition memory across the adult life span. *Journal of Gerontology: Psychological Sciences, 47,* P138–P141.

Crum, R. M., Anthony, J. C., Basset, S. S., & Folstein, M. F. (1993). Population-based norms for Mini-Mental State Examination by age and educational level. *Journal of the American Medical Association, 269,* 2386–2391.

Denney, N. W. (1989). Everyday problem solving: Methodological issues, research findings, and a model. In L. W. Poon, D. C. Rubin, & B. A. Wilson (Eds.), *Everyday cognition in adulthood and late life* (pp. 330–351). New York: Cambridge University Press.

Denney, N. W., & Heidrich, S. M. (1990). Training effects on Raven's Progressive Matrices in young, middle-aged, and elderly adults. *Psychology and Aging, 5,* 144–145.

Dikman, S., & Matthews, C. G. (1977). Effect of major motor seizure frequency upon cognitive-intellectual functions in adults. *Epilepsia, 18,* 21–29.

Dureman, I., & Sälde, H. (1959). *Psykometriska och experimental-psykologiska metoder för klinisk tillämpning.* Uppsala, Sweden: Almqvist & Wiksell.

Elder, G. H. (1979). Historical change in life patterns and personality. In P. B. Baltes & O. G. Brim (Eds.), *Life-span development and behavior* (Vol. 2, pp. 117–159). New York: Academic Press.

Elias, M. F., Wolf, P. A., D'Agostino, R. B., Cobb, J., & White, L. R. (1993). Untreated blood pressure level is inversely related to cognitive functioning: The Framingham Study. *American Journal of Epidemiology, 138,* 353–364.

Emery, O. B. (1985). Language and aging. *Experimental Aging Research, 11,* 3–60. Special Monograph Issue.

Epstein, F. H., Ostrander, L., Johnson, B. C., Payne, M. W., Hayner, N. S., Keller, J. B., & Francis, T., Jr. (1965). Epidemiological studies of cardiovascular disease in a total community: Tumseh, Michigan. *Annals of Internal Medicine, 62,* 1170–1187.

Farmer, M. E., Kittner, S. J., Abbott, R. D., Wolz, M. M., Wolf, P. A., & White, L. R. (1990). Longitudinally measured blood pressure, antihypertensive medication use, and cognitive performance: The Framingham Study. *Journal of Clinical Epidemiology, 43,* 475–480.

Flavell, J. H., & Wellman, H. M. (1977). Metamemory. In R. V. Kail, Jr. & J. W. Hagen (Eds.), *Perspectives on the development of memory and cognition* (pp. 3–34), Hillsdale, NJ: Erlbaum.

Folstein, M. F., Folstein, S. E., McHugh, P. R. (1975). "Mini-mental state". A practical method for grading the cognitive status of patients for the clinican. *Journal of Psychiatric Research, 12,* 189–198.

Fozard, J. L., Metter, E. F., & Brant, L. J. (1990). Next steps in describing aging and disease in longitudinal studies. *Journal of Gerontology: Psychological Sciences, 45,* P116–P127.

Fratiglioni, L., Grut, M., Forsell, Y., Viitanen, M., Grafström, M., Holmén, K., Eriksson, K., Bäckman, L., Ahlbom, A., & Winblad, B. (1991). Prevalence of Alzheimer's disease and other dementias in an elderly urban population: Relationship with age, sex and education. *Neurology, 41,* 1886–1892.

Fries, J. F., & Crapo, L. M. (1981). *Vitality and Ageing.* New York: Freeman.

Gallagher, D., Thompson, L., & Levy, S. (1980). Clinical psychological assessment of older adults. In L. W. Poon (Ed.), *Aging in the 1980s. Psychological issues* (pp. 19–40). Washington DC: American Psychological Association.

Gambert, S. R. (1988). Dementia secondary to metabolic and nutritional abnormalities. *Clinics in Geriatric Medicine, 4,* 831–839.

Gillund, G., & Perlmutter, M. (1988). Episodic memory and knowledge interactions across adulthood. In L. L. Light & D. M. Burke (Eds.), *Language, memory and aging* (pp. 191–208). Cambridge, UK: Cambridge University Press.

Gould, O. N., & Dixon, R. O. (1993). How we spent our vacation: Collaborative storytelling by young and old adults. *Psychology and Aging, 8,* 10–17.

Gould, O. N., Trevithick, L., & Dixon, R. O. (1991). Adult age differences in elaborations produced during prose recall. *Psychology and Aging, 6,* 93–99.

Graf, P. (1990). Life-span changes in implicit and explicit memory. *Bulletin of the Psychometric Society, 28,* 353–358.

Grant, D. A., & Berg, E. A. (1948). A behavioral analysis of the degree of reinforcement and ease of shifting to new responses in a Weigl-type card sorting problem. *Journal of Experimental Psychology, 38,* 404–411.

Grisso, T. (1986). *Evaluating competencies: Forensic assessments and instruments.* New York: Plenum.

Grut, M., Forsell, Y., Hill, R. D., Bäckman, L., & Winblad, B. (1995). *The relationship between signs of cardiovascular deficiency and cognitive performance in old age.* Manuscript submitted for publication.

Gur, R. C., Mozley, P. D., Resnick, S. M., Gottlieb, G. E., Kohn, M., Zimmerman, R., Herman, G., Atlas, S., Grossman, R., Beretta, D., Erwin, R., & Gur, R. E. (1991). Gender differences in age affect on brain atrophy measured by magnetic resonance imaging. *Proceedings of the National Academy of Sciences, 88,* 2845–2849.

Haaland, K. Y., Vranes, L. F., Goodwin, J. S., & Garry, P. J. (1987). Wisconsin Card Sort Test performance in a healthy elderly population, *Journal of Gerontology, 42,* 345–346.

Hartley, A. A. (1989). The ecology of problem solving. In L. W. Poon, D. C. Rubin, & B. A. Wilson (Eds.), *Everyday cognition in adulthood and late life* (pp. 300–309). New York: Cambridge University Press.

Hayslip, B., Jr., & Panek, P. E. (1993). *Adult development and aging* (2nd ed.). New York: HarperCollins.

Herlitz, A., Lipinska, B., & Bäckman, L. (1992). Utilization of cognitive support for episodic remembering in Alzheimer's disease. In L Bäckman (Ed.), *Memory functioning in dementia* (pp. 73–96). Amsterdam: Elsevier.

Hill, R. D., Wahlin, Å., Winblad, B., & Bäckman, L. (1995). The role of demographic and lifestyle variables in utilizing cognitive support for episodic remembering among very old adults. *Journal of Gerontology: Psychological Sciences, 50B,* P219–P227.

Horn, J. L. (1982). The theory of fluid and crystallized intelligence in relation to concepts of cognitive psychology and aging in adulthood. In F. I. M. Craik & S. Trehub (Eds.), *Aging and cognitve processes* (pp. 237–278). New York: Plenum.

Inouye, S. K., Albert, M. S., Mohs, R., Sun, K., & Berkman, L. F. (1993). Cognitive performance in a high-functioning community-dwelling elderly population. *Journal of Gerontolgy: Medical Sciences, 48,* M146–M151.

Johansson, B., Allen-Burge, R., & Zarit, S. H. (1997). Self-reports on memory functioning in a longitudinal study of the oldest old: Relation to current, prospective, and retrospective performance. *Journal of Gerontology: Psychological Sciences, 52B,* P139–P146.

Johansson, B., & Berg, S. (1992). The robustness of the terminal decline phenomenon: Longitudinal data from the digit span memory test. *Journal of Gerontology: Psychological Sciences, 44,* P184–P186.

Johansson, B. & Zarit, S. H. (1995). Prevalence and incidence of dementia in the oldest old: A longitudinal study of a population-based sample of 84–90 year-olds in Sweden. *International Journal of Geriatric Psychiatry, 10,* 359–366.

Johansson. B. & Zarit, S. H. (1997). Early cognitive markers of the incidence of dementia and mortality: A longitudinal population-based study of the oldest old. *Journal of Geriatric Psychiatry, 12,* 53–59.

Johansson, B., Zarit, S. H., & Berg, S. (1992). Changes in cognitive functioning of the oldest old. *Journal of Gerontology: Psychological Sciences, 47,* P75–P80.

Jorm, A. F., Christensen, H., Henderson, A. S., Jacomb, P. A., Korten, A. E., & Mackinnon, A. (1996). Informant ratings of cognitive decline in elderly people: Relationship to longitudinal change on cognitive tests. *Age and Ageing, 25,* 125–129.

Kahn, R. L., Zarit, S. H., Hilbert, N. M., & Niederehe, G. (1979). Memory complaint and impairment in the aged. The effect of depression and altered brain function. *Archives of General Psychiatry, 32,* 1569–1573.

Kane, R., & Kane, R. (1981). *Assessing the elderly: A*

practical guide to measurement. Lexington, MA: Lexington.

Kaszniak, A. W., & Ditraglia Christenson, G. (1995). Differential diagnosis of dementia and depression. In M. Storandt & G. R. VandeBos (Eds.), *Neuropsychological assessment of dementia and depression in older adults: A clinician's guide* (pp. 81–117). Washington, DC: American Psychological Association.

Katona, C. L. E. (1994). *Depression in old age*. Chichester, UK: Wiley.

Kausler, D. H. (1994). *Learning and memory in normal aging*. San Diego, CA: Academic Press.

Kemper, S. (1992). Language and aging. In F. I. M. Craik & T. A. Salthouse (Eds.), *The handbook of aging and cognition* (pp. 213–270). Hillsdale, NJ: Erlbaum.

Kliegl, R. L., & Baltes, P. B. (1987). Theory-guided analysis of mechanisms of development and aging through testing—The limits and research on expertise. In C. Schooler & K. W. Schaie (Eds.), *Cognitive functioning and social structure over the life course* (pp. 95–119). Norwood, NJ: Ablex.

Kohn, M. L., & Schooler, C. (1983). *Work and personality*. Norwood, NJ: Ablex.

Krauss, I. K. (1980). Between- and within-group comparisons in aging research. In L. W. Poon (Ed.), *Aging in the 1980s: Psychological issues* (pp. 542–551). Washington, DC: American Psychological Association.

Kuriansky, J., & Gurland, B. (1976). Performance test of activities of daily living. *International Journal of Aging and Human Development, 7*, 343–352.

Labouvie-Vief, G. (1982). Dynamic development and mature autonomy: A theoretical prologue. *Human Development, 25*, 161–191.

Labouvie-Vief, G. (1985). Intelligence and cognition. In J. E. Birren & K. W. Schaie (Eds.), *Handbook of psychology and aging* (pp. 500–530). New York: Van Nostrand Reinhold.

Larrabee, G. J., & Crook, T. H. (1993). Do men show more rapid age-associated decline in simulated everyday verbal memory than do women? *Psychology and Aging, 8*, 68–71.

Larsson, M., & Bäckman, L. (1993). Semantic activation and episodic odor recognition in young and older adults. *Psychology and Aging, 8*, 582–588.

LaRue, A. (1992). *Aging and neuropsychological assessment*. New York: Plenum.

Lazarus, R. S., & Folkman, S. (1984). *Stress, appraisal, and coping*. New York: Springer.

Lee, J. S. (1991). *Abstraction and aging*. New York: Springer.

Lerman, S. (1983). An experimental and clinical evaluation of lens transparency and aging. *Journal of Gerontology, 38*, 293–301.

Lezak, M. D. (1983). *Neuropsychological assessment* (2nd ed.). New York: Oxford University Press.

Lezak, M. D. (1995). *Neuropsychological assessment* (3rd ed.). New York: Oxford University Press.

Light, L. L. (1988). Language and aging: Competence versus performance, In J. E. Birren & V. L. Bengtson (Eds.), *Emergent theories of aging* (pp. 177–213). New York: Springer.

Light, L. L. (1991). Memory and aging: Four hypotheses in search of data. *Annual Review of Psychology, 42*, 333–376.

Lindenberger, U., & Baltes, P. B. (1994). Sensory functioning and intelligence in old age: A strong connection. *Psychology and Aging, 9*, 339–355.

MacKay, D. G., & Burke, D. M. (1990). Cognition and aging: A theory of new learning and the use of old connections. In T. M. Hess (Ed.), *Aging and cognition: Knowledge organization and utilization* (pp. 213–264). Amsterdam: North Holland.

Marsiske, M., Lindenberger, U., & Baltes, P. B. (1994, April). *The dedifferentiation of intelligence hypothesis revisited: From early adulthood to very old age*. Paper presented at the Cognitive Aging Conference, Atlanta, GA.

McKelvie, S. J., Standing, L., St. Jean, D., & Law, J. (1993). Gender differences in recognition memory for faces and cars: Evidence for the interest hypothesis. *Bulletin of the Psychonomic Society, 31*, 447–448.

Mennemeier, M., Garner, R. D., & Heilman, K. M. (1993). Memory, mood and measurement in hypothyroidism. *Journal of Clinical and Experimental Neuropsychology, 15*, 822–831.

Moss, M. B., Albert, M. S., & Kemper, T. L. (1992). Neuropsychology of frontal lobe dementia. In R. F. White (Ed.), *Clinical syndromes in adult neuropsychology: The practioner's handbook*. Amsterdam: Elsevier.

Neisser, U. (1978). Memory. What are the important questions? In M. M. Gruneber, P. E. Morris, & R. N. Sykes (Eds.), *Practical aspects of memory* (pp. 3–19). London: Academic Press.

Nelson, E. A., & Daneffer, D. (1992). Aged heterogeneity: Fact or fiction? The fate of diversity in gerontological research. *Gerontologist, 32*, 17–23.

Nyberg, L., Bäckman, L., Erngrund, K., Olofsson, U., & Nilsson, L.-G. (1996). Age differences in episodic memory, semantic memory, and priming: Relationships to demographic, intellectual, and biological factors. *Journal of Gerontology: Psychological Sciences, 51B*, P234–P240.

Obler, L. K., & Albert, M. L. (1985). Language skills across adulthood. In J. E. Birren & K. W. Schaie (Eds.), *Handbook of the psychology of aging* (2nd ed., pp. 463–473). New York: Van Nostrand Reinhold.

Olofsson, M., & Bäckman, L. (1993). Predictors of prose recall in adulthood and old age. *Archives of Gerontology and Geriatrics, 16*, 129–140.

Ordy, J. M., Brizzee, K. R., Beavers, T., & Medart, P. (1979). Age differences in the functional and structural organization of the auditory system in man. In J. M. Ordy & K. R. Brizzee (Eds.), *Aging: Vol. 10. Sensory systems and communication in the elderly* (pp. 153–166). New York: Raven Press.

Park, D. C. (1992). Applied cognitive aging research. In F. I. M. Craik & T. A. Salthouse (Eds.), *The handbook of aging and cognition* (pp. 449–493). Hillsdale, NJ: Erlbaum.

Parkin, A. J. (1982). Residual learning capability in organic amnesia. *Cortex, 18*, 417–440.

Perlmutter, M. (1986). A life span view of memory. In P. B. Baltes, D. Featherman, & R. Lerner (Eds.), *Advances in life-span development and behavior* (Vol. 7, pp. 271–313). Hillsdale, NJ: Erlbaum.

Raven, J. C. (1982). *Revised manual for Raven's Progressive Matrices and Vocabulary Scale*. Windsor, UK: NFER Nelson.

Reinert, G. (1970). Comparative factor analytic studies of intelligence through the human life-span. In L. R. Goulet & P. B. Baltes (Eds.), *Life-span development psychology: Research and theory* (pp. 467–484). New York: Academic Press.

Rinder, L., Roupe, S., Steen, B., & Svanborg, A. (1975). Seventy-year-old people in Gothenburg. A population study in an industrialized Swedish city. I. General presentation of the study. *Acta Medica Scandinavica, 198*, 397–407.

Robins Wahlin, T.-B., Bäckman, L., Wahlin, Å., & Winblad, B. (1993). Visuospatial functioning and spatial orientation in a community-based sample of healthy very old persons. *Archives of Gerontology and Geriatrics, 17*, 165–177.

Robins Wahlin, T.-B., Bäckman, L., Wahlin, Å., & Winblad, B. (1996). Trail Making Test performance in a community-based sample of healthy very old adults:

Effects on age on completion time, but not on accuracy. *Archives of Gerontology and Geriatrics, 22*, 87–102.

Rosow, I. (1978). What is a cohort and why? *Human Development, 21*, 65–75.

Rowe, J. W. & Kahn, R. L. (1987). Human aging: Usual and successful. *Science, 237*, 143–149.

Royall, D. A., Mahurin, R. K., & Gray, K. F. (1992). Bedside assessment of executive cognitive impairment: The executive interview. *Journal of the American Geriatrics Society, 40*, 1221–1226.

Rybash, J. M., Hoyer, W. J., & Roodin, P. (1986). *Adult cognition and aging: Developmental changes in processing, knowing and thinking*. New York: Pergamon.

Salthouse, T. A. (1983). *Adult cognition. An experimental psychology of human aging*. New York: Springer.

Salthouse, T. A. (1985). Speed of behavior and its implications for cognition. In J. E. Birren & K. W. Schaie (Eds.), *Handbook of the psychology of aging* (2nd ed., pp. 400–426). New York: Van Nostrand Reinhold.

Salthouse, T. A. (1987). The role of experience in cognitive aging. In K. W. Schaie (Ed.), *Annual review of gerontology and geriatrics* (Vol. 7, pp. 135–157). New York: Springer.

Salthouse, T. A. (1990). Cognitive competence and expertise in aging. In J. Birren & K. W. Schaie (Eds.), *Handbook of the psychology of aging* (pp. 310–319). San Diego, CA: Academic Press.

Salthouse, T. A. (1991). *Theoretical perspectives on cognitive aging*. Hillsdale, NJ: Erlbaum.

Salthouse, T. A. (1993). Speed mediation of adult age differences in cognition. *Developmental Psychology, 29*, 722–738.

Schaie, K. W. (1977–78). Towards a stage theory of adult cognitive development. *International Journal of Aging and Human Development, 8*, 129–138

Schaie, K. W. (1995). *Intellectual development in adulthood: The Seattle longitudinal study*. New York: Cambridge University Press.

Schaie, K. W. (1996). Intellectual development in adulthood. In J. E. Birren, & K. W. Schaie (Eds.), *Handbook of the psychology of aging* (4th ed., pp. 266–286). San Diego, CA: Academic Press.

Schaie, K. W., & Willis, S. L. (1993). Age difference patterns of psychometric intelligence in adulthood: Generalizability within and across ability domains. *Psychology and Aging, 8*, 44–55.

Schaie, K. W., Willis, S. H., & O'Hanlon, A. M. (1994). Perceived intellectual performance change over seven years. *Journal of Gerontology: Psychological Sciences, 49*, P108–P118.

Searight, H., & Goldberg, M. (1991). The Community Competence Scale as a measure of functional daily living skills. *Journal of Mental Health Administration, 18*, 128–134.

Shallice, T., & Burgess, P. (1991). Higher order cognitive impairments and frontal lobe lesions in man. In H. S. Levin, H. M. Eisenber, & A. I. Benton (Eds.), *Frontal lobe function and dysfunction* (pp. 125–138). New York: Oxford University Press.

Shepherd, J. (1981). Social factors in face recognition. In G. Davies, H. Ellis, & J. Shepherd (Eds.), *Perceiving and remembering faces* (pp. 55–79). New York: Academic Press.

Siegler, R. S., & Richards, D. D. (1982). The development of intelligence. In R. J. Sternberg (Ed.), *Handbook of human intelligence* (pp. 897–971). Cambridge, UK: Cambridge University Press.

Sliwinski, M., Lipton, R. B., Buschke, H., & Stewart, W. (1996). The effects of preclinical dementia on estimates of normal cognitive functioning in aging. *Journal of Gerontology: Psychological Sciences, 51B*, P217–P225.

Stankov, L. (1988). Aging, attention, and intelligence. *Psychology and Aging, 3*, 59–74.

Stine, E. A. L., Wingfield, A., & Myers, S. D. (1990). Age differences in processing information from television news: The effect of bisensory augmentation. *Journal of Gerontology: Psychological Sciences, 45*, P1–P8.

Stuss, D., & Benson, D. (1986). *The frontal lobes*. New York: Raven.

Tulving, E. (1983). *Elements of episodic memory*. Oxford, UK: Oxford University Press.

Tulving, E. (1985). How many memory systems are there? *American Psychologist, 40*, 385–398.

Van Gorp, W. G., Satz, P., & Mirushina, M. (1990). Neuropsychological processes associated with normal aging. *Developmental Neuropsychology, 6*, 279–290.

Verhaeghen, P., Marcoen, A., & Goossens, L. (1992). Improving memory performance in the aged through mnemonic training: A meta-analytical study. *Psychology and Aging, 7*, 242–251.

Wahlin, Å., Bäckman, L., Mäntylä, T., Herlitz, A., Viitanen, M., & Winblad, B. (1993). Prior knowledge and face recognition in a community-based sample of healthy, very old adults. *Journal of Gerontology: Psychological Sciences, 48*, P54–P61.

Wahlin, Å., Bäckman, L., & Winblad, B. (1995). Free recall and recognition of slowly and rapidly presented words in very old age: A community-based study. *Experimental Aging Research, 21*, 251–271.

Wahlin, Å., Hill, R. D., Winblad, B. & Bäckman, L. (in press). Effects of serum vitamin B^{12} and folate status on episodic memory performance in very old age: A population-based study. *Psychology and Aging, 11*, 487–496.

Waugh, N. C., & Norman, D. A. (1965). Primary memory. *Psychological Review, 72*, 89–104.

Weber, R. J., Brown, L. T., & Weldon, J. K. (1978). Cognitive maps of environmental knowledge and preference in nursing home patients. *Experimental Aging Research, 3*, 157–174.

Wechsler, D. (1955). *Manual for the Wechsler Adult Intelligence Scale*. New York: Psychological Corporation.

Wechsler, D. (1981). *Manual for the Wechsler Adult Intelligence-Scale Revised*. New York: Psychological Corporation.

Welford, A. T. (1977). Motor performance. In J. E. Birren, & K. W. Schaie (Eds.), *Handbook of the psychology of aging* (pp. 450–496). New York: Van Nostrand Reinhold.

West, R. L., Crook, T. H., & Barron, K. L. (1992). Everyday memory performance across the life span: Effects of age and noncognitive individual differences. *Psychology and Aging, 7*, 72–82.

Willis, S. L. (1996). Everyday problem solving. In J. E. Birren, & K. W. Schaie (Eds.), *Handbook of the psychology of aging* (4th ed., pp. 287–307). San Diego, CA: Academic Press.

Yussen, S. R., & Kane, P. T. (1983). Children's ideas about intellectual ability. In R. L. Leahy (Ed.), *The child's construction of social inequality* (pp. 109–134). New York: Academic Press.

Zarit, S. H. (1979). Helping an aging patient to cope with memory problems. *Geriatrics, April*, 82–90.

Zarit, S. H., Johansson, B., & Berg, S. (1993). Functional impairment and co-disability in the oldest old: A multidimensional approach. *Journal of Aging and Health, 5*, 291–305.

Zelinski, E. M., Gilewski, M. J., & Schaie, K. W. (1993). Individual differences in cross-sectional and three year longitudinal memory performance across the adult life span. *Psychology and Aging, 8*, 176–186.

7.03
Social Relationships and Adaptation in Late Life

FRIEDER R. LANG
Freie Universität Berlin, Germany
and
LAURA L. CARSTENSEN
Stanford University, CA, USA

7.03.1 INTRODUCTION

The role of social relationships in late-life adaptation has stimulated much social gerontological and psychological research since the 1950s (Cumming & Henry, 1961; Havighurst & Albrecht, 1953; Lee, 1985; Osgood, 1989) and generated considerable debates about theoretical models of social aging. Disengagement theorists, for example, have claimed that social withdrawal reflects an older individual's adaptive response to personal loss and to social forces such as age stereotypes and restrictive social practices (Cumming & Henry, 1961; Maddox, 1963; Pratt & Norris, 1994). Activity theorists, in contrast, have argued that successful adaptation in later life requires older people to be sociall active (Havighurst, Neugarten, & Tobin, 1968; Lemon, Bengtson, & Peterson, 1972). From a life-course perspective,

Atchley (1993) stated that individuals in old age prefer those social interactions and social activities that allow for continuity of their life-long roleidentities, experiences, and competencies. Rosow (1975, 1982) claimed that loss of social roles is inevitable in late life and adaptive social aging occurs when older people engage in social activities with age peers. Despite the great diversity in existing theoretical and empirical models of social aging, it has been widely acknowledged that the rules, mechanisms, and functions of social relationships in later life are better understood within a life-span perspective (Antonucci & Akiyama, 1995; Carstensen, 1993a; Marsiske, Lang, Baltes, & Baltes, 1995; Schulz & Rau, 1985). Socioemotional selectivity theory has emphasized and elaborated the role of life-long adaptive and motivational mechanisms that regulate social contact and social relationships (Carstensen, 1987, 1993a, 1995). According to the theory, during early phases of life, preferences for social contacts with others are instigated very frequently by information-seeking goals, yet social contacts in later life are more often determined by emotion-regulatory goals (Carstensen, 1993a, 1995). Empirical findings suggest that older people select and manage their social relationships such that attainment of emotional benefits and emotional goals is maximized or enhanced (Fredrickson & Carstensen, 1991; Lang & Carstensen, 1994; Lang, Staudinger, & Carstensen, in press; Lang & Tesch-Römer, 1993). In addition, structural and functional aspects of social networks appear to follow predictable life course patterns (Antonucci & Akiyama, 1995; Kahn & Antonucci, 1980; Lang & Carstensen, 1994). Social adaptation in later life can also be understood within the framework of the model of selective optimization with compensation (Baltes & Carstensen, 1996, Marsiske et al., 1995). In order to adapt successfully to the constraints of later life, older individuals have to first select meaningful social goals and social resources within the limits of their social-relational contexts. Such selection may then, subsequently, serve compensatory or optimizing purposes in achieving relevant social goals. Compensation, for example, pertains to seeking social support, for example, when adjusting to functional or personal loss. Optimization relates to relational enhancement mechanisms such as generativity or reciprocity (Lang & Baltes, 1997).

Social relationships are dynamic by nature. They vary from person to person, from situation to situation, and from one instance of interaction to the next instance of interaction (e.g., Caspi, Bolger, & Eckenrode, 1987). How adaptive a specific social transaction is thus depends on the situational and relational context as well as on the individual's needs and preferences. For example, a confidant's advice and support to someone who struggles with a decision may be quite supportive and useful during a specific decision-making process but the same advice may be inadequate and even disturbing after the decision has been made. In this example, the adaptive outcome of social contact depends largely on the confidant's empathy and knowledge of the individual's decisional process (e.g., Hogg & Heller, 1990). In more general terms, the adaptivity of social relationships is determined by the extent to which social-relational contexts reflect the individual's social needs and capacities. Such a match between person and context characteristics plays a critical role in understanding the older person's social adaptivity (e.g., Kahn, 1979; Lawton, 1989), and will be discussed in greater detail below.

In this chapter, normative changes in the characteristics of social relationships and social networks across adulthood focusing on close family and friendship relationships are addressed. Then empirical evidence for health-related functions of social support and social relationships underscoring the influence of the older individuals' social needs and preferences in adaptive relational outcomes is reviewed. Next the issue of negative aspects and negative outcomes of social relationships in later life is addressed. Negative aspects of social relationships often have been related to facets of the individual's social relationships, such as ineffective, inadequate, or unpleasant social resources (e.g., Rook & Pietromonaco, 1987) including even physical abuse (Pillemer & Finkelhor, 1988). However, negative aspects of social relationships also may be related to maladaptive social behaviors or characteristics of the older individual such as excessive autonomy needs (e.g., Baltes & Silverberg, 1994) or misanthropy (e.g., Schütze & Lang, 1995). Finally, in Section 7.03.4, findings on the age-, health-, and relation-specific aspects of social relationships are discussed in the light of some more recent theoretical perspectives on individuals' adaptive social behaviors and relational management in later life drawing on socioemotional selectivity theory (Carstensen, 1995) and the convoy model of social relationships (Antonucci & Akiyama, 1995).

7.03.2 AGE-RELATED CHANGES OF SOCIAL-RELATIONAL CONTEXTS

Many changes in the structural or functional characteristics in the social worlds of older people are associated with particular age-specific experiences such as retirement (Bosse, Aldwin, Levenson, Spiro, & Mroczek, 1993; Carp, 1972; Havighurst, Munnichs, Neugarten, & Thomae, 1969) and adult children leaving home, marrying, and eventually having children of their own (Lowenthal, Thurnher, & Chiriboga, 1976; Miller & Cavanaugh, 1990; White & Edwards, 1990). In addition, experiencing the loss of a spouse, close relative, or friend inevitably changes the resources available to the older person (Garrett, 1987; Lopata, 1986; Morgan, 1989). While there is strong evidence that people have fewer social contacts and social relationships in later life as compared to earlier life phases (Gordon & Gaitz, 1976; Harvey & Singleton, 1989; Heller & Mansbach, 1984; Lawton, Moss, & Fulcomer, 1987; Lee & Markides, 1990; Lowenthal et al., 1976; Palmore, 1981), there are also consistent reports suggesting that the majority of old and even very old people are well integrated into family and friendship networks (e.g., Antonucci & Akiyama, 1995; Bowling & Browne, 1991; Levitt, Weber, & Guacci, 1993).

In the United States and in Europe, most older people above 65 years report having 5–15 important or close social partners in their social network (Antonucci & Akiyama, 1987; 1995; Dykstra, 1993; House & Kahn, 1985; Lang & Carstensen, 1994; Lang, Staudinger, & Carstensen, 1996; Stacey-Konnert & Pynoos, 1992). Empirical findings regarding social network size in early and middle adulthood are less consistent but generally range from 15 to 35 network members (e.g., Antonucci & Akiyama, 1994; Carstensen & Lang, in preparation; Van Sonderen, Ormel, Brilman & Van Linden, 1990; Wellman, 1979). Compared to social networks of young or middle-aged adults, older people report a greater percentage of family members and fewer friends or acquaintances in their social networks (Antonucci & Akiyama, 1987; 1995; Babchuk, 1978–79; Levitt et al., 1993; Stacey-Konnert & Pynoos, 1992). Indeed, while many friendships with peers are lost due to death (Garrett, 1987; Johnson & Troll, 1994; Roberto & Stanis, 1994), there is also some indication that older people selectively maintain contacts with close friends rather than less meaningful friends or acquaintances in old age (Bowling & Browne, 1991; Carstensen, 1992; Lang & Carstensen, 1994).

Although the risk of social isolation or feeling lonely may increase in very old age (Larson, 1990; Mullins, Sheppard, & Andersson, 1991), this does not seem to characterize later life phases in general (Revensen & Johnson, 1984; Schultz & Moore, 1988; Shute & Howitt, 1990) and varies across individuals depending on specific relational contexts such as widowhood or marital break-up (Dykstra, 1995; Ferraro & Barresi, 1982; Keith, 1986), marital crisis (Tornstam, 1992), living alone (Henderson, Scott, & Kay, 1986), childlessness (Lang, 1994; Page & Cole, 1991), filial neglect (Connidis & McMullin, 1993; Lang, 1994), or death of close friends (Roberto & Stanis, 1994). Obviously, the social networks of people who are widowed, who have never married, or who are childless differ in many respects from those older people who have lived with their spouse for many decades or who have reared children that have eventually become independent adults (e.g., Connidis & McMullin, 1994; Dykstra, 1993; Lang, 1994). Some older individuals have divorced (e.g., Hammond & Muller, 1992), others have faced the loss of a spouse or close intimates (Dean, Matt, & Wood, 1992; Morgan, 1989), or even an adult child (Moss, Lesher, & Moss, 1986–87; Rubin, 1991–92). The majority of people over 65 years of age have experienced the death of a sibling (Moss & Moss, 1989). Some have focused their social worlds on the maintenance of friendship relationships (Armstrong & Goldsteen, 1990; Johnson & Troll, 1994; Roberto & Scott, 1987), while for others close ties with family members prevail (Field & Minkler, 1988; Field, Minkler, Falk, & Leino, 1993; Johnson & Troll, 1992). Such pervasive multifacetness and heterogeneity in the structure of interpersonal contexts in late life is also reflected in the specific demands and potentials of older peoples' family and friendship relationships.

7.03.2.1 Family Relationships

In general, family relations prove to be reliable and stable sources of social support and social embeddedness in old and very old age, even when relatively little effort is made to keep in touch or to maintain the relationship (Carstensen, 1993b; Crohan & Antonucci, 1989; Field & Minkler, 1993). The close family is most often named as a source of meaningful social contact or social support in old age (Caplan, 1982; Depner & Ingersoll-Dayton, 1985; Dykstra, 1993; Hogan, 1995; Sussman, 1985). Findings from the Berkeley Intergenerational Study have revealed that contacts and feelings of closeness in family relationships are stable or even increase in old age (Field & Minkler, 1988, 1993). This seems to be true for marital relationships and parent–child relationships although less so for sibling relationships (Cicirelli, 1989; Connidis, 1989; Scott, 1990), which are discussed later in this chapter.

7.03.2.1.1 Marriage and intimate relationships

When older people are married or live with an intimate partner, the relationship is mostly described as an important source of meaningful and satisfactory social contact in everyday life (Alwin, Converse, & Martin, 1985; Huyck, 1995). Partners are most often named as social supporters and caregivers when functional losses occur (Brody, 1985; Chappell, 1991; Connidis & McMullin, 1994; Hess & Soldo, 1985). In addition, there is consistent empirical evidence showing that older people are, on average, quite satisfied with their marriages (Brubaker, 1990; Herman, 1994; Levenson, Carstensen, & Gottman, 1993). Later life couples have fewer conflicts and experience more pleasure in sharing intimate and intergenerational experiences or activities than middle-aged couples (Levenson, Carstensen, & Gottman, 1993). Older couples also express more affection than younger couples (Carstensen, Gottman, & Levenson, 1995; Levenson, Carstensen, & Gottman, 1994). Such evidence may also suggest a survival of the fittest marriages, that is, those which have stood the test of time. Moreover, interindividual differences also matter. Empirical evidence suggests that extraversion and neuroticism are associated with marital stability (Cramer, 1993; Kurdek, 1991).

Overall, long-term marital relationships have been demonstrated consistently to be stable and reliable sources of positive and gratifying social experiences. Next to marital relationships, adult children and their families frequently are nominated as the second most important source of emotionally meaningful contact and social support in late life (Chappell, 1991; Dykstra, 1993; Eggebeen, 1992; Hogan, 1995).

7.03.2.1.2 Adult children and grandchildren

Contrary to the popular lore about older parents being abandoned and neglected by their adult children (Shanas, 1980; Steinmetz, 1988), there is considerable empirical evidence showing that adult children not only stay in contact with their parents (Hagestad, 1987), but they continue to share close emotional relationships with them (Field & Minkler, 1988). Frequently they exchange support (Eggebeen & Hogan, 1990; Hogan, 1995; Lang, 1996; Rossi & Rossi, 1990), and are, second only to spouses, the principle caregivers of frail elderly parents (Brody, 1985; Chappell, 1990; Horowitz, 1985; Mancini & Blieszner, 1989).

Typically, older parents also experience the developmental task of grandparenthood that demands the acquisition of a new social role (Kivnick, 1982) and the development of an individual style of grandparenting (Sticker, 1991). Grandparenthood is associated with many changes in the socioemotional worlds of older people such as increased contact and satisfaction with adult children (Aldous, 1987), increase in intergenerational giving (Eggebeen & Hogan, 1990; Tinsely & Parke, 1987), and becoming the keepers of meaning and conveyers of the family tradition (Ramirez-Barranti, 1985; Bengtson, 1985; Hagestad, 1985; Lang & Baltes, 1997). While grandparenthood is often associated with positive experiences and social satisfaction (Kennedy, 1992; Sticker, 1991), grandchildren are rarely named as support providers before they reach early adulthood (Hodgson,1992; Langer, 1990; Markides, Boldt, & Ray, 1986).

7.03.2.1.3 Older siblings

In many ways, social ties with siblings are unique in later adulthood. Older siblings share life-long biographical and historical experiences and are often the only social partners who have known the older individual as a child or adolescent (Cicirelli, 1995; Gold, 1987). Thus, older siblings share an exclusive biographical and sociohistorical knowledge of one another. However, compared to most other close family relationships, social contact frequencies and support exchanges among older siblings are typically limited to times of crises or increased need (Avioli, 1989; Connidis, 1994) unless other intimates such as spouses (O'Bryant, 1988; Wilson, Calsyn, & Orlofsky, 1994) or adult children are unavailable (Connidis & Davis, 1992; Ikels, 1988). As is true for most other social relationships as well, siblings interact more often when they live in close geographical proximity to one another (Connidis & Davis, 1992; Scott, 1983).

However, it is the quality and emotional closeness of sibling relationships that contributes to well-being rather than the quantitative aspects of contact or support exchange (Wilson, Calsyn, & Orlofsky, 1994). These associations are consistently found to be stronger for relationships with sisters or a same-sex sibling as opposed to relationships of sisters with their brothers (Cicirelli, 1989; Connidis, 1989; Pulakos, 1987). Although sibling relationships in later life are often continued sources of conflict and rivalry (Bedford, 1995; Goetting, 1986), older adults may be more discriminating in their choice of social partners in an effort to ensure emotionally gratifying contact with siblings.

7.03.2.2 Friendship Relations

In contrast to social relationships that are legally defined or determined by kinship, friendship is characterized by the voluntary involvement of two or more partners with one another (Adams & Blieszner, 1994; Blau, 1973; Ishii-Kuntz, 1990). Failures to abide by normative expectations in friendships (Roberto & Scott, 1986a, 1986b) in contrast to parent–child relationships, for example, leads to dissolution of the friendship. In addition, longitudinal findings suggest that while the relevance of family roles remains quite stable in old age, the significance of other social roles seems to decrease (Field & Minkler, 1993; Lehr & Minnemann, 1987). Some friendships dissipate and those that remain consist predominantly of friends who have known each other for a relatively long period of time (e.g., Lowenthal, Thurnher, & Chiriboga, 1976).

Notably, friendship relationships have been shown consistently to be associated with higher social satisfaction than relationships with family members who are not living in the same household (Chappell & Badger, 1989; Larson, Mannell, & Zuzanek, 1986, Mullins & Mushel, 1992). One possible explanation for this is that friends are often discharged from tasks that are related to instrumental support exchange and, thus, are less likely to be burdened by caregiving than are family members. In contrast, friends are often named as confidants of old people (Keith, Hill, Goudy, & Powers, 1984; Strain & Chappell, 1982) and are associated with pleasant interactions such as social companionship (Crohan & Antonucci, 1989; Rawlins, 1992). In this respect, friends might play a moderating role in older people's social networks by counterbalancing sometimes difficult or strained family relationships (Johnson, 1983) and by providing opportunities for social integration in the community (Peters & Kaiser, 1985).

When it comes to supportive transactions among friends, satisfaction with friendship is associated with the perceived equity of the exchange (Roberto, 1989; Roberto & Scott, 1986a; Rook, 1989). Nonreciprocal exchanges among friends seem to have even more detrimental effects than among family members (Antonucci & Jackson, 1990). Interestingly, though, close or "best" friends appear to be exceptions (Armstrong & Goldsteen, 1990). Older individuals who reflect their best friends' needs and welfare in their thinking (i.e., communal orientation) report greater satisfaction with their friendships than those who focus on the equity or comparibility of exchanged benefits with their friends (i.e., exchange orientation; Jones & Vaughan, 1990).

In sum, friendship and family relationships are associated with distinct social resources and specific functions that cannot be easily substituted for one another (Litwak, 1985). However, there is also evidence that when specific types of relationships such as spouse or children are unavailable, other relatives or friends appear to assume their functions (Cantor, 1979; Chatters, Taylor, & Jackson, 1986). In general, there is much evidence that older people are satisfied with both their family relationships and their friendships (Field & Minkler, 1988; Herzog & Rodgers, 1981; Ryff, 1989).

7.03.3 HEALTH-RELATED ASPECTS OF SOCIAL RELATIONSHIPS

There is widespread agreement that social relationships provide a fundamental resource for late-life adaptation. However, the underlying mechanisms and health functions of social resources are not fully understood (House, Umberson, & Landis, 1988). Social support has been proposed generally to exert a direct protective effect on health or well-being, while stressor-specific support of others may operate as a buffer when adverse or stressful events occur (Cohen & Wills, 1985; Schwarzer & Leppin, 1991). Others have proposed more complex patterns of associations in which specific types of social resources—such as emotional, instrumental, or tangible support (Rook & Pietromonaco, 1987)—are expected to have specific effects on health or well-being for specific individuals in specific situations (Gottlieb, 1983; House & Kahn, 1985; House et al., 1988; Kessler & McLeod, 1985). However, the age-specific needs and capacities of older support recipients and their social partners are often not well integrated in theoretical models of adaptivity in later life (see also Baltes & Carstensen, 1996; Carstensen & Lang, 1997; Staudinger, Marsiske, & Baltes, 1995). Indeed, considerable empirical evidence may serve to underscore the notion that age-specific social preferences and social belief systems (e.g., social self-efficacy; Lang, Featherman, & Nesselroade, in press) contribute to the adaptive functions of social support and social contact in later life.

The most convincing evidence for positive effects of social support and social networks on health comes from a variety of longitudinal studies of mortality in later life. The interested reader is referred to several excellent reviews of empirical findings about associations of social resources with mortality (Atkins, Kaplan, & Toshima, 1992; Schwarzer & Leppin, 1991), physical health (Antonucci & Jackson, 1987;

Schwarzer & Leppin, 1991), immunologic functioning (Antonucci & Jackson, 1987; Kennedy, Kiecolt-Glaser, & Glaser, 1990), disease course (Kriegsman, Penninx, & van Eijk, 1995), recovery from illness (Reifman, 1995), adjustment to cancer (Helgeson & Cohen, 1996), depression and mental health (Gotlib & Whiffen, 1992; Schwarzer & Leppin, 1992), and well-being (Bowling, 1994; Kessler & McLeod, 1985). It should be noted, however, that some reviews have reported minimal or even no impact of social support on health or well-being (Ganster & Victor, 1988; Schulz & Rau, 1985; Wallston, Alagna, DeVellis, & DeVellis, 1983) and some have also pointed to the potential negative effects of social relationships (Rook, 1984; Rook & Pietromonaco, 1987). In the following, health effects of social relationships are distinguished as they pertain to the relational contexts of older people, on the one hand, and as they pertain to relational behaviors, on the other, such as older individuals' styles or strategies of relating to others, such as selecting social partners, relying on others, reciprocating support, and enhancing social relationships.

7.03.3.1 Social Relationships and Health: Evidence for Positive Effects

Epidemiological studies in the United States and Europe have consistently found associations between the individual's risk of premature mortality and social resources or social contexts. For example, having close confidants or intimate social partners has been found repeatedly to be associated with increased longevity (Berkman, 1985; Berkman & Syme, 1979; Broadhead et al., 1983; Hammer, 1983; Hanson, Isacsson, Janzon, & Lindell, 1990; Orth-Gomer & Johnson, 1987; Steinbach, 1992; Sugisawa, Liang, & Liu, 1994). In the Terman Gifted Study, having a stable long-term marriage predicted increased longevity above and beyond gender, childhood personality, and health behaviors, while the risk of premature mortality was highest among those who had experienced divorce or separation before age 40 (Friedman et al., 1995). Separation and divorce are critical non-normative life events that may affect longevity. When individuals do not develop new intimate relationships after separation or divorce, they are at greater risk of premature mortality (Tucker, Friedman, Wingard, & Schwartz, 1996).

Furthermore, increased social network size and frequency of social contacts reduce the risk of mortality (Cohen, Teresi, & Holmes, 1986–87; Olsen, Olsen, Gunner-Svensson, & Waldstrom, 1991). However, social resources seem to affect morbidity differentially, among men and women (Bryant & Rakowski, 1992; Shye, Mullooly, Freeborn, & Pope, 1995). For example, while premature mortality is related to marital status among men (Berkman & Syme, 1979; Schoenbach, Kaplan, Fredman, & Kleinbaum, 1986), womens' chance of survival is better determined by size of social network (Shye et al., 1995), level of social activity, and church attendance (Berkman & Syme, 1979; House, Robbins, & Metzner, 1982).

In an Israeli five-year incidence study on adult men, high family conflict and low spousal support were related to increased risk of angina pectoris (Medalie & Goldbourt, 1976). In a Danish 14-year follow-up study of mortality, the perceived quality of social resources rather than quantitative characteristics of social networks were associated with increased longevity (Olsen et al., 1991). Generally, there is much empirical evidence that the perceived or subjective quality of social support or social contact are associated more strongly with adaptive outcomes than any other aspect or measure of social support (Antonucci & Jackson, 1987; Dunkel-Schetter & Bennett, 1990; Schwarzer & Leppin, 1991). This further underscores the qualification that social relationships are most effective when they are congruent with the individual's competence and social preferences (Carstensen, 1987; Carstensen & Lang, 1997). For example, in old age declines in health status are associated with receiving help and support from sources that are increasingly distant from the older person (Stoller & Pugliesi, 1988). This means that emotional or instrumental social support may often come from social partners who are not emotionally meaningful to the older person and may thus create unease or enhance feelings of dependence in the older individual.

When changes in health status occur, individuals may change their apprehension of available social relationships and social support (e.g., Gotlib & Whiffen, 1992; Wilcox, Kasl, & Berkman, 1994). When the individual's level of functioning and competence change, the individual may also adjust their preferences for specific social partners and for specific functions of social interactions. However, such changes in social preferences or needs may also affect the adequacy and satisfaction with previously available social resources. Research on social support has often neglected the fact that individuals change their social preferences and social behaviors in the course of physical or mental health crises, even when examined in prospective studies, where social support can be measured before and after health changes occur (e.g., Holahan, Moos, Holahan, & Brennan,

1995; Wilcox, Kasl, & Berkman, 1994). In fact, the benefits and positive outcomes of receiving social support may depend on the older individual's competence to utilize social resources in adaptive ways (Hansson & Carpenter, 1994; Lang, 1996; Thomae, 1994). Findings from empirical studies of health and well-being that do not consider changes in the individual's social needs and preferences may underestimate the actual impact of social resources.

7.03.3.2 The Negative Side of Social Relationships

Since the early 1980s, the perspective of social relationships as a uniformly positive resource has been challenged by conceptual and empirical work that demonstrates that positive relational outcomes can be neutralized or even reversed by negative aspects of social relationships, such as relational strain (Rook, 1984, 1987a), overprotective or unsolicited support (Thompson & Sobolow-Shubin, 1993a, 1993b), daily relational hassles (Bolger & Kelleher, 1993), and violence or physical abuse (Pillemer & Finkelhor, 1988; Pillemer & Suitor, 1992). Another, often overlooked, source of negative experience in social relationships pertains to the experience or anticipation of personal loss that is relatively common in later life (Garrett, 1987; Lopata, 1986; Morgan, 1989).

While negative aspects of social relationships, in theory, are often exclusively discussed in respect to the social behaviors of others (Rook & Pietromonaco, 1987), empirical studies on negative interactions have often focused exclusively on subjective evaluations of social support to the older individual (e.g., Schuster, Kessler, & Aseltine, 1990). Although an individual's negative relational experiences may be difficult to empirically disentangle from social (dis-)satisfaction or perceived support (in-)adequacy, this is crucial for an understanding of the individual's role in dealing with negative contents of social interactions. How an older individual responds to a specific threat or strain in a concrete social relationship may determine the individual's satisfaction or affect as much as the negative event itself. For example, conflict or friction among spouses may be easily resolved when both partners are satisfied with their marriage but may have detrimental effects and even predict separation when marital satisfaction is low (e.g., Carstensen et al., 1995; Gottman & Levenson, 1992; Levenson et al., 1993).

Most negative aspects of social relationships typical in later life may be associated with intensive emotional turmoil that demands efficient types of affective regulation on the part of the older individual. In the following, four sources of potential negative aspects of social relationships in later life are distinguished. They are: (i) dysfunctional social support, such as undesirable, ineffective, or excessive support; (ii) unpleasant or overdemanding social contact; (iii) violence or neglect; and (iv) anticipation or experience of personal loss of others.

7.03.3.2.1 Dysfunctional social support

While there is convincing empirical evidence that social support does contribute to life quality and well-being in later life, there is also a growing body of empirical studies showing that social relationships not only provide gratification but also entail risks and costs for the individual (for reviews see Jung, 1990; Rook & Pietromonaco, 1987; Shinn, Lehmann, & Wong, 1984). Failures to provide social support have been related to a variety of characteristics of the support process such as undesirable social contact (Cutrona, Cohen, & Igram, 1990; Rose, 1993), lack of empathy and sensitivity (Wortman & Lehman, 1985), grudgingly given support (Coyne, 1976), interpersonal betrayal (Hansson, Jones, & Fletcher, 1990), emotional overinvolvement (Coyne, Wortman, & Lehmann, 1988), overprotection (Thompson & Sobolow-Shubin, 1993a, 1993b), and the reinforcement of dependent behaviors (Baltes, 1995).

Negative aspects of social relationships have been shown consistently to operate relatively independently of personality or situational characteristics (Finch, Okun, Barrera, Zautra, & Reich, 1989). Furthermore, empirical evidence suggests that negative experiences in supportive interactions are more strongly associated with well-being or mental health than perceived positive instances of social support (Finch et al., 1989; Okun, Melichar, & Hill, 1990; Rook, 1984; Schuster et al., 1990). However, there is no consistent evidence that detrimental effects of negative social support are enhanced dramatically in the absence of positive social support (Schuster et al.) or in the presence of negative events (Okun et al., 1990). Typically, negative and positive social interactions are only mildly or not at all correlated (Finch et al.; Okun et al.; Rook, 1984; Shinn et al., 1984). It has been suggested (Schuster et al.; Shinn et al.) that such a dissociation of positive and negative aspects may parallel findings on independence of positive and negative affect (e.g., Watson, Clark, & Tellegen, 1988). However, no study, to the best of our knowledge, has examined the age-differential effects of positive and negative supportive interactions on the experience of positive and negative affect in daily life.

Empirical studies of the experience of negative supportive interactions typically have focused on the individual's subjective experience of such negative interaction. However, it seems plausible that older individuals may have idiosyncratic responses to negative events in their close relationships and may develop individual strategies of avoiding or managing negative aspects of close relationships (e.g., Carstensen et al., 1995). Moreover, many negative aspects of dysfunctional social support may also be related to the older individual's social contacts and social preferences. For example, a failure to communicate wishes or needs may be as much responsible for inefficient or inadequate social support as a social partners' lack of social abilities to "do the right thing" (e.g.,Query & James, 1989). It has also been suggested that individuals do not rely on others when they cannot reciprocate received benefits in order to avoid feelings of shame or guilt (Fisher, Nadler, & Whitcher-Alagna, 1982; Riley & Eckenrode, 1986; Shumaker & Jackson, 1979)

7.03.3.2.2 Unpleasant and demanding social contacts

Conflicts, demands, and criticism are part and parcel of even the best close social relationships and may even increase over time (Rook & Pietromonaco 1987; Antonucci, 1985). In addition, personal relationships are not always stable and reliable but to some extent are also characterized by unpredictability and fluctuations (e.g., Lang, Featherman, & Nesselroade, in press).

Although empirical research on unpleasant and demanding aspects of social relationships in later life remains scarce, there is some evidence that older adults may differ from younger adults in respect to how they react and deal with relational conflict or friction (e.g., Carstensen et al., 1995). Older people may be more skilled in avoiding unpleasant or overly demanding situations with social partners about whom they feel less strongly or positive. For example, it has been shown that lack of equity or reciprocity expectations in older adult's friendships are very likely to lead to dissatisfaction or even dissolution of the relationship (Roberto & Scott, 1986a, 1986b).

There is some evidence that when individuals hold negative views toward others they have a greater risk of premature mortality (Barefoot et al., 1987) and are more vulnerable to depression or other form of negative affect when confronted with demands, criticism, or rejection (Smith, 1992). For example, spouses of depressed partners are less supportive, more critical, hostile, and ambivalent towards their partners (Hautzinger, Linden, & Hoffman, 1982; Ruscher & Gotlib, 1988; for a review, see Gotlib & Hooley, 1988). Personality characteristics and relational styles may thus conjointly influence the way individuals react to unpleasant social encounters (Hansson & Carpenter, 1994). However, although personality characteristics are relatively stable over the life course (Costa & McCrae, 1994), their impact in determining outcomes of social interactions and social adaptation may well change with age and may account for fewer outcomes in later adulthood (Lang et al., in press). In other words, older people may be at greater risk of experiencing negative effects when confronted with unavoidable, unpleasant,or demanding social behaviors of others.

7.03.3.2.3 Violence and neglect: the relational dynamics of caregiving

Violent or neglectful behaviors are the most obvious and dramatic negative aspects of social relationships in later life. In the United States, estimates of incidence of elder abuse range from seven hundred thousand to one million people older than 65 years (Hansson & Carpenter, 1994). Violence or neglect occurs mostly in relationships with social partners who share a household (Pillemer & Finkelhor, 1988). Indeed, social contexts of caregiving children or spouses may be experienced as extremely stressful and frustrating for caregivers as well as older individuals (Franks & Stephens, 1996; Schulz, Tompkins, & Rau, 1988; Walker, Martin, & Jones, 1992). Caregiver stress (for reviews: Pearlin, Mullan, Semple, & Skaff, 1990; Schulz, Visintainer, & Williamson, 1990) has been reported to be associated with increased depression and emotional turmoil (Pruchno, Peters, & Burant, 1995; Townsend & Franks, 1995), social isolation, and the lack of social support (Johnson & Catalano, 1983; George & Gwyther, 1986).

In addition, the relational dynamics of caregiving may lead to further escalation of hostility and aggression in the care receiver as well as in the caregiver. Older individuals who receive care must also come to terms with their lack of autonomy and dependence on the caregiver (Baltes & Silverberg, 1994).

7.03.3.2.4 Anticipation or experience of relational loss

Finally, experiencing the deaths of close friends and relatives is normative in late life

(Holmes & Rahe, 1967; Johnson & Troll, 1994). Most individuals over 65 years have experienced losses of close friends, siblings, or of partners during late life and also struggle with the anticipatory loss of other close social partners (Garrett, 1987; Lopata, 1986; Morgan, 1989).

Despite empirical evidence for the negative impact of widowhood on the social world, however, research suggests a more differentiated perspective on adjustment to widowhood (e.g., Ferraro & Farmer, 1995). Prior to widowhood, many spouses endure extended periods when their partners suffer from severe illness and require considerable care (Bass & Bowman, 1990; Bass, Bowman, & Noelker, 1991; Mullan, 1992). Subsequently, as painful as widowhood may be, it can also entail a sense of relief that the spouse's suffering has finally come to an end and the widowed spouse regains freedom to engage in more pleasant activities.

Due to women's longer life expectancy and the traditional age differences among married couples, widowhood is a normative experience among married women. It is a less common experience for married men. In addition, widowhood seems to be related to gender-differentiated demands and needs. Adjustment to widowhood is more strongly related to social compensation among widows than among widowers (Ferraro & Farmer, 1995). Typically, widows are threatened by financial losses following widowhood, whereas men are at risk if they have difficulties with keeping up an independent household (Umberson, Wortman, & Kessler, 1992). In addition, widowhood is associated with a higher mortality risk for widowers than for widows (Bowling, 1988-89; Bowling & Windsor, 1995).

7.03.3.3 Managing Social Resources

A review of empirical studies on differential effects of positive and negative aspects of supportive relationships on late-life adaptation suggests that positive outcomes of social resources are largely determined by the extent to which social resources actually meet the older individual's social preferences and needs. For example, it has been reported consistently, that perceived adequacy of social support is more strongly associated with adaptive outcomes than any other aspects of social support. However, the cognitive and behavioral strategies in supportive interactions that determine and influence subjective support adequacy are not well understood. Few empirical studies have examined cognitive or behavioral correlates of perceived social support adequacy in adulthood (e.g., Dunkel-Schetter, Folkman, & Lazarus, 1987; Röhrle, 1994) or old age (Seeman & Berkman, 1988), let alone considered age-related changes in motivational or emotional determinants of managing social support. Empirical evidence for changed social preferences towards greater emphasis on emotionally meaningful social contacts in late adulthood (Carstensen, 1995; Fredrickson & Carstensen, 1990) suggests that the adequacy and impact of social contact and social support on well-being in later life depends on emotion-regulatory aspects of social relationships such as emotional closeness (Lang & Carstensen, 1994), intimacy (Babchuk & Anderson,1989), generativity (McAdams, de St. Aubin, & Logan, 1993), functional specificity (Felton & Berry, 1992), and trust (Holmes, 1991; Thomae, 1994). There is also empirical evidence that older people benefit from actively engaging in support-seeking behaviors (Filipp & Aymanns, 1987), and from reciprocating support to others (Jung, 1990; Krause, Herzog, & Baker, 1992; Lang, 1996). Others have focused on the personality characteristics of older people that were shown to be closely associated with increased levels of relational competence (Hansson & Carpenter, 1994) related to the initiation, maintenance, and enhancement of social relationships or relational outcomes (Carpenter, 1993; Mariske et al., 1995). Moreover, feelings of control in salient social roles (such as spouse, parent, or grandparent) have been shown to buffer deleterious effects of stressful life events on life satisfaction (Krause, 1994).

The adaptive management of social resources in later life is also illustrated by empirical evidence for the learned dependency model developed by Baltes and her colleagues (Baltes, 1995; Baltes, Neumann, & Zank, 1994). This line of observational research has revealed that dependent behaviors of older ,nursing home residents are more often positively reinforced by responsiveness and social contact than independent behaviors. Subsequent intervention studies demonstrated that independent behaviors of residents increased when staff members and other social partners were trained to be responsive to independent behaviors (Baltes et al.). The initiation of such dependence-support scripts in nursing home settings has been conceptualized as an adaptive behavioral strategy by which older people regulate and optimize the available resources in their social environment (Baltes, 1995). In this case, relinquishing independence is seen as a "proxy control" strategy where the individual gains control in particular domains of functioning through other persons, thereby exerting an indirect influence over the environment (Bandura, 1982; Baltes, 1995). Proxy control may be an important mechanism by which older individuals can compensate for the loss of primary control and enhance the perceived adequacy of social resources (Heckhausen & Lang, 1996).

Moreover, most personal relationships go through times of conflict or periods of relationship crises that must be mastered if social partners are to maintain their relationships (Antonucci, 1985; Duck, 1986). Successfully managing both the stable and varying, positive, and negative aspects of family ties or friendships is likely to be a fundamental requisite for maintaining social adaptivity throughout adulthood and late life (Lang et al., in press; Marsiske et al., 1995; Morgan, 1990).

7.03.4 THEORETICAL PERSPECTIVES ON THE MANAGEMENT OF SOCIAL RELATIONSHIPS

As people grow old, their social relationships and social networks undergo considerable change as a result of both changing relational contexts in later life as well as changes in the individual's social behaviors and preferences. In this chapter, literature showing age-related changes in relational contexts as well as age-related differences in individuals' social motivations and social contacts has been discussed. In the remainder of this chapter, we will summarize and integrate the emerging picture of normal aging in social relationships and propose a common theoretical framework of socioemotional selectivity and social adaptation. It is concluded that people select, mold, and manage their social relationships in accordance with their needs, preferences, and competencies. However, the extent to which an individual can exert control over their social relationships is constrained by the structural and functional characteristics of their social context.

Greater emphasis has been placed on the individual's goals and behaviors when dealing with others (Baltes & Carstensen, 1996; Carstensen, 1993a, 1995; Marsiske et al., 1995). It has been suggested, for example, that the adaptivity of social interactions does not depend solely on the behaviors and competencies of the individual's social partners but also on the individual's own social behaviors and competence (Hansson & Carpenter, 1994; Marsiske et al., 1995). Older individuals, as much as younger individuals, actively contribute to the positive and negative outcomes of their social relationships by selecting and maintaining relationships with particular social partners as well as influencing the specific social transactions that occur within a given social relationship (Lang & Baltes, in press). Thus, when dealing with others, older individuals actively contribute to the maximization of positive gratification or benefits and minimization of negative experience. For example, older individuals do not just receive social support, they also provide support to other people, often to those people with whom they have close relationships or friendships for many years.

7.03.4.1 Socioemotional Selectivity Theory: Emotion Regulation in Late Life

According to socioemotional selectivity theory (Carstensen, 1987, 1991, 1992, 1993a), basic functions of social interaction, such as regulating desired emotional states and acquiring knowledge about oneself or the world, differ in respect to their relative importance for determining social preferences across the life span. For example, Carstensen (1993a) argues that emotional regulation becomes more important in old age because a more limited future alters the likelihood that long-term goals will be achieved. Hence, emphasis is shifted to achieving short-term goals in the immediate social context that are mostly emotional rather than informational.

Socioemotional selectivity theory provides a theoretical framework in which most of the above-mentioned empirical findings on age-related changes and health-related functions of social relationships can be considered. Older people narrow the breadth of their social lives and social participation in order to intensify their engagement in a narrow range of social functions, focusing on close emotional relationships with peers as well as with younger social partners from whom they derive a sense of meaning in life. Reduced social contact in late life, according to this model, reflects the older individual's changed needs and motivations. Indeed, the profile of empirical findings reviewed suggests that it is not the frequency of social interaction or the number of network partners but rather the quality, emotional meaningfulness, and functional adequacy of enduring close ties that contribute to well-being in late life (Beckman, 1981; Ishii-Kuntz, 1990; Lee & Markides, 1990; Lowenthal & Haven, 1968; Rook, 1984).

7.03.4.2 Social Convoy and Support Efficacy: Maintaining Competence in Late Life

The social convoy model of social relations (Antonucci, 1985, 1990, 1991; Antonucci &

Akiyama, 1987a, 1995; Kahn & Antonucci, 1980) describes a conceptual framework for age-related changes in structural and functional characteristics of social networks. Social convoys serve as a metaphorical illustration of the dynamic and age-related changes in social networks over the life span. Throughout life, individuals construct and maintain social relationships with others who also undergo similar changes in social preferences and social behaviors. This also implies that individuals become increasingly aware of specific strengths and weaknesses of their convoy members over time.

This ever-increasing knowledge base allows people to better select particular social network members for particular functions. In other words, people learn over time who best to turn to when emotional support is needed, which social partners are best able to help with activities of daily living, and who is best suited to help in times of crisis. In short, accumulated expertise about others and about relationship rules grows over a lifetime, further guiding and refining access to potential functions of the social world. Through repeated interactions with others, for example, people learn how to avoid critical or unpleasant issues that could result in conflict or negative outcomes. The importance of social convoys to psychological status may be particularly important in old age when many social structural features of the environment (e.g., work) disappear and self-defining roles (e.g., parent) become less active at an instrumental level.

In addition to the social convoy model, the support-efficacy model of social relationships (Antonucci & Jackson, 1987; Lang, Featherman, & Nesselroade, in press) extends the perspective to the individual's competence and self-efficacy in utilizing social resources. Rather than construing social support as a unidirectional process, the support-efficacy model characterizes social support as a process that depends on the personal characteristics of a target individual and support-giver within a specific social opportunity structure. The support-efficacy model is truly relational in that social support is conceptualized as a social transaction of at least two interaction partners who share a specific relationship. In the support-efficacy model, the support-receiver is considered an active agent in the social support process who exerts influence on when and from whom social support is received. On the one hand, social support can compensate for deficits in competence and thus contribute to the older person's adjustment. For example, Hobfoll (Hobfoll, 1989; Hobfoll & Freedy, 1990) has shown that the more social and personal resources are available, the better older people compensate for age-related losses. On the other hand, relying on social support resources also places specific demands on the older individual such as the normative obligation to reciprocate received supports (Antonucci & Jackson, 1987; Gouldner, 1960; Rook, 1987b; Wentowski, 1981).

7.03.5 CONCLUSIONS AND OUTLOOK

In this chapter, it has been argued that the interplay of changes in relational contexts and relational behaviors in later life may determine negative and positive outcomes of social resources. Thus, social adaptivity in later life depends not just on characteristics of the older individual's relational contexts but also on the older individual's needs and preferences within a given structure of relational opportunities. Negative outcomes of social relationships may be a function of a mismatch between the older individual's relational preferences and individuals' actual relational contexts (Lang & Baltes, in press)

Older individuals contribute actively to the positive and negative outcomes of their social relationships, not only in terms of whom they choose to interact with but also in terms of how they engage in specific relational behaviors. Thus, an older individual may contribute actively to the maximization of positive relational outcomes and the minimization of negative relational outcomes. For example, older individuals are not simply active in help-seeking and solicitation of social support from others (Nadler, 1991), they are also support providers to others with whom they have entertained relationships for many years. Providing social support may be seen as the most pervasive illustration of the individual's active and optimizing role in social relationships. Giving support entails social rewards such as feeling needed, trusted or relied upon by others (Thomae, 1994). This also addresses the transactional nature of social relationships. In most cases, when social partners seek or utilize the older individual's advice or other forms of support, this also conveys some appraisal of the older person's competence and thus contributes to feelings of control and social connectedness. Finally, giving support may also enhance the receiver's willingness to reciprocate support in future and, thus, enhance the stability and closeness of the supportive relationship. In this sense, increasing opportunities for older people to provide social support to other people may also support social functioning in later life.

7.03.6 REFERENCES

Adams, R. G., & Blieszner, R. (1994). An integrative conceptual framework for friendship research. *Journal of Social and Personal Relationships, 11,* 163–184.

Aldous, J. (1987). New views on the family life of the elderly and the near-elderly. *Journal of Marriage and the Family, 49,* 227–234.

Alwin, D. F., Converse, P. E., & Martin, S. S. (1985). Living arrangements and social integration. *Journal of Marriage and the Family, 47,* 319–334.

Antonucci, T. C. (1985). Personal characteristics, social support, and social behavior. In R. H. Binstock & E. Shanas (Eds.), *Handbook of aging and the social sciences* (2nd ed., pp. 94–128). New York: Van Nostrand Reinhold.

Antonucci, T. C. (1990). Social supports and social relationships. In R. H. Binstock & L. K. George (Eds.), *Handbook of aging and the social sciences.* (3rd ed., pp. 205–226). San Diego, CA: Academic Press.

Antonucci, T. C. (1991). Attachment, social support, and coping with negative life events in mature adulthood. In E. M. Cummings, A. L. Greene, & K. H. Karraker (Eds.), *Life-span developmental psychology: Perspectives on stress and coping* (pp. 261–276). Hillsdale, NJ: Lawrence Erlbaum.

Antonucci, T. C., & Akiyama, H. (1987). Social networks in adult life and a preliminary examiation of the convoy model. *Journals of Gerontology, 42,* 519–527.

Antonucci, T. C., & Akiyama, H. (1994). Convoys of attachment and social relations in children, adolescents, and adults. In F. Nestmann & K. Hurrelmann (Eds.), *Social networks and social support in childhood and adolescence* (pp. 37–52). Berlin: de Gruyter.

Antonucci, T. C., & Akiyama, H. (1995). Convoys of social relations: Family and friendships within a life span context. In R. Blieszner & V. H. Bedford (Eds.), *Handbook of aging and the family* (pp. 355–371). Westport, CT: Greenwood Press.

Antonucci, T. C., & Jackson, J. S. (1987). Social support, interpersonal efficacy, and health: A life course perspective. In L. L. Carstensen & B. A. Edelstein (Eds.), *Handbook of clinical gerontology* (pp. 291–311) New York: Pergamon.

Armstrong, M. J., & Goldsteen, K. S. (1990). Friendship support patterns of older American women. *Journal of Aging Studies, 4,* 391–404.

Atchley, R. C. (1993). Continuity theory and the evolution of activity in later adulthood. In J. R.. Kelly (ed.), *Activity and aging: Staying involved in later life* (Suppl. pp. 5–16). Newbury Park, CA: Sage.

Atkins, C. J., Kaplan, R. M., & Toshima, M. T. (1992). Close relationships in the epidemiology of cardiovascular disease. In. W. H. Jones & D. Perlman (Eds.), *Advances in personal relationships* (Vol. 3, pp. 207–231). London: Kingsley.

Avioli, P. S. (1989). The social support functions of siblings in later life: A theoretical model. *American Behavioral Scientist, 33,* 45–57.

Babchuck, N. (1978–79). Aging and primary relations. *International Journal of Aging and Human Development, 9,* 137–151.

Babchuk, N., & Anderson, T. B. (1989). Older widows and married women: Their intimates and confidants. *International Journal of Aging and Human Development, 28,* 21–35.

Baltes, M. M. (1995). Dependency in old age: Gains and losses. *Current Directions in Psychological Science, 4,* 14–19.

Baltes, M. M., & Carstensen, L. L. (1996). The process of successful aging. *Ageing and Society, 16,* 397–422.

Baltes, M. M., Neumann, E. M., & Zank, S. (1994). Maintenance and rehabilitation of independence in old age: An intervention program for staff. *Psychology and Aging, 9,* 179–188

Baltes, M. M., & Silverberg, S. B. (1994). The dynamics between dependency and autonomy: Illustrations across the life-span. In D. L. Featherman, R. M. Lerner, & M. Perlmutter (Eds.), *Life-span development and behavior* (Vol. 12, pp. 41–90). Hillsdale, NJ: Erlbaum.

Bandura, A. (1982). Self-efficacy mechanism in human agency. *American Psychologist, 37,* 122–147.

Barefoot, J. C., Siegler, I. C., Nowlin, J. B., Peterson, B. L., Haney, T. L., & Williams, R. B. (1987). Suspiciousness, health, and mortality: A follow-up study of 500 older adults. *Psychosomatic Medicine, 49,* 450–457.

Bass, D. M., & Bowman, K. (1990). The transition from caregiving to bereavement: The relationship of care-related strain and adjustment to death. *The Gerontologist, 30,* 35–44.

Bass, D. M., Bowman, K., & Noelker, L. S. (1991). The influence of caregiving and bereavement support on adjusting to an older relative's death. *The Gerontologist, 31,* 32–42.

Beckman, L. J. (1981). Effects of social interaction and children's relative inputs on older women's psychological well-being. *Journal of Personality and Social Psychology, 41,* 1075–1086.

Bedford, V. H. (1995). Sibling relationships in middle and old age. In R. Blieszner & V. H. Bedford (Eds.), *Handbook of aging and the family* (pp. 201–222). Westport, CT: Greenwood Press.

Bengtson, V. L. (1985). Diversity and symbolism in grandparental roles. In V. L. Bengtson & J. F. Robertson (Eds.), *Grandparenthood* (pp. 11–26). Beverly Hills, CA: Sage.

Berkman, L. F. (1985). The relationship of social networks and social support to morbidity and mortality. In S. Cohen & S. L. Syme (Eds.), *Social support and health* (pp. 241–262). New York: Academic Press.

Berkman, L. F., & Syme, S. L. (1979). Social networks, host resistance, and mortality: A nine-year follow-up study of Alameda County residents. *American Journal of Epidemiology, 109,* 186–204.

Blau, Z.S. (1973). *Old age in a changing society.* New York: Franklin Watts.

Bolger, N., & Kelleher, S. (1993). Daily life in relationships. In S. Duck (Eds.), *Social context and relationships* (pp. 100–108). Newbury Park, CA: Sage.

Bosse, R., Aldwin, C. M., Levenson, M. R., Spiro A. III, & Mroczek, D. K. (1993). Change in social support after retirement: Longitudinal findings from the normative aging study. *Journal of Gerontology: Psychological Sciences, 48,* P210–P217.

Bowling, A. (1988–89). Who dies after widow(er)hood? A discriminant analysis. *Omega: Journal of Death and Dying, 19,* 135–153.

Bowling, A. (1994). Social networks and social support among older people and implications for emotional well-being and psychiatric morbidity. *International Review of Psychiatry, 6,* 41–58.

Bowling, A., & Browne, P. D. (1991). Social networks, health, and emotional well-being among the oldest old in London. *Journal of Gerontology: Psychological Sciences, 46,* S20–32.

Bowling, A., & Windsor, J. (1995). Death after widow(er)-hood: An analysis of mortality rates up to 13 years after bereavement. *Omega: Journal of Death and Dying, 31,* 35–49.

Broadhead, W. E., Kaplan, B. H., James, S. A., Wagner, E. H., Schoenbach, V. J., Grimson, R., Heyden, S., Tibblin, G., & Gehlback, S. H. (1983). The epidemiologic evidence for a relationship between social support and health. *American Journal of Epidemiology, 117,* 521–537.

Brody, E. M. (1985). Parent care as a normative family stress. *Gerontologist, 25,* 19–29.

Brubaker, T. H. (1990). Families in later life: A burgeoning research area. *Journal of Marriage and the Family, 52*, 959–981.

Bryant, S., & Rakowski, W. (1992). Predictors of mortality among elderly African-Americans. *Research on Aging, 14*, 50-67.

Cantor, M. H. (1979). Neighbors and friends: An overlooked resource in the informal support system. *Research on Aging, 1*, 434–463.

Caplan, G. (1982). The family as a support system. In H. I. McCubbin, A. E. Cauble & J. E. Patterson (Eds.), *Family stress, coping, and social support* (pp. 200–220). Springfield, IL: Thomas.

Carp, F. M. (Ed.) (1972). *Retirement*. New York: Behavioral Publications.

Carpenter, B. N. (1993). Relational competence. In D. Perlman & W. H. Jones (Eds.), *Advances in personal relationships* (Vol. 4, pp. 1–28). London: Kingsley.

Carstensen, L. L. (1987). Age-related changes in social activity. In L. L. Carstensen & B. A. Edelstein (Eds.), *Handbook of clinical gerontology* (pp. 222–237). New York: Pergamon.

Carstensen, L. L. (1991). Socioemotional selectivity theory: Social activity in life-span context. *Annual Review of Gerontology and Geriatrics, 11*, 195–217.

Carstensen, L. L. (1992). Social and emotional patterns in adulthood: Support for socioemotional selectivity theory. *Psychology and Aging, 7*, 331–338.

Carstensen, L. L. (1993a). Motivation for social contact across the life span: A theory of sociomotional selectivity. *Nebraska symposium on motivation* (pp. 209–254). Lincoln, NE: University of Nebraska Press.

Carstensen, L. L. (1993b). Perspective on research with older families: Contributions of older adults to families and to family theory. In P. Cowan, D. Field, D. Hansen, A. Skolnick, & G. E. Swanson (Eds.), *Family, self, and society: Toward a new agenda for family research* (pp. 353–359). Hillsdale, NJ: Lawrence Erlbaum.

Carstensen, L. L. (1995). Evidence for a life-span theory of socioemotional selectivity. *Current directions in Psychological Science, 5*, 151–156.

Carstensen, L. L., & Lang, F. R. (in preparation). *Social preferences and social contact behavior from early to late adulthood.* Stanford University.

Carstensen, L. L., & Lang, F. R. (in press). Social relationships in context and as context: Social support and the maintenance of competence in old age. In S. Willis, K. W. Schaie, & M. Hayward (Eds.), *Societal mechanisms for maintaining competence in old age* (pp. 207–222). New York: Springer.

Carstensen, L. L., Gottman, J. M., & Levenson, R. W. (1995). Emotional behavior in long-term marriage. *Psychology and Aging, 10*, 140–149.

Caspi, A., Bolger, N. & Eckenrode, J. (1987). Linking person and context in the daily stress process. *Journal of Personality and Social Psychology, 52*, 184–195.

Chappell, N. L. (1990). Aging and social care. In R. H. Binstock & L. K. George (Eds.), *Handbook of aging and the social sciences* (3rd ed., pp. 438–454). San Diego, CA: Academic Press.

Chappell, N. L. (1991). Living arrangements and sources of caregiving. *Journal of Gerontology: Social Sciences, 46*, S1–8.

Chappell, N. L., & Badger, M. (1989). Social isolation and well-being. *Journal of Gerontology: Social Sciences, 44*, 5169–5176

Chatters, L. M., Taylor, R. J., & Jackson, J. S. (1986). Aged blacks' choices for an informal helper network. *Journal of Gerontology, 41*, 94–100.

Cicirelli, V. G. (1989). Feelings of attachment to siblings and well-being in later life. *Psychology and Aging, 4*, 211–216.

Cicirelli, V. G. (1995). *Sibling relationships across the life span.* New York : Plenum.

Cohen, C. I., Teresi, J., & Holmes, D. (1986–87). Social networks and mortality in an inner-city elderly population. *International Journal of Aging and Human Development, 24*, 257–269.

Cohen, S., & Wills, T. A. (1985). Stress, social support, and the buffering hypothesis. *Psychological Bulletin, 98*, 310–357.

Connidis, I. A. (1989). Siblings as friends in later life. *American Behavioral Scientist, 33*, 81–93.

Connidis, I. A. (1994). Sibling support in older age. *Journals of Gerontology: Social Sciences, 49*, S309–S317.

Connidis, I. A., & Davis, L. (1992). Confidants and companions: Choices in later life. *Journal of Gerontology: Social Sciences, 47*, S115–122.

Connidis, I. A., & McMullin, J. A. (1993). To have or have not: Parent status and the subjective well-being of older men and women. *The Gerontologist, 33*, 630–636.

Connidis, I. A., & McMullin, J. A. (1994). Social support in older age: Assessing the impact of marital and parent status. *Canadian Journal on Aging, 13*, 510–527.

Costa, P. T., & McCrae, R. R. (1994). Set like plaster: Evidence for the stability of adult personality. In T. F. Heatherton & J. L. Weinberger (Eds.), *Can personality change?* (pp. 21–40). Washington, DC: APA.

Coyne, J. C. (1976). Depression and the response of others. *Journal of Abnormal Psychology, 85*, 186–193.

Coyne, J. C., Wortman, C. B., & Lehmann, D. R. (1988). The other side of support. Emotional overinvolvement and miscarried helping. In B. H. Gottlieb (Ed.), *Marshaling social support. Formats, processes, and effects* (pp. 305–330). Newbury Park, CA: Sage.

Cramer, D. (1993). Personality and marital dissolution. *Personality and Individual Differences, 14*, 605–607.

Crohan, S. E., & Antonucci, T. C. (1989). Friends as a source of social support in old age. In R. G. Adams & R. Blieszner (Eds.), *Older adult friendship: Structure and process* (pp. 129–146). Newbury Park, CA: Sage.

Cumming, E., & Henry, W. E. (1961). *Growing old: The process of disengagement.* New York: Basic Books.

Cutrona, C. E., Cohen, B. B., & Igram, S. (1990). Contextual determinants of the perceived supportiveness of helping behaviors. *Journal of Social and Personal Relationships, 7*, 553–562.

Dean, A., Matt, G. E., & Wood, P. (1992). The effects of widowhood on social support from significant others. *Journal of Community Psychology, 20*, 309–325.

Depner, C. E., & Ingersoll-Dayton, B. (1985). Conjugal social support: Patterns in later life. *Journal of Gerontology, 40*, 761–766.

Duck, S. (1986). *Human relationships: An introduction to social psychology.* London: Sage.

Dunkel-Schetter, C., & Bennett, T. L. (1990). Differentiating the cognitive and behavioral aspects of social support. In B. R. Sarason, I. G. Sarason, & G. R. Pierce (Eds.), *Social support: An interactional view* (pp. 267–296). New York: Wiley.

Dunkel -Schetter, C., Folkman, S., & Lazarus, R. S. (1987). Correlates of social support receipt. *Journal of Personality and Social Psychology, 53*, 71–80.

Dykstra, P. A. (1993). The differential availability of relationships and the provision and effectiveness of support to older adults. *Journal of Social and Personal Relationships, 10*, 355–370.

Dykstra, P. A. (1995). Loneliness among the never and formerly married: The importance of supportive friendships and a desire for independence. *Journals of Gerontology: Series B, Psychological and Social Sciences, 50B*, S321–S329.

Eggebeen, D. J. (1992). From generation unto generation: Parent-child support in aging American families. *Generations, 16*, 45–49.

Eggebeen, D. J., & Hogan, D. P. (1990). Giving between the generations in American families. *Human Nature, 1,* 211–232.

Felton, B. J., & Berry, C. A. (1992). Do the sources of the urban elderly's social support determine its psychological consequences? *Psychology & Aging, 7,* 89–97.

Ferraro, K. F., & Barresi, C. M. (1982). The impact of widowhood on the social relations of older people. *Research on Aging, 4,* 227–247.

Ferraro, K. F., & Farmer, M. M. (1995). Social compensation in adulthood and later life. In R. Dixon & L. Bäckman (Eds.), *Compensating for psychological deficits and declines* (pp. 127–145). Hillsdale, NJ: Erlbaum.

Field, D., & Minkler, M. (1988). Continuity and change in social support between young-old and old-old or very-old age. *Journals of Gerontology: Psychological Sciences, 43* (4), P100–106.

Field, D., & Minkler, M. (1993). The importance of family in advanced old age: The family is "forever" In P. Cowan, D. Field, D. Hansen, A. Skolnick, & G. E. Swanson (Eds.), *Family, self, and society: Toward a new agenda for family research* (pp. 331–351). Hillsdale, NJ: Lawrence Erlbaum.

Field, D., Minkler, M., Falk, R. F., & Leino, E. V. (1993). The influence of health on family contacts and family feelings in advanced old age: A longitudinal study. *Journal of Gerontology: Psychological Sciences, 48,* P18–P28.

Filipp, S. H., & Aymanns, P. (1987). Die Bedeutung sozialer und personaler Ressourcen in der Auseinandersetzung mit kritischen Lebensereignissen [The significance of social and personal resources in dealing with critical life events]. *Zeitschrift fur Klinische Psychologie, 16,* 383–396.

Finch, J. F., Okun, M. A., Barrera, M., Zautra, A., & Reich, J. W. (1989). Positive and negative social ties among older adults: Measurement models and the prediction of psychological distress and well-being. *American Journal of Community Psychology, 17,* 585–605.

Fisher, J. D., Nadler, A., & Whitcher-Alagna, S. (1982). Recipient reactions to aid. *Psychological Bulletin, 91,* 27–54.

Franks, M. M., & Stephens, M. A. P. (1996). Social support in the context of caregiving: Husbands' provision of support to wives involved in parent care. *Journals of Gerontology: Psychological Sciences, 51B,* P43–P52.

Fredrickson, B. L., & Carstensen, L. L. (1990). Choosing social partners: How old age and anticipated endings make people more selective. *Psychology and Aging, 5,* 335–347.

Friedman, H. S., Tucker, J. S., Schwartz, J. E., Tomlinson-Keasy, C., Martin, L. R., Wingard, D. L., & Criqui, M. H. (1995). Psychosocial and behavioral predictors of longevity: The aging and death of the Termites. *American Psychologist, 50,* 69–78.

Ganster, D. C. , & Victor, B. (1988). The impact of social support on mental and physical health. *British Journal of Medical Psychology, 61,* 17–36.

Garrett, J. E. (1987). Multiple losses in older adults. *Journal of Gerontological Nursing, 13,* 8–12.

George, L. K., & Gwyther, L. P. (1986). Caregiver well-being: A multidimensional examination of family caregivers of demented adults. *Gerontologist, 26,* 253–259.

Goetting, A. (1986). The developmental tasks of siblingship over the life cycle. *Journal of Marriage and the Family, 48,* 703–714.

Gold, D. T. (1987). Siblings in old age: Something special. *Canadian Journal on Aging, 6,* 199–215.

Gordon, C., & Gaitz, C. (1976). Leisure and lives. In R. Binstock & E. Shanas (Eds.), *Handbook of aging and the social sciences* (Vol. 1, pp. 310–341). New York: Van Nostrand Reinhold.

Gotlib, I. H., & Hooley, J. M. (1988). Depression and marital distress: Current status and future directions. In S. Duck (Ed.), *Handbook of personal relationships: Theory, research and interventions* (pp. 543–570). Chichester, UK: Wiley.

Gotlib, I. H., & Whiffen, V. E. (1992). The interpersonal context of depression. In W. H. Jones & D. Perlman (Eds.), *Advances in personal relationships* (Vol. 3, pp. 177–206). London: Kingsley.

Gottlieb, B. H. (1983). Social support as a focus for integrative research in psychology. *American Psychologist, 38,* 278–287.

Gottman, J. M., & Levenson, R. W. (1992). Marital processes predictive of later dissolution: Behavior, physiology, and health. *Journal of Personality and Social Psychology, 63,* 221–233.

Gouldner, A. W. (1960). The norm of reciprocity: A preliminary statement. *American Sociological Review, 25,* 161–178.

Hagestad, G. O. (1985). Continuity and connectedness. In V. L. Bengtson & J. F. Robertson (Eds.), *Grandparenthood* (pp. 31–48). Beverly Hills, CA: Sage.

Hagestad, G. O. (1987). Parent-child relations in later life: Trends and gaps in past research. In J. B. Lancaster, J. Altmann, A. S. Rossi, & L. R. Sherrod (Eds.), *Parenting across the life span: Biosocial dimensions.* New York: Aldine de Gruyter.

Hammer, M. (1983). "Core" and "extended" social networks in relation to health and illness. *Social Science and Medicine, 17,* 405–411.

Hammond, R. J., & Muller, G. O. (1992). The late-life divorced: Another look. *Journal of Divorce & Remarriage, 17,* 135–150.

Hanson, B. S., Isacsson, S.-O., Janzon, L., & Lindell, S.-E. (1990). Social network and social support influence mortality in elderly men. *Advances, 7,* 16–18.

Hansson, R. O., & Carpenter, B. N. (1994). *Relationships in old age: Coping with the challenge of transition.* New York: Guilford.

Hansson, R. O., Jones, W. H., & Fletcher, W. L. (1990). Troubled relationships in later life: Implications for support. *Journal of Social and Personal Relationships, 7,* 451–463.

Harvey, A. S., & Singleton, J. F. (1989). Canadian activity patterns across the life span: A time budget perspective. *Canadian Journal on Aging, 8,* 268–285.

Hautzinger, M., Linden, M., & Hoffman, N. (1982). Distressed couples with and without a depressed partner: An analysis of their verbal interaction. *Journal of Behavior Therapy and Experimental Psychology, 13,* 307–314.

Havighurst, R. J., & Albrecht, R. (1953). *Older people.* New York: Longmans.

Havighurst, R., Neugarten, B., & Tobin, S. (1968). Disengagement and patterns of aging. In B. Neugarten (Ed.), *Middle age and aging* (pp. 161–172). Chicago, IL: University of Chicago Press.

Havighurst, R., Munnichs, J. M. A., Neugarten, B., & Thomae, H. (Eds.) (1969), *Adjustment to retirement: A crossnational study.* Assen,The Netherlands: Van Gorcum.

Heckhausen, J., & Lang, F. R. (1996). Social construction in old age: Normative conceptions and interpersonal processes. In G. R. Semin & K. Fiedler (Eds.), *Applied social psychology* (pp. 374–398). London: Sage.

Helgeson, V. S., & Cohen, S. (1996). Social support and adjustment to cancer: Reconciling descriptive, correlational, and intervention research. *Health Psychology, 15,* 135–148.

Heller, K., & Mansbach, W. E. (1984). The multifaceted nature of social support in a community sample of elderly women. *Journal of Social Issues, 40,* 99–113.

Henderson, A. S., Scott, R., & Kay, D. W. (1986). The

elderly who live alone: Their mental health and social relationships. *Australian and New Zealand Journal of Psychiatry, 20,* 202–209.

Herman, S. M. (1994). Marital satisfaction in the elderly. *Gerontology and Geriatrics Education, 14,* 69–79.

Herzog, R. A., & Rodgers, W. L. (1981). Age and satisfaction: Data from several large surveys. *Research on Aging, 3,* 142–165.

Hess, B. B., & Soldo, B. J. (1985). Husband and wife networks. In W. J. Sauer & R. T. Coward (Eds.), *Social support networks and care of the elderly: Theory, research, and practice* (pp. 67–92). New York: Springer.

Hobfoll, S. E. (1989). Conservation of resources. A new attempt at conceptualizing stress. *American Psychologist, 44,* 513–524.

Hobfoll, S. E., & Freedy, J. R. (1990). The availability and effective use of social support. *Journal of Social and Clinical Psychology, 9,* 91–103.

Hodgson, L. G. (1992). Adult grandchildren and their grandparents: Their enduring bond. *International Journal of Aging and Human Development, 34,* 209–225.

Hogan, D. P. (1995). Sources of emergency help and routine assistance in old age. *Social Forces, 73,* 917–936.

Hogg, J. R., & Heller, K. (1990). A measure of relational competence for community-dwelling elderly. *Psychology and Aging, 5,* 580–588.

Holahan, C. J., Moos, R. H., Holahan, C. K., & Brennan, P. L. (1995). Social support, coping, and depressive symptoms in a late-middle-aged sample of patients reporting cardiac illness. *Health Psychology, 14,* 152–163.

Holmes, J. G. (1991). Trust and the appraisal process in close relationships. In W. H. Jones & D. Perlman (Eds.), *Advances in personal relationships: A research annual* (Vol. 2, pp. 57–104). London, Kingsley.

Holmes, T., & Rahe, R. (1967). The social readjustment rating scale. *Journal of Psychosomatic Research, 11,* 213–218.

Horowitz, A. (1985). Family caregiving to the frail elderly. In C. Eisdorfer (Ed.), *Annual review of gerontology and geriatrics* (Vol. 5, pp. 194–246). New York: Springer.

House, J. S., & Kahn, R. L. (1985). Measures and concepts of social support. In S. Cohen & S. L. Syme (Eds.), *Social support and health* (pp. 83–105). New York: Academic Press.

House, J. S., Robbins, C., & Metzner, H. M. (1982). The association of social relationships and activities with mortality: Prospective evidence from the Tecumset Community Health Study. *American Journal of Epidemiology, 116,* 123–140.

House, J. S., Umberson, D., & Landis, K. R. (1988). Structures and processes of social support. *Annual Review of Sociology, 14,* 293–318.

Huyck, M. H. (1995). Marriage and close relationships of the marital kind. In R. Blieszner & V. H. Bedford (Eds.), *Handbook of aging and the family* (pp. 181–200). Westport, CT: Greenwood Press.

Ikels, C. (1988). Delayed reciprocity and the support networks of the childless elderly. *Journal of Comparative Family Studies, 19,* 99–112.

Ishii-Kuntz, M. (1990). Social interaction and psychological well-being: Comparison across stages of adulthood. *International Journal of Aging and Human Development, 30,* 1, 15–36.

Johnson, C. L. (1983). Fairweather friends and rainy day kin: An anthropological analysis of old age friendship in the United States. *Urban Anthropology, 12,* 103–123.

Johnson, C. L., & Catalano, D. J. (1983). A longitudinal study of family support to impaired elderly. *The Gerontologist, 23,* 612–618.

Johnson, C. L., & Troll, L. E. (1992). Family functioning in late late life. *Journals of Gerontology: Social Sciences, 47,* S66–S72.

Johnson, C. L., & Troll, L. E. (1994). Constraints and facilitators to friendships in late life. *The Gerontologist, 34,* 79–87.

Jones, D. C., & Vaughan, K. (1990). Close friendships among senior adults. *Psychology and Aging, 5,* 451–457.

Jung, J. (1990). The role of reciprocity in social support. *Basic and Applied Social Psychology, 11,* 243–253.

Kahn, R. L. (1979). Aging and social support. In M. W. Riley (Ed.), *Aging from birth to death: Interdisciplinary perspectives* (pp. 77–91). Boulder, CO: Westview Press.

Kahn, R. L., & Antonucci, T. C. (1980). Convoys over the life course. Attachment, roles and social support. In P. B. Baltes & O. G. Brim (Eds.), *Life-span development and behavior* (pp. 254–283). New York: Academic Press.

Keith, P. M. (1986). Isolation of the unmarried in later life. *Family Relations: Journal of Applied Family and Child Studies, 35,* 389–395.

Keith, P. M., Hill, K., Goudy, W. J., & Powers, E. A. (1984). Confidants and well-being: A note on male friendship in old age. *The Gerontologist, 24,* 318– 320.

Kennedy, G. E. (1992). Quality in grandparent/grandchild relationships. *International Journal of Aging and Human Development, 35,* 83–98

Kennedy, S., Kiecolt-Glaser, J. K., & Glaser, R. (1990). Social support, stress, and the immune system. In B. R. Sarason, I. G. Sarason, G. R. Pierce (Eds.), *Social support: An interactional view* (pp. 253–266). New York: Wiley.

Kessler, R. C., & McLeod, J. D. (1985). Social support and mental health in community samples. In S. Cohen & S. L. Syme (Eds.). *Social support and health* (pp. 219–240). New York: Academic Press.

Kivnick, H. Q. (1982). *The meaning of grandparenthood.* Ann Arbor, MI: UMI Research Press.

Krause, N. (1994). Stressors in salient social roles and well-being in later life. *Journal of Gerontology: Psychological Sciences, 49,* P137–148.

Krause, N., Herzog, A. R., & Baker, E. (1992). Providing support to others and well-being in later life. *Journals of Gerontology, 47,* P300–P311.

Kriegsman, D. M. W., Penninx, B. W. H. J., & van Eijk, J. T. M. (1995). A criterion-based literature survey of the relationship between family support and incidence and course of chronic disease in the elderly. *Family Systems Medicine, 13,* 39–68.

Kurdek, L. A. (1991). Marital stability and changes in marital quality in newly wed couples: A test of the contextual model. *Journal of Social and Personal Relationships, 8,* 27–48.

Lang, F. R. (1994). *Die Gestaltung informeller Hilfebeziehungen im hohen Alter - Die Rolle von Elternschaft und Kinderlosigkeit* [Social support management in late life- The role of parenthood and childlessness]. Berlin: Edition Sigma (Max-Planck-Institut für Bildungsforschung, Studien und Berichte, Band 59).

Lang, F. R. (1996). Social support relationships of parents and non-parents in old and very old age. In H. Mollenkopf (Ed.), *Elderly people in industrialised societies: Social integration in old age by or despite technology* (pp. 43–54). Berlin: Edition Sigma.

Lang, F. R., & Baltes, M. M. (1997). Brauchen alte Menschen junge Menschen? Überlegungen zu den Entwicklungsaufgaben imhohen Lebensalter [Do older people need young people? Considerations about the developmental tasks in late life]. In L. Krappmann (Ed.), *Alt und Jung: Spannungen und solidaritaet zwischen den Generationen* (pp. 161–184). Frankfurt: Campus.

Lang, F. R., & Baltes, M. M. (in press). Being with people and being alone in late life: Costs and benefits for everyday functioning. *International Journal of Behavioral Development.*

Lang, F. R., & Carstensen, L. L. (1994). Close emotional relationships in late life: Further support for proactive aging in the social domain. *Psychology and Aging, 9,* 315–324.

Lang, F. R., Featherman, D. L., & Nesselroade, J. R. (in press). Social self efficacy and short-term variability in personal relationships: The MacArthur Successful Aging Studies. *Psychology and Aging.*

Lang, F. R., Staudinger, U. M., & Carstensen, L. L. (1996). Perspectives on socioemotional selectivity in late life: How personality does (and does not) make a difference. *Journal of Gerontology: Psychological Science.*

Lang, F. R., & Tesch-Römer, C. (1993). Erfolgreiches Altern und soziale Beziehungen: Selektion und Kompensation im sozialen Kontaktverhalten [Successful aging and social relationships: Selection and compensation in social contact behavior]. *Zeitschrift für Gerontologie, 26,* 321–329.

Langer, N. (1990). Grandparents and adult grandchildren: What do they do for one another? *International Journal of Aging and Human Development, 31,* 101–110.

Larson, R. W. (1990). The solitary side of life: An examination of the time people spend alone from childhood to old age. *Developmental Review, 10,* 155–183.

Larson, R., Mannell, R., & Zuzanek, J. (1986). Daily well-being of older adults with friends and family. *Psychology and Aging, 1,* 117–126.

Lawton, M. P. (1989). Behavior-relevant ecological factors. In K. W. Schaie & C. Schooler (Eds.), *Social structure and aging: Psychological processes* (pp. 57–78). Hillsdale, NJ: Lawrence Erlbaum.

Lawton, M. P., Moss, M., & Fulcomer, M. (1986–87). Objective and subjective uses of time by older people. *International Journal of Aging and Human Development, 24,* 171–188.

Lee, G. R. (1985).Theoretical perspectives on social networks. In W. J. Sauer & R. T. Coward (Eds.), *Social support networks and the care of the elderly: Theory, research, and practice* (pp. 21–37). New York: Springer.

Lee, D. J., & Markides, K. S. (1990). Activity and mortality among aged persons over an eight-year period. *The Journals of Gerontology: Social Sciences, 45,* S39–S42.

Lehr, U., & Minnemann, E. (1987). Veränderung von Quantität und Qualität sozialer Kontakte vom 7. bis 9. Lebensjahrzehnt [Changes of quantity and quality of social contact from the 7th to the 9th decade of life]. In U.Lehr & H. Thomae (Eds.), *Formen seelischen Alterns. Ergebnisse der Bonner Gerontologischen Längsschnittstudie* (pp. 80–91). Stuttgart: Enke.

Lemon, B. W., Bengtson, V. L., Peterson, I. A. (1972). An exploration of the activity theory of aging: Activity types and life satisfaction among inmovers to a retirement community. *Journal of Gerontology, 27,* 511–523.

Levenson, R. W., Carstensen, L. L., & Gottman, J. M. (1993). Long-term marriage: Age, gender, and satisfaction. *Psychology and Aging, 8,* 301–313.

Levenson, R. W., Carstensen, L. L.. & Gottman, J. M. (1994). The influence of age and gender on affect, physiology, and their interrelations: A study of long-term marriages. *Journal of Personality and Social Psychology, 67,* 56–68.

Levitt, M. J., Weber, R. A., & Guacci, N. (1993). Convoys of social support: An intergenerational analysis. *Psychology and Aging, 8,* 323–326.

Litwak, E. (1985). *Helping the elderly.* New York: Guilford.

Lopata, H. Z. (1986). Becoming and being a widow: Reconstruction of the self and support systems. *Journal of Geriatric Psychiatry, 19,* 203–214.

Lowenthal, M. F., & Haven, C. (1968). Interaction and adaptation: Intimacy as a critical variable. *American Sociological Review, 33,* 20–30.

Lowenthal, M. F., Thurnher, M., & Chiriboga, D. (1976). *Four stages of life : A comparative study of women and men facing transitions.* San Francisco: Jossey-Bass.

Maddox, G. L. (1963). Activity and morale: A longitudinal study of selected elderly subjects. *Social Forces, 42,* 195–204.

Mancini, J. A. & Blieszner, R. (1989).Aging parents and adult children: Research themes in intergenerational relations. *Journal of Marriage and the Family, 51,* 275–290.

Markides, K. S., Boldt, J. S., & Ray, L. A. (1986). Sources of helping and intergenerational solidarity: A three-generations study of Mexican Americans. *Journal of Gerontology, 41,* 506–511.

Marsiske, M., Lang, F. R., Baltes, P. B., & Baltes, M. M. (1995). Selective optimization with compensation: Life-span perspectives on successful human development. In R. Dixon & L. Bäckman (Eds.), *Compensating for psychological deficits and declines* (pp. 35–79). Hillsdale, NJ: Erlbaum.

McAdams, D. P. , de St. Aubin, E., & Logan, R. L. (1993). Generativity among young, midlife, and older adults. *Psychology and Aging, 8,* 221–230.

Medalie, J., & Goldbourt, V. (1976). Angina pectoris among 10,000 men: Psychosocial and other risk factors as evidenced by a multivariate analysis of a five-year incidence study. *American Journal of Medicine, 60,* 910–924.

Miller, S. S., & Cavanaugh, J. C. (1990). The meaning of grandparenthood and its relationship to demographic, relationship, and social participation variables. *Journals of Gerontology: Psychological Sciences, 45,* P244–P246.

Morgan, D. L. (1989). Adjusting to widowhood: Do social networks really make it easier? *The Gerontologist. 29,* 101–107.

Morgan, D. L. (1990). Combining the strengths of social networks, social support, and personal relationships. In S. Duck & R. C. Silver (Eds.), *Personal relationships and social support* (pp. 190–215). Newbury Park, CA: Sage.

Moss, M. S., Lesher, E., & Moss, S. Z. (1986–87). Impact of the death of an adult child on elderly parents: Some observations. *Omega: Journal of Death and Dying, 17,* 209–218.

Moss, S. Z., & Moss, M. S. (1989). The impact of the death of an elderly sibling. *American Behavioral Scientist, 33,* 94–106.

Mullan, J. T. (1992). The bereaved caregiver: A prospective study of changes in well-being. *The Gerontologist, 32,* 673–683.

Mullins, L. C., & Mushel, M. (1992). The existence and emotional closeness of relationships with children, friends, and spouses: The effect of loneliness among older persons. *Research on Aging, 14,* 448–470.

Mullins, L. C., Sheppard, H. L., & Andersson, L. (1991). Loneliness and social isolation in Sweden: Differences in age, sex, labor force status, self-rated health, and income adequacy. *Journal of Applied Gerontology, 10,* 455–468.

Nadler, A. (1991). Help-seeking behavior: Psychological costs and instrumental benefits. In M. S. Clark (Ed.), *Prosocial behavior* (pp. 290–311). Newbury Park, CA: Sage.

O'Bryant, S. L. (1988). Sibling support and older widows' well-being. *Journal of Marriage and the Family, 50,* 173–184.

Okun, M. A., Melichar, J. F., & Hill, M. D. (1990). Negative daily events, positive and negative social ties, and psychological distress among older adults. *The Gerontologist, 30,* 193–199.

Olsen, R. B., Olsen, J., Gunner-Svensson, F., & Waldstrom, B. (1991). Social networks and longevity: A 14 year follow-up study among elderly in Denmark. *Social Science and Medicine, 33,* 1189–1195.

Orth-Gomer, K., & Johnson, J. V. (1987). Social network interaction and mortality: A six-year follow-up study of a random sample of the Swedish population. *Journal of Chronic Diseases, 40,* 949–957.

Osgood, N. J. (1989). Theory and research in social gerontology. In N. J. Osgood & A. H. L. Sontz (Eds.), *The science and practice of gerontology. A multidisciplinary guide* (pp. 55–87). New York: Greenwood Press.

Page, R. M., & Cole, G. E. (1991). Demographic predictors of self-reported loneliness in adults. *Psychological Reports, 68,* 939–945.

Palmore, E. (1981). *Social patterns in normal aging: Findings from the Duke Longitudinal Study.* Durham, NC: Duke University Press.

Pearlin, L. I., Mullan, J. T., Semple, S. J., & Skaff, M. M. (1990). Caregiving and the stress process: An overview of concepts and their measures. *The Gerontologist, 30,* 583–594.

Peters, G. R., & Kaiser, M. A. (1985). The role of friends and neighbors in providing social support. In W. J. Sauer & R. T. Coward (Eds.), *Social support networks and care of the elderly: Theory, research, and practice* (pp. 123–158). New York: Springer.

Pillemer, K., & Finkelhor, D. (1988). The prevalence of elder abuse: A random sample survey. *The Gerontologist, 28,* 51–57.

Pillemer, K., & Suitor, J. J. (1992). Violence and violent feelings: What causes them among family caregivers? *Journals of Gerontology, 47,* S165–S172.

Pratt, M. W., & Norris, J. E. (1994). *The social psychology of aging.* Oxford: Blackwell.

Pruchno, R. A., Peters, N. D., & Burant, C. J. (1995). Mental health of coresident family caregivers: Examination of a two-factor model. *Journal of Gerontology: Psychological Sciences, 50B,* P247–P256.

Pulakos, J. (1987). Brothers and sisters: Nature and importance of the adult bond. *Journal of Psychology, 121,* 521–522.

Query, J. L., & James, A. C. (1989). The relationship between interpersonal communication competence and social support among elderly support groups in retirement communities. *Health Communication, 1,* 165–184.

Ramirez-Barranti, C. C. (1985). The grandparent-grandchild relationship: Family resource in an era of voluntary bonds. *Family Relations: Journal of Applied Family and Child Studies, 34,* 343–352.

Rawlins, W. K. (1992). *Friendship matters. Communication, dialectics, and the life course.* New York: de Gruyter.

Reifman, A. (1995). Social relationships, recovery from illness, and survival: A literature review. *Annals of Behavioral Medicine, 17,* 124–131.

Revenson, T. A., & Johnson, J. (1984). Social and demographic corelates of loneliness in late life. *American Journal of Community Psychology, 12,* 71–85.

Riley, D., & Eckenrode, J. (1986). Social ties: Subgroup differences in costs and benefits. *Journal of Personality and Social Psychology, 51,* 770–778.

Roberto, K. A. (1989). Exchange and equity in friendships. In R. G. Adams & R. Blieszner (Eds.), *Older adult friendship: Structure and process* (pp. 147–165) London: Sage.

Roberto, K. A., & Scott, J. P. (1986a). Equity Considerations in the friendships of older adults. *Journal of Gerontology, 41,* 241–247.

Roberto, K. A., & Scott, J. P. (1986b). Friendships of older men and women: Exchange patterns and satisfaction. *Psychology and Aging, 1,* 103–109.

Roberto, K. A., & Scott, J. P. (1987). Friendships in late life: A rural–urban comparison. *Lifestyles, 8,* 16–26.

Roberto, K. A., & Stanis, P. I. (1994). Reactions of older women to the death of their close friends. *Omega: Journal of Death and Dying, 29,* 17–27.

Röhrle, B. (1994). *Soziale Netzwerke und soziale Unterstützung [Social networks and social support].* Munich: Beltz.

Rook, K. S. (1984). The negative side of social interaction: Impact on psychological well-being. *Journal of Personality and Social Psychology, 46,* 1097–1108.

Rook, K. S. (1987a). Social support versus companionship: Effects on life stress, loneliness, and evaluations by others. *Journal of Personality and Social Psychology, 52,* 1132–1147.

Rook, K. S. (1987b). Reciprocity of social exchange and social satisfaction among older women. *Journal of Personality and Social Psychology, 52,* 145–154.

Rook, K. S. (1989). Strains in older adults' friendship. In R. G. Adams & R. Blieszner (Eds.), *Older adult friendship: Structure and process* (pp. 166–194). Newbury Park, CA: Sage.

Rook, K. S., & Pietromonaco, P. (1987). Close relationships: Ties that heal or ties that bind. In W. H. Jones & D. Perlman (Eds.), *Advances in personal relationships* (Vol. 1, pp. 1–35). Greenwich, CT: JAI Press.

Rose, J. H. (1993). Interactions between patients and providers: An exploratory study of age differences in emotional support. *Journal of Psychosocial Oncology, 11,* 43–67.

Rosow, I. (1975). *Socialization to old age.* Berkeley, CA: University of California Press.

Rosow, I. (1982). Intergenerational perspectives on aging. In G. Lesnoff-Caravaglia (Ed.), *Aging and the human condition* (pp. 40–53). New York: Human Sciences Press.

Rossi, A., & Rossi, P. (1990). *Of human bonding: Parent child-relations across the life course.* Hawthorne, NY: Aldine and Gruyter.

Rubin, S. S. (1991–92). Adult child loss and the two track model of bereavement. *Omega: Journal of Death and Dying, 24,* 183–202.

Ruscher, S. M., & Gotlib, I. H. (1988). Marital interaction patterns of couples with and without a depressed partner. *Behavior Therapy, 19,* 455–470.

Ryff, C. D. (1989). Beyond Ponce de Leon and life satisfaction: New directions in quest of successful aging. *International Journal of Behavioral Development, 12,* 35–55.

Schoenbach, V. J., Kaplan, B. H., Fredman, L., & Kleinbaum, D. G. (1986). Social ties and mortality in Evans County, Georgia. *American Journal of Epidemiology, 123,* 577–591.

Schultz, N. R. & Moore, D. (1988). Loneliness: Differences across three age levels. *Journal of Social and Personal Relationships, 5,* 275–284.

Schulz, R., & Rau, M. T. (1985). Social support through the life course. In S. Cohen & S. L. Syme (Eds.), *Social support and health* (pp. 129–149). New York: Academic Press.

Schulz, R., Tompkins, C. A., & Rau, M. T. (1988). A longitudinal study of the psychosocial impact of stroke on primary support persons. *Psychology and Aging, 3,* 131–141.

Schulz, R., Visintainer, P., Williamson, G. M. (1990). Psychiatric and physical morbidity effects of caregiving. *Journals of Gerontology, 45,* P181–P191.

Schuster, T. L., Kessler, R. C., & Aseltine, R. H. (1990). Supportive interactions, negative interactions, and depressed mood. *American Journal of Community Psychology, 18,* 423–438.

Schütze, Y., & Lang, F. R. (1995). Integration in family, kinship and friendship networks. In H. Mollenkopf (Ed.), *Elderly people in industrialized societies* (pp. 25 – 41). Berlin: Sigma.

Schwarzer, R., & Leppin, A. (1991). Social support and health: A theoretical and empirical overview. *Journal of Social and Personal Relationships, 8,* 99–127.

Schwarzer, R., & Leppin, A. (1992). Social support and mental health: A conceptual and empirical overview. In L. Montada, S.-H. Filipp & M. J. Lerner (Eds.), *Life crises and experiences of loss in adulthood* (pp. 435–458). Hillsdale, NJ: Erlbaum.

Scott, J. P. (1983). Siblings and other kin. In T. Brubaker (Ed.), *Family relationships in later life* (pp. 47–62). Newbury Park, CA: Sage.

Scott, J. P. (1990). Sibling interaction in later life. In T. H. Brubaker (Ed.), *Family relationships in later life* (2nd ed., Suppl., pp. 86–99). Beverly Hills, CA: Sage.

Seeman, T. E., & Berkman, L. F. (1988). Structural characteristics of social networks and their relationships with social support in the elderly: Who provides support? *Social Science and Medicine, 26,* 737–749.

Shanas, E. (1980). Older people and their families: The new pioneers. *Journal of Marriage and the Family, 42,* 9–15.

Shinn, M., Lehmann, S., & Wong, N. W. (1984). Social interaction and social support. *Journal of Social Issues, 40,* 55–76.

Shumaker, S., & Jackson, J. S. (1979). The aversive effects of nonreciprocated benefits. *Social Psychology Quarterly, 42,* 148–158.

Shute, R. & Howitt, D. (1990). Unraveling paradoxes in loneliness: Research and elements of a social theory of loneliness. *Social Behaviour, 5,* 169–184.

Shye, D., Mullooly, J. P., Freeborn, D. K., Pope, C. R. (1995). Gender differences in the relationship between social network support and mortality: A longitudinal study of an elderly cohort. *Social Science and Medicine, 41,* 935–947.

Smith, T. W. (1992). Hostility and health: Current status of a psychosomatic hypothesis. *Health Psychology, 11,* 139–150.

Stacey-Konnert, C., & Pynoos, J. (1992). Friendship and social networks in a continuing care retirement community. *Journal of Applied Gerontology, 11,* 298–313.

Staudinger, U. M., Marsiske, M., & Baltes, P. B. (1995). Resilience and reserve capacity in later adulthood: Potentials and limits of development across the life span. In D. Cicchetti & D. Cohen (Eds.), *Developmental psychopathology* (Vol. 2, pp. 801–847). New York: Wiley.

Steinbach, U. (1992). Social networks, institutionalization, and mortality among elderly people in the United States. *Journals of Gerontology: Social Sciences, 47,* S183–S190.

Steinmetz, S. K. (1988). Parental and filial relationships: Obligation, support and abuse. In S. K. Steinmetz (Ed.), *Family support systems across the life span* (pp. 165–182). New York: Plenum.

Sticker, E. J. (1991). The importance of grandparenthood during the life cycle in Germany. In P. K. Smith (Ed.), *The psychology of grandparenthood. An international perspective* (pp. 32–49). London: Routledge.

Stoller, E. P., & Pugliesi, K. L. (1988). Informal networks of community-based elderly: Changes in composition over time. *Research on Aging, 10,* 499–516.

Strain, L. A., & Chappell, N. L. (1982). Confidants. Do they make a difference in quality of life? *Research on Aging, 4,* 479–502.

Sugisawa, H., Liang, J., & Liu, X. (1994). Social networks, social support, and mortality among older people in Japan. *Journals of Gerontology: Social Sciences, 49,* S3–S13.

Sussman, M. B. (1985). The family life of old people. In R. H. Binstock & E. Shanas (Eds.), *Handbook of aging and the social sciences* (2nd ed., pp. 415–449). New York: Van Nostrand Reinhold.

Thomae, H. (1994). Trust, social support, and relying on others. *Zeitschrift für Gerontologie, 27,* 103–109.

Thompson, S. C., & Sobolew-Shubin, A. (1993a). Overprotective relationships: A nonsupportive side of social networks. *Basic and Applied Social Psychology, 14,* 363–383.

Thompson, S. C., & Sobolew-Shubin, A. (1993b). Perceptions of overprotection in ill adults. *Journal of Applied Social Psychology, 23,* 85–97.

Tinsley, B. J., & Parke, R. D. (1987). Grandparents as interactive and social support agents for families with young infants. *International Journal of Aging and Human Development, 25,* 259–277.

Tornstam, L. (1992). Loneliness in marriage. *Journal of Social and Personal Relationships, 9,* 197–217.

Townsend, A. L., & Franks, M. M. (1995). Binding ties: Closeness and conflict in adult children's caregiving relationships. *Psychology and Aging, 10,* 343–351.

Tucker, J. S., Friedman, H. S., Wingard, D. L., & Schwartz, J. E. (1996). Marital history at midlife as a predictor of longevity: Alternative explanations to the protective effect of marriage. *Health Psychology, 15,* 94–101.

Umberson, D., Wortman, C. B., & Kessler, R. C. (1992). Widowhood and depression: Explaining long-term gender differences in vulnerability. *Journal of Health & Social Behavior, 33,* 10–24.

Van Sonderen, E., Ormel, J., Brilman, E., & van Linden van den Heuvell, C. (1990). Personal network delineation: A comparison of the exchange, affective and role-relation approach. In K. C. P. M. Knipscheer & T. C. Antonucci (Eds.), *Social network research* (pp. 101–120). Amsterdam: Swets & Zeitlinger.

Walker, A. J., Martin, S. S., & Jones, L. L. (1992). The benefits and costs of caregiving and care receiving for daughters and mothers. *Journal of Gerontology: Social Sciences, 47,* S130–139.

Wallston, B. S., Alagna, S. W., DeVellis, B. M., DeVellis, R. F. (1983). Social support and physical health. *Health Psychology, 2,* 367–391.

Watson, D., & Clark, L. A. (1992). Affects separable and inseparable: On the hierarchical arrangement of the negative affects. *Journal of Personality and Social Psychology, 62,* 489–505.

Watson, D., Clark, L. A., & Tellegen, A. (1988). Development and Validation of Brief Measures of Positive and Negative Affect: The PANAS Scales. *Journal of Personality and Social Psychology, 54,* 1063–1070.

Wellman, B. (1979). The community question: The intimate networks of East Yorkers. *American Journal of Sociology, 84,* 1201–1231.

Wentowski, G. J. (1981). Reciprocity and the coping strategies of older people: Cultural dimenions of network building. *The Gerontologist, 21,* 600–609.

White, L., & Edwards, J. N. (1990). Emptying the nest and parental well-being: An analysis of national panel data. *American Sociological Review, 55,* 235–242.

Wilcox, V. L., Kasl, S. V., & Berkman, L. F. (1994). Social support and physical disability in older people after hospitalization: A prospective study. *Health Psychology, 13,* 170–179.

Wilson, J. G., Calsyn, R. J., & Orlofsky, J. L. (1994). Impact of sibling relationships on social support and morale in the elderly. *Journal of Gerontological Social Work, 22,* 157–170.

Wortman, C. B., & Lehman, D. R. (1985). Reactions to victims of life crisis: Support attempts that fail. In I. G. Sarason & B. R. Sarason (Eds.), *Social support: Theory, research and application* (pp. 463–489). Dordrecht: Martinus Nijhoff.

7.04
Sexuality

SUSANNE ZANK
Freie Universität Berlin, Germany

7.04.1 INTRODUCTION

Historical, societal, and demographic changes have led to the rise of gerontology. This comparatively new science already provides an impressive amount of empirical data, which contradict some common stereotypes of old age and aging. Results include, for example, developmental capacity even in the very old, tremendous interindividual differences, different developmental processes in distinct domains within an individual and the important role individual biography plays in the aging process (Baltes & Baltes, 1990; Birren & Schaie, 1985;

Kruse, 1989; Lehr & Thomae, 1987; Mayer & Baltes, 1996).

It is interesting to note, however, that there is a considerable lack of sound studies on sexuality and aging. The scientific community considers the study of sexual behavior a very difficult task which is fascinating but somewhat unseemly, especially with elderly subjects. This attitude might be caused to some extent by the unconscious resistance of scientists to exploring the sexual secrets of their parents. This problem was precisely described by the comedian Sam Levinson: "When I first found out how babies were born, I couldn't believe it. To think that my mother and father could do such a thing." Then, after a moment's reflection: "My father—maybe: but my mother—never!" (O'Donohue, 1987, p. 69).

This anecdote also reflects the conception of women as almost asexual beings, which might be one reason for the fact that gerontological knowledge about elderly sexuality refers predominantly to males. Since elderly females considerably outnumber males, due to the longer life expectancy of women, this focus on male sexual functioning is especially puzzling. It might mirror the societal "double standard of aging" (Sontag, 1972) which means that older women are perceived as being unattractive and asexual much earlier than men.

Many reviews comment on the myths of geriatric sexuality (O'Donohue, 1987; Spence, 1992). These myths suggest that elderly people are not sexually capable, not desirable, and not desirous. Such societal attitudes and stereotypes have various negative consequences for those who are affected. Mild sexual alterations might lead to panic and severe performance anxiety because they are misinterpreted as the beginning of the unavoidable end of sexuality. Many older people feel guilty or are ashamed because of their ongoing sexual interest and behavior, and this may result in total suppression of any sexual feelings (Renshaw, 1983).

Empirical data show that these attitudes are myths and do not reflect reality. Most elderly people are interested in sex and capable of sexual performance until very old age. Combating these myths, however, has led to the establishment of equally incorrect countermyths (Gatz, 1987). These countermyths almost deny any changes of sexual desire and performance with age. They establish an ideal which is a projection of middle-aged values and can be equally harmful (Thomas, 1982). Rappoport (1977) hints at this problem by saying "All we want from gerontology is eternal youth" (p. 207). Unfortunately, the unsatisfactory database on elderly sexuality provides support for truth in the myth as in the countermyth.

7.04.1.1 Reviews and Surveys

There are numerous review articles on sexuality and aging which seem to outnumber original research reports (e.g., Byers, 1983; Capuzzi, 1982; Corby & Zarit, 1983; Datan & Rodeheaver, 1983; Garza & Dressel, 1983; Genavay, 1982; Hermanova, 1983; Hodson & Skeen, 1994; Kay & Neelley, 1982; Kellett, 1993; Kirkpatrick, 1980, Laws, 1980; Libman, 1989; Ludeman, 1981; Luria & Meade, 1984; O'Donohue, 1987; Renshaw, 1983; Robinson, 1983; Starr, 1985; Sviland, 1981; Traupmann, 1984; Turner & Adams, 1983; Von Sydow, 1992a; Weg, 1983; Weiler, 1981; White, 1982). These authors usually review results of the most important studies, which were conducted in the USA and will be described in the following.

Alfred C. Kinsey and his colleagues interviewed 17 500 men and women (Kinsey, Pomeroy & Martin, 1948; Institute for Sex Research, 1953). Their sample was not representative but this was the first study to investigate sexual behaviors from childhood to old age, and it therefore represented a remarkable first attempt to understand human sexual behaviors. Cross-sectional data were collected with structured and standardized interviews. Unfortunately, only 126 males and 56 females over 60 were included in the study, and only 10 females were over 70. More recently, a new report from the Kinsey institute was published which described data gathered in 1970 from extensive interviews with more than 3000 men and women (Klassen, Williams, & Levitt, 1989). This study was restricted to sexual attitudes and did not report data on sexual behaviors.

Other important sources of information are the two Duke University Longitudinal Studies. These results are also rather old, but still very valuable, because they are the only ones which stem from longitudinal data (George & Weiler, 1981; Pfeiffer, Verwoerdt, & Wang 1968; Verwoerdt, Pfeiffer, & Wang, 1969a, 1969b). In the first study, data on sexuality were collected as part of a medical interview, and in the second study a self-administered questionnaire was used. Neither sample was representative (Weiler, 1981). Over the three measures of the first Duke Longitudinal Study the number of subjects aged over 60 declined from 254 to 126 (Verwoerdt et al., 1969a, 1969b). In the second Duke Longitudinal Study a sample of 502 men and women aged 46–71 years was drawn; 348 persons completed all four waves of data collection, but data were only reported about those 278 subjects who remained married throughout the study. Forty-eight subjects were older than 66 years at the beginning of the six-year inquiry (George & Weiler, 1981).

Most of the above mentioned reviews could not discuss the results of the more recent studies (Brecher, 1984; Janus & Janus, 1993; Laumann, Gagnon, Michael, & Michels, 1994; Starr & Weiner, 1981). Starr and Weiner (1981) investigated 800 subjects over 60 in senior centers who attended lectures on sexuality and aging. Of the 4246 subjects who participated in the Consumer Union survey, 2622 subjects were over age 60. Subjects were a self-selected sample of readers of the Consumer Report (Brecher, 1984). Janus and Janus (1993) investigated 2765 subjects with questionnaires "distributed to subjects at a wide variety of sites" (p. 3) in a cross-sectional study between 1988 and 1992; 441 of the subjects were older than 65. The samples of these three studies were also not representative. In a very carefully designed study with a representative sample Laumann et al. (1994) collected 3432 questionnaires about sexual practices in the USA. Unfortunately, they only included subjects aged between 18 and 59.

European studies are not very often reported in the US literature because they are rarely translated. Consequently, the considerable differences between results of US and European studies are not discussed (Von Sydow, 1992a). The following non-American studies are published in English. Persson (1980) selected a representative sample of 70-year-old people in Gothenburg, Sweden. Subjects were invited to take part in a health control, 85% accepted, and 166 men and 266 women were interviewed. Bergström-Walan and Nielsen (1990) drew a random sample of citizens aged 60–80 of Stockholm, Sweden. They mailed 1574 questionnaires, and 509 were returned. Antonovsky, Sadowsky, and Maoz (1990) interviewed 177 men and 121 women from a nonrepresentative sample in Israel. Data included current sexual activities and retrospective reports about past sexual experience.

Taken together, epidemiological knowledge on sexuality and aging is grounded on rather few studies. The database for men is somewhat better, because there are some studies on male sexual behavior only (e.g., Mulligan & Moss, 1991; Schiavi, 1990; Weizmann & Hart, 1987). White (1982) cited 10 studies which investigated exclusively males, while only three studies exclusively focused on females. The following section will briefly review the major epidemiological results on sexual activities. Data are extremely heterogeneous and therefore very difficult to interpret. Some scientific objections against uncautious generalization of available data will be raised.

7.04.2 EPIDEMIOLOGY

7.04.2.1 Sexual Behavior of Elderly Females

Studies in the USA have shown that 70–90% of females aged between 60 and 90 were sexually active (Adams & Turner, 1985; Brecher, 1984; Starr & Weiner, 1981). Sexual activity in these studies referred to intercourse and masturbation. German studies reported, however, that 45%–55% of females aged 50 to 60 were sexually active, and up to 3% of women over 70 years (Tümmers, 1976; Weissbach-Rieger & Franke 1987a; 1987b; Wickert, 1983).

Data on activity in sexual intercourse varied between 15 and 90% for women aged 50 to 59, and between 0 and 66% for women older than 70 years. Frequency of intercourse was reported between once a week and once per month, with a decline with age (Bergström-Walan & Nielsen, 1990; Brecher, 1984; Christenson & Johnson, 1973; George & Weiler, 1981; Janus & Janus, 1993; Institute for Sex Research, 1953; Pfeiffer, Verwoerdt, & Davis, 1972; Starr & Weiner, 1981). Bretschneider and McCoy (1988) investigated very old subjects between 80 and 102 with an average of 86.1 years; of the interviewed women, 70% no longer had intercourse.

Of women over 50 years, 10–50% masturbated, and between 0 and 49% females over 70 years reported this activity. Masturbation was reported much more frequently in US than in European studies (Adams & Turner, 1985; Aresin, 1980; Bergström-Walan & Nielsen, 1990; Brecher, 1984; Bretschneider & McCoy, 1988; Institute for Sex Research, 1953; Schneider, 1980; Starr & Weiner, 1981).

Questions about sexual enjoyment or achieving orgasm were rare. Of women in all age groups, 9–26% reported that they never achieved orgasm (Hite, 1976; Institute for Sex Research, 1953; Janus & Janus, 1993; Laumann et al., 1994). Studies about elderly females revealed that about 70% of the American subjects reported sexual enjoyment but only 20% of subjects aged over 80 (Brecher, 1984; Starr & Weiner, 1981). In an Israeli sample, 43% of women over 65 reported that they were not very satisfied. Of these subjects, 14% recalled that they were not very satisfied between 20 and 30 years, and 28% were not very satisfied in their fifties (Antonovsky et al., 1990). The rate of women who never or rarely reacted with orgasm remained stable at roughly 21% between 40 and 59 years (Laumann et al., 1994) but seemed to increase over 70 years (Bergström-Walan & Nielsen, 1990; Brecher, 1984).

Between 4 and 19% of the subjects reported that they had homosexual contacts at least once in their life and 1–5% stated an ongoing relationship (Adams & Turner, 1985; Brecher,

1984, Hagstad & Janson, 1984). Data from a representative study of subjects aged between 18 and 59 years showed that 4% had same-gender sex partners, 1.3% during the last year (Laumann et al., 1994).

7.04.2.2 Sexual Behavior of Elderly Males

Between 60% and 90% of men aged over 60 and between 48% and 79% over 70 report being sexual active. Over 80% of men in their sixties and 75% in their seventies reported a strong or moderate interest in sex (Brecher, 1984; Pfeiffer, Verwoerdt & Wang, 1968; Verwoerdt et al., 1969a, 1969b).

Between 64% and 89% of men aged over 60 reported having sexual intercourse, with 24%–69% reporting weekly or higher frequency sexual intercourse (Antonovsky et al., 1990; Bergström-Walan & Nielsen, 1990; Brecher, 1984; Janus & Janus, 1993; Weizmann & Hart, 1987). Between 46 and 62% of men over 70 years reported having intercourse (Brecher, 1984; Bretschneider & McCoy, 1988; Persson, 1980).

Between 45 and 59% of elderly males reported that they never masturbate, and 28%–44% reported masturbating at least weekly (Bergström-Walan, 1990; Brecher, 1984; Janus & Janus, 1993; Weizmann & Hart, 1987).

There seems to be a decline in orgasm with age in men. Janus and Janus (1993) reported that 77% of men between age 51 and 64 always experienced orgasm, but only 55% over age 65. Mulligan and Moss (1991) claimed that ability to experience orgasm declined from 61% in the 60–69 year olds to 21% in men aged over 90. Brecher (1984) reported that 85% of men in their sixties and 70% in their seventies always reached orgasm. In comparison, an average of 8% of men between 18 and 59 years were unable to experience orgasm (Laumann et al., 1994).

7.04.2.3 Critique of Epidemiological Studies

7.04.2.3.1 Methodological problems

(i) Sample

There are hardly any representative studies and samples are often very small. Taken together, our knowledge on sexuality and aging is based on roughly 7000 subjects. Discrepancies between European and US data cannot be interpreted because of small sample sizes. Furthermore, the age of subjects ranges between 60 and 100 years, spanning 40 years. This means that sample sizes (e.g., for 60 and 80 years olds) become extremely small for different age groups. From a gerontological perspective, 60-year-old subjects differ markedly from 80-year-olds.

Relying on epidemiological data which stem from nonrepresentative samples can be very misleading. Greeley (1994) compared results from Janus and Janus (1993) with data from the General Social Survey (GSS), which was based on a national household probability sample. The comparison was made about percentages of people having sex at least once a week. Janus and Janus (1993) reported that 81% of men aged between 51 and 64 and 69% of men over 65 had sex at least once a week. The GSS data claimed only 43% of men between age 51 and 64, and 17% over 65 had sex at least once a week. For women, Janus and Janus (1993) reported that 65% aged between 51 and 64 and 74% over 65 had sex at least once a week. GSS results showed that 25% of women between 51 and 64, and 6% over 65 had sex that often (Greeley, 1994, cited in Laumann et al., 1994).

(ii) Research design

Most of the studies used a cross-sectional design. Longitudinal designs are essential, however, to describe intra-individual changes. Cross-sectional data are very often interpreted as if they are longitudinal (Institute for Sex Research, 1953; Kinsey et al., 1948). George and Weiler (1981) reported from their longitudinal study that sexual behavior was remarkably stable over the six years of their study. Their data suggested that differences between age-groups reflected cohort-related rather than age-related effects. Liberation of sexual moral attitudes or changes in age-related stereotypes may even enhance cohort differences in the future.

(iii) Data collection

Most studies used questionnaires or standardized interviews. These methods assume that the meaning of questions will be the same for respondents and scientists. Von Sydow (1992b) conducted an interview study with 91 females and found that seven did not know the term orgasm. Five other women of this sample claimed that a woman needs to have an orgasm in order to become pregnant. Finally, the important Duke longitudinal study (George & Weiler, 1981; Pfeiffer et al. 1968; Verwoerdt et al., 1969a, 1969b) collected data on general medical problems. The medical context for exploring sexuality may not support open answers about sex, especially with many subjects suffering from chronic illness. Furthermore, structured interviews in the first study were conducted by male interviewers which may have caused some reluctance to self-disclose among older women in the 1950s (Pfeiffer & Davis, 1972; Starr, 1985; Verwoerdt et al., 1969a, 1969b).

7.04.2.3.2 Theoretical problems

Every study on human sexuality shows that men are sexually more active than women. This seems to be true for every age group, for intercourse and, especially, for masturbation (Brecher, 1984; Institute for Sex Research, 1953; Janus & Janus, 1993; Kinsey et al., 1948; Klassen et al., 1989; Laumann et al., 1994). Although physiological results indicate higher potency of female response in terms of orgasmic potential in comparison with men (Masters & Johnson, 1966, 1981), women seem not to use this potential. This appears to be particularly true for elderly females and raises the question whether research efforts have met the sexual, social, and psychological reality of older women.

(i) Intercourse

Older widowed women outnumber widowed men approximately 5:1, which means that in basically monogamous societies most women do not have many opportunities for intercourse (Malatesta, Chambless, Pollack, & Cantor, 1988). Therefore, higher frequencies of having intercourse in males do not prove age-related differences of sexual interests between men and women. Pfeiffer and Davis (1972) found that past sexual enjoyment, marital status, and age were significant determinants of female sexual behavior. Antonovsky et al. (1990) reported that marital status alone explained 25% of the variance of sexual activities in women. A representative study of 460 subjects aged over 60 in Germany showed that gender differences diminished when "availability of a partner" was statistically controlled (Brähler & Unger, 1994). Interestingly, investigations of couples revealed that both men and women agreed that they ceased intercourse because of the male (Persson, 1980; Pfeiffer et al., 1968; Von Sydow, 1993).

Differences in intercourse rates for younger age-groups are surprising because theoretically women and men should report the same amount of intercourse altogether. An explanation could be exaggeration of males or understatement of females. Another explanation could be visits to prostitutes by men.

(ii) Orgasm

Examining intercourse ignores information about individual feelings and quality of experience. Men and women can have intercourse without enjoyment or orgasm, but this happens far more often to women than to men (Laumann et al., 1994; Leiblum & Rosen, 1989b; McConaghy, 1993). The fact that important studies did not explore sexual enjoyment or orgasm but focus on intercourse (e.g., George & Weiler, 1981; Pfeiffer, Verwoerdt, & Wang 1969; Verwoerdt et al., 1969a, 1969b) reveals that research has been biased by a male point of view. The occurrence of orgasm would be a clear indicator of satisfying sexual experience and would provide solid ground for the prediction of future sexual interests (Laws, 1980). Fortunately, more recent studies have considered this aspect.

(iii) Interest in sexual activities

Many (male) scientists have investigated interest in intercourse and interpreted their results as representing interest in all sexual activities. Presumably, this has led to invalid results. Studies have shown that, in contrast to men, many women prefer other sexual activities to intercourse, like manual or oral stimulation (Denney, Field, & Quadagno, 1984; Von Sydow, 1993). The clitoris and penis are homologous organs which need stimulation for orgasm. During intercourse the penis is directly, and the clitoris indirectly stimulated. Most women need additional clitoral stimulation to achieve orgasm (Masters & Johnson, 1966; McConaghy, 1993), which explains their preferences. If true gender differences with regard to sexual interests exist they are probably due to different experiences of pleasure and orgasm during the life course (Laws, 1980).

(iv) Sexual experience and relationship

Research efforts have focused heavily on sexual performance and ignored the phenomenology of sexual experiences, namely, the subjective meaning, and relational quality of the experience. Starr (1985) reported that 75% of his subjects aged over 60 indicated that their sexual feelings were as good as or even better than in younger years. They stressed the quality of their sexual experiences instead of quantity. This seems especially true for women for whom the emotional aspect of a sexual relationship are more important than for many men (Luria & Meade, 1984).

Taken together, our knowledge about human sexual behavior and experience in the elderly is sparse. Most of the studies reveal considerable methodological and conceptual weaknesses. Nevertheless, results are often cited and generalized, supporting myths (especially for elderly women) and countermyths on aging and sexuality. Many studies have no theoretical framework. A developmental perspective of aging individuals and couples is clearly lacking in most studies. The following section will focus on physiological changes in healthy elderly people and on psychological aspects of aging and sexuality. Another focus will be on the effects of chronic illnesses on sexual functioning, because the prevalence of chronic illness increases with advancing age.

7.04.3 AGE-RELATED CHANGES IN SEXUAL FUNCTIONING

Most of the epidemiological data suggest that there is a decrease in sexual interest and sexual behavior as one ages. It is often argued that this decline is due to biological changes in sexual response capacity. Age-related biological changes in capacity are difficult to determine because changes in sexual functioning are confounded by the effects of chronic diseases, medication, and cultural expectations. Moreover, Winn and Newton (1982) have documented examples of cultural influences on sexual response capacity. They studied data of the Human Relations Area Files of about 106 preindustrial and traditional societies all over the world. For 28 cultures, data on sexual activities in males were available. In 70% of these societies, older men had little or no reduction in sexual behavior until the age of 75. Twenty-six cultures provided data about female sexuality, and 84% of these data reported continued sexual interest and activity in old females which often included having intercourse with younger men. This study gives some evidence that biological changes do not necessarily lead to a reduction in sexual interest and sexual behavior. Facts about physiological changes will be briefly reviewed in the following. Detailed information is provided by McConaghy (1993), Morley (1991), Sarrel (1990), Schiavi (1990), and Schiavi and Segraves (1995).

7.04.3.1 Physiological Changes

7.04.3.1.1 Physiological changes in females

Menopause is associated with marked hormonal changes, namely, a decrease in estrogen production by the ovaries. There is an ongoing controversy about how the hormonal changes affect female sexuality (for a methodological review and meta-analysis see Myers, 1995). It was thought that decline in sexual activity was related directly to decline in sexual hormones, but estrogen and progesterone levels did not predict women's sexual functioning in the laboratory (Roughan, Kaiser, & Morley, 1993). Estrogen deficiency is responsible, however, for decreased elasticity of the vaginal walls, atrophy of vaginal epithelium, diminished vaginal lubrication, and increased fragility of the vaginal skin (Goldstein & Teng, 1991; Leiblum, 1990; Masters & Johnson, 1966, 1981; Morley, 1991; Morley & Kaiser, 1989; Roughan et al., 1993; Schiavi & Segraves, 1995; Wise, 1989). These changes are probably responsible for coital pain, which is more often reported by postmenopausal women. Estrogen replacement therapy is very successful in treating these vaginal changes.

Although Masters and Johnson (1966, 1981) studied only 11 women aged over 60, their description of physiological changes in healthy women proved to be accurate and their data have been supported by findings from self-report surveys (Bachman & Leiblum, 1991; Dennerstein, Smith, Morse, & Burger, 1994; Hagstad, 1988; McCoy & Davidson, 1985; Morley, 1991). Physiological changes in female sexuality include decreased congestion of the labia minora, decreased separation of the labia majora, decreased vaginal lubrication, decreased orgasmic platform contraction, and occasional painful spastic contractions of the uterus. Furthermore, the breasts become less vasocongested and nipple erection is less likely to occur. Masters and Johnson (1981) reported that aging women require more time in precoital stimulation until lubrication develops sufficiently. Orgasmic duration and intensity may be reduced but the capacity for multiple orgasms remains.

There is some ongoing controversy as to whether women suffer sexual dysfunction following hysterectomy. Bernhard (1986) analyzed 18 studies and detected numerous methodological and measurement problems. Eicher (1994a, 1994b) reviewed research outcomes and concluded that older studies reported negative, and newer studies positive, consequences for female sexuality. He argued that this change is due to better information, sexual behavior advice, and historical changes in attitudes towards sexuality. Results from a recent longitudinal study with 104 women revealed that half of the women reported improvement after surgery and 21% reported poorer sexual functioning. Preoperative sexual activity was the best predictor of postoperative sexuality (Helström, Lundberg, Sörbom, & Bäckström, 1993).

Dennerstein et al. (1994) reported a study with 2001 randomly selected Australian women aged between 45 and 55 years. The natural menopause transition was clearly associated with declining sexual interest, decreased likelihood of intercourse, and increased likelihood of unusual pain during intercourse. Hällström and Samuelsson (1990) reported data from 497 subjects with a male partner who were interviewed twice within seven years. At first interviews, subjects were aged 38, 46, 50, or 54. Of the total sample, 27% reported a decrease in sexual desire and 10% experienced an increase in desire. Age-group differences were marginal. Antonovsky et al. (1990) conducted retrospective interviews with 121 women and 177 men between the ages of 65 and 85. The women reported a marked decrease in sexual desire and sexual satisfaction in comparison to their twenties, thirties, and fifties. McCoy and Davidson (1985) conducted a longitudinal study and reported a significant decrease in coital frequency and sexual thoughts in the postmenopausal compared to the premenopausal period. The decline in coital frequency was related to testosterone rather than to estrogen levels. Sarrel (1982) described sex problems after menopause in 50 couples (e.g., loss of orgasmic response in female partner, erectile difficulties in male partner) who participated in a sex counseling program. Dyspareunia in women was often followed by erectile difficulties in men.

In contradiction to the reviewed data, which support a decline hypothesis, Starr (1985) claimed that "the Starr–Weiner data indicate that women over 60 are more orgasmic than when they were younger" and that "most investigators report that sexual response remains the same or improves after menopause" (Starr, 1985, p. 102). Epidemiological data from a representative cross-sectional study clearly suggested that the number of women who never experience orgasm remained fairly stable until the age of 70 (Laumann et al., 1994). These data do not answer the question, however, whether orgasmic women increase their capacity to orgasm after menopause.

7.04.3.1.2 Physiological changes in males

Men do not undergo a clearly marked, obvious change such as females experience with menopause. Nevertheless, there is a remarkable change in hormone production as well; namely, a decrease in testosterone and bioavailable testosterone in the majority of males (Morley & Kaiser, 1989). Decrease in testosterone production has led to the hypothesis that androgen deficiency contributes to the decline in sexual desire and activity in older men (Schiavi, 1990). Remarkably few studies, however, assessed the role of gonadal hormones on age-related changes.

Schiavi and colleagues investigated 77 healthy, married men aged 45–74 and their partners. The sample was drawn via media announcements. Couples underwent an extensive interview together as well as separately. Data gathering included psychosexual, psychiatric, and marital information as well as a battery of psychological tests. The male subjects were additionally studied in a sleep laboratory for four nights. Electroencephalogram, eye movements, muscle tone, and penile tumescence were monitored. Data revealed that age was negatively correlated with bioavailable testosterone. Bioavailable testosterone showed significant associations with sexual desire, arousal, and activity measures. Furthermore, results showed age-related changes in nocturnal penile tumescence. Frequency, duration, and rigidity of this reaction decreased with increasing age. Finally, age was significantly negatively correlated with sexual desire, sexual arousal, and sexual activity, but there were no age differences in degree of enjoyment of marital sexuality. Increased age was also correlated with erectile difficulties (erectile rigidity, loss of erection during sex) and retarded ejaculation (Schiavi, 1990; Schiavi, Mandeli, & Schreiner-Engel, 1994; Schiavi, Mandeli, Schreiner-Engel, & Chambers, 1991; Schiavi, Schreiner-Engel, White, & Mandeli, 1991).

Masters and Johnson (1981) described four variations in basic sexual physiology in males who were past their mid-fifties. First, it takes longer to achieve full penile engorgement and requires more direct stimulation. Second, there is a reduction of expulsive pressure. Third, there is a reduction of the volume of seminal fluid expelled. Fourth, there is a reduction or loss of ejaculatory demand. Weiss and Mellinger (1990) stated that there are only one or two expulsive contractions of the urethra instead of four major contractions in younger men. Seminal fluid is expelled with less force, which diminishes the sensation of passage through the urethra. There is, rather, a seepage of semen which reduces the intense sensation of ejaculatory inevitability. After ejaculation, the refractory period increases with age. Many men cannot have another erection for 12–24 hours. Further physiological changes include less nipple erection; less, or absence of, flushing of neck, trunk, shoulders, thighs, and forearms; scrotal integument becomes thinner and inelastic; rapid detumescence after orgasm (Weiss & Mellinger, 1990).

7.04.3.2 Psychological Aspects

Modern developmental psychology emphasizes that development is not limited to childhood or youth but continues over the life course. This life-span perspective views development as a product of an interplay between biological, cultural, and psychological influences, that is, individuals interact with their environment continuously over the life course (Baltes, 1987; Baltes, Reese, & Lipsitt, 1980).

Cultural influences change considerably with time. This fact can be illustrated by a closer look at elderly subjects who were investigated, at age 70 in 1980. These subjects were born in 1910. Their parents grew up in the Victorian century. This means that these subjects were exposed to very strict societal norms regarding sexuality during their childhood and adolescence. Masturbation was forbidden and considered to be extremely harmful. Sexual feelings for decent women were unthinkable. Freud's theories and discoveries, especially his description of sexual feelings in children, were regarded as tremendously scandalous in Vienna at the beginning of the century (Freud, 1964). Despite short periods with less restricted sexual norms (e.g., in Berlin during the 1920s), sexuality remained a tabooed, guilt- and shame-laden topic for many years. Considerable changes began with the pioneering work of Kinsey and his colleagues (Institute for Sex Research, 1953; Kinsey et al., 1948) who provided the first published survey of sexual behavior. Masters and Johnson (1966) followed with serious information about "human sexual response." Their work was a breakthrough for the acknowledgment of female sexuality. At the same time the development of the contraceptive pill, the ideas of the hippie movement, and later feminism, contributed to the liberation of sexuality. During the 1980s, the threat of AIDS reduced sexual freedom. The above-mentioned subjects who were 70 years old in 1980 experienced all these influences, but the development of their sexual identity was strongly influenced by Victorian moral standards. The fading of sexuality over ontogenetic time might be, therefore, a product of socialization rather than of biology (Traupmann, 1984).

In addition, cultural influences are very important for age-graded behavior expectations and societal values in general. Modern Western societies are dominated by youth orientation, and sexuality is linked to it. Firm and slim bodies, smooth skin, health, energy, career orientation, money, and luxury are highly valued. All these characteristics are directly or indirectly related to youth, sexual attractiveness, and potency. Elderly people have the difficult task of coping with these societal norms which threaten their self-esteem.

Elderly homosexuals suffer from multiple myths and stereotypes. These stereotypes include that aging gays are oversexed, frustrated, unable to have a lasting relationship, and have an extreme youth orientation (Pope & Schulz, 1990). McDougall (1993) described these myths, and stressed cohort differences between younger and older gays. Elderly gays are used to hiding their sexual preferences, in contrast to younger ones who have benefited more from the gay liberation movement in the 1970s. Cruikshank (1990) reviewed gerontological studies about aging lesbians and gays, and concluded that there were more positive outcomes than expected. Friend (1990) presented a "theory of successful aging" (p. 99) for lesbian and gay individuals. He theorized that the tough lifelong reality with numerous experiences of discrimination leads to the development of a strong ego in gays. They are thus better prepared to cope with the demands and humiliating experiences of aging than the heterosexual elderly.

For women, cultural pressure is particularly damaging because esthetic and erotic feelings in Western societies lead to old women being considered as repulsive (Sontag, 1972). Whereas wrinkles and gray hair are an interesting and attractive sign of experience in men, they are a symbol of decaying beauty and femininity in women. A marriage of an older man and a young woman is a sign of vigor and vitality in the man, but when an older woman marries a young man, it is generally disapproved or even judged as pathological. An illustration of this humiliating experience for women is provided by Thomas Mann. Being himself in his late seventies, he wrote a story about a 50-year-old woman who fell in love with a young man. With his deep psychological understanding of human conflicts he described desire, restriction, and a "betrayal by nature" of this woman (Mann, 1953).

Men also have to face cultural pressures. Male identity and masculinity is directly linked to sexual performance demands. Books, stories, movies, and television shows project a "fantasy model of sex: It's two feet long, hard as steel, and can go all night" (Zilbergeld, 1992, p. 30). The penis is expected to function automatically whenever its owner wishes to use it, regardless of any other conditions. Older men who feel a normal need for more direct stimulation or experience erectile weaknesses can be threatened to the core of their identity. As a 51-year-old man put it: "You want to know how I feel, I'll tell you. I feel like an absolute nothing. I know I can satisfy her in other ways and I do, but that's not the point. I feel like shit, like the center has been taken out of me" (Zilbergeld, 1992, p. 36). Unfortunately, because of this culturally shared fantasy model of male sexuality, many women interpret occasional lack of erection as if they were rejected, not desired, not loved, or not attractive enough. Women have difficulties understanding the intense threat that erectile problems pose for men because they have no parallel experience. The female gender identity will not be questioned by any sexual dysfunction because it is not linked to sexual performance. In addition, women can almost always perform sexually: they can have intercourse without being aroused and can fake enjoyment, but there is no way to fake an erection.

These cultural influences, shared and gender-specific ones, are of considerable importance for psychosocial development and well-being in the elderly (Rosenmayr, 1995). Aging individuals as well as aging couples have to cope with various developmental tasks. Robert Peck (1956) described three phases of development in late adulthood: ego differentiation versus work-role preoccupation, body transcendence versus body preoccupation, and ego transcendence versus ego preoccupation. The first phase refers to coping with retirement. The crucial question is whether a person can derive self-esteem from activities other than work. The second phase means coping with physical decline and health problems. The last stage is very similar to Erikson's (1950) description of ego integrity vs. ego despair as the outcomes of the final developmental task in old age. Acceptance of one's unique life with unchangeable failures and the realization of death are the most important challenges of this stage. These difficult tasks represent a threat to normal narcissism and can have pathological consequences (Eckert, 1984; Liptzin, 1984). Kernberg (1977) described the difference as follows:

> It is part of normal narcissism to love oneself, to be satisfied with one's own appearance, and to wish to be accepted, liked, and loved for what one is. The problem begins when a highly ideal, beautiful and triumphant image of the self linked to childhood or youth becomes an indispensable precondition for self-acceptance and for trusting that one will be accepted by others: this usually reflects a deep devaluation or depreciation of one's self, a sense of loathing and distrust for one's present appearance and value, which can only be compensated for by the eternal looks of triumphant adolescence. (pp. 27–28)

Coping with the narcissistic wounds of aging is a major task for every individual. Fortunately, empirical data indicate that most elderly people manage well and retain positive self-esteem and life satisfaction (Bengtson, Reedy, & Gordon, 1985; Costa et al., 1987; Staudinger, Freund, Linden, & Maas, 1996).

Intimacy and intimate relationships seem to be especially important for coping with the demands of aging (Weiss, 1983, see also Chapter 3, this volume). Intrapsychic changes and role transitions additionally challenge the aging couple. Two examples are marital life after children have left the household, and the retirement of one or both partners. As one woman commented on her stress with the retirement of her husband: "I married my husband for better or for worse, but not for lunch" (Leiblum & Segraves, 1989, p. 377).

Life-span development of gender identity and the concept of androgynization with age has important implications for the individual as well as for the interindividual dynamic of couples and their sexuality (Livson, 1983). Jung (1933) reasoned that role demands in early adulthood require development of selective domains and that older people show greater awareness of aspects of their self which were suppressed earlier. "The man discovers his tender feelings and the woman her sharpness of mind" (p. 108).

Colarusso and Nemiroff (1981) theorized that oedipal issues might reawaken because of illness and death of parents. Therefore, internal representations of parents may change and alter the adult's self-concept. This change in personality may also effect sexual feelings insofar that long-standing relationships are higher valued than short-term sexual gratification (Nadelson, 1984).

Finally, aging couples have to face possible dependency of one partner due to chronic illness, and separation through death. Coping with increasing losses of significant others is one of the most difficult tasks for elderly people. Death of the partner means for many traditionally oriented women, besides many other losses, the end of any sexual activity (Malatesta et al., 1988).

7.04.3.3 Health-related Changes

One major problem in examining age-related changes is that the distinction between age-related and health-related changes is almost impossible. Chronic illnesses increase markedly with age and most diseases have a direct or indirect effect on sexual functioning. Thus, it is not aging per se, but comorbid illness that may cause an increase in sexual dysfunction (Schover, 1989, 1992; Spence, 1992). Some authors claim, however, that health aspects tend to be overestimated with regard to sexuality (Fooken, 1994). Common chronic diseases will be briefly reviewed in this section. An excellent overview about geriatric sexuality and chronic diseases is provided by Mooradian (1991). Additional information is given by Burgener and Logan (1989), Gupta (1990), Kaiser (1991), Liptzin (1984), Majerovitz and

Revenson (1994), and Sjögren, Damber, and Liliequist (1983).

7.04.3.3.1 Diabetes mellitus

The prevalence of diabetes for Caucasians aged over 65 in the USA is 7% for men and 9% for women. For the black population aged over 65, it is 12% for men and 15% for women (Zemel, 1988). Diabetes is an important cause of sexual dysfunction. Orgasmic impairments are experienced by 18%–35% of women. Impotence, retrograde ejaculation, premature ejaculation, and oligospermia are reported for men. At 65 years of age, up to 75% of diabetic men are impotent (Mooradian, 1991; Newman & Bertelson, 1986; Zemel, 1988).

7.04.3.3.2 Cardiovascular disease

Prevalence of this disease increases with age, and the disease causes over 50% of deaths in individuals aged over 64 (Wise, 1989). Both organic and psychological factors affect the sexuality of individuals suffering from cardiovascular disease. Orgasmic difficulties in women as well as erectile dysfunction and premature ejaculation in men are reported (Wise, Epstein, & Ross, 1992). Following coronary bypass surgery, the sexual desire of women appears to decline, while an increase in performance anxiety is common in men. Survivors of myocardial infarction often report anxiety and depression. Fear of sudden death during intercourse often leads to impotence. Patients are assured that they can have intercourse without any risk when they can climb two flights of stairs or can vigorously walk around a block without chest discomfort (Mooradian, 1991; Relf, 1991; Wise, 1989). This rule of thumb ignores interindividual differences in patients and, additionally, poses a psychological dilemma. Patients are allowed to resume sex but they have to watch cautiously for any signs of recurring angina. This anxious self-observation contradicts the "letting go" which is part of successful sexual experiences (Thienhaus, 1988).

7.04.3.3.3 Cancer

This disease continues to be the most dreaded diagnosis, which often leads to depression and anxiety. For most patients their initial question concerns survival. Cancer and its treatment has an intense influence on individual identity and self-esteem, and it can have negative effects on desire, arousability, and orgasm in females and males (Gendel, 1986; Kaiser, 1992; Schover, 1988a, 1988b; Schover, Evans, & Von Eschenbach, 1987; Schover, Schain, & Montague, 1989; Shell & Smith, 1994).

In women, breast and gynecological cancer and its treatment can have tremendously deleterious effects on self-image and sexual functioning. One out of nine American and European women experience breast cancer and the incidence is increasing (Kaplan, 1992). Schover et al. (1995) compared psychosocial adjustment, body image, and sexual function for 72 women who had experienced partial mastectomy and 146 women who had undergone immediate breast reconstruction after partial mastectomy. Contrary to expectations, the two groups did not differ in psychosocial adjustment to the illness, with fewer than 20% of subjects reporting poor adjustment. Women who had been treated with chemotherapy had more sexual dysfunction, poorer body image, and more psychological distress. Margolis, Goodman, and Rubin (1990) compared 22 patients who had experienced radical mastectomy with 32 women who had undergone lumpectomy combined with radiation therapy. Patients who had experienced mastectomy felt less attractive, less desirable, and experienced less sexual enjoyment than prior to treatment. Patients who had undergone radiation therapy reported no changes in these domains. Kaplan (1992) stated that all current treatments for breast cancer can have negative effects on female sexuality but that these side-effects are widely ignored by clinicians and scientists.

In men, the effects of prostate cancer on sexual functioning vary with treatment. Radical prostatectomy results in impotence in up to 85% of cases, but only 5% of patients reported impotence after transurethral resection; 80% of these patients stated, however, retrograde ejaculation which can reduce enjoyment (Mooradian, 1991; Wise et al., 1992). Penile cancer is a rare malignancy. Opjordsmoen, Waehre, Aass, and Fossa (1994) reported Norwegian data on 30 men. Their results indicate that radiotherapy preserves sexuality better than surgery or laser treatment. Partial or total penectomy severely reduces sexual interest and ability of performance.

Colon cancer often reduces sexual functioning because of psychological problems. Surgery may lead to an ostomy, and fear of stool leakage and odor may inhibit sexual responses (Kinn & Öhmann, 1986; Mooradian, 1991; Wise et al., 1992).

7.04.3.3.4 Renal failure

Many patients with decreased renal functioning report sexual difficulties. This disease is associated with various hormonal changes which may influence sexual potency (Mooradian, 1991; Wise et al., 1992).

7.04.3.3.5 Dementia

The prevalence of dementia is about 5% in individuals aged over 65, and 20% in persons over 85 (Helmchen et al., 1996; Henderson, 1986). Cognitive and personality changes of patients lead to considerable conflict, burden, and grief in relationships. Patients with Alzheimer's or multi-infarct dementia, however, may have an increase in libido, very often accompanied by inappropriate sexual behavior like exposure, public masturbation, or sexual harassment of caregivers (Mooradian, 1991). Litz, Zeiss, and Davies (1990) described psychotherapy with a man who experienced erectile dysfunction because of dramatic changes in his wife's sexual behavior due to Alzheimer's disease. Fedoroff, Peyser, Franz, and Folstein (1994) reported high frequency of sexual disorders in patients with Huntington's disease.

7.04.3.3.6 Depression

Next to dementia, depression is the second important psychiatric disease in the elderly (Helmchen et al., 1996; Henderson, 1986). Loss of libido is a common symptom of depression. Depression can be secondary to sexual dysfunction especially in men. These patients recover from depressive symptoms when sexual potency is improved. Unfortunately, mental health professionals often ignore elderly sexuality (Liptzin, 1984).

7.04.3.3.7 Use of medication

Treatment of chronic diseases almost always requires medication which may have considerable side effects on sexuality. Of the prescribed drugs, 31% are consumed by only 11.7% of the population, (i.e., elderly patients aged over 65) (Mooradian, 1991). Antihypertensive agents, major tranquilizers, minor tranquilizers, antidepressants, and miscellaneous other drugs may cause sexual dysfunction. Antihypertensive agents are probably responsible for the majority of dysfunction. They can lead to impotence, anorgasmia, and ejaculatory disturbances (Segraves & Segraves, 1992).

7.04.3.3.8 Institutionalization

Nursing home residents are often chronically ill and, therefore, dependent on caregivers (Baltes, 1996). Opportunities to express sexual feelings are often restricted because of three factors: disease-related sexual dysfunction, disapproval of sexuality by staff members, and lack of privacy (Hodson & Skeen, 1994; McCartney, Izeman, Rogers, & Cohen, 1987;Mulligan & Modigh, 1991; White, 1982). Nevertheless, institutionalized elderly people do have sexual needs and engage in sexual behaviors (Bretschneider & McCoy, 1988; White, 1982). This fact has been increasingly accepted by nursing staff, and the linkage between knowledge and attitudes towards elderly sexuality in staff has been explored (Commons, Bohn, Godon, Hauser, & Gutheil, 1992; Hillman & Stricker, 1994).

Summarizing age-related changes in sexual functioning, it seems obvious that sexuality in the elderly is not the same as in younger adults. Shaping interests in and capacity for sexual performance of older people, biology does play a role as well as socialization, individual biography with its unique events and experiences, and societal expectations. On the one hand, data show that healthy elderly people can have a satisfying sex life. On the other hand, sexual dysfunction increases with age due to the increase of chronic diseases and its treatment.

7.04.4 SEXUAL DISORDERS AND TREATMENT

Sexual functioning is often classified around three sexual response phases: desire, arousal, and orgasm (American Psychiatric Association [APA], 1994; Schiavi & Segraves, 1995). Sexual desire and sexual arousal are closely connected and the distinction between them raises scientific difficulties. Desire refers to the intensity of sexual drive whereas sexual arousal includes a subjective sense of sexual excitement. Orgasm is defined as being the peak of sexual pleasure and the release of sexual tension. Women are capable of multiple orgasms which can be experienced at the clitoral or the vaginal site. Some women experience them both, sometimes in a blended form, which are reported to be the most intense (McConaghy, 1993).

The following refers to the *Diagnostical and statistical manual of mental disorders* (4th ed.) (*DSM-IV*, APA,1994) classification. It will focus on sexual dysfunction and its treatment. The second and third group of sexual disorders, namely the paraphilias and the gender identity disorders, are not discussed here. A key diagnostic issue is the distinction between sexual disorders as the primary diagnosis versus loss of sexual functioning due to other medical or psychiatric conditions. The *DSM-IV* stresses this point by defining exclusion criteria for sexual desire disorders, sexual arousal disorders, and orgasm disorders as "the sexual dysfunction is not better accounted for by another Axis 1 disorder (except another sexual dysfunction) and is not due exclusively to the direct physiological effects of a substance (e.g., a drug of abuse, a medication) or a general medical condition" (p. 498). Other Axis 1 disorders include major depressive disorder and post-traumatic stress disorder. Sexual dysfunction in the elderly patient is often a secondary diagnosis, caused by chronic illness (Gupta, 1990; Kaiser, 1991; Leiblum & Segraves, 1989; Renshaw, 1984; Weiss & Mellinger, 1990).

Treatment of sexual disorders has changed considerably since the pioneering reports of Masters and Johnson (1966) about their success rates after two weeks of treatment, which had led to tremendous optimism with regard to sex therapy. Unfortunately, reports of successful treatment procedures had often to be corrected because long-term evaluations of the techniques failed to reveal long-term positive outcomes (Dekker & Everaerd, 1983; Fichten, Libman, & Brender, 1986; Kilmann et al., 1986). Therefore, optimism has diminished and sexual difficulties are regarded as complex problems which are the consequence of biological, psychological, cultural, and interpersonal influences. Since the late 1980s, four trends have been identified (Leiblum & Rosen, 1989b).

(i) Increased attention towards biological and medical causes, especially in the diagnosis of erectile difficulties. Vascular, hormonal, and neurological procedures have been developed in order to detect organic factors (Davidson & Rosen, 1992; Melman, 1992; Schiavi, 1992; Segraves & Segraves, 1992; Tiefer & Melman, 1989). The increased age of patients asking for sex therapy has contributed to this trend (Leiblum & Rosen, 1989b).

(ii) Increased pharmacological interventions. Again, erectile difficulties are one focus of attention. Antidepressant and antianxiety drugs are prescribed even for men with psychogenic erectile failures, which was unthinkable in the past. Kaplan and colleagues suggest pharmacotherapy in the treatment of sexual phobias and sexual aversion in addition to her psychodynamically and behavioral-oriented sex therapy (Kaplan, Fyer, & Novick, 1982; Leiblum & Rosen, 1989b; Othmer & Othmer, 1987). This trend is in line with the medical disease model and societal expectations that a sick body is like a machine and should be made to function again as quickly as possible.

(iii) Concentration on desire disorders. On the one hand, clinicians report the growing number of couples presenting desire discrepancies, with usually one partner reporting low desire (Leiblum & Rosen, 1988). On the other hand, there are case reports about sexual addicts or hyperactive sexual interest (Goodman, 1993).

(iv) A therapeutic shift from behavioral to interpersonal system concepts and psychodynamic object-relations theories. Short-term behavioral sex therapies, although successful in some cases, failed with many individuals and with complex problems (Bagarozzi, 1987; Kaplan, 1974, 1977; Leiblum & Rosen, 1992). Intrapsychic difficulties in attachment, dependency, and commitment as well as interpersonal systemic issues have become the focus of attention (Bagarozzi, 1987; Brown & Field, 1988; Leiblum & Rosen, 1992; Levay, 1983; McCarthy, 1984; Talmadge & Talmadge, 1986).

7.04.4.1 Sexual Desire Disorders

These disorders are hypoactive sexual desire disorder (HSDD) and sexual aversion disorder. HSDD is defined as:

> persistently or recurrently deficient (or absent) sexual fantasies and desire for sexual activity. The judgment of deficiency or absence is made by the clinician, taking into account factors that affect sexual functioning, such as age, sex, and the context of the person's life. (APA, 1994, p. 498)

This definition has been frequently criticized because it does not give clear-cut criteria such as length of time, and is therefore highly subjective (LoPiccolo, 1985). Nevertheless, clinicians agree that low or absent desire is one of the most prevalent psychosexual problems seen by them (Leiblum & Rosen, 1988; Rosen & Leiblum, 1989). Desire disorders are believed to be highly refractory to treatment because they are supposed to be a symptom of severe intrapsychic conflicts. Radin (1989) provided a theoretical and clinical understanding of this disorder proposing that preoedipal factors and psychological defense mechanisms that originated during the pregenital years play a significant role in the etiology. Schreiner-Engel and Schiavi (1986) tried to prove the assumption of severe underlying psychopathology. They compared 46 couples with one partner who had inhibited sexual desire with 36 controls. Results showed that individuals with inhibited desire had a history of major and/or intermittent depression twice as high as controls. Furthermore, depressive disorder coincided or preceded sexual dysfunction.

Donahey and Carroll (1993) raised the question whether there is in fact an increase in hypoactive sexual desire, or whether individuals or couples define this as a problem because sexual functioning has become very important in Western cultures. They reported that biological, psychological, and interpersonal factors have been discussed in the etiology of hypoactive sexual desire and that these factors are assumed to affect men and women equally. Donahey and Carroll (1993) hypothesized that hypoactive sexual desire develops and manifests itself differently for men and women. They investigated 47 males and 22 females and found that women reported more stress, and that they were less satisfied with their marriages. The authors suggested that treatment for women should focus more on psychological symptomatology and relationship issues. LoPiccolo (1985) noted that low sexual desire is inconsistent with the cultural expectation and fantasy of male sexuality. Therefore, it is an interesting phenomenon but empirical data are lacking.

Kaplan & Owett (1993) contributed an important physiological reason for inhibited desire in females. They showed that a loss of androgens is associated with a marked decrease in sexual desire and libido. This observation should be further investigated, because the Kaplan and Owett data stem from cancer patients who underwent chemotherapy and, thus, other explanations for decreased interest in sex are also plausible.

The differentiation between sex therapy and psychotherapy has become increasingly difficult. One reason for this change is the growing interest in sexual desire disorders. Many authors have argued that chronic desire disorders can only be treated within individual psychotherapy, in particular psychodynamic approaches, psychoanalysis, and object-relations therapy (Kaplan, 1977; Levay, 1983; Levine, 1988; Radin, 1989; Scharff; 1988; Talmadge & Talmadge, 1986).

Other authors have argued for cognitive-behavioral or systemic-interactional approaches. The necessity of exploring sexual scripts in order to understand sexual fantasies, unreal ideals, and false beliefs has been stressed (Lazarus, 1988; LoPiccolo & Stock, 1986; McCarthy, 1984; Rosen & Leiblum, 1988; 1989). Furthermore, the couple's relationship has to be examined carefully. For example, inhibited sexual desire in one individual can be a very effective means for regulating power distribution (Bagarozzi, 1987).

Some authors have suggested pharmacotherapy for treatment of low desire. Despite some successful reports, results have not been convincing (Leiblum & Rosen, 1989; Segraves, 1988).

Sexual aversion disorder is defined as "persistent or recurrent extreme aversion to, and avoidance of, all (or almost all) genital sexual contact with a sexual partner" (APA, 1994, p. 500). This syndrome occurs in both females and males. Crenshaw (1985) differentiated between primary and secondary aversion. Primary aversion is characterized by a negative response to any sexual interactions from the earliest memories to the present and is often combined with other dysfunction. A psychosexual trauma like incest or child molestation is frequently found. Secondary aversion is acquired, which means that sexuality was found pleasurable in the past. In the beginning of the disorder individuals may function well sexually when they get involved in sexual activities. The differentiation between the two desire disorders is often difficult. There are no special treatment suggestions.

7.04.4.2 Female Disorders

LaFerla (1984) listed a number of factors contributing to female sexual dysfunction in desire and orgasmic response. He differentiated psychosocial and organic factors. Psychosocial factors are relationship issues, negative past experiences, and depression as well as drug and alcohol abuse. Organic factors are chronic illness, pregnancy, pharmacological agents, and endocrine alterations.

7.04.4.2.1 Arousal disorder

For females, arousal disorder means a "persistent or recurrent inability to attain, or to maintain until completion of the sexual activity, an adequate lubrication-swelling response of sexual excitement" (APA, 1994, p. 502). The excitement phase in elderly women is much slower than in younger ones. Whereas in young women lubrication occurs after 10–15 seconds, it requires at least five minutes in the postmenopausal women (Gupta, 1990). However, this change is normal and cannot be considered a disorder. Some women produce insufficient vaginal lubrication altogether, and they may need artificial lubricants.

7.04.4.2.2 Orgasmic disorder

The female orgasmic disorder is defined as a:

> persistent or recurrent delay in, or absence of, orgasm following a normal sexual excitement phase. Women exhibit wide variability in the type or intensity of stimulation that triggers orgasm. The diagnosis of female orgasmic disorder should be based on the clinician's judgment that the woman's orgasmic capacity is less than would be reasonable for her age, sexual experience, and the adequacy of sexual stimulation she receives. (APA, 1994, p. 506).

Orgasmic disorder is still one of the most frequent sexual dysfunctions in women. It is divided into primary and secondary anorgasmia. Primary anorgasmia refers to women who have never experienced an orgasm, secondary anorgasmia refers to women who sometimes or in specific situations (e.g., masturbation) react orgasmically. Empirical data from cross-sectional studies suggest that the rate of women who never or rarely react with orgasm decreases from 50% in young adulthood to 21% at the age of 40 (McConaghy, 1993), remains fairly stable with 21% between the ages of 40 and 59 (Laumann et al., 1994), and increases to 28% over the age of 70 (Bergström-Walan & Neilsen, 1990; Brecher, 1984). Nevertheless, these data are difficult to evaluate. Concerns about women's orgasm are a rather new phenomenon. Women can have an orgasm in the same amount of time as men, and they can achieve multiple orgasms. Personal history, relationship difficulties, lack of education, and lack of knowledge about sexuality may be reasons for the inhibition of the orgasmic response. Very little is known about factors that contribute to orgasmic capacity. The neurophysiological basis of human orgasm is underexplored (Heiman & Grafton-Becker, 1989).

Treatment approaches of this disorder depend on the theoretical orientation of the therapist. Three major approaches are psychoanalytic, cognitive-behavioral, and systemic theory. Psychoanalytic psychotherapy does not focus on symptom removal but on working through underlying conflicts that lead to the symptom. Once these conflicts are understood and worked through, symptoms disappear. Kaplan (1974, 1977) combined a psychodynamic approach with behavioral sex therapy elements.

Cognitive-behavioral therapy depends on learning theory and tries to promote cognitive as well as behavioral changes. Behavioral exercises, like directed masturbation, partner stimulation, and Kegel exercises, are frequently used. Whereas directed masturbation seems to be successful in treatment of primary anorgasmia, its long-term effectiveness in treating secondary anorgasmia is questionable (Fichten, Libman, & Brender, 1986; Kilmann et al., 1986; Kuriansky, Sharpe, & O'Connor, 1982; Nairne & Hemsley, 1983; Wakefield, 1987).

Systemic therapists concentrate on the couple as a system and do not focus on the individual woman with anorgasmia. Her dysfunction is regarded as a problem of the system. Thus, therapists focus on interactional patterns. Heimann and Grafton-Becker (1989) suggested an integrated theory and practice that combines the theoretical and practical elements of psychoanalytic, cognitive-behavioral, and systemic theories.

7.04.4.2.3 Sexual pain disorders

Dyspareunia and vaginismus are sexual pain disorders. Dyspareunia is a "recurrent or persistent genital pain associated with sexual intercourse in either a male or a female" (APA, 1994, p. 513). This disorder can have organic and/or psychological causes. Careful assessment and diagnosis is very important (Sandberg & Quevillon, 1987). Lazarus (1989) described three psychological factors, namely traumatic (e.g., rape), developmental (e.g., religious taboos) and relational (e.g., resentment, insufficient sexual stimulation through partner). Unsatisfactory relationships are the major reason for this dysfunction. After a careful multimodal assessment, treatment depends on the identified cause and may consist of different methods (e.g., relationship enhancement, social skills training, imagery techniques, systematic desensitization, and sensate focus).

Vaginismus is defined as a "recurrent or persistent involuntary spasm of the musculature of the outer third of the vagina that interferes with sexual intercourse" (APA, 1994, p. 515). Women with vaginismus may function sexually without difficulties except their inability to have intercourse. Different psychological theories agree that anxiety is the core of these spastic contractions. Treatment very often consists of the gradual insertion of objects in the vagina. Dilators with increasing size are frequently used. Examples of treatment with different outcomes are discussed by Leiblum, Pervin, and Campell (1989).

7.04.4.3 Male Disorders

7.04.4.3.1 Arousal disorder

For males, arousal disorder is defined as erectile disorder: "Persistent or recurrent inability to attain, or to maintain until completion of the sexual activity, an adequate erection" (APA, 1994, p. 504). Erectile difficulties increase with age and they are the major sexual problem of elderly males (Kaiser, 1991; Levine, 1992; Nelson, 1987; Rosen & Leiblum, 1992a, 1992b; Segraves & Segraves, 1992; Weiss & Mellinger, 1990).

For many years psychological factors have been perceived as major causes of erectile difficulties, and organic causes have been widely overlooked. Recent work has focused on differential diagnosis of physiological and psychological factors (Kinder & Curtiss, 1988; LoPiccolo, 1985). Levine (1992) suggested four categories for classification: psychogenic, organic, mixed, and idiopathic (when the professional cannot identify the cause with certainty). Disease or drug-related erectile failures are common in elderly men but psychogenic factors may work in addition.

Intensive research efforts have focused on the determinants of erectile dysfunction. In addition, numerous treatment approaches have been tried (Rosen & Leiblum, 1992). Modern psychotherapeutic treatment concentrates on the systemic function of erectile difficulties (Althof, 1989; Levine, 1992; Leiblum & Rosen, 1992; LoPiccolo, 1992; Speckens et al., 1995).

Surgical treatment has become very important in recent years. There is surgical correction of reversible dysfunction and, in cases of nonreversibility, penile prosthesis can be implanted. Implant devices have, however, considerable risks and disadvantages, and careful consideration has to precede surgery (LoPiccolo & Stock, 1986; Melman & Tiefer, 1992). Injection therapy and vacuum devices are also widely used (Althof & Turner, 1992; Kaplan, 1990).

7.04.4.3.2 Orgasmic disorders

In males, there are two orgasm disorders, namely the male orgasmic disorder and premature ejaculation. Male orgasmic disorder is defined as a "persistent or recurrent delay in, or absence of, orgasm following a normal sexual excitement phase during sexual activity that the clinician, taking into account the person's age, judges to be adequate in focus, intensity, and duration" (APA, 1994, p. 509). This disorder is not often seen in a clinical context. Apfelbaum (1989) proposed that the retarded ejaculator is more responsive to his own stimulation and experiences hostility towards his partner. The patient has to become aware of his distance and anger before he can make any progress.

Premature ejaculation is defined as a "persistent or recurrent ejaculation with minimal sexual stimulation before, on, or shortly after penetration and before the person wishes it" (APA, 1994, p. 511). This disorder is more common in younger men and its treatment seems to be very effective. Information about different treatment techniques are given by LoPiccolo (1985), LoPiccolo and Stock (1986), and McCarthy (1989).

7.04.4.4 Special Issues in Treatment with Elderly Patients

Basically, there are no differences between sexual difficulties and dysfunction between younger and older adults. Nevertheless, there are some issues which should be considered. First, biological changes with age and health-related factors have to be explored thoroughly. Second, cohort experiences and values have to be considered. Third, life events and circumstances have to be evaluated (Leiblum & Segraves, 1989; LoPiccolo, 1991).

Physiological and health-related changes have been previously described in this chapter. Clinical observations about the behavior of hundreds of elderly men, women, and couples who have sought help for sexual difficulties revealed adaptation processes to the major physiological changes. Kaplan (1990) summarized that couples who have a good and intimate relationship, who care for each other and each other's pleasure, and who are sexually open and free of severe conflicts, can adapt to these changes very successfully. She described the following coping mechanisms that may help to maintain sexual functioning:

(i) *Diminished sexual desire.* This problem may occur in either one or both partners and can be overcome with the help of fantasies or erotica. Testosterone replacement is helpful in some cases. Treatment of possible depression or substance abuse might be necessary.

(ii) *Higher penile threshold for mental and physical stimulation/delayed lubrication.* These problems can be solved with partner-provided, extended physical stimulation. Erotica or fantasy and more rapid love making are helpful. Morning sex is recommended because elderly men function better in the morning due to higher testosterone levels.

(iii) *Vaginal dryness and atrophy; dyspareunia.* Use of lubricants prior to coitus and/or estrogen replacement are beneficial. Intercourse on a regular basis and dilators may be useful.

(iv) *Softer penile erections.* Coital positions which facilitate intromission (e.g., stuffing) are recommended. Stimulation, enjoyment, and orgasms by manual or oral practices should be emphasized.

(v) *Lengthened male refractory period.* This causes less frequent intercourse. Quality vs. quantity of experience should be emphasized.

(vi) *Physical mobility and pain.* Analgesics taken before sexual activity or a hot bath to reduce stiffness may help. A side-by-side-position is often more comfortable.

Counseling or treatment should be done cautiously. Very often, information about age-related changes and "permission giving" of new experiences (e.g., more manual or oral stimulation, fantasies, new positions) are helpful. Keeping in mind cohort differences, the therapist should carefully evaluate the patient's value system and possible shame reactions before any suggestions are made. Middle-class values of younger adults are easily imposed and might substantially harm the elderly patient. For example, masturbation, oral sex, or the use of a vibrator may be common practices for sex therapists but not necessarily for a couple born in the countryside in the 1920s.

In some cases, sexual dysfunction of elderly patients has a severe underlying conflict. For example, meeting the psychosocial crises of ego integrity or ego despair may result in sexual dysfunction (Fagan, Meyer, & Schmidt, 1986). In these cases individual psychotherapy should be considered. Contrary to common beliefs and stereotypes of many psychotherapists of all theoretical backgrounds, psychotherapy can be very successful with elderly patients (Radebold, 1992; Smyer, Zarit, & Qualls, 1990). It is important, however, that psychotherapists of elderly people have some gerontological and historical knowledge, and that they are aware of special countertransference issues (Apfel, Fox, Isberg, & Levine, 1984; Radebold, 1992).

Finally, it has to be recognized that sexual behavior is not easily modifiable. Sexual anxiety, which is believed to be the core of most sexual dysfunction (Patterson & O'Gorman, 1989), has "an important adaptive feature of human sexual behavior" (Cole, 1985, p. 337). Cole presented a critical review about sex therapy and its outcome research. He concluded that sex therapy has intrinsic limitations which have to be accepted. Vandereycken (1987) argued in addition that sexual lust has turned from a taboo into a "must." The establishment of new behavioral demands should certainly not be the result of gerontological research and psychotherapy with elderly people. Therefore, careful and critical reflection of scientific data and therapeutic aims is crucial.

7.04.5 CONCLUSION

This chapter has examined literature on sexuality and aging. In spite of the growing body of research on old age and aging, there is a considerable lack of sound studies in the context of sexuality and aging, particularly with respect to elderly women. Epidemiological data have been presented and their methodological and theoretical problems described. Age-related physiological changes in women and men were examined. It is important to differentiate between normal age-related changes and health-related problems. Chronic disease increases with age, but deleterious effects on sexual enjoyment are due to disease, and not to aging *per se*. Sexual disorders of desire, arousal, and orgasm as well as treatment approaches have been described. Finally, sexuality of the elderly individual should be embedded in a life-span developmental perspective. The important role that the individual biography plays in the aging process is an accepted fact in modern gerontology. Further research should pay more attention to intra-individual development. Many research results (e.g., differences in sexual activities between men and women) may be due to cohort effects and not to biological factors.

7.04.6 REFERENCES

Adams, C. G., & Turner, B. F. (1985). Reported change in sexuality from young adulthood to old age. *The Journal of Sex Research*, *21*(2), 126–141.

Althof, S. E. (1989). Psychogenic impotence: Treatment of men and couples. In S. R. Leiblum & R. C. Rosen (Eds.), *Principles and practice of sex therapy: Update for the 1990s* (2nd ed., pp. 237–265). New York: Guilford Press.

Althof, S. E., & Turner, L. A. (1992). Self-injection therapy and external vacuum devices in the treatment of erectile dysfunction: Methods and outcome. In R. C. Rosen & S. R. Leiblum (Eds.), *Erectile disorders: Assessment and treatment* (pp. 283–309). New York: Guilford Press.

American Psychiatric Association. (1994). *Diagnostic and statistical manual of mental disorders* (4th ed.). Washington, DC: Author.

Antonovsky, H., Sadowsky, M., & Maoz, B. (1990). Sexual activity of aging men and women: An Israeli study. *Behavior, Health, and Aging*, *1*(3), 151–161.

Apfel, R. J., Fox, M., Isberg, R. S., & Levine, A. R. (1984). Countertransference and transference in couple therapy: Treating sexual dysfunction in older couples. *Journal of Geriatric Psychiatry*, *17*(2), 203–214.

Apfelbaum, B. (1989). Retarded ejaculation: A much-misunderstood syndrome. In S. R. Leiblum & R. C. Rosen (Eds.), *Principles and practice of sex therapy: Update for the 1990s* (2nd ed., pp. 168–206). New York: Guilford Press.

Aresin, L. (1980). Sexualverhalten nach dem 60. Lebensjahr. *Zeitschrift für Alternsforschung*, *35*, 55–58.

Bachmann, G. A., & Leiblum, S. R. (1991). Sexuality in sexagenarian women. *Maturitas*, *13*(1), 43–50.

Bagarozzi, D. A. (1987). Marital/family developmental theory as a context for understanding and treating inhibited sexual desire. *Journal of Sex and Marital Therapy*, *13*(4), 276–285.

Baltes, M. M. (1996). *The many faces of dependency in old age*. Cambridge, UK: Cambridge University Press.

Baltes, P. B. (1987). Theoretical propositions of life-span developmental psychology: On the dynamics between growth and decline. *Developmental Psychology*, *23*, 611–626.

Baltes, P. B. & Baltes, M. M. (Eds.) (1990). *Successful aging: Perspectives from the behavioral sciences*. Cambridge, UK: Cambridge University Press.

Baltes, P. B., Reese, H. W., & Lipsitt, L. P. (1980). Life-span developmental psychology. *Annual Review of Psychology*, *31*, 65–110.

Bengston, V. L., Reedy, M. N., & Gordon, C. (1985). Aging and self-conceptions: Personality processes and social contents. In J. E. Birren & K. W. Schaie (Eds.). *Handbook of the psychology of aging* (2nd ed., pp. 544–593). New York: Van Nostrand Reinhold.

Bergström-Walan, M.-B., & Nielsen, H. H. (1990). Sexual expression among 60–80-year-old men and women: A sample from Stockholm, Sweden. *The Journal of Sex Research*, *27*(2), 289–295.

Bernhard, L. (1986). Methodology issues in studies of

sexuality and hysterectomy. *The Journal of Sex Research, 22*(1), 108–128.
Birren, J. E. & Schaie, K. W. (Eds.) (1985). *Handbook of the psychology of aging* (2nd ed.). New York: Van Nostrand Reinhold.
Brähler, E., & Unger, U. (1994). Sexuelle Aktivität im höheren Lebensalter im Kontext von Geschlecht, Familienstand und Persönlichkeitsaspekten—Ergebnisse einer repräsentativen Befragung. (Sexual activity in old age in context of gender, marital status and personality—Results of a representative study). *Zeitschrift für Gerontologie, 27* ,110–115.
Brecher, E. M. (1984). *Love, sex and aging: A Consumer Union report.* Boston: Little Brown.
Bretschneider, J. G., & McCoy, N. L. (1988). Sexual interest and behavior in healthy 80- to 102-year-olds. *Archives of Sexual Behavior, 7*(2), 109–129.
Brown, R. A., & Field, J. R. (Eds.) (1988). *Treatment of sexual problems in individual and couples therapy.* New York: PMA.
Burgener, S., & Logan, G. (1989). Sexuality concerns of the post-stroke patient. *Rehabilitation Nursing, 14*(4), 178–181.
Byers, J. P. (1983). Sexuality and the elderly. *Geriatric Nursing, 4,* 293–297.
Capuzzi, D. (1982). Sexuality and aging: An overview for counselors. *Personnel and Guidance Journal, 61,* 31–35.
Christenson, C., & Johnson, A. B. (1973). Sexual patterns in a group of older never married women. *Journal of Geriatric Psychiatry, 6*(1), 80–98.
Colarusso, C., & Nemiroff, R. (1981). *Adult development: A new dimension in psychodynamic theory and practice.* New York: Plenum.
Cole, M. (1985). Sex therapy: A critical appraisal. *British Journal of Psychiatry, 147,* 337–351.
Commons, M. L., Bohn, J. T., Godon, L. T., Hauser, M. J., & Gutheil, T. G. (1992). Professional's attitudes towards sex between institutionalized patients. *American Journal of Psychotherapy, 46*(4), 571–580.
Corby, N., & Zarit, J. M. (1983). Old and alone: The unmarried in later life. In R. B. Weg (Ed.), *Sexuality in the later years. Roles and behavior* (pp. 131–145). New York: Academic Press.
Costa, P. T., Jr., Zondermann, A. B., McCrae, R. R., Cornoni-Huntley, J., Locke, B. Z., & Barbano, H. E. (1987). Longitudinal analyses of psychological well-being in a national sample: Stability of mean levels. *Journal of Gerontology, 42,* 50–55.
Crenshaw, T. L. (1985). The sexual aversion syndrome. *Journal of Sex and Marital Therapy, 11*(4), 285–292.
Cruikshank, M. (1990). Lavender and gray: A brief survey of lesbian and gay aging studies. *Journal of Homosexuality, 20*(3/4), 77–87.
Datan, N., & Rodeheaver, D. (1983). Beyond generativity: Toward a sensuality of later life. In R. B. Weg (Ed.), *Sexuality in the later years. Roles and behavior* (pp. 280–288). New York: Academic Press.
Davidson, J. M., & Rosen, R. C. (1992). Hormonal determinants of erectile function. In R. C. Rosen & S. R. Leiblum (Eds.), *Erectile disorders: Assessment and treatment* (pp. 72–95). New York: Guilford.
Dekker, J., & Everaerd, W. (1983). A long-term follow-up study of couples treated for sexual dysfunctions. *Journal of Sex and Marital Therapy, 9*(2), 99–113.
Dennerstein, L., Smith, A. M. A., Morse, C. A., & Burger, H. G. (1994). Sexuality and the menopause. *Journal of Psychosomatic Obstetrics and Gynaecology, 15,* 59–66.
Denney, N. W., Field, J. K., & Quadagno, D. (1984). Sex differences in sexual needs and desires. *Archives of Sexual Behavior, 13,* 233–245.
Donahey, K. M., & Carroll, R. A. (1993). Gender differences in factors associated with hypoactive sexual desire. *Journal of Sex and Marital Therapy, 19*(1), 25–40.
Eckert, J. W. (1984). "Clinical perspectives on sexuality in older patients": Discussion. *Journal of Geriatric Psychiatry, 17*(2), 183–188.
Eicher W. (1994a). Hysterektomie und Sexualität (I). Eine Standortbestimmung. *Sexualmedizin, 5,* 144–148.
Eicher W. (1994b). Hysterektomie und Sexualität (II). Eine Standortbestimmung. *Sexualmedizin, 6,* 176–180.
Erikson, E. H. (1950). *Childhood and Society.* New York: Norton.
Fagan, P. J., Meyer, J. K., & Schmidt, C. W. (1986). Sexual dysfunction within an adult developmental perspective. *Journal of Sex and Marital Therapy, 12*(4), 243–257.
Fedoroff, J. P., Peyser, C., Franz, M. L., & Folstein, S. E. (1994). Sexual disorders in Huntington's disease. *The Journal of Neuropsychiatry and Clinical Neurosciences, 6,* 147–153.
Fichten, C. S., Libman, E., & Brender, W. (1986). Measurement of therapy outcome and maintenance of gains in the behavioral treatment of secondary orgasmic dysfunction. *Journal of Sex and Marital Therapy, 12*(1), 22–34.
Fooken, I. (1994). Sexuality in later years: The impact of health and body image in a sample of older women. *Patient Education and Counseling, 23*(3) 227–233.
Freud, S. (1964). Drei Abhandlungen zur Sexualtheorie. (Three contributions to the theory of sex). *Gesammelte Werke.* (Vol. V, pp. 27–145). Frankfurt, Germany: Fischer. (Original work published 1905).
Friend, R. A. (1990). Older lesbian and gay people: A theory of successful aging. *Journal of Homosexuality, 20*(3–4), 99–118.
Garza, J. M. & Dressel, P. L. (1983). Sexuality and later-life marriages. In: T. H. Brubaker (Ed.), *Family relationships in later life* (pp. 91–108). Beverly Hills, CA: Sage.
Gatz, M. (1987). *Adult development and aging: Growing older in a contingent and noncontingent world.* Presented at the Association for Advancement of Behavior Therapy annual convention, Boston.
Gendel, E. S. (1986). Self-esteem and sexuality in older patients with cancer. *Frontiers of radiation therapy and oncology, 20,* 166–172.
Genevay, B. (1982). In praise of older women. In M. Kirkpatrick (Ed.), *Women' s sexual experience. Explorations of the dark continent* (pp. 87–101). New York: Plenum.
George, L. K., & Weiler, S. J. (1981). Sexuality in middle and late life: The effects of age, cohort and gender. *Archives of General Psychiatry, 38,* 919–923.
Goldstein, M. K., & Teng, N. N. H. (1991). Gynecological factors in sexual dysfunction of the older women, *Clinics in Geriatric Medicine, 7*(1), 41–61.
Goodman, A. (1993). Diagnosis and treatment of sexual addiction. *Journal of Sex and Marital Therapy, 19*(3), 225–251.
Greeley, A. M. (1994). Janus report. *Contemporary Sociology.* Forthcoming.
Gupta, K. (1990). Sexual dysfunction in elderly women. *Clinics in Geriatric Medicine, 6*(1), 197–203.
Hagstad, A. (1988). Gynecology and sexuality in middle-aged women. *Women and Health, 13,* 57–80.
Hagstad, A., & Janson, P. O. (1984). Sexuality among Swedish women around forty: An epidemiological survey. *Journal of Psychosomatic Obstetrics and Gynaecology, 3,* 191–203.
Hällström, T., & Samuelsson, S. (1990). Changes in women's sexual desire in middle life: The longitudinal study of women in Gothenburg. *Archives of Sexual Behavior, 19*(3), 259–268.
Heiman, J. R., & Grafton-Becker, V. (1989). Orgasmic disorders in women. In S. R. Leiblum & R. C. Rosen (Eds.), *Principles and practice of sex therapy: Update for the 1990s* (2nd ed., pp. 51–88). New York: Guilford.
Helmchen, H., Baltes, M. M., Geiselmann, B., Kanowski,

S., Linden, M., Reischies, F. M., Wagner, M., & Wilms, H.-U. (1996). Psychische Erkrankungen im Alter. In K. U. Mayer & P. B. Baltes (Eds.), *Die Berliner Altersstudie* (pp. 185–219). Berlin, Germany: Akademie Verlag.

Helmström, L. , Lundberg, P. O., Sörbom, D., & Bäckstrom, T. (1993). Sexuality after hysterectomy: A factor analysis of women's sexual lives before and after subtotal hysterectomy. *Obstetrics and Gynecology, 81*(3), 357–362.

Henderson, A. S. (1986). Epidemiology of mental illness. In H. Häfner, G. Moschel & N. Sartorius (Eds.), *Mental Health in the Elderly. A Review of the Present State of Research* (pp. 29–34). Berlin, Germany: Springer-Verlag.

Hermanova, H. M. (1983). Human sexuality and aging. In M. Bergener, U. Lehr, E. Lang, & R. Schmitz-Scherzer (Eds.), *Aging in the eighties and beyond* (pp. 324–332). New York: Springer.

Hillman, J. L., & Stricker, G. (1994). A linkage of knowledge and attitudes toward elderly sexuality: Not necessarily a uniform relationship. *The Gerontologist, 34*(2), 256–260.

Hite, S. (1976). *The Hite report*. New York: Dell.

Hodson, D. S., & Skeen, P. (1994). Sexuality and aging: The hammerlock of myths. *Journal of Applied Gerontology, 13*(3), 219–235.

Institute for Sex Research (1953). *Sexual behavior in the human female*. Philadelphia: Saunders.

Janus, S. S., & Janus, C. L. (1993). *The Janus report on sexual behavior*. New York: Wiley.

Jung, C. G. (1933). *Modern Man in Search of a Soul*. New York: Harcourt Brace.

Kaiser, F. E. (1991). Sexuality and impotence in the aging man. *Clinics in Geriatric Medicine, 7*(1), 63–72.

Kaiser, F. E. (1992). Sexual function and the older cancer patient. *Oncology*, 6(2), 112–118.

Kaplan, H. S. (1974). *The new sex therapy*. New York: Brunner/Mazel.

Kaplan, H. S. (1977). Hypoactive sexual desire. *Journal of Sex and Marital Therapy, 3*, 3–9.

Kaplan, H. S. (1990). The combined use of sex therapy and intrapenile injections in the treatment of impotence. *Journal of Sex and Marital Therapy, 16*(4), 195–207.

Kaplan, H. S. (1992). A neglected issue: The sexual side effects of current treatments for breast cancer. *Journal of Sex and Marital Therapy, 18*(1), 3–19.

Kaplan, H. S., Fyer, A. J., & Novick, A. (1982). The treatment of sexual phobias: The combined use of antipanic medication and sex therapy. *Journal of Sex and Marital Therapy, 8*(1), 3–28.

Kaplan, H. S., & Owett, T. (1993). The female androgen deficiency syndrome. *Journal of Sex and Marital Therapy, 19*(1), 3–24.

Kay, B., & Neelley, J. N. (1982). Sexuality and aging: A review of current literature. *Sexuality and Disability, 5*(1), 38–46.

Kellett, J. M. (1993). Sexuality in later life. *Reviews in Clinical Gerontology, 3*(3), 309–314.

Kernberg, O. F. (1977). Normal psychology of the aging process revisited-II. Discussion. *Journal of Geriatric Psychiatry, 10*, 27–45.

Kilmann, P. R., Boland, J. P., Norton, S. P., Davidson, E., & Caid, C. (1986). Perspectives of sex therapy outcome: a survey of AASECT providers. *Journal of Sex and Marital Therapy, 12*(2), 116–138.

Kilmann, P. R., Mills, K. H., Caid, C., Davidson, E., Bella, B., Milan, R., Drose, G., Boland, J., Follingstad, D., Montgomery, B., & Wanlass, R. (1986). Treatment of secondary orgasmic dysfunction: An outcome study. *Archives of Sexual Behavior, 15*(3), 211–229.

Kinder, B. N., & Curtiss, G. (1988). Specific components in the etiology, assessment, and treatment of male sexual dysfunction: Controlled outcome studies. *Journal of Sex and Marital Therapy, 14*(1), 40–48.

Kinn, A.-C., & Öhman, U. (1986). Bladder and sexual function after surgery for rectal cancer. *Diseases of the Colon and Rectum, 29*, 43–48.

Kinsey, A. C., Pomeroy, W. B., & Martin, C. R. (1948). *Sexual behavior in the human male*. Philadelphia: Saunders.

Kirkpatrick, M. (1980). *Women's sexual development: Explorations of inner space*. New York: Plenum.

Klassen, A. D., Williams, C. J., & Levitt, E. E. (1989). *Sex and morality in the US. An empirical inquiry under the auspices of the Kinsey institute*. Middletown, CT: Wesleyan University Press.

Kruse, A. (1989). Psychologie des Alters. In: K. P. Kisker, H. Lauter, J.-E. Meyer, C. Müller & E. Strömgren (Eds.), *Psychiatrie der Gegenwart 8, Alterspsychiatrie*. (pp. 1–58). Berlin, Germany: Springer-Verlag.

Kuriansky, J. B., Sharpe, L., & O'Connor, D. (1982). The treatment of anorgasmia: Long-term effectiveness of a short-term behavioral group therapy. *Journal of Sex and Marital Therapy, 8*(1), 29–43.

LaFerla, J. J. (1984). Inhibited sexual desire and orgasmic dysfunction in women. *Clinical Obstetrics and Gynecology, 27*(3), 738–749.

Laumann, E. O., Gagnon, J. H., Michael, R. T., & Michels, S. (1994). *The social organization of sexuality. Sexual practices in the United States*. Chicago: University of Chicago Press.

Laws, J. L. (1980). Female sexuality through the life-span. In P. B. Baltes & O. G. Brim, (Eds.), *Life-span development and behavior* (Vol. 3, pp. 207–252). New York: Academic Press.

Lazarus, A. A. (1988). A multimodal perspective on problems of sexual desire. In S. R. Leiblum & R. C. Rosen (Eds.), *Sexual desire disorders* (pp. 145–167). New York: Guilford Press.

Lazarus, A. A. (1989). Dyspareunia: A multimodal psychotherapeutic perspective. In S. R. Leiblum & R. C. Rosen (Eds.), *Principles and practice of sex therapy: Update for the 1990s* (2nd ed., pp. 89–112). New York: Guilford.

Lehr, U. & Thomae, H. (Eds.) (1987), *Formen seelischen Alterns: Ergebnisse der Bonner Längsschnittstudie (BOLSA)*. Stuttgart, Germany: Enke.

Leiblum, S. R. (1990). Sexuality and the mid-life woman. Special issue: Women at midlife and beyond. *Psychology of Women Quarterly, 14*, 495–508.

Leiblum, S. R., Pervin, L. A., & Campbell, E. H. (1989). The treatment of vaginismus: Success and failure. In S. R. Leiblum & R. C. Rosen (Eds.), *Principles and practice of sex therapy: Update for the 1990s* (2nd ed., pp. 113–138). New York: Guilford Press.

Leiblum S. R., & Rosen, R. C. (Eds.) (1988). *Sexual desire disorders*. New York: Guilford Press.

Leiblum, S. R. & Rosen, R. C. (1989a). Introduction: Sex therapy in the age of Aids. In S. R. Leiblum & R. C. Rosen (Eds.), *Principles and practice of sex therapy: Update for the 1990s* (2nd ed., pp. 1–16). New York: Guilford Press.

Leiblum, S. R., & Rosen, R. C. (Eds.). (1989b). *Principles and practice of sex therapy: Update for the 1990s* (2nd ed.). New York: Guilford Press.

Leiblum, S. R., & Rosen, R. C. (1992). Couples therapy for erectile disorders: Observations, obstacles, and outcomes. In R. C. Rosen & S. R. Leiblum (Eds.), *Erectile disorders: Assessment and treatment* (pp. 226–254). New York: Guilford Press.

Leiblum, S. R., & Segraves, R. T. (1989). Sex therapy with aging adults. In S. R. Leiblum & R. C. Rosen (Eds.), *Principles and practice of sex therapy: Update for the 1990s* (2nd ed., pp. 352–381). New York: Guilford Press.

Levay, A. N. (1983). Personality change in sex therapy. *Journal of the American Academy of Psychoanalysis, 11*(3), 425–433.

Levine, S. B. (1988). Intrapsychic and individual aspects of sexual desire. In S. R. Leiblum & R. C. Rosen (Eds.), *Sexual desire disorders* (pp. 21–44). New York: Guilford Press.

Levine, S. B. (1992). Intrapsychic and interpersonal aspects of impotence: Psychogenic erectile dysfunction. In R. C. Rosen & S. R. Leiblum (Eds.), *Erectile disorders: Assessment and treatment.* (pp. 198–225). New York: Guilford Press.

Libman, E. (1989). Sociocultural and cognitive factors in aging and sexual expression: Conceptual and research issues. *Canadian Psychology/Psychologie Canadienne, 30*(3), 560–567.

Liptzin, B. (1984). Clinical perspectives on sexuality in older patients. *Journal of Geriatric Psychiatry, 17* (2), 167–188.

Litz, B. T., Zeiss, A. M., & Davies, H. D. (1990). Sexual concerns of male spouses of female Alzheimer's disease patients. *The Gerontologist, 30*(1), 113–116.

Livson, F. B, (1983). Gender identity: A life-span view of sex-role development. In R. B. Weg (Ed.), *Sexuality in the later years: Roles and behavior* (pp. 105–127). New York: Academic Press.

LoPiccolo, J. (1985). Diagnosis and treatment of male sexual dysfunction. *Journal of Sex and Marital Therapy, 11*(4), 215–232.

LoPiccolo, J. (1991). Counseling and therapy for sexual problems in the elderly. *Clinics in Geriatric Medicine, 7*(1), 161–179.

LoPiccolo (1992). Postmodern therapy for erectile failure. In R. C. Rosen & S. R. Leiblum (Eds.), *Erectile disorders: Assessment and treatment* (pp. 171–197). New York: Guilford Press.

LoPiccolo, J., & Stock, W. E. (1986). Treatment of sexual dysfunction. *Journal of Consulting and Clinical Psychology, 54*(2), 158–167.

Ludeman, K. (1981). The sexuality of the older person: Review of the literature. *The Gerontologist, 21*(2), 203–208.

Luria, Z., & Meade, R. G. (1984). Sexuality in the middle-aged woman. In: G. Baruch & R. Brooks-Gunn (Eds.), *Women in mid-life* (pp. 371–397). New York: Plenum.

Majerovitz, S. D., & Revenson, T. A. (1994). Sexuality and rheumatic disease: The significance of gender. *Arthritis-Care Research, 7*(1), 29–34.

Malatesta, V. J., Chambless, D. L., Pollack, M, & Cantor, A. (1988). Widowhood, sexuality and aging: A life span analysis. *Journal of Sex and Marital Therapy, 14*(1), 49–62.

Mann, T. (1953). Die Betrogene. (The black swan). In T. Mann. *Gesammelte Werke*. Bd. 8. Frankfurt, Germany: Fischer.

Margolis, G., Goodman, R. L., & Rubin, A. (1990). Psychological effects of breast-conserving cancer treatment and mastectomy. *Psychosomatics, 31*(1), 33–39.

Masters, W. H., & Johnson, V. E. (1966). *Human sexual response*. Boston: Little Brown.

Masters, W. H., & Johnson, V. E. (1981). Sex and the aging process. *Journal of the American Geriatrics Society, 19*(9), 385–390.

Mayer, K. U., & Baltes, P. B. (Eds.) (1996) . *Die Berliner Altersstudie*. Berlin, Germany: Akademie Verlag.

McCarthy, B. W. (1984). Strategies and techniques for the treatment of inhibited sexual desire. *Journal of Sex and Marital Therapy, 10*(2), 97–104.

McCarthy, B. W. (1989). Cognitive-behavioral strategies and techniques in the treatment of early ejaculation. In S. R. Leiblum & R. C. Rosen (Eds.), *Principles and practice of sex therapy: Update for the 1990s* (2nd ed., pp. 141–167). New York: Guilford Press.

McCartney, J. R., Izeman, H., Rogers, D., & Cohen, N. (1987). Sexuality and the institutionalized elderly. *Journal of the American Geriatrics Society, 35*, 331–333.

McConaghy, N. (1993). *Sexual behavior: Problems and management*. New York: Plenum.

McCoy, N. L. , & Davidson, J. M. (1985). A longitudinal study of the effects of menopause on sexuality. *Maturitas, 7*, 203–210.

McDougall, G. J. (1993). Therapeutic issues with gay and lesbian elders. Special issue: The forgotten aged: Ethnic, psychiatric and societal minorities. *Clinical Gerontologist, 14*(1), 45–57.

Melman, A. (1992). Neural and vascular control of erection. In R. C. Rosen & S. R. Leiblum (Eds.), *Erectile disorders: Assessment and treatment.* (pp. 55–71). New York: Guilford Press.

Melman, A., & Tiefer, L. (1992). Surgery for erectile disorders: Operative procedures and psychological issues. In R. C. Rosen & S. R. Leiblum (Eds.), *Erectile disorders: Assessment and treatment* (pp. 255–282). New York: Guilford Press.

Mooradian, A. D. (1991). Geriatric sexuality and chronic diseases. *Clinics in Geriatric Medicine, 7*(1), 113–131.

Morley, J. E. (1991). Endocrine factors in geriatric sexuality. *Clinics in Geriatric Medicine, 7*(1), 85–93.

Morley, J. E., & Kaiser, F. E. (1989). Sexual function with advancing age. *Medical Clinics of North America, 73*(6), 1483–1495.

Mulligan, T., & Modigh, A. (1991). Sexuality in dependent living situations. *Clinics in Geriatric Medicine, 7*(1), 153–160.

Mulligan, T., & Moss, C. R. (1991). Sexuality and aging in male veterans: A cross-sectional study of interest, ability, and activity. *Archives of Sexual Behavior, 20*(1), 17–25.

Myers, L. S. (1995). Methodological review and meta-analysis of sexuality and menopause research. *Neuroscience and Biobehavioral Reviews, 19*(2), 331–341.

Nadelson, C. C. (1984). Geriatric sex problems: Discussion. *Journal of Geriatric Psychiatry, 17*(2), 139–148.

Nairne, K. D., & Hemsley, D. R. (1983). The use of directed masturbation training in the treatment of primary anorgasmia. *British Journal of Clinical Psychology, 22*, 283–294.

Nelson, R. P. (1987). Male sexual dysfunction: Evaluation and treatment. *Southern Medical Journal, 80*, 69–74.

Newman, A. S., & Bertelson, A. D. (1986). Sexual dysfunction in diabetic women. *Journal of Behavioral Medicine, 9*(3), 261–270.

O'Donohue, W. T. (1987). The sexual behavior and problems of the elderly. In L. Carstensen & B. Edelstein (Eds.), *Handbook of clinical gerontology* (pp. 66–75). New York: Pergamon.

Opjordsmoen, S., Waehre, H., Aass, N., & Fossa, S. D. (1994). Sexuality in patients treated for penile cancer: patients' experience and doctors' judgment. *British Journal of Urology, 73*, 554–560.

Othmer, E., & Othmer, S. C. (1987). Effect of buspirone on sexual dysfunction in patients with generalized anxiety disorder. *Journal of Clinical Psychiatry, 48*, 201–203.

Patterson, D. G., & O'Gorman, E. C. (1989). Sexual anxiety in sexual dysfunction. *British Journal of Psychiatry, 155*, 374–378.

Peck, R. C. (1956). Psychological developments in the second half of life. In B. L. Neugarten (Ed.), *Middle age and aging* (pp. 88–92). Chicago: University of Chicago Press.

Persson, G. (1980). Sexuality in a 70-year-old urban population. *Journal of Psychosomatic Research, 24*, 335–342.

Pfeiffer, E., & Davis, G. C. (1972). Determinants of sexual behavior in middle and old age. *Journal of the American Geriatrics Society, 20*(4), 151–158.

Pfeiffer, E., Verwoerdt, A. & Davis, G. C. (1972). Sexual behavior in middle life. *American Journal of Psychiatry, 128*, 1262–1267.

Pfeiffer, E., Verwoerdt, A., & Wang, H. S. (1968). Sexual

behavior in aged men and women. Observations on 254 community volunteers. *Archives of General Psychiatry, 19*, 753–758.

Pfeiffer, E., Verwoerdt, A., & Wang, H. S. (1969). The natural history of sexual behavior in a biologically advantaged group of aged individuals. *Journal of Gerontology, 24*, 193–198.

Pope, M., & Schulz, R. (1990). Sexual attitudes and behavior in mid-life and aging homosexual males. *Journal of Homosexuality, 20*(3-4), 169–177.

Radebold, H. (1992). *Psychodynamik und Psychotherapie Älterer*. Berlin: Springer-Verlag.

Radin, M. M. (1989). Preoedipal factors in relation to psychogenic inhibited sexual desire. *Journal of Sex and Marital Therapy, 15*(4), 255–268.

Rappoport, L. (1977). Aging as oppression. *Human Development, 20*, 204–209.

Relf, M. V. (1991). Sexuality and the older bypass patient. *Geriatric Nursing, 12*(6), 294–296.

Renshaw, D. C. (1983). Sex, intimacy, and the older woman. *Women and Health, 8*, 43–54.

Renshaw, D. C. (1984). Geriatric sex problems. *Journal of Geriatric Psychiatry, 17*(2), 123–138.

Robinson, P. K. (1983). The sociological perspective. In R. B. Weg, (Ed.), *Sexuality in the later years* (pp. 81–103). New York: Academic Press.

Rosen, R. C., & Leiblum, S. R. (1988). A sexual scripting approach to problems of desire. In S. R. Leiblum & R. C. Rosen (Eds.), *Sexual desire disorders* (pp. 168–191). New York: Guilford Press.

Rosen, R. C., & Leiblum, S. R. (1989). Assessment and treatment of desire disorders. In S. R. Leiblum & R. C. Rosen (Eds.), *Principles and practice of sex therapy: Update for the 1990s* (2nd ed., pp. 19–47). New York: Guilford Press.

Rosen, R. C., & Leiblum, S. R. (Eds.) (1992a). *Erectile disorders: Assessment and treatment*. New York: Guilford Press.

Rosen, R. C., & Leiblum, S. R. (1992b). Erectile disorders: An overview of historical trends and clinical perspectives. In R. C. Rosen & S. R. Leiblum (Eds.), *Erectile disorders: Assessment and treatment* (pp. 3–26). New York: Guilford Press.

Rosenmayr, L. (1995). Eros und Liebe im Alter. In M. M. Baltes & L. Montada. *Produktives Leben im Alter* (pp. 258–289). Frankfurt, Germany: Campus.

Roughan, P. A., Kaiser, F. E., & Morley, J. E. (1993). Sexuality and the older women. *Clinics in Geriatric Medicine, 9*(1), 87–106.

Sandberg, G., & Quevillon, R. B. (1987). Dyspareunia: an integrated approach to assessment and diagnosis. *Journal of Family Practice, 24*(1), 66–70.

Sarrel, P. M. (1982). Sex problems after menopause: A study of fifty married couples treated in a sex counseling programme. *Maturitas, 4*, 231–237.

Sarrel, P. M. (1990). Sexuality and menopause. *Obstetrics and Gynecology, 75* (Suppl. 4), 26S–35S.

Scharff, D. E. (1988). An object relations approach to inhibited sexual desire. In S. R. Leiblum & R. C. Rosen (Eds.), *Sexual desire disorders* (pp. 45–74). New York: Guilford Press.

Schiavi, R. C. (1990). Sexuality and aging in men. *Annual Review of Sexual Research, 1*, 227–249.

Schiavi, R. C. (1992). Laboratory methods for evaluating erectile dysfunction. In R. C. Rosen & S. R. Leiblum (Eds.), *Erectile disorders: Assessment and treatment*. (pp. 141–170). New York: Guilford Press.

Schiavi, R. C., Mandeli, J. & Schreiner-Engel, P. (1994). Sexual satisfaction in healthy aging men. *Journal of Sex and Marital Therapy, 20*(1), 3–13.

Schiavi, R. C., Mandeli, J., Schreiner-Engel, P., & Chambers, A. (1991). Aging, sleep disorders, and male sexual function. *Biological Psychiatry, 30*, 15–24.

Schiavi, R. C., Schreiner-Engel, P., White, D., & Mandeli, J. (1991). The relationship between pituitary–gonadal function and sexual behavior in healthy aging men. *Psychosomatic Medicine, 53*, 363–374.

Schiavi, R. C., & Segraves, R. T. (1995). The biology of sexual function. *Psychiatric Clinics of North America: Clinical Sexuality, 18*(1), 7–23.

Schneider, H. D. (1980). Sexualverhalten in der zweiten Lebenshälfte: Ergebnisse sozialwissenschaftlicher Forschung. Stuttgart, Germany: Kohlhammer.

Schover, L. (1988a). *Sexuality and cancer: For the man who has cancer and his partner*. New York: American Cancer Society.

Schover, L. (1988b). *Sexuality and cancer: For the woman who has cancer and her partner*. New York: American Cancer Society.

Schover, L. R. (1989). Sexual problems in chronic illness. In S. R. Leiblum & R. C. Rosen (Eds.), *Principles and practice of sex therapy: Update for the 1990s* (2nd ed., pp. 319–351). New York: Guilford Press.

Schover, L. R. (1992). Erectile failure and chronic illness. In R. C. Rosen & S. R. Leiblum (Eds.), *Erectile disorders: Assessment and treatment* (pp. 341–367). New York: Guilford Press.

Schover, L. R., Evans, R. B., & Von Eschenbach, A. C. (1987). Sexual rehabilitation in a cancer center: Diagnosis and outcome in 384 consultations. *Archives of Sexual Behavior, 16*(6), 445–461.

Schover, L. R., Schain, W. S., & Montague, D. K. (1989). Sexual problems of patients with cancer. In V. T. DeVita, S. Hellman, & S. A. Rosenberg (Eds.), *Cancer: Principles and practice of oncology* (3rd ed., pp. 2206–2225). Philadelphia: Lippincott.

Schover, L. R., Yetman, R. J., Tuason, L. J., Meisler, E., Esselstyn, C. B., Hermann, R. E., Grundfest-Broniatowski, S., & Dowden, R. V. (1995). Partial mastectomy and breast reconstruction: A comparison of their effects on psychosocial adjustment, body image, and sexuality. *Cancer, 75*(1), 54–64.

Schreiner-Engel, P., & Schiavi, R. C. (1986). Lifetime psychopathology in individuals with low sexual desire. *The Journal of Nervous and Mental Disease, 174*(11), 646–651.

Segraves, R. T. (1988). Drugs and desire. In S. R. Leiblum & R. C. Rosen (Eds.), *Sexual desire disorders* (pp. 313–347). New York: Guilford Press.

Segraves, R. T., & Segraves, K. B. (1992). Aging and drug effects on male sexuality. In R. C. Rosen & S. R. Leiblum (Eds.), *Erectile disorders: Assessment and treatment*. (pp. 96–138). New York: Guilford Press.

Shell, J. A., & Smith, C. K. (1994). Sexuality and the older person with cancer. *Oncology Nursing Forum, 21*(3), 553–558.

Sjögren, K., Damber, J.-E., & Liliequist, B. (1983). Sexuality after stroke with hemiplegia. I: Aspects of sexual dysfunction. *Scandinavian Journal of Rehabilitation Medicine, 15*, 55–61.

Smyer, M. A., Zarit, S. H., & Qualls, S. H. (1990). Psychological intervention with the aging individual. In J. E. Birren & K. W. Schaie (Eds.), *Handbook of the Psychology of Aging* (3rd ed., pp. 375–403). San Diego, CA: Academic Press.

Sontag, S. (1972). The double standard of aging. *Saturday Review, 55*, 29–38.

Speckens, A. E. M., Hengeveld, M. W., Lycklama à Nijeholt, G., van Hemert, A. M., & Hawton, K. E. (1995). Psychosexual functioning of partners of men with presumed non-organic erectile dysfunction: Cause or consequence of the disorder? *Archives of Sexual Behavior, 24*(2), 157–172.

Spence, S. H. (1992). Psychosexual dysfunction in the elderly. *Behaviour Change, 9*(2), 55–64.

Starr, B. D. (1985). Sexuality and aging. *Annual Review of*

Gerontology and Geriatrics, 5, 97–126.
Starr, B. D., & Weiner, M. B. (1981). *The Starr–Weiner report on sex and sexuality in the mature years*. New York: McGraw-Hill.
Staudinger, U. M., Freund, A. M., Linden, M., & Maas, I. (1996). Selbst, Persönlichkeit und Lebensgestaltung im Alter: Psychologische Widerstandsfähigkeit und Vulnerabilität. In K. U. Mayer & P. B. Baltes. *Die Berliner Altersstudie* (pp. 321–350). Berlin, Germany: Akademie Verlag.
Sviland, M. (1981). Sexuality and intimacy in later life. In: R. Kastenbaum (Ed.), *Old age in the new scene* (pp. 15–26). New York: Springer.
Talmadge, L. D., & Talmadge, W. C. (1986). Relational sexuality: An understanding of low sexual desire. *Journal of Sex and Marital Therapy, 12*(1), 3–21.
Thienhaus, O. J. (1988). Practical overview of sexual function and advancing age. *Geriatrics, 43*(8), 63–67.
Thomas, L. E. (1982). Sexuality and aging: Essential vitamin or popcorn? *The Gerontologist, 22*(3), 240–243.
Tiefer, L., & Melman, A. (1989). Comprehensive evaluation of erectile dysfunction and medical treatments. In S. R. Leiblum & R. C. Rosen (Eds.), *Principles and practice of sex therapy* (2nd ed., pp. 207–236). New York: Guilford Press.
Traupmann, J. (1984). Does sexuality fade over time? A look at the question and the answer. *Journal of Geriatric Psychiatry, 17*(2), 149–159.
Tümmers, H. (1976). Sozialpsychologische Aspekte der Sexualität im Alter.Cologne, Germany: Bühlau.
Turner, B. F., & Adams, C. G. (1983) . The sexuality of older women. In E. W. Markson (Ed.), *Older women—Issues and perspectives* (pp. 55–72). Lexington, KY: Lexington.
Vandereycken, W. (1987). On desire, excitement, and impotence in modern sex therapy. *Psychotherapy and Psychosomatics, 47*, 175–180.
Verwoerdt, A., Pfeiffer, F. & Wang, H. S. (1969a). Sexual behavior in senescence. I. Changes in sexual activity and interest of aging men and women. *Journal of Geriatric Psychiatry, 2*, 163–180.
Verwoerdt, A., Pfeiffer, F. & Wang, H. S. (1969b). Sexual behavior in senescence. II. Patterns of sexual activity and interest. *Geriatrics, 24*, 137–154.
Von Sydow, K. (1992a). Weibliche Sexualität im mittleren und höheren Erwachsenenalter: Übersicht über vorliegende Forschungsarbeiten. (Female sexuality in middle and old age: Research review). *Zeitschrift für Gerontologie, 25*, 113–127.
Von Sydow, K. (1992b). Eine Untersuchung zur weiblichen Sexualität im mittleren und höheren Erwachsenenalter (A study on female sexuality in middle and old age). *Zeitschrift für Gerontologie, 25*, 105–112.
Von Sydow, K. (1993). *Lebenslust: Weibliche Sexualität von der frühen Kindheit bis ins hohe Alter*. Bern, Switzerland: Huber.
Wakefield, J. C. (1987). The semantics of success: Do masturbation exercises lead to partner orgasm? *Journal of Sex and Marital Therapy, 13*(1), 3–14.
Weg, R. B. (Ed.) (1983). *Sexuality in the later years: Roles and behavior*. New York: Academic Press.
Weiler, S. J. (1981). Aging and sexuality and the myth of decline. In R. W. Fogel, E. Hatfield, S. B. Kiesler, & E. Shanas (Eds.), *Aging: Stability and change in the family* (pp. 317–327). New York: Academic Press.
Weiss, L. J. (1983). Intimacy and adaptation. In R. B. Weg (Ed.), *Sexuality in the later years: Roles and behavior* (pp. 147–166). New York: Academic Press.
Weiss, J. N., & Mellinger, B. C. (1990). Sexual dysfunction in elderly men. *Clinics in Geriatric Medicine, 6*(1), 185–196.
Weissbach-Rieger, A., & Franke, B. (1987a). Partnerbeziehung, Sexualität und Sexualverhalten bei älteren Frauen und Männern nach dem 55. Lebensjahr (1.+2. Mitteilung). *Zeitschrift für Alternsforschung, 42*(4), 203–209.
Weissbach-Rieger, A., & Franke, B. (1987b). Partnerbeziehung, Sexualität und Sexualverhalten bei älteren Frauen und Männern nach dem 55. Lebensjahr (3. Mitteilung). *Zeitschrift für Alternsforschung, 42*(4), 211–213.
Weizmann, R., & Hart, J. (1987). Sexual behavior in healthy married elderly men. *Archives of Sexual Behavior, 16*(1), 39–44.
White, C. B. (1982). Sexual interest, attitudes, knowledge, and sexual history in relation to sexual behavior in the institutionalized aged. *Archives of Sexual Behavior, 11*(1), 11–21.
Wickert, J. (1983). *Partnerschaft im Alter. Auswertung der Ergebnisse einer Längsschnittstudie* (Berichte aus dem Institut für Psychologie). Cologne, Germany: Universität Köln, Erziehungswissenschaftliche Fakultät.
Winn, R. L., & Newton, N. (1982). Sexuality in aging: A study of 106 cultures. *Archives of Sexual Behavior, 11*(4), 283–298.
Wise, T. N. (1989). Sexuality in the aging individual: A biopsychosocial perspective. *Issues in the Geriatric Psychiatry, 19*, 53–66.
Wise, T. N., Epstein, S., & Ross, R. (1992). Sexual issues in the medically ill and aging. *Psychiatric Medicine, 10*(2), 169–180.
Zemel, P. (1988). Sexual dysfunction in the diabetic patient with hypertension. *The American Journal of Cardiology, 61*, 27–33.
Zilbergeld, B. (1992). The man behind the broken penis: Social and psychological determinants of erectile failure. In R. C. Rosen & S. R. Leiblum (Eds.), *Erectile disorders: Assessment and treatment* (pp. 27–51). New York: Guilford Press.

7.05
Bereavement

DALE A. LUND
University of Utah, Salt Lake City, UT, USA

7.05.1 INTRODUCTION

Issues about death surround everyone's daily lives, yet most people neglect to use these opportunities to improve their understanding of grief. A plane carrying hundreds of passengers crashes in the Florida swamps and Americans watch with interest on television and read in newspapers and magazines about the loss of lives, grieving families, heroic workers trying to retrieve bodies, and the need for improved safety standards in the airline industry. Another assisted suicide is described in the media but very few people ever discuss the grief of the family members. The evening news regularly reports on the victims of gang-related murders that occurred the previous night. Local newspaper obituaries include another person who has died from AIDS. Each of these four examples contain in-depth stories of human emotion and relationships in the lives of the victims and survivors, yet most passive onlookers fail to realize that they will share many of the same emotional and social experiences that these distant "people in the news" have had to encounter. While most people never experience horrendous or public deaths nearly everyone will have several personal bereavement experiences during their lives. Individuals could benefit from learning more about death and grief by more closely examining some of these news events and people and assessing their own personal feelings and reactions. Instead, most people only learn about death, grief, loss, and bereavement when they have no other choice because it is now their own personal experience.

In order better to describe the complexities of the bereavement process and how we might best assist those who have the greatest difficulty, this chapter will summarize and highlight some of the most basic and essential knowledge available. The chapter begins with a review and discussion of the many common but highly diverse bereavement experiences that occur throughout the life course. Although the primary focus is on bereavement in later life it is necessary to place these losses in the context of the entire life course because earlier experiences continue to impact coping strategies used in late life. Bereavement is also examined in a multidimensional context because it can affect nearly every aspect of a person's life. Knowledge about grief and bereavement comes from a variety of experts and sometimes the information is contradictory or inconsistent, so it is important to understand the advantages and limitations from these diverse sources. This section is presented along with a discussion of the benefits from integrating theory, research, and clinical practice to achieve a better understanding of the bereavement process. Reviewed next are the most common features of the long-term process and predictors of who is most likely to have the greatest difficulty. The chapter ends with a review of the most promising ways to intervene to assist those in greatest need, and some additional comments about the need to be creative and collaborate with others from a variety of different disciplines.

Many people use the terms bereavement, grief, and mourning as though they were interchangeable or have the same meaning. This is not the case. All three of these terms are highly interrelated but it is important to note that each has a unique meaning.

Bereavement is the broadest or most general of the three terms because it refers to both the situation and the long-term process of adjusting to the death of someone to whom a person feels close (Lund, 1993). The term also has been used in reference to losses other than death, such as the loss of a home or personal belongings because of a fire or a natural disaster. It is more common, however, to use the term bereavement in situations following the death of a friend or relative, or even an animal companion. Grief and mourning are more specific in their meaning because they refer to different aspects of the overall bereavement process. Grief refers specifically to the affective or emotional responses that people often experience during the early phases of the bereavement process. These feelings frequently include disbelief, confusion, shock, numbness, sadness, and sometimes anger and guilt. Feeling abandoned, lonely, or depressed, and being preoccupied with thoughts of the deceased person and the events surrounding the death are often components of grief (Parkes, 1987).

It is common for bereaved persons to feel a wide range of emotions that come and go quickly and then reappear many months or even years later. These grief-related feelings do not come as a set package to all bereaved persons. Each person experiences a relatively unique array of emotions with varying levels of intensity and duration. Culture plays a major role in shaping how people experience and express bereavement because it provides the beliefs, values, and norms that guide behavior (Lund, 1989b). Most professionals use the term mourning to refer to the commonly accepted or culturally patterned ways people behave and express themselves during the adjustment process (Lund, 1993). Mourning refers to such behaviors as crying; missing work; altering daily routines; attending funerals, cremations, and burials; following standards for dress and appearance; and participating in other rituals that are influenced by the surrounding culture. Each culture has traditions to determine the most appropriate ways to behave (Chigier, 1988; Stroebe & Stroebe, 1987). Some cultures avoid open displays of sadness yet others expect the bereaved to be vocal and demonstrative (Irish, Lundquist, & Nelsen, 1993). Each of these three related terms will be further clarified later in this chapter along with discussion of the many commonalities and diverse ways that people experience bereavement.

7.05.2 LIFELONG BEREAVEMENT EXPERIENCES

Throughout the life course nearly everyone experiences many kinds of losses that require them to make adjustments. Infants become temporarily separated from parents and siblings when they leave the familiar surroundings of the home to attend day care and school. With increasing numbers of dual-career couples, children are leaving their homes at much younger ages to spend much of their weekday time away from both parents. Children also lose toys, clothes, pets, and valued belongings. With increased geographic mobility it is becoming common for children to move several times from one neighborhood to another, changing friends and familiar surroundings with each move. Young adults have lost relationships with teachers, clubs, organizations, and peers, as they advance from elementary grades, through high school and college. In later life adults continue to lose more friendships and relationships because of relocations, deaths, and retirement. With divorce rates near 50% in the USA (Hess, Markson, & Stein, 1996), millions are experiencing the loss of marital relationships, parents, and family life. Due to physiological changes associated with aging, people often lose hair, hearing, sight, muscle tone, independence, and mobility. In short, people who are fortunate to live long lives will experience many significant losses. Each loss has the potential of disrupting patterns of behavior, initiating grief-related feelings and requiring adjustments, but also adding to the course of human development.

Older adults have many opportunities to develop their coping skills or become overwhelmed by life's cumulative losses. It is much easier to understand how people cope with their current bereavement situations if one recognizes how they have managed their previous losses. For example, in the case of older bereaved spouses, effective interventions need to take into account how they experienced relocation, physical, and relationship losses earlier in their life (Lund, 1989a). If they relied on task-oriented strategies in handling these previous situations then a similar approach might be effective again. At the same time we need to appreciate the uniqueness of each loss or bereavement experience and not assume that the loss of personal belongings is the same as a divorce or death of a parent. While sadness might be a grief response common to both relocation and the death of a parent, it is unlikely that anger or guilt would be equally present in both situations (Farnsworth, Pett, & Lund, 1989).

The field of gerontology has been redefined since the late 1970s to give greater recognition to aging as a lifelong process (Hooyman & Kiyak, 1996). Rather than being exclusively focused on older adults, it recognizes that aging occurs throughout the life course but the primary focus still remains on later life. The most common death-related losses of interest to gerontologists are the deaths of parents, spouses, siblings, and friends. Much of the information in this chapter is based on spousal bereavement in later life because more gerontological research has focused on this particular loss. Children's death-related bereavement experiences are most likely to result from the death of a neighbor, parent, older relative, or school classmate. Some experts have described the death of a parent as the loss of our past, the death of a spouse or sibling as the loss of the present, and the death of a child as a loss of part of our future (Leming & Dickinson, 1990; Schiff 1977; Staudacher, 1987). Again, early and consistent experiences with death-related losses can shape subsequent attitudes and ways of coping well into later life (Lund, 1993). For example, the young boy who is told to be strong and not to cry after his father's death might easily grow up to be the unexpressive and isolated widower in later life.

Although statistics cannot capture the full essence of the bereavement process they are very helpful in documenting the commonality and expectedness of the experience. Each year approximately eight million Americans experience the death of an immediate family member. Even though suicides are underreported in the USA roughly 27 000 are reported each year. Over 400 000 of the deaths are children and youths under the age of 25. Also, each year there are at least 800 000 new widows and widowers (Osterweis, Solomon, & Green, 1984).

The death of a spouse is an increasingly common experience among aging adults, particularly women. The 1990 Census revealed that only 1% of the population between ages 18 and 54 were widowed, but 34% of those 65 and over and 67% of those 85 and over were widowed. A gender difference becomes increasingly apparent in the later years of life. After age 65, nearly 49% of the women but only 14% of men were widowed. After age 85, 80% of women and 43% of men were widowed (US Bureau of the Census, 1991). These high percentages actually underestimate the number of persons who experience the death of a spouse because they do not include those who remarried. In short, death-related bereavement is a common and expected experience for older adults.

7.05.3 BEREAVEMENT IN A MULTIDIMENSIONAL CONTEXT

One of the major reasons why bereavement has become such an important topic to clinicians, researchers, health professionals, clergy, and educators is the growing recognition that the adjustment process can impact virtually every aspect of a person's life (Lund, 1989b; Shuchter, 1986; Shuchter & Zisook, 1993). This pervasive and multidimensional nature of bereavement means that the coping process can affect emotions, spirituality, identity, social interactions and relationships, sexuality and intimacy, work productivity, financial stability, health, and even death. Clinicians and others who are interested in providing assistance to the bereaved need to recognize the broad range of possible effects and determine the extent to which bereavement is the cause of the difficulty. For example, patterns of interaction in family life can be radically altered when someone dies. Family meals, and other daily rituals related to getting ready for work, school, or church are affected by the absence of the deceased family member. Worden (1991) presents this difficulty as one of four tasks of mourning. He refers to this as the need to adjust to an environment in which the deceased is missing. These tasks of mourning are discussed in more detail later in this chapter. In the case of spousal bereavement survivors often change their self-concept to an "uncoupled identity" because they now carry out their daily life alone rather than as part of a couple (Lund, Caserta, Dimond, & Gray, 1986). Our society places great importance on adults doing many activities as couples rather than doing them alone. Imagine the difficulty of a bereaved spouse going alone to a movie or restaurant after many years of always doing these things with their husband or wife. Bereaved persons may also lose their appetite and motivation to remain physically active so nutrition, exercise, and physical well-being can be essential parts of the coping process (Lund, 1989a).

The multidimensional nature of bereavement is evident in the topics that professionals from different disciplines choose for special attention. Sociologists often examine bereavement's impact on family life, interactions, life satisfaction, and the role of culture and socioeconomic characteristics in shaping these bereavement outcomes. Finding differences among men and women, rich and poor, and diverse ethnic groups are common concerns for sociologists. Psychologists frequently examine the emotions of grief, depression, morale, and identity, and how previous relationships and the personality of the bereaved influence their coping strategies. Social workers are likely to assess family functioning and the need for, and effectiveness of, specific community services. Nurses and other health professionals are often concerned about the mental and physical well-being of bereaved persons. Economists are usually interested in the financial stability of bereaved persons and their families. Because many women in the USA do not have the same level of retirement and other financial benefits as men, they are much more likely to suffer economically during widowhood (Caserta, Lund, & Dimond, 1989). Each discipline and professional group adds a unique focus to examining bereavement experiences, and collectively, we better understand the many ways that bereavement can affect our lives. Clinicians interested in further reading about the many dimensions of grief and bereavement should read Shuchter (1986), Worden (1991), and Stroebe, Stroebe, and Hansson (1993b). These references also include recommendations based on international research studies.

The multidimensional nature of bereavement cannot be understood without an awareness that bereavement takes place within a broad context that varies from person to person. Although there are many common reactions and feelings that most people experience during the course of bereavement, there also are many unique experiences that may not be widely shared. For example, some bereaved persons feel intense guilt and anger while others feel a general sense of relief because the deceased is no longer suffering pain and discomfort. Some are overwhelmed with sadness and immobilized by depression while others confront the loss as a challenge and opportunity for growth. In order to understand why one person manages very well and another never seems to adjust to the loss, it is necessary to examine the multidimensional nature of the context in which bereavement occurs (Cleiren, 1993; Lund, 1989b). Previous life experiences, personality traits, social support received from others, circumstances surrounding the death, and a person's competency in managing the many tasks of daily living are some of the many factors that comprise the context of bereavement. Health professionals and clinicians who work with bereaved persons are better able to provide assistance when they know more about the specific aspects of each individual's bereavement context. What helps one person may not be of much value to another.

7.05.4 EXPERTS ON BEREAVEMENT

For thousands of years the subject of death has received considerable thought and discussion but much less attention has been devoted to the subject of how death affects those who are left to grieve (Stephenson, 1985). Since the Second World War, however, we have seen a steady increase in interest and writing about bereavement. Various kinds of experts have emerged during this time, each relying on different experiences, training, and sources of knowledge. Academic disciplines, especially psychology, sociology, social work, nursing, and other behavioral and health professions have contributed attention and knowledge to the subject through the development of theory and research (Stroebe et al., 1993b). Clinicians who work directly with the bereaved have added their knowledge about ways to help those who are having the greatest difficulty (Rando, 1993; Worden, 1991). Religious leaders and clergy from various denominations have shared their experiences regarding spiritual aspects of the bereavement process (Grollman, 1977; Kushner, 1982). Local bookstores are now replete with numerous autobiographical reports written by bereaved persons who have had experiences that they want to share (Caine, 1974; Lewis, 1961). These five sources of expertise and knowledge—theory, research, clinical reports, religious views, and autobiographical accounts—each make unique contributions to our understanding of bereavement. These different sources of knowledge, however, have unique advantages and limitations that need to be recognized because they can lead to different and competing conclusions.

Some bereaved persons will automatically turn to their religious leaders or their religious beliefs for comfort and guidance. Most religions have a set of beliefs regarding the questions of ultimate meaning. What is the purpose of life? Does God or a supernatural being have a plan for each specific person? Is there special meaning in the death of the loved one? Because most religions offer answers to these and other questions, religiously oriented people can find predictability, structure, and meaning to help them during the upheaval of bereavement. Research has shown that religion and spirituality are only part of the bereavement context and that the long-term adjustment process involves much more than a religious code to follow (Faletti, Gibbs, Clark, Pruchno, & Berman, 1989; Gass, 1989a; Lund, Caserta, & Dimond, 1988). In fact, some bereaved persons report disappointment that their religious beliefs did not provide greater comfort and relief. Research has not confirmed that religious beliefs and practices are universally helpful to bereaved persons but we do know that many people turn to their spiritual views as a source of knowledge and assistance (Lund, 1989a).

Personal accounts written by bereaved persons are abundant because bereaved persons want to know how others have managed, if their experiences are unique or common, and how they can cope better with their loss. These autobiographical accounts can be useful because they offer detailed descriptions of feelings, problems, and solutions that worked for the authors. Some bereaved persons, for example, might find comfort in knowing that their feelings of anger and guilt were shared by the author and may benefit by following some of the suggestions in the book. Kushner's (1982) *When Bad Things Happen to Good People* has continued for many years to be on the best-sellers list because bereaved readers often find comfort in his expressions of anger, sadness, and even in some disappointment in his previous long-standing religious beliefs. Caution should be exercised, however, in fully relying on these autobiographical accounts because the authors' experiences may not be widely shared and their credentials are most likely in journalism rather than bereavement.

Therapists, counselors, psychologists, psychiatrists, and other clinicians have provided valuable information and insights about bereavement. Like autobiographical accounts, clinical reports often offer detailed personal descriptions of the bereavement process and suggestions for helping to alleviate some of the most difficult problems. These in-depth reports about individuals' bereavement experiences are not only interesting but they help to organize experiences of more people, identify serious but common adjustment difficulties, and inform other professionals and bereaved persons of specific intervention strategies and their potential benefits. Knowledge that comes from clinical practice, however, must be interpreted in a way that recognizes the uniqueness of the clients or patients. Those who receive counseling or professional clinical services are likely to differ in some important ways from those who never seek help (Caserta & Lund, 1992a). Bereaved persons who receive these services are more likely to be experiencing the greatest difficulty in adjusting, have less social support available to them, have financial resources adequate to pay for the services, and have a tendency to rely on others for help (Caserta & Lund, 1992a). Knowledge about bereavement based solely on information from those who sought help from clinicians does not include the experiences of the majority of bereaved persons (Lund, Dimond, & Juretich, 1985; Stroebe & Stroebe, 1987). It is equally important to know how people manage their grief on their own and to what extent they want and need help even though they do not seek professional assistance.

Theory and research have been much slower in adding to our knowledge about bereavement but their contributions have been essential. Freud (1957) was one of the earliest to theorize about bereavement. In the early 1900s Freud practiced and wrote extensively about psychoanalytic theory and applied it to understanding the feelings and thoughts that follow separation or loss of attachment. His work was followed by other theorists and eventually systematic research studies were completed. Lindemann (1944) also used a psychoanalytic framework to guide perhaps the first bereavement study in the 1940s. His study interviewed over 100 relatives of 13 people killed in a fire at the Coconut Grove night club in Boston. Research and theory related to bereavement has steadily increased since these early beginnings (Stroebe, Stroebe, & Hansson, 1993a). Numerous theories and research findings have emerged that both support and challenge what we initially believed to be true about bereavement. These early theories and more recent conceptual frameworks are discussed in greater detail later in this chapter.

Research has generated knowledge on a much broader range of bereaved persons. By collecting data from people who have not sought professional help, and including persons from varied cultures and social classes, we have learned much more about what is common and what is unique during bereavement (Caserta & Lund, 1992a). Systematic research studies, using well-developed and standardized scales, representative samples of bereaved persons, and nonbereaved control groups, have revealed findings that are inconsistent with and challenge some of the previous views based upon the other sources of knowledge (Stroebe & Stroebe, 1991; Wortman & Silver, 1989). These research findings are presented in more detail in Section 7.05.7. One of the most prominent research findings is that while bereavement is a highly stressful experience and some people report never getting over it, the majority of bereaved persons are very resilient, especially older bereaved spouses. Many bereaved persons find personal and social resources to meet their needs and manage their adjustment process. Research has also not been able to confirm that people go through specific stages as suggested by many clinicians and some theorists (Lund, Caserta, & Dimond, 1986; Shuchter & Zisook, 1993; Wortman, Silver, & Kessler, 1993). The process is much more varied and complex than the uniform and orderly course depicted in the stage theories (Bowlby, 1969). Research has revealed that not all people need to express in equal amounts their emotions outwardly to others in order to avoid a build-up of problems that will come out even worse later (Wortman & Silver, 1989). Many people who appear in control and able to manage their early grief tend to be doing very well years later (Wortman et al., 1993). Conversely, those who were doing poorly and were most expressive of their difficulties in the first several weeks were still having great difficulty two years later. These findings appear to be similar for adults of all ages (Lund, Dimond, et al., 1986; Wortman et al., 1993). In short, all five types of experts and their unique experiences and knowledge have added to a more comprehensive and useful understanding of bereavement.

7.05.5 THEORIES ABOUT BEREAVEMENT

The bereavement process is multidimensional and requires professionals from different disciplines to contribute their specific theories of human behavior to our understanding, explanation, and prediction of how people will experience this complicated process. Various conceptual frameworks have been applied to grief and bereavement, each providing a unique focus on specific parts of the bereavement context. These theories are particularly valuable if they predict adjustments and guide the development of interventions to help those in greatest need. The following sections briefly summarize some of the most prominent theories about grief and bereavement.

7.05.5.1 Psychoanalytic Theories

Most of the variations in psychoanalytic theory that have applied to bereavement emphasize the importance of recognizing the conscious and subconscious ties or attachments that the bereaved person formed with the deceased (Cleiren, 1993; Parkes, 1987; Stroebe et al., 1993a). According to this view the bereaved person must express rather than repress all of the feelings associated with the detachment or loss. Anger, guilt, fear, and love, when expressed by the bereaved, help lead to normal instead of abnormal grief. These theories also stress the importance of early childhood relationships and separations because these first experiences remain throughout life. When children have traumatic losses in early life they often form ambivalent relationships later, repress their anxieties, and have greater difficulty with grief and bereavement. Separation anxiety is seen as an instinctive reaction to loss but it is essential that the bereaved person withdraw from the deceased and form new attachments.

Freud (1957), Lindemann (1944), Bowlby (1969), Parkes (1987), and Marris (1958) are the most prominent contributors to the application of psychoanalytic theory to bereavement (Cleiren, 1993). While all theorists have their own unique interpretations they have generally agreed that grief is largely an intrapsychic process that each bereaved person must cognitively resolve in order to avoid delayed, distorted, or abnormal grief. Some of the abnormal reactions include social withdrawal, hypochondriacal symptoms, psychosomatic illnesses, and hyperactivity. Normal grief is thought to be marked by distress and impaired functioning but recovery is to be expected (Parkes, 1987). Bereaved persons usually experience a period of upset, protest, and anxiety because of the separation. They are likely to search for the deceased in familiar settings. Despair and depression can follow because the deceased person does not return. A reorganization phase occurs when grievers accept the reality of the loss, resolve the feelings of guilt and anger, restructure their lives and return to normal functioning (Parkes, 1987; Worden, 1991). These theories suggest that bereavement follows a relatively ordered progression of phases and that unresolved grief occurs when the sequence is disrupted or distorted.

7.05.5.2 Stress, Appraisal, and Coping Theories

Theories of stress, appraisal, and coping have been applied to bereavement because the death of a spouse, parent, child, or sibling is generally considered to be among the most stressful events that can ever happen. Stress exists when the demands on the individual exceed the resources readily available to meet the demands. The death of a loved one, particularly when the deceased played an important part in the daily life of the bereaved, creates stress in many ways for the survivor. Daily life is radically changed because the bereaved can no longer rely on the deceased for on-going companionship, conversation, security, guidance, comfort, love, sharing, and listening; and instrumental assistance such as financial support, transportation, and caregiving. Bereavement requires the survivor to change and adjust to an environment where the deceased is absent (Worden, 1991).

When bereavement occurs people must cognitively appraise their situation, usually consistent with their previously established patterns of dealing with stress. Cognitive appraisal means that people consciously assess their loss, try to make sense out of it, and determine the consequences that are likely to result from different courses of action. The degree of stress and subsequent adjustment difficulties is largely dependent on the bereaved person's appraisal of the situation and the coping strategies used.

The most common types of appraisal are pain, threat, challenge, and relief (Gass, 1989b). Those who primarily see the pain often focus their attention on the damage already done and expend much of their energy expressing anger, sadness, and depression, and their coping strategy often involves withdrawal, self-blame, and feeling overwhelmed. Those who see their loss as a threat are aware of the stress but are uncertain about their ability to deal with it. The death of their loved one means that they see other losses that are likely to follow. Their coping strategies usually include fear and worry about future threats to their lives. Rather than focusing their energy in broader ways to make their adjustment easier, they often engage in wishful thinking. The bereaved who see their loss as a challenge recognize the stress and the need to adapt. They assess their strengths, limitations, and needs and pursue a course of action that will allow them to learn and possibly grow from the experience. Having pride, self-confidence, motivation, and some skills in carrying out the many tasks of daily living helps the bereaved to define the situation as a challenge and follow a more problem-focused approach to adjustment (Lund, Caserta, Dimond & Shaffer, 1989). Lazarus (1966), Folkman, Lazarus, Dunkel-Schetter, De Longis, and Gruen (1986), Pearlin and Mullan (1992), and many others have advanced theory and research on stress, appraisal, and coping, and the perspective continues to make very important contributions to understanding bereavement.

7.05.5.3 Stage and Task Models

Ever since Kubler-Ross (1969) proposed the well-known stage model of the dying process, it has been applied to many discussions of how people deal with problems and life crises. The dying person was seen to pass through a naturally occurring sequence of experiences beginning with denial and progressing through anger, bargaining, depression, and eventually culminating in acceptance. Because bereaved persons and many professionals became familiar with the stage model developed by Kubler-Ross and they could see many similar emotions, thoughts, and issues expressed during the course of bereavement, it seemed only natural to apply the sequential and progressive stages to bereavement.

While research has identified and confirmed that bereaved persons experience many of the same kinds of emotions, thoughts, and behaviors presented in the stage models (Aiken, 1994; Hardt, 1978; Parkes, 1987), the overall bereavement process appears to be much less orderly, sequential, and uniform than these models suggest (Lund, Caserta, & Dimond, 1986; Wortman et al., 1993). For example, some bereaved persons report many years after the loss that they sometimes feel the sadness, pain, and regret that they experienced in the first several weeks (Lund, 1989a). The stage models have contributed to our knowledge about bereavement because they have helped to identify parts of the complex process and provided a foundation for further study.

Similar to the stage models and building on some of the concepts from other theories is the idea that adaptation requires the bereaved person to accomplish or complete specific tasks. Worden's (1991) "tasks of mourning" approach is an example. His work is based on the assumption that grief is work, requiring both emotional and physical energy to complete. He suggests that it is important for the bereaved eventually to accept the reality of the loss, to experience the pain of grief, to adapt emotionally and socially to an environment in which the deceased is missing, and to relocate psychologically the deceased person in their life and move forward. The notion of "relocating the deceased" recognizes the value of keeping memories alive and not assuming that the bereaved should forget the importance of their past relationships. While many other specific tasks can be added to his model, it does provide a very useful approach in helping bereaved persons. The task-oriented approach highlights the importance of being active and learning new skills rather than simply being passive and allowing time to pass and heal the wounds of grief. Worden's book is highly recommended reading for clinicians and researchers.

7.05.5.4 Other Theories

A wide range of theories from social, behavioral, and health sciences have been used to understand specific aspects of grief and bereavement but most of them have not been systematically tested in research. Some of the theories have received only limited attention even though they have considerable promise in explaining and predicting bereavement behaviors and helping bereaved persons through the process. For example, family and systems theories, symbolic interactionism, the health belief model, and the theory of reasoned action have much to add but have not been extensively used in research or practice.

Family and systems theories (Olson, Sprenkle, & Russell, 1979) are relevant to bereavement because bereaved people are members of nuclear and extended families and their lives take place within functioning systems. People do not live in total isolation from families, groups, and organizations, and their experiences within these units are important parts of the broader bereavement context. An 80-year-old widow is impacted by how other family members grieve the death of her husband, who also was a father, grandfather, uncle, and brother. Just like individuals, families grieve. Some family members provide strength and support to one another and other families create more conflict and tension during bereavement (Worden, 1991). Systems theory recognizes that people are parts of larger systems and individual lives consist of various functioning parts as well. Anger and depression following bereavement can easily carry over from the home to the workplace and many other social settings, thereby impacting and further complicating other relationships.

Symbolic interaction theory, which comes from the discipline of sociology, has much to offer the topic of bereavement (Lund, Caserta, Dimond, & Gray, 1986). This theory emphasizes the importance of social interactions with others and how they shape a person's self-concept or identity which in turn, influence behavior. Bereavement losses have the potential of altering a person's interactions and self-concepts and ultimately bereavement adjustments (Worden, 1991). From the field of health education, the health belief model (Rosenstock, 1990) and theory of reasoned action (Ajzen & Fishbein, 1980) are examples of conceptual frameworks relevant to bereavement. Both are applicable to examining the way bereaved persons make decisions and what they take into account to decide a course of action. Bereavement can very easily lead to neglect of one's own health. These approaches suggest that a broad range of factors including messages in the media can influence bereavement behaviors by identifying healthy behaviors to pursue and stressing the likelihood of positive outcomes that will follow. Grief requires considerable energy so good nutrition and regular exercise can be very helpful during the bereavement process (Lund, 1989a).

Finally, the most prominent theories in the field of gerontology have relevancy to understanding bereavement but they have not received much attention. Disengagement (Cumming & Henry, 1961), activity (Havighurst, 1968), continuity (Atchley, 1989), and age stratification (Riley, 1971) theories have contributions to make and hopefully, in the future, they will be examined and tested in research. Disengagement theory would suggest that those who were already gradually withdrawing from society will have less difficulty during bereavement than those who have not yet begun the process of withdrawal. The bereavement experience would not seem as abrupt to them. Activity theory would argue in favor of maintaining relatively high levels of physical activity during bereavement because it will help create greater life satisfaction and well-being. Continuity theory would suggest that the best course of action during bereavement would be to continue doing most of the things that one had always enjoyed. Age stratification theory could be used for a better understanding of why age might influence bereavement adjustments and that people in different age cohorts have different needs during stressful life transitions. An excellent reference resource for more information about these and other gerontological theories is *Social Gerontology* (Hooyman & Kiyak, 1996). In short, theory helps to inform and guide research and we need considerably more of both theory and research to improve our knowledge about grief and bereavement.

7.05.6 FEATURES OF THE BEREAVEMENT PROCESS

Research on bereavement, and particularly studies which examine predictors of outcomes, has considerably increased since the early 1980s. Some research investigators have waited many weeks and months to interview bereaved persons and others have obtained information only days after the death occurred (Stroebe & Stroebe, 1987). Nearly all of the early research studies avoided contacting bereaved persons during the first six months of the process, assuming that the bereaved persons would be too upset to participate. Later studies revealed that was not necessarily the case and by waiting too long much valuable information was lost (Lund, 1989b). Some studies followed bereaved persons for several years to examine long-term outcomes but most projects obtained information at only one point in time, providing only a limited picture of the process (Stroebe et al., 1993b). These cross-sectional studies did not adequately capture the many dynamic aspects of the process.

Only few investigators have included nonbereaved control groups, even though it is valuable to be able to compare the thoughts, feelings, and behaviors of bereaved persons with those who are not experiencing death-related bereavement (Lund, 1989a; Stroebe, Hansson, & Stroebe, 1993). In fact, nonbereaved control groups are needed to help determine what effects are most likely attributed to bereavement rather than pre-existing conditions. The ideal study design would include before and after bereavement measures to assess the effects of bereavement most directly, but these studies are expensive and lengthy. Research has also included more women than men, more adults than children, and more Caucasians than non-Caucasians. Therefore, much of what we have learned from research has been limited to specific populations. Even with these and other limitations, research has improved our understanding about grief and bereavement. It is not possible to review all or even most of these findings but five of the most important general conclusions are presented here.

First, bereavement is very stressful but many people manage their losses with considerable resiliency. In the case of spousal bereavement, the majority of research participants (72%) reported that their loss situation was the worst and most stressful thing that had ever happened to them (Lund, 1989b). The death of a child also creates stress and is particularly difficult because children are expected to live longer than their parents (Rubin, 1993). Among adults, it is disturbing when both parents are deceased because it means that their own generation in the family is now the most senior. The death of a spouse, parent, or child almost always brings out thoughts of mortality and death among the survivors. In Western culture, thoughts about the inevitability of death are usually troubling because, as mentioned in the introduction to this chapter, we have not openly discussed death. Some researchers have attempted to identify how many people continue for several years having major difficulties that interfere with their daily lives. It has been estimated that between 15 and 25% will need some kind of professional help with their bereavement adjustments (Lund, 1989a; Lund, Dimond, et al., 1986).

Even though bereavement is extremely stressful, it is somewhat surprising to know that many people are very resilient and able to restructure their lives in ways that allow them to find enjoyment again (Caserta & Lund, 1992b; Cleiren, 1993; McCrae & Costa, 1993; Murrell, Himmelfarb, & Phifer, 1988). One study (Caserta & Lund, 1992b) found that older bereaved spouses rated their stress levels in the range of 5.0–5.5 (on a 1–7 scale) during the first two years of bereavement. However, the currently married, nonbereaved control subjects indicated that their expected stress levels would range from 5.8 to 6.0 if they were in that same spousal bereavement situation (Caserta & Lund, 1992b). These data suggest that it is possible that many older adults will cope more effectively with bereavement than they expect. These research findings also help direct our attention to those 15–25% who are most distressed and unable to manage their bereavement losses alone and also recognize that not all bereaved persons will need professional assistance (Murrell et al., 1988; Wortman & Silver, 1989). These issues are discussed in further detail in the next section of this chapter.

Second, there is considerable diversity among and within bereaved persons (Levy, Martinkowski, & Derby, 1994). Not all people experience the same feelings, thoughts, and actions as they move through the process. For example, a 65-year-old widow in a research project described herself in the following way four weeks after her husband's death: "I am a very lonely person. Lousy, all washed out, despondent, feel deserted, angry, hurt, hopeless, alone, mixed-up, cannot concentrate, very emotional, very tired, cry a lot, hateful, very bitter, misfit, nobody, very miserable, very much of a loner." This same woman described herself in much the same troubled way two years into the bereavement process. She added that she was concerned about herself, and really hurt inside. She noted that she was sick of living alone and didn't care about life. In contrast, another 69-year-old widow described herself at six months after her husband's death as being "independent, excited about keeping busy, enjoying the company of others, and working in my yard and doing handiwork." Similar diversity in bereavement reactions is also found within each individual (Cleiren, 1993; Lund, Caserta & Dimond, 1993). It is not unusual to find a person simultaneously experiencing a very broad range of feelings and behaviors. For example, bereaved persons can feel angry, guilty, and lonely, yet at the same time feel personal strength and pride in how they are coping. A 70-year-old woman described herself at length as being busy, enjoying many different activities, and doing things with other people, but her final self-descriptive comment was that she still feels lonely. It is common for bereaved persons to experience simultaneously both positive and negative feelings (Lund, Caserta, & Dimond, 1986). For these reasons, it is difficult accurately to describe a bereaved person as doing very well or coping poorly. It is much more accurate to identify specific aspects or dimensions of people's lives where they are in greatest need for assistance.

Third, a theme emerging from recent studies is that of being more cautious in using the terms "normal" and "abnormal" to describe grief or bereavement experiences (Lund, 1993). Individuals may experience and express themselves in a variety of ways during bereavement. Research has shown that what would have been considered outside the realm of "normal" grief several years ago may now be considered a normal part of the process. For example, talking to a deceased spouse was previously thought to be abnormal or even pathological, but recent research findings show that this is actually a very common practice among bereaved spouses, and it is now often encouraged as a therapeutic technique related to reminiscence or relocating the deceased in the life of the bereaved (Worden, 1991). When we learn from a community-based sample of bereaved research subjects that they regularly talk out loud to their deceased spouses and appear to be coping relatively well, it suggests that the behavior is not nearly so problematic (Lund, 1989b).

Rather than applying rigid labels such as "normal" or "abnormal," it is more appropriate to use terms such as "common" or "uncommon" to describe bereavement feelings and behaviors (Lund, 1996). Bereaved persons are far less stigmatized by being told that they are experiencing some uncommon feelings than by being told, "You are abnormal." In fact, Western culture values people for being unique and different from others. Clinicians, in particular, need to be cautious not to assume that being different is abnormal.

Fourth, recent studies have revealed that the bereavement process is more like a rollercoaster ride than an orderly progression of stages with clear time frames associated with each stage (Lund, 1996; Lund et al., 1993). The bereavement roller coaster is characterized by the rapidly changing emotions of grief; meeting the challenges of learning new skills; recognizing personal weaknesses and limitations; developing new patterns of behavior; experiencing fatigue, loneliness, and helplessness; and forming new friendships and relationships.

Research has been unable to identify clear time markers associated with these many ups and downs. In fact, the highs and lows can occur within minutes, the same day, week, or month. Fortunately, most bereaved persons experience a roller coaster ride that becomes more manageable over time, with fewer abrupt highs and lows. This gradual improvement may never lead to an end or resolution (Silverman, 1986), however, because many bereaved persons report: "You never get over it—you learn to live with it."

Fifth, loneliness and problems associated with managing the tasks of daily living are two of the most common and difficult adjustments for older adults (Lund et al., 1993). These problems are even more difficult for the spousally bereaved because their daily lives are closely connected with their spouses and they frequently become dependent on each other for conversation, love, and sharing of tasks. Loneliness is problematic because it involves missing, sadness, and a void that does not go away simply by being with or among other people (Lopata, 1973; Osterweis et al., 1984; Parkes, 1987). Many bereaved persons report feeling lonely but not being alone. In the case of experiencing the death of a parent, child, or sibling who may live many miles away, the bereaved often describe how lonely they feel when they realize they can no longer call their loved one on the phone or hear their voice again. In a study by the author, 70% of the bereaved spouses reported that loneliness was their single greatest difficulty during the two years following their partners' deaths (Lund, 1989a).

Unfortunately, most older adults have not learned to do many of the tasks of daily life that are important to maintaining their health, well-being, and happiness. Many older men have not learned how to prepare meals, wash clothes, and clean house because they left these tasks to their wives. Similarly, many older women have not learned how to do home repairs, maintain or sometimes even drive an automobile, and manage finances. Research has shown that these deficiencies further complicate the bereavement process because grief requires physical and mental energy which can be additionally depleted by worrying about how these tasks will be done (Lund, Caserta, et al., 1989). The lack of skills in daily living lends itself to a promising focus for future interventions because these skills can be easily taught. Hopefully, future cohorts of men and women will be better prepared and more skilled in a much broader range of tasks of daily living.

7.05.7 PREDICTORS OF BEREAVEMENT ADJUSTMENTS

It is very common to hear people say that the passage of time will heal the wound of grief, loss, or bereavement (Parkes, 1987; Silverman, 1986). This assumption is problematic and inaccurate because it implies that little or no effort is required to cope with the situation (Worden, 1991). Simply allowing time to pass is expected to bring about successful adjustment. Although it is a fact that with the passage of time most bereaved persons experience less difficulty and make more positive adjustments, it is important to recognize that it is what people do with their time that has the most direct impact on their outcomes (Lund, 1989a). Successful adjustments require active rather than passive coping strategies. The importance of being active and taking charge is integrated within Worden's task-oriented approach to grief (1991). Worden recommends this approach to clinicians because it involves an active coping strategy that fits well into a variety of interventions and it appears to be a more effective strategy than just letting time heal a wound (Silverman, 1986).

Another similar finding supported by research is that many bereaved persons have told others that it is most helpful to take one day at a time and to remain active, busy, and socially connected with other people (Caserta, Van Pelt, & Lund, 1989). Being physically and socially active during the process can help to reduce the feelings of despair, helplessness, loneliness, and being overwhelmed that often contribute to a long-term strategy of waiting—often in vain—for time to bring about healing. In addition to these active coping strategies, recent studies have documented the importance of having social support from others and opportunities for self-expression available, especially in the early months of bereavement (Dimond, Lund, & Caserta, 1987; Lund, Dimond et al., 1986; Schuster & Butler, 1989; Thompson, Gallagher, Cover, Gilewski, & Peterson, 1989). Some of the most difficult and stressful bereavement experiences occur in the first few months when grief issues are especially intense (Wortman et al., 1993). The quality of social support from friends, neighbors, and family is more important than the quantitative dimensions of support and it appears that older spousally bereaved persons tend to rely increasingly more on neighbors and friends because they are most convenient to contact (Dimond et al., 1987; Lund, Caserta, Van Pelt, & Gass, 1990; Schuster & Butler, 1989).

Research has also shown that how a person copes with loss early in the process appears to be one of the best predictors of long-term coping (Levy et al., 1994). Those who report that they are doing quite well during the first couple of months usually cope better than others a few years later (Lund, Dimond et al., 1986; Wortman & Silver, 1989). Bereaved persons therefore are likely to benefit most from social support that they receive during the first two to eight weeks and from opportunities to express how they feel at this time. The first couple of months are most critical because that is when new patterns of behavior are developed and the adjustments that are required can be overwhelming. Early social support, therefore, is most beneficial (Schuster & Butler, 1989; Trunnell, Caserta, & White, 1992). Bereaved persons most value the support provided by those who allow them to openly express anger, sadness, and other emotions without passing along advice and counsel (Caserta, Van Pelt, & Lund, 1989; Dimond et al., 1987; Vachon & Stylianos, 1988). It is important for the bereaved to know that their reactions are common and that others respect their feelings and care about their well-being. People can be most supportive by being good listeners. This also relieves pressure that many people impose on themselves by believing that they need to say things that will make everything better. Such bereavement-eliminating messages do not exist. Self-help groups for bereaved persons provide good opportunities for self-expression, particularly for those who do not already have someone in whom they can confide (Lund & Caserta, 1992). These support groups vary considerably in quality and effectiveness but they do have the potential of providing some valuable sources of support (Lieberman, 1993).

The importance of internal coping resources is supported by research (Ben-Sira, 1983), that has focused on the role of self-esteem (Lund, Dimond et al., 1986) and self-efficacy (Bandura, 1982; Goldfried & Robins, 1982; Parkes, 1987). Both concepts represent personal coping resources that individuals develop throughout their lives. Self-esteem refers to the positive or negative judgments or evaluations that one makes about self-worth. In addition to being a husband or wife and a father or mother, we usually make assessments about being good or bad in the way we perform these roles. Self-efficacy refers to one's ability to meet the changing demands of everyday life and feeling confident to do so. Not all of us feel equally able to manage difficult and challenging situations, particularly bereavement, which requires a broad range of skills and confidence in being able to develop and use them.

The way people feel about themselves and how skilled they are in managing the many tasks of daily—living maintaining a household, paying bills, driving a car, knowing how to access resources, and so forth—will influence how effectively they adjust to the loss of a loved one (Lund, Caserta, et al., 1989). Men and women in today's older age cohort are highly deficient in predictable skills, with men not being well prepared to do shopping, cooking, and cleaning and women being unskilled in financial matters and home repairs. People who develop positive self-esteem and competencies such as social, interpersonal, and instrumental skills are likely to have more favorable bereavement outcomes than those who develop negative self-images and lack self-efficacy. The need to be skilled in the tasks of daily living is important to bereaved people of all ages (Goldfried & Robins, 1982). Worden (1991) describes one of his four tasks of mourning as adjusting to an environment in which the deceased is missing. Learning new skills is considered to be essential to this part of the adjustment process.

Self-esteem and self-efficacy are highly interrelated because people who have confidence and pride in themselves are usually more motivated to learn new skills, and the process of becoming more competent in daily life itself creates more positive self-esteem (Lund, Caserta et al., 1989). Bereaved persons with these positive characteristics are likely to cope quite well because they will not be content with a passive approach to coping and simply waiting for things to get better. People with high self-esteem are more likely to believe that they deserve to feel better and have the desire to at least try to engage in new activities and pursue interests that they have always had. Conversely, bereaved people who never developed these personal coping resources are likely to experience long-term difficulties because they are more inclined to believe that they deserve to remain depressed, lonely, and incapacitated. One research subject said, "Things are terrible, I feel awful but who cares." These people tend to feel overwhelmed and take few, if any, constructive actions on their own behalf. In short, the three best predictors of how older adults experience bereavement are self-esteem, competence in managing tasks of daily living, and opportunities for self-expression (Lund, Dimond et al., 1986). When bereaved older adults are high on these three traits they are much more likely to manage quite well, and adults who are lacking all three are at considerable risk of having long-term difficulties. These factors are likely to be similarly important to people of all ages (Lund et al., 1993).

While it is extremely difficult to summarize briefly the growing and increasingly complicated research literature regarding the many factors that might predict bereavement outcomes, it is appropriate to note that many variables that were expected to be important have not been consistently related to the adjustment process. For example, research has not found large differences in adjustments between those who experienced expected or sudden death situations (Faletti et al., 1989; Hill, Thompson, & Gallagher, 1988). The general expectation has been that it is much easier to manage a bereavement loss if it was anticipated. Unfortunately, there do not appear to be substantial benefits from knowing that a loved one is dying because when the death actually occurs it still sets in motion the most profound parts of the bereavement process which include dealing with loneliness, depression, and managing the numerous tasks of daily living. When a death is sudden and unexpected, the bereaved survivors are likely to feel more intensely the grief-related emotions, but when these gradually subside, the long-term process is quite similar to those who expected the death (Lund, 1989a). If there are benefits from anticipating the death, they are most likely to be attributed to what people do with their time while they anticipate the death. The key element to realizing any benefit is the preparation, not for the death itself, but preparation for learning to do some of the many things that will be required after the death such as learning to do the laundry, cooking, home repairs, and other tasks of daily living. Developing new skills and "having affairs in order" can be helpful to bereaved persons of all ages because energy can then be focused on the grief work that needs to be done (Worden, 1991).

Research comparing bereaved persons from different religious membership groups, with unique religious beliefs and various degrees of religiosity, has revealed that these variables might create some unique bereavement experiences but they do not predict very well the major outcomes such as depression, loneliness, morale, life satisfaction, and a variety of other physical and mental health measures (Falleti et al., 1989; Gallagher, Lovett, Hanley-Dunn, & Thompson, 1989; Lund et al., 1993). It is possible that with different measures of adjustment these religious factors might be more influential but current research points out that these and other factors may be less important than previously expected. The degree of religious activity did, however, emerge in some research to be associated with bereavement adjustment with the more religiously active coping more effectively than the less active (Lund et al., 1988). This finding is consistent with other research that has shown an advantage to bereaved persons who make an effort to remain more socially active and to keep busy (Caserta, Van Pelt, & Lund, 1989). For many older adults, their religious participation can be a very important, convenient, and consistent source of activity that offers social contact, informal support, and a meaningful use of time.

Another important finding to emerge from research is that many older spousally bereaved persons find themselves in a dilemma wherein they must make decisions either to please themselves or others (Caserta, Van Pelt, & Lund, 1989; Dimond et al., 1987; Lund et al., 1990). It is not uncommon for some adult children to exert considerable pressure on their grieving parent to sell the house, get away from the memories, move closer to others in the family, sell the car, or simply do what they expect of them. In most cases, the bereaved older adult does not want the parent/child roles to reverse where they feel pressure to do what their children want them to do (Lund et al., 1990). Most adult children typically have good intentions but sometimes get carried away with trying to take away their parent's grief and make everything instantly better. As research shows, there are no quick solutions to the many adjustments that need to be experienced.

The pressure to conform to the desires and wishes of others, including the deceased, happens often enough that it can be referred to as "grieving according to the expectations of others" or even, "grieving according to the expectations of the deceased." One very common example of doing or saying what others expect occurs when an adult child visits a grieving parent and asks how he or she is doing. Our research interviewers have heard many of these bereaved parents say that they simply tell their children that they are doing fine because they know that is what their children want and expect to hear. They say that they do not want to trouble their children with the truth. They also report feeling that they need to project an image of strength to their children, neighbors, and family. Another interesting example was a bereaved woman who told an interviewer that she wanted to continue a friendship that she had with another man but felt that others would not approve of her spending time with him. She and her deceased husband had been lifelong friends with this man and his deceased wife. They had done many things together as couples. Now that they had both been widowed they wanted to continue spending time together. This woman made it clear to the interviewer that they were "just friends, nothing sexual going on." Rather than living according to their own expectations they made the effort to conceal from others that they were spending time together. Her male friend would wait until dark to visit and would park his car around the block and sneak through a neighbor's backyard to get to her house. As she described the strategy, the interviewer noted that she was embarrassed about the behavior but did not know how she could be more open about the relationship for fear of what others might think.

The deceased often continue to play important influential roles in how the bereaved survivor makes decisions about what is appropriate or not (Troll, Miller, & Atchley, 1979). Some bereaved spouses participating in research studies have said that they were very reluctant to do things that their deceased partners would not approve and that they were struggling with a decision or had already decided in favor of their deceased spouse's wishes. Most commonly, the decisions were regarding what to do with personal belongings and household items, forming new friendships, selling the house and moving to another area, returning to old hobbies and interests, and the purchase of clothing, furniture, and automobiles. One of the more interesting examples was a widow in a research project who described the very serious dilemma that she was having while trying to decide what to do with her husband's favorite friend, the dog. She indicated that she had always hated the dog and would love to get rid of it. Now that her husband was dead she had the opportunity to give the dog away. But, as she considered her choices she now felt that her deceased husband would be very upset if she did not keep and care for his companion. The widow did not take this matter lightly and chose to keep the dog even though her preference was to end the relationship. Until they are actually in the bereavement process people do not realize how difficult some daily life decisions can become. What appear to be rather simple choices are in fact complicated by the reality that others' opinions and expectations create considerable pressure. Although statistical data are not available regarding this, it is very likely that those who are bold enough to live more according to their own expectations will make the many bereavement adjustments with greater satisfaction than those who favor doing things primarily to please others (Caserta, Van Pelt, & Lund, 1989). Many older adults will need validation that it is acceptable for them to do things consistent with their own wishes, but, at the same time, know that others may disagree with their choices. Bereaved people will need to work through these kinds of dilemmas many times and discover what works best for them.

The predictors of adjustment to bereavement are similar for both men and women and for young and older adults (Lund, Caserta, & Dimond, 1986). Age and gender are not the most influential factors in the course of bereavement (Lund et al., 1993). What is of greater importance is to develop positive feelings about oneself early in life, continue to enhance these views over the life course, and develop skills that help one to meet the changing circumstances and demands of daily living (Lund, 1989a; Worden, 1991). People with these traits are more likely than others to adjust well to nearly any major life stress or transition (Goldfried & Robins, 1982; Hooyman & Kiyak, 1996). Human development is a lifelong process. In the case of late life bereavement, the developmental process is challenged. During this transition period, the bereaved person can remain physically, psychologically, and socially disrupted or can emerge with a sense of growth from learning new skills, becoming more independent, and developing a clearer self-identity.

7.05.8 WORKING WITH THE BEREAVED

Although bereavement is one of the most stressful experiences that occur in our lives, we should not conclude that most bereaved persons will need help with their adjustment process. Research has shown that many bereaved persons do not want or need intervention services (Levy, Derby, & Martinkowski, 1993; Lund et al., 1985). Most researchers estimate that between 15 and 25% of the bereaved will experience considerable long-term difficulty and may require major forms of assistance from others (Lund, 1993). This point is important to recognize because many clinicians and other service providers assume that most older bereaved persons are depressed, socially isolated, and incapacitated by their loss. In fact, gerontologists have reminded us that the majority of older adults do not fit the general stereotypes of being dependent, frail, poor, lonely, and in poor health (Hooyman & Kiyak, 1996). The research evidence does not support these and other assumptions, although certainly some bereaved persons are depressed, isolated, and incapacitated (Wortman & Silver, 1989). In fact, as mentioned previously, older adults are quite resilient and find ways to manage the many losses that they experience throughout their lives (Cleiren, 1993; Lund, 1993; Murrell et al., 1988; Worden, 1991).

The tasks for those developing intervention services are many, and among their first should be an attempt to reach those who are at greatest risk—to seek them out rather than simply announcing the existence of the service—and encourage their participation by explaining how and why the service will be helpful. It is absolutely critical to recognize that many, perhaps most, of the potential population of bereaved persons will not want to participate (Caserta & Lund, 1993; Lund et al., 1985). This can be discouraging to those who are committed to the value of their services, but their motivation to continue their efforts will probably be less adversely affected if they anticipate the lack of enthusiasm among many potential clients. For example, only 44% of the bereaved spouses who completed a study by the author said that they would have liked the opportunity of attending self-help groups (Lund et al., 1985). Later in another study only 27% of those assigned to self-help groups actually agreed to participate (Lund, Redburn, Juretich, & Caserta, 1989). For those who need assistance but are reluctant, it is often beneficial to obtain encouragement from others in the bereaved person's network, particularly physicians and important family members and friends.

Interventions need to be available early in the bereavement process and continue over relatively long periods of time (Horacek, 1995; Schuster & Butler, 1989; Trunnell et al., 1992). As discussed previously, there is a good deal of research evidence suggesting that the first few months are the most difficult and that early adjustments will influence outcomes much later (Caserta & Lund, 1993; Wortman et al., 1993). Also, because bereavement may last for many years and some people may not be ready for early interventions, it would be most helpful to have services available over long periods of time so that they may obtain the appropriate help when they are most ready to receive and benefit from it (Faletti et al., 1989). Others may require intervention or assistance for long periods of time but dependency on any particular form of help is not desired (Silverman, 1986).

Because the impact of bereavement is multidimensional, it is imperative that interventions offer comprehensive and diverse sets of services. It is unlikely that any one intervention will be capable of providing all that is needed, but each intervention should clearly identify which needs are being targeted in relation to the overall multidimensional process so that there is an awareness of what help is not being provided. For example, the death of a spouse in later life can impact emotions, psychosocial functioning, health, family life, interpersonal relationships, work, recreation, and financial situations. Therefore, those designing interventions which provide primarily an opportunity for self-expression (such as self-help groups) should recognize that some dimensions are not likely to be addressed (Shuchter, 1986; Shuchter & Zisook, 1993). Clinicians need to be aware of the full range of services that are available in their communities so their clients can obtain a unique set of diverse services to meet their unique needs. Ideally, all communities would have available a variety of interventions or services so that each person's unique skills, resources, and circumstances could be matched to the most appropriate set of services. While this is unlikely, we can at least strive to offer interventions with the broadest scope of impact. Therefore, whenever possible, it would be worthwhile to impact several dimensions simultaneously (Shuchter, 1986) by providing opportunities for self-expression and the enhancement of self-esteem; by teaching new skills to complete the tasks of daily living; by enhancing and mobilizing already existing social support networks; by providing education and assistance regarding health, nutrition, and exercise; and by encouraging social participation. Each of the predictor variables reviewed in this chapter can be integrated within nearly every type of intervention.

Behavioral competency interventions (Ben-Sira, 1983; Hill, Lund, & Packard, 1996) that identify and provide specialized training in daily survival skills can be of great value for several reasons. First, such training equips bereaved individuals with the special expertise they need to manage the tasks that had been performed by their deceased loved one. Second, successful mastery of new skills builds self-esteem and reinforces beliefs about personal competence. Finally, the process of training provides informal opportunities for the individual to socialize and interact with others while learning important life skills. Skill training interventions offer an innovative approach with promise for helping bereaved older adults cope with issues of grief and mourning and prepare for healthy independent living.

Various intervention formats and professionals are needed to ensure that appropriate services are available. Not all people experience bereavement in the same way; similarly, not all people will use or benefit from the same interventions. In terms of format, some people will only want to have a one-on-one type of intervention. This might be because they feel the uniqueness of their situation can be dealt with more effectively one-to-one, because they are reluctant to express personal and sensitive feelings in group situations (Silverman, 1986). Others have reported that they particularly enjoyed being in a self-help group because they learned from others, recognized some commonalities in their situations, and enjoyed the socializing and friendships which developed (Lund & Caserta, 1992; Caserta & Lund, 1996).

Self-help support groups are a commonly used intervention with older adults (Lund, Redburn et al., 1989). Such groups generally consist of bereaved individuals who voluntarily meet to discuss issues and problems associated with their situation (Lieberman, 1993; Lieberman & Videka-Sherman, 1986). Participants can experience hope, learn new ideas and problem-solving strategies, improve skills for developing social relationships, become less lonely, explore new role definitions, discover that others have similar difficulties, and receive additional social support and encouragement. Belonging to a group and sharing feelings of fellowship and solidarity have been helpful to many older adults. Many of the general benefits of various self-help groups are especially relevant to bereaved older adults. Group members often discuss ways to alleviate the feelings of loneliness, social isolation, and hopelessness that accompany widowhood. Members also have opportunities to meet new people, participate in social activities, and form new friendships (Caserta & Lund, 1993). In addition, many bereaved spouses experience difficulties managing tasks of daily living such as meal preparation, house cleaning, yard maintenance, and transportation that were performed previously by the deceased spouse. Group members regularly share information, advice, and resources about these common problems. Finally, self-help groups are less expensive than most alternative services and are often attractive to individuals who are reluctant to use the services of mental health professionals and agencies. Support groups are not without their share of problems because they require clear goals, well trained leaders, and realistic expectations. Poorly run groups can become overly depressing and ineffective. Good outcomes do not often happen by chance but are the result of careful planning and good leadership (Lund, Redburn et al., 1989).

Many people have skills and expertise which are well suited for helping the bereaved. Silverman (1986), who developed the widow-to-widow program, has shown that widows are quite capable of assisting each other. An experienced widow can reveal to the new widow that she has been there and knows how it feels to grieve. Also, there are important contributions that can be made by researchers, gerontologists, psychologists, psychiatrists, physicians, social workers, nurses, occupational therapists, counselors, clergy, and many other professionals, including social scientists, lawyers, accountants, educators, and direct service providers. Again, because bereavement has a multidimensional impact, interventions can be developed by many different professional and trained team members. Other bereaved persons can provide a sharing of experiences while trained persons assist with legal, financial, health, spiritual, and educational issues. A multidimensional team approach is highly recommended because it will increase the likelihood of developing interventions which address the diversity of needs and lead to greater success.

7.05.9 SUMMARY

Bereavement is a common and natural experience that we all share. Unfortunately, many people are not well prepared for the pain, threats, and challenges that it presents. Because bereavement occurs in broader contexts, we do not all have the same personal and social resources available (Caserta & Lund, 1993), or have the same experiences and needs. What appears to help one person may have an entirely different impact on someone else. The best way to be prepared to help bereaved persons is to be educated about the process, assess the context in which it occurs, become familiar with a wide range of helping resources, and be patient, a good listener and nonjudgmental.

One final suggestion concerning future research and clinical practice is the need to be creative and work in interdisciplinary teams whenever possible. Being creative means that while looking at the same thing you are able to see something different, perhaps many different things. Good quality research and interventions are not always the result of following a "cookbook" approach where we simply look up the issue or problem and find the recipe to resolve it. In order to ask the most interesting and important research questions, decide on the best methodology, or develop and offer the most effective intervention, we need to be very creative. We need to be willing to take a risk and modify the way we mechanically make research and treatment decisions. One of the best ways to be more creative is to work in interdisciplinary teams.

Researchers and clinicians are trained within specific disciplines and learn to favor specific research designs and intervention strategies. Over time, each professional's training becomes his or her area of expertise and there is a natural tendency to define questions and issues in a way that leads to using the same methodologies and practices. Abraham Kaplan, a philosopher of science, refers to this rigidity as "the law of the instrument" (1964, p. 28). He states that if you give a young boy a hammer, everything he encounters will need pounding. If a researcher or clinician exclusively uses only one theory, one methodology, or one counseling strategy then other techniques and strategies are ignored. If they cannot become skilled with more than just a single approach to their work (the hammer) it is even more important for them to work collaboratively in interdisciplinary teams so that other tools, strategies, perspectives, and methodologies are used. One of the best ways to be creative is to assemble a team of investigators who represent diverse and needed areas of expertise. When clinicians and researchers from medicine, pharmacy, nursing, social work, social and behavioral sciences, and other disciplines work collaboratively the end results are much greater than just the sum of the parts. New methodologies, techniques, and strategies will result from the creativity that is enhanced by working in multidisciplinary teams.

Death and other bereavement-related losses will continue to surround our daily lives, offering us choices to learn from these experiences or to use them to be better prepared for our personal losses and our professional work. Although we have learned much from research and clinical practice there are substantial gaps in our knowledge. Much creative and pioneering work remains for those who have the interest, expertise and enthusiasm to learn more about grief and bereavement and to apply this knowledge to make a difference in people's lives.

7.05.10 REFERENCES

Aiken, L. R. (1994). *Dying, death and bereavement* (3rd ed.) Boston: Allyn & Bacon.

Ajzen, I., & Fishbein, M. (1980). *Understanding attitudes and predicting social behavior*. Englewood Cliffs, NJ: Prentice-Hall.

Atchley, R. C. (1989). A continuity theory of normal aging. *The Gerontologist, 29*, 183–190.

Bandura, A. (1982). Self-efficacy mechanism in human agency. *American Psychologist, 37*, 122–147.

Ben-Sira, Z. (1983). Loss, stress, and readjustment: The structure of coping with bereavement and disability. *Social Science Medicine, 17*, 1619–1632.

Bowlby, J. (1969). *Attachment and loss. Vol.1: Attachment*. New York: Basic Books.

Caine, L. (1974). *Widow*. New York: Bantam.

Caserta, M. A., & Lund, D. A. (1992a). Bereaved older adults who seek early professional help. *Death Studies, 16*(1), 17–30.

Caserta, M. S., & Lund, D. A. (1992b). Bereavement stress and coping among older adults: Expectations versus the actual experience. *Omega, 25*, 33–45.

Caserta, M. S., & Lund, D. A. (1993). Intrapersonal resources and the effectiveness of self-help groups for bereaved older adults. *The Gerontologist, 33*, 619–629.

Caserta, M. S., & Lund, D. A. (1996). Beyond bereavement support group meetings: Exploring outside social contacts among the members. *Death Studies, 20*, 537–556.

Caserta, M. S., Lund, D. A., & Dimond, M. F. (1989). Older widows' early bereavement adjustments. *Journal of Women and Aging, 1*(4), 5–27.

Caserta, M. S., Van Pelt, J., & Lund, D. A. (1989). Advice on the adjustment to loss from bereaved older adults: An examination of resources and outcomes. In D. A. Lund (Ed.), *Older bereaved spouses: Research with practical applications*. New York: Hemisphere.

Chigier, E. (1988). *Grief and bereavement in contemporary society*. London: Freund.

Cleiren, M. (1993). *Bereavement and adaptation: A comparative study of the aftermath of death*. Washington, DC: Hemisphere.

Cumming, E., & Henry, W. E. (1961) *Growing old*. New York: Basic.

Dimond, M.F., Lund, D. A., & Caserta, M. S. (1987). The role of social support in the first two years of bereavement in an elderly sample. *The Gerontologist*, 27, 599–604.

Faletti, M. V., Gibbs, J. M., Clark, M. C., Pruchno, R. A., & Berman, E. A., (1989). Longitudinal course of bereavement in older adults. In D. A. Lund (Ed.), *Older bereaved spouses: Research with practical applications* (pp. 37–51). New York: Hemisphere.

Farnsworth, J., Pett, M., & Lund, D. A. (1989). Predictors of loss management and well-being in later life widowhood and divorce. *Journal of Family Issues, 10*, 102–121.

Folkman, S., Lazarus, R. S., Dunkel-Schetter, C., De Longis, A., & Gruen, R. J. (1986). Dynamics of a stressful encounter: Cognitive appraisal, coping, and encounter outcomes. *Journal of Personality and Social Psychology, 50*, 992–1003.

Freud, S. (1957). *The Standard Edition of the Complete Psychological Works of Sigmund Freud*. London: Hogarth.

Gallagher, D., Lovett, S., Hanley-Dunn, P., & Thompson, L. W. (1989). Use of select coping strategies during late-life spousal bereavement. In D. A. Lund (Ed.), *Older bereaved spouses: Research with practical applications* (pp. 111–121). New York: Hemisphere.

Gass, K. A. (1989a). Appraisal, coping, and resources: Markers associated with the health of aged widows and widowers. In D. A. Lund (Ed.), *Older bereaved spouses: Research with practical applications* (pp. 79–94). New York: Hemisphere.

Gass, K. A. (1989b). Health of older widowers: Role of appraisal, coping, resources, and type of spouse's death. In D. A. Lund (Ed.), *Older bereaved spouses: Research with practical applications* (pp. 95–110). New York: Hemisphere.

Goldfried, M. R., & Robins, C. (1982). On the facilitation of self-efficacy. *Cognitive Therapy and Research*, 6, 361–380.

Grollman, E. A., (1977). *Living when a loved one has died*. Boston: Beacon.

Hardt, D. V. (1978). An investigation of the stages of bereavement. *Omega, 9*, 279–285.

Havighurst, R. J. (1968). Personality and patterns of aging. *The Gerontologist, 8*, 20–23.

Hess, B., Markson, E., & Stein, P. (1996). *Sociology*. Needham Heights, MA: Allyn & Bacon.

Hill, C. D., Thompson, L. W., & Gallagher, D. (1988). The role of anticipatory bereavment in older women's adjustment to widowhood. *The Gerontologist, 28*, 792–796.

Hill, R. D., Lund, D. A., & Packard, T. (1996). Bereavement. In J. I. Sheikh (Ed.), *Treating the elderly* (pp. 45–74). San Francisco: Jossey Bass.

Hooyman, N., & Kiyak, H. A. (1996). *Social gerontology: A multidisciplinary perspective*. Needham Heights, MA: Simon & Schuster.

Horacek, B. J. (1995). A heuristic model of grieving after high-grief deaths. *Death Studies, 19*, 21–31.

Irish, D. P., Lundquist, K. F., & Nelsen, V. J. (1993). *Ethnic variations in dying, death, and grief*. Washington, DC: Taylor & Francis.

Kaplan, A. (1964). *The conduct of inquiry*. San Francisco: Chandler.

Kubler-Ross, E. (1969). *On death and dying*. New York: Macmillan.

Kushner, H. S. (1982). *When bad things happen to good people*. New York: Avon.

Lazarus, R. S. (1966). *Psychological stress and the coping process*. New York: McGraw-Hill.

Leming, M. R., & Dickinson, G. E. (1990). *Understanding dying, death and bereavment*. New York: Holt, Rinehart & Winston.

Levy, L. H., Derby, J. F., & Martinkowski, K. S. (1993). Effects of membership in bereavement support groups on adaptation to conjugal bereavement. *American Journal of Community Psychology, 21*, 361–381.

Levy, L. H., Martinkowski, K.S., & Derby, J. F. (1994). Differences in patterns of adaptation in conjugal bereavement: Their sources and potential significance. *Omega, 29*, 71–87.

Lewis, C. S. (1961). *A grief observed*. Minneapolis, MN: Winston.

Lieberman, M. A. (1993). Bereavement self-help groups: A review of conceptual and methodological issues. In M. S. Stroebe, W. Stroebe, & R. O. Hansson (Eds.), *Handbook of bereavement: Theory, research, and intervention* (pp. 411–426). New York: Cambridge University Press.

Lieberman, M. A., & Videka-Sherman, L. (1986). The impact of self-help groups on the mental health of widows and widowers. *American Journal of Orthopsychiatry, 56*, 435–449.

Lindemann, E. (1944). The symptomatology and management of acute grief. *American Journal of Psychiatry, 101*, 141–48.

Lopata, H. Z. (1973). *Widowhood in an American city*. Cambridge, MA: Schenkman.

Lund, D. A. (1989a). Conclusions about bereavement in later life and implications for interventions and future research. In D. A. Lund (Ed.), *Older bereaved spouses: Research with practical applications* (pp. 217–231). New York: Hemisphere.

Lund, D. A. (1989b). *Older bereaved spouses: Research with practical applications*. New York: Hemisphere.

Lund, D. A. (1993). Widowhood: The coping response. In R. Kastenbaum (Ed.), *The encyclopedia of adult development* (pp. 537–541).Phoenix, AZ: Oryx.

Lund, D. A. (1996). Coping in later life. In K. J. Doka (Ed.), *Journeys* (pp. 1,3). Washington, DC: Hospice Foundation of America.

Lund, D. A., & Caserta, M. S. (1992). Older bereaved spouses' participation in self-help groups. *Omega, 25*, 47–61

Lund, D. A., Caserta, M. S., & Dimond, M. F. (1986). Gender differences through two years of bereavement among the elderly. *The Gerontologist, 26*(3), 314–320.

Lund, D. A., Caserta, M. S., & Dimond, M. F. (1988). A comparison of bereavement adjustments between Mormon and non-Mormon older adults. *Journal of Religion and Aging, 5*(1/2), 75–92.

Lund, D. A., Caserta, M. S., & Dimond, M. F. (1993). The course of spousal bereavement in later life. In M. S.

Stroebe, W. Stroebe, & R. O. Hansson (Eds.), *Handbook of bereavement* (pp. 240–254). New York: Cambridge University Press.

Lund, D. A., Caserta, M. S., Dimond, M. F., & Gray, R. M. (1986). Impact of bereavement on the self-conceptions of older surviving spouses: An application of the interactionist perspective. *Symbolic Interaction, 9*(2), 235–244.

Lund, D. A., Caserta, M. S., Dimond, M. F., & Shaffer, S. K. (1989). Competencies, tasks of daily living, and adjustments to spousal bereavement in later life. In D. A. Lund (Ed.), *Older bereaved spouses: Research with practical applications* (pp. 135–152). New York: Hemisphere.

Lund, D. A., Caserta, M. S., Van Pelt, J., & Gass, K. A. (1990). Stability of social support networks after later-life spousal bereavement. *Death Studies, 14*, 53–73.

Lund, D. A., Dimond, M. F., Caserta, M. S., Poulton, J. L., Johnson, R. J., & Connelly, R. J. (1986). Identifying elderly with coping difficulties after two years of bereavement. *Omega: Journal of Death & Dying, 16*(3), 213–224.

Lund, D. A., Dimond, M. F., & Juretich, M. (1985). Bereavement support groups for the elderly: Characteristics of potential participants. *Death Studies, 9*, 309–321.

Lund, D. A., Redburn, D. E., Juretich, M. S., & Caserta, M. S. (1989). Resolving problems implementing bereavement self-help groups. In D. A. Lund (Ed.), *Older bereaved spouses: Research with practical applications* (pp. 213–216). New York: Hemisphere.

Marris, P. (1958). *Widows and their families*. London: Routledge & Kegan Paul.

McCrae, R. R., & Costa, P. T. (1993). Psychological resilience among widowed men and women: A 10-year follow-up of a national sample. In M. S. Stroebe, W. Stroebe, & R. O. Hansson (Eds.), *Handbook of Bereavement: Theory, research and intervention* (pp. 196–202). New York: Cambridge University Press.

Murreli, S. A., Himmelfarb, S., & Phifer, J. F. (1988). Effects of bereavement/loss and pre-event status on subsequent physical health in older adults. *International Journal of Aging and Human Development, 27*, 89–107.

Olson, D. H., Sprenkle, D., & Russell, C. (1979). Circumplex model of marital and family systems: 1. Cohesion and adaptability dimensions, family types, and clinical applications. *Family Process, 18*, 3–28.

Osterweis, M., Solomon, F., & Green, M. (1984). *Bereavement reactions, consequences, and care*. Washington, DC: National Academy Press.

Parkes, C. M. (1987). *Bereavement: Studies of grief in adult life* (2nd ed.). Madison, WI: International Universities Press.

Pearlin, L. I., & Mullan, J. T. (1992). Loss and Stress in Aging. In M. L. Wykle, E. Kahana, & J. Kowal (Eds.) *Stress & health among the elderly* (pp. 117–132). New York: Springer.

Rando, T. A. (1993). *Treatment of complicated mourning*. Champaign, IL: Research Press.

Riley, M. W. (1971). Social gerontology and the age stratification of society. *The Gerontologist, 11*, 79–87.

Rosenstock, I. M. (1990). The health belief model: Explaining health behavior through expectancies. In K. Glanz, F. M. Lewis, & B. K. Rimer (Eds.), *Health behavior and health education* (pp. 39–62). San Francisco: Jossey-Bass.

Rubin, S. S. (1993). The death of a child is forever: The life course impact of child loss. In M. S. Stroebe, W. Stroebe, & R.O. Hansson (Eds.), *Handbook of bereavement: Theory, research, and intervention* (pp. 285–299). New York: Cambridge University Press.

Schiff, H. S. (1977). *The bereaved parent*. New York: Penguin.

Schuster, T. L., & Butler, E. W. (1989). Bereavement, social networks, social support, and mental health. In D. A. Lund (Ed.), *Older bereaved spouses: Research with practical applications* (pp. 55–68) New York: Hemisphere.

Shuchter, S. R. (1986). *Dimensions of grief: Adjusting to the death of a spouse*. San Francisco: Jossey-Bass.

Shuchter, S. R., & Zisook, S. (1993). The course of normal grief. In M. S. Stroebe, W. Stroebe, & R. O. Hansson, (Eds.), *Handbook of bereavement: Theory, research, and intervention* (pp. 23–43). New York: Cambridge University Press.

Silverman, P. R. (1986). *Widow to widow*. New York: Springer.

Staudacher, C. (1987). *Beyond grief: A guide for recovering from the death of a loved one*. Oakland, CA: New Harbinger.

Stephenson, J. S. (1985). *Death, grief and mourning: Individual and social realities*. New York: Free Press.

Stroebe, M. S., Hansson, R. O., & Stroebe, W. (1993). Contemporary themes and controversies in bereavement research. In M. S. Stroebe, W. Stroebe, & R. O. Hansson (Eds.), *Handbook of Bereavement: Theory, research, and intervention* (pp. 457–477). New York: Cambridge University Press

Stroebe, M. S., & Stroebe W. (1991). Does "grief work" work? *Journal of Consulting and Clinical Psychology, 59*, 479–482.

Stroebe, M. S., Stroebe, W, & Hansson, R. O. (1993a). Bereavement research and theory: An introduction to the handbook. In M. S. Stroebe, W. Stroebe, & R. O. Hansson (Eds.), *Handbook of Bereavement: Theory, research, and intervention* (pp. 3–22). New York: Cambridge University Press.

Stroebe, M. S., Stroebe, W., & Hansson, R. O. (Eds.) (1993b). *Handbook of Bereavement: Theory, research, and intervention*. New York: Cambridge University Press.

Stroebe, W., & Stroebe, M. (1987). *Bereavement and Health: The Psychological and physical consequences of partner loss*. London: Cambridge University Press.

Thompson, L. W., Gallagher, D., Cover, H., Gilewski, M., & Peterson, J. (1989). Effects of bereavement on symptoms of psychopathology in older men and women. In D. A. Lund. *Older bereaved spouses: Research with practical applications* (pp. 17–24). New York: Hemisphere.

Troll, L. E., Miller, S. J., & Atchley, R. C. (1979). *Families in later life*. Belmont, CA: Wadsworth.

Trunnell, E. P., Caserta, M. S., & White, G. L. (1992). Bereavement: Current issues in intervention and prevention. *Journal of Health Education, 23*, 275–280.

US Bureau of the Census (1991). Marital status and living arrangements: March 1990. *Current Population Reports, Series P–20, No. 450*. Washington, DC: Government Printing Office.

Vachon, M. L., & Stylianos, S. K. (1988). The role of social support in bereavement. *Journal of Social Issues, 44*, 175–190.

Worden, J. W. (1991) *Grief counseling and grief therapy* (2nd ed.). New York: Springer.

Wortman, C., & Silver, R. (1989). The myths of coping with loss. *Journal of Consulting and Clinical Psychology, 57*, 349–357.

Wortman, C., Silver, R., & Kessler, R. (1993). The meaning of loss and adjustment to bereavement. In M. S. Stroebe, W. Stroebe, & R. O. Hansson (Eds.), *Handbook of bereavement: Theory, research, and intervention* (pp. 349–366). New York: Cambridge University Press.

7.06
Understanding Decisional Capacity of Older Adults

LORI FRANK
MEDTAP International, Bethesda, MD, USA
and
MICHAEL SMYER
Boston College, Chestnut Hill, MA, USA

7.06.1 INTRODUCTION

With age comes increased interaction with the legal system in our society. Because of increased prevalence of cognitive impairment with age, psychologists are often expected to address legal concerns that result from potential cognitive impairment. Concerns about the capacity of the older individual to make autonomous decisions surface frequently, in part because of the greater decisional burden that age-related health problems place on older adults. Thus, assessing capacity for decision making is a large and growing area of geropsychology.

An understanding of decision-making ability of older adults is dependent upon a number of different fields of inquiry and several different areas of literature. This chapter is organized into five main sections. The first summarizes the development of the current doctrine of informed consent and the literature on informed consent with older adults is briefly reviewed. In the second, the concept of competence is examined more closely, beginning with a brief history of the development of theoretical and empirical work on decisional capacity. In section three, the forensic psychology and cognitive psychology contributions to the concept of capacity are compared. In the fourth, competence assessment is discussed. In the fifth section some of the issues raised by work with older adults is explored in the context of a specific policy, the Patient Self-determination Act. Finally, additional areas relevant to older adults' decisional capacity are highlighted.

7.06.2 INFORMED CONSENT

7.06.2.1 Brief History of the Doctrine of Informed Consent

Investigations of the adequacy of informed consent procedures usually involve reference to measurable components of the construct of "informed consent." Three components are identified in a widely accepted model of informed consent, a model which derives from legal requirements: there must be adequate disclosure of relevant information, the choice must be voluntary, and the individual must be competent to make the decision (Appelbaum and Grisso, 1988, 1995; Faden & Beauchamp, 1986). While some controversy surrounds all three of these elements, competence has been the most difficult to define and measure, and has generated the most discussion. Views of competence in the late 1990s will be examined in the next section. First, however, the development of the current view is described.

The legal history of informed consent in the USA can be traced back to eighteenth century Britain, where the King's Court ruled that medical surgery performed without the consent of the patient constituted a "tortious assault." More recently, a 1905 Minnesota case (*Mohr v. Williams*) established that surgery performed without permission constituted a battery. The significance of this ruling was that the patient, and not the physician, was to determine choices as to physical interference with an individual's body. Further affirmation of this principle of self-determination was recorded by Justice Benjamin Cardozo, in an opinion written in 1914: "every human being of adult years and sound mind has a right to determine what should be done with his own body" (*Schloendorff v. Society of New York Hospitals,* 1914).

Two cases refined the concept of "informed consent." In the 1957 case of *Salgo v. Leland Stanford Jr. Board of Trustees*, the court ruled that physicians had a duty to disclose information about the risks and alternatives of treatment. In the 1960 case of *Natanson v. Kline*, the court ruled that the patient must be provided with a certain amount of relevant information; it was no longer sufficient for the patient to consent to or decline treatment. At that time, the legal standard for the amount and kind of information provided was based on a professional practice standard and was, therefore, set by the medical community: "deviation from the standard of conduct of a reasonable and prudent medical doctor of the same school of practice as the defendant under similar circumstances."

In 1972, the case of *Canterbury v. Spence* shifted the determination of the legal standard for disclosure from the medical community to the patient. The patient was entitled to disclosure of information that any "average, reasonable patient" would require in deciding whether or not to consent to the procedure, and *not* disclosure based on a professional practice standard. This ruling is significant for its emphasis on patients' rights which, according to the court, "demands a standard set by law for physicians rather than one which physicians may or may not impose upon themselves."

By the end of the 1970s, legal developments required that patients be apprised of the nature and risks of a medical procedure by the physician. The concern of the law was that information was properly provided to the patient, the patient comprehended it, and the patient voluntarily consented to the procedure.

The cases reviewed above indicate the source of legal standards in the late 1990s for the information that providers are required to disclose, but the practical translation of these legal requirements to clinical situations is unclear. The law has paid less attention to the abilities an individual should possess in order to provide truly informed consent; such requirements are being explored more thoroughly in the field of psychology (and will be discussed more fully later).

7.06.2.2 Informed Consent and the Elderly

The elderly are a heterogeneous group (Stanley, Guido, Stanley, & Shortell, 1984), yet older adults are grouped together for the purposes of many policy initiatives. Besides policy precedent, there may be other reasons to examine older adults as a single group. In some studies, elderly subjects have demonstrated poorer comprehension of informed consent information than younger subjects (Stanley et al., 1984; Taub, 1980). Given historical differences in education level and vocabulary level between successive cohorts in the US, certain segments of the elderly population may be at increased risk for poorer comprehension of informed consent material.

To the extent that age differences continue to be manifest, and since end-of-life decisions occur more commonly among older adults than any other age group, elderly people may in fact present "unique ethical challenges" (Buehler, 1990) to health care providers. Before singling out a group for study, however, consideration must be made of the criteria involved in defining the group, and within-group heterogeneity must be acknowledged. While it is true that certain broad statements about a heterogeneous group like the elderly are of limited use (and may be ethically questionable (Cohen, 1996)), generalities do exist which justify the examination of elderly people as a separate group.

The process of obtaining informed consent from older adults may differ from obtaining informed consent from younger adults in important ways. For example, because of the prevalence of chronic medical conditions among older adults, disclosure and consent may be part of an ongoing process rather than just elements related to an acute episode. Chronic illness may change important features of the relationship between health care provider and patient for which informed consent laws were written.

Moody (1988) advocates a shift in emphasis from informed consent to the concept of "negotiated consent," in which emphasis shifts from a dichotomous variable view of consent (can the patient provide informed consent or not?) to a continuous variable view (to what extent can the patient understand this information and make an informed choice, over time?). Although originally conceived of in relation to long-term care settings, the concept of "negotiated consent" may be applicable in acute care settings as well, particularly for older adults with chronic conditions, re-admitted to the same facility multiple times.

7.06.3 COMPETENCE TO PROVIDE INFORMED CONSENT

Historically, legal applications of the term "competence" have provided inadequate specificity and have been underdetermined for research purposes (Appelbaum & Grisso, 1988). The limitations of legal conceptualizations of competence have prompted some researchers to examine the concept from a psychological perspective instead. Below, the evolution of definitions of the term "competence" are briefly reviewed. General aspects of definitions are presented first, drawing largely from the forensic psychology literature. In Section 7.06.4, contributions of forensic and cognitive psychology to thinking about competence are reviewed. The ways in which conceptualizations have been put into practice are discussed in Section 7.06.5.

7.06.3.1 Definitions of Competence

Definitions current in the late 1990s, are most readily understood when considered in relation to recent historical developments. These developments are briefly reviewed below, and Table 1 provides a summary of this discussion. As shown in the table, it is possible to trace a progression from early definitions which included a requirement that the choice be rational to later definitions which dropped the requirement for a rational choice ("Rationality" in the table) and added a requirement of awareness or insight ("Appreciation" in the table). Each of these individual definitional elements requires some explanation.

Definitions of competence have historically been tied to legal definitions of informed consent. Because proper disclosure of information is central to legal requirements for informed consent, early definitions of competence centered around understanding of the disclosed information. Roth, Meisel, and Lidz (1977) found most definitions required that "an individual must be able to comprehend the nature of the particular conduct in question and to understand its quality and its consequences" (p. 279). Appelbaum and Grisso (1988) identify understanding as "the concept referred to most often in legal cases and statutes" (p. 1635). As

Table 1 Elements of definitions of decisional competence from selected sources, 1977–1995.

	Definition Elements			
	Understanding	*Reasoning*	*Appreciation*	*Rationality*
Rationality-dependent definitions				
as noted in Roth et al. (1977)	X	X		X
Lidz et al. (1984)	X			X
Stanley et al. (1984)	X	X		X
Combination Definitions				
Miles (1989)	X		X	X
Draper and Dawson (1990)	X		X	X
Appreciation-dependent definitions				
Appelbaum and Roth (1982)	X	X	X	
Tepper and Elwork (1984)	X	X	X	
Kapp (1988)	X	X	X	
Appelbaum and Grisso (1995)	X	X	X	

Kelman (1982) states: "Voluntary, informed consent is illusory if the participants lack the capacity to evaluate the information" (p. 62). It is so central to competence, in fact, that "most researchers have implicitly assumed that an understanding of treatment information is the sole criterion of competence" (Tepper & Elwork, 1984, p. 205) . Understanding therefore appears as a standard in every definition of competence (see column 1 of Table 1). Of interest is the appearance of other standards and the rationale for their inclusion.

In general, earlier definitional systems included reference to a standard of reasonableness or rationality of the choice. Because of problems in separating politically or socially subjective standards of rationality from competence assessment, the rationality standard is often excluded from more recent systems, although rationality of the *reasons* for the choice is still included in many formulations of competence. Rationality of the reasons behind the choice requires both reasoning ability and some level of appreciation of the relevance of the decision to oneself. Rationality of reasons is a component of reasoning quality, and systems which include this criterion are listed under "Reasoning" (column 2) in Table 1. Systems which evaluate rationality of the decision itself are listed under "Rationality" (column 4). Those systems which attend to individuals' appreciation of the relevance of the information for their own situation (or at least acknowledgment of illness) are indicated under "Appreciation" (column 3).

As Table 1 indicates, definitions of competence tend to take one of two forms, labeled here as rationality-dependent and appreciation-dependent types.

7.06.3.1.1 Rationality-dependent definitions

One example of an early formulation is presented by Roth et al., (1977). They cite the following four standards as ones in use at the time of their writing: evidencing a choice, reasonableness of choice, rationality of reasons for choice (which requires an ability to understand), and actual understanding. Their presentation is not an endorsement, and in fact they point out some of the problems with each standard, particularly with the reasonableness standard.

Building from the earlier work of Roth and colleagues, Lidz et al., (1984) define competence as "the legal presumption that a patient has the capacity to comprehend the information the doctor discloses" (p.22). In addition to understanding of disclosed information, they cite rationality of the decision and rational reasoning ability as additional required elements.

Stanley et al., (1984) present a substantially similar definition to Lidz et al. they include comprehension, rationality of the choice, and quality of reasoning as required elements for competence. Of interest in their system is the criterion they use for evaluating quality of reasoning: evidence of weighing risks and benefits. This is a criterion that appears in later—and more sophisticated—systems as well.

7.06.3.1.2 Combination definitions

Like Stanley et al. (1984), Miles and Gomez Carlos (1989) define competence as "an ability to learn and repeat risks and benefits and make personal choices in light of that knowledge."

Also like Stanley et al., they include a decisional component in addition to an understanding component. Rationality of the choice is also part of his framework. An important difference, however, is that Miles and Gomez Carlos includes appreciation of the relevance of the information as a standard.

In 1990, Draper and Dawson presented their definition of competence to consent to treatment. Like Miles and Gomez Carlos's system, appreciation of the situation is included, but no reference is made to reasoning ability. Surprisingly, despite a warning to remember that "legal competence is not identical to rationality, that rationality is not a necessary condition of legal competence" (p. 286), rationality is included in their system, in which the rationality of the choice itself—rather than rationality of the reasons for the choice—is required for competence.

7.06.3.1.3 Appreciation-dependent definitions

Only those definitional systems that exclude rationality of the choice as a standard, and include appreciation of the relevance of the information for oneself are considered representative of the second definitional type, the appreciation-dependent definition. The appreciation requirement excludes as incompetent individuals with delusional thought about the relationship between the informed consent disclosure and their own lives. The appreciation-dependent definitional type is represented by the work of Appelbaum and Grisso (1995), Appelbaum and Roth (1982), Kapp (1988), and Tepper and Elwork (1984).

Most researchers agree that individuals out of touch with reality fall outside a credible definition of competence. The appreciation and rationality standards are both attempts to include a contact with reality requirement in a definition of competence. The rationality-dependent definition, by using rationality of the choice as the measure of contact with reality, allows for societal norms and evaluator subjectivity to intrude on the assessment of competence and it implicitly assumes that rationality can be objectively evaluated, or at least that there is an absolute standard of rationality. The appreciation-dependent type of definition requires no such assumptions. Competence is free to remain a relative term, accommodating idiosyncratic aspects of the individual's thinking, with the exception of delusional thinking. An individual needs to demonstrate some understanding of the disclosed information and some ability to think about that information in a rational manner. But individuals must also possess insight into the fact that informed consent represents a choice point: they must be aware that the disclosed information is relevant to the choice in question.

Kapp (1988) presents a system which includes rationality of reasons for the choice as a standard, but significantly he does not include a criterion of reasonableness of the choice. He labels his system a "functional approach" in which the focus is on individual ability. In addition to rationality of reasons, the following standards are cited as requirements: the ability to make and communicate a choice, the ability to reason about the choice, and understanding of relevant information and appreciation of the relevance of that information for oneself. Kapp's system is noteworthy because, like Appelbaum and Roth's (1982), it adds the dimension of appreciation of the situation.

Appelbaum and Grisso (1995) present an appreciation-dependent definition of competence as well. Understanding, rational manipulation of disclosed information (i.e., reasoning), and appreciation of the relevance of the disclosed information for one's own situation are all required elements. This particular definition will be discussed in greater detail in Section 7.06.5.1, below.

7.06.3.2 Other Considerations for Definitions

As discussed earlier, requiring that the reasons for a choice be rational still allows for objective assessment. Requiring that the *choice* be rational implicitly requires a subjective value judgment on the part of the assessor. Recognition of the interaction of social and legal requirements with definitions of competence represents an improvement in definitional schemes. For some, this interaction requires some means of minimizing the role of socially based values—like rationality—from competence determinations. One way is to use an individual-centered view of competence. An example of such a system is Drane's (1985) recommendation of the use of a sliding scale, in which the threshold for each of the relevant standards is a function of the nature of the situation. This relativistic position is also expressed by Katz, who recommends shared decision making (from Faden & Beauchamp, 1986); Moody's (1988) idea of "negotiated consent" (discussed above) is similarly individual-centered. In these views, an individual may be competent to make decisions at a low level, that is, when the decision does not require truly "autonomous action" (Faden & Beauchamp, 1986). Higher thresholds may be surpassed with assistance. Setting the appropriate threshold, however, involves moral judgments. While some researchers deal with the need for thresholds (e.g., Wang & Ennis, 1986), few acknowledge the dependence on socially determined, subjective standards.

A more complex view of competence is presented by Grisso (1994), in which he addresses the issue of threshold setting and subjectivity explicitly. He discusses four essential components of competence: functional, causal, interactive, and judgmental. The functional component centers around the extent to which an individual can "understand or do that which is relevant." The extent to which an individual fulfills this requirement can be assessed either functionally (in practice) or inferentially (based on clinical assessment). The causal component requires presence of a "causal explanation for any functional deficits." This component is an attempt to include objectivity in the definition. It stimulates exploration of potential causal disorders and it also brings attention to the remediability and relevance of those disorders. For example, if someone's competence is in question because of a diagnosis of Alzheimer's disease, to what extent do the consequences of that disease affect the individual's abilities? To what extent might some relevant consequences be corrected? The interactive component includes consideration of the individual's abilities in relation to the contextual demands on that individual. Grisso's interactive component is most similar to the context-specific competence described by Faden and Beauchamp (1986) and to the domain-specific competence of Sprung and Winick (1989).

Grisso's final component of competence recognizes the close relationship between individual-level and societal-level considerations. The judgmental component depends on societal norms, those criteria that society deems important in determinations of competence. The tension between societal obligations to protect individuals and societal obligations to respect individual autonomy characterize the judgmental component.

Legal and social context influences all competence-related activities. Like Grisso, Kopelman (1990) recognizes the impact of social and legal norms on definitions of competence; she states that competence cannot be defined without reference to those norms. The issue is best expressed by Faden and Beauchamp (1986) in their distinction between two senses of informed consent. To satisfy the first sense, an individual must be psychologically competent, meaning that relevant abilities are possessed. In the second sense, an individual must meet legal criteria (being over the age of majority, for example). The two senses may be assessed separately, but both are required under legal systems in the late 1990s. Their distinction between general and specific components of competence flows from this dichotomy.

Because of the confusion possible when applying general definitions of competence to specific situations, legal definitions are advancing from the general to the specific (Sullivan & Youngner, 1994). Grisso (1994) and Anderer (1990) note the trend in state statutes, and Appelbaum, Lidz, and Meisel (1987) observe that judicial decisions reflect this trend as well. The earlier definitions of competence are general, and thus are inadequate for application to specific situations. Attempts to refine and improve definitions of competence have resulted in attention to the dynamic nature of the abilities in question and their dependence on context for meaning (e.g., Grisso, 1994; Willis, 1996).

Other definitions also make the distinction between general and specific components of competence. Faden and Beauchamp (1986) say that competence is "the ability to perform a task," and this definition is invariant across all domains to which it is applied. This is the general component of the definition. They go on to note that criteria for determination of competence, however, vary by situation, and are therefore context-dependent. The dependence on context is their form of a specific component.

Sprung and Winick (1989) take a dual aspect approach to the definition of competence as well. Similar to Faden and Beauchamp's identification of a specific context-dependent competence, Sprung and Winick identify domain-specific incompetence. (Use of the term competence and incompetence is frequently mixed in most discussion, with incompetence implicitly assumed to represent the inverse of competence. This assumption remains unexamined, however, and arguably incompetence may be defined as something different from simple "noncompetence." For the purposes of this discussion, however, the focus remains on defining competence, and the term incompetence" is used only when the research in question uses that term.) However, Sprung and Winick's view differs from Faden and Beauchamp's in terms of the meaning of the general component. To Faden and Beauchamp, it is a characteristic of the definition which is general, that is, that all definitions of incompetence are similar because of their reliance on an inability. For Sprung and Winick, general incompetence means global inability. Individuals are incompetent in the general sense if they are unconscious or profoundly psychotic, for example. This latter view is more pervasive.

Lidz et al., (1984) make the distinction between two different types of incompetency in the same manner that Sprung and Winick do; general incompetence means global inability, and specific incompetence means inability to make a specific decision.

As Tepper and Elwork (1984) note, "development of an operational definition of any construct is, in part, a subjective endeavor" (p. 219), and as such will defy definitive resolution. Clearly, definitions of competence are evolving, accommodating increasing complexity and acknowledging the interaction between societal standards and individual abilities.

7.06.4 PSYCHOLOGICAL PERSPECTIVES ON COMPETENCE TO MAKE DECISIONS

In this section, psychological views of competence are examined in greater detail. The contributions of two distinct psychological perspectives to the question of competence are reviewed in detail: the forensic psychological view, which originates from legal requirements, and the cognitive psychological view, which originates from the study of human cognitive processes.

Both perspectives share a disciplinary emphasis of psychology, the science of the mind and behavior. The differences in the views will be reviewed further, but one critical distinction must be made before further examination. The forensic psychological perspective is concerned with "research that can lead to the development of improved and empirically based criteria for decision-making with respect to a number of difficult law and mental health issues" (S. Shah, quoted in Voit, 1995, p. 10). Competence questions are framed in terms of what relevant skills the law requires; the law is the springboard for investigation. In contrast, the cognitive psychological perspective is concerned with identification and measurement of cognitive processes such as problem solving, reasoning, memory, and knowledge representation (Craik & Salthouse, 1992; Datan, Rodeheaver, & Hughes, 1987). Most of the 1980s and 1990s definitions of competence reviewed above derive from a forensic psychological perspective. The next subsection expands on the meaning of a forensic psychological view, followed by a brief review of cognitive psychological perspectives on competence. Finally, the contributions of these two psychological views are compared.

7.06.4.1 Forensic Psychological Views of Competence

The forensic psychological view of competence is most often used by individuals with a combination of legal and psychological training. In most cases, these researchers have the express goal of enhancing psychological practice by attending to relevant legal issues and enhancing legal policy through empirical assessment. The forensic psychological view is distinguished from purely legal views by its emphasis on quantification of relevant variables.

One prominent feature of forensic psychological definitions is reliance on the term "decisional capacity" rather than "competence" as a means of improving specificity (Appelbaum & Grisso, 1988; President's Commission for the Study of Ethical Problems in Medicine and Biomedical and Behavioral Research, 1983). As discussed in the preceding review of definitions, a trend towards increased specificity is evident. Similarly, the American Bar Association (1991) notes the evolution in the legal concept of competence, from a global conception to a conception based on functional abilities; the American Bar Association report even recommends use of the specific term "decisional capacity" (instead of the more global term "competence") in legal contexts.

The contribution of forensic psychology to definitions of competence is evident in the review of definitions presented above. For example, the forensic psychological view has advanced definitions from a simple, global level centered around understanding to a more complex, hierarchical set of standards or component abilities. The work of Appelbaum and Grisso (1995), Appelbaum and Roth (1982), Kapp (1988), and Tepper and Elwork (1984) all represent forensic psychological views. All share a sensitivity to the process of mapping legal notions of informed consent to actual situations. One of the main contributions of this work is the foundation it lays for assessment of legally based constructs in clinical situations. The assessment approaches developed within this perspective will be reviewed later in the chapter.

7.06.4.2 Cognitive Psychological Views of Competence

Cognitive psychology has made distinct contributions to the clarification of competence. Several caveats must be noted before reviewing this literature, however. First, "competence" has numerous meanings in cognitive psychology, only some of which relate to the informed consent component of interest here. For example, the subject index of an edited volume in cognitive psychology includes a listing for "competence" but says "see also Self-efficacy" (Lachman & Barrack, 1993). Similarly, in Sternberg and Wagner's (1986) volume *Practical Intelligence*, several different types of competence are referenced in the subject index, including cognitive, social, intellectual, and interpersonal. Applying a cognitive psychology perspective to the examination of competence to provide informed consent therefore requires vigilance regarding the concepts actually being discussed.

The literature on everyday problem solving has some important parallels to the development of the concept of competence to provide informed consent. Although definitions vary slightly, in general, everyday problem solving is defined as intelligence directed at practical problems, distinct from abstract or "academic" intelligence (Sternberg & Wagner 1986). Measures of academic intelligence have been characterized as holding little intrinsic interest for the individual, being disconnected from the individual's daily experience, and often having a single correct answer (Sternberg & Wagner). In contrast, practical intelligence has as a goal "the solution of problems which challenge the well-being, needs, plans, and survival of the individual" (Charlesworth, 1976, quoted in Sternberg & Wagner, p. 52).

Willis and Schaie (1994) list the following five aspects of everyday problem solving: relevant mental abilities and skills; domain-specific knowledge; understanding of personal circumstances and of interpersonal context; attitudes, beliefs, and preferences; and integration of these dimensions. An important feature of this type of problem solving is recursiveness, that is, solutions or decisions may be arrived at in a nonlinear manner (Willis, 1996).

Two of cognitive psychology's everyday problem-solving dimensions are notably absent from forensic conceptualizations, however. Within the forensic framework, the role of attitudes, beliefs, and preferences is not addressed, nor is the potential for recursiveness in the decision process. Arguably, legal requirements necessitate a single response on a single occasion, and the importance of attitudes, beliefs, and preferences to the decision is potentially minimized by this single-time focus: each may change over time, but if a one-time decision is the focus of the law, then at most the law will be concerned with the influence of each on the present decision. A single-time focus also obviates a temporally recursive perspective.

Among the core issues addressed by cognitive psychology are memory and attention, both of which are relevant to a consideration of competence. Not surprisingly, findings from cognitive psychology are immediately applicable to competence concerns. Salthouse (1996) notes that mental screening tests are one method of assessing "cognitive competency, and indirectly the capacity to make responsible decisions" (p. 36). Using the Mini Mental State Examination (MMSE, Folstein et al., 1975) as an example, he notes that comprehension, short-term memory, and the ability to attend and concentrate are among the skills assessed by the MMSE. These skills are the minimum needed for "reasonable decision making," and thus are applicable to views of competence. Salthouse identifies the main similarities between forensic psychology and cognitive psychology views of competence when he discusses competence assessment, which he says "should not only be context-sensitive or situation-specific but should also incorporate evaluations of the individual's comprehension and reasoning relevant to the decision" (p. 13).

Advances in conceptualizations of competence have led to attempts to assess competence empirically, since assessment follows from, and in some cases feeds back to, conceptualization. Assessment of competence is considered next.

7.06.5 ASSESSMENT OF COMPETENCE

Older adults are increasingly confronted with serious health decisions, yet little normative information about the decision-making abilities of older adults exists. The growth of the elderly population in the USA and the widespread availability of life-sustaining technology underscore the need for proper assessment of medical decision-making ability.

Assessment schemes depend on definitions of competence and the standards used to operationalize the concept. Several assessment schemes are examined below, and some of their problems are explored. Table 2 presents an overview of this discussion. As the table demonstrates, all systems reviewed here include at least some aspect of "Understanding." The systems differ in their attention to the other conceptual elements. Mental status is arguably an implied component of most, especially those which address memory and language elements explicitly. The rationality and appreciation elements are discussed for each example.

7.06.5.1 Assessment of Competence to Consent to Treatment

An example of an early competence assessment scheme is that of Stanley et al., (1984). Comprehension figures prominently, as does

Table 2 Conceptual elements addressed in the empirical assessment of competence (organized by type of competence).

	Conceptual Element						
	Mental status	*Understanding*	*Memory*	*Language*	*Reasoning*	*Rationality*	*Appreciation*
Type of competence							
Consent to treatment							
Stanley et al., 1984		X			X	X	
Wang and Ennis, 1986		X	X	X			
Draper and Dawson, 1990		X				X	X
Fitten and Waite, 1990		X			X		
Freedman et al., 1991		X	X	X	X		X
Janofsky et al., 1992		X					
Appelbaum and Grisso, 1995		X	X	X	X		X
Competency to stand trial							
Golding et al., 1984	X	X	X	X			X
Civil competence							
Schwartz and Barone, 1992	X	X	X	X			
Testamentary capacity							
Spar and Garb, 1992	X	X					

"quality of reasoning" indicated by weighing of risks and benefits. Absent from their scheme, however, is attention to the appreciation of the information to the subject's own situation. Another problem is their inclusion of a reasonableness of choice standard.

Wang and Ennis (1986) developed an elaborate "cognitive competency test" which includes subtests designed to assess memory, reading skill, verbal reasoning, and spatial orientation. The test is based on their multidimensional view of cognitive skills required for competence. While their assessment scheme addresses only global competence, they do recommend combining this assessment with a more focused assessment of "mental status." However, little mention is made of matching specific situational demands with specific skill tests.

Draper and Dawson (1990) present an example of another assessment scheme: a flowchart for determination of competency. The main decision nodes occur regarding understanding of illness and treatment alternatives. Of interest is the inclusion of a question about acknowledgement of illness but one problem with this assessment scheme, in addition to extensive reliance on understanding, is the reliance on rationality of choice for competence determination.

Fitten and Waite (1990) assessed understanding of various elements of the disclosure (the condition, the treatment, risks, benefits, and alternatives) and the "quality of patient's or subject's reasoning process" (p. 1718). These authors hint at a distinction between "bureaucratic" disclosure forms and forms geared toward patient understanding, but they do not expand upon the distinction. Prompting (cuing) helped their control group more than their hospitalized group. The hospitalized sample was impaired relative to controls on weighing of alternatives.

Like Wang and Ennis (1986), Freedman, Stuss, and Gordon (1991) identify attention, language, memory, and frontal lobe function as the "cognitive functions underlying competency" and base their suggestions for assessment on these four areas. Once these abilities are established, "then issues related to judgment and awareness must be critically evaluated" (p. 207). The result is a measure of global competence to the exclusion of situation-specific abilities.

A more recent system also relies upon understanding and little else. Janofsky, McCarthy, and Folstein (1992) base their assessment scheme on a quick measure of understanding of a disclosure. Comparison is made between their test instrument, the Hopkins Competency Assessment Tool (HCAT), and a forensic psychiatrist's assessment. Several criticisms have been made of HCAT. While it does assess understanding, other domains relevant to competence are unaddressed. Both Lavin (1992) and Sales (1992) note that reasoning or rational weighing of choices is ignored. Lavin also argues that relatively stable personal values are a required component of competence, one which HCAT does not measure. Englehart (1992) notes the lack of attention to the risk–benefit ratio of the choice in question, and Kaye (1992) notes that prognosis if no treatment is undertaken is not included in the HCAT disclosure vignette. Another problem of their assessment method is the potential for subjective error with their "gold standard" of clinician judgment. Thus, at best HCAT can be considered a measure of understanding only, and not a measure of a more global concept of competence.

Some of the work reviewed above suggests another crucial element to consider when assessing competence: context. Appelbaum, Mirkin, and Bateman (1981) observed that "The stress surrounding any hospitalization, whether psychiatric or medical, may contribute to a failure of rational modes of thought, as may the necessity for making critical decisions from a position of relative ignorance about the medical issues involved" (p. 1175). Empirical evidence supports this claim. According to Fitten and Waite (1990), the context of hospitalization impaired performance in general: in their sample of older adults, 28% of the hospitalized subjects had impaired performance on a vignette decision-making task despite no evidence of cognitive impairment on a standardized mental status exam or via clinical assessment (Fitten and Waite, 1990). Dellasega, Smyer, Frank, and Brown (1996) and Frank (1995) also found evidence of decision-making impairment despite relatively high mental status exam scores among their elderly hospitalized subjects. The specific causes of impairment (e.g. the subject's illness, medical interventions) are unknown, but these studies suggest that hospitalized older adults are one group "most vulnerable to decisional impairments" (Fitten & Waite, 1990).

Consideration of context in competence assessment is also crucial in long-term care settings. Increasingly the nursing home is recognized as a setting in which decisional capacity assessments are often required, and research suggests that three-quarters of nursing home residents exhibit some decisional capacity impairments (Goodwin, Smyer, & Lair,1995). Pruchno, Smyer, Rose, Hartman-Stein, and Henderson-Laribee (1995) discuss methods that are objective, reliable, and easily administered to assess decision-making ability of residents in nursing homes.

Appelbaum and Grisso (1995) have developed three separate instruments for the purposes of assessing competence to provide informed consent, or more specifically, medical treatment decision-making capacity. The Understanding of Treatment Disclosure (UTD) assesses capacity to understand relevant information. The Perception of Disorder (POD) assesses appreciation of relevant information for the individual's own situation. The Thinking Rationally About Treatment (TRAT) assesses the individual's ability to manipulate relevant information rationally. The TRAT represents an expansion of the quality of reasoning standard that is part of Stanley et al.'s (1984) scheme. Stanley and colleagues use comparison of risks and benefits as their indicator of quality of reasoning; the TRAT goes beyond that and includes other abilities as well: consequential thinking, complexity of thinking, and the ability to generate consequences for choices. The TRAT, POD, and UTD instruments provide a consistent method for assessment based on relevant legal criteria, but have not yet been normed for use with older adults.

7.06.5.2 Assessment of Other Types of Competence

Some researchers have recognized the need to match assessment to the specific competence ability under question (Grisso, 1994; Roth et al., 1977). As demonstrated above, the law increasingly recognizes that competence is not a global construct. Instead, competence may vary by content area within an individual. It is possible to find "islands of competent functioning" (Gutheil & Bursztajn, 1986) in an otherwise incompetent individual. Attention to the context of the assessment is therefore desirable.

Civil competence, testamentary capacity, and competency to stand trial are all distinct concepts from competence to consent to treatment, but important work has been done in assessment of each of these types, and that work is relevant to the discussion here. The assessment of both civil competence and competency to stand trial share elements with several approaches to assessing capacity to consent to treatment. The Community Competence Scale-Revised (CCS-R, Schwartz & Barone, 1992) was developed to assess civil competence, and the Interdisciplinary Fitness Interview (IFI, Golding, Roesch, & Schreiber, 1984) was developed to assess competency to stand trial. Both attempt to tie mental health issues to legal requirements by including assessment of psychological functioning. The CCS-R contains 17 subscales and the IFI contains 16, so while they clearly address global aspects of competence, the high degree of detail offers the potential for quite specific applications. Further, by attending to both psychological and legal issues, they represent an attempt to bridge the divide between Faden and Beauchamp's (1986) two senses of consent and competence.

Spar and Garb (1992) state that to assess competence one must determine global mental status, assess specific aspects of mental functioning relevant to the ability in question, determine implications of those abilities for the specific context, and finally, form a diagnostic impression. Although it was developed for the assessment of testamentary capacity rather than treatment, their assessment fits well with the four components discussed by Grisso (1994): diagnostic impression addresses the causal component, determining abilities relative to context addresses the interactive component, and the functional component is implied in the assessment of mental functioning. Given their goal of presenting assessment consonant with current legal and social systems, the judgmental component is implied.

Several problems exist in most 1990s assessment schemes. First, rarely does assessment address all of the specific domains relevant to competence, that is, causal processes and interactive components as well as functional abilities. Instead, as noted above, many systems are based on assessment of global competence. Individual-centered and contextually sensitive systems are rare. Second, few authors attend to the subjective components of their assessment schemes. As with definitions of competence, some assessment schemes allow societally determined standards of reasonableness or rationality to intrude. Third, criteria for success on an ability are often set casually rather than following formal investigation. The relative weight each ability should be given in an assessment is largely neglected. Fourth, there is a dearth of norms for older populations. Thus, when gauging the functioning of older people, it is difficult to assess their relative standing.

Increasingly, psychological and legal conceptualizations of competence are being tied together. Linking the two increases complexity, but conceptualizations of competence have been improved by this increased attention to the relationship between psychological and legal issues. Rigorous investigation of definitions, standards, and assessment methods will further refine and improve our understanding of competence.

Miller and Cugliari (1990) surveyed long-term care facilities in New York State regarding treatment policies and found that only 12% of responding facilities had written guidelines for the determination of decisional capacity in 1986. By 1988 that number grew to 48%. The content of those policies varied, but of interest is the trend toward increased attention to formalizing the assessment process through guidelines. The question, however, is what should be contained in those guidelines? Additional empirical investigation of the concept of competence is required before that question can be answered.

7.06.6 COMPETENCE IN ACTION: ADVANCE DIRECTIVES

In multiple contexts, from law courts to medical clinics, competence assessment is central to the protection of autonomy and fulfillment of society's obligation to protect individuals. Every day, competence of individuals—especially older adults—is brought into question, but in the early 1990s a new area emerged making decisional competence even more prominent. Because of advances in life-sustaining technology, and because of the increased cost of these technologies, social and governmental forces recognized the need for increased attention to decision making about life-sustaining technologies. Particular attention was focused on decision making in the event that an individual becomes incompetent, increasing concern for the proper assessment of competence. Because of their relevance to decision making by older adults, developments in end-of-life decision making are reviewed below. The Patient Self-determination Act (PSDA) is used as an example of a social context in which decision-making concerns are played out.

7.06.6.1 The Patient Self-determination Act

The PSDA became effective in December 1991, and requires that all institutional Medicare and Medicaid participants address the question of advance directives (ADs) with patients (Omnibus Budget Reconciliation Act, 1990). According to regulations published by the Health Care Financing Administrations (Medicare and Medicaid Programs, 1992), all competent individuals have the right to issue ADs. The capacity of an individual to create an AD is explicitly equated with the capacity of that individual to provide informed consent for medical treatments. However, the extent to which the two capacities may differ is unknown. One study directly compared AD and medical treatment decision-making capacity (Frank, 1995). While few quantitative differences emerged, the relationships of variables like cognitive status and verbal ability to the two types of decision making differed, suggesting that the decision types may be distinct. Given the significant consequences of end-of-life decisions, closer empirical attention to differences between capacities is necessary.

The need for instruments to assess decisional capacity is acute and growing (Fitten and Waite, 1990; Stanley, Stanley, Guido & Garvin, 1988; Kapp, 1992). The hospital is the focus of most serious medical interventions and thus hospitalized older adults are often called upon to make serious medical treatment decisions. The PSDA has drawn attention to an often neglected area of treatment decisions, those centered on life-and-death concerns. The mandates of that law (specifically the requirement to address AD issues with newly admitted hospital patients) increase the prominence of the hospital as the site for such life-and-death decisions for patients. Developments in the area of assisted suicide have focused additional attention on end-of-life decisions.

7.06.6.1.1 Knowledge and attitudes of the elderly about ADs

Zweibel and Cassel (1989) report criteria that older adults use in making hypothetical end-of-life treatment decisions. Prominent among them are the desire to avoid being a burden to family, the desire to avoid living with impaired cognitive function, and the desire to avoid pain.

According to self-report data, individual characteristics that most influence preferences regarding life-sustaining treatments of hospitalized elders are personal values, religion, and personal experience with illness (self or others) (Cohen-Mansfield, Droge, & Billig, 1992). Multiple studies have found that most patients want to discuss ADs (Emanuel, Barry, Stoeckle, Ettelson, & Emanuel, 1991; Gamble, McDonald, & Lichstein 1991; Lo, McLeod, & Saika, 1986; Shmerling, Bedell, Lilienfeld, & Delbanco, 1988; Smucker et al., 1993; Wolf et al., 1991).

The validity of an individual's preference regarding life-sustaining treatment is of concern for both ethical and legal reasons. One index of the validity of patients' preferences is the stability of those preferences over time. Several studies indicate high stability over time (cited in Wolf et al., 1991). However, the effect of several specific potential influences on preferences and their stability have been studied in detail, especially depression, prognosis information, and information framing.

(i) Depression

Because of concern about the potential for depression to invalidate decisions to avoid life-sustaining treatment, the relationship of depression to preference stability has been examined. In their examination of 43 older adults admitted to an inpatient psychiatric facility for major depression, Ganzini, Lee, Heintz, Bloom, and Fenn (1994) found an association between treatment for depression and preference for life-sustaining treatment: 26% of the subjects preferred more life-sustaining treatment following treatment for depression. However, these subjects were initially rated as more severely depressed than the rest of the sample. Among individuals with less severe depression, preferences remained relatively stable. In a separate study comparing depressed and nondepressed elderly patients, Lee and Ganzini (1994) found higher variability in stated preference over time among the depressed group. Of interest is their finding that their depressed subjects did not differ from control subjects in actual choices made (in either frequency or kind). A limitation of the Lee and Ganzini study is that it does not examine the extent to which change in preference is related to relevant legal standards for informed consent, like change in level of understanding of the information and/or change in ability to manipulate the information rationally. If the mechanism of action of depression on preferences is through these abilities, then assessment of the abilities, rather than of depression *per se*, is appropriate. The relationship between the abilities and level of depression must therefore be explored.

Additional studies are required to address the role of depression in preference stability, but the influence of depression on decisional capacity itself remains to be explored.

(ii) Prognosis information

As noted by Torian, Davidson, Fillit, Fulop, and Sell (1992), Do-Not-Resuscitate (DNR) orders indicating that in the event of a cardiac arrest, health providers should not attempt to resuscitate the patient, are unique among potential advance directives because of the necessity for quick response in the case of cardiac arrest, leaving no time for a decision change. They found that the majority of frail elderly on an inpatient geriatric medicine unit express a preference to have cardiopulmonary resuscitation (CPR) performed rather than forego it. However, patients in this study were not presented with prognosis information, another potential influence on patient preferences.

In an important experimental study of patient preferences for the DNR type of advance directive, Murphy et al. (1994) report that probability of survival does in fact influence patient preferences for CPR. They questioned ambulatory geriatric patients about desire for DNR orders in three different hypothetical situations: following an accident, in the event of an acute medical illness, and in the event of chronic illness. Over 40% of their sample expressed a desire for CPR to be performed following an accident or acute illness. Only 11% would desire CPR in the event of chronic illness. Next, subjects were asked their preferences for CPR following presentation of probabilities of survival to discharge following CPR for each of the three situations. Presentation of this information reduced by half the number of patients who would request CPR. These authors conclude that once presented with probability of survival information, most patients would choose not to undergo CPR.

Murphy et al. (1994) demonstrated that preference for CPR decreased with age: once the probability of survival was discussed, only a few subjects over age 85 would opt for CPR in any of the three hypothetical situations. Clearly, potential prognosis is a crucial factor to be considered in any advance directive decision, but this study leaves the influence of mode of information presentation unexplored.

(iii) Information framing

Evidence suggests that the manner in which information is presented may exert a strong influence on preference (Mazur & Merz, 1993; Redelmeier, Rozin, & Kahneman, 1993; Tymchuk, Ouslander, Rahbar, & Fitten, 1988). For example, the following two explanations present the same outcome: (i) 90 of 100 patients survive an operation and 34 are alive after five years; (ii) 10 of 100 patients die after surgery, and 66 die by the end of five years. Subjects express a preference for the procedure associated with the first version; the procedure associated with the second version is nonpreferred. Thus subject preference for a medical procedure is dependent upon the way in which outcome statistics are framed (Redelmeier et al., 1993).

Similarly, subjects prefer zero risk to any risk when deciding between two risk reduction dilemmas, regardless of the magnitude of risk reduction for the nonzero choice (reported in Redelmeier et al., 1993). Subjects are also more averse to loss than they are enthusiastic about gains. These effects highlight just some of the ways in which framing of information can influence subject choice. Any exploration of decisional capacity must therefore attend to manner of presentation.

7.06.6.1.2 Practical and ethical aspects of implementation of the PSDA

This subsection uses the PSDA as an example to review some of the concerns relevant to older adults' decision making, including timing of decision, standards for acceptance of decision, assessment of the validity of the decision, and coercion.

As required by the PSDA, patients must be approached at admission with information about ADs. As expressed by Wolf and colleagues (1991), "Implementation may result in drowning patients in written materials on admission, [and] insensitive and ill-timed inquiry into patients' preferences"; therefore "Concern ... persists about whether the time of admission or initial receipt of treatment is an appropriate moment to broach the topic of directives" (p. 1667).

Another potential problem with PSDA implementation relates to standards for acceptance of ADs. Some authors maintain that the strictness of the standard for accepting informed consent should be directly proportional to the seriousness of the consequences of the decision (Drane, 1985).

Drane (1985) strongly supports a contextual definition of competence. He outlines three levels of standards to be used based on the situation at hand. At the lowest level, decisional consequences are minimal, and awareness and assent are all that are required of the individual. With more serious decisions, understanding and expression of a choice based on medical outcomes is required. For the most stringent level, appreciation of the situation and rationality of the decision are required.

Roth et al. (1977) also outline a context-specific standard for competency tests, based on the risk–benefit ratio of treatment and whether the patient is accepting or refusing the treatment in question. The sliding scale notion has an important limitation, however: the degree of seriousness of the decision is determined by the assessor and not by the individual being assessed.

In the course of describing a treatment refusal scenario, Drane (1985) writes: "Objectively, the standard medical treatment is preferable to what she decides" (p.20). The preference is the author's. Elsewhere, he describes a voluntary psychiatric hospitalization scenario, in which the patient's consent to hospitalization is accepted as valid at a low threshold. A "higher degree of competence" will be required, however, if "more dangerous" treatment is required (p. 18). Drane's view is that there are treatments more serious than limiting one's own freedom via hospitalization. This is the author's opinion, but certainly different individuals may have different, but potentially equally valid, ranking systems for "evils" (Culver & Gert, 1982). Fitten and Waite (1990) also acknowledge the problem of assessor perspective, stating that the threshold for competence is influenced by the assessors' view of "normality" (p. 1720).

How should clinicians rate the seriousness of the decisions included in ADs? Should a lower standard of acceptance be applied to DNR orders than to withdrawal of nutrition and hydration requests? Is the "seriousness" hierarchy of medical interventions applicable to end-of-life issues?

Discussion of attitudes of older adults towards advance directives must also include reference to the role of families in medical decision making. Families are usually included in critical decisions by health care professionals as well as by the patient (Watts, 1992). In fact, Ely, Peters, Zweig, Elder, and Schneider (1992) demonstrated that clinicians will defer to the family, even in the presence of an advance directive document. Also, most state laws regarding surrogate decision making set up explicit hierarchies based on family relationship to the patient. The role of the family in decision making by older adults will be addressed further in the next section.

Another concern about PSDA implementation relates to a unique feature of ADs: one may decide not to decide, and instead designate a proxy decision maker. Alexander Capron has written that consent requires disclosure of information because information is "necessary to make meaningful the power to decide" (quoted in Freedman, 1975). The case of proxy designation in advance directives presents a special challenge to this interpretation of informed consent. By specifying another individual to make decisions for them, individuals may be engaging in "valid yet ignorant consent" (Freedman, 1975). In addition, AD decisions may be invalid due to subtle impairments in judgment or reasoning.

A related ethical concern raised by PSDA is the threat of involuntary rationing through coercion (Callahan, 1988; Jecker, 1988). Assessment of the extent to which an older adult's decision about ADs is truly informed and voluntary is therefore an important means of avoiding coercion.

7.06.7 OTHER ISSUES

7.06.7.1 Other Considerations for Decision Making

7.06.7.1.1 The nature of preferences

Any complete consideration of medical decision making requires attention to the nature of preferences and choices. What exactly is a choice? What is the definition of a preference? Available research suggests that static preferences are a myth (Slovic, 1995). Instead, a more useful conceptualization is that of preferences that are constructed "on the spot by an adaptive decision maker" (Slovic, 1995, p. 369). As Slovic notes, "decision making is a highly contingent form of information processing, sensitive to task complexity, time pressure, response mode, framing, reference points, and numerous other contextual factors" (p. 369). Consideration of the role of the family (discussed further below) represents one step towards contextual sensitivity to the decision-making process. Other factors need to be addressed, including the formation of personal values and their relationship to medical decisions and the influence of information from different sources on values and decision outcomes.

"Negotiated consent" has been suggested as a means of supporting patient autonomy (Moody, 1988); a closely related concept is that of "participative decision making" in which patient and clinician share responsibility for each phase of the decision-making process (Ballard-Reisch, 1990). However, if one accepts the premise that individuals actually construct decisions based on a variety of factors, including information framing, information presentation, and method of response elicitation (Slovic, 1995), then negotiated consent does not necessarily bring us closer to the goal of autonomous, valid consent. The ideal of legally valid informed consent requires a full comprehension of the disclosed information by the individual. Negotiated consent puts the individual at risk of making less than legally informed and valid choices based on a variety of factors, including the individual's relationship to others involved in the decision, and the manner in which information is portrayed.

In practice, decisions are not purely rational (Appelbaum, et al. 1987). Explorations of ways to improve the informed consent process must acknowledge the multiple sources of choice construction. As discussed earlier, depression, prognosis information, and information framing are among the factors that might influence decisions. More importantly, the potential for improving the nature of informed consent must be explored. Simple remedial measures should be tested. For example, expanding explanation of alternatives and treatment choices during a disclosure may improve understanding of information (Grisso & Appelbaum, 1995), and may ultimately improve the quality of the choice rendered.

7.06.7.1.2 The role of the family

As noted above, some older adults defer consent to participate until they can consult with a family member (Gueldner & Hanner, 1989) and many studies document the tendency for older adults to rely on family members in medical treatment decision situations (High, 1993; Kapp, 1991; Zweibel & Cassel, 1989). One potential reason for this preference may be related to a general lack of familiarity among older adults with technological advances. Reasons have not been explored in depth, but the ability of older adults to consider the issues involved in end-of-life decisions needs to be measured.

Because of evidence of the preference of some older adults for family involvement, some commentators suggest that society's emphasis on individual autonomy is misplaced in the case of older adults; instead, courts should adopt a "rebuttable presumption in favor of family surrogates" (High, 1991). High argues that by favoring autonomy over family involvement, the current system denies the role of caring concern on the part of the family in decision-making, and it underestimates the role of values shared by the family unit.

Kapp (1989) points out additional problems with an individual autonomy focus for older adults. The current view simply transfers decisional authority from the institution to the patient, with the danger of condoning neglect when older adults do not exercise their autonomy sufficiently. Instead, he argues, autonomy is best blended with beneficence, with "negotiated sharing" the result. In this way the institution's obligations towards the patient are not dismissed in the name of autonomy. Kapp makes the additional point that autonomy "is the capacity for self-determination" and the individual is free to choose to exercise autonomy or not.

Of interest is that many states in the USA have a "family consent" statute in which authority for medical treatment decisions is designated to family members, in a specific order based on relationship to the patients, in the event that the patient becomes unable to make or communicate his or her own choices. The law in most states therefore recognizes the prime role of family in health care decisions for incapacitated individuals.

In practice, evidence suggests that many older adults make decisions in collaboration with others, particularly with family members (Kapp, 1991). Among the reasons why older adults may choose to share decision making is to minimize family burden (Kapp, 1991), and concern among older adults about family burden has been documented (e.g., Zweibel and Cassel, 1989). Thus, assessment approaches require sensitivity to the role of the family for a full understanding of decision making by older adults.

7.06.7.2 Directions for Future Research

Assessment of decisional capacity requires solid theoretical formulations of decisional capacity as well as construction of valid and reliable assessment instruments. In the late 1990s, most of the theoretical formulations about decisional capacity stem from the legal requirements for informed consent. Instrument development requires that theoretical formulations be translated into measurable psychological constructs. This translation has proven difficult, however, given the differences between legal traditions and psychological traditions.

Requirements of legal informed consent stipulate that treatment choices and alternatives be discussed, along with risks and benefits of treatments. The doctrine of informed consent was developed through the legal tradition, in the absence of empirical testing. If certain elements of the informed consent disclosure are more difficult than other elements (in terms of subject understanding), then the legal goal of valid, informed consent may not be being met. If portions of the informed consent disclosure are truly more difficult than other portions for subjects to understand, then remedial measures are indicated. Either the doctrine of informed consent must be reconsidered, or special attention must be given to the communication of certain elements of the disclosure. Rather than relying on a set of criteria for informed consent, perhaps health care professionals should consider a more focused question and ask "informed consent for what?"

For informed consent for research, a sliding scale has been suggested (Levine, 1995). It may be the case that such a sliding scale is appropriate for medical treatment decisions as well. For example, if individuals can understand the symptoms of their disorder and the risks and benefits of a low-risk treatment, they can be considered competent to decide whether to accept or reject that treatment. However, if understanding is intact for symptoms, risks, and benefits, but impaired for other choices or alternatives, then a limited decisional autonomy may be appropriate. The positive effect of corrected feedback on understanding of informed consent information has been documented (Taub, Kline, & Baker, 1981). The extent to which simple feedback could improve performance on these measures should be addressed.

Application of additional measurement methods could enhance understanding of decisional capacity. For example, item response theory and factor analysis could contribute to identification of the distinct latent traits measured by each instrument. The relevance of those traits to legal requirements for competence could then be quantified. These methods could also reduce respondent burden of many instruments. Improved conceptualization and measurement awaits application of advanced methodologies to this area.

In addition to making consent procedures more situation-specific, researchers should aim to make the procedures more subject-specific as well. Identifying specific predictors of performance for groups of subjects (hospitalized adults, cognitively impaired patients, etc.) represents one strategy for matching the subject and the task. Another strategy involves identification of individual-level differences, such as differences in verbal ability or level of depressive symptoms. Quantifying the effects of these differences on the informed consent process could lead to improvements in the match of individual to context.

When considering "older adults" it is necessary to remain aware of heterogeneities within the population. As Murphy et al. (1994) found, adults over the age of 85 were distinct from other older adults in terms of reaction to a CPR scenario (see Section 7.06.6 for a synopsis). Different age groups may have a different constellation of responses to decision-making tasks. Further research is needed to identify the range of responses across a broader age range.

Many studies explore decisional capacity at a single time point. However, a single-time study is inadequate for full characterization of decisional capacity for several reasons. First, many studies document the susceptibility of hospitalized older adults to transient shifts in cognitive functioning (e.g., Francis, Martin, & Kapoor, 1990). Thus the role of time in obtaining informed consent is particularly important for this population. Second, a single-time study provides no information about the developmental nature of the phenomenon under study. Both short-term changes (including those resulting from training or other intervention) and long-term changes should be explored. There may be important differences between an individual's decision making before and after a health crisis; a prospective study could address this question. A longitudinal examination of the same subjects could provide insight into another important aspect of decision-making: the relationship between the stability of patient preferences and the validity of the patient's choices. There is a growing literature on the stability of patient preference over time (e.g., Emanuel et al., 1991; Everhart and Pearlman, 1990), but few studies address both AD decision and medical treatment decision stability.

A body of research exists about adolescent treatment decision making (e.g., Ambuel & Rappaport, 1992; Ginsburg et al., 1995; Lewis, 1987; Mann, Harmoni, & Power, 1989; Scott, Repucci, & Woolard, 1995). Much could be gained theoretically and empirically by linking work on the development of decisional capacity with work on the expression of decisional capacity in later life. Also, some of the questions about the role of age and health status in decision making should be addressed.

The goal of obtaining legally and ethically valid informed consent for treatment is a worthy one, but many commentators agree that practices in the late 1990s fall short of this goal (Culver & Gert, 1982; Mazur, 1988; Rodwin, 1989; Taub, Baker, & Sturr, 1986; Tymchuk & Ouslander, 1990). Improving our understanding of the many issues involved in decision-making by older adults will improve the decision-making process. The aging of our society assures that these issues will have increasing personal and public policy relevance.

7.06.8 REFERENCES

Ambuel, B., & Rappaport, J. (1992). Developmental trends in adolescents' psychological and legal competence to consent to abortion. *Law and Human Behavior, 16*(2), 129–154.

American Bar Association. (1991). *Patient Self-determination Act. State law guide.* Washington DC: ABA Commission on Legal Problems of the Elderly.

Anderer, S. J. (1990). *Determining competency in guardianship proceedings.* Washington, DC: American Bar Association.

Appelbaum, P. S., & Grisso, T. (1988). Assessing patients' capacities to consent to treatment. *New England Journal of Medicine, 319,* 1635–1638.

Appelbaum, P. S., & Grisso, T. (1995). The MacArthur Treatment Competence Study. I. Mental illness and competence to consent to treatment. *Law and Human-Behavior, 19*(2), 105–126.

Appelbaum, P. S., Lidz, C. W., & Meisel, A. (1987). *Informed consent: Legal theory and clinical practice.* New York: Oxford University Press.

Appelbaum, P. S., Mirkin, S. A., & Bateman, A. L. (1981). Empirical assessment of competency to consent to psychiatric hospitalization. *American Journal of Psychiatry, 138*(9), 1170–1176.

Appelbaum, P., & Roth, L. H. (1982). Competency to consent to research. A psychiatric overview. *Archives of General Psychiatry, 39,* 951–958.

Ballard-Reisch, D. S. (1990). A model of participative decision making for physician–patient interaction. *Health Communication, 2*(2), 91–104.

Buehler, D. A. (1990). Informed consent and the elderly. An ethical challenge for critical care nursing. *Critical Care Nursing Clinical of North America, 2(3),* 461–471.

Callahan, J. C. (1988). Acts, omissions, and euthanasia. *Public Affairs Quarterly, 2*(3), 21–36.

Canterbury v. Spence, 464 F.2d 772, (D.C. Cir. 1972).

Cohen E. S. (1996). Resolving ethical dilemmas arising from diminished decision-making capacity of the elderly. In M. Smyer, K. W. Schaie, & M. B. Kapp. (Eds.) *Older adults' decision-making and the law* (pp. 162–174). New York: Springer.

Cohen-Mansfield, J., Droge, J. A., & Billig, N. (1992). Factors influencing hospital patients' preferences in the utilization of life-sustaining treatments. *Gerontologist, 32*(1), 89–95.

Craik, F. I. M., & Salthouse, T. (Eds.) (1992). *The handbook of aging and cognition.* Hillsdale, NJ: Erlbaum.

Culver, C. M. & Gert, B. (1982). *Philosophy in medicine. Conceptual and ethical issues in medicine and psychiatry.* New York: Oxford University Press.

Datan, N., Rodeheaver, D., & Hughes, F. (1987). Adult development and aging. In M. R. Rosenzweig & L. W. Porter (Eds.). *Annual Review of Psychology,* (Vol. 38, pp. 153–80). Palo Alto, CA: Annual Reviews Inc.

Dellasega, C., Smyer, M., Frank, L., & Brown, R. (1996). Decision-making capacity in the acutely ill elderly. In M. Smyer, K. W. Schaie, and M. B. Kapp. (Eds.) *Older adults' decision-making and the law* (pp. 112–161). New York: Springer.

Drane, J. F. (1985). The many faces of competency. *Hastings Center Report, 19*(2),17–21.

Draper, R. J., & Dawson, D. (1990). Competence to consent to treatment: A guide for the psychiatrist. *Canadian Journal of Psychiatry, 35*(4), 285–289.

Ely, J. W., Peters, P. G., Zweig, S., Elder, N., & Schneider, F. D. (1992). The physician's decision to use tube feedings: The role of the family, the living will, and the Cruzan decision. *Journal of the American Geriatrics Society, 40,* 471–475.

Emanuel, L. L., Barry, M. J., Stoeckle, J. D., Ettelson, L. M., & Emanuel, E. J. (1991). Advance directives for medical care—a case for greater use. *New England Journal of Medicine, 324,* 889–95.

Englehart, J. (1992). Assessing competency. (Letter to the editor). *Hospital and Community Psychiatry, 43*(6), 647–648.

Everhart, M. A., & Pearlman, R. A. (1990). Stability of patient preferences regarding life-sustaining treatment. *Chest, 97*(1), 159–164.

Faden, R. R., & Beauchamp, T. L. (1986). *A history and theory of informed consent.* New York: Oxford University Press.

Fitten, L. J., & Waite, M. S. (1990). Impact of medical hospitalization on treatment decision-making capacity in the elderly. *Archives of Internal Medicine, 150,* 1717–1721.

Folstein, M., Folstein, S., & McHugh, P. (1975). Mini Mental State: A practical method for grading the cognitive state of patients for the clinician. *Journal of Psychiatric Research, 12,* 189–198.

Francis, J., Martin, D., & Kapoor, W. (1990). A prospective study of delirium in hospitalized elderly. *Journal of the American Medical Association, 263*(8), 1097–1101.

Frank, L. B. (1995). *Psychological and legal considerations in the assessment of decision-making capacity of hospitalized older adults.* Pennsylvania State University. Dissertation. State College, PA.

Freedman, B. (1975). A moral theory of informed consent. *Hastings Center Report, 5(4)*, 32–39.

Freedman, M., Stuss, D. T. and Gordon, M. (1991). Assessment of competency: the role of neurobehavioral deficits. *Annals of Internal Medicine, 115*(3), 203–208.

Gamble, E. R., McDonald, P. J., & Lichstein, P. R. (1991). Knowledge, attitudes, and behavior of elderly persons regarding living wills. *Archives of Internal Medicine, 151*, 277–280.

Ganzini, L., Lee, M. A., Heintz, R. T., Bloom, J. D., & Fenn, D. S. (1994). The effect of depression treatment on elderly patients' preferences for life-sustaining medical therapy. *American Journal of Psychiatry, 151*(11), 1631–1636.

Ginsburg, K. R., Slap, G. B., Cnaan, A., Forke, C. M., Balsley, C. M., & Rouselle, D. M. (1995). Adolescents' perceptions of factors affecting their decisions to seek health care. *Journal of the American Medical Association, 273*(24), 1913–1918.

Golding, S. L., Roesch, R., & Schreiber, J. (1984). Assessment and conceptualization of competency to stand trial. Preliminary data on the Interdisciplinary Fitness Interview. *Law and Human Behavior, 8*(3/4), 321–334.

Goodwin, P. E., Smyer, M. A., & Lais, T. I. (1995). Decision-making incapacity among nursing home residents: Results from the 1987 NMES survey. *Behavioral Sciences and the Law, 13*, 405–414.

Grisso, T. (1994). Clinical assessments for legal competency of older adults. In M. Storandt & G. P. Vanden Bos (Eds.), *Neuropsychological assessment of dementia and depression in older adults: A clinician's guide* (pp. 119–139). Washington, DC: American Psychological Association.

Grisso, T., & Appelbaum, P. S. (1995). The MacArthur Treatment Competence Study: III. Abilities of patients to consent to psychiatric and medical treatments. *Law and Human Behavior, 19*(2), 149–174.

Gueldner, S. H., & Hanner, M. B. (1989). Methodological issues related to gerontological nursing research. *Nursing Research, 38*(3), 183–185.

Gutheil, T. G., & Bursztajn, H. (1986). Clinicians' guidelines for assessing and presenting subtle forms of patient incompetence in legal settings. *American Journal of Psychiatry, 143*, 1020–1023.

High, D. M. (1991). A new myth about families of older people? *Gerontologist, 31*(5), 611–618.

High, D. M. (1993). Advance directives and the elderly: A study of intervention strategies to increase use. *Gerontologist, 33*(3), 342–349.

Janofsky, J. S., McCarthy, R. J., & Folstein, M. F. (1992). The Hopkins Competency Assessment Test: A brief method for evaluating patients' capacity to give informed consent. *Hospital and Community Psychiatry, 43*(2), 132–136.

Jecker, N. S. (1988). Disenfranchising the elderly from life-extending medical care. *Public Affairs Quarterly, 2*(3), 51–58.

Kapp, M. B. (1988). Decision making by and for nursing home residents: A legal view. *Clinics in Geriatric Medicine, 4*(3), 667–679.

Kapp, M. B. (1989). Medical empowerment of the elderly. *Hastings Center Report, 19*(4), 5–7.

Kapp, M. B. (1991). Health care decision making by the elderly: I get by with a little help from my family. *Gerontologist, 31*(5), 619–623.

Kapp, M. B. (1992). *Geriatrics and the Law. Patient rights and professional responsibilities* (2nd ed.). New York: Springer.

Kaye, N. S. (1992). Assessing competency. (Letter to the editor). *Hospital and Community Psychiatry, 43*(2), 132–136.

Kelman, H. C. (1982). Ethical issues in different social science methods. In T. L. Beauchamp, R. R. Faden, R. J. Wallace, Jr., & L. Walters (Eds.), *Ethical Issues in Social Science Research* (pp. 40–98). Baltimore: Johns Hopkins University Press.

Kopelman, L. M. (1990). On the evaluative nature of competency and capacity judgments. *International Journal of Law and Psychiatry, 13*(4), 309–329.

Lachman, M., & Barrack, O. R. (1993). Planning and control processes across the life span: An overview. *International Journal of Behavioral Development, Special Issue. 16*(2), 129–384.

Lavin, M. (1992). Assessing competency (Letter to the editor). *Hospital and Community Psychiatry, 43*(2), 132–136.

Lee, M., & Ganzini, L. (1994). The effect of recovery from depression on preferences for life-sustaining therapy in older patients. *Journal of Gerontology: Medical Sciences, 49*(1), M15–M21.

Levine, R. J. (1995, January). *Proposed regulations for research involving those institutionalized as mentally infirm: A consideration of their relevance in 1994.* Paper presented at Ethics in Neurobiological Research with Human Subjects, Baltimore.

Lewis, C. C. (1987). Minors' competence to consent to abortion. *American Psychologist, 42*(1), 84–88.

Lidz, C. W., Meisel, A., Zerubavel, E., Carter, M., Sestak, R. M., & Roth, L. H. (1984). *Informed consent. A study of decision making in psychiatry.* New York: Guilford.

Lo, B., McLeod, G. A., & Saika, G. (1986). Patient attitudes to discussing life-sustaining treatment. *Archives of Internal Medicine, 146*(8), 1613–1615.

Mann, L, Harmoni, R., & Power, C. (1989). Adolescent decision making: The development of competence. *Journal of Adolescence, 12*(3), 265–278.

Mazur, D. J. (1988). Why the goals of informed consent are not realized: Treatise on informed consent for the primary care physician. *Journal of General Internal Medicine, 3*, 370–380.

Mazur, D. J., & Merz, J. F. (1993). How the manner of presentation of data influences older patients in determining their treatment preferences. *Journal of the American Geriatrics Society, 41*, 223–228.

Medicare and Medicaid Programs; Advance Directives, 57 Fed. Reg. 8194-01 (1992).

Miles, S. H., & Gomez Carlos, F. (Eds.) (1989). *Protocols for elective use of life-sustaining treatments: A design guide.* New York: Springer.

Miller, T., & Cugliari, A. M. (1990). Withdrawing and withholding treatment: policies in long-term care facilities. *Gerontologist, 30*(4), 462–468.

Mohr v. Williams, 95 Minn. 261, 104 N.W. 12 (1905).

Moody, H. R. (1988). From informed consent to negotiated consent. *Gerontologist, 28*(Supp.), 64–70.

Murphy, D. J., Burrows, D., Santilli, S., Kemp, A. W., Tenner, S., Kreling, B., & Teno, J. (1994). The influence of the probability of survival on patients' preferences regarding cardiopulmonary resuscitation. *New England Journal of Medicine, 330*, 545–549.

Natanson v. Kline, 186 Kan. 393, 350 (1960).

Omnibus Budget Reconciliation Act of 1990, Pub. L. No. 101-508, Sections 4206,4751. (1990).

President's Commission for the Study of Ethical Problems in Medicine and Biomedical and Behavioral Research (1983). *Deciding to forego life-sustaining treatment*, 51–52. Washington, DC: Government Printing Office.

Pruchno, R. A., Smyer, M. A., Rose, M. S., Hartman-Stein, P. E., & Henderson-Laribee, D. L. (1995). Competence of long-term care residents to participate in decisions about their medical care: A brief objective assessment. *The Gerontologist, 35*(5), 622–629.

Redelmeier, D. A., Rozin, P., & Kahneman, D. (1993). Understanding patients' decisions. Cognitive and emotional perspectives. *Journal of the American Medical Association, 270*(1), 72–76.

Rodwin, M. A. (1989). Physicians' conflicts of interest: The limitations of disclosure. *The New England Journal of Medicine, 321*(20), 1405–1408.

Roth, L. H., Meisel, A., & Lidz, C. W. (1977). Tests of competency to consent to treatment. *American Journal of Psychiatry, 134*(3), 279–284.

Sales, G. N. (1992). Assessing competency. (Letter to the editor.) *Hospital and Community Psychiatry, 43*(6), 646.

Salgo v. Leland Stanford Jr. University Board of Trustees, 317 P.2d 170, 181 (1957).

Salthouse, T. (1996). Commentary: A cognitive psychologist's perspective on the assessment of cognitive competency. In M. Smyer, K. W. Schaie, and M. B. Kapp (Eds.), *Older adults' decision making and the law*, (pp. 29–39). New York: Springer.

Schloendorff v Society of New York Hospitals. 211 NY 125, 126, 105, NE 92, 93. (1914).

Schwartz, J. J., & Barone, D. F. (1992). Assessing civil competence in the elderly. *Journal of Forensic Sciences, 37*(3), 938–941.

Scott, E. S., Reppucci, N. D., & Woolard, J. L. (1995). Evaluating adolescent decision making in legal contexts. *Law and Human Behavior, 19*(3), 221–244.

Shmerling, R. H., Bedell, S. E., Lilienfeld, A., & Delbanco, T. L. (1988). Discussing cardiopulmonary resuscitation: A study of elderly outpatients. *Journal of General Internal Medicine, 3*(4), 317–221.

Slovic, P. (1995). The construction of preference. *American Psychologist, 50*(5), 364–371.

Smucker, W. D., Ditto, P. H., Moore, K. A., Druley, J. A., Danks, J. H., & Townsend, A. (1993). Elderly outpatients respond favorably to a physician-initiated advance directive discussion. *Journal of the American Board of Family Practice, 6*(5), 473–482.

Spar, J. E., & Garb, A. S. (1992). Assessing competency to make a will. *American Journal of Psychiatry, 149*(2), 169–174.

Sprung, C. L., & Winick, B. J. (1989). Informed consent in theory and practice: Legal and medical perspectives on the informed consent doctrine and a proposed reconceptualization. *Critical Care Medicine, 17*(12), 1346–1354.

Stanley, B., Guido, J., Stanley, M., and Shortell, D. (1984). The elderly patient and informed consent. Empirical findings. *Journal of the American Medical Association, 252*(10), 1302–1306.

Stanley, B., Stanley, M., Guido, J., and Garvin, L. (1988). The functional competency of elderly at risk. *Gerontologist, 28*(Suppl.), 53–58.

Sternberg, R. J., & Wagner, R. K. (Eds) (1986). *Practical intelligence.* New York: Cambridge University Press.

Sullivan, M. D., & Youngner, S .J. (1994). Depression, competence, and the right to refuse lifesaving medical treatment. *American Journal of Psychiatry, 151*(7), 971–978.

Taub, H. A. (1980). Informed consent, memory and age. *Gerontologist, 20*(6), 686–690.

Taub, H. A., Baker, M. T., & Sturr, J. F. (1986). Informed consent for research. Effects of readability, patient age, and education. *Journal of the American Geriatrics Society, 34*(8), 601–606.

Taub, H. A., Kline, G. E., & Baker, M. T. (1981). The elderly and informed consent: effects of vocabulary level and corrected feedback. *Experimental Aging Research, 7*(2), 137–146.

Tepper, A. M.., & Elwork, A. (1984). Competence to consent to treatment as a psycholegal construct. *Law and Human Behavior, 8*(3/4), 205–223.

Torian, L. V., Davidson E. J., Fillit, H. M., Fulop, G., & Sell, L.L. (1992). Decisions for and against resuscitation in an acute geriatric medicine unit serving the frail elderly. *Archives of Internal Medicine, 152*(3), 561–565.

Tymchuk, A. J., & Ouslander, J. G. (1990). Optimizing the informed consent process with elderly people. *Educational Gerontology 16*, 245–257.

Tymchuk, A. J., Ouslander, J. G., Rahbar, B., & Fitten, J. (1988). Medical decision-making among elderly people in long term care. *Gerontologist, 29*(Suppl.), 59–63.

Voit, E. S. (1995). Developing a research program: Saleem Shah's leadership role at the National Institute of Mental Health. *Law and Human Behavior 19*(1), 5–14.

Wang, P. L., & Ennis, K. E. (1986). Competency assessment in clinical populations: An introduction to the Cognitive Competency Test. In P. Uzzell & Y. Gross (Eds.), *Clinical neuropsychology of intervention* (pp. 119–133). Hingham, MA: Martinus Nijhoff.

Watts, A. T. (1992). The family's will or the living will: Patient self-determination in doubt. *Journal of the American Geriatrics Society, 40*, 533–534.

Willis, S. L. (1996). Assessing everyday competence in the cognitively challenged elderly. In M. Smyer, K. W. Schaie, and M. B. Kapp (Eds.), *Older adults' decision making and the law* (pp. 87–127). New York: Springer.

Willis, S. L., & Schaie, K. W. (1994). Assessing everyday competence in the elderly. In C. B. Fisher & R. M. Lerner (Eds.), *Applied developmental psychology* (pp. 339–372). New York: McGraw Hill.

Wolf, S. M., Boyle, P., Callahan, D., Fins, J. J., Jennings, B., Nelson, J. L., Barondess, J. A., Brock, D. W., Dresser, R., Emanuel, L., Johnson, S., Lantos, J., Mason, D. R., Mezey, M., Orentlicher, D., & Rouse, F. (1991). Special report: sources of concern about the patient self-determination act. *New England Journal of Medicine, 325*, 1666–1671.

Zweibel, N. R., & Cassel, C. K. (1989). Treatment choices at the end of life: a comparison of decisions by older patients and their physician-selected proxies. *Gerontologist, 29*(5), 615–621.

7.07
Neuropsychological Assessment of the Elderly

JOHN R. CRAWFORD and ANNALENA VENNERI
University of Aberdeen, UK

and

RONAN E. O'CARROLL
University of Stirling, UK

7.07.1 THE AIMS OF NEUROPSYCHOLOGICAL ASSESSMENT

In the early days of clinical neuropsychology, most neuropsychological assessment was aimed at answering questions concerning differential diagnosis and lesion location. With the rapid advances in brain imaging technology the importance of this aim has diminished; the focus of assessment has moved to identifying the cognitive and behavioral consequences of cerebral dysfunction whether this be for rehabilitative or medico-legal purposes. However, the neuropsychologist continues to play a valuable role in these former areas, most notably in the diagnosis of dementing illnesses. In addition, although most neuropsychologists work in acute neurological/neurosurgical services or rehabilitation settings, most also take direct referrals from general medical and psychiatric services. As a result of this they are often the first to establish evidence for the presence of a neurological disorder.

Medico-legal assessments constitute a significant part of many neuropsychologists' workloads. Areas of particular relevance to the elderly in which a neuropsychological opinion is sought include issues of guardianship (e.g., is a client competent enough to manage their own financial affairs?) and fitness to hold a driving license. Other areas include personal injury litigation, fitness to plead in criminal cases (i.e., could a client with known or suspected neuropsychological deficits follow a legal argument against her/him and have an appreciation of its import), and evaluation of pleas of diminished responsibility (i.e., did pre-existing neuropsychological deficits impair a client's responsibility for her/his actions?).

In broad terms, neuropsychological assessment is aimed at answering the following questions:

(i) Which components of the cognitive system are dysfunctional, how severe is this dysfunction, and also, just as importantly, which components have been spared?

(ii) To what extent has there been change in mood, comportment, and personality; to what extent are these likely to be a direct effect of neurological damage as opposed to a psychological reaction to any injury or illness?

(iii) What are the implications of any changes in cognition, mood, and comportment for a client's every day functioning now and in the foreseeable future?

(iv) Based on the pattern of cognitive strengths and weaknesses and changes in mood and comportment, what practical advice can be given regarding the design of any formal rehabilitation and what advice can be given to the client and significant others to help them adjust to any deficits?

These questions are answered by integrating information gained from the medical notes, an interview with the client (and whenever possible a relative or close acquaintance), and the qualitative and quantitative findings from formal neuropsychological testing.

7.07.2 SOME SPECIFIC CONSIDERATIONS IN NEUROPSYCHOLOGICAL ASSESSMENT OF THE ELDERLY

There is a strong relationship between sensory deficits and cognitive function in elderly populations. For example, Lindenberger and Baltes (1994) conducted structural equation modeling of the relationship between age, cognitive test performance, and sensory functioning in an elderly sample (age range 70–103) and found that visual and auditory acuity accounted for 49% of the total and 93% of the age-related variance in cognitive performance. They evaluated a number of causal hypotheses to explain this relationship and concluded that it arose because both cognitive performance and acuity were indicators of the underlying physiological integrity of the aging brain. However, an additional possibility not considered by Lindenberger and Baltes is that sensory deficits impose an additional central processing load, resulting in poorer performance on cognitive tasks. Consistent with this possibility, Rabbit (1990) has reported that elderly subjects with 35–50 db hearing loss could repeat aloud flawlessly words read out to them but showed poor recall relative to age and IQ-matched controls with good hearing. In contrast, they had no such problem when the words were presented visually. This effect can be modeled in young subjects with good hearing when they have to process words heard through white noise. Rabbitt (1968) found that, under these conditions, the words were repeated successfully but recall was poor. It would appear, then, that the extra effort expended on making out the material places demands on processing resources which would otherwise be free for rehearsal or elaborative encoding, etc. This has far-reaching implications for the interpretation of neuropsychological test results in the elderly as evidence that clients are able to successfully to make out the stimulus materials does not rule out the possibility that their sensory deficits, rather than a higher level problem, has impaired their performance.

The presence of sensory loss should also be borne in mind when attempting to evaluate if there is dispositional change resulting from a central organic process. For example, hearing loss can lead to withdrawal from previous social activities because of frustration and the impatience of others.

Test fatigue can be an issue with the elderly and requires avoiding long test sessions. The neuropsychologist should also be sensitive to the possibility of effects arising from the order of test administration when examining test profiles. Clinicians experienced in working with individuals with dementia, particularly those in the early stages, will also be aware of their ability to "lift their game" for short periods sometimes to the frustration of their relatives who have sought an appointment because of concerns over cognitive deterioration.

As the result of more elderly people taking an increased interest in their health and the risks associated with aging, the neuropsychologist can play an important role in establishing objective evidence of adequate performance, thereby providing reassurance to clients.

Prior to 1990, there was a lack of adequate normative data on neuropsychological tests for the elderly. However, as governments have digested the implications of the change in the age structure of their populations, resources have been allocated to large-scale studies such as the Australian Longitudinal Study of Ageing (e.g., Bryan, Luszcz, & Crawford, 1997), the Cambridge Ageing Project (see Huppert, 1994), the Mayo Older Americans Normative Study (e.g., Ivnik et al., 1992), and the Canadian Study of Health and Aging (e.g., Tuokko & Woodward, 1996) among others. As a result, it will soon be possible to have better norms for the elderly than for other age groups.

The conventional approach to norming of tests is to obtain a sample which has been screened carefully to exclude potential participants with any medical conditions which may have a detrimental effect on cognitive performance. The case for an alternative approach has been well made by Huppert and colleagues. For example, Huppert (1994) has argued that "Rather than excluding individuals with risk factors which might affect performance, normalisation samples should be based on unselected population samples and the effects of these risk factors should be examined" (pp. 315–316). These two approaches are best seen as complimentary rather than competitors. Comparison of an individual's performance with conventional norms, or norms based on regression scores derived from demographic variables (i.e., age, education, current or former occupation, etc.), can address the issue of whether there is evidence of acquired impairment in a particular functional domain. The latter approach, presumably using multiple regression equations, can then potentially inform the clinician as to whether such impairment is likely to be unusual for someone with this particular combination of factors in their medical history. It should be noted, however, that this latter approach would be complex and would require very large samples.

7.07.3 THE NEUROPSYCHOLOGICAL INTERVIEW

Conducting a neuropsychological interview demands considerable empathy, tact, and intellectual effort. In many cases, the client will have multiple cognitive and physical disabilities and organically induced changes in mood and personality; they will also be attempting to cope with the often massive interpersonal and economic upheaval arising from their illness or injury. Added to this is the fact that a neuropsychological assessment can be anxiety provoking because of potential threats to self-esteem or because of its medico-legal ramifications; accordingly some clients can exhibit more concern at the prospect of such an assessment than over the lengthy and sometimes painful and bewildering physical investigations they may have to undergo.

As in all clinical interviewing, time must be spent establishing rapport and clarifying the nature and purpose of the investigation. General, open-ended, and nonthreatening questions should be employed, followed by a request for the client to describe any problems they have been experiencing in their everyday life. The client's description of these everyday problems constitutes a principal source for the generation and refinement of clinical hypotheses which will be tested in the course of the examination. Such descriptions and follow-up questions are also crucial in establishing the degree of insight the client has into the nature and severity of their deficits. Lack of insight is a major barrier to effective intervention and a client's successful adjustment. A client may exhibit a cheery disregard in the face of severe deficits coupled with grossly unrealistic expectations concerning a return to a former occupation or lifestyle; in other cases there may be a disproportionate concern with a relatively minor cognitive or physical problem when other deficits have much more serious implications.

Often, the most useful clinical information from the interview is gained by asking clients about their short-, medium-, and long-term goals and how they intend to achieve them. Answers to such questions are relevant to assessing drive, mood, planning ability, and level of insight. Inquiries about how they spend a typical day can also be employed to address these issues which have implications for the approach that should be adopted in any rehabilitation/remediation attempts. As Brooks (1989) states in this latter context, "the examiner is attempting to estimate whether the patient is a passive receptor of disability or an active fighter struggling to achieve a better outcome" (p. 66).

The neuropsychologist has a large agenda to cover in the interview and often will be under time pressure; this necessitates a structured, systematic inquiry. However, most formal neuropsychological tests also provide a structure for the client; the examiner sets out the concrete aims and rules, and largely controls the pace and order of the items administered (see the section on assessment of executive deficits for further discussion and exceptions to this). It is, therefore, important that enough of the interview is minimally structured to determine the extent to which the client initiates and organizes the discussion of topics.

A detailed educational history is important in building a picture of a client's premorbid abilities. The history should include years of schooling (with a check on whether any of these were repeat years), the nature of any tertiary education and any further study (evening classes, day release, etc.), and formal qualifications and grades achieved. The possibility that health, economic, social, or attitudinal factors may have prevented a client achieving their full educational and occupational potential should be carefully explored.

The client should be asked to describe the nature of their previous and/or current occupation with a detailed breakdown of the duties and functions performed. The nature of their work and responsibilities provides additional clues to general premorbid level of functioning but also an indication of specific premorbid cognitive skills that are likely to have been strongly developed/highly practiced. The clinician should inquire if there have been any recent changes in living circumstances, and if relevant, the work environment (i.e., introduction of new technology, reorganization of duties) as such changes can often be the catalyst which exposes problems in an individual who had previously been coping despite diminished cognitive resources.

Lezak (1995) sets out a number of fundamental questions which must be addressed prior to formal testing; these include: does the client understand the reason for referral and do they have specific questions of their own they want answered? Do they understand the uses to which the information gained from the examination may be put and who will and will not have access to it? (of particular importance in medico-legal contexts); do they know how and when feedback will be provided? Finally, do they appreciate that the assessment will largely be concerned with cognitive functioning (misperceptions abound) and are they aware of the general nature of the tests to be employed? In individuals with severe deficits the answers to these questions cannot be fully in the affirmative and it is therefore important that their relatives or guardians are briefed.

7.07.4 BASIC PSYCHOMETRIC ISSUES

7.07.4.1 The Rationale of Deficit Measurement in Clinical Practice

Attempting to detect and quantify cognitive deficits in the individual case is problematic because of the wide variability in cognitive abilities within the general population. Scores on neuropsychological measures which are average or even above average can still represent a significant impairment for an individual of high premorbid ability (and have serious implications for return to a previous lifestyle or occupation). Similarly, test scores which fall well below the mean do not necessarily reflect an acquired impairment for an individual whose premorbid resources were modest. Because of this, normative comparison standards are of limited utility in neuropsychological assessment and must be supplemented by individual comparison standards when assessing acquired deficits (Crawford, 1992; Lezak, 1983; Walsh, 1991). Ideally, this individual comparison standard can be obtained from psychological test scores obtained in the premorbid period. However, this is rarely a viable option; the amount of routine psychological testing conducted varies greatly between countries so that many individuals may have had no prior formal testing. Even where such test results exist they are often difficult or impossible to obtain, the content of the tests may have limited relevance, or they may have been administered so long ago that they are of questionable value. Because of these difficulties clinicians normally have to settle for an individual comparison standard which is based on a client's current performance. The explicit rationale here is that (i) cognitive ability measures are almost invariably positively correlated, therefore performance on one measure allows some level of prediction of performance on another, and (ii) some abilities will be preserved, or relatively so, following most neurological injuries or illnesses. Thus, the areas in which a client has performed best are used as the standards (i.e., estimates of premorbid ability) against which to compare performance on other measures. Large discrepancies between measures are taken as indicators of the presence and severity of acquired impairment (Lezak, 1991).

7.07.4.2 Converting Scores to a Common Measurement Scale

In constructing a neuropsychological profile of a client's strengths and weaknesses, most clinicians use instruments drawn from diverse sources. These instruments will differ from each other in the measurement scale used to express test scores; for some instruments no formal scaling will have been developed so that clinicians will be working from the means and standard deviations (SDs) of the raw score from normative samples. The process of assimilating the information from these tests is eased greatly if the scores are all converted to a common scale of measurement.

Converting all scores to percentiles has the important advantage that percentiles are comprehended easily by other health workers. However, because such a conversion involves an area transformation (i.e., the difference between a percentile score of 10 and 20 does not reflect the same underlying raw score difference as that between 40 and 50), they are not ideally suited to the rapid and accurate assimilation of information from a client's profile; percentiles are also inappropriate for use with many inferential statistical methods. Z scores do not suffer from these problems but have the disadvantage of including negative values and decimal places which can cause problems in communication.

One option is to convert all scores to have a mean of 100 and SD of 15 (McKinlay, 1992) as tests commonly forming a part of the neuropsychologist's armamentarium are already expressed on this scale, that is, IQs and factor score indices on the Wechsler Adult Intelligence Scale-Revised (WAIS-R; Wechsler, 1981), memory indices from the Wechsler Memory Scale-Revised (WMS-R; Wechsler, 1987), and estimates of general premorbid ability such as the National Adult Reading Test (NART; Nelson & Willison, 1991). The most common alternative is to use *T* scores (mean 50; SD = 10); the meaning of such scores are easy to communicate and are free of the conceptual baggage associated with deviation IQs.

Regardless of which method is used, the clinician must be constantly aware that the validity of any inferences regarding relative strengths and weaknesses is heavily dependent on the degree of equivalence of the normative samples for the test results compared. Although the quality of normative data for neuropsychological tests has improved markedly since the 1980s, there are still tests used in practice which are standardized on small samples of convenience, the representativeness of which are largely unknown. Thus, discrepancies in an individual's profile may in some cases be more a reflection of differences between normative samples than differences in the individual's relative level of functioning in the domains covered by the tests.

7.07.4.3 Reliability

Adequate reliability is a fundamental requirement for any instrument used in neuropsychology regardless of purpose (Franzen, 1989). However, when the concern is with assessing the cognitive status of an individual its importance is magnified, particularly as the demands of clinical practice are such that decisions, must be commonly made based on information from single administrations of each instrument.

Information on test reliability is used to quantify the degree of confidence that can be placed in test scores, for example, when comparing an individual's scores with appropriate normative data or assessing whether discrepancies between scores on different tests represent genuine differences in the functioning of the underlying components of the cognitive system as opposed to simply reflecting measurement error in the tests employed. In the latter case, that is, where evidence for a differential deficit is being evaluated, it is important to consider the extent to which the tests are matched for reliability; an apparent deficit in function A with relative sparing of function B may simply reflect the fact that the measure of function B is less reliable. This point was well made in a classic paper by Chapman and Chapman (1973) in which the performance of a schizophrenic sample on two parallel reasoning tests was examined. By manipulating the number of test items the schizophrenic sample was made to appear to have a large differential deficit on one or other of the tests.

Particular care should be taken in comparing test scores when one of the measures is not a simple score but a difference or ratio score. Such scores are used quite commonly in neuropsychological assessment; for example, in the assessment of implicit memory functioning a priming score may be derived from the difference between completion of word fragments (e.g., c–pe– / carpet) from a list that has been primed in an earlier study phase and an unprimed list (performance on the unprimed list essentially controls for individual differences in verbal ability). This priming score will have poor reliability because the measurement error associated with the two lists is additive. For example, if both lists had reliabilities of 0.75 and an intercorrelation of 0.6, the formula for the reliability of a difference score (e.g., see Crocker & Algina, 1986) reveals that the reliability of this priming score would be only 0.37. This compares unfavorably with the reliability of most explicit memory tests and raises the danger that the clinician may conclude that an individual has impaired explicit memory coupled with preserved implicit memory when the pattern may simply be an artifact of differences in reliability.

7.07.4.4 Reliable vs. Abnormal Differences

The distinction between the reliability and the abnormality of differences between test scores is an important one in clinical neuropsychology. A difference between scores normally would be considered reliable if it exceeded the 95% confidence interval for the difference, that is, a difference of this magnitude is unlikely to have arisen from measurement error in the instruments. Establishing if a difference is reliable is only the first step in neuropsychological profile analysis. There is considerable intraindividual variability in cognitive abilities in the general elderly population such that reliable (i.e., statistically significant) differences between tests of these different abilities are common. In evaluating the probability that a discrepancy reflects acquired impairment, it is important to consider the abnormality or rarity of the difference, that is, what percentage of the general (i.e., unimpaired) elderly population would be expected to exhibit a difference of this magnitude?

Base rate data, which permits the clinician to assess the abnormality of test score discrepancies, is available for some neuropsychological measures. When such data are not available, a simple formula can be used to estimate the abnormality of any discrepancy from the correlation between the two tests of interest (see Payne & Jones, 1957). It is also possible to assess the abnormality of the discrepancy between a single test and a client's mean scores on a series of measures (Silverstein, 1984).

To highlight the distinction between the reliability and abnormality of a difference take the example of a discrepancy between the General Memory and Attention/Concentration indices of the WMS-R. A discrepancy of 17 points would be necessary for a reliable difference ($p < 0.05$). Based on the average correlation between these two indices in the WMS-R standardization sample ($r = 0.51$), approximately 25% of the general population would be expected to exhibit a discrepancy of this magnitude; to be abnormal (operationally defined for the present purpose as discrepancy which would occur in less than 5% of the general population), a 29-point discrepancy would be required.

The importance of evaluating the abnormality of discrepancies through base rate data or correlational techniques cannot be overstressed. Most clinical neuropsychologists have not had the opportunity to administer neuropsychological measures to significant numbers of individuals drawn from the general elderly population. It is possible, therefore, to form a distorted impression of the degree of intrasubject variability found in unimpaired individuals. The impression is that the degree of normal variability may be underestimated leading to a danger of overinterference when working with clinical populations. For example, Matarazzo, Daniel, Prifitera, and Herman (1988) have reported that in the WAIS-R standardization sample, a sample presumed to be free of neurological or psychiatric disorder, the mean difference between an individual's highest and lowest WAIS-R subtest score was 6.7. For this difference (i.e., the subtest range to be abnormal it would have to exceed 11 Scaled score points. As subtests have an SD of 3, it can be seen that a subtest range of around 3 SDs is not unusual in individuals without acquired impairments. These considerations are just as relevant when profile analysis is carried out with more specific neuropsychological instruments. The WMS-R and WAIS-R are used here as examples simply because of the availability and quality of the relevant data.

7.07.4.5 Monitoring Change

There are many situations in which the neuropsychologist needs to measure potential changes in cognitive functioning in the elderly. Common examples would be to determine whether cognitive decline is occurring in an individual in whom a degenerative neurological process is suspected, or to determine the extent of recovery of function following a stroke or traumatic brain injury. In both these cases, neuropsychological assessment will provide useful information to assist clients, relatives, and other health professionals to plan for the future. Monitoring the cognitive effects of surgical, pharmacological, or cognitive interventions in the individual case is also an important role for the neuropsychologist. Although the aim here is most commonly to determine if there has been any improvement, the possibility of detrimental effects can also be an issue. For example, many drugs can potentially impair cognitive functioning, particularly in the elderly. Anticholinergic agents provide a good example as they are widely used in the treatment of various conditions and yet can have serious negative effects on cognition, particularly memory (Crawford, Besson, & Ebmeier, 1990).

In assessing the effectiveness of a rehabilitation effort it is often possible to obtain multiple repeated measures of an individual's performance before, during, and after intervention. A number of inferential statistical techniques can be used in this situation because there are multiple data points for the different phases (see Barlow & Hersen, 1984 for a general treatment of single-case designs). However, in general clinical practice the neuropsychologist often must come to conclusions about change from only a single retesting. This situation will also arise in rehabilitation settings; although multiple measures may have been obtained on the training task(s), the issue of the generalizability of any improvement is often addressed by comparing single before-and-after scores on related, but separate tests.

Monitoring change on the basis of a single retesting is a formidable task except in cases where the level of change has been dramatic. It is rendered more formidable by the fact that many of the standard instruments used in clinical neuropsychology (e.g., the WMS-R) do not have parallel versions. The clinician must therefore differentiate changes resulting from systematic practice effects and random measurement error from change reflecting genuine improvement or deterioration. Among other complications are the fact that (i) the magnitude of practice effects vary with the nature of the task (e.g., the Performance subtests of the WAIS-R show larger practice effects than their Verbal counterparts), (ii) the length of time that has elapsed between test and retest will influence the magnitude of effects, and (iii) a diminution of practice effects is to be expected in neurological populations given the high prevalence of memory and learning deficits, but the expected diminution is difficult to estimate for individuals.

One approach to dealing with many of these considerable interpretive problems is to gather information from test–retest studies on the relevant neuropsychological tests. Provided that such studies report the test–retest correlations, means, and SDs, regression equations can be constructed to predict performance on retest from scores at initial testing. The predicted scores are then compared with the retest scores actually obtained by the client to assess whether the observed gain or decline significantly exceeds that expected (see Knight & Shelton, 1983; McSweeny, Naugle, Chelune, & Lüders, 1993). The utility of this approach is determined by the extent and nature of retest studies available for a particular test. For example, the test–retest scores on memory tasks for an elderly client with suspected dementia could be compared with estimated retest scores derived from a healthy, elderly sample retested after a similar period to gauge how atypical any decline may be. For some questions test–retest data from a clinical sample may be used. For example, a stroke patient's scores on measures of attention or speed of processing could be compared with estimated retest scores from a stroke sample if the clinician suspects that the extent of recovery is atypical.

7.07.5 APPROACHES TO ASSESSMENT IN CLINICAL NEUROPSYCHOLOGY

Approaches to the assessment process can be characterized as falling on a continuum between what has been referred to as the "fixed, big battery" approach and a flexible, hypothesis-testing approach (Brooks, 1989; Walsh, 1991). In the former, a large comprehensive battery is routinely administered to all clients. This approach is most common in the USA and is exemplified by the Halstead–Reitan battery which consists of a large number of specific neuropsychological measures, for example, tests of tactual performance, sensory extinction, finger tapping, categorization, language functioning, etc., which are often supplemented with a full-length WAIS or WAIS-R and personality inventories (see Reitan, 1986).

In the latter approach, measures are selected to test clinical hypotheses derived from the neuropsychological literature on a client's known or suspected disorder and from information gained from the interview. The process is a dynamic one; the results of preliminary testing are used to test or modify existing hypotheses and generate new ones. As a simple example, screening measures may detect problems with the organization of visual material which are consistent with spatial and/or planning deficits; follow-up measures can then be administered to evaluate these three competing possibilities.

Proponents of the flexible approach acknowledge that there is a potential danger of failing to detect a client's difficulties in some cognitive domains if the clinician focuses too rapidly on testing inappropriate hypotheses (Miller, 1992). However, they argue that the fixed, big battery approach may represent an inefficient use of resources and is simply not an option in some hard-pressed services (Brooks, 1989; Walsh, 1991). Further, because of the time taken to complete an assessment, many of the measures may be administered by psychology assistants rather than fully accredited clinicians. It has been argued that important clinical information may therefore be missed or misinterpreted (Brooks, 1989). In the fixed, battery approach all clients and normative groups are administered the same tests, therefore services employing this approach accumulate substantial data on their measures. Such databases are tremendous clinical assets. However, the very existence of this database, and the resources expended to obtain it, may promote a reluctance to substitute existing tests with newer measures designed to reflect developments in neuropsychological knowledge.

Approaches to assessment can also be characterized by the emphasis placed on qualitative vs. quantitative evidence. The extreme quantitative pole of this dimension is characterized by a strict statistical/actuarial methodology in which comparison of a client's test scores against various cut-offs is the principal focus. At the other extreme, tests are used to reveal qualitative features of a client's behavior, the emphasis being on how a task is approached rather than on any empirical analysis of the test scores obtained. In the service of this end there may be major deviations from standardized test instructions, thus precluding statistical analysis in any case. Although there is no fundamental reason why this dimension should not be orthogonal to the fixed/flexible dimension, in practice they have tended to be correlated. The fixed, battery approach arose from researchers working in the actuarial tradition and the sheer number of measures administered almost demands the employment of actuarial indices to assist in the assimilation of the information obtained.

A strict quantitative methodology could be employed with the flexible hypothesis-testing approach. Indeed, the term hypothesis-testing might be seen as implying this and indeed influential figures in the development of this approach devoted considerable attention to quantification (e.g., Shapiro, 1973). However, many clinical proponents of this approach have tended to emphasize qualitative analysis that is, hypotheses may be expressed and tested in qualitative as well as quantitative terms (Walsh, 1991). It should be stressed that very few clinical neuropsychologists are at the extreme ends of this qualitative/quantitative dimension; qualitative observations are verified with quantitative instruments whenever possible whilst recognizing that much important information is not easily amenable to such verification.

7.07.6 SCREENING TESTS FOR MENTAL STATUS

This section will briefly review screening tests for mental status. All these Scales include questions covering basic orientation for time and place but differ in the extent to which they address other competencies. Among the most common Scales are the Mini Mental State Examination (MMSE; Folstein, Folstein, & McHugh, 1975), the Mattis Dementia Rating Scale (MDRS; Mattis, 1976), and the cognitive section (CAMCOG) of the Cambridge Mental Disorders of the Elderly Examination (CAMDEX; Roth et al., 1986). These instruments produce a global score which summarizes a patient's cognitive competence. They are brief and easy to administer and provide sufficient information for epidemiological studies, or as an index of severity of decline. They cannot be viewed as exhaustive diagnostic instruments.

The MMSE (Folstein et al., 1975) is probably the most frequently used screening Scale and is often used as part of a larger battery for a comprehensive assessment of dementia. It is a very brief and easily administered instrument and takes about 5–10 minutes in total. It tests orientation, information, and visuoconstructive abilities; total scores can range between 0 and 30. In their original study, Folstein et al. reported a high test–retest reliability of 0.83 when retesting was conducted by a different examiner, and 0.89 when the same examiner was used. High test–retest reliability, ranging from 0.8 to 0.95, has been confirmed by later studies (Anthony, Le Resche, Niaz, Van Korff, & Folstein, 1982; Dick et al., 1984). An effect of age on MMSE scores has been reported by several studies (Magni, Binetti, Bianchetti, Rozzini, & Trabucchi, 1996; Pi, Olive, & Esteban, 1994; Tombaugh & McIntyre, 1992). Furthermore, caution is required when interpreting scores obtained from poorly educated individuals. Level of education has been shown consistently to have an effect on MMSE score (Kittner et al., 1986; Kukull et al., 1994; Uhlmann & Larson, 1991).

A useful instrument for the evaluation of the mental status is the Mattis Dementia Rating Scale (MDRS) (Mattis, 1976). This Scale can take about 30–45 minutes to administer, but since items are ordered in descending order of difficulty passes on early items can shorten the time required because of discontinuation rules. The MDRS tests orientation, attention, initiation and perseveration, visuoconstructive abilities, conceptualization, and memory. Split-half reliability for this Scale is high (0.90) (Gardner, Oliver-Munoz, Fisher, & Empting, 1981). Norms are available (Montgomery, 1982); however, according to Spreen and Strauss (1991) the normative sample cannot be considered representative of the elderly population as it contained a disproportionate number of high socioeconomic status (SES), highly educated participants.

As noted, the CAMDEX (Roth et al., 1986) includes a cognitive section (CAMCOG). This Scale contains the items of the MMSE with the addition of some additional coverage of perception, memory, and abstract thinking. A study (Huppert et al., submitted) has examined the psychometric properties of the CAMCOG; the test–retest reliability of the Scale as a whole was very high (0.86), as was its internal consistency (coefficients ranged from 0.82 to 0.89). A study carried out in a group of 222 elderly people reported that CAMCOG scores are affected by age, sociocultural factors, and hearing and visual deficits (Blessed, Black, Butler, & Kay, 1991). The cognitive subScale of the Alzheimer's Disease Assessment Scale (Rosen, Mohs, & Davis, 1984) is used increasingly widely in clinical trials in DAT because of its proven sensitivity to the effects of cholinesterase inhibitors and other drugs (Schneider, 1996). It takes around an hour to administer and includes tests of word recall, orientation, naming, spoken language and comprehension, and constructional praxis.

7.07.7 MEASURES OF CURRENT INTELLECTUAL ABILITY

7.07.7.1 Use of the WAIS-R With the Elderly

The WAIS-R (Wechsler, 1981) continued to be used widely in neuropsychological assessment of all individuals of all ages. Lezak (1988a), for example, describes the Wechsler as, "the workhorse of neuropsychological assessment" and identifies it as "the single most utilized component of the neuropsychological repertory" (p. 38). A number of points should be made about the use of the WAIS-R with the elderly. First, as will be discussed later, many clinicians base their analysis of WAIS-R performance on a client's subtest profile. It is important that age-graded Scaled scores are used in this process rather than the standard Scaled scores which are not corrected for age (Lezak, 1995). Failure to use these former scores can produce a totally misleading picture of individuals' strengths and weaknesses relative to their peers; (see Crawford, 1992 p. 27). Second, as aging is associated with reduced visual acuity, it is regrettable that the stimulus materials for some of the subtests (most notably Picture Completion and Picture Arrangement) are unnecessarily small and the artwork poor.

The most obvious problem in using the WAIS-R with the elderly is that the original norms only cover those up to age 74 years. For clients over this age two sets of independently collected norms are available (Ivnik et al., 1992; Ryan, Paolo, & Brungardt, 1990). The Mayo norms were established on a sample of 512 healthy individuals from Rochester and surrounding areas in the US and covers up to age 97 years. However, many of the total subject pool were under age 74 years and were used to examine the comparability of the MAYO norms with the existing WAIS-R norms. Thus, the norms for those over age 74 years were based on a subsample of 222. The sample was relatively highly educated and had an under-representation of ethnic minorities. Two features of these norms are potentially appealing. First the norms were established using the method of overlapping midpoint age ranges described by Pauker (1988); this takes maximum advantage of the data available and, because it permits more age bands to be formed, lessens the sometimes substantial apparent improvement in scores that can occur when an individual moves from one age band to the next. As an aside, it is worth noting that, using the existing WAIS-R norms and any spreadsheet package, it is possible to go one step further and derive continuous norms for those aged under 74 years (see Zachary & Gorsuch, 1985). Second, age corrections are carried out at the subtest level rather than when converting the sum of Scaled scores to IQs. This is the same approach used for the Wechsler children's Scales; why it was not adopted for the adult Scales remains a mystery.

Ryan et al's. (1990) norms were established for two age groups, 75–79 ($n=60$) and 80 and above ($n=70$). Although this sample was somewhat smaller than the Mayo sample, it was recruited to be broadly representative of the US elderly population in terms of those demographic variables that were considered to be most pertinent to cognitive tests. Paolo and Ryan (1995) discuss the pros and cons of both samples in detail. They also provided an example subtest profile for a case aged 75 years (i.e., just outside the standard WAIS-R norms) and compared the results obtained by both sets of elderly norms and by scoring the case as if he were 74 years using the original norms. The original and Ryan norms showed much greater evidence of convergence; the Mayo norms indicated significant deficits on some Performance subtests which were not present in the other two profiles. An additional advantage of the Ryan norms is that base rate data on subtest scatter and other aspects of performance are available (e.g., Ryan & Paolo, 1992).

7.07.7.2 Analysis of Subtest Profiles

Analysis of WAIS-R performance can be based on the IQs, the subtests or scores derived from factor analysis. Authorities on the Wechsler have divided opinions on the usefulness of the summary IQs. Matarazzo and Herman (1985), for example, have suggested that the discrepancy between Verbal and Performance IQs is the best validated Wechsler index of cerebral dysfunction, whereas Lezak (1995) is dismissive of its importance. Many clinicians primarily base their interpretation of the WAIS-R on the pattern of strengths and weaknesses in a client's subtest profile (e.g., Lezak 1995; Walsh, 1991). Lezak (1988b), for example, notes that IQs can obscure clinically important strengths and weaknesses and suggests that "although the traditional scoring scheme for the Wechsler exemplifies the IQ problem, these tests also show us a way out of the problem by providing a profile of (subtest) scores" (p. 359).

A starting position in conducting such a profile analysis is to assess whether any observed subtest differences are reliable (i.e., statistically significant) as opposed to simply reflecting measurement error. The only assistance for this process provided in the WAIS-R manual appears in Table 13 (Wechsler, 1981). This table provides the critical values required for significance when comparing any subtest with any other. It is appropriate to use these critical values if and only if the clinician has made an *a priori* decision to examine the difference between only one pair of subtests out of the 55 potential comparisons that could be made. However, in practice, clinicians will want to compare more than one pair; indeed, when the client's history and behavior at interview provide insufficient grounds for forming clinical hypotheses, such comparisons will be *post hoc*. In effect, all possible comparisons are made in this situation even though the clinician will focus attention on the subtest comparisons which yielded the largest discrepancies.

The principal problem with Wechsler's approach is that it does not introduce any correction for the inflation of the Type I error rate that occurs when multiple comparisons are conducted (Crawford, 1992; Silverstein, 1982). Any attempt to overcome this problem inevitably involves striking a balance between controlling the Type I error rate while retaining reasonable power to reject the null hypothesis of no subtest differences. For example, an unsatisfactory solution would be to produce a modified table in which a Bonferroni correction was applied to derive new critical values reflecting the fact that 55 comparisons were involved. Although such an approach would control for inflation of the Type I error rate, it would result in very low power to detect subtest differences, that is, the Type II error rate (i.e., the rate of false negatives) would be unacceptably high.

Knight and Godfrey (1984) and Silverstein (1982) independently suggested a method which achieves a useful compromise between the need to minimize both Type I and Type II errors; instead of potentially comparing all subtests with each other, each subtest is compared with a client's mean subtest score. In the case of a full-length WAIS-R this reduces the number of comparisons to 11 so that, when the Bonferroni correction is applied to maintain the Type I error rate at the specified level, the loss of power to detect subtest differences is much less acute; 11 appears in the denominator rather than 55. Both authors provided a table which recorded the size of discrepancy between each subtest and an individual's mean subtest scores required for varying levels of statistical significance. This approach, when combined with equivalent tables on the abnormality of any subtest differences (see below), provides a rapid and straightforward means of analyzing a client's profile of strengths and weaknesses and therefore provides information which can be integrated usefully with other quantitative and qualitative information available to the clinician.

Crawford (1997) presented a modified table which corrects a minor error common to both of the original tables. Further tables are provided for use with any of nine short-forms of the WAIS-R, including those specifically developed for neuropsychological purposes (e.g., Reynolds, Willson, & Clark, 1983; Walsh, 1991) and those in which the selection of subtests was guided by their suitability for use with the elderly and other groups in which reduced visual acuity can be a problem (e.g., Britton & Savage, 1966; Crawford, Allan, & Jack, 1992a).

If subtest differences are found to be reliable, it is often appropriate to determine if they are also abnormal, that is, to establish how rarely differences of the magnitude observed in an individual's profile occur in the general population (see Section 7.07.4.4). Many healthy individuals have reliable strengths and weaknesses in their subtest, thus reliable differences do not imply the presence of acquired impairment. Silverstein (1984) provided a table to assess the abnormality of subtest differences. As was the case for the reliability of subtest differences, this table is used to compare each subtest with an individual's mean subtest score. Crawford, Allan, McGeorge, and Kelly (1997) adopted the same method to prepare a set of abnormality tables for use with any of the nine WAIS-R short-forms referred to earlier.

The above methods allow clinicians to test hypotheses based on clinical experience or the research literature on a client's known or suspected neurological disorder. However, the methods themselves make no *a priori* assumptions about the nature of an individual's subtest pattern. In contrast, there have also been attempts in the past to identify fixed, specific subtest patterns for differential diagnostic purposes. Most of these attempts naively aimed to identify "organicity" and hence were based on a unitary concept of brain damage which is totally discredited. Not surprisingly, empirical studies of these profiles, such as Wechsler's "Hold–Don't Hold" pattern, have been consistently disappointing (e.g., Christensen & MacKinnon, 1992; Savage, Britton, Bolton, & Hall, 1973).

A more rational and interesting attempt to identify specific subtest patterns was conducted by Fuld (1984). This approach arose from evidence implicating cholinergic dysfunction in the cognitive deficits seen in dementia of the Alzheimer type (DAT) (e.g., Perry et al., 1978; see Crawford et al., 1990 for a review). Fuld (1984) examined Drachman and Leavitt's (1974) data on the effects of scopolamine on the WAIS performance of healthy adults and reported that the age-graded subtest profile could be typified by the formula $A > B$; $B > C$, $C \leqslant D$, $A > D$ where A is the mean of Information and Vocabulary, B of Similarities and Digit Span, C of Digit Symbol and Block Design, and D is Object Assembly. Fuld reported that around a half of patients with DAT exhibited this profile, whereas it was observed in less than 7% of controls and patients with multi-infarct dementia (MID). These results provoked much interest (see Massman & Bigler, 1993 for a review). Subsequent studies have reported rates of occurrence in DAT ranging from a high of 57% (Brinkman & Braun, 1984) to a low of 7% (Logsdon, Teri, Williams, Vitiello, & Prinz, 1989). Most subsequent data on the specificity of the profile indicated that it occurred with low frequency in the healthy elderly and in neurological disorders other than DAT. However, reasonably high rates of occurrence have been reported in depression (16%) and schizophrenia (15%). A particularly disappointing set of results was reported in the previously mentioned study by Logsdon et al. (1989) in which the 7% rate of occurrence in DAT was exactly equivalent to the rates in the healthy elderly and depressed patients. Gfeller & Rankin (1991) have also reported that the profile was exhibited by 12% of cases of multi-infarct dementia, a figure which is little different from the rate found in their DAT sample (15%).

With knowledge on the extent of intraindividual variability in subtest scores (e.g., Matarazzo et al., 1988), it should not be surprising that the profile has low sensitivity for DAT. For example, it would not be uncommon for individuals to have premorbid Block Design or Digit Symbol scores which were well over one SD higher than their average subtest score; similarly, it would not be uncommon for individuals to have Information or Vocabulary scores which were substantially below their average subtest score. Thus, although these sets of subtests may be differentially affected by the onset of DAT, a massive effect would be required to reverse the premorbid pattern; accordingly, these differential effects often would be obscured in the individual case. In conclusion, the Fuld profile has little to recommend its use in clinical practice. However, it is still of some theoretical interest as scopolamine-treated healthy subjects and DAT cases are apparently the only groups studied to date in which the profile is exhibited in their respective means. This provides some support for the cholinergic hypothesis in DAT. However, it should be noted that there has been no attempt to replicate the original report on the effects of scopolamine. It would also be important to demonstrate that the profile has pharmacological specificity, that is, that a similar profile would not be observed following administration of a benzodiazepine or some other centrally active agent.

7.07.7.3 WAIS-R Factor Scores

An alternative to the analysis of both IQs and subtest discrepancies is to examine scores obtained from factor analysis of the WAIS-R (Atkinson, 1991; Canavan, Dunn, & McMillan, 1986; Crawford, Allan, Stephen, Parker, & Besson, 1989a; Kaufman, 1990). Although this suggestion has a long history (Maxwell, 1960), factor scores have not been employed widely in clinical practice or research. Factor analyses of the WAIS and WAIS-R commonly have extracted three factors: a verbal (V) factor on which Information, Vocabulary, Comprehension, and Similarities have high loadings; a perceptual–organization (PO) factor defined by high loadings from Block Design and Object Assembly (other Performance subtests have more modest loadings); and a third factor termed attention/concentration (A/C) or freedom-from-distractibility consisting of Arithmetic, Digit Span, and often Digit Symbol (Crawford et al., 1989a; Leckliter, Matarazzo, & Silverstein; 1986). The arguments in favor of using factor scores when interpreting WAIS-R performance are many and compelling. First, the IQs do not have optimal construct validity, the subtests were allocated to a Verbal and Performance Scale on intuitive grounds. Second, the factor structure of the WAIS-R appears to be very robust in that it is consistently extracted from samples from countries outwith the USA. Most crucially, it emerges when the WAIS-R scores of clinical samples are factor analyzed (e.g., Atkinson, Cyr, Doxey, & Vigna, 1989). Third, the reliabilities of factor scores are much higher than those of the individual subtests from which they are formed. Fourth, although authorities on the Wechsler have laid stress on the analysis of subtest scatter, the WAIS-R could be viewed as primarily providing broad indicators of current functioning against which more specific neuropsychological measures are compared. Again, the superior construct validity of the factorially derived composites suggest they are better suited to provide these broad intraindividual comparison standards than the IQs.

Crawford, Johnson, Mychalkiw, and Moore (in press-a) have examined the clinical utility of IQs, indices of subtest scatter, and factor scores in discriminating between healthy ($n=356$) and head-injured samples ($n=233$). The scatter indices employed were the Profile Variability Index (McLean, Reynolds, & Kaufman, 1990), which simply records the variance of an individual's subtest scores, and The Mahalanobis Distance Index (Burgess, 1991); this latter index factors in the correlation between subtests (therefore, a discrepancy involving a subtest which has a relatively low average correlation with the other subtests is given less weight than a discrepancy involving a subtest with a high correlation). Factor scores were significantly better than both the IQ Scales and the scatter indices at discriminating between healthy and impaired performance; the scatter indices essentially performed at chance levels. The extent to which these findings will generalize to neurological conditions more directly associated with the elderly (e.g., DAT, stroke, etc.) remains to be determined.

The lack of a rapid method of factor scoring the WAIS-R, combined with the absence of data with which to assess the reliability and abnormality of discrepancies between factors, acted as barriers to the effective use of factor scores in clinical practice. Both these limitations have simultaneously been rectified in a very useful paper by Atkinson (1991).

7.07.8 SPECIFIC METHODS FOR THE ESTIMATION OF PREMORBID ABILITY

The National Adult Reading Test (NART) (Nelson & Willison, 1991) is the test most widely used to estimate premorbid ability. The NART is a single word, oral reading test consisting of 50 items. All the words are irregular, that is, they violate grapheme–phoneme correspondence rules (e.g., chord). Because the words are irregular, intelligent guess work should not provide the correct pronunciation, therefore the test taps previous word knowledge; as the test only requires the reading of single words, clients do not have to analyze a complex stimulus and it is argued that the test therefore makes minimal demands on current cognitive capacity (Nelson & O'Connell, 1978). Development of the NART arose from the clinical observation that oral reading is commonly preserved in dementia (whereas reading for meaning is commonly impaired). However, the test is used to estimate premorbid ability in a wide range of conditions.

To qualify for use as a measure of premorbid ability, a test must fulfill three criteria (Crawford; 1992; O'Carroll, 1995). First, as with any psychological test, it must possess adequate reliability. The NART has high split-half reliability/internal consistency, test–retest reliability, and inter-rater reliability (Crawford, 1992). Second, it must have high criterion validity. The NART is normally used to provide an estimate of general premorbid IQ against which current performance on the WAIS-R is compared. Thus, to meet the second requirement, the NART must be capable of predicting a substantial proportion of IQ variance. There has been some confusion in the literature on how to examine this aspect of putative measures of premorbid ability (e.g., Klesges, Wilkening, & Golden, 1981), so it is worth noting that it must necessarily be studied using unimpaired rather than clinical samples. In a clinical sample, NART performance and performance on the criterion (e.g., the WAIS-R) will commonly become dissociated, indeed it is the presence of such a dissociation (i.e., a large discrepancy between estimated premorbid ability and current ability in favor of the former) that is used to infer impairment. In most studies using the WAIS or WAIS-R as the criterion variable the NART predicted well over 50% of IQ variance. For example, in one study the NART predicted 66% of WAIS IQ variance in a sample of 151 healthy subjects (Crawford, 1992).

The final criterion for a putative measure of premorbid ability is that test performance be resistant to neurological or psychiatric disorder. NART performance appears to be largely resistant to the effects of many neurological and psychiatric disorder, for example, depression, acute schizophrenia alcoholic dementia, closed head injury, and Parkinson's disease (Crawford, 1992; O'Caroll, 1995) and compares favorably with previously suggested alternative measures of premorbid ability such as the Vocabulary subtest of the WAIS or WAIS-R (e.g., Crawford et al., 1988). Mixed findings have been found in samples with probable DAT. O'Carroll, Baike, and Whittick (1987) readministered the NART to a sample of dementia cases after one year and found no change in performance despite a significant decline on measures of dementia severity. Crawford et al. (1988) found that the NART performance of DAT cases did not differ significantly from matched controls despite the presence of severe deficits on other cognitive measures and the presence of marked morphological and blood flow abnormalities on brain imaging. Stebbins, Wilson, Gilley, Bernard, and Fox (1988), in contrast, found that NART performance was impaired significantly in DAT cases classified as moderate or severe, although impairment was not in evidence in mild cases. Subsequent studies have continued to produce conflicting results in DAT (e.g., Patterson, Graham, & Hodges, 1994; Sharpe & O'Carroll, 1991) but it is becoming increasingly clear that NART performance can be impaired substantially in many cases of moderate to severe dementia. Any findings of impaired NART performance poses a threat to the validity of this approach. However, the practical implications of impaired performance in cases of severe neurological disorder are not as serious as they may appear; in such cases the presence of deficits is unfortunately only too obvious, thereby largely obviating the need for the NART or a similar instrument to assist in its detection and quantification.

Most research on the NART's ability to estimate premorbid ability has used scores on IQ tests as the criterion variable. Although this is in keeping with the notion of obtaining an estimate of general level of premorbid functioning, the NART also has the potential to provide estimates of premorbid functioning for other WAIS-R indices and for more specific neuropsychological tests. For example, Crawford, Moore, and Cameron (1992c) built a regression equation which can be used to estimate premorbid performance on the FAS verbal fluency test (see Section 7.07.13). Similarly Crawford, Obonsawin, and Allan (in press-b) have provided an equation which uses NART and age to estimate premorbid scores on the Paced Auditory Serial Addition Test (PASAT; Gronwall, 1977).

Schlosser and Ivison (1989) derived a regression equation which incorporated age and NART scores to estimate performance on the Wechsler Memory Scale (WMS). They reported that the discrepancy between current WMS performance and estimated premorbid performance was a highly successful index for the detection and quantification of memory dysfunction in DAT. O'Carroll et al. (1994) extended this work by comparing a group of DAT patients, a group of depressed patients, and a group of healthy controls on the discrepancy between NART-estimated premorbid intellectual ability and current mnemonic ability as assessed using the various indices of the WMS-R. While large mean differences were demonstrated between groups, the degree of overlap between the DAT and depressed group was large, leading them to conclude that none of the NART/WMS-R discrepancy quotients were significantly discriminating between depression and DAT to be useful in clinical practice.

A proposed modification to the NART is the Cambridge Contextual Reading Test (CCRT; Beardsall & Huppert, 1994). As its name suggests, the NART words are embedded in sentences to provide context for the examinee. Baddeley, Emslie, and Nimmo-Smith (1993) proposed another alternative reading test which they termed the Spot The Word Test (STW). STW is a lexical decision task in which the examinee has to identify the legitimate words from a series word/pseudoword pairs (e.g., stamen/floxid). Both of these new tests have considerable potential as alternatives to the NART. However, their use is mainly limited to research applications as regression equations have yet to be developed to provide estimates of premorbid ability for individuals and there is insufficient evidence on their resistance to impairment.

An entirely different approach to the estimation of premorbid ability uses demographic variables (e.g., years of education, occupational classification) as predictors. This has the advantage that the estimates it provides are entirely independent of current level of functioning (care should, however, be taken to assess whether prodromal difficulties could have led to a client's failing to achieve their educational or occupational potential). As evidence of impaired NART performance in various clinical conditions accumulates, the demographic approach may be a useful alternative method in cases where use of the NART would be inappropriate. However, the obvious disadvantage of the demographic approach is its modest criterion validity. Where WAIS or WAIS-R scores have been used as the criterion variable, regression equations based solely on demographic variables account for only 30–54% of the variance (Barona, Reynolds, & Chastain, 1984; Crawford & Allan, 1997; Crawford et al., 1989b; Wilson et al., 1978). This compares unfavorably with the NART and its variants (Crawford, 1992; O'Carroll, 1995).

7.07.9 AGING AND MEMORY

7.07.9.1 Introduction to Aging and Memory

It is a well-established phenomenon that as humans age, memory complaints increase. These subjective complaints are reflected in objective measurements of memory test performance. For example, Davis and Bernstein (1992) examined verbal memory performance, as assessed by the Auditory Verbal Learning Test (AVLT) in a sample of 474 healthy individuals ranging from those in their twenties to those in their eighties; a steady decrease in performance was observed with increasing age in those over 30 years. Free recall performance often appears to be more detrimentally affected by the aging process than recognition, although other memory processes do appear to be sensitive to age effects, for example, priming skill learning and classical conditioning (see Binks, 1989 and Schonfield, 1980 for reviews).

Shimamura (1994) proposed that age-related effects on memory may be associated with regional brain changes, that is, that problems of attention, working memory, word finding, and source memory may be related to aging effects in frontal lobe functioning, whereas problems with new learning may be related to medial temporal lobe dysfunction. Superimposed on these changes, Shimamura (1994) argued that general changes in neuronal efficiency may pervade all neural systems as a consequence of age (e.g., reduced blood flow, inability to prevent damage from oxidation, and poor metabolic uptake). It is proposed that these metabolic changes account for the pervasive finding of cognitive slowing in older individuals. It can be imagined easily how these specific age-related memory effects may act synergistically with nonspecific slowing to result in impaired performance. Evidence has shown that differing brain regions undergo differing degrees of neuronal loss with age. Many areas, such as striate-cortex and parietal cortex, do not lose an appreciable number of neurons during life. However, 15–20% of the neurons in the neo-striatum and frontal cortex are lost between young adulthood and old age (Squire, 1987). Similarly, approximately 5% of hippocampal neurons are lost per decade, so that at the age of 80 years; approximately 20–30% of hippocampal pyramidal cells will have been lost (Squire (1987). It is tempting, therefore, to link the neuronal cell loss in frontal and hippocampal regions to frontal and temporal memory systems which Shimamura (1994) has implicated in the aging process.

7.07.9.2 Age-associated Memory Impairment

Crook et al. (1986) proposed the concept of age-associated memory impairment (AAMI). The following criteria were developed:

(i) at least 50 years of age;

(ii) gradual onset of complaints of memory loss in everyday activities;

(iii) memory test performance one standard deviation below the mean of young adults on standardized tests of recent memory with adequate normative data;

(iv) adequate intellectual function (e.g., Scaled score of at least nine on WAIS-R vocabulary);

(v) absence of dementia (i.e., Mini-Mental Status Examination score of 24 or above); and

(vi) exclusion criteria, delirium, neurological disorder, cerebrovascular pathology, head injury, etc.

However, it is clear that a vast number of elderly people would meet these criteria, particularly the reference to scoring one standard deviation below memory test scores for young adults; indeed by definition over 16% of young adults would meet this criterion. This led to the proposed diagnostic category being severely criticized (e.g., O'Brien & Levy, 1992). Partly as a consequence of this type of criticism, AAMI was not included in the *Diagnostic and Statistical Manual of Mental Disorders* (*4th ed., DSM-IV*) of the American Psychiatric Association. Some skeptics felt that the condition may have been invented in order to legitimize pharmaceutical treatment of this new disorder. However, it is clear that aging is associated with significant impairment of memory functioning and more needs to be known about this naturally occurring phenomenon rather than labeling it as a categorical disorder. Caine (1992) has proposed that instead of the term AAMI, age-related cognitive decline (ARCD) should be discussed and researched and this has been included in *DSM-IV* (code 780.9).

7.07.9.3 Does Memory Functioning in Dementia Represent Accelerated Aging?

In many studies, the finding that memory after a delay is poorer in the elderly than in young subjects has usually been attributed to an acquisition deficit rather than to faster rate of forgetting. For many years, a controversy has raged over whether dementia (particularly of the Alzheimer type) represents accelerated aging effects or whether it represents a quite separate clinical entity (Huppert, 1994). In an important study, Huppert and Kopelman (1989) found that normal aging produces a mild acquisition deficit as well as a significant increase in forgetting rate, and the rapid rate of forgetting in the elderly cannot be attributed simply to differences in the initial level of acquisition. In a comparison of normal aging with dementia, normal aging produced a mild acquisition deficit and a slight increase in the rate of forgetting, whereas dementia superimposes a severe acquisition defect but no further effect on forgetting rate (Huppert & Kopelman, 1989). In their study, Greene, Baddely, and Hodges (1996) employed the Doors and People test (Baddeley, Emslie, & Nimmo-Smith, 1994; see below) in a comparison of early DAT patients vs. elderly controls. They concluded that the episodic memory deficit in DAT is general in nature and primarily reflects impaired learning rather than accelerated forgetting or disrupted retrieval. Thus, memory functioning in dementia appears to be qualitatively different from that observed in "normal" aging.

7.07.9.4 Commonly Used Memory Tests: Implications for use with Elderly Subjects

In the following sections several commonly used clinical memory measures will be outlined briefly and evaluated, with a particular emphasis on the appropriateness of their use with the elderly. For further details, the interested reader is referred to Lezak (1995) and Spreen and Strauss (1991). Unfortunately, pressure of space precludes coverage of all but a few of the most widely used instruments.

7.07.9.4.1 The Auditory Verbal Learning Test

The auditory verbal learning test (AVLT; Rey, 1964) is one of the most widely used word learning tests in clinical research and practice. Five presentations of a 15-word list are given, each followed by attempted recall. This is followed by a second 15-word list (list B), followed by recall of list A, and delayed recall and recognition are also tested. A key feature of the AVLT (and its successor, the California Verbal Learning Test) is that it affords the opportunity to measure rate of learning, as opposed to recall of a single stimulus, or series of stimuli. An equivalent form of AVLT has been provided by Crawford, Stewart, and Moore (1989c). Because of the rather abstract nature of the test, that is, 15 unconnected words and repetition over five trials, this can be a rather stressful measure for an elderly individual of failing cognitive abilities. The initial normative data that was referred to widely was rather limited (Lezak, 1983). However, the situation has improved, with excellent norms for the elderly provided by Geffen, Moar, O'Hanlon, Clark, and Geffen (1990), Ivnik et al. (1992), and Tuokko and Woodward (1996). The normative data on this test has also been reviewed by D'Elia, Boone, and Mitrushimo (1995). For a detailed review of the AVLT, see Peaker and Stewart (1989).

7.07.9.4.2 The California Verbal Learning Test

In an attempt to expand upon the assessment of learning and retrieval strategies, the California Verbal Learning Test (CVLT) evolved from the AVLT and was developed to provide an instrument "reflecting the multifactorial ways in which examinees learn, or fail to learn, verbal material. The CVLT's assessment of learning strategies, processes, and errors is designed for use in both clinical and research practice" (Delis, Kramer, Kaplan, & Ober, 1987). A variety of memory measures are obtainable from this measure including short- and long-term free recall and recognition, serial learning curves, learning strategy (i.e., semantic vs. serial clustering), etc. The CVLT also has the added advantage of presenting the stimuli in an everyday, relatively nonthreatening manner, that is, learning two shopping lists. The reliability data for the principal measures appear to be adequate although some of the scores which are derived from them have poor reliability. The normative database consists of 273 neurologically intact individuals, 104 males, 169 females, with a mean age of 58.9 (15.4) years. This mean age for controls is considerably higher than that normally employed for psychometric test development. However, the control subjects were recruited from several research projects and the authors state "in order to make the best use of the data while giving due regard to the varying number of cases at each age and sex, smoothed age curves were fitted to the raw data using multiple regression" (Delis et al., 1987, p. 35). This curve-fitting procedure for normative data has been criticized (see Elwood, 1991).

7.07.9.4.3 The Wechsler Memory Scale-Revised

The WMS-R (Wechsler, 1987) is generally considered to be a considerable improvement on its predecessor, the WMS. The WMS-R includes new subtests such as figural memory, visual paired associates, and visual memory span. As Mayes and Warburg (1990) comment, "the revised WMS therefore appears (potentially) to be considerably more satisfactory in a number of respects than its older brother—particularly in respect of normative data, information of standardization, validity and reliability, scoring criteria (especially logical memory), range of memory functions sampled and provision for clinical interpretation of test rests. This has been achieved at the cost of increased administration time, particularly if the Delayed Recall is tested, abandonment of provision of an equivalent alternate form, and increased cost of the test." For elderly subjects, however, the Delayed Recall Test requires an attempt to reach a criterion on both verbal and visual paired associates. This can lead to repeated experience of failure over six trials which can provoke distress in elderly individuals. In addition, the scoring of the tapping forwards and backwards subtest leads to considerable anxiety on the part of many psychologists as they find it an extremely difficult subtest to score. However, preliminary data on the inter-rater reliability of this subtest appears to be satisfactory (O'Carroll & Badenoch, 1994).

The normative sample consists of 316 subjects in six age groups, selected to be representative of the US population in terms of race, geographic region, education, and IQ. Elwood (1991) points out that the normative sample of 316 "seems hardly adequate for the standardization sample, given the broad age range of its target population. In relative terms, comparison between the WMS-R sample and the 2000 subjects used for the WAIS-R is striking" (p. 185). It is important to note that the WMS-R standardization sample systematically excluded subjects in the age range of 45–54 years using interpolated values in their place.

Given that the WMS-R is one of the most widely used memory tests, it would be expected that the normative sample would be representative of the general population. However, Huppert (1994) has pointed out that examiners were instructed to screen potential examinees for a list of several medical factors which may affect cognitive performance and has suggested that, not only were these criteria poorly specified, they almost certainly excluded a high percentage of normal nondemented older individuals. As she states, "this has serious consequences for the use of these norms in assessing whether or not an individual's memory performance is below that expected for their age. The effect will be to over-estimate the number of elderly people with clinically significant memory impairment" (p. 315). A further brief discussion of this issue can be found in Section 7.07.2.

7.07.9.4.4 The Rivermead Behavioural Memory Test

The Rivermead Behavioural Memory Test (RBMT) was designed specifically to try to detect impairment of everyday memory function by providing test items that resembled activities in everyday life, for example, remembering to deliver a message, remembering to retrieve a personal belonging after an interval, etc. The RBMT has the advantage of having four matched parallel versions, thus allowing for repeated assessment to determine the effects of disease progression and/or clinical intervention. An additional important advantage of the RBMT is the careful work the authors have undertaken in order to ensure the measure's validity. They assessed validity in three ways: (i) by demonstrating a high correlation between the RBMT and other standard memory tests; (ii) by demonstrating a high correlation between RBMT scores and subjective ratings of memory impairment; and (iii) most importantly, by demonstrating a high correlation between RBMT score and observer ratings of memory lapses (Wilson, Cockburn, Baddeley, & Hiorns 1989). Such a rigorous approach to demonstrating the ecological validity of a memory measure is both unusual and welcome.

In general, the RBMT is well tolerated by elderly individuals on account of its "everyday feel" and the fact that it consists of a number of brief, relatively nonthreatening subtests. The initial normative data were provided from 118 subjects aged 16–69 years. However, a supplement to the manual provides details of elderly healthy subject's performance and is, therefore, a welcome addition to the clinical neuropsychologist's armamentarium for the assessment of memory in the elderly adult. Cockburn and Smith (1989) recruited 119 people aged between 70 and 94 years, with a mean age of 80.5 years. In order to provide as random a sample as possible, every fourth name of people born in or before 1917 was taken separately from anyone from the age/sex register of a five-doctor general practice that covered both urban and rural areas. Such a detailed attempt to recruit a truly "normative" elderly sample is welcome. Furthermore, the authors determined that age and general intellectual ability were significant correlates of Rivermead performance. Accordingly, they developed useful tables for determining abnormal memory scores in relation to age and estimated premorbid intellectual level. This additional work renders the RBMT one of the best memory measures for use in an elderly sample. Furthermore, the nonthreatening nature of the stimulus materials makes it more user-friendly for an elderly sample than many of its competitors. A limitation of the RBMT is that it may be rather insensitive to mild impairments of memory. Following on from this, ceiling effects may be encountered in mildly impaired patients, making any positive effects of intervention difficult to demonstrate.

7.07.9.4.5 The Rey Complex Figure Test

This test has been used widely (Rey, 1964), particularly because of the dearth of adequate visuospatial memory tests. A complicated figure is presented and the subject is requested to copy it. The original and copy are then removed and the subject is asked to draw the figure again from memory, after varying delay intervals. As Mayes and Warburg (1990) point out there have been many variants on administration and scoring criteria; and the available norms, particularly for elderly samples, have been rather limited. Spreen and Strauss (1991), however, provide normative data from the age ranges 60–85 years. While this is a welcome addition, the numbers in each respective age band are again limited. For example, in the 70+ age range, the sample size is $n = 10$. This obviously makes clinical interpretation somewhat difficult.

7.07.9.4.6 The Recognition Memory Test

The recognition memory test (RMT) is a widely used instrument, particularly in amnesia research (Warrington, 1984). It consists of two subtests, recognition memory for 50 words and recognition memories for 50 faces. Following presentation of the words and faces, the testee is required to perform an immediate two-choice recognition task and is generally considered to be less stressful and anxiety provoking than many other memory measures. The normative data consists of 310 control in-patients without cerebral disease, aged 18–70 years. As Nelson (1990) points out in a review of the RMT, "This test can only be used with subjects up to the age of 70 because of the unknown effects of normal aging on the test scores past this age."

7.07.9.4.7 The Doors and People Test

The Doors and People Test was devised in order to provide comparable measures of visual and verbal memory that test both recall and recognition, that does not provide floor or ceiling effects and includes both learning and forgetting measures (Baddeley et al., 1994). The test comprises four sections: a doors test, where single doors have to be recognized against three competing distracters; a shapes test, where diagrams have to be reproduced from memory; a names test, which is a verbal recognition test; and finally, the peoples test, where the subject is required to learn an association between a series of photographs and names. Normative data from 238 subjects is provided, in five age bands (16–31, 32–47, 48–63, 64–79, 80–97). In fact, one of the stated aims was that doors and people should "provide an unstressful test that is acceptable to a wide range of subjects, extending from patients suffering from dementia or dense amnesia to healthy young normal subjects" (Baddeley et al., p. 4). However, some elderly, cognitively impaired subjects may find this test quite demanding.

7.07.10 ASSESSING LANGUAGE DYSFUNCTION

In normal aging, deterioration of language has been considered to be either very marginal or a consequence of deterioration of other cognitive functions. Although the majority of elderly people do not develop any gross language disturbance, close scrutiny suggests that some subtle changes are indeed present (Kemper, 1992). In contrast, language deficits are a very pronounced aspect of cognitive deterioration in DAT. Aspects of language may also be disrupted by other forms of cortical and subcortical dementias (e.g., fronto-temporal dementias, Huntington disease, Parkinson's disease, vascular dementia, etc.).

Given the frequency of occurrence of language disorders after degenerative neurological diseases associated with old age, language should be investigated in depth. In the following sections, the most frequent language disturbances encountered either in normal aging or as a consequence of degenerative disorders will be reviewed briefly and suggestions made about appropriate assessment procedures. The examination of language competence should include assessment of verbal expression (naming, vocabulary, discourse and verbal fluency, repetition, prosody), verbal academic skills (reading, writing, spelling), and verbal comprehension (syntax, idioms, and proverb interpretation). As yet there is no comprehensive battery specifically designed for assessing language abilities in the elderly, therefore clinicians often fall back on general aphasia batteries. This can be problematic as the norms for the elderly are limited. In addition there is a need to derive individual comparison standards when assessing language function because of the large degree of variability in premorbid competence (see Section 7.07.4.1). Therefore, examiners should devote time in their initial interview to inquire about factors such as educational level, previous occupation, and reading habits.

7.07.10.1 Naming

Everybody has personal experience of looking for the name of an object, having a very strong feeling of exactly knowing what one wants to say but being unable to recall the correct word. This phenomenon is often referred to as "tip of the tongue." Word finding difficulty is the most common language symptom experienced by healthy people over 60 (Burke, Mackay, Worthley, & Wade, 1991). It is experienced occasionally by young people, but aging seems to exacerbate the problem. The standard task for assessing word finding abilities is confrontation naming, in which subjects are required to name a given object, or more commonly, to name objects depicted in line drawings. One of the most popular tests is the Boston Naming Test (BNT) (Kaplan, Goodglass, & Weintraub, 1983). The original version of this test included 85 items (Kaplan, Goodglass, & Weintraub, 1978); however, the shortened version produced in 1983 is used more frequently. This test consists of 60 line drawings of objects of graded difficulty, ranging from very common objects (e.g., a tree) to less familiar objects such as an abacus. Although the original normative data are scanty, several studies have provided supplementary norms; these studies have been reviewed comprehensively by D'Elia et al. (1995). Data collected from a large sample of 750 older adults (over the age of 55 years) showed that performance on the BNT was influenced by age which accounted for more than 10% of the raw score variance (Ivnik, Malec, Smith, Tangalos, & Petersen, 1996).

A study carried out with patients showed that correlation between the two (long and short) forms of the test and two 42-item forms (obtained by dividing the original test into two nonoverlapping forms) ranged from 0.96 to 0.92 (Huff, Collins, Corkin, & Rosen, 1986). A study (Mitrushina & Satz, 1995) carried out with healthy elderly individuals has reported that repeated testing with the BNT reveals a high stability of scores over time, suggesting a lack of practice effects.

Naming may also be assessed using the Object Naming Test (Newcombe, Oldfield, Ratcliff, & Wingfield, 1971) or the Graded Naming Test (Warrington, 1984). A detailed examination of naming should also include naming of actions (verbs), body parts, and colors. Naming of actions may be tested by means of formal action naming tests (McCarthy & Warrington; 1986; Obler & Albert, 1978). As an alternative, the Boston Diagnostic Aphasia Examination (Goodglass & Kaplan, 1987) provides a comprehensive examination of naming abilities. However, this test is time-consuming and is best suited to highly experienced examiners; furthermore, there is limited normative data for the healthy elderly.

Confrontation naming studies based on the BNT indicate that there is an increase in the variability of scores among apparently healthy individuals in their 60s, thereby suggesting impairment in a subset of this age group (Van Gorp, Satz, Kiersch, & Henry, 1986). There is consistent evidence of a steep decline in the late 70s (Goodglass, 1980; Mitrushina & Satz, 1995). This decline is evident with both low-frequency nouns and verbs but is more marked in the former (Obler, Albert, & Goodglass, 1981). Poor scores on confrontation naming can arise because of a failure to give any response or because of incorrect responses. Increases in the number of errors on confrontation naming tasks were observed in a couple of studies that compared the performance of over 80-year-old subjects with younger subjects (60- and 70-year-olds) (Albert, Heller, & Milberg, 1988; Borod, Goodglass, & Kaplan, 1980). Obler and Albert (1985) analyzed the qualitative features of errors made by the elderly and noted that they tend to be characterized by the use of circumlocutions.

Naming can also be studied using verbal fluency tasks which require the generation of words from semantic or phonemic cues. These tasks are reviewed in Section 7.07.13.2. Two hypotheses have been put forward to explain the naming problems that occur with normal aging. One argues for a degradation in the structure of lexical knowledge, whilst the other argues for an impairment in retrieval mechanisms (see Light, 1992 for a review). Experimental evidence shows that semantic priming effects are virtually identical for young and healthy older adults (Balota & Duchek, 1988; Burke, White, & Diaz, 1987; Monti et al., 1996); further, in naming tasks, performance both of young and old subjects is enhanced more by phonological cues than by semantic cues (Nicholas, Obler, Albert, & Goodglass, 1985). These findings suggest that structural semantic knowledge of words is intact and that a deficit of retrieval or access to this knowledge may be responsible for word-finding difficulties.

The situation is more complicated when trying to understand the severe word-finding difficulties that occur in DAT. Conflicting explanations have been provided for this, and evidence in favor of an access or retrieval deficit (Kempler, 1988; Neils, Brennan, Cole, Boler, & Gerdeman, 1988), or evidence of a structural disruption (Hodges, Patterson, Graham, & Dawson, 1996; Kempler, Andersen, & Henderson, 1995; Nebes, Brady, & Huff, 1989) has been reported. Further, in demented people, failure on confrontation naming could be due to visuoperceptual deficits that result in failure to identify and recognize an object, as suggested either by the fact that performance improves when additional sensory cues are provided (Barker & Lawson, 1968) or by the fact that errors consist of naming objects which are visually rather than semantically related to the target.

7.07.10.2 Vocabulary

As discussed earlier, structural knowledge about words does not change greatly in the normal elderly population, and vocabulary scores do not typically decrease in the normal aged (Salthouse, 1988), rather they may increase, albeit modestly. This evidence supports the notion of a preserved structural knowledge of words in the normal aged population. The most widely used instrument for the assessment of vocabulary ability is the Vocabulary subtest of the WAIS-R (Wechsler, 1981) which consists of 35 items organized in order of increasing difficulty. Performance on this test is greatly influenced by education (Malec, Ivnik, Smith, & Tangalos, 1992) and socio-cultural factors (Huttenlocher, Haight, & Bryk, 1991) rather than age. A test–retest reliability coefficient of 0.71 has been reported in a study of the healthy elderly (Snow, Tierney, Zorzitto, Fisher, & Reid, 1989).

7.07.10.3 Discourse

The assembling of a meaningful and well-structured discourse requires lexical and syntactic competence, including a knowledge of pragmatics (i.e., discourse structure and rules), adequate sequencing skills, including the ability to integrate concepts within and between sentences, and adequate working memory capacity. Material from the clinical interview can be used to assess the quality of discourse and this can be supplemented by asking a patient to describe a standard picture or relate a well-known story (e.g., Little Red Riding Hood). As a standard picture, the Cookie Theft Picture of the Boston Diagnostic Aphasia Examination (Goodglass & Kaplan, 1983) may be used. The examiner should assess whether the production is assembled coherently, if elements are connected and sequenced in the appropriate order, whether an individual makes correct use of reference pronouns, and whether appropriate elements are produced. Performance should also be evaluated in terms of the complexity of sentences, grammar and syntax, and richness of vocabulary.

Aging does not have macroscopic effects on discourse; some subtle deficits, however, may be present in the use of pronouns in discourse, with older subjects using pronouns without specifying their referent in spontaneous speech, a situation that especially involves memory (Pratt, Boyes, Robins, & Manchester, 1989). It has also been reported that deficits on discourse production reflect changes in those macrolinguistic skills that require integration of linguistic and nonlinguistic cognitive processes rather than language-specific cognitive processes (Glosser & Deser, 1992). It was observed that elderly subjects did not differ from young subjects on microlinguistic aspects such as syntactic complexity, lexical production, and use of lexical cohesive ties; however, older individuals failed to refer coherently to the general topic. Discourse production is impaired significantly in patients with DAT, even in the very early stages, and is characterized by incoherence and emptiness of speech; spontaneous speech therefore remains fluent but carries less information (Giles, Patterson, & Hodges, 1996; Ripich & Terrell, 1988).

7.07.10.4 Verbal Comprehension

Comprehension is usually well preserved in healthy elderly individuals, and apparent deficits are often simply a reflection of poor auditory acuity (see Section 7.07.2). The most common test of verbal comprehension is the Token Test (De Renzi & Vignolo, 1962). The original version of this test consists of 62 items but a 36-item short-form (De Renzi & Faglioni, 1978) is more commonly used in clinical practice. The materials consist of tokens which differ in color, shape (squares and circles), and size (large and small). The examinee has to follow verbal instructions which increase in complexity from simple commands (e.g., "Touch a circle," "Touch the red circle") to commands such as "Before touching the yellow circle, pick up the red square." The test authors recommend that scores be adjusted for years of education. Adjusted scores of 25–28 are regarded as indicating mild comprehension problems and 17–27 moderate problems; scores below this are classified as severe or very severe. This test is extremely sensitive to impairment of linguistic processes. De Renzi and Faglioni (1978) reported a true positive classification rate of 93% when assessed against results from an extensive aphasia examination; the true negative rate was 95%.

Test–retest reliability with aphasic patients is very high, ranging from 0.92 to 0.96 (Gallagher, 1979; Orgass, 1976). There are inconsistent reports about the effects of age and education on performance, some suggesting a moderate increase in number of errors with aging (see Lezak, 1995).

Memory and attention play an important role in performance on comprehension tests. For example, working memory load is high on the later items of the Token Test. Therefore, results obtained from measures of attention and memory must be integrated with the results from tests of comprehension when reaching a formulation regarding the nature of an individual's difficulties.

7.07.11 ASSESSING VISUOPERCEPTUAL DYSFUNCTION

Visuoperceptual deficits represent a very common finding in sufferers of degenerative cortical illnesses. A comprehensive evaluation of visuoperceptual abilities should include assessment of color perception, visual recognition, visual organization, and visual interference. A first step in assessing visuoperceptual functions should be to test for the presence of unilateral neglect; this topic is covered in Section 7.07.12.1.

7.07.11.1 Visual Recognition

Evaluation of visual recognition abilities includes assessment of several aspects. It includes, first of all, assessment of perception of angulation. The most widely used test in this case is the Judgment of Line Orientation Test (Benton, Hannay, & Varney, 1975). This test includes 30 pairs of angled lines to be matched with the corresponding lines in a radially arranged 11-line display. An advantage of this test over many clinical tests used to assess visuospatial functioning is that it imposes minimal demands on praxic, mnestic, or executive functions. The norms include correction factors for age and education but are based on only 144 subjects. Age effects on this test have been confirmed by Eslinger and Benton (1983); test–retest reliability over a one-year delay in an elderly sample was modest ($r = 0.59$) (Levin et al., 1991).

The recognition of objects depicted under conventional and unusual views should be examined. Warrington and Taylor's (1973) Unusual Views Test can be used for the latter. Assessment of visual recognition also includes testing of face recognition abilities. For this purpose the Benton Facial Recognition Test (BFRT) (Benton, Hamser, Varney, & Spreen, 1983; Benton & Van Allen, 1968) may be administered. The original version of this test includes 22 items; it is a matching task rather than a true recognition task since it requires matching a front-view photograph of a target face to a matrix of faces photographed either in front-view, three-quarter-view, or under different lighting conditions. Norms are available up to the age of 74 years. Some degree of age-related decline in performance on this test has been observed (Benton, Eslinger, & Damasio, 1981) and the norms have correction factors for age and education. Further evidence of age-associated impairment at several stages of the face recognition process has been reported (Maylor, 1990). It should be noted that prosopagnosics can perform within normal limits on the BFRT. However, they take an inordinate amount of time per trial as their performance is characterized by a piecemeal strategy in which each feature of the target face is compared with each feature of the faces in the matrix (Ellis, 1992).

7.07.11.2 Visual Organization

Making sense out of fragmented, incomplete, or ambiguous figures requires intact visual organization abilities. Those abilities may be tested using tasks such as the Street Completion Test (Street, 1931) or the Hooper Visual Organization Test (HVOT) (Hooper, 1983). The HVOT requires examinees to name 30 fragmented objects. Test–retest reliability in an elderly sample was 0.68 (Levin et al., 1991) and the original norms cover up to age 68 years. Studies which have investigated this task in elderly subjects (55–92 years of age) indicate that performance drops off significantly with age (Farver & Farver, 1982; Montgomery & Costa, 1973; Villardita, Cultrera, Cupone, & Mejia, 1985).

7.07.11.3 Visuoconstructional Ability

Visuoconstructional abilities are usually assessed by means of copying or free drawing. The Rey-Osterreith Complex Figure (Osterreith, 1944) is the most widely used copying test (for further details see Section 7.07.9.4.5). The Block Design subtest of the WAIS-R may be used for assessing two-dimensional constructional abilities.

7.07.11.4 Visual Interference

Visual interference may be evaluated by means of the Hidden Figures Test (Gottschaldt, 1928) which requires a subject to recognize a simpler figure, hidden in a more complex one, by marking its outline. Normative data up to the age of 79 years are provided in Spreen and Strauss (1991). Another useful and well-known task for assessing visual interference is the Overlapping Figure Test (Poppelreuter, 1917). An effect of normal aging on performance on this test has been reported in a recent study (Della Sala, Laiacona, Trivelli, & Spinnler, 1995) in which severely impaired performance was observed in a sample of patients with DAT.

7.07.12 ASSESSMENT OF ATTENTION

7.07.12.1 Unilateral Neglect

Unilateral cerebral lesions (especially right parietal lesions) often results in unilateral neglect. Neglect labels a phenomenon that involves lack of awareness of stimuli appearing on the side contralateral to the cerebral lesion. It is accepted widely that neglect is not a unitary phenomenon and evidence of dissociations across modalities within the same patient and between patients have been reported (Halligan & Robertson, 1992).

Assessment of neglect should explore representational and motor abilities as well as visuospatial abilities. Personal (relating to the subjects body), peripersonal (within arms length), and extrapersonal space should be investigated. A dissociation between personal peripersonal space and extrapersonal space has been illustrated by Halligan and Marshall (1991) who described a case with severe neglect in the former spheres but who nevertheless failed to exhibit neglect for distant experimental stimuli and could aim successfully at areas on a dart board which were to the left of the midline.

The most frequently administered test for assessing visuospatial exploration is the Albert Test (Albert, 1973) which consists of 40 lines drawn out at various angles on a sheet of paper; the subject's task is to cross out all of them. Normal subjects usually perform flawlessly on this test. Neglect may also be assessed using the Bells Test (Gauthier, Dehaut, & Joanette, 1989) that includes 315 silhouettes of common objects, of which 35 are bells; the subject's task is to search for the bells. Normative data (including data from subjects aged 50–89 years) are available for this test, and no more than three bells are usually missed by normal elderly subjects. Test–retest reliability over a two-week period was reported as 0.69.

Line Bisection is also a widely used task for assessing neglect; it requires a subject to divide horizontal lines at the center point. Performance on this task can be highly variable, and it is advisable to acquire data from multiple trials. Patients with right hemisphere lesions show a right-deviation error of the bisection point, that increases as a function of the length of the line (Halligan & Marshall, 1989).

Representational neglect, that involves mental imagery, may be assessed by asking a patient to describe a well-known scene from a particular perspective. A patient may fail to recall objects on the left but recall the same objects when asked to imagine the scene from the opposite perspective (Bisiach & Luzzatti, 1978).

A comprehensive battery for testing visual neglect has been assembled by Wilson, Cockburn, and Halligan (1987). This battery is called the Behavioural Inattention Test (BIT) and includes conventional tests (star cancellation, letter cancellation, figure copying, line crossing, line bisection, and representational drawing) and behavioral subtests (picture scanning, telephone dialing, menu reading, article reading, telling and setting the time, coin sorting, address and sentence copying, map navigation, and card sorting). The test manual reports impressively high coefficients for inter-rater reliability (0.99), test–retest reliability (0.99) and parallel form reliability (0.91). Among the six conventional tests included in the battery, star cancellation had substantially greater sensitivity than the other tests (Halligan & Marshall, 1988) (see Figure 1).

Although many studies have explored the performance of normal subjects on some of the tests commonly used to assess neglect, relatively little is known about the effect of normal aging and dementia on these tasks. Neglect is seldom found in DAT, despite the frequency of visuoperceptual disorders in this condition; Huff et al. (1987) reported an incidence of 3% based on 95 cases. A high incidence of neglect has been reported by one study of visuospatial ability in DAT (Freedman & Dexter, 1991). These authors concluded that neglect in DAT may not be an unusual phenomenon but could often be missed because of a failure to conduct a detailed assessment. However, it should be noted that neglect was considered to be present if the discrepancies between errors on left- vs. right-sided stimuli on visuospatial tasks exceeded control values (these control values were simple difference scores). As there typically will be a high number of errors on visuospatial tasks in DAT cases, and often they will exhibit considerable intrasubject variability, these results may be an artifact of Freedman and Dexter's (1991) scoring methods. This alternative explanation is strengthened by the fact that the number of cases classified as exhibiting right-sided neglect was exactly equivalent to the number classified as exhibiting left-sided neglect (right-sided neglect is relatively rare). When looking at individual reports of cases of DAT displaying neglect, only three cases have been reported (Ishiai, Okiyama, Koyama, & Seki, 1996; Pentore & Venneri, (1994). Pentore and Venneri (1994) in their study reported two patients with DAT of moderate severity who manifested neglect in the later stages; one of these patients manifested motor neglect in addition to visuospatial neglect. Such limited evidence may lead to the conclusion that neglect in DAT is actually rather rare. This would be in accord with the fact that neglect is generally observed after unilateral lesions, while DAT, although it may present some degree of asymmetry at onset, involves bilateral degeneration (see Kirk & Kertesz, 1991, for further discussion).

7.07.12.2 The Anterior Attention System

The anterior attention system is considered to underlie performance on tasks of sustained, divided, and selective attention (Posner & Petersen, 1990). Such attentional problems are common and debilitating features of many neurological and psychiatric disorders associated with aging (Crawford, McKinlay, & Parker, 1992b; Lezak, 1995; Walsh, 1991). However, the assessment of attentional dysfunction is a problematic area in clinical neuropsychology as many potentially useful tasks used in experimental studies have not been translated into practical clinical instruments. Many existing tests do not reflect theoretical knowledge on attention and its fractionation (Posner & Petersen, 1990) and, in many cases, are poorly standardized (Lezak, 1995). An additional consideration is that tests such as the PASAT, which have proved valuable in work with younger clinical populations because of their demonstrated sensitivity and predictive validity, are too demanding to be suitable for use with the majority of elderly clients. Because of space limitations, we will limit coverage to a single battery, the Test of Everyday Attention

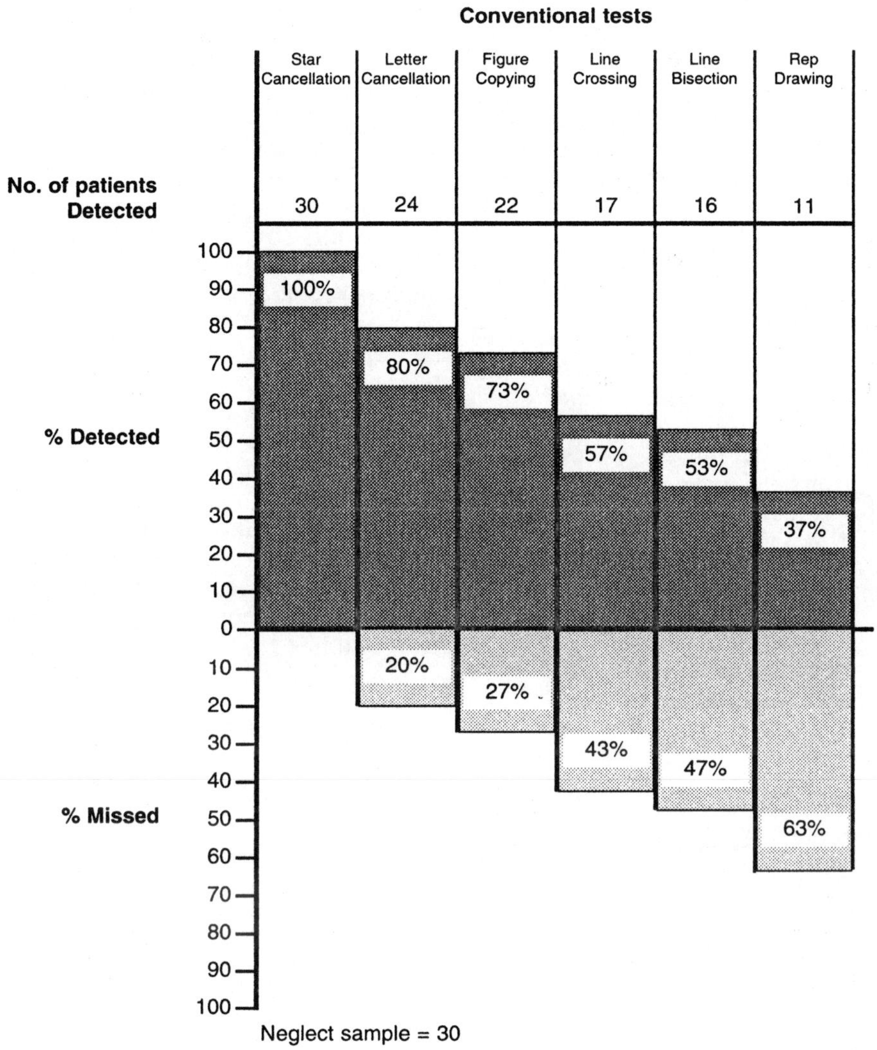

Figure 1 The relative sensitivities of the six conventional screening tests of the Behavioral Inattention Test (reproduced from Hallingan & Robertson, 1992).

(TEA) (Robertson, Ward, Ridgeway, & Nimmo-Smith, 1994; Robertson, Ward, Ridgeway, & Nimmo-Smith, 1996).

TEA is a welcome development as it attempts to overcome some of the aforementioned problems in the assessment of attentional dysfunction. It consists of eight subtests, standardized to have means of 10 and SDs of 3, which measure sustained, selective, and divided attention. For example, in the Map Search subtest, which was designed as a measure of visual selective attention, the examinee has to search for symbols (e.g., a knife and fork representing eating facilities) on a tourist map of a city. The Elevator Counting subtest, which was designed to measure sustained attention, is a tone counting task in which the examinee is asked to imagine they are in an elevator in which the floor indicator has failed (thus counting the tones is the only way to establish which floor the elevator is on). A related subtest, designed to measure auditory selective attention, requires the examinee to ignore distracter tones which are of a higher pitch.

The TEA was normed on 154 healthy participants aged 18–80 years. In addition to reflecting current thinking on the fractionation of attention, it is designed to be ecologically valid, that is, many of the subtests are designed to mimic everyday activities. Another advantage is that it has three parallel versions; this avoids the interpretative problems encountered when attempting to measure change using the same test materials.

Crawford, Somerville, and Robertson (1997) have prepared tables which allow clinicians to examine a client's relative strengths and weaknesses on the TEA (in terms of the reliability and abnormality of subtests deviations from the subtest mean), thereby supplementing the conventional normative comparison standards presented in the test manual with individual comparison standards.

7.07.13 ASSESSMENT OF EXECUTIVE FUNCTIONS

Executive deficits arising from damage to the prefrontal cortex and related structures can have a much more profound effect on a client's prospects for successful adjustment and independent living than the more circumscribed deficits arising from posterior cortical lesions. However, these problems have proven difficult to quantify and as such can be regarded as constituting the most problematic area in neuropsychological assessment. For example, reviews of tests such as the Wisconsin Card Sorting Test (Grant & Berg, 1948; Heaton, 1981), which are aimed specifically at capturing the core cognitive problems (e.g., planning deficits, underutilization of feedback, etc.), indicate that existing indices are of limited utility when used with individuals (Mountain & Snow, 1993; Reitan & Wolfson, 1994). Thus, considerable reliance must be placed on careful scrutiny of a client's approach to a range of tasks to identify these cognitive difficulties.

7.07.13.1 Frontal Hypotheses

Executive deficits are thought to underlie many of the behavioral disturbances seen in neurological disorders associated with increasing age. One of the more obvious examples is Parkinson's disease (PD). Executive deficits would be expected in PD on pathophysiological grounds as the basal ganglia, which are deprived of dopaminergic innervation because of degeneration in the substantia nigra, have strong reciprocal connections with the frontal cortex. In addition, the ventral tegmental area, which provides a direct dopaminergic innervation of the prefrontal cortex, also deteriorates in PD (see Crawford, Besson & Ebmeier, 1990 for brief review). There is neuropsychological evidence which suggests that executive deficits are an early feature in PD and that these deficits qualify as differential deficits in executive functioning (Lees & Smith, 1983). Indeed, it has been argued that fronto-executive dysfunction provides a parsimonious explanation for all of the cognitive deficits observed in nondemented Parkinson's cases (Della Sala, 1988). This is an extreme position but it is interesting to note that Bondi, Kaszniak, Bayles, and Vance (1993) have demonstrated that deficits in other cognitive domains were no longer significant after partialing out performance on tests of executive function.

It has also been proposed that normal aging is associated with a selective decline in fronto-executive function (Dempster, 1992). Daigneault, Braun, and Whitaker (1992), for example, note that "The currently dominant neuropsychological model of normal brain aging postulates that cognitive functions dependent on the integrity of the prefrontal brain regions are among the first to deteriorate" (p. 99). This frontal hypothesis stems from indications that age-related changes in the neuroanatomy and neurochemistry of the brain are more pronounced in the frontal lobes than in other cortical areas (Fuster, 1989) and from demonstrations of age-related deficits on neuropsychological tasks sensitive to frontal dysfunction (Daigneault & Braun; 1993; Daigneault et al., 1992; Mittenberg, Seidenberg, O'Leary, & DiGiulio, 1989). However, there is only limited evidence that such deficits qualify as differential deficits (i.e., that they significantly exceed the deficits found in other cognitive domains).

7.07.13.2 Verbal Fluency

Verbal fluency tests, and in particular initial letter fluency, are widely used as tests of executive dysfunction (Parker & Crawford; 1992; Walsh, 1991). Initial letter fluency, also referred to as the Controlled Oral Word Association Test (COWAT) (Benton; 1969) or phonemic fluency, requires the generation of words from initial letters (normally F, A, and S or C, F, and L) under time constraints (normally 60 seconds per letter, although 90 seconds is also used). Fluency tests are reliable, quick to administer, and even patients with quite severe deficits can understand the task requirements. In an area replete with failures to replicate, studies of initial letter fluency have been remarkably consistent in demonstrating impaired fluency following left or bilateral damage (Benton, 1968; Bornstein, 1986; Miceli, Caltagirone, Gainotti, Masullo, & Silveri, 1981; Miller, 1984; Milner, 1964). In view of the above, fluency tests are among the most useful tests in the clinician's armamentarium.

Performance on verbal fluency tasks reflects the integrity of the semantic system (i.e., the system responsible for storage of words and their associations), the efficiency of retrieval strategies, and the efficiency of self-monitoring and inhibition of inappropriate responses. In an early influential paper, Perret (1974) reported significant deficits on initial letter fluency in patients with focal frontal lesions whilst noting that semantic or category fluency (i.e., generating exemplars from categories such as animals, fruits, etc.) often failed to expose deficits (Newcombe, 1969). Perret (1974) and others have argued that the differential sensitivity of initial letter fluency to frontal dysfunction stems from the fact that in everyday life words are retrieved predominantly on the basis of their meaning. Thus, initial letter fluency is relatively novel and places greater demands on strategy generation and inhibition of semantic associates. In contrast, semantic fluency places greater demands on the integrity of the semantic system. Hodges, Salmon, and Butters, (1990), for example, is one of many studies in which there was evidence of a differential deficit in semantic fluency vs. initial letter fluency in DAT. This is consistent with other evidence indicating that deterioration of the semantic system is a marked feature of DAT (e.g., Grober, Buschke, Kawas, & Fuld, 1985).

Further support for this distinction comes from dual task studies of initial letter and semantic fluency in healthy participants. Martin, Wiggs, Lalonde, and Mack (1994) demonstrated that a secondary task involving motor sequencing (designed to activate frontal cortex) produced a differential deficit in initial letter fluency, whereas a secondary task involving semantic decisions regarding visual stimuli (designed to activate posterior cortex) produced a differential deficit in semantic fluency.

Some very useful normative data for the elderly have been published. Ivnik et al., (1996) present age- and education-based norms based on 743 elderly participants using the COWAT (i.e., the letters C, F, and L with 60 seconds per trial). Particularly positive features of these data are the age range covered (55–97 years) and the fact that most participants were also administered other commonly used neuropsychological instruments. This latter feature makes the data useful when attempting to construct a profile of a client's relative strengths and weaknesses as raw scores are converted to a common Scale and there is no worry that observed discrepancies are artifacts of differences between normative samples (see Section 7.07.4.2). Kozora and Cullum (1995) have published elderly norms for initial letter fluency (F, A, and S) and semantic fluency covering the age range 50–90 years. The semantic fluency test used was the supermarket item list from the Mattis Dementia Rating Scale (Mattis, 1988).

Errors on verbal fluency tasks have been afforded great significance in both the research literature and in advice offered to clinicians (Walsh, 1991). Perseverative errors (repeating a word produced previously) and rule-break errors (e.g., producing a proper noun or a word beginning with the wrong letter on initial-letter fluency trials) have been regarded as evidence of disinhibition or a failure of self-monitoring (Crowe, 1992; Walsh, 1991). Crowe (1992) has produced data to suggest that such errors tend to be associated with orbito-frontal damage, whereas impoverished but legitimate output is more indicative of damage to the lateral convexity.

Given the importance attached to such errors, there is surprisingly little normative data on errors to assist clinicians interpret an individual client's performance. Kozora and Cullum's (1995) study provided means and ranges for perseverative and rule-break errors. Although the mean and modal rates were low in all age bands, a finding consistent with a COWAT normative study conducted by Ruff, Light, Parker, and Levin (1996), the ranges are quite substantial (e.g., 0–15 in the 50–59 age group). It would be useful to know how many errors are required to exceed the 85th or 95th percentiles of the healthy population but there is no relevant published data.

There is a strong relationship between verbal fluency and general verbal ability in the general population. For example, Miller (1984) reported a correlation of 0.87 between initial letter fluency and Verbal IQ in a healthy sample ($N = 30$). Crawford, Obonsawin, and Bremner (1993) reported a lower but still substantial correlation of 0.64 between Wechsler Verbal IQ in a sample of 144 healthy participants. This indicates that an individual's premorbid verbal ability must be considered as an important factor when interpreting fluency performance in clinical populations. This was graphically illustrated by Borkowski, Benton, and Spreen (1967) who reported that the fluency performance of a "brain-damaged" sample of above average verbal IQ was significantly higher than the performance of healthy subjects of below average verbal IQ. Crawford et al. (1992c) have provided a NART-based regression equation which provides an estimate of a client's premorbid fluency performance (see Section 7.07.8 for details of the NART). This equation was derived from a healthy sample ($N = 142$) with an age range of 16–88 years.

7.07.13.3 Nonverbal Fluency

A number of attempts have been made to develop methods of assessing nonverbal fluency. Jones-Gotman and Milner (1977) developed a task they termed Design Fluency which requires examinees to draw abstract (nonsense) designs under a time constraint. This test can capture the lack of creativity and spontaneity and the perseverative tendencies which are often striking clinical features of patients with frontal damage. The disadvantages of this test include the lack of adequate normative data, the highly subjective nature of scoring, and the fact that it can be difficult to maximize cooperation, either because clients fail to grasp the nature of the task or view it as odd and lacking in relevance.

Ruff and colleagues (Ruff, 1988; Ruff, Light, & Evans, 1987) have developed a figural fluency test (hereafter RFFT) which requires the examinee to join up a repeating sequence of dots such that each design formed is unique. The procedure removes subjectivity from scoring as each design is unequivocally unique, a perseveration, or (more rarely) an error. The RFFT was normed on a sample of 358 healthy individuals with an age range of 16–70 years. Group studies of clinical populations indicate that the RFFT is sensitive to anterior cerebral damage, particularly in the right hemisphere (Lee et al., 1997; Ruff, Allen, Farrow, Nieemann, & Wylie, 1994). For example, Lee et al. found that 35% of designs produced by a group with right frontal lesions were perseverations, a figure which substantially exceeded the rate in right temporal (14%) and left frontal (17%) cases.

Motor slowing is a common consequence of cerebral damage and should be considered as a factor when interpreting the number of legitimate designs produced on the RFFT. Ruff, Evans, and Marshall (1986) have reported that significant RFFT deficits are observed in neurological samples after controlling for motor speed using a finger-tapping test. However, the appropriateness of finger-tapping as a control measure could be questioned. Crawford, Wright, and Bate (1995) used a simple motor task which required subjects to join repeated pairs of dots; the motor demands of this task are very similar to the RFFT but it does not require the generation of designs. They reported that the RFFT deficit in a head-injured sample did not significantly exceed the deficit on the motor task.

7.07.13.4 Behavioral Assessment of the Dysexecutive Syndrome

A very useful battery for assessing executive problems has been developed (Wilson, Alderman, Burgess, Emslie, & Evans, 1996; Wilson, Evans, Emslie, Alderman, & Burgess, in press). The Behavioral Assessment of the Dysexecutive Syndrome (BADS) battery consists of six subtests and was normed on a sample of 216 healthy participants with an age range of 16–87 years. As was noted previously, many of the formal neuropsychological tests can fail to detect executive problems because they are highly structured. Shallice and Burgess (1991) note "The patient typically has a single explicit problem to tackle at any one time ... the trials tend to be very short ... task initiation is strongly prompted by the examiner and what constitutes successful trial completion is clearly characterized" (pp. 727–728). Although some of the tests reviewed above clearly attempt to deviate from this formula, the BADS represents the most ambitious and systematic attempt to date to capture the core elements of dysexecutive syndromes.

The BADS subtests include the Rule Shifts Cards Test in which a previously established response set (responding "yes" to red cards, "no" to black) has to be inhibited in favor of responding in terms of whether or not a card matches the color of the card immediately preceding it. The Action Program Test is a planning task in which the solution requires the client to utilize various everyday materials (e.g., plastic, cork, and wire). The Modified Six Elements Test (see Shallice & Burgess, 1991) assesses scheduling and time management by requiring clients to tackle three different tasks within the time limit; there are two versions of each task and the rules prohibit tackling these contiguously.

The inter-rater reliability of the BADS is excellent; correlations between raters ranged from a low of 0.88 on one index from the Modified Six Elements Test, to unity, or near unity, on most of the other tasks. Test–retest reliability coefficients obtained from a small subset of the standardization sample (retested over a 6–12 month interval) ranged from modest to poor but this, in part, reflects the effects of range restriction.

A useful supplement to the formal BADS subtests is the Dysexecutive Questionnaire (DEX). The DEX covers dispositional and cognitive changes and comes in two forms, one for completion by the client, the other by a relative or carer. A provisional factor analysis indicates that the DEX measures three broad factors labeled as "Behavior," "Cognition," and "Emotion." Large discrepancies between client and carer reports of change are common when working with clients who have executive problems. The DEX provides one means of quantifying this lack of insight; DEX results can also form a basis for discussion when counseling clients and their families.

The DEX has been used to examine the relationship between carers' ratings of executive problems and formal test scores. Multiple regression analyses found that BADS scores were the only significant predictors of rated problems from among a set of measures which included traditional "frontal" tasks and measures of current and premorbid general intellectual ability.

7.07.14 THE DIFFERENTIAL DIAGNOSIS OF DEMENTIA VS. DEPRESSION

The differential diagnosis of dementia vs. depression has been described as "probably the knottiest problem of differential diagnosis" (Lezak, 1995), yet is a common reason for elderly patient referral to clinical psychologists. Depression is the functional disorder which can most closely resemble the early stages of a dementing condition. It is vitally important for an accurate differential diagnosis to be made because as Woods and Britton (1985) point out, "Depression can be treated; dementia typically leads to therapeutic despair." Des Rosiers (1992) reviewed 18 studies and reported that, on average, 10% of cases initially diagnosed as organic dementia were later rediagnosed as depression. In practice, the diagnosis of dementia vs. depression is made by drawing on information from a wide variety of sources, that is, previous history, informant's account, phenomenology, brain scan measures, blood biochemistry, etc. Problems emerge, however, when an individual presents with no well-documented history and no useful informant information.

Huppert (1994) has pointed out that in most studies where an early DAT group has been compared with a control group, it is likely that the controls vary from the demented subjects in ways which are rarely specified. For example, as the normal controls are usually community volunteers, they are less likely to have mobility problems than sensory deficits and are more likely to be in good health. The patients usually have been referred to specialists which means that dementia is sufficiently severe to have come to specialist attention, and second, that the patients who see specialists may not be representative of all demented subjects. As Huppert (1994) states "one implication of these considerations is that observed differences are likely to be an exaggeration (if not a distortion) of the performance which would be seen in a genuinely representative sample" (p. 295).

7.07.14.1 Delayed Verbal Recall Impairment as an Indicator of Early DAT?

Over the years there have been many attempts at using memory tests to help distinguish between dementia and depression. In order to highlight the problems associated with this approach, in the following section the Delayed Word Recall test will be used as an example.

In two studies by the consortium to establish a registry for DAT (CERAD), the investigators reported that delayed verbal recall was a highly sensitive indicator of early DAT (Morris et al., 1989; Welsh, Butters, Hughes, Mohs, & Heyman, 1992). In DAT, there appears to be a rapid rate of forgetting within the first 5–10 minutes following acquisition (Butters et al., 1988; Hart, Smith, & Swash, 1988) but a relatively normal rate of forgetting thereafter (Corkin et al., 1984; Kopelman, 1985). Knopman and Ryberg (1989) suggested that elaborative encoding may provide a substantial benefit in normal elderly individuals but not to patients with DAT. They proposed that the optimum memory test procedure for the early diagnosis of DAT should involve: (i) a study phase in which subjects were required to engage in elaborative encoding; (ii) a filled delay interval; and (iii) a test phase which involved free recall. Accordingly, Knopman and Ryberg (1989) developed the Delayed Word Recall test (DWR). Ten nouns are presented on cards, one at a time (chimney, salt, harp, button, meadow, train, flower, finger, rug, book). For each word, the subject is asked to read out the word and try to remember it and then to make up a sentence using the word. When all 10 words have been presented, the complete procedure is repeated, with subjects instructed to produce an alternative sentence. Following a five minute filled delay, free recall for the 10 words in the list is tested. Based on the delayed free recall cut-off score of less than or equal to 2 out of 10 = DAT, Knopman and Ryberg (1989) reported an overall predictive accuracy of 95% in a group of DAT patients vs. elderly control subjects. This is an extremely impressive degree of between-group separation.

In a follow-up study, Coen et al. (1996) compared a group of mildly demented DAT patients with individually matched healthy controls and found that the DWR recall measure achieved 98% overall accuracy (i.e., almost perfect between-group separation). In an extension to the original DWR, Coen et al. included a four-choice recognition memory test and, using a cut-off score of less than or equal to 9 out of 10 = DAT, greater than nine = controls, they reported that the recognition measure yielded a sensitivity of 98%, specificity of 95%, and an overall accuracy of 96%. Taken together, the results of the Knopman and Ryberg (1989) and Coen et al. studies suggests that the DWR is an extremely promising measure to aid in the early detection of DAT.

However, for any neuropsychological test index to have clinical utility, the method must be shown clearly to identify patients suffering from DAT without producing false-positives from an elderly depressed comparison group. Unfortunately, too many studies have appeared which have focused on the simple comparison between DAT and very healthy controls, and this criticism can be leveled at the Knopman and Ryberg (1989) and Coen et al. studies.

O'Carroll, Conway, Ryman, and Prentice (1997) attempted to test the utility of the DWR in separating patients with DAT from patients with major depression. Fifty patients with DAT were compared with 50 patients who fulfilled *DSM-IV* criteria for a major depressive episode. While there were highly significant differences in mean free recall and recognition scores, the between-group overlap was large (e.g., see Figure 2 for free recall results—very similar results were obtained for recognition). Put simply, if the recommended cut-off point for free recall of 2 or less out of 10 = DAT is adopted, 44% depressed patients would be misclassified as suffering from DAT. Using the less than 10 recommended cut-off score for recognition score, 48% of depressed patients would be misclassified as suffering from DAT. This study highlights the degree of cognitive impairment which often presents in elderly depressed patients which can masquerade as "pseudo-dementia" (Robbins, Joyce, & Sahakian, 1992).

7.07.14.2 Kendrick Cognitive Tests for the Elderly

The Kendrick Cognitive Tests for the Elderly (KCTE) comprise two components, a pictorial memory task (the Object Learning Test or OLT) and the Digit Copying Test (DCT). The principle underlying the use of the KCTE in differential diagnosis lies in the expected pattern of visual memory and psychomotor speed in depression vs. dementia. According to Kendrick, Gibson, and Moyes (1979), both DCT and OLT should be affected in primary dementia and not in depression. An innovation of the Kendrick test is the requirement that the measures be readministered six weeks following the initial assessment. desRosiers (1992) describes this requirement as somewhat less than practical. However, in our opinion, repeat neuropsychological assessment in cases where diagnosis is in doubt represents good clinical practice.

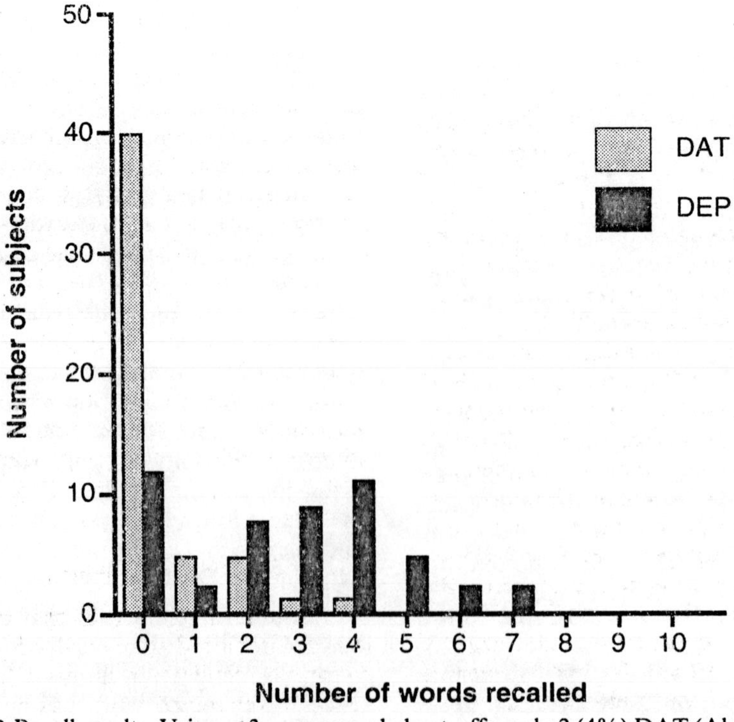

Figure 2 DWR Recall results. Using < 3 recommended cut-offs, only 2 (4%) DAT (Alzheimer) sujects would be misclassified, but 22 (44%) DEP (Depressed) would be classed as DAT (reproduced from O'Carroll et al., 1997).

One of the strongest claims regarding the KCTE is that "it has been found possible to discriminate absolutely between dementias and non-dementing subjects" (Kendrick et al., 1979, p. 329). The literature on the Kendrick test is well reviewed by desRosiers (1992). Some reports have confirmed the utility of the KCTE in differentiating a depressed sample from a demented sample. However, as is usually the case in studies of this sort, the samples consist of very well-defined groups where differential diagnosis is not a problem (Knight & Moroney, 1985). As desRosiers (1992) cautions, the validity of the KCTE should best be examined in patients for whom diagnosis is still ambiguous. A further point to consider when considering the theoretical foundation of the KCTE is the assumption that in depression, psychomotor speed, and mnemonic function are not as detrimentally affected as in early DAT. However, in depressive pseudodementia, it is precisely because both domains are seriously impaired that diagnostic difficulties arise.

7.07.14.3 Effortful vs. Automatic Processing and Memory

Weingartner, Cohen, Bunney, Ebert, and Kaye (1982) proposed that tasks that are normally accomplished automatically and require little cognitive capacity are particularly useful in distinguishing progressive dementia patients from depressed patients. Weingartner (1984, 1986) reported that depressed patients experienced difficulty on memory tasks that require elaborate or effortful organization and processing of material to be remembered, but that they do not show problems in memory tasks on which "automatic" memory encoding is presumed to be involved. In contrast, it is postulated that demented patients have difficulty with both automatic and effortful processing. In line with this proposal, Weingartner, Cohen, Murphy, Martello, and Gerdt (1981) reported that depressed patients demonstrate impairments on delayed free recall (effortful) with no impairment on recognition memory (relatively automatic), whereas demented patients perform poorly in both conditions. However, Lachner, Satzger and Engel (1994) have provided evidence which challenges the Weingartner model. They compared three groups (demented, depressed, and healthy subjects) who were in their 70s on five verbal recall and two recognition memory tasks. They found that both delayed recall and recognition after long delay were the measures which best discriminated between the demented and the depressed patient groups. It is interesting to note that the recognition measure was more discriminating than free recall, selective reminding, or serial learning, all presumably more "effortful" than a recognition task.

Lachner et al. (1994) point out that the labeling of some cognitive tasks as effortful vs. automatic is often ambiguous, and propose sensibly that "In future research, the tasks cognitive capacity requirements should be examined empirically to avoid inconsistencies by subjectively estimating capacity demands" (Lachner et al., p. 10). A particular advantage of the Lachner et al. study is their comparison of severely depressed psychiatric inpatients with a demented patient sample where 60% were still capable of independently running their household, as it is this type of comparison of mildly demented and severely depressed patients that is of particular clinical interest with regard to the problem of differential diagnosis.

7.07.14.4 Is Poor Memory Test Performance in Elderly Depressed Patients an Artifact of Poor Motivation?

In commenting on the relatively poor performance of many depressed patients with standard neuropsychological measures, many writers have attributed this impairment to the nonspecific effects of motivational deficits. Few studies have tested this hypothesis experimentally. One notable exception is the study of Richards and Ruff (1989), who randomly assigned two groups of subjects, depressed and nondepressed, to either motivation or nonmotivation conditions (motivation involved encouragement, a monitory incentive and performance feedback). Richards and Ruff (1989) reported that motivation (as measured by improvement on a simple card-sorting task) was enhanced for the subjects in the motivation condition. Crucially, motivation did not significantly affect neuropsychological test performance and the authors concluded that although depressed patients may be less motivated, this reduced motivation does not fully account for the observed cognitive impairments in depression.

7.07.14.5 Future Directions

The literature indicates that demented subjects are impaired at any task which requires the conscious recollection of newly learned material. However, much work has been carried out attempting to evaluate whether specific aspects of memory functioning are disproportionately impaired in early DAT. Divided attention tasks are particularly sensitive to DAT, that is, tasks where subjects are required to divide their attention during learning (e.g., performing a digit span test while keeping a stylus on a target on a pursuit rotor task). This would appear to be a particular deficit in "working memory," that is, the ability to hold information in a short-term store or carrying out the other processing operations (Baddeley & Wilson, 1986). Additionally, prospective memory tasks appear to be particularly impaired in early DAT. Huppert and Beardsall (1993) administered a variety of memory tasks and found that even patients with minimal dementia were disproportionately impaired on prospective memory tasks (e.g., remembering to ask for a belonging back at the end of the Rivermead Behavioural Memory Test). In the search for particularly dementia-sensitive screening tasks, a combination of divided attention and prospective memory tasks may well be worthy of further investigation.

7.07.14.6 Recommendations and Conclusions for the Differential Diagnosis of Dementia vs. Depression

Sweet, Newman, and Bell (1992) made several useful recommendations to facilitate the differential diagnosis of depressed patients from demented patients. First, they recommend administering neuropsychological measures that assess domains which the literature indicate are particularly discriminating, notably psychomotor retardation, recognition vs. recall, and easy vs. difficult paired associated learning. Second, they recommend utilization of measures of affective status (e.g., the Beck Depression Inventory or the Geriatric Depression Rating Scale). They also propose seeking collateral information through interviewing the spouse or significant other. Third, when evidence of depression is found, customary cognitive "cut-off" scores may be misleading and they propose using more stringent criteria (e.g., an additional standard deviation away from normal performance). Fourth, with depressed patients, they caution against diagnosing brain dysfunction based only on findings such as mild attentional or memory problems. For example, as psychomotor retardation in depression can easily result in a markedly impaired performance on the Stroop task (Trenerry, Crosson, DeBoe, & Leber, 1989), many depressed patients fall within the recommended cut-off score used to indicate "brain damage."

Sweet et al. (1992) also urge against differentiating depression from brain damage after only a single session with the patient and propose seeing the patient on more than one day and, if in doubt, readministering at least a portion of the measures on a second testing session (this would be in accord with the protocol of the Kendrick Cognitive Tests for the Elderly). Sweet et al. conclude "In the event that a diagnostic conclusion regarding brain dysfunction in the depressed patient appears unclear, despite all your best efforts, recommend a re-evaluation of the depressed patient after a period of pharmacological or psychotherapeutic intervention" (p. 41). This is a recommendation that is fully endorsed. Neuropsychological measures should be used in conjunction with information derived from a variety of sources (e.g., relatives and clinical history). Developments in neuroimaging precision suggest that an *in vivo* maker for DAT may become available (Jobst et al., 1994).

Given the potentially catastrophic outcome of misclassifying a treatable, depressed patient as having DAT, it has to be concluded that the available evidence indicates that no single neuropsychological measure can be recommended for use in the individual case to confidently separate early DAT from major depression in an elderly population. However, neuropsychological measures may offer useful information that can be integrated with data gathered from a variety of sources. In particular, accurate objective quantification of change over time is one of the key areas where detailed assessment of cognitive functioning can provide important diagnostic information. Furthermore, changes in neuropsychological status can offer a useful measure of treatment response in both dementia and depression.

7.07.15 REFERENCES

Albert, M. L. (1973). A simple test of visual neglect. *Neurology*, *23*, 658–664.

Albert, M. S., Heller, H. S., & Milberg, W. (1988). Changes in naming ability with age. *Psychology and Aging*, *3*, 173–178.

Anthony, J. C., Le Resche, L., Niaz, U., Von Korff, M. R., & Folstein, M. F. (1982). Limits of the Mini-Mental-State as a screening test for dementia and delirium among hospital patients. *Psychological Medicine*, *12*, 397–408.

Atkinson, L. (1991). Some tables for statistically based interpretation of WAIS-R factor scores. *Psychological Assessment*, *3*, 288–291.

Atkinson, L., Cyr, J. J., Doxey, N. C. S., & Vigna, C. M. (1989). Generalizability of WAIS-R factor structure within and between populations. *Journal of Clinical Psychology*, *45*, 124–129.

Baddeley, A., Emslie, H., & Nimmo-Smith, I. (1993). The Spot-the-Word Test: A robust estimate of verbal intelligence based on lexical decision. *British Journal of Clinical Psychology*, *32*, 55–65.

Baddeley, A., Emslie, H., & Nimmo-Smith, I. (1994). *Doors*

and people: A test of visual and verbal recall and recognition. Bury St. Edmunds, UK: Thames Valley Test Company.

Baddeley, A., & Wilson, B. (1986). Dementia and working memory. *Quarterly Journal of Experimental Psychology, 38*(A), 603–618.

Balota, D. A., & Duchek, J. M. (1988). Age related differences in lexical access, spreading activation, and simple pronunciation. *Psychology and Aging, 3,* 84–93.

Barker, M. G., & Lawson, J. S. (1968). Nominal aphasia in dementia. *British Journal of Psychiatry, 114,* 1351–1356.

Barlow, D. H., & Hersen, M. (1984). *Single case experimental designs: strategies for studying behavior change* (2nd ed.). New York: Pergamon.

Barona, A., Reynolds, C. R., & Chastain, R. (1984). A demographically based index of premorbid intelligence for the WAIS-R. *Journal of Consulting and Clinical Psychology, 52,* 885–887.

Beardsall, L., & Huppert, F. A. (1994). Improvement in NART word reading in demented and normal older persons using the Cambridge Contextual Reading Test. *Journal of Clinical and Experimental Neuropsychology, 16,* 232–242.

Benton, A. L. (1968). Differential behavioral effects in frontal lobe disease. *Neuropsychologia, 6,* 53–60.

Benton, A. L. (1969). Development of a multilingual aphasia battery: Progress and problems. *Journal of the Neurological Sciences, 9,* 39–48.

Benton, A. L., Eslinger, P. J., & Damasio, A. R. (1981). Normative observations of neuropsychological test performances in old age. *Clinical Neuropsychology, 3,* 33–42.

Benton, A. L., Hamser, K. D. S., Varney, N. R., & Spreen, O. (1983). *Contributions to neuropsychological assessment.* New York: Oxford University Press.

Benton, A. L., Hannay, H. J., & Varney, N. R. (1975). Visual perception of line direction in patients with unilateral brain disease. *Neurology, 25,* 907–910.

Benton, A. L., & Van Allen, M. W. (1968). Impairment in facial recognition in patients with cerebral disease. *Cortex, 4,* 344–358.

Binks, M. (1989). Changes in mental functioning associated with normal ageing. In R. Tallis (Ed.), *The clinical neurology of old age* (pp. 27–39). Chichester, UK: Wiley.

Bisiach, E., & Luzzatti, C. (1978). Unilateral neglect of representational space. *Cortex, 14,* 129–133.

Blessed, G., Black, S. E., Butler, T., & Kay, D. W. K. (1991). The diagnosis of dementia in the elderly a comparison of CAMCOG (the cognitive section of CAMDEX), the AGECAT program, DSM-III, The Mini-Mental State Examination and some short rating Scales. *British Journal of Psychiatry, 159,* 193–198.

Bondi, M. W., Kaszniak, A. W., Bayles, K. A., & Vance, K. T. (1993). Contributions of frontal system dysfunction to memory and perceptual abilities in Parkinson's disease. *Neuropsychology, 7,* 89–102.

Borkowski, J. G., Benton, A. L., & Spreen, O. (1967). Word fluency and brain damage. *Neuropsychologia, 5,* 135–140.

Bornstein, R. A. (1986). Contribution of various neuropsychological measures to detection of frontal lobe impairment. *International Journal of Clinical Neuropsychology, 8,* 18–22.

Borod, J. C., Goodglass, H., & Kaplan, E. (1980). Normative data on the Boston Diagnostic Aphasia Examination, Parietal Lobe Battery, and the Boston Naming Test. *Journal of Clinical Neuropsychology, 2,* 209–215.

Brinkman, S. D., & Braun, P. (1984). Classification of dementia patients by a WAIS profile related to central cholinergic deficiencies. *Journal of Clinical Neuropsychology, 6,* 393–400.

Britton, P. G., & Savage, R. D. (1966). A short form of the WAIS for use with the aged. *British Journal of Psychiatry, 112,* 417–418.

Brooks, D. N. (1989). Closed head trauma: assessing the common cognitive problems. In M. D. Lezak (Ed.), *Assessment of the behavioral consequences of head trauma. Frontiers of Clinical Neuroscience* (Vol. 7, pp. 61–85). New York: Liss.

Bryan, J., Luszcz, M. A., & Crawford, J. R. (1997). Verbal knowledge and speed of information processing as mediators of age differences in verbal fluency performance among older adults. *Psychology and Aging, 12,* 473–478.

Burgess, A. (1991). Profile analysis of the Wechsler Intelligence Scales: a new index of subtest scatter. *British Journal of Clinical Psychology, 30,* 257–263.

Burke, D. M., Mackay, D. G., Worthley, J. A., & Wade, E. (1991). On the tip of the tongue: what causes word finding failures in young and older adults? *Journal of Memory and Language, 30,* 542–579.

Burke, D. M., White, H., & Diaz, D. L. (1987). Semantic priming in young and older adults: evidence for age-constancy in automatic and attentional processes. *Journal of Experimental Psychology: Human Perception and Performance, 13,* 79–88.

Butters, B., Salmon, D. P., Cullum, C. M., Cairns, P., Troster, A. I., & Jacobs, D. (1988). Differentiation of amnesic and demented patients with the Wechsler Memory Scale-Revised. *Clinical Neuropsychologist, 2,* 133–148.

Caine, E. D. (1992). *Nomenclature and diagnosis of cognitive disorders: a US perspective.* Paper presented at the Abstract from Age-related Cognitive Disorders Conference, Nice, France.

Canavan, A. G. M., Dunn, G., & McMillan, T. M. (1986). Principal components of the WAIS-R. *British Journal of Clinical Psychology, 25,* 81–35.

Chapman, L. J., & Chapman, J. P. (1973). Problems in the measurement of cognitive deficit. *Psychological Bulletin, 79,* 380–385.

Christensen, H., & MacKinnon, A. (1992). Wechsler intelligence scale profiles in Alzheimer type dementia and healthy ageing. *International Journal of Geriatric Psychiatry, 7,* 241–246.

Cockburn, J., & Smith, P. T. (1989). *The Rivermead Behavioural Memory Test (Suppl. 3: Elderly people).* Bury St. Edmunds, England: Thames Valley Test Company.

Coen, R. F., Swanwick, G. R. J., Maguire, C., Kirby, M., Lawlor, B. A., Walsh, J. B., & Coakley, D. (1996). Memory impairment in Alzheimer's disease: replication and extension of the delayed word recall (DWR) test. *Irish Journal of Psychological Medicine, 13,* 55–58.

Corkin, S., Growdon, J., Nissen, M. J., Huff, F. J., Freed, D. M., & Sagar, H. J. (1984). Recent advances in the neuropsychological study of Alzheimer's disease. In R. J. Wurtman, S. Corkin, & J. H. Growdon, (Eds.), *Advances in basic research and therapies* (pp. 75–94). New York: Centre for Brain Sciences and Metabolism Trust.

Crawford, J. R. (1992). Current and premorbid intelligence measures in neuropsychological assessment. In J. R. Crawford, D. M. Parker & W. McKinlay, (Eds.), *A handbook of neuropsychological assessment* (pp. 21–49). Hove, UK: Erlbaum.

Crawford, J. R. (1997). WAIS-R short-forms: Assessing the statistical significance of subtest differences. *British Journal of Clinical Psychology, 36,* 601–608.

Crawford, J. R., & Allan, K. M. (1997). Estimating premorbid IQ with demographic variables: regression equations derived from a U.K. sample. *The Clinical Neuropsychologist, 11,* 192–197.

Crawford, J. R., Allan, K. M., & Jack, A. M. (1992a). Short-forms of the UK WAIS-R: regression equations and their predictive accuracy in a general population sample. *British Journal of Clinical Psychology, 31*, 191–202.

Crawford, J. R., Allan, K. M., McGeorge, P., & Kelly, S. M. (1997). Base rate data on the abnormality of subtest scatter for WAIS-R short-forms. *British Journal of Clinical Psychology, 36*, 433–444.

Crawford, J. R., Allan, K. M., Stephen, D. W., Parker, D. M., & Besson, J. A. O. (1989a). The Wechsler Adult Intelligence Scale-Revised (WAIS-R): Factor structure in a UK sample. *Personality and Individual Differences, 10*, 1209–1212.

Crawford, J. R., Besson, J. A. O., & Ebmeier, K. P. (1990). Dementia: The role of neurotransmitter deficits. In T. G. Dinan (Ed.), *Principles and practice of biological psychiatry* (pp. 105–133). London: Clinical Neuroscience Publishers.

Crawford, J. R., Besson, J. A. O., & Parker, D. M., (1988). Estimation of permorbid intelligence in organic conditions. *British Journal of Psychiatry, 153*, 178–181.

Crawford, J. R., Johnson, D. A., Mychalkiw, B., & Moore, J. W. (in press-a). WAIS-R performance following closed head injury: A comparison of the clinical utility of summary IQs, factor scores and subtest scatter indices. *The Clinical Neuropsychologist, 11*.

Crawford, J. R., Moore, J. W., & Cameron, I. M. (1992c). Verbal fluency: a NART-based equation for the estimation of premorbid performance. *British Journal of Clinical Psychology, 31*, 327–329.

Crawford, J. R., Obonsawin, M. C., & Allan, K. M. (in press-b). PASAT and components of WAIS-R performance: Convergent and discriminant validity. *Neuropsychological Rehabilitation*.

Crawford, J. R., Obonsawin, M. C., & Bremner, M. (1993). Frontal lobe impairment in schizophrenia: Relationship to intellectual functioning. *Psychological Medicine, 23*, 787–790.

Crawford, J. R., Parker, D. M., & McKinlay, W., & (Eds.). (1992b). *A handbook of neuropsychological assessment*. Hove, UK: Erlbaum.

Crawford, J. R., Sommerville, J., & Robertson, I. H. (1997). Assessing the reliability and abnormality of subtest differences on the Test of Everyday Attention. *British Journal of Clinical Psychology, 36*, 609–617.

Crawford, J. R., Stewart, L. E., Cochrane, R., Foulds, J., Besson, J. A. O., & Parker, D. M. (1989b). Estimating premorbid IQ from demographic variables: a regression equation derived from a UK sample. *British Journal of Clinical Psychology, 28*, 275–278.

Crawford, J. R., Stewart, L. E., & Moore, J. W. (1989c). Demonstration of savings on the AVLT and development of a parallel form. *Journal of Clinical and Experimental Neuropsychology, 11*, 975–981.

Crawford, J. R., Wright, R., & Bate, A. (1995). Verbal, figural and ideational fluency in CHI. *Journal of the International Neuropsychological Society, 1*, 321.

Crocker, L. M., & Algina, J. (1986). *Introduction to classical and modern test theory*. New York: Holt, Rhinehart & Winston.

Crook, T., Bartus, R. T., Ferris, S. H., Whitehouse, P., Cohen, G. D., & Gershon, S. (1986). Age-associated memory impairment: proposed diagnostic criteria and measures of clinical change: Report of a National Institute of Mental Health Work Group. *Developmental Neuropsychology, 2*, 261–276.

Crowe, S. F. (1992). Dissociation of two frontal lobe syndromes by a test of verbal fluency. *Journal of Clinical and Experimental Neuropsychology, 14*, 327–339.

Daigneault, S., & Braun, C. M. J. (1993). Working memory and the self-ordered pointing task: Further evidence of early prefrontal decline in normal aging. *Journal of Clinical and Experimental Neuropsychology, 15*, 881–895.

Daigneault, S., Braun, C. M. J., & Whitaker, H. A. (1992). Early effects of normal aging on perserverative and non-perseverative prefrontal measures. *Developmental Neuropsychology, 8*, 99–114.

Davis, H. P., & Bernstein, P. A. (1992). Age-related changes in explicit and implicit memory. In L. R. Squire & N. Butters (Eds.), *Neuropsychology of memory* (2nd ed., pp. 249–261). New York: Guilford Press.

De Renzi, E., & Faglioni, P. (1978). Normative data and screening power of a shortened version of the Token Test. *Cortex, 14*, 41–49.

De Renzi, E., & Vignolo, L. A. (1962). The Token Test: A sensitive test to detect disturbances in aphasics. *Brain, 85*, 665–678.

D'Elia, L. F., Boone, K. B., & Mitrushima, A. M. (1995). Handbook of normative data for neuropsychological assessment. New York: Oxford University Press.

Delis, D. C., Kramer, J. H., Kaplan, E., & Ober, B. A. (1987). *California Verbal Learning Test—Adult Version: Research Edition Manual Version 1*. San Antonio, CA: The Psychological Corporation.

Della Sala, S. (1988). Cognitive deficits of Parkinsonians and Occam's Razor. *Europa Medicophysica, 24*, 1–22.

Della Sala, S., Laiacona, M., Trivelli, C., & Spinnler, H. (1995). Poppelreuter-Ghent overlapping figures test. Its sensitivity to age, and its clinical use. *Archives of Clinical Neuropsychology, 10*(6), 511–534.

Dempster, F. N. (1992). The rise and fall of the inhibitory mechanism: Toward a unified theory of cognitive development and aging. *Development Review, 12*, 45–75.

desRosiers, G. (1992). Primary or depressive dementia: Psychometric assessment. *Clinical Psychology Review, 12*, 307–343.

Dick, J. P. R., Guiloff, R. J., Stewart, A., Blackstock, J., Bielawska, C., Paul, E. A., & Marsden, C. D. (1984). Mini Mental State Examination in neurological patients. *Journal of Neurology, Neurosurgery, and Psychiatry, 47*, 496–499.

Drachman, D. A., & Leavitt, J. (1974). Human memory and the cholinergic system: A relationship to aging? *Archives of Neurology, 30*, 113–121.

Ellis, H. D. (1992). Assessment of deficits in facial processing. In J. R. Crawford, D. M. Parker, & W. W. McKinlay (Eds.), *A handbook of neuropsychological assessment* (pp. 141–150). Hove, UK: Lawrence Erlbaum.

Elwood, R. W. (1991). The Wechsler Memory Scale-Revised: Psychometric characteristics and clinical application. *Neuropsychology Review, 2*, 179–201.

Eslinger, P. J., & Benton, A. L. (1983). Visuoperceptual performance in aging and dementia. Clinical and theoretical implications. *Journal of Clinical Neuropsychology, 5*, 213–220.

Farver, P. F., & Farver, T. B. (1982). Performance of normal older adults on tests designed to measure parietal lobe functions. *American Journal of Occupational Therapy, 36*, 444–449.

Folstein, M. F., Folstein, S. E., & McHugh, P. R. (1975). Mini-Mental-State: A practical method for grading the cognitive state of patients for the clinician. *Journal of Psychiatry Research, 12*, 189–198.

Franzen, M. D. (1989). *Reliability and validity in neuropsychological assessment*. New York: Plenum.

Freedman, L., & Dexter, L. E. (1991). Visuospatial ability in cortical dementia. *Journal of Clinical and Experimental Neuropsychology, 13*(5), 677–690.

Fuld, P. A., (1984). Test profile of cholinergic dysfunction and of Alzheimer-type dementia. *Journal of Clinical Neuropsychology, 6*, 380–392.

Fuster, J. M. (1989). *The prefrontal cortex* (2nd ed.). New York: Raven Press.

Gallagher, A. J. (1979). Temporal reliability of aphasic performance on the Token Test. *Brain and Language, 7*, 34–41.

Gardner, R., Oliver-Munoz, S., Fisher, L., & Empting, L.

(1981). Mattis Dementia Rating Scale: Internal reliability study using a diffusely impaired population. *Journal of Clinical Neuropsychology, 3*, 271–275.
Gauthier, L., Dehaut, F., & Joanette, Y. (1989). The Bells Test: A quantitative and qualitative test for visual neglect. *International Journal of Clinical Neuropsychology, 11*, 49–54.
Geffen, G., Moar, K. J., O'Hanlon, A. P., Clark, C. R., & Geffen, L. B. (1990). Performance measures of 16- to 86-year-old males and females on the Auditory Verbal Learning Test. *Clinical Neuropsychologist, 4*, 45–63.
Gfeller, J. D., & Rankin, E. J. (1991). The WAIS-R profile as a cognitive marker of Alzheimer's Disease: A misguided venture? *Journal of Clinical and Experimental Neuropsychology, 13*, 629–636.
Giles, E., Patterson, K., & Hodges, J. R. (1996). Performance on the Boston Cookie Theft Picture Description Task in patients with early dementia of the Alzheimer's type: Missing information. *Aphasiology, 10*, 395–408.
Glosser, G., & Deser, T. (1992). A comparison of changes in macrolinguistic and microlinguistic aspects of discourse production in normal aging. *Journals of Gerontology, 47*, 266–272.
Goodglass, H. (1980). Naming disorders in aphasia and ageing. In L. K. Obler & M. L. Albert (Eds.), *Language and communication in the elderly* (pp. 37–45). Lexington, MA: Heath.
Goodglass, H., & Kaplan, E. (1983). *Boston Diagnostic Aphasia Examination (BDAE)*. Philadelphia: Lea & Febiger.
Goodglass, H., & Kaplan, E. (1987). *The assessment of aphasia and related disorders* (2nd ed.). Philadelphia: Lea & Febiger.
Gottschaldt, K. (1928). Uber den Einfluss der Erfahrung auf die Wahrnehmung von Figuren. *Psychologische Forschung, 18*, 18–317.
Grant, D. A., & Berg, E. A. (1948). A behavioural analysis of degree of reinforcement and ease of shifting to new responses in a Weigl-type card-sorting problem. *Journal of Experimental Psychology, 38*, 404–411.
Greene, J. D. W., Baddeley, A. D., & Hodges, J. R. (1996). Analysis of the episodic memory deficit in early Alzheimer's disease: Evidence from the Doors and People Test. *Neuropsychologia, 34*, 537–551.
Grober, E., Buschke, H., Kawas, C., & Fuld, P. (1985). Impaired ranking of semantic attributes in dementia. *Brain and Language, 26*, 276–286.
Gronwall, D. (1977). Paced auditory serial-addition task: a measure of recovery from concussion. *Perceptual and Motor Skills, 44*, 367–373.
Halligan, P. W., & Marshall, J. C. (1988). How long is a piece of string? A study of line bisection in a case of visual neglect. *Cortex, 24*, 321–328.
Halligan, P. W., & Marshall, J. C. (1989). Line bisection in visuo-spatial neglect: Disproof of a conjecture. *Cortex, 25*, 517–521.
Halligan, P. W., & Marshall, J. C. (1991). Left neglect for near but not far space in man. *Nature, 350*, 498–500.
Halligan, P. W., & Robertson, I. H. (1992). The assessment of unilateral neglect. In J. R. Crawford, D. M. Parker, & W. W. McKinlay (Eds.), *A handbook of neuropsychological assessment* (pp. 151–175). Hove, UK: Lawrence Erlbaum.
Hart, S., Smith, C. M., & Swash, M. (1988). Word fluency in patients with early dementia of Alzheimer type. *British Journal of Clinical Psychology, 27*, 115–124.
Heaton, R. K. (1981). *Wisconsin Card Sorting Test manual.* Odessa, FL: Psychological Assessment Resources.
Hodges, J. R., Patterson, K., Graham, N., & Dawson, K. (1996). Naming and knowing in dementia of Alzheimer's type. *Brain and Language, 54*, 302–325.
Hodges, J. R., Salmon, D. P., & Butters, N. (1990). Differential impairment of semantic and episodic memory in Alzheimer's and Huntington's diseases: A controlled prospective study. *Journal of Neurology, Neurosurgery and Psychiatry, 53*, 1089–1095.
Hooper, H. E. (1983). *Hooper Visual Organization Test (VOT)* Los Angeles: Western Psychological Services.
Huff, F. J., Boller, F., Lucchelli, F., Querriera, R., Beyer, J., & Belle, S. (1987). The neurologic examination in patients with probably Alzheimer's disease. *Archives of Neurology, 44*, 929–932.
Huff, F. J., Collins, C., Corkin, S., & Rosen, T. J. (1986). Equivalent forms of the Boston Naming Test. *Journal of Clinical and Experimental Psychology, 8*, 556–562.
Huppert, F. A. (1994). Memory function in dementia and normal aging: Dimension or dichotomy? In F. A. Huppert, C. Brayne, & D. W. O'Connor (Eds.), *Dementia and normal aging* (pp. 291–330). Cambridge: Cambridge University Press.
Huppert, F. A., & Beardsall, L. (1993). Prospective memory impairment as an early indicator of dementia. *Journal of Clinical and Experimental Neuropsychology, 15*, 805–821.
Huppert, F. A., Jorm, A. F., Brayne, C., Girling, D. M., Barkley, C., Beardsall, L., & Paykel, E. S. (submitted). Psychometric properties of the CAMCOG and its efficacy in the diagnosis of dementia.
Huppert, F. A., & Kopelman, M. D. (1989). Rates of forgetting in normal ageing: A comparison with dementia. *Neuropsychologia, 27*, 849–860.
Huttenlocher, J., Haight, W., & Bryk, A. (1991). Early vocabulary growth: Relation to language input and gender. *Developmental Psychology, 27*, 236–248.
Ishiai, S., Okiyama, R., Koyama, Y., & Seki, K. (1996). Unilateral spatial neglect in Alzheimer's disease. A line bisection study. *Acta Neurologica Scandinavica, 93*, 219–224.
Ivnik, R. J., Malec, J. F., Smith, G. E., Tangalos, E. G., & Petersen, R. C. (1996). Neuropsychological tests' norms above age 55: COWAT, BNT, MAE Token, WRAT-R reading, AMNART, STROOP, TMT, and JLO. *The Clinical Neuropsychologist, 10*, 262–278.
Ivnik, R. J., Malec, J. F., Smith, G. E., Tangalos, E. G., Peterson, R. C., Kokmen, E., & Kurland, L. T. (1992). Mayo's older Americans normative studies: WAIS-R norms for ages 56 to 97. *The Clinical Neuropsychologist, 6*, 1–30.
Jobst, K. A., Smith, A. D., Szatmari, M., Esiri, M. M., Jaskowski, A., Hindley, N., McDonald, B., & Molyneux, A. J. (1994). Rapidly progressing atrophy of medial temporal lobe in Alzheimer's disease. *Lancet, 343*, 829–830.
Jones-Gotman, M., & Milner, B. (1977). Design fluency: The invention of nonsense drawings after focal frontal lesions. *Neuropsychologia, 15*, 653–674.
Kaplan, E. F., Goodglass, H., & Weintraub, S. (1978). *The Boston Naming Test.* (Experimental ed.). Boston: Kaplan & Goodglass.
Kaplan, E. F., Goodglass, H., & Weintraub, S. (1983). *The Boston Naming Test* (2nd ed.). Philadelphia: Lea & Febiger.
Kaufman, A. S. (1990). *Assessing adolescent and adult intelligence.* Boston: Allyn & Bacon.
Kemper, S. (1992). Language and aging. In F. I. M. Craik & T. A. Salthouse (Eds.), *The handbook of aging and cognition* (pp. 213–272). Hillsdale, NJ: Erlbaum.
Kempler, D. (1988). Lexical and pantomime abilities in Alzheimer's disease. *Aphasiology, 2*, 147–159.
Kempler, D., Andersen, E. S., & Henderson, V. W. (1995). Linguistic and attentional contributions to anomia in Alzheimer's disease. *Neuropsychiatry, Neuropsychology, and Behavioural Neurology, 8*(1), 33–37.
Kendrick, D. C., Gibson, A. J., & Moyes, I. C. A. (1979). The revised Kendrick Battery: Clinical studies. *British*

Journal of Social and Clinical Psychology, 18, 329–340.

Kirk, A., & Kertesz, A. (1991). On drawing impairment in a Alzheimer's disease. *Archives of Neurology, 48*, 73–77.

Kittner, S. J., White, L. R., Farmer, M. E., Wolz, M, Kaplan, E., Moes, E., Brody, J. A., & Feinleib, M. (1986). Methodological issues in screening for dementia: The problem of education adjustment. *Journal of Chronic Diseases, 39*, 163–170.

Klesges, R. C., Wilkening, G. N., & Golden, C. J. (1981). Premorbid indices of intelligence: A review. *Clinical Neuropsychology, 3*, 32–39.

Knight, R. G., & Godfrey, H. P. D. (1984). Assessing the significance of differences between subtests on the Wechsler Adult Intelligence Scale-Revised. *Journal of Clinical Psychology, 40*, 808–810.

Knight, K. R., & Moroney, B. (1985). An investigation of the validity of the Kendrick Battery for the detection of dementia in the elderly. *International Journal of Clinical Psychology, 7*, 147–151.

Knight, R. G., & Shelton, E. J. (1983). Tables for evaluating predicted retest changes in Wechsler Adult Intelligence Scale scores. *British Journal of Clinical Psychology, 22*, 77–81.

Knopman, D. S., & Ryberg, S. (1989). A verbal memory test with high predictive accuracy for dementia of the Alzheimer type. *Archives of Neurology, 46*, 141–145.

Kopelman, M. D. (1985). Rates of forgetting in Alzheimer-type dementia and Korsakoff's syndrome. *Neuropsychologia, 23*, 623–638.

Kozora, E., & Cullum, C. M. (1995). Generative naming in normal aging: Total output and qualitative changes using phonemic and semantic constraints. *The Clinical Neuropsychologist, 9*, 313–320.

Kukull, W. A., Larson, E. B., Teri, L., Bowen, J., McCormick, W., & Pfanschmidt, M. L. (1994). The Mini-Mental State Examination score and the clinical diagnosis of dementia. *Journal of Clinical Epidemiology, 47*, 1061–1067.

Lachner, G., Satzger, W., & Engel, R. R. (1994). Verbal memory tests in the differential diagnosis of depression and dementia: discriminative power of seven test variations. *Archives of Clinical Neuropsychology, 9*, 1–13.

Leckliter, I. N., Matarazzo, J. D., & Silverstein, A. B. (1986). A literature review of factor analytic studies of the WAIS-R. *Journal of Clinical Psychology, 42*, 332–342.

Lee, G. P., Strauss, E., Loring, D. W., McCloskey, L., Haworth, J. M., & Lehman, R. A. W. (1997). Sensitivity of figural fluency on the Five Point Test to focal neurological dysfunction. *The Clinical Neuropsychologist, 11*, 59–68.

Lees, A. J., & Smith, E. (1983). Cognitive deficits in the early stages of Parkinson's disease. *Brain, 106*, 257–270.

Levin, B. E., Llabre, M. M., Reisman, S., Weiner, W. J., Sanchez Ramos, J., Singer, C., & Brown, M. C. (1991). Visuospatial impairment in Parkinson's disease. *Neurology, 41*, 365–369.

Lezak, M. D. (1983). *Neuropsychological assessment* (2nd ed.). New York: Oxford University Press.

Lezak, M. D. (1988a). Neuropsychological tests and assessment techniques. In F. Boller & J. Grafman (Eds.), *Handbook of neuropsychology* (Vol. 1, pp. 47–68). Amsterdam: Elsevier.

Lezak, M. D. (1988b). IQ: R.I.P. *Journal of Clinical & Experimental Neuropsychology, 10*, 351–361.

Lezak, M. D. (1991). Identifying neuropsychological deficits. In R. G. Lister & H. J. Weingartner (Eds.), *Perspectives on cognitive neuroscience* (pp. 357–367). New York: Oxford University Press.

Lezak, M. D. (1995). *Neuropsychological assessment* (3rd ed.). New York: Oxford University Press.

Light, L. L. (1992). The organization of memory in old age. In F. I. Craik & T. A. Salthouse (Eds.), *The handbook of aging and cognition* (pp. 111–166). Hillsdale, NJ: Erlbaum.

Lindenberger, U., & Baltes, P. B. (1994). Sensory functioning and intelligence in old age: A strong connection. *Psychology and Aging, 3*, 339–355.

Logsdon, R. G., Teri, L., Williams, D. E., Vitiello, M. V., & Prinz, P. N. (1989). The WAIS-R profile: a diagnostic tool for Alzheimer's disease? *Journal of Clinical and Experimental Neuropsychology, 11*, 892–898.

Magni, E., Binetti, G., Bianchetti, A., Rozzini, R., & Trabucchi, M. (1996). Mini Mental State Examination. A normative study in Italian elderly population. *European Journal of Neurology, 3*(3), 198–202.

Malec, J. F., Ivnik, B. J., Smith, G. E., Tangalos, G. G. (1992). Mayo's older American normative studies: Utility of corrections for age and education for the WAIS-R. *The Clinical Neurospychologist, 6* (Suppl.), 31–47.

Martin, A., Wiggs, C. L., Lalonde, F., & Mack, C. (1994). Word retrieval to letter and semantic cues: a double dissociation in normal subjects using interference tasks. *Neuropsychologia, 32*, 1487–1494.

Massman, P. J., & Bigler, E. D. (1993). A quantitative review of the diagnostic utililty of the WAIS-R Fuld profile. *Archives of Clinical Neuropsychology, 8*, 417–428.

Matarazzo, J. D., Daniel, M. H., Prifitera, A., & Herman, D. O. (1988). Inter-subtest scatter in the WAIS-R standardization sample. *Journal of Clinical Psychology, 44*, 940–950.

Matarazzo, J.D., & Herman, D. O. (1985). Clinical uses of the WAIS-R: Base rates of differences between VIQ and PIQ in the WAIS-R standardisation sample. In B. Wolman (Ed.), *Handbook of intelligence: Theories, measurement and applications* (pp. 899–932). New York: Wiley.

Mattis, S. (1976). Mental status examination for organic mental syndrome in the elderly patient. In L. Bellack & T. B. Karasu (Eds.), *Geriatric psychiatry* (pp. 77–121). New York: Grune & Stratton.

Mattis, S. (1988). *Dementia Rating Scale*. Odessa, FL: Psychological Assessment Resources.

Maxwell, A. E. (1960). Obtaining factor scores on the Wechsler Adult Intelligence Scale. *Journal of Mental Science, 106*, 1060–1062.

Mayes, A., & Warburg, R. (1990). Memory assessment in clinical practice and research. In J. R. Crawford, D. M. Parker, & W. W. McKinlay (Eds.), *A handbook of neuropsychological assessment* (pp. 73–101). Hove, UK: Erlbaum.

Maylor, E. A. (1990). Recognizing and naming faces. Aging, memory retrieval, and the tip of the tongue state. *Journal of Gerontology, 45*(6), 215–226.

McCarthy, R. A., & Warrington, E. K. (1986). Visual associative agnosia: A clinico-anatomical study of a single case. *Journal of Neurology, Neurosurgery and Psychiatry, 49*, 1233–1240.

McKinlay, W. W. (1992). Assessment of the head-injured for compensation. In J. R. Crawford, D. M. Parker, & W. W. McKinlay (Eds.), *A handbook of neuropsychological assessment* (pp. 381–392). Hove, UK: Erlbaum.

McLean, J. E., Reynolds, C. R., & Kaufman, A. S. (1990). WAIS-R subtest scatter using the profile variability index. *Psychological Assessment: A Journal of Consulting and Clinical Psychology, 2*, 289–292.

McSweeny, A. J., Naugle, R. I., Chelune, G. J., & Lüders, H. (1993). "T Scores for Change": an illustration of a regression approach to depicting change in clinical neuropsychology. *The Clinical Neuropsychologist, 7*, 300–312.

Miceli, G., Caltagirone, C., Gainotti, G., Masullo, C., & Silveri, M. C. (1981). Neuropsychological correlates of localized cerebral lesions in nonaphasic brain-damaged patients. *Journal of Clinical Neuropsychology, 3*, 53–63.

Miller, E. (1984). Verbal fluency as a function of a measure of verbal intelligence and in relation to different types of cerebral pathology. *British Journal of Clinical Psychology, 23*, 53–57.

Miller, E. (1992). Some basic principles of neuropsychological assessment. In J. R. Crawford, D. M. Parker, & W. W. McKinlay (Eds.), *A handbook of neuropsychological assessment* (pp. 7–20). Hove, UK: Lawrence Erlbaum.

Milner, B. (1964). Some effects of frontal lobectomy in man. In J. M. Warren & K. Alkert (Eds.), *The frontal granular cortex and behaviour* (pp. 313–331). New York: McGraw-Hill.

Mitrushina, M., & Satz, P. (1995). Repeated testing of normal elderly with the Boston Naming Test. *Aging: Clinical and Experimental Research, 7*(2), 123–127.

Mittenberg, W., Seidenberg, M., O'Leary, D. S., & DiGiulio, D. V. (1989). Changes in cerebral functioning associated with normal aging. *Journal of Clinical and Experimental Neuropsychology, 11*, 918–932.

Montgomery, K., & Costa, L. (1973). *Neuropsychological test performance of a normal elderly sample.* Paper presented at the Annual Meeting of the International Neuropsychological Society, Mexico City, Mexico.

Montgomery, K. M. (1982). *A normative study of neuropsychological test performance of a normal elderly sample.* Unpublished Master's thesis, University of Victoria, British Columbia, Canada.

Monti, L. A., Reminger, S. L., Gabrieli, J. D. E., Rinaldi, J. A., Wilson, R. S., & Fleischman, D. A. (1996). Differential effects of aging and Alzheimer's disease on conceptual implicit and explicit memory. *Neuropsychology, 10*, 101–112.

Morris, J. C., Heyman, A., Mohs, R. C., Hughes, J. P., van Belle, G., Fillenbaum, G., Mellits, E. D., & Clark, C. (1989). The consortium to establish a registry for Alzheimer's disease (CERAD) 1. Clinical and neuropsychological assessment of Alzheimer's disease. *Neurology, 39*, 1159–1165.

Mountain, M. A., & Snow, W. G. (1993). Wisconsin Card Sorting Test as a measure of frontal pathology: A review. *The Clinical Neuropsychologist, 7*, 108–118.

Nebes, R. D., Brady, C. G., & Huff, F. J. (1989). Automatic and attentional mechanisms of semantic priming in Alzheimer's disease. *Journal of Clinical and Experimental Neuropsychology, 11*, 219–230.

Neils, J., Brennan, M. M., Cole, M., Boller, F., & Gerdeman, B. (1988). The use of phonemic cueing with Alzheimer's disease patients. *Neuropsychologia, 26*, 351–354.

Nelson, H. E. (1990). Review of the Recognition Memory Test. In J. R. Beech & L. Harding (Eds.), *Assessment of the elderly* (pp. 126–127). Windsor, UK: NFER-Nelson.

Nelson, H. E., & O'Connell, A. (1978). Dementia: the estimation of pre-morbid intelligence levels using the new adult reading test. *Cortex, 14*, 234–244.

Nelson, H. E., & Willison, J. (1991). *National Adult Reading Test manual* (2nd ed.). Windsor: NFER-Nelson.

Newcombe, F. (1969). *Missile wounds of the brain: A study of psychological deficits.* London: Oxford University Press.

Newcombe, F., Oldfield, R. C., Ratcliff, G. G., & Wingfield, A. (1971). Recognition and naming of object-drawing by men with focal brain wounds. *Journal of Neurology, Neurosurgery and Psychiatry, 34*, 329–340.

Nicholas, M., Obler, L., Albert, M., & Goodglass, H. (1985). Lexical retrieval in healthy aging. *Cortex, 21*, 595–606.

Obler, L., & Albert, M. (1978). *Action Naming Test.* (Experimental ed.). Boston: VA Medical Center.

Obler, L. K., & Albert, M. L. (1985). Language skills across adulthood. In J. Birren & K. W. Schaie (Eds.), *The psychology of aging* (pp. 134–156). New York: Van Nostrand Reinhold.

Obler, L., Albert, M., & Goodglass, H. (1981). *Word finding difficulties in aging and dementia.* Paper presented at the Proceedings of the Gerontology Society of America Meetings. Toronto, ON.

O'Brien, J. T., & Levy, R. (1992). Age associated memory impairment. *British Medical Journal, 304*, 5–6.

O'Carroll, R. (1995). The assessment of premorbid ability: A critical review: *Neurocase, 1*, 83–89.

O'Carroll, R. E., & Badenoch, L. D. (1994). The inter-rater reliability of the Wechsler Memory Scale-Revised Visual Memory test. *British Journal of Clinical Psychology, 33*, 208–210.

O'Carroll, R. E., Baikie, E. M., & Whittick, J. E. (1987). Does the National Adult Reading Test hold in dementia? *British Journal of Clinical Psychology, 26*, 315–316.

O'Carroll, R. E., Conway, S., Ryman, A., & Prentice, N. (1997). Performance on the Delayed Word Recall Test (DWR) fails to clearly differentiate between depression and Alzheimer's disease in the elderly. *Psychological Medicine, 27*, 967–971.

O'Carroll, R. E., Curran, S. M., Ross, M., Murray, C., Riddle, W., Moffoot, A. P. R., Ebmeier, K. P., & Goodwin, G. M. (1994). The differentiation of major depression from dementia of the Alzheimer-type using within-subject neuropsychological discrepancy analysis. *British Journal of Clinical Psychology, 33*, 23–32.

Orgass, B. (1976). Eine Revision des Token Test II. Validitatsnachweis, Normierung und Standardisierung. *Diagnostica, 22*, 141–156.

Osterreith, P. A. (1944). Le test de copie d'une figure complexe. *Archives de Psychologie, 30*, 206–256.

Paolo, A. M., & Ryan, J. J. (1995). Selecting WAIS-R norms for persons 75 years and older. *The Clinical Neuropsychologist, 9*, 44–49.

Parker, D. M., & Crawford, J. R. (1992). Assessment of frontal lobe function. In J. R. Crawford, D. M. Parker, & W. W. McKinlay (Eds.), *A handbook of neuropsychological assessment* (pp. 267–291). Hove, UK: Lawrence Erlbaum.

Patterson, K., Graham, N., & Hodges, J. R. (1994). Reading in dementia: A preserved ability? *Neuropsychology, 8*, 395–407.

Pauker, J. D. (1988). Constructing overlapping cell tables to maximise the clinical usefulness of normative test data: rationale and an example from neuropsychology. *Journal of Clinical Psychology, 44*, 930–933.

Payne, R. W., & Jones, G. (1957). Statistics for the investigation of individual cases. *Journal of Clinical Psychology, 13*, 115–121.

Peaker, A., & Stewart, L. E. (1989). Rey's Auditory Verbal Learning Test: A review. In J. R. Crawford & D. M. Parker (Eds.), *Developments in clinical and experimental neuropsychology* (pp. 219–236). New York: Plenum.

Pentore, R., & Venneri, A. (1994). Visuo-spatial neglect in Alzheimer's disease. *Journal of Neurology, 241*(Suppl. 1), 57–58.

Perret, E. (1974). The left frontal lobe of man and the suppression of habitual responses in verbal categorical behaviour. *Neuropsychologia, 12*, 323–330.

Perry, E. K., Tomlinson, B. E., Blessed, G., Bergmann, K., Gibson, P. H., & Perry, R. H. (1978). Correlation of cholinergic abnormalities with senile plaques and mental test scores in senile dementia. *British Medical Journal, 2*, 1457–1459.

Pi, J., Olive, J. M., & Esteban, M. (1994). Mini Mental State examination: Association of the score obtained with the age and degree of alphabetization in an elderly population. *Medicina Clinica, 103*(17), 641–644.

Poppelreuter, W. (1917). *Die psychischen Schadigungen durch Kopfschuss im Kriege.* Leipzig: Leopold Voss.

Posner, M. I., & Petersen, S. E. (1990). The attention system of the human brain. *Annual Review of Neuroscience, 13*, 25–42.

Pratt, M. W., Boyes, C., Robins, S., & Manchester, J. (1989). Telling tales: Aging, working memory, and the narrative cohesion of story retellings. *Developmental Psychology, 25*, 628–635.

Rabbitt, P. (1990). Applied cognitive gerontology: Some problems, methodologies and data. *Applied Cognitive Psychology, 4*, 225–246.

Rabbitt, P. M. A. (1968). Channel capacity, intelligibility and immediate memory. *Quarterly Journal of Experimental Psychology, 20*, 241–248.

Reitan, R. M. (1986). Theoretical and methodological bases of the Halstead-Reitan Test Battery. In I. Grant & K. M. Adams (Eds.), *Neuropsychological assessment of neuropsychiatric disorders* (pp. 3–30). New York: Oxford University Press.

Reitan, R. M., & Wolfson, D. (1994). A selective and critical review of neuropsychological deficits and the frontal lobes. *Neuropsychology Review, 4*, 161–198.

Rey, A. (1964). *L'examen clinique en psychologie*. Paris: Presses Universitaires de France.

Reynolds, C. R., Willson, V. L., & Clark, P. L. (1983). A four-test short form of the WAIS-R for clinical screening. *Clinical Neuropsychology, 5*, 111–116.

Richards, P. M., & Ruff, R. M. (1989). Motivational effects on neuropsychological functioning: Comparison of depressed versus nondepressed individuals. *Journal of Consulting and Clinical Psychology, 57*, 396–402.

Ripich, D. N., & Terrell, B. Y. (1988). Patterns of discourse: Cohesion and coherence in Alzheimer's disease. *Journal of Speech and Hearing Disorders, 53*, 8–15.

Robbins, T. W., Joyce, E. M., & Sahakian, B. J. (1992). Neuropsychology and imaging. In E. S. Paykel (Ed.), *Handbook of affective disorders* (2nd ed., pp. 289–309). Edinburgh, UK: Churchill Livingstone.

Robertson, I. H., Ward, T., Ridgeway, V., & Nimmo-Smith, I. (1994). *The Test of Everyday Attention*. Bury St. Edmunds, UK: Thames Valley Test Company.

Robertson, I. H., Ward, T., Ridgeway, V., & Nimmo-Smith, I. (1996). The structure of normal human attention: The Test of Everyday Attention. *Journal of the International Neuropsychological Society, 2*, 525–534.

Rosen, W. G., Mohs, R. C., & Davis, K. L. (1984). A new rating scale for Alzheimer's disease. *American Journal of Psychiatry, 141*, 1356–1364.

Roth, M., Tym, E., Mountjoy, C. Q., Huppert, F. A., Hendrie, J., Verma, S., & Goddard, R. (1986). CAMDEX: A standardized instrument for the diagnosis of mental disorder in the elderly with special reference to the early detection of dementia. *British Journal of Psychiatry, 149*, 698–709.

Ruff, R. M. (1988). *Ruff Figural Fluency Test administration manual*. San Franscisco: Neuropsychological Resources.

Ruff, R. M., Allen, C. C., Farrow, C. E., Nieemann, H., & Wylie, T. (1994). Figural fluency: Differential impairment in patients with left versus right frontal lobe lesions. *Archives of Clinical Neuropsychology, 9*, 41–56.

Ruff, R. M., Evans, R., & Marshall, L. F. (1986). Impaired verbal and figural fluency after head injury. *Archives of Clinical Neuropsychology, 1*, 87–102.

Ruff, R. M., Light, R. H., & Evans, R. (1987). The Ruff Figural Fluency Test: A normative study with adult. *Developmental Neuropsychology, 3*, 37–51.

Ruff, R. M., Light, R. H., Parker, S. B., & Levin, H. S. (1996). Benton Controlled Oral Word Association Test: Reliability and updated norms. *Archives of Clinical Neuropsychology, 11*, 329–338.

Ryan, J. J., & Paolo, A. M. (1992). Base rates of intersubtest scatter in the old age standardization sample of the WAIS-R. *Archives of Clinical Neuropsychology, 7*, 515–522.

Ryan, J. J., Paolo, A. M., & Brungardt, T. M. (1990). Standardization of the Wechsler Adult Intelligence Scale-Revised for persons 75 years and older. *Psychological Assessment, 2*, 404–411.

Salthouse, T. A. (1988). Effects of aging on verbal abilities: Examination of the psychometric literature. In L. L. Light & D. M. Burke (Eds.), *Language, memory, and aging* (pp. 17–35). Cambridge: Cambridge University Press.

Savage, R. D., Britton, P. G., Bolton, N., & Hall, E. H. (1973). *Intellectual functioning in the aged*. London: Methuen.

Schlosser, D., & Ivison, D. (1989). Assessing memory deterioration with the Wechsler Memory Scale, the National Adult Reading Test, and the Schonell Graded Word Reading Test. *Journal of Clinical and Experimental Neuropsychology, 11*, 785–792.

Schneider, L. S. (1996). An overview of rating scales used in dementia research. *Alzheimer Insights, 2*(3), 1–7.

Schonfield, A. E. D. (1980). Learning, memory and aging. In J. E. Birren & R. B. Sloane (Eds.), *Handbook of mental health and aging* (pp. 214–244). Englewood Cliffs, NJ: Prentice-Hall.

Shallice, T., & Burgess, P. W. (1991). Deficits in strategy application following frontal lobe damage in man. *Brain, 114*, 727–741.

Shapiro, M. B. (1973). Intensive assessment of the single case. In P. E. Mittler (Ed.), *The psychological assessment of mental and physical handicaps* (pp. 645–666). London: Tavistock.

Sharpe, K., & O'Carroll, R. (1991). Estimating premorbid intellectual level in dementia using the National Adult Reading Test: A Canadian study. *British Journal of Clinical Psychology, 30*, 381–384.

Shimamura, A. P. (1994). Neuropsychological perspectives on memory and cognitive decline in normal human aging. *The Neurosciences, 6*, 387–394.

Silverstein, A. B. (1982). Pattern analysis as simultaneous statistical inference. *Journal of Consulting and Clinical Psychology, 50*, 234–240.

Silverstein, A. B. (1984). Pattern analysis: The question of abnormality. *Journal of Consulting and Clinical Psychology, 52*, 936–939.

Snow, W. G., Tierney, M. C., Zorzitto, M. L., Fisher, R. H., & Reid, D. W. (1989). WAIS-R test-retest reliability in a normal elderly sample. *Journal of Clinical and Experimental Neuropsychology, 11*, 423–428.

Spreen, O., & Strauss, E. (1991). *A compendium of neuropsychological tests. Administration, norms, and commentary*. New York: Oxford University Press.

Squire, L. R. (1987). *Memory and brain*. Oxford: Oxford University Press.

Stebbins, G. T., Wilson, R. S., Gilley, D. W., Bernard, B. A., & Fox, J. H. (1988). Use of the National Adult Reading Test to estimate premorbid IQ in dementia. *The Clinical Neuropsychologist, 4*, 18–24.

Street, R. F. (1931). *A Gestalt Completion Test*. New York: Bureau of Publications, Teachers College, Columbia University.

Sweet, J. J., Newman, P., & Bell, B. (1992). Significance of depression in clinical neuropsychological assessment. *Clinical Psychology Review, 12*, 21–45.

Tombaugh, T. N., & McIntyre, N. J. (1992). The Mini Mental State Examination. A comprehensive review. *Journal of American Geriatrics Society, 40*(9), 922–935.

Trenerry, M. R., Crosson, B., DeBoe, J., & Leber, W. R. (1989). *Stroop Neuropsychological Screening Test Manual*. Odessa, FL: Psychological Assessment Resources Inc.

Tuokko, H., & Woodward, T. S. (1996). Development and validation of a demographic correction system for neuropsychological measures used in the Canadian Study of Health and Aging. *Journal of Clinical and Experimental Neuropsychology, 18*, 479–616.

Uhlmann, R. F., & Larson, E. B. (1991). Effect of education on the Mini-Mental State Examination as a screening test for dementia. *Journal of American Geriatric Society, 39*, 876–880.

Van Gorp, W. G., Satz, P., Kiersch, M. E., & Henry, R. (1986). Normative data on the Boston Naming Test for a group of normal older adults. *Journal of Clinical and Experimental Neuropsychology, 8*, 702–705.

Villardita, C., Cultrera, S., Cupone, V., & Mejia, R. (1985). Neuropsychological test performances and normal aging. *Archives of Gerontology and Geriatrics, 4*, 311–319.

Walsh, K. W. (1991). *Understanding brain damage: A primer of neuropsychological evaluation.* (2nd ed.). Edinburgh, Scotland: Churchill Livingstone.

Warrington, E. K. (1984). *Recognition memory test.* Windsor: Nelson.

Warrington, E. K., & Taylor, A. M. (1973). Contribution of the right parietal lobe to object recognition. *Cortex, 9*, 152–164.

Wechsler, D. (1981). *Wechsler Adult Intelligence Scale-Revised.* New York: The Psychological Corporation.

Wechsler, D. (1987). *Wechsler Memory Scale-Revised.* New York: The Psychological Corporation.

Weingartner, H. (1984). Psychobiological determinants of memory failures. In L. R. Squire & N. M. Butters (Eds.), *Neuropsychology of Memory* (pp. 203–212). New York: Guildford Press.

Weingartner, H. (1986). Automatic and effort-demanding cognitive processes in depression. In L. W. Poon (Ed.), *Handbook for clinical memory assessment of older adults* (pp. 218–225). Washington, DC: American Psychological Association.

Weingartner, H., Cohen, R. M., Bunney, W. E., Ebert, M. H., & Kaye, W. (1982). Memory-learning impairments in progressive dementia and depression. *American Journal of Psychiatry, 139*, 135–136.

Weingartner, H., Cohen, R. M., Murphy, D. L., Martello, J., & Gerdt, C. (1981). Cognitive processes in depression. *Archives of General Psychiatry, 38*, 42–47.

Welsh, K. A., Butters, N., Hughes, J. P., Mohs, R. C., & Heyman, A. (1992). Detection and staging of dementia in Alzheimer's disease. Use of the neuropsychological measures developed for the consortium to establish a registry for Alzheimer's disease. *Archives of Neurology, 49*, 448–452.

Wilson, B. A., Alderman, N., Burgess, P., Emslie, H., & Evans, J. J. (1996). *Behavioural Assessment of the Dysexcutive Syndrome.* Bury St Edmunds, England: Thames Valley Test Company.

Wilson, B. A., Cockburn, J., & Halligan, P. (1987). *Behavioural Inattention Test.* Bury St. Edmunds, UK: Thames Valley Test Company.

Wilson, B. A., Cockburn, J. M., Baddeley, A. D., & Hiorns, R. (1989). The development and validation of a test battery for detecting and monitoring everyday memory problems. *Journal of Clinical and Experimental Neuropsychology, 11*, 855–870.

Wilson, B. A., Evans, J. J., Emslie, H., Alderman, N., & Burgess, P. (in press). The development of an ecologically valid test for assessing patients with a dysexecutive syndrome. *Neuropsychological Rehabilitation.*

Wilson, R. S., Rosenbaum, G., Brown, G., Rourke, D., Whitman, D., & Grisell, J. (1978). An index of premorbid intelligence. *Journal of Consulting and Clinical Psychology, 46*, 1554–1555.

Woods, R. T., & Britton, P. G. (1985). *Clinical psychology with the elderly.* London: Croom Helm.

Zachary, R. A., & Gorsuch, R. L. (1985). Continuous norming: Implications for the WAIS-R. *Journal of Clinical Psychology, 41*, 86–94.

7.08
Anxiety Disorders

MELINDA A. STANLEY
University of Texas Medical School, Houston, TX, USA
and
J. GAYLE BECK
State University of New York at Buffalo, NY, USA

7.08.1 INTRODUCTION

Significant progress has been made since the late 1960s with regard to understanding and treating anxiety disorders (Barlow, 1988; Beidel & Turner, 1991). It is now well known that these conditions can have a profound impact on social and occupational functioning, and lifetime prevalence rates have indicated that anxiety disorders are one of the two most common forms of psychiatric disturbance (Robins et al, 1984). The body of knowledge currently available regarding anxiety disorders, however, is focused largely on the younger adult population. Although the need to expand this work to older adults has been emphasized repeatedly (Cartensen, 1988; Hersen & Van Hasselt, 1992; Salzman & Lebowitz, 1991), very little attention had been paid to the nature and treatment of anxiety disorders in this segment of the population. In the late 1990s, a small body of literature has begun to accumulate (Beck & Stanley, 1997; Stanley & Beck, in press). This work will be reviewed here, with particular focus on the prevalence, onset and associated risk factors, psychopathology and differential diagnosis, measurement, and treatment of anxiety in elderly people.

7.08.2 PREVALENCE

7.08.2.1 Anxiety Disorders

The National Institute of Mental Health (NIMH) Epidemiological Catchment Area (ECA) survey documented a one-month prevalence rate of 5.5% for anxiety disorders in older adults (age 65 years or older) (Regier et al., 1988; Regier, Narrow, & Rae, 1990). This figure is slightly lower than the 7.3% rate noted for younger adults, a pattern that mirrors another epidemiological report from Canada (Bland, Newman, & Orn, 1988). Although these figures suggest gradually decreasing rates of clinical anxiety disorders over the life span, they nonetheless indicate that anxiety in elderly people is a significant mental health problem. In fact, in the ECA study, anxiety disorders occurred more than twice as often as affective disorders in older adults, with a frequency four to eight times greater than major depression (Regier et al., 1988; Weissmann et al., 1985). Given the significant attention that has already been focused on depression as a major health problem in the elderly (Reynolds, Lebowitz, & Schneider, 1993), the ECA data emphasize the need for further study of older adults with anxiety problems, particularly those with symptoms which interfere with daily functioning.

The majority of anxiety disorders assigned to older adults within the ECA survey were classified as phobias (4.8%), including agoraphobia, social phobia, and simple phobia. Much lower prevalence rates were documented for obsessive-compulsive disorder (OCD; 0.8%) and panic disorder (PD; 0.1%). At the Yale University site, wherein older adults were oversampled, prevalence rates were similar (Weissmann et al., 1985). In particular, six-months figures showed an overall rate of 4.6% for anxiety disorders among elderly people, again with the majority classified as patients with phobic disorders (3.9%) and many fewer individuals with OCD (0.7%) or PD (0.1%). Additional analyses of the New Haven data indicated that prevalence rates were higher among homebound elderly people (that is, those confined to homes, beds, or chairs) relative to community residents with more freedom of movement, although these differences may have been related to poorer physical health status among the homebound individuals (Bruce & McNamara, 1992).

Even though the ECA data suggested that anxiety disorders pose a significant mental health problem for elderly people, it is important to note that these figures may have underestimated the percentage of older adults with significant anxiety problems. First, many individuals in this age group tend to underreport or deny psychological symptoms (Lasoski; 1986; Oxman, Barrett, Barrett, & Gerber, 1987). Second, prevalence figures were based on interviews with individuals residing in the community, and it has been demonstrated that rates of anxiety disorders may be much higher among institutionalized elderly people (Bland et al., 1988). Given the significant percentage of elders who reside in institutionalized settings, prevalence figures may seriously underrepresent the scope of anxiety disorders in older populations. Finally, Wave 1 of the survey, which produced the overall 5.5% rate, failed to consider prevalence of post-traumatic stress disorder (PTSD) and generalized anxiety disorder (GAD). GAD was excluded because it had not been recognized as a distinct psychiatric disorder at the time (American Psychiatric Association, 1980). Wave 2 of the study, however, which occurred approximately one year later, queried a subset of the original participants about the symptoms of PTSD and GAD. Only total population estimates for PTSD have been published (Helzer, Robins, & McEvoy, 1987), but six-month and lifetime prevalence rates of 1.9% and 4.6% were noted for GAD in the elderly (Blazer, George, & Hughes, 1991). These rates, although striking as they are presented, also may have underestimated the true prevalence of GAD given that hierarchical diagnostic criteria required exclusion of GAD if any other *Diagnostic and statistical manual of mental disorders* (*3rd ed.*) (*DSM-III*) diagnosis was present. As such, all individuals with diagnoses of major depression or PD, for example, who may also have met criteria for GAD, were not included in the published prevalence rates.

In addition to the data provided by the ECA study, at least seven other random sample community surveys from the US, Canada, and the UK have provided prevalence figures for anxiety problems in older adults (defined here as age 60 years or older; see review by Flint, 1994). Some of these studies surveyed all adults over age 18 but reported separate prevalence figures for older and younger groups, while others examined anxiety only in elderly samples. Across the studies, overall prevalence rates for anxiety disorders ranged from 0.7% to 18.6%. Figures presented separately for specific groups of disorders varied as follows: phobic disorders, 0.0%–10.0%; GAD, 0.7%–7.1%; OCD, 0.0%–1.5%; and PD, 0.1%–1.0% (Flint, 1994). These data generally are consistent with ECA findings that phobias and GAD are most common, although specific figures varied widely given the range of survey methods, case definitions, and diagnostic procedures used to establish diagnoses. For example, some diagnoses were based on self-report measures and others on semistructured clinical interviews. Some studies utilized widely accepted standards for case definition, while others relied on more idiosyncratic diagnostic criteria. In light of these methodological variations, ECA data probably represent the best figures currently available to estimate the prevalence of anxiety disorders in elderly people, despite criticisms that have been leveled at ECA methodology including variations in interview procedures at different sites, the use of lay interviewers rather than trained clinicians, and low sensitivity for diagnostic procedures (Beidel & Turner, 1991; McNally, 1994).

7.08.2.2 Anxiety Symptoms

Another collection of studies has addressed the prevalence of distressing anxiety symptoms in elderly people rather than anxiety disorder diagnoses *per se*. These reports have assessed the frequency and/or severity of symptoms using standardized self-report inventories such as the Hopkins Symptom Checklist (Derogatis, Lipman, Rickels, Uhlenhuth, & Covi, 1973) and the State-Trait Anxiety Inventory (Spielberger, Gorsuch, & Lushene, 1970). In these surveys, cut-off scores based on standard deviations from mean scores in normal and psychiatric samples of older adults were established to define cases of elevated anxiety. This type of methodology has suggested that up to 20% of elderly people in the community report significant levels of anxiety (Feinsen & Thoits, 1986; Himmelfarb & Murrell, 1984). Significant anxiety has also been reported for 8–11% of elders assessed in primary care settings in both the US (Oxman et al., 1987) and Hong Kong (Wong & Pan, 1994). When relevant comparisons have been made, patterns again fail to confirm the notion of increasing anxiety over the life span given lower prevalence of distressing anxiety in older than younger adults (Feinsen & Thoits, 1986; Oxman et al., 1987). Although these figures disallow differential diagnosis that would separate anxiety symptoms resulting from various medical and/or psychiatric conditions (see Section 7.08.4), they nonetheless confirm that a substantial number of elders report distressing anxiety symptoms.

7.08.3 ONSET AND ASSOCIATED RISK FACTORS

7.08.3.1 Age of Onset

It has been suggested from the younger adult literature that age of onset for anxiety disorders may be based at least to some degree on developmental stage (Beidel & Turner, 1991). For example, the onset of specific phobias seems to mirror the progression of developmentally appropriate normal fears through childhood; that is, animal phobias are often first noticed between the ages of four and seven, when animal fears are common (Marks & Gelder, 1996; Ost, 1987), and phobias of natural disasters and health-related situations frequently begin among older elementary school children at the ages when these fears are commonly reported (Barrios, Hartmann, & Shigetomi, 1981). Likewise, the age of onset for social phobia is typically in early to late adolescence when the establishment of social relationships is a critical developmental task (Beidel & Turner, 1991). These patterns suggest that some phobias reported by older adults may represent fears which originated in earlier developmental stages and continued through later adulthood, while others may have developed more recently from concerns that are developmentally appropriate for older adults, for example, fears of falling (Downton & Andrews, 1990). In fact, available data regarding age of onset for phobias in elderly people are mixed, suggesting the possibility of varying periods of onset for different fears. In a British survey of older adults, Lindesay (1991) reported that specific phobias generally had their onset during childhood, a finding that is consistent with data from the younger adult literature (Thyer, Parrish, Curtis, Nesse, & Cameron, 1985). Alternatively, data from the the US ECA study implied that many phobias reported by older adults were of recent onset (Eaton et al., 1989). Similarly, Lindesay reported that agoraphobic fears (e.g., of enclosed places crowds, public transportation, going away from home) among elderly people most often were of recent onset. However, many of these "agoraphobic" fears began after an episode of physical illness or trauma. As such, the fears may have represented realistic or excessive fears of physical limitations rather than anticipation of panic, suggesting that a diagnosis of specific phobia might have been more appropriate for consideration than agoraphobia (see McNally (1994) for a discussion of this diagnostic issue in younger adults). In addition, a high incidence of depression in Lindesay's sample suggested that "agoraphobic" fears may have been associated with a social withdrawal characteristic of a depressive clinical picture (Flint, 1994).

In light of these inconsistent findings and important differential diagnosis issues, as well as the influential role played by developmental stages in the origin of phobias, further investigation is needed to understand patterns of onset for different types of phobias reported by elderly people. In this area, the important differentiation of realistic versus excessive fear is central, particularly given developmentally appropriate fears that may be characteristic of normal aging.

The age of onset for GAD among elderly people appears to have a bimodal distribution. In Wave 2 of the US ECA study, 39% of participants reported duration of GAD for 21 years or more (Blazer et al., 1991). For these individuals, GAD may have been conceptualized best as a personality disturbance rather than an Axis I disorder, a perspective that has received some attention in the literature of the 1990s (Sanderson & Wetzler, 1991). For another 52% of participants, the onset of GAD was reported within five years of the interview. For this subset of older adults, GAD may have begun as a reaction to stressful life events, a pattern that has been documented in both younger and older adults (Blazer, Hughes, & George, 1987; Ganzini, McFarland, & Culter, 1990). In particular, younger adult men and women interviewed in Wave 2 of the ECA survey experienced a threefold increase in risk for GAD in the year following one or more unexpected, negative, and important life events (Blazer et al., 1987). In a separate sample of older adults, an increased incidence of GAD was reported during the 20 months following a catastrophic financial loss (Ganzini et al., 1990). In this sample, 27% of participants reported symptoms meeting criteria for GAD during the postloss period relative to 10% of elders in a control sample during this same time.

A bimodal pattern of onset for GAD was also reported in a sample of older adults recruited for participation in a treatment study (Beck, Stanley, & Zebb, 1996a). A comparison of clinical features (e.g., anxiety, depression, specific fears) in patients with onset of GAD in childhood (before age 15) and those reporting onset in middle adulthood (after age 39) revealed very few differences. The impact of age of onset on treatment response was not studied, however, given inadequate sample sizes.

Given that prevalence rates for PD and OCD in older adults are quite low, few data are available to address the onset of these syndromes. Although ECA data indicated that neither of these disorders typically began in older age (Eaton et al., 1989), a retrospective chart review of 51 elderly clinic patients with panic disorder revealed that over half reported onset at age 60 years or later (Raj, Covea, & Dagon, 1993). Related case reports have also suggested that panic disorder may begin in later life (Luchins & Rose, 1989; Sheikh, King, & Taylor, 1991). However, conclusions about time and mode of onset for PD and OCD will require greater study.

The potential role of stressful life events in the development of anxiety in later life has already been noted (Ganzini et al., 1990). It has also been demonstrated in studies of Holocaust survivors and World War Two prisoners of war that stress-related symptoms of PTSD can persist into old age (Kluznick, Speed, Van Valkenberg, & Magraw, 1986; Kuch & Cox, 1992). However, no data are available regarding onset of PTSD in elderly people. Given the number of traumatic life events that can occur for older adults (e.g., elder abuse, muggings, motor vehicle accidents), onset of PTSD symptoms in later life is of significant interest and importance. Relevant to this issue are published findings suggesting that prior experience with trauma can serve to "inoculate" older adults against the anxiety-related effects of natural disasters (Norris & Murrell, 1988). The more general role of prior stress as a buffer against the development of PTSD in late life will need to be considered.

7.08.3.2 Associated Risk Factors

7.08.3.2.1 Gender

As has been shown repeatedly among younger adults, ECA data demonstrated that elderly women are at greater risk of experiencing anxiety disorders than elderly men, with a ratio of approximately 2:1 among adults over age 65 (Regier et al., 1988; Regier et al., 1990; Weissman et al., 1985). In a similar Canadian survey (Bland et al., 1988), older women residing in the community were 1.5 times more likely to be diagnosed with an anxiety disorder than men in the same age group. In an institutionalized subgroup of participants surveyed for this study, women were five times as likely to be assigned an anxiety disorder diagnosis as men. However, figures from both of these studies failed to address the prevalence and/or gender distribution of GAD. Two studies relevant to this issue have suggested that elderly women are approximately two to nine times more likely than elderly men to meet criteria for this disorder (Flint, 1994). In Wave 2 of the ECA survey, prevalence rates for GAD within gender were presented separately for black and nonblack participants (Blazer et al., 1991). These figures indicated that elderly black women were 12 times more likely to be assigned a diagnosis of GAD than black men in the same age group. Nonblack elderly women also were more likely to be diagnosed with GAD than their nonblack male counterparts, with a ratio of 4:1.

With regard to the prevalence of notable anxiety symptoms instead of disorders, women have also been identified more often than men to have significant anxiety according to preestablished cutoff scores on standardized self-report instruments (Himmelfarb & Murrell, 1984). Similarly, elderly women reported greater overall fearfulness than elderly men on a standardized measure of specific fears (Liddell, Lockes & Burman, 1991). Thus, epidemiological data overall indicate that women are at greater risk of experiencing problematic anxiety than men among the older adult population.

7.08.3.2.2 Ethnicity

Another potential risk factor for the experience of anxiety in elderly people is ethnicity, although the impact of this variable has been understudied. In the ECA survey, problems with sampling strategies for some minority groups were noted across all age groups (Beidel & Turner, 1991), making it difficult to draw even general conclusions from these data. Moreover, very few ECA data relevant to ethnicity have been provided separately by age. Among the elderly people interviewed through the New Haven site, Weissman et al. (1985) noted that rates of cognitive impairment were higher in blacks than whites, although other *DSM-III* disorders were less prevalent among blacks, relative to whites. However, no data were presented regarding the distribution of anxiety disorders among these groups. In Wave 2 of the survey, prevalence rates for GAD in elderly people were presented by both ethnicity and gender, as noted earlier, with figures suggesting the highest rate among black women (3.7%). Rates for the other groups were as follows: nonblack women (2.7%), black men (0.3%), and nonblack men (0.7%).

In studies examining prevalence rates for anxiety symptoms rather than disorders, nonsignificant correlations between ethnicity and anxiety severity have been reported (Feinson & Thoits, 1986; Himmelfarb & Murrell, 1984). However, in one of these reports, minority groups were underrepresented (Feinson & Thoits, 1986), and in the other, the ethnic distribution of the sample was unspecified (Himmelfarb & Murrell, 1984). Given the very limited data available to address this issue, as well as significant methodological problems evident in the reports that are accessible, the potential role of ethnicity as a risk factor for the experience of anxiety in later life is unclear and requires future study.

7.08.3.2.3 Other risk factors

Other potential risk factors for the experience of anxiety in elderly people relate to marital status, income, and level of education. In particular, fewer anxiety symptoms have been reported by married older adults relative to unmarried older persons, including all individuals not married at the time of assessment (Feinsen & Thoits, 1986). A more complicated interaction between marital status and gender was reported in another study, with highest levels of anxiety occurring among never-married men and the least amount of anxiety within a group of never-married women (Himmelfarb & Murrell, 1984). Significant negative correlations have also been noted between income and anxiety among the elderly (Feinsen & Thoits, 1986; Himmelfarb & Murrell, 1984; Liddell et al., 1991), and in some reports, between level of education and anxiety severity (Himmelfarb & Murrell, 1984; Liddell et al., 1991). In general, these patterns are similar to those reported in younger adults with anxiety disorders (Regier et al., 1990).

7.08.4 PSYCHOPATHOLOGY AND DIFFERENTIAL DIAGNOSIS

Significant advances have been made in understanding the nature and experience of anxiety in younger adults (see Barlow, 1988; Beidel & Turner, 1991; Rapee & Barlow, 1991 for reviews of this literature). However, whether this knowledge applies directly to the experience of anxiety among elderly people is unknown. Of crucial importance to this issue are descriptions of the specific nature of anxiety in older adults with and without psychiatric disorders, the relationship between anxiety and medical problems common in older adults, and the overlap between anxiety and sleep disturbance, depression, and cognitive impairment, in particular, memory. These issues are reviewed here.

7.08.4.1 Nature of Anxiety

A small body of literature has begun to address potential differences in the experience of anxiety across the life span. As noted earlier, the prevalence of anxiety disorders seems to decrease with age, but also of interest are potential differences in the qualitative experience of anxiety from younger to older adulthood. In one relevant empirical examination, Lawton, Kleban, and Dean (1993) examined potential differences in the factor structure and prevalence of affect across three age groups: younger adults (ages 18–30), middle-aged adults (ages 31–59), and older adults (age 60 and over). Although a six-factor structure was evident for each group in initial exploratory analyses, subsequent confirmatory analyses revealed differences in the loading sizes, factor correlations, and residual correlations across the three groups. The primary differences occurred between younger and older adults with regard to factors assessing positive affect and depression, but differences between these two groups were also evident on the anxiety-guilt factor. In particular, affect terms assessing guilt (e.g., ashamed, guilty, worried, blamed) were more salient to this factor for younger adults than for the older group. As suggested by the authors, this difference may indicate that older adults grew up before "guilt became fashionable" (p. 174). Consequently, they may experience anxiety more directly than younger adults who make cognitive connections between anxiety and guilt (Lawton et al., 1993). Other analyses revealed that older adults reported less of almost every negative emotional state, including anxiety, than participants in the other two groups. Fewer differences between groups were evident with regard to the experience of positive affect. These data suggest that affect terms may have different meanings across the life span and that the experience of anxiety may vary in important ways with age. As such, theoretical and empirical knowledge regarding the experience of anxiety among younger adults cannot be extrapolated directly to an older population.

Another group of studies has addressed the nature of fears and worries among older adults living in the community. As noted earlier, a developmental examination of normal fears is needed as a baseline against which to understand the experience of problematic anxiety. For older adults, as with individuals in any other age group, it is necessary to differentiate maladaptive anxiety from realistic fears that accompany a particular developmental stage, in this case, aging. It is also important, however, for practitioners not to overattribute anxiety and fears in elderly people to the normal aging process and in so doing, overlook or ignore treatable psychological symptoms (Weiss, 1994). In either case, the experience of anxiety as it accompanies the normal aging process needs to be understood clearly.

The majority of work addressing the nature of normal fears among elderly people has focused on worry, probably because generalized anxiety is one of the most common forms of anxiety in this age group (Blazer et al., 1991). In one community survey of adults ages 25–64, Person and Borkovec (1995) classified participants' worries or concerns into five categories: family–home–interpersonal, illness–health–injury, work–school, finances, and miscellaneous. Comparisons of worries reported by younger (age 25–64) and older (age 65 and over) adults revealed that elderly people worried most about health and least about work, whereas younger adults were most concerned about family and finances. These data suggested that worry content across age groups was representative of changing life circumstances. Similar findings were reported in another community survey of worries in younger and older adults (Powers, Wisocki, & Whitbourne, 1992). In particular, the elderly reported few worries overall, with significantly fewer worries about social events and financial issues than a college-age comparison group. Older adults worried most about health, although scores in this domain were not significantly different from the younger sample.

In an assessment study with 94 older adults characterized via semistructured interview to be free of any psychiatric diagnoses, scores on standardized self-report measures of worry, state and trait anxiety, specific fears, and obsessive-compulsive symptoms were significantly lower than normal mean scores reported in other samples of younger adults (Stanley, Beck, & Zebb, 1996). These data accentuate the need for age-appropriate norms to interpret scores on self-report measures of anxiety symptoms and are consistent with prior findings suggesting that severity of anxiety seems to decrease with age.

The fact that older age is not necessarily associated with increasing anxiety should not detract from the impact that problematic anxiety can have in this population. In one of the first studies to examine the clinical characteristics of anxiety disorders in elderly people, 44 older adults with GAD (diagnosed according to semistructured interview and *DSM-III-R* criteria) were compared with a sample free of psychiatric diagnoses who were equivalent with regard to age, gender, level of education, and ethnicity (Beck et al., 1996a). Analyses revealed that GAD was associated with increased levels of worry, anxiety, social fears, and depression, with scores on these measures comparable to younger samples of GAD patients. Similarly, Raj et al. (1993) reported that clinical characteristics of a group of elderly patients with PD were similar to those reported in younger samples with the same diagnosis. As such, although the overall severity and frequency of fears and worries may decrease over the life span, anxiety disorders appear to be associated with similar clinical features regardless of age. However, additional data with groups of elderly patients meeting criteria for various anxiety disorders are needed to replicate and expand these findings.

7.08.4.2 Anxiety and Medical Problems

The overlap between medical and psychological problems is a highly salient issue for practitioners working with older adults. In fact, it has been suggested that these two areas are so closely interwoven that treatment of mental health problems is impossible without knowledge of medical illnesses common among the elderly (Frazer, 1995). As noted by Frazer, the relationship between physical and psychological symptoms or disorders can occur for at least three reasons: medical illnesses can mimic and/or cause psychological difficulties, the two types of symptoms can coexist, and psychological disturbance can potentially leave one vulnerable for development of physical difficulties. Katz (1996), in a 1995 presidential address to the American Association for Geriatric Psychiatry, noted that the significant degree of interrelatedness between psychological and medical difficulties among elderly people should serve a central role in the development of public policy and the design of health care services for the elderly. In this domain, a reasonable amount of attention has focused on the comorbidity between medical disease and depression (Katz, 1996), but less work has addressed the relationship between physical illness and anxiety.

It is of particular importance to consider the overlap of anxiety and medical disease, given that older adults often attribute anxiety-related symptoms such as agitation, fears, or aches and pains to physical illness, thereby denying or underreporting psychological difficulties (Gurian & Miner, 1991). Furthermore, a range of medical conditions can create anxiety-like symptoms, in particular, cardiovascular disease, chronic obstructive pulmonary disease, hyperthyroidism, and visual and auditory impairments. (Cohen, 1991). Limited empirical data have addressed the nature of the overlap between physical illness and anxiety, although a few studies have explored the prevalence of anxiety symptoms in samples of older adults presenting to medical clinics or hospitals.

As noted earlier, prevalence rates of 8–11% for anxiety disorders were reported among elderly outpatients (age 55 years and over) in a rural US group practice (Oxman et al., 1987). Case identification in this study was based on symptom checklist scores that were at least two standard deviations above a mean. Given apparent differences in prevalence rates for anxiety in urban and rural settings (Blazer et al., 1991), along with the restricted ability of self-report inventories to identify diagnosable cases, the data from this report are somewhat limited. In another survey of Italian medical inpatients, 40% of adults over age 60 reported moderate to high levels of distress on an anxiety symptom checklist (Magni, Schifano, deDominicis, & Belloni, 1988). Severity of anxiety was not associated with the classification of medical problems as being acute or chronic, but scores on a phobia subscale were significantly higher for patients with central nervous system disturbances than for those with other diseases. Again, although these data provide an interesting pattern of results, conclusions are limited given reliance solely on a self-report symptom checklist to evaluate anxiety.

In two other studies, elderly medical patients were evaluated to examine the relationship between complaints of postural disturbance (dizziness, fear of falling) and anxiety. In one of these, 203 adults age 75 and over were recruited from four general medical practices in Manchester, UK (Downton & Andrews, 1990). In this sample, dizziness and fear of falling were associated with higher levels of anxiety, and symptoms were more severe for participants who had actually experienced a fall within the previous 12 months. It is interesting to note that 42% of the sample reported restricted activity due to fear of falling, a behavioral pattern that requires differentiation from agoraphobic fears reported in older adults (Beck & Stanley, 1997). In another report, 37.5% of 56 older adults (age 60 and over) who presented to a dizziness clinic were diagnosed with at least one *DSM-III-R* Axis I disorder (Sloane, Hartman, & Mitchell, 1994). The most frequent diagnoses in this group were anxiety disorders, depression, and adjustment disorders. Older adults with chronic dizziness also scored significantly higher on a symptom checklist of anxiety than a matched group of healthy adults. In a follow-up study of stroke survivors, prevalence rates of 5% and 19% for anxiety disorders were reported for elderly men and women at four months post-stroke (Burvill et al., 1995). When hierarchical rules for diagnosing *DSM-III* disorders were suspended, rates were 12% and 28% for men and women, respectively. Participants with anxiety disorders at the time of stroke were identified via retrospective interview. When these individuals were excluded, prevalence rates for men and women were 9% and 20%, figures that far outweigh general population estimates for older adults.

These data suggest that elderly patients presenting for medical treatment frequently have disturbing symptoms of anxiety. As such, it is important for medical practitioners to be aware of the signs and symptoms of anxiety and to provide appropriate treatment or referrals when needed. Likewise, it is important for mental health care providers to be cognizant of medical causes or correlates of anxiety (Stanley & Beck, in press). In this latter domain, epidemiological data from a British survey documented that older adults with phobic disorders reported significantly more physical symptoms than control participants (Lindesay, 1991). In particular, adults with phobic disorders more frequently reported the experience of palpitations, dyspnea, dysphagia, abdominal pain, bowel problems, giddiness, tinnitus, and joint swelling within the three months prior to interview. In another community survey, a strong positive correlation ($r = 0.60$) was observed between severity of anxiety and physical health problems (Himmelfarb & Murrell, 1984). Given a reported low correlation between age and physical health, however, the authors concluded that the observed relationship between anxiety and physical condition was not mediated only by age. Multivariate examination of this issue appears warranted, as bivariate correlations do not reveal complex patterns of interrelationships among variables. In a study of institutionalized elders living in nursing homes or congregate housing, significant associations were also observed between anxiety and physical health, with more anxious residents reporting more severe renal problems and other gastrointestinal and urninary difficulties (Parmelee, Katz, & Lawton, 1992).

Taken together, these data strongly support the importance of considering the overlap between anxiety symptoms and medical health problems. To determine appropriate diagnoses and treatment approaches, close attention to both of these areas is paramount, with careful focus on differential diagnosis issues. It seems clear that any evaluation of older adults presenting for either psychological or medical help should include detailed assessments in both domains.

7.08.4.3 Anxiety and Sleep Disturbance

Sleep disturbance, in particular insomnia, is a frequent problem among older adults (Engle-Friedman & Bootzin, 1991) and in fact, is the topic of Chapter 14, this volume. Of interest here, however, is the potential overlap between sleep disturbance and anxiety. Sleep difficulties in elderly people are often viewed as part of the normal aging process and thereby overlooked or underdiagnosed, as are many other symptoms reported frequently in this group (Morin & Gramling, 1989). However, sleep disturbance can lead to changes in mood and conversely, stress and psychopathology can create disruptions in normal sleep patterns (Engle-Friedman & Bootzin, 1991). Thus, an examination of the overlap between sleep difficulties and anxiety is of relevance.

Insomnia has been associated with increases in a variety of self-reported psychological symptoms, including introversion, anxiety, neuroticism, and depression (Engle-Friedman & Bootzin, 1991). When relevant comparisons of older and younger adults have been undertaken, elders reporting sleep disturbance have endorsed fewer symptoms of anxiety, depression, and other psychopathology than younger individuals with similar difficulties (Bliwise, Bliwise, & Dement, 1985; Roehrs, Lineback, Zorick, & Roth, 1982; Roehrs, Zorick, Sicklesteel, Wittig, & Roth, 1983). Morin and Gramling (1989) suggested a number of possible explanations for this pattern, including differences in typical problematic sleep patterns across the two groups (i.e., older adults more often report trouble maintaining rather than initiating sleep) and the tendency of older adults to focus on physical rather than psychological symptoms. Nonetheless, at least two recent studies have demonstrated a significant relationship between sleep difficulties and increased anxiety among the elderly.

In the first of these, Morin and Gramling (1989) assessed 42 adults age 60 and over who responded to media advertisements for participants with chronic sleep difficulties. These individuals were compared on a variety of sleep and mood measures with a control group of 30 individuals matched for age, gender, education, and marital status. Results demonstrated increased levels of anxiety and depression in the self-reported insomniac group relative to the comparison group without sleep difficulties. However, scores on mood measures within the poor sleeper group were not in the pathological range, suggesting to the authors that sleep disturbance alone may not be a good indicator of psychological problems among elderly people. In a more recent study, Friedman, Brooks, Bliwise, and Yesavage (1993) extended these findings by including an objective measure of sleep, in particular a wrist actigraph. Twenty-seven older community volunteers with sleep complaints were assessed on measures of state and trait anxiety and depression. They were also asked to complete daily sleep logs for a period of two weeks and to wear a wrist actigraph continuously for a period of three days. Results demonstrated no correlation between state anxiety and any measure of sleep. However, trait anxiety correlated positively with two self-reported sleep measures: amount of time spent awake after first falling asleep, and total time spent in bed. Trait anxiety also correlated in a significant positive way with total sleep time as determined by the actigraph. The positive correlation between anxiety and total sleep time was unexpected, although the authors noted that the actigraph may have overestimated sleep time for participants who spent a lot of time lying awake and motionless in bed. They also suggested that more anxious adults may have perceived their sleep to be worse than it actually was.

In addition to the mixed data regarding anxiety in older adults with sleep complaints, it is of interest to note that some treatment studies for sleep disorders in elderly people have examined the impact of relaxation treatment (Friedman, Bliwise, Yesavage, & Salom, 1991) or have included relaxation as part of a multicomponent treatment package (Morin, Colecchi, Ling, & Sood, 1995). The impact of relaxation for reducing anxiety is well-known, although studies addressing the utility of these interventions for sleep disturbance failed to include measures of anxiety that might have addressed the impact of treatment on coexistent psychological symptoms. In another study of psychosocial treatment for insomnia that omitted an anxiety-reduction component (Morin, Kowatch, Barry, & Walton, 1993), no impact of treatment on anxiety was noted. However, given the apparent overlap between symptoms of anxiety and sleep difficulties for at least some patients, it will be of interest for future treatment studies of both anxiety and insomnia to examine more regularly transfer effects to the nontarget set of symptoms.

7.08.4.4 Anxiety and Depression

The overlap between anxiety and depression is an issue of longstanding importance within psychology and psychiatry given the high rates of coexistence for these conditions regularly reported among younger adults (Cloninger, 1990; Copp, Schwiderski, & Robinson, 1990; Feldman, 1993). In fact, six-month prevalence data from the ECA survey documented that one-fifth of individuals with an anxiety disorder also had symptoms that met criteria for an affective disorder (Regier et al., 1990). Conversely, one-third of those assigned an affective disorder diagnosis also were given at least one anxiety disorder diagnosis (Regier et al., 1990). Given these high rates of coexistence, further understanding of the nature of this overlap is warranted among elderly people.

ECA data regarding the coexistence of anxiety and affective disorders were not presented separately for the elderly. Nonetheless, recent reviews have highlighted the significant overlap between these sets of diagnoses and symptoms in this segment of the population (Alexopoulos, 1991; Flint, 1994). With regard to data addressing coexistence of assigned diagnoses, it has been reported that over 90% of older adults from the community who reported symptoms appropriate for a diagnosis of GAD also met criteria for depression (Lindesay, Briggs, & Murphy, 1989). In this same community sample, almost 40% of individuals with a phobia diagnosis were also assigned a diagnosis of depression according to the *International classification of disease (8th ed.)* (*ICD-8*) criteria assessed via semi-structured interview. In another study conducted via retrospective chart review (Raj et al., 1993), 45% of elderly clinic patients with PD diagnosed according to *DSM-III-R* also met criteria for coexistent major depression. In an examination of 44 older adults with a principal *DSM-III-R* diagnosis of GAD (Beck et al., 1996a), approximately 15% met criteria for a coexistent affective disorder. When older adults with affective disorders have been evaluated, over one-third have met criteria for a coexistent anxiety disorder diagnosis (Alexopoulos, 1991). Thus, rates of overlap between anxiety and affective disorders among the elderly are high.

Other reports have addressed the degree of overlap between symptoms of anxiety and depression, rather than prevalence of coexistent disorders *per se*. In these studies, significant positive associations between symptoms of anxiety and depression have been observed in community samples of older adults (Lindesay et al., 1989; Ben-Arie, Swartz, & Dickman, 1987), institutionalized elderly people (Parmelee et al., 1992), and older clinic patients (Alexopoulos, 1991). In the authors' own investigation of older adults with GAD, higher levels of depressive symptoms were also evident relative to a matched control sample (Beck et al., 1996a).

In a longitudinal study of 1070 older adults from the community, 702 of whom were interviewed twice over a three-year interval, Larkin et al (1992) reported some covariance between anxiety and depressive symptoms assessed in the context of "neurotic" conditions. These data highlight further the significant overlap between anxiety and depression among the elderly, and may even be interpreted to support some indistinguishability among these two sets of symptoms (Beck & Stanley, 1997). However, data reviewed below attest to the ability of clinicians to differentiate and diagnose both types of disorders reliably among elderly samples (see Section 7.08.5).

7.08.4.5 Anxiety and Cognitive Impairment

Normal age-related changes in cognitive functioning have been studied extensively (see Chapter 2, this volume), and a relatively large body of work has examined the impact of depression on cognitive performance among elderly people (see Chapters 9 and 10, this volume). Results of this latter research have demonstrated moderate relationships between depression and cognitive impairment that are influenced by sample characteristics and the measures selected to evaluate cognitive function (Burt, Zembar, & Niederehe, 1995; Poon, 1992). Less work has examined the overlap between anxiety and cognitive functioning, and results of available studies are mixed and limited by a number of methodological problems. In particular, wide ranges of both anxiety and cognitive measures have been used, limiting the ability to generalize findings across studies. In addition, the majority of studies have been conducted with community volunteers recruited for participation in studies of memory. No studies to date have examined cognitive function among older adults who report significant anxiety symptoms or who meet diagnostic criteria for anxiety disorders. Nonetheless, among older adult volunteers, some relationships have been demonstrated between increased anxiety and decreased cognitive performance, most often related to memory.

In one early report, 67 women volunteers over age 65 were administered measures of anxiety, verbal and nonverbal memory, and self-reported memory complaints in a single testing session (West, Boatwright, & Schleser, 1984). Results demonstrated significant negative correlations between state anxiety and measures of nonverbal memory (recall for sequences of related or unrelated numbers), although no similar relationship was demonstrated between anxiety and memory for lists of related or unrelated words. Higher state anxiety was also related to increased memory complaints, although life satisfaction was a stronger predictor of perceived memory abilities.

In another study of community volunteers, ages 60–79, significant negative correlations were noted between state anxiety and cognitive performance measured by a Piagetian problem-solving task and the Wechsler Adult Intelligence Scale Similarities subtest (LaRue & D'Elia, 1985). In this report, correlations between anxiety and cognitive function were stronger among younger adults (r = 0.24–0.46), ages 40–59, relative to older adults (r = 0.09–0.29). Hill and Vandervoort (1992) reported a significant negative association between state anxiety and performance on a verbal memory task for a group of 74 older adult volunteers, age 60 years and older. However, it is important to note that the measure of anxiety in this study was administered after participants were given feedback about their cognitive performance. As such, feedback that performance had been poorer than expected might have created elevated levels of anxiety. In another comparison, significant negative correlations were observed between measures of verbal recall and anxiety, depression, and social withdrawal for older adult volunteers, ages 60–78 (Deptula, Singh, & Pomara, 1993). In this group, ratings of social withdrawal accounted for a significantly larger proportion of the variance in memory scores than both anxiety and depression. In a younger group of adults assessed in the same study (ages 19–35), no significant relationships were observed between any measure of affect and memory.

In addition to these studies demonstrating significant, albeit moderate, relationships between anxiety and cognitive performance, another small set of reports has examined the impact of anxiety reduction treatment on memory. In the earliest of these, 26 older adult volunteers, ages 59–85, were recruited for a memory improvement study (Yesavage, Rose, & Spiegel, 1982). Participants with evidence of dementia or significant depression were excluded, and four weekly sessions of relaxation training were provided. Anxiety measures were taken at pretreatment, and verbal recall was measured before and after relaxation induction during session three. Results revealed significant positive correlations between two measures of anxiety and improvement in recall following relaxation. In other words, participants with increased anxiety before treatment improved more on the recall task following relaxation. In a second study, Yesavage and Jacob (1984) provided training in both relaxation and mnemonic procedures for a group of 25 older adults, ages 61–82. Results revealed improvement in memory following the combined intervention and significant negative correlations between anxiety and recall at post-treatment.

In general, this small body of literature suggests some potentially important overlap between anxiety and cognitive function. However, further studies are needed to examine cognitive performance in older adults with well-diagnosed anxiety disorders relative to carefully selected control participants. In addition, broad-based and well-standardized measures of both anxiety and cognitive function need to be used.

7.08.5 MEASUREMENT

Severity of anxiety can be measured in a variety of ways, including clinician ratings, standardized self-report instruments, behavioral observation, and psychophysiological recording. Among younger adults, strategies for the evaluation of anxiety within each of these domains have received extensive study, and many well-established measures are currently available (Nietzel, Bernstein, & Russell, 1988). However, as has been suggested elsewhere (Hersen & Van Hasselt, 1992, Hersen, Van Hasselt, & Goreczny, 1993), the same type of work is needed to establish the utility of a range of anxiety measures for use with elderly people. In fact, the development of psychometrically sound assessment tools for evaluating anxiety in this population will be the cornerstone of future research examining the psychopathology and treatment of older anxious adults.

At least two general approaches have been taken in the initial development of anxiety measures for older adults. In one of these, the utility of measures developed with younger samples has been assessed with older participants. This approach is economical and allows for direct comparisons of clinical features in younger and older groups. However, such a strategy may fail to take into account phenomenological features of anxiety that are particularly salient for older adults (e.g., worries about health), and may overlook potentially important discriminations between anxiety and related difficulties (e.g., medical problems, depression) (Hersen et al., 1993; Sheikh, 1991). Given these limitations, an alternative approach involves the development of unique measures of anxiety for use among the elderly. This method is more costly in terms of time and expense, but it allows for more specialized assessment. Both of these strategies have been used to produce a small amount of work focused on the development of assessment technques for measuring anxiety in older adults.

7.08.5.1 Clinician-rated Measures

Clinician-rated instruments have been used routinely among younger adults to diagnose anxiety disorders and evaluate the severity of anxiety symptoms. With regard to establishing anxiety disorder diagnoses, recent data have suggested that two semistructured interviews used routinely among younger adults can also be used reliably in elderly samples. First, the Anxiety Disorders Interview Schedule-Revised (ADIS-R; DiNardo, Moras, Barlow, Rapee, & Brown, 1993) was used by the authors and colleagues in a set of studies designed to examine the nature and treatment of GAD among adults ages 55 and over (Beck et al., 1995, 1996a; Stanley, Beck, & Glassco, 1996; Stanley et al., 1996). Estimates of interrater reliability for use of this measure indicated 100% agreement for principal diagnoses of *DSM-III-R* GAD (although this may have been due at least in part to extensive telephone screening of participants prior to ADIS-R administration), as well as perfect agreement for coexistent diagnoses of social phobia, simple phobia, and panic disorder ($\kappa = 1.00$). Moderate reliability was noted for the diagnosis of major depression ($\kappa = 0.58$). Although these data were obtained with only 28% of the total sample ($n = 14$ of 50), the figures nonetheless suggest that the ADIS-R can be a useful tool for the diagnosis of anxiety and affective disorders among older samples. Future studies will need to address the utility of the ADIS-IV (Brown, DiNardo, & Barlow, 1994), which was recently created to conform with *DSM-IV* criteria (American Psychiatric Association, 1994).

Another set of studies examined the utility of the structured clinical interview for *DSM-III-R* (SCID, Spitzer, Williams, Gibbon, & First, 1988) among older adults (Segal, Hersen, Van Hasselt, Kabacoff, & Roth, 1993; Segal, Kabacoff, Hersen, Van Hasselt, & Ryan, 1995). This interview covers a broader range of potential psychiatric disorders than the ADIS, and data have supported its use for the diagnosis of anxiety, affective, and somatoform disorders in older samples. In particular, the SCID was administered to two sets of adults ages 55 years and older, with all interviews reviewed by a second clinician to evaluate interrater agreement for any diagnostic category with a base rate over 10%. Kappa coefficients indicated adequate agreement for the broad categories of anxiety disorders (0.73–0.77) and somatoform disorders (0.84–1.00), as well as the more specific diagnoses of major depression (0.70–0.79) and panic disorder (0.80). These data suggest that the SCID can also be useful for the diagnosis of anxiety disorders among the elderly. It is important to note, however, that all data examining the reliability of the ADIS and SCID have utilized videotaped interviews which may heighten interrater agreement given that reliability raters are able to hear the interviewer's questions at key decision points of the interview. In this regard, future studies should address the reliability of the interviews when administered separately by two different clinicians.

Other clinician-rated instruments focus on the severity of anxiety symptoms, irrespective of psychiatric diagnosis. The most well-known of these instruments is the Hamilton Anxiety Rating Scale (HARS, Hamilton, 1959), a 14-item measure used routinely in studies of anxiety in younger adults. Although the potential utility of the HARS among the elderly has been questioned due to its emphasis on somatic symptoms (Sheikh, 1991), a report by the authors and colleagues provided support for its use among older adults (Beck, Stanley, & Zebb, 1996b). In particular, interrater agreement for the HARS was adequate among a subgroup of older adults with GAD. Additionally, the instrument successfully discriminated the patient sample from a matched group of normal control participants without psychiatric diagnoses, with near perfect classification. The patient and control groups were both selected based on administration of the ADIS-R, and normative data for the HARS were provided for each. As such, this instrument is a potentially viable measure for evaluating anxiety severity in older adults. However, correlations between the HARS and the Hamilton Rating Scale for Depression (HRSD, Hamilton, 1960) were high (Beck et al, 1996b), and the utility of these measures for discriminating between anxiety and depression among the elderly warrants further study. Revisions in both the HARS and HRSD have been proposed in an attempt to improve internal consistency and discriminant validity (Riskind, Beck, Brown, & Steer, 1987). However, these reconstructed scales continue to share considerable variance among older adults (Beck et al. 1996b), a finding that has also been documented in younger samples (Moras, Di-Nardo, & Barlow, 1992).

7.08.5.2 Self-report Measures

A wide range of psychometrically sound self-report measures are available to assess anxiety in young and middle-aged adults, although only a small body of literature has examined the utility of these same measures with older samples. Moreover, much of this work is limited due to heterogeneous samples of participants, omission of standardized diagnostic procedures for group assignment, and potentially confounding variables including medication use and poor physical health (Hersen & Van Hasselt, 1992).

The earliest studies attempting to document the utility of standardized anxiety questionnaires among older adults evaluated the psychometric properties of the Spielberger State-Trait Anxiety Inventory (STAI; Spielberger et al., 1970). In an initial report, the STAI was administered along with the STAI for Children (STAIC; Spielberger, Edwards, Lushene, Montouri, & Platzek, 1973) to a group of adults, ages 55–87, who were participating in a mental health gerontology program. (Patterson, O'Sullivan, & Spielberger, 1980). The STAIC was included given that its simpler verbage and format were thought to be appropriate for some individuals who experienced difficulty with the STAI. Results provided support for the convergent and divergent validity of both instruments. Given that the STAI and STAIC were significantly and positively correlated, the authors recommended that these instruments could be used as parallel forms for the evaluation of anxiety in older adults (Patterson et al., 1980). However, the small and heterogeneous nature of the sample, as well as the inclusion of some participants who were heavily medicated, limits these conclusions (Hersen & van Hasselt, 1992). In addition, variations in item content and format between the STAI and STAIC limit the potential utility of these measures as parallel forms.

In another study with the STAI, the trait scale was administered to two large samples of geriatric inpatients and community residents (Himmelfarb & Murrell, 1983). Adequate internal consistency was evident in both groups, and convergent validity was demonstrated by significant correlations between the STAI trait scale and other measures of negative affect and life satisfaction. STAI scores were significantly different between the inpatient and community groups, even when variance accounted for by age, gender, health, and marital status was removed. However, the most potent predictors of group membership were measures of depression and life satisfaction, with the STAI trait scale providing no additional contribution to the differentiation of groups. The implications of these findings for the utility of the STAI in discriminating anxious and nonanxious elders are limited, however, given that the patient group was not selected to represent individuals with primary anxiety difficulties. In fact, both groups were heterogeneous and standardized diagnostic procedures were not used.

More recently, the authors and colleagues investigated the psychometric properties of the STAI in 50 older adults with GAD and a control group of 94 older adults with no diagnosable psychiatric difficulties (Stanley et al., 1996). Participants in both groups were identified based on the ADIS-R, and data provided support for the internal consistency of both STAI subscales in each group. Test–retest reliability, assessed in a subset of the normal control group, was strong for the trait subscale, but only moderate for the state subscale, as expected. Convergent validity for the STAI was evident in the control group, but mixed results in this regard were apparent among participants with GAD, suggesting some degree of independence among different types of anxiety symptoms within this group. In general, although methodological limitations of these reports preclude definitive conclusions, the STAI appears to be a potentially useful measure of anxiety among elderly people.

Other self-report measures that have been examined in samples of older adults include Hopkins Symptom Checklist (SCL-90, Derogatis et al., 1973), the Self-Rating Anxiety Scale (SAS, Zung, 1971), the Penn State Worry Questionnaire (PSWQ, Meyer, Miller, Metzger, & Borkovec, 1990), the Padua Inventory (PI, Sanavio, 1988), and the Fear Questionnaire (FQ, Marks & Mathews, 1979). Data addressing the SCL-90 and SAS are limited to descriptive reports of SCL-90 scores in a group of 178 elderly hospital patients (Magni & De Leo, 1984) and SAS scores for 92 older adults from the community (Zung, 1980). Thus, conclusions about the utility of these measures are tentative at best.

More thorough psychometric data addressing the potential use of the PSWQ, PI, and FQ are available from data collected by the authors and colleagues in their study of the nature and treatment of GAD among the elderly (Beck et al., 1995; Stanley et al., 1996). The PSWQ is a 16-item scale designed to evaluate the tendency to worry, irrespective of worry content; the PI is a 60-item questionnaire that evaluates obsessive-compulsive symptoms; and the FQ is a 15-item instrument measuring severity of specific fears. All of these instruments have strong psychometric properties when used to assess various aspects of anxiety among younger adults. One purpose of the authors' work was to assess whether psychometric characteristics of these measures would be similar in older adult groups. As noted previously, two samples of older adults were selected via diagnostic interview for this set of studies, one characterized by the presence of GAD and the other with no diagnosable psychiatric complaints. Participants with GAD were administered the questionnaires as part of a larger pretreatment battery; normal control participants received financial compensation for completion of the instruments.

In general, results supported the utility of the PSWQ and the PI (Beck et al., 1995; Stanley et al., 1996). In particular, estimates of internal consistency were adequate for both measures in each participant group, with the exception of the PI behavior control subscale in the normal control group. This subscale measures fears of losing control over motor behavior, a symptom that was only seldom endorsed in this group. Thus, a restricted range of scores in the control group probably created subscale instability in this instance. Adequate convergent validity was demonstrated for the PSWQ and the PI in both participant groups. Factor analysis of the PSWQ suggested a two-factor structure in both groups, with one factor assessing a tendency to worry and a second factor estimating the absence of worry (Beck et al., 1995). Similar analyses were not conducted for the PI given inadequate sample sizes (Stanley et al., 1996). The test–retest reliability of the PI, assessed in a subsample of the normal control group, demonstrated that the total score and scores on the contamination and behavior control subscales assessed stable, trait-like features ($r > 0.70$), while scores on the mental control and checking subscales ($r = 0.61$, 0.64) estimated more statelike clinical symptoms. In general, however, these initial data supported the utility of the PSWQ and the PI in anxious and nonanxious elders.

On the other hand, data for the FQ suggested that alternative measures of specific fears should be investigated for use with the elderly (Stanley et al., 1996). In particular, estimates of internal consistency were mixed in both groups of participants, a finding that is unexpected given the construction of the FQ and the stable nature of phobic fear. Test–retest reliablility (as above, assessed in a subgroup of the normal control sample) was poor and suggested the possibility of regression to the mean over a two to four week interval. In addition, the FQ failed to correlate significantly with other measures of anxiety, indicating poor convergent validity. Furthermore, item content was not selected to probe specific fears of particular relevance for the elderly. As such, the FQ does not appear to be a viable measure of specific fears among older adults.

As an alternative to examining the psychometric properties of measures that are well-established for younger groups, at least one measure of anxiety has been developed specifically with older adults in mind. Wisocki and colleagues created the Worry Scale (WS, Wisocki, Handen, & Morse, 1986), a 35-item questionnaire, to assess worries of particular significance for older adults, namely, concerns about financial, health, and social issues. Initial normative data and support for concurrent validity of the WS were provided by Wisocki and colleagues (Powers et al., 1992; Wisocki, 1988; Wisocki et al., 1986). In the authors' own work described above (Stanley et al., 1996), the WS also demonstrated good internal consistency and generally adequate test–retest reliability. The only exception to the latter was poor stability for the health subscale, potentially due to the sensitivity of this measure to real physical complaints which may vary over time. Finally, the WS demonstrated adequate convergent validity. In this regard, the measure seems to hold promise for the evaluation of worry in older adults.

7.08.5.3 Behavioral Observation

Behavioral observation has been described as an essential component for the evaluation of fear and anxiety (Last & Hersen, 1988). Despite the availability of various systematic schemes for behavioral observation of anxiety among younger adults (Nietzel et al., 1988), only case studies have provided any such approaches for the assessment of anxiety in elderly people. In one report, Turner, Hersen, Bellack, and Wells (1979) described a behavioral observation scheme for monitoring ritualistic handwashing and associated symptoms in a 66-year-old woman with OCD. Behavioral observations were made on an inpatient unit by research assistants three times a day, with measures estimating mean time spent washing and percentage of observation periods in which washing occurred. In another case report, Junginger and Ditto (1984) measured the frequency and nature of checking behaviors in a 65-year-old woman receiving inpatient psychiatric treatment for OCD and major depression. However, no standardized approaches for the behavioral observation of anxiety symptoms in older adults have been developed, and the need for further research in this area has been highlighted (Hersen et al., 1993). In particular, reliable systems for the observation of behavior in clinical and naturalistic settings are needed.

7.08.5.4 Psychophysiological Assessment

As noted by Hersen et al., (1993) psychophysiological responses to stress may be expected to change with increasing age. In particular, changes in cardiovascular variables over the life span have been reported, with older anxious adults showing increased cardiovascular reactivity (Hersen et al., 1993). However, hypothesized age-related changes in physiological functioning are not well-documented, and psychophysiological assessment of anxiety is an issue that has yet to be addressed within the older adult literature. Of interest here will be comparisons of baseline arousal in older anxious and nonanxious adults, as well as potentially differential responses to stressors and feared stimuli (Hersen et al., 1993). In general, the inclusion of physiological measures should be considered carefully, as the use of psychophysiological assessment has not always yielded useful information about the nature and treatment of anxiety (Barlow & Maser, 1984).

7.08.6 TREATMENT

7.08.6.1 Utilization of Services

It is well-documented that mental health resources are severely underutilized by the elderly (Arean, 1993; Lasoski, 1986; Smyer & Gatz, 1995). Overall, it appears that only about one-third of older adults in need of mental health care actually see a mental health professional; the other two-thirds either receive no care or obtain services from primary care physicians (Smyer & Gatz, 1995). Low rates of referral for psychiatric or psychological services have also been reported among primary care physicians who treat older adults (Smyer & Gatz, 1995).

More specific data relevant to treatment of anxiety disorders among elderly people are similarly disconcerting. For example, Blazer et al. (1991) reported that only 38% of older adults with GAD indicated use of outpatient mental health services during the year before they were interviewed. Even lower rates of mental health care were reported in the ECA study, with less than 1% of older adults with agoraphobia and only 2% of those with other phobias indicating that they had sought sevices from a mental health professional during the previous six months (Thompson et al., 1988). A larger percentage of elders with phobic disorders reportedly had sought help for mental health problems from other sources (e.g., clergy, general physicians), but rates of help-seeking overall were still significantly lower among older adults than in the group of adults between the ages of 25 and 64 (Thompson et al., 1988).

A number of explanations have been posited to account for these low rates of mental health care among the elderly. First, older adults themselves are reluctant to define their difficulties in terms of psychological problems, and they are often hesitant to seek social services of any kind (Lasoski, 1986; McCarthy, Katz, & Foa, 1991). Additionally, older adults may be fearful of the implications of their symptoms and perceive that mental health services will be of no real benefit (Smyer & Gatz, 1995). Problems in daily living, such as transportation difficulties and financial limitations, may also contribute to low rates of mental health care services sought by the elderly. Second, problems within the health care community can also be identified. For example, relatively few treatment providers with adequate training are available to provide services to older adults, and outreach and/or publicity of services are often limited (Lasoski, 1986; McCarthy et al., 1991). In addition, negative attitudes about the aging process, and perceptions that the signs and symptoms of anxiety are due merely to normal aging and are therefore irreversible, may create a tendency to ignore or misdiagnose mental health problems among elderly people (Smyer & Gatz, 1995; Weiss, 1994).

Despite the low rates of services sought by elders, a growing body of literature has begun to address the efficacy of both pharmacological and psychosocial interventions for anxiety problems. Much of this literature is limited by serious methodological problems, but growing interest in the nature and treatment of anxiety in this population suggests that notable advances in the area will be made in the early years of the twenty-first century.

7.08.6.2 Pharmacological Interventions

Given that much of the mental health care sought by older adults is provided through primary care physicians, (Blazer et al., 1991; McCarthy et al., 1991; Smyer & Gatz, 1995), it is not surprising that treatment for anxiety most often involves the use of medication, usually the benzodiazepines. Among older adults, use of the benzodiazepines occurs far more frequently than in younger samples. (Blazer et al., 1991; Salzman, 1991). Clinical recommendations for the use of benzodiazepines among the elderly, however, are not based on well-controlled treatment trials. Although some data have suggested the utility of a variety of benzodiazepines, all studies available in the late 1990s are limited by serious methodological problems (Cohn, 1984; Salzman, 1991). For example, patients generally were not selected via any systematic diagnostic procedure. As such, generalization of conclusions is limited by the heterogeneous nature of the study samples. Relatedly, patients with anxiety symptoms or disorders were not well-differentiated from participants with anxiety secondary to depression or medical illness, nor was anxiety always distinguished from behavioral agitation associated with cognitive impairment. Finally, the studies varied significantly with regard to outcome criteria, treatment duration, and the use of concommitant medications.

Despite the severe methodological limitations of the outcome literature, recommendations regarding the use of benzodiazepines are fairly consistent, with the suggestion that compounds with short half-lives be used for as brief a duration as possible (Fernandez, Levy, Lachar, & Small, 1995; Markovitz, 1993; Weiss, 1994). Benzodiazepine doses recommended for older adults are also generally lower than those prescribed for younger adults given altered pharmacokinetic properties that lead to increased therapeutic and adverse effects (Lader, 1986). In general, strategies for benzodiazepine use have been recommended based on studies addressing the utility of anxiolytics in younger adults, the pharmacokinetic properties of the medications in nonsymptomatic older samples, and anxiolytic toxicity among the elderly (Salzman, 1991).

Problems with the use of benzodiazepines among the elderly are noted routinely, with some authors even suggesting that psychosocial interventions be considered in conjunction with a pharmacological approach (Lader, 1986; Wengel, Burke, Ranno, & Roccaforte, 1993). Given the increased sensitivity to these medications generally observed in older adults, adverse events of particular concern include cognitive impairment (e.g., amnesia, delayed recall, confusion, disorientation), agitation (which may exacerbate anxiety symptoms), respiratory depression, and psychomotor slowing which may lead to increased rates of falls and hip fractures (Weiss, 1994; Wengel et al., 1993). Increased rates of medical illness among older adults also raise the issue of potentially harmful drug interactions.

Thus, although the benzodiazepines are recommended routinely for the treatment of anxiety among the elderly, the literature upon which clinical recommendations are made is quite limited and the increased risk of potentially serious adverse effects warrants caution in using these compounds. Other medications may be considered as alternatives, although again, the relevant treatment literature is quite limited in scope. For example, clinical recommendations have suggested the use of buspirone as an alternative to benzodiazepines for the treatment of anxiety in older adults, given its apparently equivalent therapeutic effects without significant potential for serious adverse effects, tolerance, or withdrawal (Weiss, 1994). However, the treatment literature has documented the efficacy of buspirone only in a number of open trials (Salzman, 1991), and other more well-controlled research will need to substantiate these clinical claims. Likewise, clinical recommendations have suggested the potential utility of beta blockers and antidepressants for the treatment of anxiety among the elderly (Fernandez et al., 1995; Markowitz, 1993), but these suggestions are based only on literature documenting the efficacy of these compounds in younger anxious adults. Future studies will need to address directly the efficacy of these medications in well-diagnosed samples of older adults.

7.08.6.3 Psychosocial Interventions

The consideration of psychosocial treatments as an adjunct or alternative to the use of medication for the treatment of psychiatric disturbance in the elderly is an important but understudied issue. In general, it has been noted that many of the basic clinical skills useful for the treatment of younger adults are appropriate for therapeutic work with elderly people (Taylor & Hartman Stein, 1995). However, variations in technique or approach are often necessary to address the special needs of an older population. In particular, the importance of assessing both patients' and family members' beliefs about mental health problems and their treatment has been noted, as well as the need to educate both of these groups about the nature of psychosocial treatment (Arean, 1993; Gallagher-Thompson & Thompson, 1995). In addition, differences in learning strategies and sensory function between older and younger adults need to be considered, with recommendations suggesting that therapy with elderly people occur at a slower pace and include increased use of visual and written aids (Gallagher-Thompson & Thompson, 1995; Smyer, Zarit, & Qualls, 1990) Group approaches have also been recommended to reduce cost and increase social contact and support (Arean, 1993; Yost, Beutles, Corbishley & Allender, 1986) and regular contact with the patient's primary care physician has been suggested (Arean, 1993; Gallagher-Thompson & Thompson, 1995).

In addition to these general recommendations, the older adult literature includes a number of well-controlled clinical trials documenting the specific efficacy of psychosocial treatment for depression (Arean et al., 1993, Thompson, Gallagher, & Breckenridge, 1987; see Chapter 9, this volume). However, much less attention has been paid to the development of psychosocial treatments for anxiety among the elderly, and the need for further work in this domain has been noted repeatedly (Cartensen, 1988, Hersen & Van Hasselt, 1992; Niederehe, Cooley, & Teri, 1995). Given the voluminous body of work documenting the efficacy of cognitive behavioral treatments for anxiety in younger adults (Barlow, 1988, Beidel & Turner, 1991) it is not surprising that initial attempts to establish psychosocial interventions for older adults have focused on these approaches. However, the available literature is limited largely to clinical case studies and group comparisons with community volunteers reporting general anxiety symptoms.

A relatively large group of case studies has examined the use of cognitive behavioral interventions that have been demonstrated efficacious in younger adult samples. In particular, interventions including exposure, response prevention, relaxation training, and cognitive restructuring have been utilized to treat elderly patients with a range of anxiety disorders, such as GAD (King & Barrowclough, 1991), PD (Swales, Solfvin, & Sheikh, 1996), specific phobias (Thyer, 1981), and OCD (Calamari, Faber, Hitsman; & Poppe, 1994; Carmin, Ownby, & Pollard, 1995; Rowan, Holborn, Walker, & Siddiqui, 1984) The efficacy of cognitive behavioral interventions with a wide range of anxiety difficulties suggests strongly the utility of further work in this domain. However, conclusions from these reports alone can be drawn only cautiously given the absence of appropriate methodological controls.

Other more controlled research has examined the utility of cognitive behavior therapy (CBT) for the reduction of anxiety symptoms in nonclinical, community volunteers. In one of the earliest of these studies, DeBerry (1982) compared the effects of two versions of relaxation training with an attention control condition in a sample of older adult women volunteers with various anxiety complaints. Results demonstrated the efficacy of both relaxation training conditions, relative to the control group, on measures of state and trait anxiety. In a similar comparison, 24 older community volunteers reporting both anxiety and depressive symptoms were assigned randomly to receive relaxation training, CBT for depression, or a nonspecific control condition (Sallis, Lichstein, Clarkson, Stalgaitis, & Campbell, 1983). Results revealed significant reductions in both anxiety and depression across all treatment groups.

In a subsequent study, another community group of older adults with anxiety symptoms received relaxation training, cognitive restructuring, or an attention control condition

(DeBerry, Davis, & Reinhard, 1989). In this comparison, only relaxation training was effective in decreasing state anxiety, although trait anxiety and symptoms of depression were reduced at post-treatment across all conditions. In a more recent comparison with a larger group of community volunteers, the effects of progressive and imaginal relaxation training were examined relative to a wait-list control condition (Scogin, Rickard, Keith, Wilson & McElreath, 1992). Both types of relaxation training led to significant decreases in anxiety, relative to the control group, and treatment gains were maintained at one year follow-up (Rickard, Scogin, & Keith, 1994).

These studies together suggest that CBT, in particular relaxation training, may be beneficial for the treatment of anxiety in older adults. However, the sample sizes in many of these reports were small, and participants were not evaluated for the presence of diagnosable anxiety pathology. Only recently has a preliminary empirical trial examined the utility of cognitive behavioral interventions in older adults with well-diagnosed anxiety disorders.

In this comparison, the efficacy of CBT was evaluated relative to a nondirective supportive psychotherapy condition in a sample of 48 older adults with a principal diagnosis of GAD (Stanley et al., 1996). Treatment in both conditions was administered in a small group format over a period of 14 weeks. CBT followed the treatment approach described by Craske, Barlow, and O'Leary (1992) and included relaxation training, cognitive therapy, and systematic exposure to worry-related situations. Modifications to this treatment model included the use of a group format, as well as increased use of visual and written aids (e.g., outlines of session topics, written instructions for homework and monitoring assignments). Results revealed significant decreases at post-treatment for participants in both treatment conditions on self-report and clinician-rated measures of worry, anxiety, and depression. CBT also produced significant improvement in severity of specific fears, although psychometric limitations of the FQ restrict the conclusions which can be made in this regard. Results of a six month follow-up evaluation revealed maintenance of treatment gains in both conditions, with some continued improvement in severity of worry over time. Correlational analyses suggested that pretreatment severity of anxiety and ratings of treatment credibility were significant predictors of outcome. As such, these data further substantiate the potential utility of CBT (and other psychosocial interventions) for the treatment of anxiety among the elderly. However, study conclusions are limited given the omission of a no-treatment or wait-list control condition. Future research will need to replicate these findings in a better controlled design.

7.08.7 SUMMARY

Anxiety disorders are the most prevalent of all psychiatric conditions among elderly people and they pose a major public health problem for this population. Nevertheless, research addressing the prevalence, nature, and treatment of these conditions among elderly is in an infancy stage. No data are available regarding the prevalence of PTSD among the elderly, and the clinical picture of many anxiety syndromes in this segment of the population is as yet unclear. Much of the available literature is limited due to the significant dearth of well-established measures of anxiety among elderly people and the failure to utilize strict diagnostic criteria in the selection of clinical groups. The utility of measures already established for use with younger groups deserves further study in this regard. Additionally, new instruments that target specifically the unique features of anxiety among elderly people will need to be developed. In this domain, the focus will need to be not only on self-report instruments, but also on systematic methods of behavioral observation, clinician rating, and psychophysiological assessment. The development of more refined measures will assist in clarifying the difference between anxiety disorders and other syndromes that may produce similar clinical features, including depression, various medical conditions, sleep disorders, and cognitive dysfunction.

With the establishment of psychometrically sound assessment tools, more sophisticated treatment research should emerge. Pharmacological trials might focus on the relative efficacy of various antianxiety and antidepressant medication, and psychosocial treatment comparisons should evaluate further the utility of CBT and alternative interventions in well-diagnosed groups of older patients. Emphasis in all of these investigations should be given not only to the effects of treatment on symptom reduction, but also to the transfer effects of the interventions on associated clinical features, physical health, and social functioning. Durability of treatment response following both pharmacological and psychosocial treatments will need to be examined with well-controlled evaluations over long-term follow-up intervals, and findings will need to be generalized to patients recruited from a variety of settings (e.g., psychiatric clinics, primary care clinics) and from diverse sociocultural backgrounds.

7.08.8 REFERENCES

Alexopoulos, G. S. (1991). Anxiety and depression in the elderly. In C. Salzman & B. D. Lebowitz (Eds.), *Anxiety in the elderly: Treatment and research* (pp. 63–77). New York: Springer.

American Psychiatric Association (1980). *Diagnostic and statistical manual of mental disorders* (3rd ed.). Washington, DC: Author.

American Psychiatric Association (1994). *Diagnostic and statistical manual of mental disorders* (4th ed.). Washington, DC: Author.

Arean, P. A. (1993). Cognitive behavioral therapy with older adults. *The Behavior Therapist, 16*, 236–239.

Arean, P. A., Perri, M. G., Nezu, A. M., Schein, R. L., Christopher, F., & Joseph, T. X. (1993). Comparative effectiveness of social problem-solving therapy and reminiscence therapy as treatments for depression in older adults. *Journal of Consulting and Clinical Psychology, 61*, 1003–1010.

Barlow, D. H. (1988). *Anxiety and its disorders: The nature and treatment of anxiety and panic*. New York: Guilford.

Barlow, D. H., & Maser, J. D. (1984). Psychopathology in anxiety disorders. *Journal of Behavioral Assessment, 6*, 331–348.

Barrios, B. A., Hartmann, D. B., & Shigetomi, C. (1981). Fears and anxieties in children. In E. J. Mash & L. G. Terdal (Eds.), *Behavioral assessment of childhood disorders* (pp. 259–304). New York: Guilford Press.

Beck, J. G., & Stanley, M. A. (1997). Anxiety disorders in the elderly: The emerging role of behavior therapy. *Behavior Therapy, 28*, 83–100

Beck, J. G., Stanley, M. A., & Zebb, B. J. (1995). Psychometric properties of the Penn State Worry Questionnaire in older adults. *Journal of Clinical Geropsychology, 1*, 33–42.

Beck, J. G., Stanley, M. A., & Zebb, B. J. (1996a). Characteristics of generalized anxiety disorder in older adults: A descriptive study. *Behaviour Research and Therapy, 34*, 225–234.

Beck, J. G., Stanley, M. A., & Zebb, B. J. (1996b, August). *How do the Hamilton Scales perform with geriatric GAD patients*? Presented at the Annual Convention for the American Psychological Association, Toronto, ON, Canada.

Beidel, D. C., & Turner, S. M. (1991). Anxiety disorders. In M. Hersen & S. M. Turner (Eds.), *Adult psychopathology and diagnosis* (pp. 226–278). New York: Wiley.

Ben-Arie, O., Swartz, L., & Dickman, B. J. (1987). Depression in the elderly living in the community: Its presentation and features. *British Journal of Psychiatry, 150*, 169–174.

Bland, R. C., Newman, S. C., & Orn, H. (1988). Prevalence of psychiatric disorders in the elderly in Edmonton. *Acta Psychiatrica Scandanavia (Suppl.), 338*, 57–63.

Blazer, D., George, L. K., & Hughes, D. (1991). The epidemiology of anxiety disorders: An age comparison. In C.. Salzman & B. D. Lebowitz (Eds.), *Anxiety in the elderly: Treatment and research* (pp. 17–30). New York: Springer.

Blazer, D., Hughes, D., & George, L. K. (1987). Stressful life events and the onset of a generalized anxiety syndrome. *American Journal of Psychiatry, 144*, 1178–1183.

Brown, T. A., DiNardo, P. A., & Barlow, D. H. (1994). *Anxiety Disorders Interview Schedule for DSM-IV*. Albany, NY: Graywinds.

Bliwise, N. G., Bliwise, D. L., & Dement, W. C. (1985). Age and psychopathology in insomnia. *Clinical Gerontologist, 4*, 3–9.

Bruce, M. L., & McNamara, R. (1992). Psychiatric status among the homebound elderly: An epidemiologic perspective. *Journal of the American Geriatrics Society, 40*, 561–566.

Burt, D. B., Zembar, M. J., & Niederehe, G. (1995). Depression and memory impairment: A meta-analysis of the association, its pattern, and specificity. *Psychological Bulletin, 117*, 285–305.

Burvill, P. W., Johnson, G. A., Jamrozik, K. D., Anderson, C. S., Stewart-Wynne, E. G., & Chakera, T. M. H. (1995). Anxiety disorders after stroke: Results from the Perth Community Stroke Study. *British Journal of Psychiatry, 166*, 328–332.

Calamari, J. E., Faber, S. D., Hitsman, B. L., & Poppe, C. J. (1994). Treatment of obsessive compulsive disorder in the elderly: A review and case example. *Journal of Behavior Therapy and Experimental Psychiatry, 25*, 95–104.

Carmin, C. N., Ownby, R. L., & Pollard, C. A. (1995, November). *Effects of cognitive behavioral treatment of obsessive compulsive disorder in geriatric versus younger adult patients*. Presented at the Annual Convention of the Association for Advancement of Behavior Therapy, Washington, DC.

Carstensen, L. L. (1988). The emerging field of behavioral gerontology. *Behavior Therapy, 19*, 259–281.

Cloninger, C. R. (1990). Comorbidity of anxiety disorders. *Journal of Psychopharmacology, 10*, 43–46.

Cohen, G. D. (1991). Anxiety and general medical disorders. In C. Salzman & B. D. Lebowitz (Eds.), *Anxiety in the elderly: Treatment and research* (pp. 47–62). New York: Springer.

Cohn, J. B. (1984). Double-blind safety and efficacy comparison of alprazolam and placebo in the treatment of anxiety in geriatric patients. *Current Therapeutic Research, 35*, 100–112.

Copp, J. E., Schwiderski, U. E., & Robinson, D. S. (1990). Symptom comorbidity in anxiety and depressive disorders. *Journal of Clinical Psychopharmacology, 10*, 52–60.

Craske, M. G., Barlow, D. H., & O'Leary, T. (1992). *Mastery of your anxiety and worry*. Albany, NY: Graywind.

DeBerry, S. (1982). The effects of meditation–relaxation on anxiety and depression in a geriatric population. *Psychotherapy: Theory, Research, and Practice, 19*, 512–521.

DeBerry, S., Davis, S., & Reinhard, K. E. (1989). A comparison of meditation–relaxation and cognitive behavioral techniques for reducing anxiety and depression in a geriatric population. *Journal of Geriatric Psychiatry, 22*, 231–247.

Deptula, D., Singh, R., & Pomara, N. (1993). Aging, emotional states, and memory. *American Journal of Psychiatry, 150*, 429–434.

DiNardo, P. A., Moras, K., Barlow, D. H., Rapee, R. M., & Brown, T. A. (1993). Reliability of DSM-III-R anxiety disorder categories: Using the Anxiety Disorders Interview Schedule—Revised (ADIS-R). *Archives of General Psychiatry, 50*, 251–256.

Downton, J. H., & Andrews, K. (1990). Postural disturbance and psychological symptoms amongst elderly people living at home. *International Journal of Geriatric Psychiatry, 5*, 93–98.

Eaton, W. M., Kramer, M., Anthony, J. C., Dryman, A., Shapiro, S., & Locke, B. Z. (1989). The incidence of specific DIS/DSM-III mental disorders: Data from the NIMH Epidemiologic Catchment Area Program. *Acta Psychiatrica Scandanavia, 79*, 163–178.

Engle-Friedman, M., & Bootzin, R. (1991). Insomnia as a problem for the elderly. In P. A. Wisocki (Ed.), *Handbook of clinical behavior therapy with the elderly client: applied clinical psychology* (pp. 273–298). New York: Plenum.

Feinson, M. C., & Thoits, P. A. (1986). The distribution of

distress among elders. *Journal of Gerontology, 41*, 225–233.

Feldman, L. A. (1993). Distinguishing depression and anxiety in self-report: Evidence from confirmatory factor analysis on nonclinical and clinical samples. *Journal of Consulting and Clinical Psychology, 61*, 631–638.

Fernandez, F., Levy, J. K., Lachar, B. L., & Small, G. W. (1995). The management of depression and anxiety in the elderly. *Journal of Clinical Psychiatry, 56*, 20–29.

Flint, A. J. (1994). Epidemiology and comorbidity of anxiety disorders in the elderly. *American Journal of Psychiatry, 151*, 640–649.

Frazer, D. W. (1995). The medical issues in geropsychology training and practice. In B. G. Knight, L. Teri, P. Wohlford, & J. Santos (Eds.), *Mental health services for older adults: Implications for training and practice in geropsychology* (pp. 63–71). Washington, DC: American Psychological Association.

Friedman, L., Bliwise, D. L., Yesavage, J. A., & Salom, S. R. (1991). A preliminary study comparing sleep restriction and relaxation treatments for insomnia in older adults. *Journal of Gerontology, 46*, 1–8.

Friedman, L., Brooks, J. O., Bliwise, D. L., & Yesavage, J. A. (1993). Insomnia in older adults: Relations to depression and insomnia. *American Journal of Geriatric Psychiatry, 1*, 153–159.

Gallagher-Thompson, D., & Thompson, L. W. (1995). Efficacy of psychotherapeutic interventions with older adults. *The Clinical Psychologist, 48*, 24–30.

Ganzini, L., McFarland, B. H., & Culter, D. (1990). Prevalence of mental disorders after catastrophic financial loss. *Journal of Nervous and Mental Disease, 178*, 680–685.

Gurian, B. S., & Miner, J. H. (1991) Clinical presentation of anxiety in the elderly. In C. Salzman & B. D. Lebowitz (Eds.), *Anxiety in the elderly: Treatment and research* (pp. 31–44). New York: Springer.

Hamilton, M. (1959). The assessment of anxiety states by rating. *British Journal of Medical Psychology, 32*, 50–55.

Hamilton, M. (1960). A rating scale for depression. *Journal of Neurology, Neurosurgery, & Psychiatry, 23*, 56–62.

Helzer, J. E., Robins, L. N., & McEvoy, L. (1987). Post-traumatic stress disorder in the general population: Findings of the Epidemiologic Catchment Area survey. *The New England Journal of Medicine, 317*, 1630–1634.

Hersen, M., & Van Hasselt, V. B. (1992). Behavioral assessment and treatment of anxiety in the elderly. *Clinical Psychology Review, 12*, 619–640.

Hersen, M., Van Hasselt, V. B., & Goreczny, A. J. (1993). Behavioral assessment of anxiety in older adults: Some comments. *Behavior Modification, 17*, 99–112.

Hill, R. D., & Vandervoort, D. (1992). The effects of state anxiety on recall performance in older learners. *Educational Gerontology, 18*, 597–605.

Himmelfarb, S., & Murrell, S. A. (1983). Reliability and validity of five mental health scales in older persons. *Journal of Gerontology, 38*, 333–339.

Himmelfarb, S., & Murrell, S. A. (1984). The prevalence and correlates of anxiety symptoms in older adults. *The Journal of Psychology, 116*, 159–167.

Junginger, J., & Ditto, B. (1984). Multitreatment of obsessive-compulsive checking in a geriatric patient. *Behavior Modification, 8*, 379–390.

Katz, I. R. (1996). On the inseparability of mental and physical health in aged persons: Lessons from depression and medical comorbidity. *The American Journal of Geriatric Psychiatry, 4*, 1–16.

Lader, M. (1986). The use of hypnotics and anxiolytics in the elderly. *International Clinical Psychopharmacology, 1*, 273–283.

King, P., & Barrowclough, C. (1991). A clinical pilot study of cognitive-behavioral therapy for anxiety disorders in the elderly. *Behavioural Psychotherapy, 19*, 337–345.

Kluznick, J. C., Speed, N., Van Valkenberg, C., & Magraw, R. (1986). Forty-year follow-up of United States prisoners of war. *American Journal of Psychiatry, 143*, 1443–1446.

Kuch, K., & Cox, B. J. (1992). Symptoms of PTSD in 124 survivors of the Holocaust. *American Journal of Psychiatry, 149*, 337–340.

Larkin, B. A., Copeland, J. R. M., Dewey, M. E., Davidson, I. A., Saunders, P. A., Sharma, V. K., McWilliam, C., & Sullivan, C. (1992). The natural history of neurotic disorder in an elderly urban population: Findings from the Liverpool Longitudinal Study of Continuing Health in the Community. *British Journal of Psychiatry, 160*, 681–686.

LaRue, A., & D'Elia, L. F. (1985). Anxiety and problem solving in middle-aged and elderly adults. *Experimental Aging Research, 11*, 215–220.

Lasoski, M. C. (1986). Reasons for low utilization of mental health services by the elderly. In T. L. Brink (Ed.), *Clinical gerontology: A guide to assessment and intervention* (pp. 1–18). New York: Haworth.

Last, C. G., & Hersen, M. (Eds.) (1988). *Handbook of anxiety disorders*. New York: Pergamon.

Lawton, M. P., Kleban, M. H., & Dean, J. (1993). Affect and age: Cross-sectional comparisons of structure and prevalence. *Psychology and Aging, 8*, 165–175.

Liddell, A., Locker, D., & Burman, D. (1991). Self-reported fears (FSS-II) of subjects aged 50 years and over. *Behaviour Research and Therapy, 29*, 105–112.

Lindesay, J. (1991). Phobic disorders in the elderly. *British Journal of Psychiatry, 159*, 531–541.

Lindesay, J., Briggs, K., & Murphy, E. (1989). The Guy's/Age Concern Survey: Prevalence rates of cognitive impairment, depression and anxiety in an urban elderly community. *British Journal of Psychiatry, 155*, 317–329.

Luchins, D. J., & Rose, R. P. (1989). Late-life onset of panic disorder with agoraphobia in three patients. *American Journal of Psychiatry, 146*, 920–921.

Magni, G., & De Leo, D. (1984). Anxiety and depression in geriatric and adult medical inpatients: A comparison. *Psychological Reports, 55*, 607–612.

Markovitz, P. J. (1993). Treatment of anxiety in the elderly. *Journal of Clinical Psychiatry, 54*, 64–68.

Marks, I. M., & Gelder, M. G. (1966). Different ages of onset in varieties of phobia. *American Journal of Psychiatry, 123*, 218–221.

Marks, I. M., & Mathews, A. M. (1979). Brief standardized self-rating for phobic patients. *Behaviour Research and Therapy, 17*, 263–267.

McCarthy, P. R., Katz, I. R., & Foa, E. B. (1991). Cognitive-behavioral treatment of anxiety in the elderly: A proposed model. In C. Salzman & B. D. Lebowitz (Eds.), *Anxiety in the elderly: Treatment and research* (pp. 197–214). New York: Springer.

McNally, R. J. (1994). *Panic disorder: A critical analysis*. New York: Guilford Press.

Meyer, T. J., Miller, M. L., Metzger, R. L., & Borkovec, T. D. (1990). Development and validation of the Penn State Worry Questionnaire. *Behaviour Research and Therapy, 28*, 487–495.

Moras, K., DiNardo, P. A., & Barlow, D. H. (1992). Distinguishing anxiety and depression: Re-examination of the reconstructed Hamilton Scales. *Psychological Assessment, 4*, 224–227.

Morin, C. M., Colecchi, C. A., Ling, W. D., & Sood, R. K. (1995). Cognitive behavior therapy to facilitate benzodiazepine discontinuation among hypnotic-dependent patients with insomnia. *Behavior Therapy, 26*, 733–745.

Morin, C. M., & Gramling, S. E. (1989). Sleep patterns and aging: Comparison of older adults with and without insomnia complaints. *Psychology and Aging, 4*, 290–294.

Morin, C. M., Kowatch, R. A., Barry, T., & Walton, E. (1993). Cognitive-behavior therapy for late-life insomnia. *Journal of Consulting and Clinical Psychology, 61*, 137–136.

Niederehe, G., Cooley, S. G., & Teri, L. (1995). Research and training in clinical geropsychology: Advances and current opportunities. *The Clinical Psychologist, 48*, 37–44.

Nietzel, M. T., Bernstein, D. A., & Russell, R. L. (1988). Assessment of anxiety and fear. In A. S. Bellack & M. Hersen (Eds.), *Behavioral assessment: A practical handbook*, (3rd ed., pp. 280–312). New York: Pergamon.

Norris, F. H., & Murrell, S. A. (1988). Prior experience as a moderator of disaster impact on anxiety symptoms in older adults. *American Journal of Community Psychology, 16*, 665–683.

Ost, L. G. (1987). Age of onset in different phobias. *Journal of Abnormal Psychology, 96*, 223–229.

Oxman, T. E., Barrett, J. E., Barrett, J., & Gerber, P. (1987). Psychiatric symptoms in the elderly in a primary care practice. *General Hospital Psychiatry, 9*, 167–173.

Parmelee, P. A., Katz, I. R., & Lawton, M. P. (1992). Anxiety and its association with depression among institutionalized elderly. *American Journal of Geriatric Psychiatry, 1*, 46–58.

Patterson, R. L., O'Sullivan, M. J., & Spielberger, C. D. (1980). Measurement of state and trait anxiety in elderly mental health clients. *Journal of Behavioral Assessment, 2*, 89–97.

Person, D. C., & Borkovec, T. D. (1995, August). *Anxiety disorders among the elderly: Patterns and issues.* Paper presented at the annual meeting of the American Psychological Association, New York.

Poon, L. W. (1992). Toward an understanding of cognitive functioning in geriatric depression. *International Psychogeriatrics, 4*, 241–266.

Powers, C. B., Wisocki, P. A., & Whitbourne, S. K. (1992). Age differences and correlates of worrying in young and elderly adults. *The Gerontologist, 32*, 82–88.

Raj, B. A., Covea, M. H., & Dagon, E. M. (1993). The clinical characteristics of panic disorder in the elderly: A retrospective study. *Journal of Clinical Psychiatry, 54*, 150–155.

Rapee, R. M., & Barlow, D. H. (1991). *Chronic anxiety: Generalized anxiety disorder and mixed anxiety-depression.* New York: Guilford Press.

Regier, D. A., Boyd, J. H., Burke, J. D., Rae, D. S., Myers, J. K., Kramer, M., Robins, L. N., George, L. K., Karno, M., & Locke, B. Z. (1988). One-month prevalence of mental disorders in the United States: Based on five epidemiologic catchment area sites. *Archives of General Psychiatry, 45*, 977–986.

Regier, D. A., Narrow, W. E., & Rae, D. S. (1990). The epidemiology of anxiety disorders: The Epidemiologic Catchment Area (ECA) experience. *Journal of Psychatric Research, 24*, 3–14.

Reynolds, C. F., Lebowitz, B. D., & Schneider, L. S. (1993). The NIH Consensus Development Conference on the diagnosis and treatment of depression in late life: An overview. *Psychopharmacology Bulletin, 29*, 83–85.

Rickard, H. C., Scogin, F., & Keith, S. (1994). A one-year follow-up of relaxation training for elders with subjective anxiety. *The Gerontologist, 34*, 121–122.

Riskind, J. H., Beck, A. T., Brown, G. B., & Steer, R. A. (1987). Taking the measure of anxiety and depression: Validity of the reconstructed Hamilton Scales. *Journal of Nervous and Mental Disease, 175*, 474–479.

Robins, L. N., Helzer, J. E., Weissman, M. M., Orvaschel, H., Gruenberg, E., Burke, J. D., & Regier, D. A. (1984). Lifetime prevalence of specific psychiatric disorders in three sites. *Archives of General Psychiatry, 41*, 949–958.

Roehrs, T., Lineback, W., Zorick, F., & Roth, T. (1982). Relationship of psychopathology to insomnia in the elderly. *Journal of the American Geriatrics Society, 30*, 312–315.

Roehrs, T., Zorick, F., Sicklesteel, J., Wittig, R., & Roth, T., (1983). Age-related sleep–wake disorders at a sleep disorder center. *Journal of the American Geriatrics Society, 31*, 364–370.

Rowan, V. C., Holborn, S. W., Walker, J. R., & Siddiqui, A. R. (1984). A rapid multi-component treatment for an obsessive-compulsive disorder. *Journal of Behavior Therapy and Experimental Psychiatry, 15*, 347–352.

Sallis, J. F., Lichstein, K. L., Clarkson, A. D., Stalgaitis, S., & Campbell, M. (1983). Anxiety and depression management for the elderly. *International Journal of Behavioral Geriatrics, 1*, 3–12.

Salzman, C. (1991). Pharmacologic treatment of the anxious elderly patient. In C. Salzman & B. D. Lebowitz (Eds.), *Anxiety in the elderly: Treatment and research* (pp. 149–173). New York: Springer.

Salzman, C., & Lebowitz, B. D. (1991). *Anxiety in the elderly: Treatment and research.* New York: Springer.

Sanavio, E. (1988). Obsessions and compulsions: The Padua Inventory. *Behaviour Research and Therapy, 26*, 169–177.

Sanderson, W. C., & Wetzler, S. (1991). Chronic anxiety and generalized anxiety disorder: Issues in comorbidity. In R. M. Rapee & D. H. Barlow (Eds.), *Chronic anxiety: Generalized anxiety disorder and mixed anxiety-depression* (pp. 119–135). New York: Guilford Press.

Scogin, F., Rickard, H. C., Keith, S., Wilson, J., & McElreath, L. (1992). Progressive and imaginal relaxation training for elderly persons with subjective anxiety. *Psychology and Aging, 7*, 419–424.

Segal, D. L., Hersen, M., Van Hasselt, V. B., Kabacoff, R. I., & Roth, L. (1993). Reliability of diagnosis in older psychiatric patients using the Structured Clinical Interview for DSM-III-R. *Journal of Psychopathology and Behavioral Assessment, 15*, 347–356.

Segal, D. L., Kabacoff, R. I., Hersen, M., Van Hasselt, V. B., & Ryan, C. F. (1995). Update on the reliability of diagnosis in older psychiatric outpatients using the Structured Clinical Interview for DSM-III-R. *Journal of Clinical Geropsychology, 1*, 313–321.

Sheikh, J. I. (1991). Anxiety rating scales for the elderly. In C. Salzman & B. D. Lebowitz (Eds.), *Anxiety in the elderly: Treatment and research* (pp. 251–265). New York: Springer.

Sheikh, J. I., King, R. J., & Taylor, C. B. (1991). Comparative phenomenology of early onset versus later onset panic attacks: A pilot survey. *American Journal of Psychiatry, 148*, 1231–1233.

Sloane, P. D., Hartman, M., & Mitchell, C. M. (1994). Psychological factors associated with chronic dizziness in patients aged 60 and older. *Journal of the American Geriatric Society, 42*, 847–852.

Smyer, M. A., & Gatz, M. (1995). The public policy context of mental health care for older adults. *The Clinical Psychologist, 48*, 31–36.

Smyer, M. A., Zarit, S. H., & Qualls, S. H. (1990). Psychological intervention with the aging individual. In J. E. Birren & K. W. Schaie (Eds.), *Handbook of the psychology of aging* (3rd ed., pp. 375–403). San Diego, CA: Academic Press.

Spielberger, C. D., Edwards, C. D., Lushene, R. E., Montouri, J., & Platzek, D. (1973). *STAIC: Preliminary manual for the State-Trait Anxiety Inventory for children.* Palo Alto, CA: Consulting Psychologists Press.

Spielberger, C., Gorsuch, R., & Lushene, R. (1970). *Manual for the State-Trait Anxiety Inventory.* Palo Alto, CA: Consulting Psychologists Press.

Spitzer, R. L., Williams, J. B. W., Gibbon, M., & First, M. B. (1988). *Structured Clinical Interview for DSM-III-R—Patient Edition (SCID-P 6/1/88).* New York: Biometrics Research Department, New York State Psychiatric Institute.

Stanley, M. A., Beck, J. G., & Glassco, J. D. (1996).

Generalized anxiety in older adults: Treatment with cognitive-behavioral and supportive approaches. *Behavior Therapy, 27,* 565–581.

Stanley, M. A., & Beck, J. G. (in press). Anxiety disorders. In M. Hersen and V. B. Van Hasselt (Eds.). *Handbook of clinical geropsychology,* New York: Plenum.

Stanley, M. A., Beck, J. G., & Zebb, B. J. (1996). Psychometric properties of four anxiety measures in older adults. *Behaviour Research and Therapy, 34,* 827–838.

Swales, P. J, Solfvin, J. F., & Sheikh, J. I. (1996). Cognitive-behavioral therapy in older panic disorder patients. *The American Journal of Geriatric Psychiatry, 4,* 46–60.

Taylor, G. P., & Hartman-Stein, P. E. (1995). Providing psychological services to older adults: Opportunities for psychologists to sail beyond the sunset. *The Clinical Psychologist, 48,* 5–11.

Thompson, J. W., Burns, B. J., Bartko, J., Boyd, J. H., Taube, C. A., & Bourdon, K. H. (1988). The use of ambulatory services by persons with and without phobia. *Medical Care, 26,* 183–198.

Thompson, L. W., Gallagher, D., & Breckenridge, J. S. (1987). Comparative effectiveness of psychotherapies for depressed elders. *Journal of Consulting and Clinical Psychology, 55,* 385–390.

Thyer, B. A. (1981). Prolonged *in vivo* exposure therapy with a 70-year-old woman. *Journal of Behavior Therapy and Experimental Psychiatry, 12,* 69–71.

Turner, S. M., Hersen, M., Bellack, S., & Wells, K. C. (1979). Behavioral treatment of obsessive-compulsive neurosis. *Behaviour Research and Therapy, 17,* 95–106.

Weiss, K. J. (1994). Management of anxiety and depression syndromes in the elderly. *Journal of Clinical Psychiatry, 55,* 5–12.

Weissman, M. M., Myers, J. K., Tischler, G. L., Holzer, C. E., Leaf, P. J., Orvaschel, H., & Brody, J. A. (1985). Psychiatric disorders (DSM-III) and cognitive impairment among the elderly in a US urban community. *Acta Psychiatrica Scandanavia, 71,* 366–379.

Wengel, S. P., Burke, W. J., Ranno, A. E., & Roccaforte, W. H. (1993). Use of benzodiazepines in the elderly. *Psychiatric Annals, 23,* 325–331.

West, R. L., Boatwright, L. K., & Schleser, R. (1984). The link between memory performance, self-assessment, and affective status. *Experimental Aging Research,* 10, 197–200.

Wisocki, P. A. (1988). Worry as a phenomenon relevant to the elderly. *Behavior Therapy, 19,* 369–379.

Wisocki, P. A., Handen, B., & Morse, C. K. (1986). The Worry Scale as a measure of anxiety among homebound and community active elderly. *The Behavior Therapist, 9,* 91–95.

Wong, M. T. H., & Pan, P. C. (1994). Patterns of psychogeriatric referral and attendance at three different settings in Hong Kong. *International Psychogeriatrics, 6,* 199–208.

Yesavage, J. A., & Jacob, R. (1984). Effects of relaxation and mnemonics on memory, attention and anxiety in the elderly. *Experimental Aging Research, 10,* 211–214.

Yesavage, J. A., Rose, T. L., & Spiegel, D. (1982). Relaxation training and memory improvement in elderly normals: Correlation of anxiety ratings and recall improvement. *Experimental Aging Research, 8,* 195–198.

Yost, E. B., Beutler, L. E., Corbishley, M. A., & Allender, J. R. (1986). *Group Cognitive Therapy: A treatment approach for depressed older adults.* New York: Pergamon.

Zung, W. W. K. (1971). A rating instrument for anxiety disorders. *Psychosomatics, 12,* 371–379.

Zung, W. W. K. (1980). How normal is anxiety? *Current Concepts.* Kalamazoo, MI: Scope.

7.09
Mood Disorders in Late Life

AMY FISKE, JULIA E. KASL-GODLEY, and MARGARET GATZ
University of Southern California, Los Angeles, CA, USA

7.09.1 INTRODUCTION

This chapter provides an overview of mood disorders in older adults. Issues addressed include: How well does the current diagnostic system map onto the types of affective disorders that are observed among older adults? How frequent are mood disorders among older adults? What is the connection of depression to suicide among older adults? What interventions are effective for preventing depression in old age, for alleviating episodes of depression, and for maintaining improvement and thwarting recurrence? Additionally, what is known about etiology is explored, emphasizing the complex influences that link affective symptoms, physical illness, and cognitive dysfunction. This material is then used to inform the discussion of assessment and treatment.

Although the relative proportions are unclear, a key differentiation is between depressive disorders that represent a continuation of conditions from earlier in the life cycle and disorders with first onset in old age. Throughout the chapter, therefore, this differentiation will be maintained, although regrettably the literature frequently does not provide sufficient information to divide the data in this manner.

The mood disorders include depressive disorders, both major depressive disorder and dysthymic disorder, and bipolar disorders. There is minimal literature on mania or bipolar illness in old age. Instead, gerontological researchers have paid most attention to either major depression or subsyndromal symptom constellations. While the task is to encompass all mood disorders, the emphases reflect the differential availability of literature.

Finally, attention is called to the importance of this material, given the common image of depression as characteristic of old age and the frequency with which depressive symptoms are used as outcome measures in research on aging.

7.09.2 DEFINITION AND CLASSIFICATION

Definitional problems underlie debates about prevalence and etiology. For this reason, different classification systems are reviewed and the effect of differences in criteria on decisions about diagnosis and rates of disorder is explored. The most commonly accepted classifications of mood disorders are those in the *Diagnostic and statistical manual of mental disorders* (*4th Edition; DSM-IV*; American Psychiatric Association, 1994) and the *International classification of disease* (*10th Edition*; *ICD-10*; World Health Organization, 1992). These include depressive disorders (major depressive disorder and dysthymic disorder) and bipolar disorders. It is not clear, however, how fully these conventional diagnostic categories represent the experience of affective disorders among older adults. For this reason, descriptions of several subtypes of depression are also presented that may better capture the syndromes prevalent in late life.

7.09.2.1 Standardized Classification Systems

7.09.2.1.1 DSM-IV

Major depressive disorder is defined in the *DSM-IV* by the presence most of the day, nearly every day, of dysphoria (depressed mood), anhedonia (diminished interest or pleasure in all or nearly all activities), appetite or weight disturbance, sleep disturbance, psychomotor agitation or retardation, loss of energy, worthlessness or guilt, inability to concentrate, and/or recurrent thoughts of death or suicide. At least five symptoms must be present, of which one must be either dysphoria or anhedonia. Symptoms attributed to uncomplicated bereavement, the direct physiological effects of a medical condition, or use of a substance (including medications), are excluded. A diagnosis of depressive disorder is made, however, if symptoms in a bereaved person persist longer than two months or include marked functional impairment, morbid preoccupation with worthlessness, suicidal ideation, psychotic symptoms, or psychomotor retardation.

Dysthymic disorder is characterized by chronicity and a lower level of severity than major depression. Depressive symptoms must be present for at least two years. If criteria for both major depressive and dysthymic disorder are met, both diagnoses are assigned, a condition commonly referred to as double depression.

Bipolar-I disorder is marked by alternating major depressive and manic episodes, resulting in impaired functioning. If the manic episodes are briefer and do not interfere with functioning (i.e., hypomanic episodes), the diagnosis of bipolar-II is assigned. Hypomanic episodes alternating with dysthymic symptoms are classified as cyclothymic disorder.

Depressive symptoms that do not meet the above diagnostic criteria, but can be attributed to a specific stressor, may be classified as adjustment disorder with depressed mood.

7.09.2.1.2 ICD-10

There is much similarity between *ICD-10* and *DSM-IV* for mood disorders. Depressive disorders are classified by severity, with moderate and severe equivalent to the *DSM-IV* category of major depressive disorder, and mild episode more closely resembling the provisional category of minor depression in the appendix of *DSM-IV*. *ICD-10* criteria for bipolar affective disorder, dysthymia, and cyclothymia are equivalent to the corresponding *DSM-IV* categories.

7.09.2.1.3 Earlier versions of DSM *and* ICD

Much of the currently available research on mood disorders is based on earlier versions of *DSM* and *ICD*, including *DSM-III* (American Psychiatric Association, 1980), *DSM-III-R* (American Psychiatric Association, 1987), *ICD-9-CM* (Commission on Professional Hospital Activities, 1978), and *ICD-9* (World Health Organization, 1977), or on the Research Diagnostic Criteria (RDC; Spitzer, Endicott, & Robins, 1978). The RDC influenced changes appearing in *DSM-III*, which was published shortly thereafter. RDC mood disorder classifications include: major depressive disorder, minor depressive disorder, bipolar with mania (bipolar-I), bipolar with hypomania (bipolar-II), and intermittent depressive disorder. Changes in *DSM* categories since 1980 have been minimal, while some *ICD* classifications have been completely reworked during this time frame.

In the *DSM*, criteria for mood disorder have become somewhat more stringent with later revisions. A requirement that symptoms be clinically significant or cause impaired social, occupational, or other functioning was introduced in the *DSM-III-R* for dysthymia and in the *DSM-IV* for major depressive disorder. This criterion could affect diagnosis in older adults disproportionally, who may be less likely to engage in social or occupational roles in which impaired functioning could be observed. There have been significant changes in the specification of melancholic features, with *DSM-IV* criteria more closely resembling *DSM-III* than *DSM-III-R*. Bipolar-II disorder was added to *DSM-IV* as a new classification.

Perhaps the greatest changes have occurred between *ICD-9* and *ICD-10*. In the earlier version, mood disorders were classified as either a neurotic disorder or an affective psychosis. Since diagnostic criteria were not specified in detail in *ICD-9*, precise comparisons of classifications are not possible. Affective psychosis approximates the *ICD-10* category of depressive disorder with somatic symptoms, while a neurotic depression would be diagnosed in *ICD-10* as either depressive disorder without somatic symptoms or dysthymia. Due to the differences between classification systems (particularly between *ICD-9* and all other systems), caution should be exercised when comparing results of studies that were not based on a common rubric.

7.09.2.2 Symptom Presentation in Late Life

Although some scholars emphasize similarities between older and younger individuals in the experience of depressive symptoms, there is also an accumulating body of research identifying differences in symptom presentation in late life (for a review, see Caine, Lyness, King, & Connors, 1994). The most frequent differences include: lower prevalence of dysphoria, fewer ideational symptoms (e.g., guilt, suicidal ideation), and increases in selected somatic symptoms.

Several authors have reported a decreased likelihood of dysphoria as a symptom of depression in old age (e.g., Kongstvedt & Sime, 1992). In the Epidemiologic Catchment Area (ECA) sample, Gallo, Anthony, and Muthén (1994) found that older individuals were less likely to endorse an item comprising dysphoria or anhedonia than younger respondents with the same level of overall depression. Using a self-report symptom checklist, Gatz and Hurwicz (1990) found that depressed mood was neither higher nor lower in older adults; however, the older adults in their sample were less likely than other age groups to endorse items on a well-being subscale. Consequently, these authors speculate that older adults may be more likely to experience a lack of positive feelings than active negative feelings.

Age differences in ideational symptoms among depressed patients have been described by Musetti et al. (1989) and Small, Komanduri, Gitlin, and Jarvik (1986). They found lower levels of guilt and lower levels of a factor including self-blame and suicidal ideation. Even though older adults are more likely to complete acts of suicide than younger individuals (Gulbinat, 1996), they appear to be less likely to display suicidal ideation (Blazer, Bachar, & Hughes, 1987; Brown, Sweeney, Loutsch, Kocsis, & Frances, 1984). Brown et al. noted that lower levels of guilt were characteristic of late-onset cases.

The central question about somatic symptoms in depressed older adults is whether they are reliable indicators of depression or merely an artifact of the high comorbidity of physical illness in this age group. Blazer et al. (1987) found that older adults with melancholia were more likely than younger adults to have weight loss and constipation. In patients with major depression, older adults have been found more likely to have delusions, agitation, appetite disturbance, initial insomnia, and hypochondriasis than younger patients (Brodaty et al. 1991; Brown et al. 1984). No difference in somatic symptom presentation was found between early- and late-onset cases. Other investigators have found no age differences in somatic symptoms or preoccupation with physical health, either in depressed psychiatric patients (Kongstvedt & Sime, 1992) or among male patients with medical problems (Koenig, Cohen, Blazer, Krishnan, & Silbert, 1993). Using self-report depression symptom instruments, Kessler, Foster, Webster, and House (1992) found similar relationships with age for both mood and somatic symptom subscales. Finally, Davidson, Feldman, and Crawford (1994) found that physically disabled older adults who scored high on the somatic factor tended to score high on the other factors as well.

Regardless of how common or uncommon specific symptoms are in older adults, it is also important to know which of them are useful prognostically. The particular symptoms that best distinguish depressed from nondepressed older individuals seem to include loss of interest, lack of energy, sleep disturbance, suicidal thoughts, and feeling blue (Koenig et al., 1993; Norris, Snow-Turek, & Blankenship, 1995). Fatigue and changes in appetite and sexual activity did not, and may reflect physical comorbidity or normal aging.

7.09.2.3 Subtypes

Knowledge of the depressive symptoms most frequently experienced by older adults informs the discussion of several subtypes of depression or symptom constellations thought to be relevant in later life. The subtypes reviewed here include ones that can be accommodated within the diagnostic rubric (melancholia and delusional depression), experimental diagnostic categories (minor depression and mixed anxiety–depression), and other syndromes that may occur in older adults (masked depression, depletion syndrome, and hopelessness depression). There is also considerable convergence across many of these entities.

7.09.2.3.1 Melancholic

In the *DSM-IV*, individuals with a unique pattern of symptoms, including nearly complete loss of pleasure in most activities, lack of reactivity to pleasurable stimuli, a distinct quality of mood, depression worse in the morning, early waking, psychomotor retardation or agitation, weight loss, and excessive guilt, are diagnosed with major depressive disorder with melancholic features. At least one of the first two symptoms must be present. The criteria for melancholia in *ICD-10*, referred to as "somatic symptoms," includes the same symptom pattern as "melancholic features" in *DSM-IV* with the exception of distinct quality of depressed mood and excessive guilt. The term "endogenous" has also been used to refer to melancholic depression.

7.09.2.3.2 Delusional depression

Delusional depression is a depressive disorder with the presence of mood-incongruent delusions. It is diagnosed in *DSM-IV* and *ICD-10* by specifying psychotic features/symptoms. In

ICD-10, psychotic symptoms are further classified as mood-congruent or incongruent. There is mixed evidence concerning the relationship between delusional depression and age of onset. Meyers, Greenberg, and Mei-Tal (1985) found delusional depression to be more common in later-onset cases and in late-onset endogenous depression (Meyers, Kalayam & Mei-Tal, 1984). As mentioned earlier, Brodaty et al. (1991) found delusions to be more common in older adults than in younger adults. Nelson, Conwell, Kim, and Mazure (1989) and Baldwin (1995), on the other hand, found no such association.

7.09.2.3.3 Minor depression

As a result of concerns regarding the validity of diagnostic categories for older adults, the 1991 Consensus Conference on Depression in Late Life issued a call for research on "minor (subsyndromal) depression" (Blazer, 1994). Standardized study criteria for minor depression, included in the appendix of *DSM-IV*, are the same as those for major depressive disorder but require fewer symptoms. A similar definition has been referred to as "subdysthymic depression" (Mossey, Knott, Higgins, & Talerico, 1996) or simply "depressive symptoms" (Newmann, 1989; Wells et al., 1989). Several authors have used the term "minor depression," but defined it more inclusively, capturing dysthymia and adjustment disorder with depressed mood as well as dysphoria (Beekman et al., 1995; Koenig & Blazer, 1992; Parmelee, Katz, & Lawton, 1989).

Beekman et al. (1995) found that risk factors for major depression (family history of depression, previous episodes of depression) differed from those for minor depression (being unmarried, having smaller networks of social contacts, living in a large city, chronic disease, and functional limitations). These authors concluded that major depression may be more chronic, while minor depression may be more reactive to stressors. Although minor depression requires fewer symptoms than major depression, and the name implies a syndrome with lesser severity, the Medical Outcomes Study (Wells et al., 1989) revealed that even depressive symptoms in the absence of a depressive disorder were associated with more functional disability than most physical illnesses studied.

7.09.2.3.4 Mixed anxiety–depressive disorder

Another experimental category added to *DSM-IV* that may be relevant to older adults is mixed anxiety–depressive disorder. This proposed disorder is characterized by a combination of subsyndromal depression and anxiety symptoms. The research criteria require a persistent or recurrent dysphoric mood lasting at least one month, with at least four of these additional symptoms: difficulty concentrating, sleep disturbance, fatigue or low energy, irritability, worry, tearfulness, hypervigilance, anticipating the worst, hopelessness, or low self-esteem. Although mixed anxiety-depression was found in one study to be more prevalent in younger than in older age groups (Blazer et al., 1988), this subtype merits further research in an older population due to the obvious overlap between the specified symptoms and those found commonly in depressed older adults.

7.09.2.3.5 Masked depression

A further term used for older individuals is masked depression (Blumenthal, 1980). Also known as somatic depression, masked depression refers to a predominance of somatic symptoms without mood-related symptoms. As the term "masked" implies, diagnosis can be difficult due to the absence of the dysphoric mood that characterizes depression.

7.09.2.3.6 Depletion syndrome

Fogel and Fretwell (1985) proposed depletion syndrome as a new subtype of depression, characterized by predominant somatic and vegetative symptoms in depressed older adults with good premorbid psychosocial functioning and no evidence of psychosis. Newmann, Klein, Jensen, and Essex (1996) have pursued this concept, identifying a set of symptoms that occur together more frequently in older adults than in younger individuals. This constellation of symptoms differs from the depression syndrome in that self-deprecating feelings (self-blame and inappropriate guilt) are not present, dysphoric mood items are less prominent, and enervation, loss of interest in things, hopelessness, and loss of appetite are more prominent. Although sleep disturbance is associated with depletion syndrome, it does not include early morning awakening. Newmann et al. characterize this syndrome as "quieter" than major depression. In a longitudinal study, they found that individuals with depletion syndrome were more likely to die before the next time of measurement than those with depressive syndrome, suggesting that depletion syndrome may be related to a wearing down process. It is important to note that the only research on this subtype to date has been in a female population.

7.09.2.3.7 *Hopelessness depression*

This subtype was developed in younger populations (Abramson, Metalsky, & Alloy, 1989). Like depletion syndrome, it is characterized by decreased motivation, lack of energy, apathy, and psychomotor retardation, as well as by sad affect. Thus, applicability of this conceptualization to older adults seems warranted.

7.09.2.4 Categorical vs. Dimensional Systems

Although the focus has been on various categories used to describe mood disorders in older adults, depression has also been conceptualized as a continuum. Caine et al. (1994) recommend the use of a dimensional descriptive system encompassing the full range of mood syndromes and comorbid medical conditions. Unlike categorical diagnostic methods, depressive symptom checklists yield a rating on a continuous scale and are inclusive in approach. In general, scores relating to the presence or severity of individual symptoms are summed to provide a single rating of level of depressive symptomology. Since no symptoms are excluded due to etiology (e.g., bereavement, physical illness), a more complete picture of distress is provided.

7.09.3 PREVALENCE

7.09.3.1 Rates of Mood Disorders

Studies measuring depressive disorders have found a relatively low prevalence in late life. In a review of earlier studies, Kay and Bergmann (1980) concluded that the prevalence of depressive neuroses ranged from 4 to 9%, and that field surveys on affective psychoses were too limited to yield reliable information. Table 1 summarizes studies of the prevalence of mood disorders in late life that employed representative sampling methods and large sample sizes. The one-year prevalence of major depression among individuals aged 65 years and older ranges from a reported low of 0.9% in the ECA survey in the US (Weissman, Bruce, Leaf, Florio, & Holzer, 1991) to a high of 5.7% in a study of ethnic Chinese living in Singapore (Kua, 1992), with more studies finding rates at the low end of this range. Fewer studies have specifically measured rates of dysthymia in an older population. Due to the chronic nature of this disorder, only lifetime rates have been reported. Weissman and Myers (1978) found a 1.8% lifetime prevalence of dysthymic disorder among older adults using RDC. In the more recent ECA study, based on *DSM-III* criteria, Weissman et al. (1991) reported an overall rate of dysthymic disorder of 1.7% among those aged 65 years or older. Studies of bipolar disorder in older adults are even more rare. According to ECA data, one-year prevalence rates of bipolar disorder ranged from 0 to 0.4% across study sites, for an overall prevalence of 0.1%. Establishing the prevalence of other diagnostic subtypes, such as minor depression, is complicated by varying definitions of these entities.

7.09.3.2 Presence of Depressive Symptoms

Several studies have measured the prevalence of clinically significant depressive symptoms, without tying symptoms to diagnostic criteria for a depressive disorder. Rates of mood disorders suggested through the use of clinical cutoffs on depressive symptom checklists are shown in Table 2 for adults aged 65 years and older. These rates range from 9.0 to 16.9%. Rates found by these studies are generally high compared to studies using diagnostic criteria, as would be expected, since summary scores cannot distinguish between individuals with a disorder and those with subsyndromal levels of symptoms.

7.09.3.3 Age and Depression

In general, epidemiological studies have found lower rates of depressive disorders in older adults compared to other age groups, whereas studies measuring depressive symptoms have found elevated levels in late life, particularly after age 75 years (see Newmann, 1989, for a review). This outcome lends support to the notion that the symptoms experienced by older individuals may not map well onto existing diagnostic criteria.

The association between age and depression is further complicated by the consistent finding that older individuals report a lower lifetime prevalence of depression compared to younger individuals (Weissman et al., 1991). Since older adults have had more years in which to experience depressive episodes, this finding is remarkable. Several possible explanations have been posited. Some researchers have suggested that later-born generations in the twentieth century have experienced progressively higher rates of depression than those born earlier (e.g., Klerman et al., 1985). This cohort effect could explain relatively low rates of depression among those now old, and would predict that rates of depression in late life would rise as successive generations enter old age. A second hypothesis suggests that lifetime prevalence rates are

Table 1 Prevalence of affective disorders in late life.

Authors	*Study*	*Sample*	*N*	*Age range*	*Measures*	*Diagnostic criteria*	*Major depression*	*Minor depression*	*Dysthymia*	*Bipolar disorder*
Baltes et al. (1993); Wernicke and Linden (1994)	Berlin Aging Study	Stratified random (West Berlin)	156	70+	GMS-A, HAS	*DSM-III-R*	4.8%			
Beekman et al. (1995)	Longitudinal Aging Study, Amsterdam	Stratified random (Netherlands)	3056	55–85	DIS, CES-D (16+)	*DSM-III*	2.0% m = 1.4% f = 2.6%	12.9% m = 9.8% f = 15.7%		
Copeland, Dewey, et al. (1987)		Random[b] (Liverpool)	1070	65+	GMS-A AGECAT		2.9% m = 1.7% f = 3.6%	8.3% m = 5.9% f = 9.9%		
Copeland, Gurland, et al. (1987)	US–UK Cross-National Project	Random (London[b] New York)	841	65+	GMS-A AGECAT		2.5% m = 1.3% f = 3.2%	m = 11.8% f = 17.3%		
Henderson et al. (1993)	Canberra-Queanbeyan Study of the Elderly	Random community and institutional samples (Australia)	848	70+	Canberra Interview for the Elderly	*DSM-III-R* *ICD-10*	*DSM*: 1.0% m = 0.4% f = 1.5% *ICD*: 3.3%[a] m = 2.2%[a] f = 3.9%[a]			
Kua (1992)		Stratified random (Singapore)	612	65+	AGMS-A AGECAT	*ICD-9*	5.7%			
Matt, Dean, Wang, and Wood (1992)		Stratified probability (Albany, New York)	1131	50+	SCL-90	*DSM-III-R*	3.9% m = 3.2% f = 4.4%			

Table 1 (continued).

Authors	*Study*	*Sample*	*N*	*Age range*	*Measures*	*Diagnostic criteria*	*Major depression*	*Minor depression*	*Dysthymia*	*Bipolar disorder*
O'Hara, Kohout, and Wallace (1985)		Entire population of two rural counties (Iowa)	3159	65+	CES-D	RDC	1.2%	9.0%		
Uhlenhuth, Balter, Mellineger, Cisin, and Clinthorne (1983)		National probability (US)	798	65–79	HSCL	*DSM-III*	5.1%[c]			
Weissman and Myers (1978)		Stratified random (New Haven)	110	66+	SADS, project specific scale	RDC	5.4%	2.7%	1.8%	
Weissman et al. (1988, 1991)	Epidemiologic Catchment Area (ECA)	Area probability		65+	DIS	*DSM-III*	0.9%, m = 0.4% f = 1.4%		m = 1.0% f = 2.3%	0.1%
		(New Haven)		2576			m = 0.8% f = 1.8%		m = 1.4% f = 3.1%	0.1%
		(Baltimore)		923			m = 0.3% f = 1.5%		m = 0.6% f = 1.3%	0.0%
		(St. Louis)		576			m = 0.1% f = 0.6%		m = 0.5% f = 1.6%	0.4%
		(Central NC)		1240			m = 0.1% f = 1.2%		m = 0.3% f = 2.5%	0.1%
		(Los Angeles)		386			m = 0.7% f = 1.2%		m = 2.5% f = 2.4%	0.0%

[a]Includes mild, moderate, and severe depression. [b]Sampling frame—general medical practice patient lists. [c]Includes dysthymia.
GMS-A, Geriatric Mental State Schedule-Abbreviated; HAS, History and Aetiology Schedule; DIS, Diagnostic Interview Schedule; CES-D, Center for Epidemiological Studies—Depression Scale; AGECAT, Automated Geriatric Examination for Computer-Assisted Taxonomy; SCL-90, Symptom Checklist 90; RDC, Research Diagnostic Criteria; HSCL, Hopkins Symptom Checklist; SADS, Schedule for Affective Disorders and Schizophrenia; m, male; f, female.

Table 2 Prevalence of clinically significant depressive symptoms in late life.

Authors	*Study*	*Sample*	*N*	*Age range*	*Measures*	*Above cutoff*
Berkman et al. (1986)	EPESE/Yale Health and Aging Study	Probability, noninstitutionalized (New Haven)	2806	65+	CES-D (16+)	16.4% m = 11.3% f = 19.2%
Blazer et al. (1991)	EPESE/Duke	Stratified random (North Carolina)	4163	65+	modified CES-D (9+)	9.0% m = 6.4% f = 10.7%
Eaton and Kessler (1981)	HANES	National cluster probability (US)	338[a]	65+	CES-D (16+)	14.8%
Frerichs et al. (1981)		Area probability (Los Angeles)	126	66+	CES-D (16+)	16.7%
Fuhrer et al. (1992)	Paquid	Stratified random, noninstitutionalized (France)	2792	65+	CES-D (m = 17+, f = 23+)	13.4% m = 12.8% f = 13.8%
Gatz Johansson, Pedersen, Berg, and Reynolds (1993)	SATSA	Population-based, twins (Sweden)	1193	50–59 60–69 70–79 80+	CES-D (16+)	20% 24% 25% 28%
Kennedy et al. (1989)		Random (urban community, USA)	2137	65+	CES-D (16+)	16.9% m = 11.1% f = 19.9%
Lindesay Briggs, and Murphy (1989)	Guy's/Age Concern	Random, noninstitutional (inner city London)	890	65+	CARE (13+)	4.3% m = 2.8%, f = 5.3%
					(8+)	13.5%, m = 8.4%, f = 16.9%
Murrell et al. (1983)		Stratified area probability (Kentucky)	2517	55+	CES-D (20+)	m = 13.7% f = 18.2%
O'Hara et al. (1985)		Entire population of two rural counties (Iowa)	3159	65–105	CES-D (16+)	9.0% m = 7.3% f = 10.0%
Stallones et al. (1990)		Stratified probability, noninstitutionalized (US)	1232	65+	CES-D (16+)	9.9%

[a]Reported total $n = 2867$, 11.8% aged 65+ years.

EPESE, Established Populations for Epidemiologic Studies of the Elderly; CES-D, Center for Epidemiologic Studies—Depression Scale; HANES, Health and Nutrition Examination; SATSA, Swedish Adoption/Twin Study of Aging; CARE, Comprehensive Assessment and Referral Evaluation; m, male; f, female.

selectively biased in old age, with forgetting of symptoms exacerbated by cognitive impairment. In fact, research has found lifetime prevalence rates to be fairly unreliable at all ages (Kendler, Neale, Kessler, Heath, & Eaves, 1993). A third factor is selective mortality. Since depression has been associated with increased risk of mortality (Burvill, & Hall, 1994), depressed individuals would be less likely than nondepressed individuals to survive into old age. However, Klerman and Weissman (1889) argued that selective mortality is insufficient to explain observed differences, since a strong association between depressive disorders and subsequent death has not been consistently demonstrated.

It is not clear what proportion of depression in older adults within the community represents late-onset cases. Two studies of consecutive psychiatric admissions found approximately half to have first onset after the age of 60 years (Meyers et al., 1985; Steingart & Herrmann, 1991).

7.09.3.4 Gender

Studies of mixed age populations have consistently found the prevalence of major depressive disorders to be higher in women than in men. This sex difference is also evident for older adults. In both the ECA data (Weissman et al., 1991) and the Canberra study (Henderson et al., 1993), the rate of major depressive disorder in older women was 3.5 times the rate for older men. Evidence indicates, however, that this difference diminishes, or even reverses, in extreme old age. Equal prevalence rates for men and women with major depression were found by Girling et al. (1995) for individuals over 77 years and by Forsell, Jorm, von Strauss, and Winblad (1995) for nonagenarians. Wallace and O'Hara (1992) found that the sex difference on the Center for Epidemiologic Studies—Depression scale (CES-D) diminished in older age and was reversed in individuals aged 85 years and older.

In contrast to the sex ratio for major depressive disorder, bipolar disorder seems to occur with equal frequency in men and in women in mixed-age samples and in old age (Weissman et al., 1984).

7.09.3.5 Ethnicity/Race

Few studies report rates of mood disorders in older adults by race or ethnicity. Blazer, Burchett, Service, and George (1991) reported no differences between Black and non-Black older adults on a modified CES-D. In a national probability sample of older adults, Stallones, Marx, and Garrity (1990) found no differences in rates of major depression for Black and White men, but Black women were nearly twice as likely to have major depressive disorder as White women. Both Frerichs, Aneshensel, and Clark (1981) and Kemp, Staples, and Lopez-Aqueres (1987) found Latino older adults in Los Angeles to have especially elevated rates of depression. The authors suggest that income and education levels may account for ethnic differences. In the latter report, rates were highest among non-English speaking individuals, raising issues both of translation of terms and cultural understanding of the meaning of symptoms.

7.09.3.6 Special Populations

7.09.3.6.1 Medical inpatients and outpatients

The prevalence of mood disorders is higher in medical outpatients, medical inpatients, and residents of long-term care facilities than in the general population (see review by Koenig & Blazer, 1992). The few studies examining depressive disorders among older adult outpatients have reported widely varying rates. Barrett, Barrett, Oxman, and Gerber (1988) found major depression or minor episodic depression in 5.6% of patients over age 65 years in a general medical practice, with an additional 7.9% showing masked depression. In contrast, two studies of Veterans Administration (VA) outpatient clinic populations found rates of major depression of 23% (Norris, Gallagher, Wilson, & Winograd, 1987) and 31% (Okimoto et al., 1982).

Studies of older medical inpatients have yielded rates of major depression ranging generally from 6 to 13%, with an additional 15–30% displaying dysthymia, adjustment disorder, depressive disorders not otherwise specified, or dysphoria (Koenig & Blazer, 1992). As with outpatient samples, the highest rates of depression among older adult inpatients have been found in a VA setting. Kitchell, Barnes, Veith, Okimoto and Raskind (1982) found major depressive disorder in 45% of a sample of veterans.

7.09.3.6.2 Long-term care facilities

Studies of depression in institutional settings have found 6–16% meeting *DSM* criteria for major depression, and an additional 25–35% diagnosed with another type of depressive disorder or significant dysphoria (Henderson et al., 1993; Koenig & Blazer, 1992). Both Parmelee et al. (1989) and Mann, Graham, and Ashby 1984) found an approximately doubled risk among newly admitted residents compared to veteran residents or intrainstitution transfers.

Although few studies have examined rates of bipolar disorder in institutional settings, the ECA found a rate of 9.7% in nursing homes compared to a rate of major depression of 16.2% (Weissman et al., 1991).

7.09.3.6.3 Caregivers

Depressive disorders and depressive symptoms have been found in a high proportion of older adult caregiver samples, although methodological issues make comparisons with the general population difficult. In studies using diagnostic criteria ascertained by clinical interview, rates of depressive disorders among caregivers range from 23 to 46%, while virtually all studies measuring depressive symptoms have found elevated levels in this group (Schulz & Williamson, 1994). A problem with research on caregivers is lack of representative sampling, since most samples are drawn from individuals who have sought help (e.g., support group members) and therefore may be more distressed.

7.09.4 ETIOLOGICAL AND CORRELATED FACTORS

This section reviews factors that are related to clinically diagnosed depression and severity of depressive symptoms. Some of these variables are generally regarded as risk factors. However, the terminology of risk factors implies a temporal and causal relationship, whereas the terminology of correlated factors allows for reversed causal order, feedback mechanisms, or that both depression and the respective factor are the outcome of the same process. Variables encompassed in this section include physical health, cognitive dysfunction, interpersonal relations and stressful life events, and genetic risk.

When considering etiological and correlated factors, it is important to keep in mind that not all older adults who experience one or more of these factors necessarily become depressed. Why are some individuals vulnerable and others apparently resilient? Coping styles, perceived control and efficacy, and social support are among the variables that have been shown to mediate the relationship. These are relevant protective factors when designing preventive interventions and useful variables in accounting for individual differences in response to physical illness, interpersonal loss, and cognitive impairment.

7.09.4.1 Physical Health

Physical health status, which can be defined in terms of medical conditions and associated medication use, functional disability, pain, and subjective perceptions of poor health, has been found to be correlated with depression (Forsell et al., 1995; Heikkinen, Berg, & Avlund, 1995; Kennedy et al., 1989; Stallones et al., 1990). This is one of the most well-established correlations in studies of mood and aging. Several explanations for this association exist: physical illness and/or its treatment induce biological changes that trigger depressive symptoms; the same physiological factors underlie physical illness and depression; depression leads to physical illness by creating vulnerabilities, possibly neuroimmune, or by undermining self-care efforts such as medication compliance; physical illness is a stressful experience with which people have difficulty coping; or physical illness and depression co-occur as independent conditions. Thus, the powerful relationship between physical illness, associated conditions such as reduced activity, functional disability and perceptions of health, and depressive symptoms could reflect interdependence and continuing feedback loops of biological changes and psychological factors.

Biological changes induced by neurochemical, neuroanatomical, and functional alterations can create a liability for depression or for mania (see Ferrier & McKeith, 1991, and Leuchter, 1994, for reviews; Conn, 1989; Shulman, Tohen, Satlin, Mallya, & Kalunian, 1992). Preexisting disease processes, such as Parkinson's disease, medical conditions, such as hypothyroidism, or focal lesions may also induce affective changes (see Rubin, 1994 for review; Ferrier & McKeith, 1991). Cerebrovascular disease, including stroke and more minor insults such as deep white matter changes and lacunar infarcts, are particularly likely to precipitate depression (Lawlor & Anderson, 1995; Robinson & Starkstein, 1990), and vascular disease has a notable relationship with late-onset depression (Baldwin & Tomenson, 1995). Use of prescription medications for these conditions may precipitate or aggravate depression (Kinzie, Lewinsohn, Maricle, & Teri, 1986), as may psychotropic medications (Forsell et al., 1995).

Once present, depressive symptoms can worsen morbidity in medically ill individuals (Rapp, Smith, & Britt, 1990). This worsening may reflect a depression-induced vulnerability, a shared process, or a reaction to illness and disability. For example, stroke-induced paralysis could reduce mobility and increase dependence that has a negative impact on social and emotional functioning. Lyness, Caine, Conwell, King, and Cox (1993) found that in both younger and older depressed inpatients, physical disability was associated with depressive symptoms independent of, and likely additive to, medical illness. This finding is consistent with the conclusion that physical disability is associated with depressive symptomology across a range of physical conditions (Turner & Beiser, 1990), some of which do not have a purported biological basis for depression.

However, depression has also been found to increase risk of disability in individuals in the absence of significant health problems or disability (Bruce, Seeman, Merrill, & Blazer, 1994). Perceptions of health may be an important moderating variable given that perceived poor health or disability, irrespective of objective health status, can create depressogenic effects (Williamson & Schulz, 1992b). However, depressive symptoms also can influence self-perceived physical function (Cress et al., 1995).

The presence of pain contributes to the association between depression, disability, and medical illness. The association among illness, pain, disability, and depression has been examined in both community and institutionalized samples. In a community sample, Williamson and Schulz (1992a) found pain related to depression through its association with activity restriction. In institutionalized older adults, Parmelee, Katz, and Lawton (1991) found pain to serve as an independent predictor of depression.

7.09.4.2 Cognitive Dysfunction

Depression has been found to be associated with varying degrees of cognitive dysfunction. Three primary associations seem to exist: (i) memory loss can lead to depression; (ii) depression can be accompanied by cognitive impairment that is reversible, at least temporarily, in that it lifts when the depression is treated (referred to as "pseudodementia" or "depression related cognitive dysfunction"); and (iii) depression can co-occur with dementia, where depression represents a prodromal symptom, a comorbid condition possibly reflecting similar physiological factors, or a reaction to the dementia. The possibility of these variations, expanded below, underscores the difficulty in differentiating depression and dementia diagnostically.

Depression does not seem to be associated with a global decline in cognition. When an effect is observed, it tends to be limited to circumscribed deficits in specific domains, that is, executive functions and right-hemisphere tasks, although findings are equivocal across studies and among different measures of the same domain (see La Rue, 1992, for a review). For example, depressed middle-aged and older adults have been found to show deficits in nonverbal memory, select frontal lobe skills (Boone et al., 1994), and visual-spatial tasks (Lyness, Eaton, & Schneider, 1994), which Boone et al. interpret as premature "aging" of cognitive abilities. In contrast, O'Hara, Hinrichs, Kohout, Wallace, and Lemke (1986) found no significant verbal memory impairment in depressed elderly community-residing older adults. These findings are important because complaints about memory frequently accompany depression in older adults (O'Connor, Pollitt, Roth, Brook, & Reiss, 1990), and depression can affect concentration and hence performance on cognitive test batteries (Poon, 1992). Demonstrable cognitive deficits are observed more often among very severely depressed patients than in community samples. One study of older adult depressed inpatients found that impairment in learning and memory was related to longer duration of depression (La Rue, Goodman, & Spar, 1992). Further, elderly inpatients with psychotic features show poorer cognitive functioning than depressed patients without psychotic features (Kunik, Champagne, Harper, & Chacko, 1994).

The added difficulty with these studies is that it is possible that some of the more severe depressed patients are actually early dementia cases. Longitudinal follow-up suggests that a majority of cognitively impaired depressed patients who regain premorbid cognitive function after the depression is treated will develop dementia if followed long enough (Kral & Emery, 1989) and that degree of cognitive impairment in depression may predict who will develop dementia (Alexopolous, Meyers, Young, Mattis, & Kakuma, 1993). Various characteristics have been suggested to distinguish patients whose cognitive symptoms are due to depression alone from patients who are becoming demented, especially motivational disturbances and vegetative symptoms (Forsell, Jorm, & Winblad, 1994; Lazarus, Newton, Cohler, Lesser, & Schweon, 1987). History may be even more helpful than current features (see Kaszniak & Christenson (1994) for a comprehensive discussion of differential diagnosis).

Finally, there can be multiple, shared, or reciprocal causes. Although little is known about the cognitive dysfunction of depressed, demented individuals, there is some suggestion that depression worsens the cognitive impairment (Fitz & Teri, 1994). Moreover, demented patients with co-occurring depression show some cognitive improvement when depression is treated (Greenwald et al., 1989). Gross cognitive impairment concomitant with later age of onset of depression may suggest a shared biological vulnerability (Steingart & Herrmann, 1991). Awareness of deficits caused by dementia may engender dysthymia (Migliorelli et al., 1995; Seltzer, Vasterling, & Buswell, 1995). Some observers feel that depressed mood correlates negatively with degree of impairment, which intimates the role of awareness, although others have found no association between awareness and illness (Ballard, Cassidy, Bannister, & Mohan, 1993).

7.09.4.3 Interpersonal Relationships and Stressful Life Experiences

Both diagnosed depression and depressive symptoms have been found to be related to interpersonal difficulties (Hinrichsen & Zweig, 1994). This association may reflect three primary processes: (i) depression strains and disrupts interpersonal relationships, (ii) depression influences an individual's perception of social relationships; and (iii) unsupportive, demanding, sparse or nonreciprocal, nonequitable interpersonal interactions precipitate depression. Whether or not depression is an outcome of these processes seems to be determined, in part, by an individual's level of assertiveness (Kogan, Van Hasselt, Hersen, & Kabacoff, 1995), self-efficacy, or personal control (Krause, Hertzog, & Baker, 1992), degree of social embeddedness (Adelmann, 1994) and concurrent stressors.

What is known about interpersonal difficulties of depressed older adults tends to be derived from studies of social support that often are examined in the context of stressful life events. These events provide the occasion for emotional support and tangible assistance (Dean, Kolody, & Wood, 1990; Russell & Cutrona, 1991). Stressful life experiences include discrete, disruptive negative life events, chronic strains, and daily hassles. They may or may not be predictable or under a person's control. Often a discrete event precipitates chronic strains or hassles. Some common events with which older adults often must cope are widowhood, deaths of family and friends, caregiving, and the need for institutionalization. These events have been found to be associated with depression (see Murrell & Meeks, 1992 for a review). Declining health, increasing disability, and cognitive dysfunction are also stressful experiences that have been discussed earlier.

As with declining health and cognitive dysfunction, the causal direction of the association between stressful experiences, disrupted interpersonal relationships, and depression is controversial. However, a likely shared mechanism for depression is the depletion of resources (Hobfoll & Wells, in press). Identity, independence, and perceived control or efficacy can be threatened. Stressful experiences may result in disrupted relationships. Depressed individuals may act in ways that alienate their support network, or losses in a support network can precipitate depression. These processes all have implications for psychotherapeutic intervention.

One of the most important loss events is bereavement. Depressive symptoms following loss of spouse vary in relation to characteristics of the death (Gilewski, Farberow, Gallagher, & Thompson, 1991), quality of the relationship and degree of attachment with the deceased (Levy, Martinowski, & Derby, 1994; Murrell & Himmelfarb, 1989), concurrent stressors (Levy et al., 1994), timing and type of social support received (Schuster & Butler, 1989), and perceived competencies (Lund, Caserta, Dimond, & Shaffer, 1989).

Depressive symptoms or bereavement-related depression have been distinguished from grief, or the psychological and physiological reactions to the loss (Marwit, 1991), although both responses are time-limited. However, sometimes grief becomes complicated and the individual fails to return to preloss levels of well-being (Prigerson et al., 1995). Symptoms include crying, being stunned by loss, searching and yearning for the deceased, disbelief about the death, and preoccupation with thoughts of the deceased.

The distinction between grief and depression may explain some inconsistencies in previous studies on depression and loss events. Few investigations have examined the relationship between complicated grief and depression. Gilewski et al. (1991) found that levels of depression at the time of bereavement predicted subsequent adjustment. Hays, Kasl, and Jacobs (1994) and Lichtenstein, Gatz, Pedersen, Berg, and McClearn (1996) observed elevated depressive symptoms prior to the actual loss, with no significant difference between the period directly before the death and the period right after the loss. This pattern seems to be consistent with anticipatory grieving, a process that others have suggested may facilitate adaptation to bereavement (Levy et al., 1994).

7.09.4.4 Genetic Risk

Heritability of major depressive disorder has been studied using family, twin, and adoption designs in younger adults but not in older adults. It is generally accepted that there is some genetic involvement in etiology, that recurring episodes of depression suggest a more heritable form of the disorder, and that early-onset depression has greater genetic determination than late-onset depression (Moldin, Reich, & Rice, 1991). Baldwin and Tomenson (1995) found family history of depression in about a third of early-onset cases compared with 5% of late-onset cases (mean age of onset = 74 years).

In adult samples, Torgersen (1986) reported concordance rates of 27% for monozygotic (MZ) and 12% for dizygotic (DZ) twin pairs from a Norwegian sample and he estimated the heritability of major depression to be 54%. In a Danish twin sample, Bertelsen, Harvald, and Hauge (1977) found concordance rates for unipolar depression of 39% for MZ and 12.5% for DZ pairs. In the Swedish Adoption/Twin Study of Aging, with twin pairs all aged 50 and older, concordance rates for scoring 16 or higher on the CES-D were 33% in MZ and 12% in DZ pairs (Gatz, 1992). Using a British twin register, McGuffin, Katz, Watkins, and Rutherford (1996) reported concordance rates of 46% in MZ and 20% in DZ pairs for *DSM-IV* diagnosed major depression, resulting in heritability estimates of 48–75% dependent upon true population prevalence.

Heterogeneity in etiology is likely. Torgersen (1986) found that, while partners of probands with major depression were apt to have major depression, dysthymic disorder, or depressive adjustment disorder, concordance rates for dysthymic disorder were low in both MZ and DZ twin pairs. Kendler, Neale, Kessler, Heath, and Eaves (1992), using adult twins, suggest that genetic liability to major depression and to generalized anxiety disorder is influenced by the same genetic factors but different environmental experiences.

Consistent with the notion that genetic factors for early-onset depression are distinct from those for late-onset depression, van Ojen et al. (1995a, 1995b) found that older adults with depression accompanied by cognitive impairment were likely to have no history of psychiatric illness themselves and a family history of dementia or of Down's syndrome rather than a family history of depressive disorder. Those depressed older adults who reported both personal and family history of mental illness did not have impaired cognitive performance.

More than major depression, manic-depressive disorder has generally been regarded as running in families, and twin studies have suggested greater genetic influence for bipolar than for unipolar disorder (Bertelsen et al., 1977; Torgersen, 1986). Shulman et al. (1992) found that elderly patients admitted to a hospital for mania were more likely to have a family history suggestive of genetic predisposition compared with elderly admissions for major depression.

7.09.5 ASSESSMENT

In this section the focus is on psychometric properties, measurement efficiency, and measurement invariance of instruments used to assess depression. There follows a discussion on how validity is influenced by uncertainties about the diagnostic criteria in older adults and whether depression is the same across age and within different subgroups, defined by gender, ethnicity, or comorbid conditions (for other reviews and recommendations about measuring depression in older adults, see Pachana, Gallagher-Thompson, & Thompson, 1994, and Scogin 1994).

The efficiency of an assessment instrument can be gauged in terms of several metrics. Sensitivity is proportion of correctly identified depressed cases; specificity is proportion of nondepressed cases correctly identified; positive predictive power (PPP) is probability that a score at or above the clinical cutoff will correspond to a diagnosis of depression; negative predictive power (NPP) is probability that a score below the cutoff will correspond to the absence of a diagnosis of depression. PPP and NPP are influenced by population prevalence. The efficiency of any given cutoff will change with the base rate for depression. Because base rates are known to vary with cognitive impairment, physical illness and gender, efficiency can be affected. Variability in efficiency will also result when there are differences between groups in the underlying construct.

Assessment instruments are grouped on the basis of whether they are self-report or interview-based and by the population with whom they were developed. Interview-based measures include observer-rated measures and structured interviews. Structured interviews have two general formats: one applies diagnostic algorithms upon completion; the second incorporates the algorithms into the structure of the interview (i.e., if a required criterion is not met, the remaining questions are skipped).

7.09.5.1 Self-report Instruments

7.09.5.1.1 Depression scales developed with mixed-age samples

The Beck Depression Inventory (BDI; Beck, Ward, Mendelson, Mock, & Erbaugh, 1961) includes 21 items, each including four alternative statements ranging in order of severity from zero to three. Conventional cutoffs are 0–9 for normal range, 10–18 for mild to moderate depression, 19–29 for moderate to severe depression, and 30–63 for severe depression (Beck, Steer, & Garbin, 1988). For the 13-item short form (Beck & Beck, 1972), 0–4 corresponds to none or minimal depression, 5–7 to mild depression, 8–15 to moderate depression, and 16 or higher to severe depression.

The BDI has demonstrated test–retest and split-half reliability as well as concurrent validity with older adults (see Gallagher, 1986). With a cutoff of 10, the BDI has shown good efficiency with older depressed psychiatric outpatients (100% sensitivity, 96% specificity, 100% PPP, 100% NPP; Olin, Schneider, Eaton, Zemansky, & Pollock, 1992). In a sample seeking outpatient mental health services, Kogan, Kabacoff, Hersen, and Van Hasselt (1994) found that a cutoff of 22 maximized efficiency, yielding 64% sensitivity and 73% specificity.

The BDI has good efficiency in older medical outpatients (Rapp, Parisi, Walsh, & Wallace, 1988) and medical inpatients (Norris et al., 1987). Cognitively impaired individuals have been found to have difficulty comprehending the format (Lyons, Strain, Hammer, Ackerman & Fulop, 1989) and the BDI may be less sensitive to detecting major depression in older men when compared with older women (Allen-Burge, Storandt, Kinscherf, & Rubin, 1994).

The other conspicuous feature of the BDI lies in its inclusion of somatic symptoms. Zemore and Eames (1979) demonstrated that age differences on the BDI could be explained entirely by the somatic symptoms, with no age differences on the more cognitive symptoms.

The Zung Self-rating Depression Scale (SDS; Zung, 1965) contains 20 items, 10 worded positively, and 10 negatively. Items are on a one to four scale; raw scores are converted into a percentage by dividing the sum of all questions by 0.80. Conventional cutoffs are 25–43 for no depression, 50–59 for mild to moderate depression, 60–69 for moderate to severe depression, and 70 or over for severe depression (Zung, 1967). Older adults have shown higher normal baseline scores than the validation sample (Zung, 1967) which may be attributed to the large number of items about somatic symptoms (Berry, Storandt, & Coyne, 1984). Reliability has been found to be moderate or low, particularly among the oldest old, and sex and age differences in factor structure have been suggested (Kivela & Pahkala, 1986; Kivela & Pahkala, 1987; McGarvey, Gallagher, Thompson, & Zelinski, 1982). In medically ill inpatients, the SDS has been found to have a 58% sensitivity and 87% specificity using a cutoff score of 60 (Kitchell et al., 1982) in comparison with an 82% sensitivity–87% specificity in medical outpatients (Okimoto et al., 1982). A 10-item interviewer-assisted form has been developed and validated for older adults (Tucker, Ogle, Davison, & Eilenberg, 1986). A cutoff score above 70 is recommended for the 10-item form.

The Center for Epidemiological Studies—Depression Scale (CES-D; Radloff, 1977) is a 20-item measure designed for large-scale epidemiological surveys. It can be self-administered, by paper-and-pencil or using computer speech recognition (Muñoz, Gonzales, & Starkweather, 1995), or used in an interview, face-to-face or by telephone (George, Blazer, Hughes & Fowler, 1989). Four items are worded positively and are reverse scored; these items have a particularly high rate of omission or response bias (Callahan & Wolinsky, 1994; Gatz & Hurwicz, 1990). Scores range from zero to 60. A score of 16 or more is used as the conventional cutoff for clinical depression, although a cutoff score of 20 may have increased efficiency with older adults (see Radloff & Teri, 1986; Murrell, Himmelfarb, & Wright, 1983). Several shorter forms have been developed specifically for use with older adults by collapsing response categories and giving only 10 or 11 of the items (Andresen, Malmgren, Carter, & Patrick, 1994; Kohout, Berkman, Evans, & Cornoni-Huntley, 1993). The CES-D has probable measurement invariance across age (Hertzog, Van Alstine, Usala, Hultsch, & Dixon, 1990), culture (Heikkinen et al., 1995), and physical health or disability (Davidson et al., 1994). Although the same broad factors emerge, there are differences across gender and ethnic or racial subgroups with respect to factor loadings and placement of specific items on factors. Garcia and Marks (1989) and Callahan and Wolinsky (1994) emphasize that these differences imply sociocultural differences in the expression of depression.

Two self-report forms of the observer-rated Hamilton Rating Scale for Depression (HRSD) have been developed: the Carroll Rating Scale for Depression (CRS; Carroll, Feinberg, Smouse, Rawson, & Greden 1981; Feinberg, Carroll, Smouse, & Rawson, 1981; Smouse, Feinberg, Carroll, Park, & Rawson, 1981) and the Hamilton Depression Inventory (HDI; Reynolds & Kobak, 1991). In the CRS, 52 "yes/no" items replace the HRSD severity ratings. A score of 10 is the recommended clinical cutoff. Koenig, Meador, Cohen, and Blazer (1988, 1992) examined a 12-item short version of the CRS in medical inpatients

(BCDRS; Duke Depression Evaluation Schedule for the Elderly, 1988). A cutoff of six yielded the best efficiency.

The Inventory to Diagnose Depression (IDD; Zimmerman & Coryell, 1987; Zimmerman, Coryell, Corenthal, & Wilson, 1986) is a 22-item instrument designed to diagnose major depressive disorder according to *DSM-III* criteria and to provide information about symptom severity and duration. Although the IDD has been used with older adults, psychometric properties are unknown.

7.09.5.1.2 Instruments devised specifically for use with older adults

The Geriatric Depression Scale (GDS; Yesavage et al., 1983) includes 30 "yes/no" items, 10 reverse scored. A cutoff of 11 demonstrates good sensitivity (84%) and specificity (95%; Yesavage et al.) and adequate hit rates (17% false-negative rate, 18% false-positive rate; Dunn & Sacco, 1989) in community-dwelling older adults; good overall efficiency in psychiatric outpatients preselected for major depression (96% sensitivity, 96% specificity, 96% PPP, 96% NPP; Olin et al., 1992); and good sensitivity (89%) but poorer specificity (75%) and positive predictive value (27%) in older medical inpatients when compared with psychiatric interview (Koenig et al., 1988; Koenig, et al., 1992). Others suggest a cutoff of 14–16 for best efficiency (Burke, Houston, Boust, & Roccaforte, 1989; Kogan et al., 1994). Other evidence suggests that the GDS maintains its reliability and validity when administered over the telephone (Burke, Roccaforte, Wengel, Conley, & Potter, 1995).

The GDS has been found less effective in the detection of major depression in older men when compared with older women (Allen-Burge et al., 1994). It appears to be reliable and valid for older, medically ill outpatients (Norris et al., 1987), hospitalized individuals (Lyons et al., 1989; Rapp et al., 1988), and noncognitively impaired nursing home residents (Lesher, 1986), although some items are sensitive to health status (Fischer, Rolnick, Jackson, Garrard, & Luepke, 1996). There is some suggestion that it is insensitive to detecting minor depression (Harper, Kotik-Harper, & Kirby, 1990; Parmelee et al., 1989). Some older respondents have expressed dissatisfaction with the "yes/no" format (Fischer et al., 1996).

Use of the GDS in cognitively-impaired older adults is equivocal. When identifying depression in mildly to moderately demented individuals, Lichtenberg, Marcopulos, Steiner, and Tabscott (1992) found that a cutoff of 11 yielded good sensitivity (82%) and specificity (88%). With geriatric assessment center clients, Burke, Nitcher, Roccaforte, and Wengel (1992) found that a cutoff of 14 yielded the highest combined sensitivity (70%) and specificity (78%). Other studies show that the GDS does little better than chance as a screening measure for depression in cognitively-impaired individuals (Burke et al., 1989; Kafonek et al., 1989).

A 15-item short form of the GDS (Lesher & Berryhill, 1994; Sheikh & Yesavage, 1986) retains the same "yes/no" format and the same ratio of positively- and negatively-worded items. A cutoff of five is recommended. The GDS short form has good efficiency with medically ill skilled nursing facility residents (Baker & Miller, 1991) and older primary care surgery attenders (sensitivity 91%, specificity 72%, NPP 94%; D'ath, Katona, Mullan, Evans, & Katona, 1994), but poorer efficiency in ethnically heterogeneous populations (Cwikel & Ritchie, 1988) and in cognitively-impaired individuals (Burke, Roccaforte, & Wengel, 1991; Lesher & Berryhill, 1994).

7.09.5.1.3 Multidimensional measures with depression subscales

The 567-item Minnesota Multiphasic Personality Inventory-2 (MMPI-2; Butcher, Dahlstrom, Graham, Tellegen, & Kaemmer, 1989) includes a 57-item depression scale. Little is known about the measurement properties of the MMPI-2-D with older adults. One 15-item short form of the MMPI-D was developed and construct-validated using a sample of older adult male inpatients (Dush & Hutzell, 1986). Another short form has been used for detecting depression in cognitively-impaired older adults (Ward, Wadsworth, & Peterson, 1994).

The Symptom Checklist 90—Revised (SCL-90-R; Derogatis, 1977), as well as its precursors, the SCL-90 and the Hopkins Symptom Checklists (HSCL), assess distress on a wide range of psychiatric symptoms. The depression subscale on the SCL-90-R comprises 13 items. A 53-item short version of the SCL-90, entitled the Brief Symptom Inventory (BSI; Derogatis & Melisaratos, 1983), includes the depression dimension, reduced to six items. Norms have been published for use with community-dwelling older adults (Hale, Cochran, & Hedgepeth, 1984) and with caregivers (Anthony-Bergstone, Zarit, & Gatz, 1988). The BSI depression subscale excludes all somatic items. For medically ill patients, high false-negative rates have been reported, particularly those with minor depression (Harper et al., 1990).

Other self-report mood instruments that sometimes appear in the literature are the Multiple Affect Adjective Check List (MAACL:

Zuckerman & Lubin, 1965; MAACL-R: Zuckerman & Lubin, 1985) and the Profile of Mood States (POMS; McNair, Lorr, & Droppleman, 1971/1981/1992) or a shortened form (Guadagnoli & Mor, 1989). Properties with older adults are not well known.

7.09.5.2 Observer-rated Inventories

The Hamilton Rating Scale for Depression (Hamilton, 1960; Hamilton, 1967) is a 17-item instrument that was designed to measure frequency and intensity of depressive symptoms in individuals with major depressive disorder. Ratings are made using either a five- or a three-point scale, yielding total scores from zero to 61. Conventional clinical cutoff scores range from 14 to 20, with 17 being the most common in pharmacological research (see Reynolds & Kobak, 1991). The HRSD has demonstrated reliability, validity, and efficiency in older adults (Stukenberg, Dura, & Kiecolt-Glaser, 1990).

Cognitively-impaired, medically ill older adults have shown difficulty understanding, responding to, and completing the questions (Baker & Miller, 1991) and use of the HRSD for identifying depression in demented individuals has mixed results (Lichtenberg et al., 1992; Vida, Des Rosiers, Carrier, & Gauthier, 1994a). With a cutoff of 17, the HRSD showed 9% sensitivity and 92% specificity in mild to severely demented hospitalized patients. However, a cutoff of seven maximized efficiency, yielding 90% sensitivity and 63% specificity. A structured interview guide has been developed for the HRSD (SIGH-D; Williams, 1988) to standardize the way in which rating information is obtained; its use in older adults is unknown.

Another observer-rating inventory that more often appears in European literature is the Montgomery–Åsberg Depression Rating Scale (MADRS; Montgomery & Åsberg, 1979).

The Geriatric Depression Rating Scale (GDRS; Jamison & Scogin, 1992) was developed specifically for older adults. It includes 29 of the 30 items on the GDS and six somatic items to conform to RDC criteria. A cutoff of 20 can be used to discriminate depressed and nondepressed individuals (88% sensitivity, 82% specificity).

7.09.5.3 Structured Interviews

7.09.5.3.1 Instruments designed for mixed ages

The Present State Examination (PSE; Wing, Birley, Cooper, Graham, & Issacs, 1967) uses a standardized question format from which a computer program (CATEGO) yields behavioral syndromes that approximate the *ICD* diagnostic categories.

The Schedule for Affective Disorders and Schizophrenia (SADS; Endicott & Spitzer, 1978) is a semistructured interview developed in conjunction with the RDC. There are three versions: regular SADS, which queries severity of symptoms during the preceding week and at the time when they were the most severe during the current episode; lifetime version (SADS-L); and the version for measuring change (SADS-C). The SADS has been used with older adults. Efficiency is good (82% sensitivity and 93% specificity; Gallagher, Breckenridge, Steinmetz & Thompson, 1983) when compared with the BDI as a criterion measure.

The National Institute of Mental Health Diagnostic Interview Schedule (DIS; Robins, Helzer, Croughan, & Ratcliff, 1981) is a structured interview used in the ECA. Both current and lifetime diagnoses using *DSM-III* and RDC criteria can be made by computer.

The Composite International Diagnostic Interview (CIDI; Robins et al., 1988) was designed for cross-cultural epidemiologic and comparative studies of psychopathology in general populations, whereas its companion, the Schedules for Clinical Assessment in Neuropsychiatry (SCAN), was intended for use in clinical samples. The CIDI is constructed in diagnostic modules that can be extracted and administered on their own. These modules yield both *DSM-III-R* and PSE principal diagnoses, each with its own set of diagnostic computer programs. CIDI short screening scales are available for quicker administration (Kessler & Mroczek, 1993).

The Structured Clinical Interview for *DSM-III-R* (SCID; Spitzer, Williams, Gibbon, & First, 1992) provides current and lifetime diagnoses. It has been revised for *DSM-IV*. It is intended to be administered by clinicians and makes allowance for clinical judgement in modifying and supplementing the interview (Spitzer et al.). Use of information from multiple sources to inform rating decisions is encouraged. There are two versions of the SCID: the SCID-P (Patient) and the SCID-NP (Nonpatient). The major depression module of the SCID-P has been studied with older adults (Segal, Herzen, Van Hasselt, Kabacoff, & Roth, 1993).

7.09.5.3.2 Instruments designed for older adults

The Geriatric Mental State examination (GMS; Copeland et al., 1976) is a semistructured interview from which the AGECAT computer program is used to assign diagnoses and confidence ratings for each diagnosis.

Many of the 541 items were derived from the PSE. AGECAT depression diagnoses have been shown to have a sensitivity of 80%, a specificity of 89%, and a PPP of 71% in physically ill hospitalized older adults (Ames, Flynn, Tuckwell, & Harrigan, 1994).

The Geriatric Mental State Schedule-Depression Scale (GMSS-DS; Ravindran, Welburn, & Copeland, 1994) is a 33-item rating scale derived from the GMS, designed to be sensitive to symptomatic changes in depression with treatment in older adults.

The Comprehensive Assessment and Referral Evaluation (CARE; Gurland et al., 1977–78) uses a shortened form of the GMS as part of a comprehensive assessment package of health and social problems of elderly community residents. There is a 19-item depression/demoralization scale on the CORE–CARE (Golden, Teresi, & Gurland, 1984). The GMS–AGECAT and CARE are used in differential diagnosis of depression and dementia.

7.09.5.4 Assessing Depression in Cognitively-impaired Older Adults

Measures developed specifically to assess depression in cognitively-impaired individuals tend to use simple formats and to incorporate informant information and direct behavior observations. Information from collaterals has been demonstrated to provide an accurate, independent indicator of depression (Gilley et al., 1995; Logsdon & Teri, 1995), although discrepancies from patient report or unavailability of a collateral can pose problems in interpretation (Gilley et al.; Moye, Robiner, & Mackenzie, 1993; Ott & Fogel, 1992; Teri & Wagner, 1991).

Measures include the Cornell Scale for Depression in Dementia (CSDD; Alexopoulos, Abrams, Young, & Shamoian, 1988), the National Institute of Mental Health Dementia Mood Assessment Scale (DMAS; Sunderland et al., 1988), Columbia University Scale for Psychopathology in Alzheimer's disease (CUSPAD; Devanand et al., 1992), Canberra Interview for the Elderly (CIE; MacKinnon et al., 1993), Cambridge Mental Disorders of the Elderly Examination (CAMDEX; Roth et al., 1986), the Neurobehavioral Rating Scale (NRS; Sultzer, Levin, Mahler, High, & Cummings, 1992), and the Psychogeriatric Assessment Scales (PAS; Jorm et al., 1995).

The overlap of symptoms of depression and dementia raises difficult questions for the diagnostician. Vida, Des Rosiers, Carrier, and Gauthier (1994b) examined the validity of RDC criteria for major and minor depression in individuals with Alzheimer's disease (AD). They found that three criteria were not associated with major depression (difficulty with concentration or thinking, excessive self-reproach or guilt, anhedonia or apathy), whereas nonverbal manifestations of depression, resentfulness, irritability, anger or complaining, and demandingness or clinging dependency, showed the strongest association with major depressive disorder. Diagnostic criteria for minor depression remained valid.

7.09.5.5 Assessing Depression in Older Adults with Poor Physical Health

Assessment of depression in individuals with comorbid medical illness or disability has been an area of focused attention because of ambiguity in the interpretation of somatic symptoms. Several strategies have been undertaken: (i) development of new instruments, (ii) development of instruments that eliminate somatic symptoms or substitute cognitive/affective symptoms for somatic ones, and (iii) use of alternative diagnostic schemes that count all criterion-related symptoms and do not require judgments about etiology.

Koenig, Cohen, Blazer, Meador, and Westlund (1992) developed a scale with 11 items derived from the GDS and the CRS, selected for their predictive validity in medically ill individuals. When examined in a sample of men over age 65 years admitted to a medical and neurological VA service, a cutoff score of three yielded a sensitivity of 83% and specificity of 77%. The scale showed moderate correlations with other self-report measures. Evans (1993) developed the 15-item Evans Liverpool Depression Rating Scale (ELDRS) for detection of depression in physically ill older adults. It obtains both patient and collateral information in "yes/no" format. The ELDRS has been found to have adequate interrater reliability and good efficiency using a cutoff of 5/6 (sensitivity of 88–91% and specificity of 85–96%).

Rapp and Vrana (1989) examined the sensitivity and specificity of conventional SADS/RDC depression diagnoses, which exclude somatic symptoms judged to be secondary to organic condition, compared with a modification of the RDC that reassigned diagnoses after substituting nonsomatic symptoms for somatic symptoms. Fully 96% of individuals were classified the same way with both sets of criteria; the alternative criteria showed 87% sensitivity and 100% specificity. Eliminating the somatic symptoms without replacement, however, resulted in poorer classification. Koenig, Pappas, Holsinger, and Bachar (1995) evaluated the reliability of six diagnostic strategies varying in inclusivity. Some strategies eliminated fatigue and anorexia. Some replaced four somatic symptoms (fatigue, anorexia/weight loss, psychomotor retardation, impaired concentration) with four cognitive/affective symptoms (irritability, tearfulness, social withdrawal, feeling punished). When structured interviews were used, clinicians were able to determine reliably whether major depression was present regardless of diagnostic strategy. These studies suggest that there is no advantage to abandoning the *DSM-IV* in medically ill older adults, but that modified criteria may be easier and more accurate than the conventional system requiring judgments about the cause of somatic symptoms.

7.09.6 SUICIDE

A discussion of affective disorders in late life would be incomplete without consideration of suicide among this population. Death by suicide is more common among older adults than at any other age. Although most depressed older adults do not commit suicide, many older adults who do commit suicide are depressed.

7.09.6.1 Rates

The suicide rate for older adults in most countries is higher than that of any other age group (Gulbinat, 1996). Among nations reporting to the World Health Organization, rates of suicide for older men are up to seven times higher than adolescent male suicide rates (Gulbinat, 1996). Male suicides among all ages are two to three times more frequent than female suicides (Gulbinat, 1996). Rates also vary by race and ethnic background. In the US, suicide rates are highest among Native Americans and Whites, followed by people of Asian origin and Blacks, with people of Latino origin having lower rates of suicide than non-Latino origin. Gender, racial, and ethnic differences in suicide rates are most pronounced among older adults (McIntosh, 1992).

7.09.6.2 Methods

Methods used by older adults to commit suicide are generally less amenable to intervention than those used by younger age groups (De Leo & Diekstra, 1990). In the US, guns are used to commit suicide more frequently than any other method, both by men and women (Kaplan, Adamek, & Johnson, 1994; McIntosh, 1992). This is true of all ages, but to the greatest extent in late life. In Finland, hanging is the leading method of suicide for all ages, with the proportion of suicides using this method greatest in old age. In most Western countries, over 85% of older adult suicides involve hanging, poisoning, or drowning, with hanging more common in men and poisoning more characteristic of women (De Leo & Diekstra, 1990). In Japan, the most frequently used methods in late life are hanging, drowning, and jumping.

A unique feature of older adult suicide is the small window of opportunity for intervention. The ratio of attempted to completed suicides among older adults has been estimated at 4:1, whereas this ratio among all ages is estimated at 20:1, and among youth it is thought to be as high as 200:1 (McIntosh, 1992; Parkin & Stengel, 1965). This difference could reflect several factors: the selection of less reversible means, which in itself can be a sign of increased lethality of intent, decreased powers of recuperation (Lindesay, 1991), or isolation from rescue. Older adults have also been found to be less likely to express suicidal ideation than younger adults (Blazer et al., 1987), a factor further complicating assessment efforts.

7.09.6.3 Depression and Suicide

Depression and suicide are linked closely throughout the lifespan. Individuals who are depressed are more likely to commit suicide, and individuals who committed suicide were more likely to have been depressed. On a neurobiological level, the same serotonin pathways have been implicated in depression and suicide, particularly in violent suicides (Åsberg, Nordström, & Träskman-Bendz, 1986). Moreover, the association between depression and suicide is strongest in late life.

In a review of follow-up studies, Miles (1977) concluded that 15% of depressed individuals of all ages would eventually die by suicide. Gardner, Bahn, and Mack (1964) calculated suicide rates for individuals with affective psychosis to be 207/100 000 for those under age 55 years and 475/100 000 for those aged 55 years or older. Psychological autopsy studies in England and the US have found evidence for affective disorders in 83–87% of older adults who committed suicide (Barraclough, Bunch, Nelson, & Sainsbury, 1974; Conwell, Olsen, Caine, & Flannery, 1991), while a psychological autopsy study in Finland found depressive disorders in 67% of suicides who were over age 60 years (Henriksson, Marttunen et al., 1995). Substance use disorders are also prevalent in older suicides (either alone or comorbid with affective disorders), but they are less common than among younger suicides (see Conwell & Brent, 1995, for a review; Henriksson, Marttunen et al., 1995). Although differential mortality could be an alternative explanation for the lower rates of substance use disorders among older adult suicides, this would not explain the higher rates of affective disorders. As Conwell and Brent (1995) concluded, since affective disorders are less prevalent in late life but more common among older completed suicides, older adults who are depressed seem to be at higher risk of suicide than depressed younger adults.

7.09.6.4 Hopelessness

Hopelessness has been studied extensively as a possible correlate of suicide. Hopelessness has been linked to suicidal ideation (Wetzel, Margulies, Davis, & Karam, 1980) and completed suicides (Beck, Steer, Kovacs, & Garrison, 1985; Fawcett et al., 1990).

7.09.6.5 Issues in Late Life Suicide

A growing literature has documented the phenomenon that older adults who commit suicide frequently have seen a physician within a short interval before the suicidal death. In psychological autopsy studies of older adult suicides, Conwell et al. (1991) found that 75% had seen their physician within a month of the suicide. Takahashi et al. (1995) found that older adult inpatients on a psychiatric ward who were admitted after a suicide attempt were three times more likely to have seen a physician within the previous two weeks than older psychiatric inpatients who had not made a suicide attempt.

Another important issue concerns suicide among the medically ill. Suicides in this population have been described as rational, particularly in the presence of chronic pain or a poor prognosis (Battin, 1991). Although few studies have explored suicidal behavior in chronic or terminally ill individuals, the existing research indicates that depressive disorders are prominent in these cases (Henriksson, Isometsä, et al., 1995; Leibenluft & Goldberg, 1988). This result highlights the need to assess carefully for affective disorders and for suicide risk in medically ill individuals. Since pain has been associated with depressive disorders (Parmelee et al., 1991), effective treatment of pain may be an avenue for reducing both depression and suicide risk among medically ill older adults.

7.09.6.6 Assessment and Treatment

Assessment of suicide risk in older adults is an inexact science. Although older adults are at highest risk of suicide, most suicide research has focused on younger populations. There is ample reason, however, to doubt that findings would necessarily translate to an older suicidal population. As discussed earlier, older adult suicides differ in several important ways from younger suicides, including a higher degree of lethality and decreased likelihood of expressed suicidal ideation. There are no widely accepted assessment instruments validated with older individuals (for approaches to suicide risk assessment in this population, see Wolfe, Morrow, & Frederickson, 1995).

Even less research is available on the efficacy of interventions for suicidal older adults, or indeed for suicidal individuals of any age. In the absence of such information, the most promising approach in working with suicidal individuals with affective disorders is the effective treatment of these affective disorders.

7.09.7 COURSE OF DEPRESSION

In monitoring the course of depression, individuals can be classified as recovered (partial or full remission), relapsed, or chronic (nonremitted). Some have suggested that older adults show worse prognosis both in terms of lower rates of recovery and greater chance of relapse, but differences in study designs or sample characteristics make alternative explanations replete. When the differences are controlled, age in and of itself seems to have little prognostic value. Hinrichsen (1992) examined recovery and relapse rates in elderly depressed inpatients and compared them with those observed in a mixed age sample, using the same diagnostic and follow-up methods and the same uncontrolled treatment approach. He found that the rates were comparable: by one year after hospital admission, 59% of the elderly individuals achieved full or partial sustained recovery, 13% recovered and subsequently relapsed into the same condition as the index episode, and 28% never recovered. The figures for the mixed age sample were 58%, 16%, and 26%, respectively.

Kennedy, Kelman, and Thomas (1991) examined factors that contributed to chronicity, remission, and emergence of depressive symptoms in elderly community residents. Baseline health status was less predictive than change in health. Declining health and increasing disability were associated with chronicity, whereas improved health was associated with remission. This association could reflect a psychological reaction to decline or a more general wearing down process.

Diagnosed depression and depressive symptoms are associated with increased risk of mortality in institutionalized and inpatient samples (Evans, 1993; Parmelee, Katz, & Lawton, 1992) and in community residents (Thomas, Kelman, Kennedy, Ahn, & Yang, 1992). However, the explanation remains unclear. For example, the increased mortality may be related to the presence of cognitive impairment, that is, a comorbid dementia (Snowdon & Lane, 1995).

Burvill and colleagues examined mortality rates in a cohort of elderly depressed inpatients at the time of the index depressive episode, one year later, and then at five years (Burvill & Hall, 1994). Poor outcome of the index episode after one year (i.e., "depressive invalids" who had moderate symptoms of depression but not enough to merit diagnosis of major depression, continuously ill, or demented) was associated with increased mortality over the subsequent four years. Individuals most at risk of death were those who, on entry into study, were male, aged 75 years or older, had a diagnosis of major depression without melancholia or psychosis, and had substantial health and mobility problems.

Evans (1993), in contrast, found that one year death rates of depressed patients 12 months after inpatient treatment did not differ significantly from those of psychologically well individuals. Only timing of deaths varied, with most deaths occurring in the first three months for depressed individuals compared to being evenly distributed in the nondepressed group.

7.09.8 TREATMENT APPROACHES

The array of treatments provided to depressed older adults largely parallels those used to treat depression in adults generally. These can be divided into psychosocial treatments, predominantly psychotherapy, and somatic treatments, that is, psychopharmacological treatments and electroconvulsive therapy (ECT). There do appear to be some age differences in the distribution of treatments. For example, psychosocial interventions based on life review or reminiscence are exclusive to older adults. ECT has registered an increase in its use, disproportionately accounted for by older adults (Warren & Levy, 1991).

The literature is just beginning to have sufficient information to give good guidance. In the past, studies have not always distinguished between treating a disorder and endeavoring to raise scores on depression self-report scales for community volunteers who were not necessarily depressed to begin with. In fact, this failure may contribute to a misperception perpetuated by the Consensus Development Conference Statement (Friedhoff, 1994) that psychotherapy is for mild (nonserious) depression, while somatic treatments are for true depression. Because the topic of the chapter is mood disorders, for the purposes of discussing efficacy of treatment, the focus is on studies with individuals who have a diagnosed disorder. However, to reflect interest in variations of disorder observed in older adults, literature concerning subdysthymic disorder is included.

7.09.8.1 Psychotherapeutic Interventions

Psychosocial treatments for depression encompass psychodynamic psychotherapy, brief psychodynamic therapy, interpersonal therapy, behavior therapy, cognitive and cognitive behavior therapy, life review, marital and family therapy, and group therapy (which can be psychodynamic or cognitive-behavioral). Empirical evidence to date suggests that efficacy of treatments for older adults is basically similar to efficacy for adults generally. However, the fact that older adults are not routinely included in evaluations of interventions is disturbing, for example, the Treatment of Depression Collaborative Research Program (Elkin et al., 1989).

There are several available reviews of psychological treatments for depression, including Scogin and McElreath's (1994) meta-analysis and chapters by Futterman, Thompson, Gallagher-Thompson, and Ferris (1995), Niederehe (1994), Smyer, Zarit, and Qualls (1990), Teri, Curtis, Gallagher-Thompson, and Thompson (1994), and Wolfe, Morrow, and Frederickson (1995). Clinical psychologists have placed more explicit attention on identifying those interventions that are supported empirically, and on establishing criteria by which to make this judgment (Chambless et al., 1996; Gatz et al., in press). While not directly employing this framework, treatments that are supported by good empirical designs are emphasized (e.g., randomized controlled trial).

7.09.8.1.1 Cognitive-behavior therapy

The rationale for behavioral therapy for depression is found in Lewinsohn, Muñoz, Youngren, and Zeiss (1996), and the rationale for cognitive therapy in Beck, Rush, Shaw, and Emery (1979). Behavior therapy teaches the role of reduced reinforcement in creating and maintaining depression, methods to increase pleasant events, relaxation techniques (Bernstein & Borkovec, 1973), and problem-solving skills (Nezu, Nezu, & Perri, 1989). Cognitive therapy teaches the importance of negative, pervasive attributions about oneself, the world, and the future in determining one's mood, and offers methods to monitor and challenge these thoughts. In both cases, the treatment was developed for adults in general. In studying the effectiveness of these therapies, sometimes the two are contrasted with one another; sometimes a combined cognitive-behavioral therapy is compared with another treatment. In practice, it is probably most common to combine elements of both behavioral and cognitive treatments, and the outcome research does not lead us to differentiate among these approaches.

Adaptations for older adults include changing pleasant events lists to be more appropriate to the activities in which older adults are likely to engage and resolving practical barriers such as mobility and vision limitations (Rybarczyk et al., 1992). These adaptations seem unlikely to interfere with comparisons of treatment outcome across age groups.

Gallagher and Thompson have conducted a series of studies that provide the clearest evidence for the efficacy of cognitive and behavioral treatments for patients meeting diagnostic criteria for major depressive disorder. The first study (Gallagher & Thompson, 1982) compared individual cognitive, behavioral, and supportive/insight therapy; the second (Thompson, Gallagher, & Breckenridge, 1987) compared individual cognitive, behavioral, and brief dynamic therapy with a waiting list control group also included in the design. Treatment lasted 20 sessions. At post-test, all therapies registered improvement on self-report and observer-rated scales and on proportions of patients diagnosed as depressed; all therapies were more effective than the control group. At follow-up assessment a year after termination of treatment, in the first study, maintenance of gains was superior for the behavioral and cognitive groups compared with those who had received supportive/insight therapy (Gallagher & Thompson, 1983). In the second study, there was no difference among treatments (Gallagher-Thompson, Hanley-Peterson, & Thompson, 1990).

Two other research groups have included psychopharmacological conditions, but permit evaluation of the psychotherapy component. Beutler et al. (1987) compared various combinations of cognitive therapy and alprazolam (Xanax). Cognitive therapy was administered in small groups. All four groups (including the placebo) improved on both BDI and HRSD. The placebo group and the medication-only group showed less steep improvement on the BDI and a reversal to baseline levels at follow-up.

Steuer et al. (1984) compared cognitive-behavioral to psychodynamic psychotherapy administered in groups. Participants had volunteered for a drug study (Jarvik, Mintz, Steuer, & Gerner, 1982), and psychotherapy groups were by and large filled by those for whom pharmacologic treatment was contraindicated due to a chronic physical disease or to a medication being used to treat such a condition. Periodic assessments over the nine months of psychotherapeutic treatment showed significant improvement on self- and observer-rated scales for both modalities. On the BDI, cognitive-behavioral treatment was superior to psychodynamic. Riskind, Beck, and Steer (1985) used Steuer et al.'s data to demonstrate that nearly 50% of the cognitive therapy patients were either in remission or only mildly depressed at the conclusion of treatment.

These studies have not been replicated by large numbers of other laboratories. Campbell (1992) found significant reductions in depression after individual cognitive therapy combined with reminiscence in comparison with a psychological placebo (a crafts group) and to an untreated control group. Improvement was measured with the Zung SDS and with thought diaries. Arean et al. (1993) compared problem-solving group therapy, group reminiscence therapy, and a waiting list control group. Individuals in both the problem-solving and reminiscence group showed reductions in depression (assessed with HRSD, BDI, GDS) in comparison with the control group, with extent of improvement at post-test and maintenance of gain better for the problem-solving therapy than for reminiscence. Problem-solving therapy was also applied successfully by Hussian and Lawrence (1981) with mildly to severely depressed nursing home residents.

All of these outcome studies had similar exclusion criteria: nonsuicidal, nonpsychotic, no cognitive impairment, or alcohol abuse. In addition, many potential participants with chronic physical illnesses were *de facto* excluded because these studies typically relied on community samples who could come to the facility where treatment was being administered. However, it should not be concluded that depression was not severe. For example, in Thompson et al. (1987), mean BDI was 23.5 at pretest; mean HSRD was 19.1. In Beutler et al. (1987), mean HSRD at pretest was 22.0 across all groups, mean BDI (on the 13-item form) was 11.3. In Steuer et al. (1984), mean BDI (on the 13-item form) was 15.3; mean HSRD was 18.7.

Dropout rates are not always easy to discern from published descriptions. Thompson et al. (1987) report that they had four patients drop out of behavioral (14%), four from psychodynamic (14%), and 10 from cognitive therapy (27%). Dropping out reflected expressed dissatisfaction or more ambiguous causes, such as the client's declaring transportation problems or physical illness. Beutler et al. (1987) reported dropout at 13% in the first four weeks; thereafter, it was 67% for medication and 31% for cognitive therapy, with or without medication. Side effects of the drugs was a key factor for most. Steuer et al. (1984) found dropout rate to be 39% across both types of psychotherapies, with no difference between them, but only 9% before the 12th week.

7.09.8.1.2 Brief psychodynamic, interpersonal, and life review therapies

Brief psychodynamic and interpersonal therapies have resulted in a clinical literature describing special aspects of their application to older adults. For interpersonal therapy, a manual has been prepared for older adults (described in Reynolds et al., 1992). The most salient difference is in the nature of the interpersonal problems. Life review traces its conceptual roots to Erik Erikson's description of the eighth stage in the life cycle, where the individual deals with the achievement of ego integrity. Butler (1974) has provided a framework for making this task more intentional and more therapeutic. There is no comparable therapy for younger adults.

Thompson et al. (1987), Gallagher and Thompson (1982), and Steuer et al. (1984), already described, all showed brief psychodynamic therapy or supportive/insight therapy to be generally equivalent to cognitive-behavioral approaches, sometimes not on all measures or after extended follow-up. Schneider, Sloane, Staples, and Bender (1986) found interpersonal therapy (IPT) to be as effective as nortriptyline and superior to placebo control, indicated by 58% improvement on HDRS for drug and 64% for psychotherapy; in addition, dropout rate was lower for IPT than for medication.

Reynolds et al. (1992) tested the efficacy of IPT combined with nortriptyline, IPT alone, nortriptyline alone, and placebo as a maintenance treatment for depression. Participants were older adult patients who had already been treated in the acute and continuation phases by combined IPT and nortriptyline. No one started maintenance treatment unless they had already improved. Of patients who began the study, there was 19% attrition before the end of the continuation phase, and 16% of those who completed treatment did not improve. Preliminary results showed that 24% of those shifted to placebo suffered relapse, with no significant difference for those in IPT or not in IPT.

A variant of IPT, interpersonal counseling (IPC), has also been used with subsyndromal dysthymia. Mossey et al. (1996) compared IPC to usual care for recently discharged medical patients with GDS scores in excess of 10 at two occasions before treatment began, but who did not meet diagnostic criteria for major depressive disorder. Follow-up at 2–3 months after completing 10 sessions of IPC indicated that those receiving IPC had significantly lower depressive symptoms than the control group.

Fry (1983) compared life review to unstructured reminiscence and found both superior to an attention placebo. Haight (1992) compared reminiscence, using structured life review devised by the author to standardize the intervention, to a friendly visitor program (attention control) and to a no-treatment group. She found improved psychological well-being that was maintained at follow-up but no significant change on Zung SDS. In neither of these studies were *DSM* diagnoses used to screen participants. Haight's sample was homebound and therefore assumed to be at elevated risk of depression.

With participants diagnosed with major depressive disorder, Arean et al. (1993), as has been described, found life review superior to a waiting list control but not to problem-solving therapy. In a nursing home sample, Dhooper, Green, Huff, and Austen-Murphy (1993) found a combined life review and problem-solving group superior to a control group, with depression measured with the Zung SDS. Niederehe (1994) cautions not only has most of the research on life review been conducted with minimally symptomatic samples, but also the technique could have negative effects with individuals who do have major depressive disorder.

7.09.8.1.3 Support groups and psychoeducational interventions for depression in caregivers of dementia patients

A population that has received special attention are caregivers of older adults, especially of older adults with AD. As noted already, caregivers are subject to increased risk of depression as well as more general strain and burden. Moreover, depression often accompanies dementia; thus, both the older adult with dementia and the caregiver are appropriate targets for treatment.

A meta-analysis of interventions for caregiver distress (Knight, Lutzky, & Macofsky-Urban, 1993) concluded that these interventions did have a respectable effect on mood and burden. Although outcome measures often include measures of depression, participants do not always meet criteria for depressive disorder. Elements of intervention with caregivers typically include emotional support and sharing of common experiences, training in problem solving and stress reduction, and education about the disease and community resources. The component concerned with problem solving and stress reduction tends to build on a behavioral model of treatment for depression. Using this framework, for example, Gallagher-Thompson (1994) developed a treatment manual and curriculum, called "Coping with the Blues." She and her colleagues reported significant reduction of depression on the BDI (Lovett & Gallagher, 1988).

An additional element is added by Teri, Logsdon, Wagner, and Uomoto (1994), whose model is to involve both the caregivers and dementia patients. The intervention explicitly teaches the caregivers to use a behavioral model with the dementia patient, focused on the role of pleasant events in maintaining a positive emotional state.

7.09.8.2 Pharmacological Interventions

The most common psychopharmacological treatment for depression in older adults has been the tricyclic antidepressants, amitriptyline (Elavil), imipramine (Tofranil), desipramine (Norpramin), protriptyline (Vivactyl), and nortriptyline (Pamelor). Tricyclics all have anticholinergic side effects, related to degree of muscarinic blockage, manifesting both centrally (delirium, confusion) and peripherally (urinary retention, tachycardia, orthostatic hypotension). The older drugs in this category, such as amitriptyline and imipramine, have more severe side effects, while nortriptyline is regarded as perhaps causing the least orthostatic hypotension, and desipramine is least anticholinergic (Jenike, 1989; Salzman, 1994). Age-related changes in drug metabolism by the liver and in neurotransmitters may also lead to greater sensitivity to both therapeutic and side effects (Naranjo, Herrmann, Mittmann, & Bremner, 1995). The effect of concurrent medications can also be substantial (Reynolds, Schneider, Lebowitz, & Kupfer, 1994). The reason that orthostatic hypotension is a concern lies in risk of falls. One report suggests that risk of hip fracture is tripled by the use of tricyclic antidepressants (Ray, Griffin, Schaffner, Baugh, & Melson, 1987). Cardiac side effects are also a concern (Glassman & Roose, 1994).

Newer, or second-generation, antidepressants with atypical structure, such as trazodone (Desyrel), may be especially sedating although having fewer anticholinergic effects and cardiac side effects. Other newer medications are selective serotonin-reuptake inhibiting (SSRI) antidepressants, for example, fluoxetine (Prozac) and sertraline (Zoloft). These do not have the same cholinergic side effects as tricyclics, however, their cardiac side effects have not received sufficient study (Reynolds et al., 1994). It has been reported that substitution of SSRIs for tricyclics is occurring at a slower rate for patients aged 65 years and older than for patients younger than 65 years (Klawansky, 1994), although the picture may be changing and different settings may have different prescribing habits.

Monoamine oxidase inhibitors also present side effects, including orthostatic hypotension (Naranjo et al., 1995). Lithium, which is commonly used to treat bipolar disorder, requires particularly careful regulation of dosage in older adults, and creates a particular risk of neurotoxicity when the patient is demented (Jenike, 1989).

In their review of drug studies through 1986, Gerson, Plotkin, and Jarvik (1988) conclude that remission rates on the HRSD among those with major depressive disorder averaged 51% across different drugs, predominantly tricyclic antidepressants, with no obvious advantage for one drug over another. This contrasts with a mean improvement of 20% for those on placebo. Dropout rates were 19% for those in the active drug conditions and 31% for those in the placebo condition (average = 21%). Side effects were described as a major impediment.

Klawansky (1994) collected all available randomized controlled trials through 1991 for meta-analysis. Drugs were more effective than placebo and also had more side effects. There was no overall difference in dropout rates between tricyclics and placebo. Those on medication mainly dropped out because of side effects and those in the placebo condition, due to lack of benefit. In comparisons of fluoxetine to tricyclics, dropout was less for those assigned to the fluoxetine condition.

As with psychotherapeutic studies, psychopharmacologic studies tend to feature time-limited treatments and to exclude patients who have various complications. By default, those excluded are often the oldest patients. There is almost no literature on patients aged 80 years and older (Salzman, 1994). In these respects, research may match poorly with actual practice. Thus, it is of interest to look at Katz, Simpson, Curlik, Parmelee, and Muhly (1990), who conducted a double-blind study of nortriptyline with nursing home and congregate housing residents. After excluding those who had contraindications (22%), or refused, or met some other exclusion criterion, patients who completed the drug treatment improved significantly on the HRSD but not on the GDS relative to the placebo control group. Still, of patients given active medication, 11 of 32 (34%) had some sort of adverse event, acknowledging that it is impossible to accurately distinguish side effects from unrelated medical events. Nortriptyline has also been studied with patients who have both depression and dementia (Salzman, 1994), a group for whom cognitive side effects are a particular concern.

Comparisons of pharmacotherapy to psychotherapy are limited. In Jarvik et al. (1982), although assignment to drug and to psychotherapy was not random, the authors note that (i) more patients dropped out of the drug conditions than group therapy, (ii) improvement for psychotherapy tended to be more homogeneous, while improvement for the drug conditions was bimodal, with patients either responding or failing to respond, (iii) group therapy was significantly more effective than placebo drug. Given the concern with side effects among older adults, the recommendation of Wexler and Cicchetti (1992) seems sensible; that is, begin with psychotherapy, and if it is not effective, add medication.

7.09.8.3 Electroconvulsive Therapy

Treatment with electroconvulsive therapy (ECT) is attractive when side effects of medications are of particular concern or the patient has not responded to medication, or when there is particular urgency. Many argue that ECT is actually safer than drugs. The short-term efficacy of ECT with older adults is well accepted (Sackheim, 1994). Relapse does tend to be high, which has led to studies of continuation and maintenance ECT (e.g., Zorumski, Rubin, & Burke, 1988). While drugs are used commonly to prevent relapse after ECT, the same reasons for not turning to drugs in the acute phase would also be applicable when considering drugs for this role.

Rate of complications does increase with age, although ECT is used in those over age 80 years (Cattan et al., 1990). The main side effects are cardiovascular, with these complications generally accounting for ECT-related mortality. Cognitive side effects are a major concern, including the fact that confusion can lead to falls. Brief confusion directly after treatment is standard. Duration of amnesia varies. Severity of cognitive sequelae appears to be related to mode of administration. It is also not established whether those who already have cognitive dysfunction are particularly at risk of cognitive complications, especially lasting or severe effects, if their depression is treated with ECT. However, ECT is used in mixed depression and dementia (Liang, Lam, & Ancill, 1988).

While ECT advocates argue that the treatment is underused, there are three other implications of this literature. First, improved recognition of depression could lead to its earlier treatment, so that cases do not take on the urgency that more often results in referral for ECT. Second, since side effects do seem so dependent on technique, monitoring of side effects and relapse is advisable not only in controlled trials in academic clinical centers, but also at sites where ECT is often administered, such as private not-for-profit and private for-profit hospitals (Sackheim, 1994). Third, treatments to prevent relapse should incorporate more psychotherapy and more environmental manipulation, including work with the family and social networks.

7.09.8.4 Concluding Comment

It is difficult to discuss treatment without also discussing problems in getting the older adult to treatment (Estes, 1995). Older adults tend to be seen by a primary care physician who either does not notice depression or elects not to treat it. The older adult may contribute by failing to seek treatment for symptoms of depression, or by not mentioning the symptoms to the primary care physician. Reasons suggested for failure to recognize depression include: comorbidity with physical health problems, which become the focus of treatment; lack of training in geriatrics; older adults' reticence to discuss emotional distress; older adults' attribution of the symptoms to normal aging. As a consequence, much depression may go untreated, may not be treated until it becomes severe, or may be mistreated, for example, with anxiolytics or with sleeping pills, until it becomes severe and gives the false impression of intractability and hopelessness. If the depression is recognized by the primary care physician, it may be easiest to treat it with drugs, like the patient's physical conditions are being treated, particularly because the depression may have notable somatic manifestations. Referral to specialists is uncommon. Because of delays in initiating treatment, by the time that treatment is begun, the depressed older adult may more often seem like a psychiatric emergency, posing a danger to him or herself explicitly via creating fears of suicide or implicitly by extreme lack of self-care (e.g., not eating). These delays are combined with a greater background chance of physical frailty, so that the individual may not be physically as capable of enduring an episode of depression. This systemic context may lead to greater emphasis on somatic solutions.

7.09.9 PREVENTION

Prevention of depression is of keen interest because research results about risk and protective factors can inform preventive intervention strategies. Risk and protective factors, both established and putative, are suggested by the literature on correlated and etiological influences. In turn, this literature betokens key points of intervention for any preventive efforts.

The Institute of Medicine (Mrazek & Haggerty, 1994) recommends distinguishing universal, selective, and indicated preventive measures. Indicated interventions are directed toward individuals who may have symptoms that foreshadow disorder or some kind of marker that may indicate a predisposition. Selective preventive interventions are targeted to subgroups who may have an elevated risk. Universal measures are targeted to the general public. These distinctions can usefully be applied to older adults (Smyer, 1995).

7.09.9.1 Indicated Preventive Measures

Screening and outreach are core tools for indicated preventive intervention. One of the best indicators of risk of future depression is depressive symptoms. Using Epidemiologic Catchment Area survey data, Horwath, Johnson, Klerman, and Weissman (1992) demonstrated that incidence of first-onset major depression was significantly increased in individuals who reported depressive symptoms when interviewed the previous year. Indeed, over half of new cases of major depression were associated with a history of depressive symptoms. These findings provide a strong empirical rationale for depression symptom screening, for example, national depression awareness days.

Unfortunately, screening for depression, especially in older adults, is not practiced widely. Dorfman et al. (1995) used a computer-assisted questionnaire with depression items from the CES-D supplemented by a second instrument. Among a sample of generally healthy community-dwelling adults aged 65 years and older, they found that nearly three-quarters of those with major depression were not being treated. However, when these individuals were referred to a mental health professional, two-thirds did seek help. These results illustrate both the failure to screen, since these individuals had not heretofore been identified as having depressive disorder, and the fact that screening can be effective in getting people with significant distress linked to treatment.

The high rate of depressive symptoms and disorder among medical patients suggests that primary care practitioners are uniquely well positioned to conduct screening for depression. However, underrecognition of psychiatric conditions by primary care physicians in outpatient and inpatient settings is well demonstrated (Jorm, 1995; Rapp et al., 1988). In a sample of older individuals of Latino origin in Southern California, Kemp et al. (1987) found that none of the respondents who scored as depressed on the screening instrument reported receiving any treatment for depression. Notably, 90% had seen a physician within the past year, where there could have been an opportunity for screening to occur. Mann (1995) determined that primary care physicians were unaware of their patient's depression in two out of every three cases where the patient was in fact pervasively depressed. The pivotal role of the primary care practitioner is further supported by evidence that some three-quarters of elderly persons who kill themselves have recently seen a physician (Conwell et al., 1991).

These observations have led to strong recommendations that health service providers be trained to screen for depression as a condition of licensure or certification (White House Mini-Conference on Emerging Issues in Mental Health and Aging, 1995). Methods for improving the recognition of depression by primary care physicians have been evaluated, including visits to the physician's office analogous to visits by drug industry representatives, during which the physician is presented with a list of questions to use in making a diagnosis (Pond, Mant, Kehoe, Hewitt, & Brodaty, 1994).

Outreach programs to older adults aim to make it easier for the older adult who does have symptoms of depression to connect with someone who can offer assistance. Waters (1995) emphasizes the use of alternative settings, not only health care clinics, but also neighborhood centers, senior centers, religious institutions, community organizations, educational institutions, as locations where mental health care is available. Raschko (1985) established the Gatekeepers program, in which he trained meter readers, letter carriers, bank tellers, and others who might have contact with older individuals who lived alone, so that they became referral sources.

Once individuals with symptoms of depression are identified, Horwath et al. (1992) caution that most will not go on to become clinically depressed. Therefore, these authors suggest, it would be premature to use antidepressant medication to treat depressive symptoms. There may also be reluctance to see a mental health professional. Thus, Breckenridge, Zeiss, and Thompson (1987) developed a nine-week Life Satisfaction Course for older adults who have depressive symptoms but do not meet criteria for major depression. The course is built on Lewinsohn's psychoeducational model (Lewinsohn et al., 1986). This group (Thompson, Gallagher, Nies, & Epstein, 1983) has also offered Coping with Depression classes for older adults, targeted towards those who were clinically depressed. Participation in these classes resulted in improvement on measures of depression and life satisfaction.

7.09.9.2 Selective Preventive Interventions

Selective interventions are directed toward subgroups who have an elevated risk of depression. Research on risk factors for depression suggests what some of those subgroups may be. Phifer and Murrell (1986) found that an increase in CES-D scores from below 16 to 20 or higher was predicted by depressive symptoms six months earlier, poor health, loss events, and low social support, with support functioning both additively and interactively. In the Western Collaborative Group Study of older men, increase on the CES-D was predicted by poor perceived health and stroke, while physical exercise was protective (McElroy, Carmelli, Swan, & LaRue, 1995). It is often observed that the rate of mood disorders in stroke patients is high, and that depression can interfere with cognitive and functional recovery.

A major loss event is spousal bereavement. One of the best known prevention programs is "Widow-to-Widow," developed by Silverman (1969) and sponsored by the American Association of Retired Persons (AARP). Vachon et al. (1980) showed, in a controlled study, that fewer depressive symptoms were experienced by program participants than by the control group. Vachon and Stylianos (1988) have suggested ways to identify which bereaved individuals may be at greater risk of distress based on the adequacy of their social support network, and they propose that friends and family of the bereaved could be taught to distinguish helpful from unhelpful methods of support.

Among medical patients, strategies to prevent depression can include treatment of pain and maintenance of good nutrition (Katz, Streim, & Parmelee, 1994). In cognitively intact or mildly demented patients admitted to long-term care facilities, it has been suggested that prevention of depression may be accomplished through fostering social support in the setting, maximizing opportunities for autonomy and control, and promoting coping skills with respect to institutional life (Foster & Cataldo, 1994). However, there is not good research on the effectiveness of psychotherapeutic interventions with the physically ill or with those in long-term care settings (Jorm, 1995).

A final typical target for selective preventive interventions are caregivers of demented or physically incapacitated older adults. Meta-analysis suggests that psychoeducational support groups are effective in alleviating burden (Knight et al., 1993).

7.09.9.3 Universal Preventive Interventions

Universal preventive programs include public education campaigns and various wellness programs (Waters, 1995). Prevention research programs under this heading present major methodological problems, particularly with respect to demonstrating decreased incidence of a specific mental disorder (Mrazek & Haggerty, 1994). A central consideration should be linking the knowledge base about risk and protective factors to educational strategies for older adults and those who work with them (Smyer, 1995).

7.09.10 CONCLUSION

Old age is not characterized by depression. When depression is experienced, the most frequent mood disorders seem to be those about which least is known. Some of the newer diagnostic categories or symptom clusters, that is, minor depression, depletion syndrome, hopelessness depression, are promising descriptors.

Gerontological literature often blurs the distinction between depression as a clinical entity and depression as an expression of negative affect and hence a convenient indicator of well-being in old age. This blurring may contribute to the misconception that depression is an inevitable accompaniment of aging, brought on by the various losses and indignities, and also by the conviction that depression is underdiagnosed among older adults. Blurring also occurs in the literature on prevention, where distinctions often are poorly drawn between programs to augment well-being and programs where prevention of mood disorder is legitimately realized.

Stress does predict depression. Yet, despite the chronic illnesses and psychosocial strains that frequently distinguish old age, most older people manage without becoming depressed. Physical illness and cognitive dysfunction are major correlated factors for depression in old age. These factors help to account for age differences in presentation and appear to be of etiological significance. For example, there may be a general wearing down process underlying depression, physical symptoms (often cardiovascular), and functional decrements. For late-onset depression, with no previous episodes at younger ages, the depression often foreshadows dementia. Depression in old age also has important consequences with respect to both morbidity and mortality.

Numerous assessment instruments are available, with relative levels of use and sanction not necessarily reflective of existing empirical evidence as to measurement efficiency. The problems with depression scales reflect the nature of depression in old age, that is, the need to evaluate syndromes other than major depression and issues of differentiating depressive disorders among those who are physically or cognitively frail.

Although suicide is a relatively rare event, and most people who are depressed do not commit suicide, the risk of a completed suicide is highest in old age. This is an area where proper assessment and intervention can make a difference.

Psychotherapy works rather well with older adults, and there is empirical and practical guidance available about the best approaches. Somatic approaches have been overemphasized in the treatment of depression in late life. Although they appear to be effective for acute treatment, evidence is not unambiguous that they are more effective than psychotherapy. The guideline that psychopharmacology should be used with severe depression while psychotherapy should be used with mild depression does not accurately reflect the research. In studies of both drugs and psychotherapy, the patients tend to be young old, less physically ill, and more compliant. Risks of pharmacotherapy are higher in older individuals due to greater likelihood of comorbid medical conditions, greater likelihood of interaction with other medications, and greater sensitivity to dosage levels. Moreover, somatic treatments have no lasting effect on dysfunctional thoughts and nonhelpful or depopulated social networks. There is need for evaluations of combined treatments that reflect actual clinical practice, greater attention to dropouts and those who relapse, and studies of depressed patients with concurrent medical conditions. Better outreach and early assessment can also reduce the need for urgent intervention.

Finally, promising approaches to prevention of depression among older adults lie in training those in a position to screen for symptoms, targeting the most vulnerable segments of the older population, and disseminating knowledge about risk and protective factors.

7.09.11 REFERENCES

Abramson L. Y., Metalsky G. I., & Alloy L. B. (1989). Hopelessness depression: A theory-based subtype of depression. *Psychological Review, 96*, 358–372.

Adelmann, P. K. (1994). Multiple roles and psychological well-being in a national sample of older adults. *Journal of Gerontology: Social Sciences, 49*, 277–285.

Alexopoulos, G. S., Abrams, R. C., Young, R. C., & Shamoian, C. A. (1988). Cornell Scale for Depression in Dementia. *Biological Psychiatry, 23*, 271–284.

Alexopoulos, G. S., Meyers, R. S., Young, R. C., Mattis, S., & Kakuma, T. (1993). The course of geriatric depression with "reversible dementia": A controlled study. *American Journal of Psychiatry, 150*, 1693–1799.

Allen-Burge, R., Storandt, M., Kinscherf, D. A., & Rubin, E. H. (1994). Sex differences in the sensitivity of two self-report depression scales in older depressed inpatients. *Psychology and Aging, 9*, 443–445.

American Psychiatric Association (1980). *Diagnostic and statistical manual of mental disorders* (3rd ed.). Washington, DC: Author.

American Psychiatric Association (1987). *Diagnostic and statistical manual of mental disorders* (3rd ed., Rev.). Washington, DC: Author.

American Psychiatric Association (1994). *Diagnostic and statistical manual of mental disorders* (4th ed.). Washington, DC: Author.

Ames, D., Flynn, E., Tuckwell, V., & Harrigan, S. (1994). Diagnosis of psychiatric disorder in elderly general and geriatric hospital patients: AGECAT and *DSM-III-R* compared. *International Journal of Geriatric Psychiatry, 9*, 627–633.

Andresen E. M., Malmgren J. A., Carter W. B., & Patrick, D. L. (1994). Screening for depression in well older adults: Evaluation of a short form of the CES-D. *American Journal of Preventive Medicine, 10*, 77–84.

Anthony-Bergstone, C. R., Zarit, S. H., & Gatz, M. (1988). Symptoms of psychological distress among caregivers of dementia patients. *Psychology and Aging, 3*, 245–248.

Arean, P. A., Perri, M. G., Nezu, A. M., Schein, R. L., Christopher, F., & Joseph, T. X. (1993). Comparative effectiveness of social problem-solving therapy and reminiscence therapy as treatments for depression in older adults. *Journal of Consulting and Clinical Psychology, 61*, 1003–1010.

Åsberg, M., Nordström, P., Träskman-Bendz, L. (1986). Cerebrospinal fluid studies in suicide: An overview. *Annals of the New York Academy of Sciences, 487*, 243–255.

Baker, F. M., & Miller, C. L. (1991). Screening a skilled nursing home population for depression. *Journal of Geriatric Psychiatry and Neurology 4*, 218–221.

Baldwin, R. C. (1995). Delusional depression in elderly patients: Characteristics and relationship to age at onset. *International Journal of Geriatric Psychiatry, 10*, 981–985.

Baldwin, R. C., & Tomenson, B. (1995). Depression in later life: A comparison of symptoms and risk factors in early and late onset cases. *British Journal of Psychiatry, 167,* 649–652.

Ballard, C. G., Cassidy, G., Bannister, C., & Mohan, R. N. C. (1993). Prevalence, symptom profile and aetiology of depression in dementia sufferers. *Journal of Affective Disorders, 29,* 1–6.

Baltes, P. B., Mayer, K. U., Helmchen, H., & Steinhagen-Thiessen, E. (1993). The Berlin Aging Study (BASE): Overview and design. *Ageing and Society, 13,* 485–515.

Barraclough, B., Bunch, J., Nelson, B., & Sainsbury, P. (1974). A hundred cases of suicide: Clinical aspects. *British Journal of Psychiatry, 125,* 355–373.

Barrett, J. E., Barrett, J. A., Oxman, T. E., & Gerber, P. D. (1988). The prevalence of psychiatric disorders in a primary care practice. *Archives of General Psychiatry, 45,* 1100–1106.

Battin, M. P. (1991). Rational suicide: How can we respond to a request for help? Special Issue: Suicide in the Elderly. *Crisis, 12,* 73–80.

Beck, A. T., & Beck, R. W. (1972). Screening depressed patients in family practice: a rapid technique. *Postgraduate Medicine, 52*(6), 81–85.

Beck, A. T., Rush, A. J. Shaw, B. F., & Emery, G. (1979). *Cognitive therapy for depression.* New York: Guilford Press.

Beck, A. T., Steer, R. A., & Garbin, M. G. (1988). Psychometric properties of the Beck Depression Inventory: Twenty-five years of evaluation. *Clinical Psychology Review, 8,* 77–100.

Beck, A. T., Steer, R. A., Kovacs, M., & Garrison, B. (1985). Hopelessness and eventual suicide: A 10-year prospective study of patients hospitalized with suicidal ideation. *American Journal of Psychiatry, 142,* 559–563.

Beck, A. T., Ward, C. H., Mendelson, M., Mock, J., & Erbaugh, J. (1961). An inventory for measuring depression. *Archives of General Psychiatry, 4,* 53–63.

Beekman, A. T. F., Deeg, D. J. H., van Tilburg, T., Smit, J. H., Hooijer, C., & van Tilburg, W. (1995). Major and minor depression in later life: A study of prevalence and risk factors. *Journal of Affective Disorders, 36,* 65–75.

Berkman, L. F., Berkman, C. S., Kasl, S., Freeman, D. H., Jr., Leo, L., Ostfeld, A. M., Cornoni-Huntley, J., & Brody, J. A. (1986). Depressive symptoms in relation to physical health and functioning in the elderly. *American Journal of Epidemiology, 124,* 372–388.

Bernstein, D. A., & Borkovec, T. D. (1973). *Progressive relaxation training: A manual for the healing professions.* Champaign, IL: Research Press.

Berry, J. M., Storandt, M., & Coyne, A. (1984). Age and sex differences in somatic complaints associated with depression. *Journal of Gerontology, 39,* 465–467.

Bertelsen A., Harvald B., & Hauge M. A. (1977). A Danish twin study of manic-depressive disorders. *British Journal of Psychiatry, 130,* 330–351.

Beutler, L. E., Scogin, F., Kirkish, P., Schretlen, D., Corbishley, A., Hamblin, D., Meredith, K., Potter, R., Bamford, C. R., & Levenson, A. I. (1987). Group cognitive therapy and alprazolam in the treatment of depression in older adults. *Journal of Consulting and Clinical Psychology, 55,* 550–556.

Blazer, D. G., (1994). Epidemiology of late life depression. In L. S. Schneider, C. F. Reynolds, III, B. D. Lebowitz, & A. J. Friedhoff (Eds.), *Diagnosis and treatment of depression in late life: Results of the NIH Consensus Development Conference* (pp. 9–19). Washington, DC: American Psychiatric Press.

Blazer, D., Bachar, J. R., & Hughes, D. C. (1987). Major depression with melancholia: A comparison of middle-aged and elderly adults. *Journal of the American Geriatrics Society, 35,* 927–932.

Blazer, D. G., Burchett, B., Service, C., & George, L. K. (1991). The association of age and depression among the elderly. An epidemiological exploration. *Journals of Gerontology: Medical Sciences, 46,* M210–M215.

Blazer, D., Swartz, M., Woodbury, M., Manton, K. G., Hughes, D., & George, L. K. (1988). Depressive symptoms and depressive diagnoses in a community population: Use of a new procedure for analysis of psychiatric classification. *Archives of General Psychiatry, 45,* 1078–1084.

Blumenthal, M. D. (1980). Depressive illness in old age: Getting behind the mask. *Geriatrics, 35,* 34–43.

Boone, K. B., Lesser, I., Miller, B., Wohl, M., Berman, N., Lee, A. & Palmer, B. (1994). Cognitive functioning in a mildly to moderately depressed geriatric sample: Relationship to chronological age. *Journal of Neuropsychiatry and Clinical Neurosciences, 6,* 267–272.

Breckenridge, J. S., Zeiss, A. M., & Thompson, L. W. (1987). The Life Satisfaction Course: An intervention for the elderly. In R. F. Muñoz (Ed.), *Depression prevention: Research directions* (pp. 185–196). Washington, DC: Hemisphere Publishing.

Brodaty, H., Peters, K., Boyce, P., Hickie, I., Parker, G., Mitchell, P., & Wilhelm, K. (1991). Age and depression. *Journal of Affective Disorders, 23,* 137–149.

Brown, R. P., Sweeney, J., Loutsch, E., Kocsis, J., & Frances, A. (1984). Involutional melancholia revisited. *American Journal of Psychiatry, 141,* 24–28.

Bruce, M. L., Seeman, T. E., Merrill, S. S., & Blazer, D. G. (1994). The impact of depressive symptomatology on physical disability: MacArthur studies of successful aging. *American Journal of Public Health, 84,* 1796–1799.

Burke, W. J., Houston, M. J., Boust S. J., & Roccaforte, W. H. (1989). Use of the Geriatric Depression Scale in dementia of the Alzheimer's type. *Journal of the American Geriatrics Society, 37,* 856–860.

Burke, W. J., Nitcher, R. L., Roccaforte, W. H., & Wengel, S. P. (1992). A prospective evaluation of the Geriatric Depression Scale in an outpatient geriatric assessment center. *Journal of the American Geriatrics Society, 40,* 1227–1230.

Burke, W. J., Roccaforte, W. H., & Wengel, S. P. (1991). The short form of the Geriatric Depression Scale: A comparison with the 30-item form. *Journal of Geriatric Psychiatry and Neurology, 4,* 173–178.

Burke, W. J., Roccaforte, W. H., Wengel, S. P., Conley, D. M., & Potter, J. F. (1995). The reliability and validity of the Geriatric Depression Rating Scale administered by telephone. *Journal of the American Geriatric Society, 43,* 674–679.

Burvill, P. W., & Hall, W. D. (1994). Predictors of increased mortality in elderly depressed patients. *International Journal of Geriatric Psychiatry, 9,* 219–227.

Butcher, J. N., Dahlstrom, W. G., Graham, J. R., Tellegen, A., & Kaemmer, B. (1989). *Minnesota Multiphasic Personality Inventory-2 (MMPI-2): Manual for administration and scoring.* Minneapolis, MN: University of Minnesota Press.

Butler, R. N. (1974). Successful aging and the role of the life review. *Journal of the American Geriatric Society, 22,* 529–535.

Caine, E. D., Lyness, J. M., King, D. A., & Connors, B. A. (1994). Clinical and etiological heterogeneity of mood disorders in elderly patients. In L. S. Schneider, C. F. Reynolds, III, B. D. Lebowitz, & A. J. Friedhoff (Eds.), *Diagnosis and treatment of depression in late life: Results of the NIH Consensus Development Conference* (pp. 23–53). Washington, DC: American Psychiatric Press.

Callahan, C. M., & Wolinsky, F. D. (1994). The effect of gender and race on the measurement properties of the CES-D in older adults. *Medical Care, 32,* 341–356.

Campbell, J. M. (1992). Treating depression in well older adults: Use of diaries in cognitive therapy. *Issues in Mental Health Nursing, 13,* 19–29.

Carroll, B. J., Feinberg, M., Smouse, P. E., Rawson, S. G., & Greden, J. F. (1981). The Carroll Rating Scale for Depression I. Development, reliability and validation. *British Journal of Psychiatry, 138,* 194–200.

Cattan R. A., Barry P. P., Mead G., Reefe W. E., Gay A., & Silverman M. (1990). Electroconvulsive therapy in octogenerians. *Journal of the American Geriatrics Society, 38,* 753–758.

Chambless, D. L., Sanderson, W. C., Shoham, V., Johnson, S. B., Pope, K. S., Crits-Christoph, P., Baker, M., Johnson, B., Woody, S. R., Suie, S., Beutler, L., Williams, D. A., & McCurry, S. (1996). An update on empirically validated therapies. *The Clinical Psychologist, 49*(2), 5–18.

Commision on Professional Hospital Activities (1978). *ICD-9-CM. The international classification of diseases: Clinical modifications* (9th Rev.). Ann Arbor, MI: Author.

Conn, D. K. (1989). Neuropsychiatric syndromes in the elderly: An overview. In D. K. Cohen, A. Grek, & J. Sadavoy (Eds.), *Psychiatric consequences of brain disease in the elderly: A focus on management* (pp. 1–49). New York: Plenum.

Conwell, Y., & Brent, D. (1995). Suicide and aging I: Patterns of psychiatric diagnosis. *International Psychogeriatrics, 7,* 149–164.

Conwell, Y., Olsen, K., Caine, E. D., & Flannery, C. (1991). Suicide in later life: Psychological autopsy findings. *International Psychogeriatrics, 3,* 59–66.

Copeland, J. R. M., Dewey, M. E., Wood, N., Searle, R., Davidson, I. A., & McWilliam, C. (1987). Range of mental illness among the elderly in the community: Prevalence in Liverpool using the GMS-AGECAT package. *British Journal of Psychiatry, 150,* 815–823.

Copeland, J. R. M., Gurland, B. J., Dewey, M. E., Kelleher, M. J., Smith, A. M. R., & Davidson, I. A. (1987). The distribution of dementia, depression and neurosis in elderly men and women in an urban community: Assessed using the GMS-AGECAT package. *International Journal of Geriatric Psychiatry, 2,* 177–184.

Copeland, J. R. M., Kelleher, M. J., Kellett, J. M., Gourlay, A. L., with Gurland, B. J., Fleiss, J. L., & Sharpe, L. (1976). A semi-structured clinical interview for the assessment of diagnosis and mental state in the elderly: the Geriatric Mental State Schedule I. Development and reliability. *Psychological Medicine, 6,* 439–449.

Cress, M. E., Schechtman, K. B., Mulrow, C. D., Fiatarone, M. A., Gerety, M. B., & Buchner, D. M. (1995). Relationship between physical performance and self-perceived physical function. *Journal of the American Geriatrics Society, 43,* 93–101.

Cwikel, J., & Ritchie, K. (1988). The short GDS: Evaluation in a heterogeneous, multilingual population. *Clinical Gerontologist, 8,* 63–83.

D'Ath, P., Katona, P., Mullan, E., Evans, S., & Katona, C. (1994). Screening, detection and management of depression in elderly primary care attenders. I: The acceptability and performance of the 15 item Geriatric Depression Scale (GDS15) and the development of short versions. *Family Practice, 11,* 260–266.

Davidson, H., Feldman, P. H., & Crawford, S. (1994). Measuring depressive symptoms in the frail elderly. *Journal of Gertontology: Psychological Sciences, 49,* 159–164.

Dean, A., Kolody, B., & Wood, P. (1990). Effects of social support from various sources on depression in elderly persons. *Journal of Health and Social Behavior, 31,* 148–161.

De Leo, D., & Diekstra, R. F. W. (1990). *Depression and suicide in late life.* Lewiston, NY: Hogrefe & Huber.

Derogatis, L. R. (1977). *SCL-90: Administration, scoring and procedures manual I for the R (revised) version.* Baltimore, MD: Johns Hopkins University School of Medicine.

Derogatis, L. R., & Melisaratos, N. (1983). The Brief Symptom Inventory: An introductory report. *Psychological Medicine, 13,* 595–605.

Devanand, D. P., Miller, L., Richards, M., Marder, K., Bell, K., Mayeux, R., & Stern, Y. (1992). The Columbia University Scale for Psychopathology in Alzheimer's Disease. *Archives of Neurology, 49,* 371–376.

Dhooper, S. S., Green, S. M., Huff, M. B., & Austen-Murphy, J. (1993). Efficacy of a group approach to reducing depression in nursing home elderly residents. *Journal of Gerontological Social Work, 20,* 87–100.

Dorfman, R. A., Lubben, J. E., Mayer-Oakes, A., Atchison K., Schweitzer S. O., DeJong, F. J., & Matthias, R. E. (1995). Screening for depression among a well elderly population. *Social Work, 40,* 295–304.

Duke Depression Evaluation Schedule for the Elderly (1988). Center for the Study of Depression in Later Life, Department of Psychiatry, Duke University Medical Center, Durham, NC.

Dunn, V. K., & Sacco, W. P. (1989). Psychometric evaluation of the Geriatric Depression Scale and the Zung Self-Rating Scale using an elderly community sample. *Psychology and Aging, 4,* 125–126.

Dush, D. M., & Hutzell, R. R. (1986). A brief MMPI depression scale for the elderly. *Clinical Gerontologist, 5,* 175–185.

Eaton, W. W., & Kessler, L. G. (1981). Rates of symptoms of depression in a national sample. *American Journal of Epidemiology, 114,* 528–538.

Elkin, I., Shea, M. T., Watkins, J. T., Imber, S. D., Sotsky, S. M., Collins, J. F., Glass, D. R., Pilkonis, P. A., Leber, W. R., Doherty, J. P., Fiester, S. J., & Parloff, M. B. (1989). NIMH Treatment of Depression Collaborative Research Program: General effectiveness of treatments. *Archives of General Psychiatry, 46,* 971–982.

Endicott, J., & Spitzer, R. L. (1978). A diagnostic interview. The Schedule for Affective Disorders and Schizophrenia. *Archives of General Psychiatry, 35,* 837–844.

Estes, C. L. (1995). Mental health services for the elderly: Key policy elements. In M. Gatz (Ed.), *Emerging issues in mental health and aging* (pp. 303–327). Washington, DC: American Psychological Association.

Evans, M. E. (1993). Depression in elderly physically ill inpatients: A 12-month prospective study. Special issue: Affective disorders: Current and future perspectives. *International Journal of Geriatric Psychiatry, 8,* 587–592.

Fawcett, J., Scheftner, W. A., Fogg, L., Clark, D. C., Young, M. A., Hedeker, D., & Gibbons, R. (1990). Time-related predictors of suicide in major affective disorder. *American Journal of Psychiatry, 147,* 1189–1194.

Feinberg, M., Carroll, B. J., Smouse, P. E., & Rawson, S. G. (1981). The Carroll Rating Scale for Depression: III. Comparison with other rating instruments. *British Journal of Psychiatry, 138,* 205–209.

Ferrier, I. N., & McKeith, I. G. (1991). Neuroanatomical and neurochemical changes in affective disorders in old age. Special Issue: Affective disorders in old age. *International Journal of Geriatric Psychiatry, 6,* 445–451.

Fischer, L. R., Rolnick, S. J., Jackson, J., Garrard, J., & Luepke, L. (1996). The Geriatric Depression Scale: A content analysis of respondent comments. *Journal of Mental Health and Aging, 2,* 125–135.

Fitz, A. G., & Teri, L. (1994). Depression, cognition, and functional ability in patients with Alzheimer's disease. *Journal of the American Geriatric Society, 42,* 186–191.

Fogel, B. S., & Fretwell, M. (1985). Reclassification of depression in the medically ill elderly. *Journal of the American Geriatrics Society, 33,* 446–448.

Forsell, Y., Jorm, A. F., von Strauss, E., & Winblad, B.

(1995). Prevalence and correlates of depression in a population of nonagenarians. *British Journal of Psychiatry, 167,* 61–64.

Forsell, Y., Jorm, A. F., & Winblad, B. (1994). Association of age, sex, cognitive dysfunction, and disability with major depressive symptoms in an elderly sample. *American Journal of Psychiatry, 151,* 1600–1604.

Foster, J. R., & Cataldo, J. K. (1994). Protection from clinical depression in medical long-term care facilities: Evidence for psychologic adaptation in cognitively intact patients. *International Journal of Geriatric Psychiatry, 9,* 115–125.

Frerichs, R. R., Aneshensel, C. S., & Clark, V. A. (1981). Prevalence of depression in Los Angeles County. *American Journal of Epidemiology, 113,* 691–699.

Friedhoff, A. J. (1994). Consensus Development Conference Statement: Diagnosis and treatment of depression in late life. In L. S. Schneider, C. F. Reynolds, III, B. D. Lebowitz, & A. J. Friedhoff (Eds.), *Diagnosis and treatment of depression in late life: Results of the NIH Consensus Development Conference* (pp. 493–511). Washington, DC: American Psychiatric Press.

Fry, P. S. (1983). Structured and unstructured reminiscence training and depression among the elderly. *Clinical Gerontologist, 1,* 15–37.

Fuhrer, R., Antonucci, T. C., Gagnon, M., Dartigues, J.-F., Barberger-Gateau, P., & Alperovitch, A. (1992). Depressive symptomatology and cognitive functioning: An epidemiological survey in an elderly community sample in France. *Psychological Medicine, 22,* 159–172.

Futterman, A., Thompson, L., Gallagher-Thompson, D., & Ferris, R. (1995). Depression in later life: Epidemiology, assessment, etiology, and treatment. In E. E. Beckham & W. R. Leber (Eds.), *Handbook of depression* (2nd ed., pp. 494–525). New York: Guilford Press.

Gallagher, D. (1986). The Beck Depression Inventory and older adults: Review of its development and utility. *Clinical Gerontologist, 5,* 149–163.

Gallagher, D., Breckinridge, J., Steinmetz, J., & Thompson, L. (1983). The Beck Depression Inventory & Research Diagnostic Criteria: Congruence in an older population. *Journal of Consulting and Clinical Psychology, 51,* 945–946.

Gallagher, D. E., & Thompson, L. W. (1982). Treatment of major depressive disorder in older adult outpatients with brief psychotherapies. *Psychotherapy: Theory, Research and Practice, 19,* 482–490.

Gallagher, D. E., & Thompson, L. W. (1983). Effectiveness of psychotherapy for both endogenous and nonendogenous depression in older adult outpatients. *Journal of Gerontology, 38,* 707–712.

Gallagher-Thompson, D. (1994). Clinical intervention strategies for distressed caregivers: Rationale and development of psychoeducational approaches. In E. Light, G. Niederehe, & B.D. Lebowitz (Eds.), *Stress effects on family caregivers of Alzheimer's patients: Research and interventions* (pp. 260–277). New York: Springer.

Gallagher-Thompson, D. E., Hanley-Peterson, P., & Thompson, L. W. (1990). Maintenance of gains versus relapse following brief psychotherapy for depression. *Journal of Consulting and Clinical Psychology, 58,* 371–374.

Gallo, J. J., Anthony, J. C., & Muthén, B. O. (1994). Age differences in the symptoms of depression: A latent trait analysis. *Journal of Gerontology: Psychological Sciences, 49,* P251–P264.

Garcia, M., & Marks, G. (1989). Depressive symptomatology among Mexican-American adults: An examination with the CES-D Scale. *Psychiatry Research, 27,* 137–148.

Gardner, E. A., Bahn, A. K., Mack, M. (1964). The relationship between premature deaths and affective disorders. *British Journal of Psychiatry, 115,* 1277–1282.

Gatz, M. (1992, December 14). *Depression and dementia studies in twins.* Berlin: Department of Psychiatry, Free University, and Max Planck Institute.

Gatz, M., Fiske, A., Fox, L., Kaskie, B., Kasl-Godley, J. E., McCallum, T. J., & Wetherell, J. (in press). Empirically-validated psychological treatments for older adults. *Journal of Mental Health and Aging.*

Gatz, M., & Hurwicz, M. (1990). Are old people more depressed? Cross-sectional data on Center for Epidemiological studies depression scale factors. *Psychology and Aging, 5,* 284–290.

Gatz, M., Johansson, B., Pedersen, N., Berg, S., & Reynolds, C. (1993). A cross-national self-report measure of depressive symptomatology. *International Psychogeriatrics, 5,* 147–156.

George, L. K., Blazer, D. G., Hughes, D. C., & Fowler, N. (1989). Social support and the outcome of major depression. *British Journal of Psychiatry, 154,* 478–485.

Gerson, S. C., Plotkin, D. A., & Jarvik, L. F. (1988). Antidepressant drug studies, 1964 to 1986: Empirical evidence for aging patients. *Journal of Clinical Psychopharmacology, 8,* 311–322.

Gilewski, M. J., Farberow, N. L., Gallagher, D. E., & Thompson, L. W. (1991). Interaction of depression and bereavement on mental health in the elderly. *Psychology and Aging, 6,* 67–75.

Gilley, D. W., Wilson, R. S., Fleischman, D. A., Harrison, D. W., Goetz, C. G., & Tanner, C. M. (1995). Impact of Alzheimer's Type Dementia and information source on the assessment of depression. *Psychological Assessment, 7,* 42–48.

Girling, D. M., Barkley, C., Paykel, E. S., Gehlhaar, E., Brayne, C., Gill, C., Methewson, D., & Huppert, F. A. (1995). The prevalence of depression in a cohort of the very elderly. *Journal of Affective Disorders, 34,* 319–329.

Glassman, A. H., & Roose, S. P. (1994). Risks of antidepressants in the elderly: Tricyclic antidepressants and arrhythmia-revising risks. *Gerontology, 40*(Suppl. 1), 15–20.

Golden, R. R., Teresi, J. A., & Gurland, B. J. (1984). Development of indicator scales for the comprehensive assessment and referral evaluation (CARE) interview schedule. *Journal of Gerontology, 39,* 138–146.

Greenwald, B. S., Kramer-Ginsberg, E., Marin, D. B., Laitman, L. B., Hermann, C. K., Mohs, R. C., & Davis, K. L. (1989). Dementia with coexistent major depression. *American Journal of Psychiatry, 146,* 1472–1478.

Guadagnoli, E., & Mor, V. (1989). Measuring cancer patients' affect: Revision and psychometric properties of the profile of mood states (POMS). *Psychological Assessment: A Journal of Consulting and Clinical Psychology, 2,* 150–154.

Gulbinat, W. H. (1996). The epidemiology of suicide in old age. *Archives of Suicide Research, 2,* 31–42.

Gurland, B., Kuriansky, J., Sharpe, L., Simon, R., Stiller, P., & Birkett, P. (1977–78). The Comprehensive Assessment and Referral Evaluation (CARE): Rationale, development and reliability. *International Journal of Aging and Human Development, 8,* 9–42.

Haight, B. K. (1992). Long-term effects of a structured life review process. *Journal of Gerontology, 47,* P312–P315.

Hale, W. D., Cochran, C. D., & Hedgepeth, B. E. (1984). Norms for the elderly on the Brief Symptom Index. *Journal of Consulting and Clinical Psychology, 52,* 321–322.

Hamilton, M. (1960). A rating scale for depression. *Journal of Neurology, Neurosurgery, and Psychiatry, 23,* 56–62.

Hamilton, M. (1967). Development of a rating scale for primary depressive illness. *British Journal of Social and Clinical Psychology, 6,* 278–296.

Harper, R. G., Kotik-Harper, D., & Kirby, H. (1990). Psychometric assessment of depression in an elderly general medical population: Over- or underassessment?

The Journal of Nervous and Mental Disease, 178, 113–119.

Hays, J. C., Kasl, S. V., & Jacobs, S. C. (1994). The course of psychological distress following threatened and actual conjugal bereavement. *Psychological Medicine, 24,* 917–927.

Heikkinen R.-L., Berg S., & Avlund K. (1995). Depressive symptoms in late life. *Journal of Cross-Cultural Gerontology, 10,* 315–330.

Henderson, A. S., Jorm, A. F., MacKinnon, A., Christensen, H., Scott, L. R., Korten, A. E., & Doyle, C. (1993). The prevalence of depressive disorders and the distribution of depressive symptoms in later life: A survey using Draft *ICD-10* and *DSM-III-R. Psychological Medicine, 23,* 719–729.

Henriksson, M. M., Isometsä, E. T., Hietanen, P. S., Aro, H., & Lönnqvist, J. K. (1995). Mental disorders in cancer suicides. *Journal of Affective Disorders, 36,* 11–20.

Henriksson, M. M., Marttunen, M. J., Isometsä, E. T., Heikkinen, M. E., Aro, H. M., Kuoppasalmi, K. I., & Lönnqvist, J. K. (1995). Mental disorders in elderly suicide. *International Psychogeriatrics, 7,* 275–286.

Hertzog, C., Van Alstine, J., Usala, P. D., Hultsch, D. F., Dixon, R. (1990). Measurement properties of the Center for Epidemiological Studies Depression Scale (CES-D) in older populations. *Psychological Assessment: A Journal of Consulting and Clinical Psychology, 2,* 64–72.

Hinrichsen, G. A. (1992). Recovery and relapse from major depressive disorder in the elderly. 144th Annual Meeting of the American Psychiatric Association (1991, New Orleans, LA.). *American Journal of Psychiatry, 149,* 1575–1579.

Hinrichsen, G. A., & Zweig, R. (1994). Family issues in late-life depression. *Journal of Long-Term Home Health Care, 13,* 4–15.

Hobfoll, E., & Wells, J. D. (in press). Conservation of resources, stress, and aging: Why do some slide and some spring? In J. Lomranz (Ed.), *Handbook of aging and mental health.* New York: Plenum.

Horwath, E., Johnson, J., Klerman, G. L., & Weissman, M. M. (1992). Depressive symptoms as relative and attributable risk factors for first-onset major depression. *Archives of General Psychiatry, 49,* 817–823.

Hussian, R. A., & Lawrence, P. S. (1981). Social reinforcement of activity and problem-solving training in the treatment of depressed institutionalized elderly patients. *Cognitive Therapy and Research, 5,* 57–69.

Jamison, C., & Scogin, F. (1992). Development of an interview-based geriatric depression rating scale. *International Journal of Aging and Human Development, 35,* 193–204.

Jarvik, L. F., Mintz, J., Steuer, J. L., & Gerner, R. (1982). Treating geriatric depression: A 26-week interim analysis. *Journal of the American Geriatric Society, 30,* 713–717.

Jenike, M. A. (1989). Treatment of affective illness in the elderly with drugs and electroconvulsive therapy. *Journal of Geriatric Psychiatry, 22,* 77–112.

Jorm, A. F. (1995). The epidemiology of depressive states in the elderly: Implications for recognition, intervention, and prevention. *Social Psychiatry and Psychiatric Epidemiology, 30,* 53–59.

Jorm, A. F., MacKinnon, A. J., Henderson, A. S., Scott, R., Christensen, H., Korten, A. E., Cullen, J. S., & Mulligan, R. (1995). The Psychogeriatric Asssessment Scales: a multidimensional alternative to categorical diagnoses of dementia and depression in the elderly. *Psychological Medicine, 25,* 447–460.

Kafonek, S., Ettinger, W. H., Roca, R., Kittner, S., Taylor, N., & German, P. S. (1989). Instruments for screening for depression and dementia in a long-term care facility. *Journal of the American Geriatrics Society, 37,* 29–34.

Kaplan, M. S., Adamek, M. E., & Johnson, S. (1994). Trends in firearm suicide among older American males: 1979–1988. *The Gerontologist, 34,* 59–65.

Kaszniak, A. W., & Christenson, G. D. (1994). Differential diagnosis of dementia and depression. In M. Storandt & G. R. Vanden Bos (Eds.), *Neuropsychological assessment of dementia and depression in older adults: A clinician's guide.* Washington, DC: American Psychological Association.

Katz, I. R., Simpson, G. M., Curlik, S. M., Parmelee, P. A., & Muhly, C. (1990). Pharmacologic treatment of major depression for elderly patients in residential care settings. *Journal of Clinical Psychiatry, 51* (Suppl. 7), 41–47.

Katz, I. R., Streim, J., & Parmelee, P. (1994). Prevention of depression, recurrences, and complications in late life. *Preventive Medicine: An International Journal Devoted to Practice and Theory, 23,* 743–750.

Kay, D. W. K., & Bergmann, K. (1980). Epidemiology of mental disorders among the aged in the community. In J. E. Birren & R. B. Sloane (Eds.), *Handbook of mental health and aging* (pp. 34–56). Englewood Cliffs, NJ: Prentice Hall.

Kemp, B. J., Staples, F., & Lopez-Aqueres, W. L. (1987). Epidemiology of depression and dysphoria in an elderly Hispanic population: Prevalence and correlates. *Journal of the American Geriatrics Society, 35,* 920–926.

Kendler, K. S., Neale, M. C., Kessler, R. C., Heath, A. C., & Eaves, L. J. (1992). Major depression and generalized anxiety disorder: Same genes, (partly) different environments? *Archives of General Psychiatry, 49,* 716–722.

Kendler, K. S., Neale, M. C., Kessler, R. C., Heath, A. C., & Eaves, L. J. (1993). The lifetime history of major depression in women: Reliability of diagnosis and heritability. *Archives of General Psychiatry, 50,* 863–870.

Kennedy, G. J., Kelman, H. R., & Thomas, C. (1991). Persistence and remission of depressive symptoms in late life. *American Journal of Psychiatry, 148,* 174–178.

Kennedy, G. J., Kelman, H. R., Thomas, C., Wisniewski, W., Metz, H., & Bijur, P. E. (1989). Hierarchy of characteristics associated with depressive symptoms in an urban elderly sample. *American Journal of Psychiatry, 146,* 220–225.

Kessler, R. C., Foster, C., Webster, P. S., & House, J. S. (1992). The relationship between age and depressive symptoms in two national surveys. *Psychology and Aging, 7,* 119–126.

Kessler, R., & Mroczek, D. (1993). *UM-CIDI Short-Form* [Memo]. Ann Arbor, MI: University of Michigan.

Kinzie, J. D., Lewinsohn, P., Maricle, R., & Teri, L. (1986). The relationship of depression to medical illness in an older community population. *Comprehensive Psychiatry, 27,* 241–246.

Kitchell, M. A., Barnes, R. F., Veith, R. C., Okimoto, J. T., & Raskind, M. A. (1982). Screening for depression in hospitalized geriatric medical patients. *Journal of the American Geriatrics Society, 30,* 174–177.

Kivela, S., & Pahkala, K. (1986). Sex and age differences of factor pattern and reliability of the Zung Self-Rating Depression Scale in a Finnish elderly population. *Psychological Reports, 59,* 587–597.

Kivela, S., & Pahkala, K. (1987). Factor structure of the Zung Self-rating Depression Scale among a depressed elderly population. *International Journal of Psychology, 22,* 289–300.

Klawansky, S. (1994). Meta-analysis on the treatment of depression in late life. In L. S. Schneider, C. F. Reynolds, III, B. D. Lebowitz, & A. J. Friedhoff (Eds.), *Diagnosis and treatment of depression in late life: Results of the NIH Consensus Development Conference* (pp. 333–352). Washington, DC: American Psychiatric Press.

Klerman, G. L., Lavori, P. W., Rice, J., Reich, T., Endicott, J., Andreasen, N. C., Keller, M. B., & Hirschfield, R. M. A. (1985). Birth-cohort trends in rates of major depressive disorder among relatives of patients with affective disorder. *Archives of General Psychiatry, 42,* 689–693.

Klerman, G. L., & Weissman, M. M. (1989). Increasing rates of depression. *Journal of the American Medical Association, 261,* 2229–2235.

Knight, B. G., Lutzky, S. M., & Macofsky-Urban, F. (1993). A meta-analytic review of interventions for caregiver distress: Recommendations for future research. *Gerontologist, 33,* 240–248.

Koenig, H. G., & Blazer, D. G. (1992). Epidemiology of geriatric affective disorders. *Clinics in Geriatric Medicine, 8,* 235–251.

Koenig, H. G., Cohen, H. J., Blazer, D. G., Krishnan, K. R. R., & Sibert, T. E. (1993). Profile of depressive symptoms in younger and older medical inpatients with major depression. *Journal of the American Geriatrics Society, 41,* 1116–1176.

Koenig, H. G., Cohen, H. J., Blazer, D. G., Meador, K. G., & Westlund, R. (1992). A brief Depression Scale for use in the medically ill. *International Journal of Psychiatry in Medicine, 22,* 183–195.

Koenig, H. G., Meador, K. G., Cohen, H. J., & Blazer, D. G. (1988). Self-rated depression scales and screening for major depression in the older hospitalized patient with medical illness. *Journal of the American Geriatrics Society, 36,* 699–706.

Koenig, H. G., Meador, K. G., Cohen, H. J., & Blazer, D. G. (1992). Screening for depression in hospitalized elderly medical patients: Taking a closer look. *Journal of the American Geriatrics Society, 40,* 1013–1017.

Koenig, H. G., Pappas, P., Holsinger, T., & Bachar, J. R. (1995). Assessing diagnostic approaches to depression in medically ill older adults: How reliably can mental health professionals make judgments about the cause of symptoms? *Journal of the American Geriatrics Society, 43,* 472–478.

Kogan, E. S., Kabacoff, R. I., Hersen, M., & Van Hasselt, V. B. (1994). Clinical cutoffs for the Beck Depression Inventory and the Geriatric Depression Scale with older adult psychiatric outpatients. *Journal of Psychopathology and Behavioral Assessment, 16,* 233–242.

Kogan, E. S., Van Hasselt, V. B., Hersen, M., & Kabacoff, R. I. (1995). Relationship of depression, assertiveness, and social support in community-dwelling older adults. *Journal of Clinical Geropsychology, 1,* 157–163.

Kohout, F. J., Berkman, L. F., Evans, D. A., & Cornoni-Huntley, J. (1993). Two shorter forms of the CES-D depression symptoms index. *Journal of Aging and Health, 5,* 179–193.

Kongstvedt, S. J., & Sime, W. (1992). Diagnosis of depression in early- and late-onset geriatric depression: An evaluation of commonly used self-assessment measures. *Behavior, Health and Aging, 2,* 133–148.

Kral, V. A., & Emery, O. B. (1989). Long-term follow-up of depressive pseudodementia of the aged. *Canadian Journal of Psychiatry, 34,* 445–446.

Krause, N., Herzog, A. R., & Baker, E. (1992). Providing support to others and well-being in later life. *Journal of Gerontology: Psychological Sciences, 47,* 300–311.

Kua, E. H. (1992). A community study of mental disorders in elderly Singaporean Chinese using the GMS-AGE-CAT package. *Australian and New Zealand Journal of Psychiatry, 26,* 502–506.

Kunik, M. E., Champagne, L., Harper, R. G., & Chacko, R. C. (1994). Cognitive functioning in elderly depressed patients with and without psychosis. *International Journal of Geriatric Psychiatry, 9,* 871–874.

La Rue, A. (1992). *Aging and neuropsychological assessment.* New York: Plenum.

La Rue, A., Goodman, S., & Spar, J. E. (1992). Risk factors for memory impairment in geriatric depression. *Neuropsychiatry, Neuropsychology, and Behavioral Neurology, 5,* 178–184.

Lawlor, B. A., & Anderson, M. C. (1995). The neurobiology of late-life depression: Impact of silent cerebrovascular disease. *Human Psychopharmacology, 10,* S223–S227.

Lazarus, L. W., Newton, N., Cohler, B., Lesser, J., & Schweon, C. (1987). Frequency and presentation of depressive symptoms in patients with primary degenerative dementia. *American Journal of Psychiatry, 144,* 41–45.

Leibenluft, E., & Goldberg, R. L. (1988). The suicidal, terminally ill patient with depression. *Psychosomatics, 29,* 379–386.

Lesher, E. L. (1986). Validation of the Geriatric Depression Scale among nursing home residents. *Clinical Gerontologist, 4,* 21–28.

Lesher, E. L., & Berryhill, J. S. (1994). Validation of the Geriatric Depression Scale—Short form among inpatients. *Journal of Clinical Psychology, 50,* 256–260.

Leuchter, A. F. (1994). Brain structural and functional correlates of late life depression. In L. S. Schneider, C. F. Reynolds, III, B. D. Lebowitz, & A. J. Friedhoff (Eds.), *Diagnosis and treatment of depression in late life: Results of the NIH Consensus Development Conference* (pp. 117–130). Washington, DC: American Psychiatric Press.

Levy, L. H., Martinkowski, K. S., & Derby, J. F. (1994). Differences in patterns of adaptation in conjugal bereavement: Their sources and potential significance. *Omega: Journal of Death and Dying, 29,* 71–87.

Lewinsohn, P., Muñoz, R., Youngren, M. A., & Zeiss, A. (1986). *Control your depression.* Englewood Cliffs, NJ: Prentice Hall.

Liang, R. A., Lam, R. W., & Ancill, R. J. (1988). ECT in the treatment of mixed depression and dementia. *British Journal of Psychiatry, 152,* 281–284.

Lichtenberg, P. A., Marcopulos, B. A., Steiner, D. A., & Tabscott, J. A. (1992). Comparison of the Hamilton Depression Rating Scale and the Geriatric Depression Scale: Detection of depression in dementia patients. *Psychological Reports, 70,* 515–521.

Lichtenstein, P., Gatz, M., Pedersen, N. L., Berg, S., & McClearn, G. E. (1996). A cotwin-control study of response to widowhood. *Journal of Gerontology: Psychological Sciences, 51B,* P279–P289.

Lindesay, J. (1991). Suicide in the elderly. *International Journal of Geriatric Psychiatry, 6,* 355–361.

Lindesay, J., Briggs, K., & Murphy, E. (1989). The Guy's/Age Concern Survey: Prevalence rates of cognitive impairment, depression and anxiety in an urban elderly community. *British Journal of Psychiatry, 155,* 317–329.

Logsdon, R. G., & Teri, L. (1995). Depression in Alzheimer's Disease patients: Caregivers as surrogate reporters. *Journal of the American Geriatrics Society, 43,* 150–155.

Lovett, S., & Gallagher, D. (1988). Psychoeducational interventions for family caregivers: Preliminary efficacy data. *Behavior Therapy, 19,* 321–330.

Lund, D. A., Caserta, M. S., Dimond, M. F., & Shaffer, S. K. (1989). Competencies, tasks of daily living, and adjustments to spousal bereavement in later life. In D. A. Lund (Ed.), *Older bereaved spouses: Research with practical applications* (pp. 135–152). Series in Death Education, Aging, and Health Care. New York: Hemisphere Publishing.

Lyness, J. M., Caine, E. D., Conwell, Y., King, D. A., & Cox, C. (1993). Depressive symptoms, medical illness, and functional status in depressed psychiatric inpatients. *American Journal of Psychiatry, 150,* 910–915.

Lyness, S. A., Eaton, E. M., & Schneider, L. S. (1994). Cognitive performance in older and middle-aged depressed outpatients and controls. *Journal of Gerontology: Psychological Sciences, 49,* 129–136.

Lyons, J. S., Strain, J. J., Hammer, J. S., Ackerman, A. D., & Fulop, G. (1989). Reliability, validity, and temporal stability of the Geriatric Depression Scale in hospitalized elderly. *International Journal of Psychiatry in Medicine, 19,* 203–209.

MacKinnon, A., Christensen, H., Cullen, J. S., Doyle, C. J., Henderson, A. S., Jorm, A. F., Korten, A. E., & Scott, L. R. (1993). The Canberra Interview for the Elderly: Assessment of its validity in the diagnosis of dementia and depression. *Acta Psychiatrica Scandinavica, 87,* 146–151.

Mann, A. H. (1995). Future directions for the specialty of old age psychiatry: Some suggestions for debate. *International Journal of Geriatric Psychiatry, 10,* 87–91.

Mann, A., Graham, N., & Ashby, D. (1984). Psychiatric illness in residential homes for the elderly: A survey in one London borough. *Age and Ageing, 13,* 257–265.

Marwit, S. J. (1991). *DSM-II-R,* grief reactions and a call for revision. *Professional Psychology: Research and Practice, 22,* 75–79.

Matt, G. E., Dean, A., Wang, B., & Wood, P. (1992). Identifying clinical syndromes in a community sample of elderly persons. *Psychological Assessment, 4,* 174–184.

McGuffin, P., Katz, R., Watkins, S., & Rutherford, J. (1996). A hospital-based twin register of the heritability of *DSM-IV* unipolar depression. *Archives of General Psychiatry, 53,* 129–136.

McElroy, M. R., Carmelli, D., Swan, G. E., & LaRue, A. (1995). Risk factors for the onset of depressive symptoms in older men: A 5-year follow-up of the Western Collaborative Group Study. Paper presented at the Gerontological Society of America, Los Angeles, CA.

McGarvey, B., Gallagher, D., Thompson, L. W., & Zelinski, E. (1982). Reliability and factor structure of the Zung Self-rating Depression Scale in three age groups. *Essence, 5,* 141–158.

McIntosh, J. L. (1992). Epidemiology of suicide in the elderly. In A. A. Leenaars, R. Maris, J. L. McIntosh, & J. Richman (Eds.), *Suicide and the older adult* (pp. 15–35). New York: Guilford Press.

McNair, D. M., Lorr, M., & Droppleman, L. F. (1971/1981/1992). *Manual for the Profile of Mood States.* San Diego, CA: Educational and Industrial Testing Service.

Meyers, B. S., Greenberg, R., & Mei-Tal, V. (1985). Delusional depression in the elderly. In C. A. Shamoian (Ed.), *Treatment of affective disorders in the elderly.* Washington, DC: American Psychiatric Press.

Meyers, B. S., Kalayam, B., & Mei-Tal, V. (1984). Late-onset delusional depression: A distinct clinical entity? *Journal of Clinical Psychiatry, 45,* 347–349.

Migliorelli, R., Teson, A., Sabe, L., Petracchi, M., Leiguarda, R., & Starkstein, S. E. (1995). Prevalence and correlates of dysthymia and major depression among patients with Alzheimer's disease. *American Journal of Psychiatry, 152,* 37–44.

Miles, C. P. (1977). Conditions predisposing to suicide: A review. *Journal of Nervous and Mental Disease, 164,* 231–246.

Moldin, S. O., Reich, T., & Rice, J. P. (1991). Current perspectives on the genetics of unipolar depression. *Behavior Genetics, 21,* 211–242.

Montgomery, S. A., & Åsberg, M. (1979). A new depression scale designed to be sensitive to change. *British Journal of Psychiatry,* 134, 382–389.

Mossey, J. M., Knott, K. A., Higgins, M., & Talerico, K. (1996). Effectiveness of a psychosocial intervention, interpersonal counseling, for subdysthymic depression in medically ill elderly. *Journal of Gerontology: Medical Sciences, 51A,* M172–M178.

Moye, J., Robiner, W. N., & Mackenzie, T. B. (1993). Depression in Alzheimer patients: Discrepancies between patient and caregiver reports. *Alzheimer Disease and Associated Disorders, 7,* 187–201.

Mrazek, P. J., & Haggerty, R. J. (Eds.). (1994). *Reducing risks for mental disorders: Frontiers for preventive intervention research.* Washington, DC: National Academy Press.

Muñoz, R. F., Gonzalez, G. M., & Starkweather, J. (1995). Automated screening for depression: Toward culturally and linguistically appropriate uses of computerized speech recognition. *Hispanic Journal of Behavioral Sciences, 17,* 194–208.

Murrell, S. A., & Himmelfarb, S. (1989). Effects of attachment, bereavement, and pre-event conditions on subsequent depressive symptoms in older adults. *Psychology and Aging, 4,* 166–172.

Murrell, S. A., Himmelfarb, S., & Wright, K. (1983). Prevalence of depression and its correlates in older adults. *American Journal of Epidemiology, 117,* 173–185.

Murrell, S. A. & Meeks, S. (1992). Depressive symptoms in older adults: Predispositions, resources, and life experiences. In K. W. Schaie & M. P. Lawton (Eds.), *Annual review of gerontology and geriatrics* (Vol. 11, pp. 261–275). New York: Springer.

Musetti, L., Perugi, G., Soriani, A., Rossi, V. M., Cassano, G. B., & Akiskal, H. S. (1989). Depression before and after age 65: A re-examination. *British Journal of Psychiatry, 155,* 330–336.

Naranjo C. A., Herrmann N., Mittmann N., & Bremner K. E. (1995). Recent advances in geriatric psychopharmacology. *Drugs and Aging, 7,* 184–202.

Nelson, J. C., Conwell, Y., Kim, K., & Mazure, C. (1989). Age at onset in late-life delusional depression. *American Journal of Psychiatry, 146,* 785–786.

Newmann, J. P. (1989). Aging and depression. *Psychology and Aging, 4,* 150–165.

Newmann, J. P., Klein, M. H., Jensen, J. E., & Essex, M. J. (1996). Depressive symptom experiences among older women: A comparison of alternative measurement approaches. *Psychology and Aging, 11,* 112–126.

Nezu, A. M., Nezu, A. M., & Perri, M. G. (1989). *Problem-solving therapy for depression: Theory, research, and clinical guidelines.* New York: Wiley.

Niederehe G. T. (1994). Psychosocial therapies with depressed older adults. In L. S. Schneider, C. F. Reynolds, III, B. D. Lebowitz, & A. J. Friedhoff (Eds.), *Diagnosis and treatment of depression in late life: Results of the NIH Consensus Development Conference* (pp. 293–315). Washington DC: American Psychiatric Press.

Norris, J. T., Gallagher, D. E., Wilson, A., & Winograd, C. H. (1987). Assessment of depression in geriatric medical outpatients: The validity of two screening measures. *Journal of the American Geriatrics Society, 35,* 989–995.

Norris, M. P., Snow-Turek, A. L., & Blankenship, L. (1995). Somatic depressive symptoms in the elderly: Contribution or confound? *Journal of Clinical Geropsychology, 1,* 5–17.

O'Connor, P. W., Pollitt, P. A., Roth, M., Brook, C. P. B., & Reiss, B. B. (1990). Memory complaints and impairment in normal depressed and demented elderly persons identified in a community survey. *Archives of General Psychiatry, 47,* 224–227.

O'Hara, M. W., Hinrichs, J. V., Kohout, F. J., Wallace, R. B., & Lemke, J. H. (1986). Memory complaint and memory performance in the depressed elderly. *Psychology and Aging, 3,* 208–214.

O'Hara, M. W., Kohout, F. J., & Wallace, R. B. (1985). Depression among the rural elderly: A study of prevalence and correlates. *Journal of Nervous and Mental Disease, 173,* 582–589.

Okimoto, J. T., Barnes, R. F., Veith, R. C., Raskind, M. A., Inui, T. S., & Carter, W. B. (1982). Screening for depression in geriatric medical patients. *American Journal of Psychiatry, 139,* 799–802.

Olin, J. T., Schneider, L. S., Eaton, E. M., Zemansky, M. F., & Pollock, V. E. (1992). The Geriatric Depression Scale and the Beck Depression Inventory as screening instruments in an older adult outpatient population. *Psychological Assessment, 4,* 190–192.

Ott, B. R. & Fogel, B. S. (1992). Measurement of depression in dementia: Self vs. clinician rating. *International Journal of Geriatric Psychiatry, 7,* 899–904.

Pachana, N. A., Gallagher-Thompson, D., & Thompson, L. W. (1994). Assessment of depression. In M. P. Lawton & J. A. Teresi (Eds.), *Focus on assessment techniques.* New York: Springer.

Parkin, D., & Stengel, E. (1965). Incidence of suicidal attempts in an urban community. *British Medical Journal, 2,* 133–138.

Parmelee, P. A., Katz, I. R., & Lawton, M. P. (1989). Depression among institutionalized aged: Assessment and prevalence estimation. *Journal of Gerontology: Medical Sciences, 44,* M22–M29.

Parmelee, P. A., Katz, I. R., & Lawton, M. P. (1991). The relation of pain to depression among institutionalized aged. *Journal of Gerontology: Psycholoical Sciences, 46,* P15–P21.

Parmelee, P. A., Katz, I. R., & Lawton, M. P. (1992). Depression and mortality among institutionalized aged. *Journal of Gerontology: Psychological Sciences, 47,* P3–P10.

Phifer, J. F., & Murrell, S. A. (1986). Etiologic factors in the onset of depressive symptoms in older adults. *Journal of Abnormal Psychology, 95,* 282–291.

Pond, C. D., Mant, A., Kehoe, L., Hewitt, H., & Brodaty. (1994). General practitioner diagnosis of depression and dementia in the elderly: Can academic detailing make a difference? *Family Practice, 11,* 141–147.

Poon, L. W. (1992). Toward an understanding of cognitive functioning in geriatric depression. *International Psychogeriatrics, 4* (Suppl. 2), 241–266.

Prigerson, H. G., Frank, E., Kasl, S. V., Reynolds, C. F., Anderson, B., Zubenko, G. S., Houck, P. R., George, C. J., & Kupfer, D. J. (1995). Complicated grief and bereavement-related depression as distinct disorders: Preliminary empirical validation in elderly bereaved spouses. *American Journal of Psychiatry, 152,* 22–30.

Radloff, L. S. (1977). The CES-D Scale: A self-report depression scale for research in the general population. *Applied Psychological Measurement, 1,* 385–401.

Radloff, L. S., & Teri, L. (1986). Use of the Center for Epidemiological Studies-Depression Scale with older adults. *Clinical Gerontologist, 5,* 119–136.

Rapp, S. R., Parisi, S. A., Walsh, D. A., & Wallace, C. E. (1988). Detecting depression in elderly medical inpatients. *Journal of Consulting and Clinical Psychology, 56,* 509–513.

Rapp, S. R., Smith, S. S., & Britt, M. (1990). Identifying comorbid depression in elderly medical patients: Use of the extracted Hamilton Depression Rating Scale. *Psychological Assessment, 2,* 243–247.

Rapp, S. R., & Vrana, S. (1989). Substituting nonsomatic for somatic symptoms in the diagnosis of depression in elderly male medical patients. *American Journal of Psychiatry, 146,* 1197–1200.

Raschko, R. (1985). Systems integration at the program level: Aging and mental health. *Gerontologist, 25,* 460–463.

Ravindran, A. V., Welburn, K., & Copeland, J. R. (1994). Semi-structured depression scale sensitive to change with treatment for use in the elderly. *British Journal of Psychiatry, 164,* 522–527.

Ray, W. A., Griffin, M. R., Schaffner, W., Baugh, D. L., & Melson. (1987). Psychotropic drug use and the risk of hip fracture. *New England Journal of Medicine, 316,* 363–369.

Reynolds, C. F., III, Frank, E., Perel, J. M., Imber, S. D., Cornes, C., Morycz, R. K., Mazumdar, S., Miller, M. D., Pollock, B. G., Rifai, A. H., Stack, J. A., George, C. J., Houck, P. R., & Kupfer, D. J. (1992). Combined pharmacotherapy and psychotherapy in the acute and continuation treatment of elderly patients with recurrent major depression: A preliminary report. *American Journal of Psychiatry, 149,* 1687–1692.

Reynolds, W. M., & Kobak, K. A. (1991). *Hamilton Depression Inventory: A self-report version of the Hamilton Depression Rating Scale.* Odessa, FL: Psychological Assessment Resources.

Reynolds, C. F., Schneider, L. S., Lebowitz, B. D., & Kupfer, D. (1994). Treatment of depression in elderly patients: Guidelines for primary care. In L. S. Schneider, C. F. Reynolds, III, B. D. Lebowitz, & A. J. Friedhoff (Eds.), *Diagnosis and treatment of depression in late life: Results of the NIH Consensus Development Conference* (pp. 463–490). Washington, DC: American Psychiatric Press.

Riskind, J. H., Beck, A. T., & Steer, R. A. (1985). Cognitive-behavioral therapy in geriatric depression: Comment on Steuer et al. *Journal of Consulting and Clinical Psychology, 53,* 944–945.

Robins, L. N., Helzer, J. E., Croughan, J., & Ratcliff, K. S. (1981). National Institute of Mental Health Diagnostic Interview Schedule: Its history, characteristics, and validity. *Archives of General Psychiatry, 38,* 381–389.

Robins, L. N., Wing, J., Wittchen, H. U., Helzer, J. E., Babor, T. F., Burke, J., Farmer, A., Jablenski, A., Pickens, R., Regier, D. A., Sartorius, N., & Towle, L. H. (1988). The Composite International Diagnostic Interview. An epidemiological instrument suitable for use in conjunction with different diagnostic systems and in different cultures. *Archives of General Psychiatry, 45,* 1069–1077.

Robinson, R. G., & Starkstein, S. E. (1990). Current research in affective disorders following stroke. *Journal of Neuropsychiatry, 2,* 1–14.

Roth, M., Tym, E., Mountjoy, C. Q., Huppert, F. A., Hendrie, H., Verma, S., & Goddard, R. (1986). CAMDEX: A standardized instrument for the diagnosis of mental disorder in the elderly with special reference to the early detection of dementia. *British Journal of Psychiatry, 149,* 698–709.

Rubin, R. T. (1994). Neuroendocrine aspects of stress in major depression. In R. P. Lieberman & J. Yager (Eds.), *Stress in psychiatric disorders.* New York: Springer.

Russell, D. W., & Cutrona, C. E. (1991). Social support, stress, and depressive symptoms among the elderly: Test of a process model. *Psychology and Aging, 6,* 190–201.

Rybarczyk, B., Gallagher-Thompson, D., Rodman, J., Zeiss, A., Gantz, F. E., & Yesavage, J. (1992). Applying cognitive-behavioral psychotherapy to the chronically ill elderly: Treatment issues and case illustration. *International Psychogeriatrics, 4,* 127–140.

Sackeim, H. A. (1994). Use of electroconvulsive therapy in late-life depression. In L. S. Schneider, C. F. Reynolds, III, B. D. Lebowitz, & A. J. Friedhoff (Eds.), *Diagnosis and treatment of depression in late life: Results of the NIH Consensus Development Conference* (pp. 259–277). Washington, DC: American Psychiatric Press.

Salzman, C. (1994). Pharmacological treatment of depression in elderly patients. In L. S. Schneider, C. F. Reynolds, III, B. D. Lebowitz, & A. J. Friedhoff (Eds.), *Diagnosis and treatment of depression in late life: Results of the NIH Consensus Development Conference* (pp. 181–244). Washington, DC: American Psychiatric Press.

Schneider L. S., Sloane R. B., Staples F. R., & Bender M. (1986). Pretreatment orthostatic hypotension as a predictor of response to nortriptyline in geriatric depression. *Journal of Clinical Psychopharmacology, 6,* 172–176.

Schulz, R., & Williamson, G. M. (1994). Health effects of caregiving: Prevalence of mental and physical illness in Alzheimer's caregivers. In E. Light, G. Niederehe, & B. D. Lebowitz (Eds.), *Stress effects on family caregivers of*

Alzheimer's patients (pp. 38–63). New York: Springer.
Schuster, T. L., & Butler, E. W. (1989). Bereavement, social networks, social support, and mental health. In D. A. Lund (Eds.), *Older bereaved spouses: Research with practical applications* (pp. 55–68). New York: Hemisphere Publishing.
Scogin, F. R. (1994). Assessment of depression in older adults: A guide for practitioners. In M. Storandt & G. R. Vanden Bos (Eds.), *Neuropsychological assessment of dementia and depression in older adults: A clinician's guide* (pp. 61–80). Washington, DC: American Psychological Association.
Scogin, F., & McElreath, L. (1994). Efficacy of psychosocial treatments for geriatric depression: A quantitative review. *Journal of Consulting and Clinical Psychology, 62,* 69–74.
Segal, D. L., Hersen, M., Van Hasselt, V. B., Kabacoff, R. I., & Roth, L. (1993). Reliability of diagnosis in older psychiatric patients using the Structured Clinical Interview for DSM-III-R. *Journal of Psychopathology and Behavioral Assessment, 15,* 347–356.
Seltzer, B., Vasterling, J. J., & Buswell, A. (1995). Awareness of deficit in Alzheimer's disease: Associations with psychiatric symptoms and other disease variables. *Journal of Clinical Geropsychology, 1,* 79–87.
Sheikh, J. I., & Yesavage, J. A. (1986). Geriatric Depression Scale (GDS): Recent evidence and development of a shorter version. *Clinical Gerontologist, 5.* 165–173.
Shulman, K. I., Tohen, M., Satlin, A., Mallya, G., & Kalunian, D. (1992). Mania compared with unipolar depression in old age. *American Journal of Psychiatry, 149,* 341–345.
Silverman, P. R. (1969). The Widow-to-Widow Program: An experiment in preventive intervention. *Mental Hygiene, 53,* 333–337.
Small, G. W., Komanduri, R., Gitlin, M., & Jarvik, L. (1986). The influence of age on guilt expression in major depression. *International Journal of Geriatric Psychiatry, 1,* 121–126.
Smouse, P. E., Feinberg, M., Carroll, B. J., Park, & Rawson, S. G. (1981). The Carroll Rating Scale for Depression: II. Factor Analysis of the feature profiles. *British Journal of Psychiatry, 138,* 201–204.
Smyer, M. A. (1995). Prevention and early intervention for mental disorders of the elderly. In M. Gatz (Ed.), *Emerging issues in mental health and aging* (pp. 163–182). Washington, DC: American Psychological Association.
Smyer, M. A., Zarit, S. H., & Qualls, S. H. (1990). Psychological intervention with the aging individual. In J. E. Birren & K. W. Schaie (Eds.), *Handbook of the psychology of aging* (3rd ed.). San Diego, CA: Academic Press.
Snowdon, J., & Lane, F. (1995). The Botany Survey: A longitudinal study of depression and cognitive impairment in an elderly population. *International Journal of Geriatric Psychiatry, 10,* 349–358.
Spitzer, R. L., Endicott, J., & Robins, E. (1978). Research Diagnostic Criteria: Rationale and reliability. *Archives of General Psychiatry, 35,* 773–782.
Spitzer, R. L., Williams, J. B. W., Gibbon, M., & First, M. B. (1992). The structured clinical interview for *DSM-III-R* (SCID) I: History, rationale, and description. *Archives of General Psychiatry, 49,* 624–629.
Stallones, L., Marx, M. B., & Garrity, T. F. (1990). Prevalence and correlates of depressive symptoms among older U. S. adults. *American Journal of Preventive Medicine, 6,* 295–303.
Steingart, A., & Herrmann, N. (1991). Major depressive disorder in the elderly: The relationship between age of onset and cognitive impairment. *International Journal of Geriatric Psychiatry, 6,* 593–598.
Steuer, J. L., Mintz, J., Hammen, C. L., Hill, M. A., Jarvik, L. F., McCarley, T., Motoike, P., & Rosen, R. (1984). Cognitive-behavioral and psychodynamic group psychotherapy in treatment of geriatric depression. *Journal of Consulting and Clinical Psychology, 52,* 180–189.
Stukenberg, K. W., Dura, J. R., & Kiecolt-Glaser, J. K. (1990). Depression screening scale validation in an elderly, community-dwelling population. *Psychological Assessment, 2,* 134–138.
Sultzer, D. L., Levin, H. S., Mahler, M. E., High, W. M., & Cummings, J. L. (1992). Assessment of cognitive, psychiatric, and behavioral disturbances in patients with dementia: the Neurobehavioral Rating Scale. *Journal of the American Geriatrics Society, 40,* 549–555.
Sunderland, T., Alterman, I. S., Yount, D., Hill, J. L., Tariot, P. N., Newhouse, P. A., Mueller, E. A., Mellow, A. M., & Cohen, R. M. (1988). A new scale for the assessment of depressed mood in demented patients. *American Journal of Psychiatry, 145,* 955–959.
Takahashi, Y., Hirasawa, H., Koyama, K., Asakawa, O., Kido, M., Onose, H., Udagawa, M., Ishikawa, Y., & Uno, M. (1995). Suicide and aging in Japan: An examination of treated elderly suicide attempters. *International Psychogeriatrics, 7,* 239–251.
Teri, L., Curtis, J., Gallagher-Thompson, D., & Thompson, L. (1994). Cognitive-behavior therapy with depressed older adults. In L. S. Schneider, C. F. Reynolds, III, B. D. Lebowitz, & A. J. Friedhoff (Eds.), *Diagnosis and treatment of depression in late life: Results of the NIH Consensus Development Conference* (pp. 279–291). Washington, DC: American Psychiatric Press.
Teri L., Logsdon R., Wagner A., & Uomoto J. (1994). The caregiver role in behavioral treatment of depression in dementia patients. In E. Light, G. Niederehe, & B. D. Lebowitz (Eds.), *Stress effects on family caregivers of Alzheimer's patients: Research and interventions* (pp. 185–204). New York: Springer.
Teri, L., & Wagner, A. W. (1991). Assessment of depression in patients with Alzheimer's disease: Concordance among informants. *Psychology and Aging, 6,* 280–285.
Thomas, C., Kelman, H. R., Kennedy, G. J., Ahn, C., & Yang, C. (1992). Depressive symptoms and mortality in elderly persons. *Journal of Gerontology: Social Sciences, 47,* 80–87.
Thompson, L. W., Gallagher, D. E., & Breckinridge, J. S. (1987). Comparative effectiveness of psychotherapies for depressed elders. *Journal of Consulting and Clinical Psychology, 55,* 385–390.
Thompson, L. W., Gallagher, D. E., Nies, G., & Epstein, D. (1983). Evaluation of the effectiveness of professionals and nonprofessionals as instructors of "Coping with Depression" classes for elders. *Gerontologist, 23,* 390–396.
Torgersen, S. (1986). Genetic factors in moderately severe and mild affective disorders. *Archives of General Psychiatry, 43,* 222–226.
Tucker, M. A., Ogle, S. J., Davison, J. G., Eilenberg, M. D. (1986). Development of a brief screening test for depression in the elderly. *Journal of Clinical Experimental Gerontology, 8,* 173–190.
Turner, R. J., & Beiser, M. (1990). Major depression and depressive symptomology among the physically disabled: Assessing the role of chronic stress. *Journal of Nervous and Mental Disease, 178,* 343–350.
Uhlenhuth, E. H., Balter, M. B., Mellinger, G. D., Cisin, I. H., & Clinthorne, J. (1983). Symptom checklist syndromes in the general population: Correlations with psychotherapeutic drug use. *Archives of General Psychiatry, 40,* 1167–1173.
Vachon, M. L. S., Sheldon, A. R., Lancee, W. J., Lyall, W. A. L., Roger, J., & Freeman, S. J. J. (1980). A controlled study of self-help intervention for widows. *American Journal of Psychiatry, 137,* 1380–1384.

Vachon, M. L. S., & Stylianos, S. K. (1988). The role of social support in bereavement. *Journal of Social Issues, 44,* 175–190.
van Ojen, R., Hooijer, C., Bezemer, D., Jonker, C., Lindeboom, J., & van Tilburg, W. (1995a). Late-life depressive disorder in the community: I. The relationship between MMSE score and depression in subjects with and without psychiatric history. *British Journal of Psychiatry, 166,* 311–315.
van Ojen, R., Hooijer, C., Bezemer, D., Jonker, C., Lindeboom, J., & van Tilburg, W. (1995b). Late-life depressive disorder in the community: II. The relationship between psychiatric history, MMSE and family history. *British Journal of Psychiatry, 166,* 316–319.
Vida, S., Des Rosiers, P., Carrier, L., & Gauthier, S. (1994a). Depression in Alzheimer's disease: Receiver operating characteristics analysis of the Cornell Scale for Depression in Dementia and the Hamilton Depression Scale. *Journal of Geriatric Psychiatry and Neurology, 7,* 159–162.
Vida, S., Des Rosiers, P., Carrier, L., & Gauthier, S. (1994b). Prevalence of depression in Alzheimer's disease and validity of research diagnostic criteria. *Journal of Geriatric Psychiatry and Neurology, 7,* 238–244.
Wallace, J., & O'Hara, M. W. (1992). Increases in depressive symptomatology in the rural elderly: Results from a cross-sectional and longitudinal study. *Journal of Abnormal Psychology, 101,* 398–404.
Ward, L. C., Wadsworth, A. P., & Peterson, L. P. (1994). Concurrent validity of measures of anxiety, depression, and somatization in elderly, demented, male patients. *Clinical Gerontologist, 15,* 3–13.
Warren, C. A., & Levy, K. A. (1991). Electroconvulsive therapy and the elderly. *Journal of Aging Studies, 5,* 309–327.
Waters, E. (1995). Let's not wait 'till it's broke: Interventions to maintain and enhance mental health in late life. In M. Gatz (Ed.), *Emerging issues in mental health and aging* (pp. 183–209). Washington, DC: American Psychological Association.
Weissman, M. M., Bruce, M. L., Leaf, P. J., Florio, L. P., & Holzer, C., III. (1991). Affective disorders. In L. N. Robins & D. A. Regier (Eds.), *Psychiatric disorders in America* (pp. 53–80). New York: Free Press.
Weissman, M. M., Leaf, P. J., Holzer, C. E., Myers, J. K., & Tischler, G. L. (1984). The epidemiology of depression: An update on sex differences in rates. *Journal of Affective Disorders, 7,* 179–188.
Weissman, M. M., Leaf, P. J., Tischler, G. L., Blazer, D. G., Karno, M., Bruce, M. L., & Florio, L. P. (1988). Affective disorders in five United States communities. *Psychological Medicine, 18,* 141–153.
Weissman, M. M., & Myers, J. K. (1978). Affective disorders in a US urban community: The use of Research Diagnostic Criteria in an epidemiological survey. *Archives of General Psychiatry, 35,* 1304–1311.
Wells, K. B., Stewart, A., Hays, R. D., Burnam, M. A., Rogers, W., Daniels, M. Berry, S., Greenfield, S., & Ware, J. (1989). The functioning and well-being of depressed patients: Results from the Medical Outcomes Study. *Journal of the American Medical Association, 262,* 914–919.
Wernicke, T. F., & Linden, M. (1994). Clinical recognition and drug treatment of depression in cases found by standardized assessment. *Pharmacopsychiatry, 27* (Suppl.), 54–57.
Wetzel, R. D., Margulies, T., Davis, R., & Karam, E. (1980). Hopelessness, depression, and suicide intent. *Journal of Clinical Psychiatry, 41,* 159–160.
Wexler, B. E., & Cicchetti, D. V. (1992). The outpatient treatment of depression: Implications of outcome research for clinical practice. *Journal of Nervous and Mental Disease, 180,* 277–286.
White House Mini-Conference on Emerging Issues in Mental Health and Aging. (1995). Resolutions of the White House Mini-Conference on Emerging Issues in Mental Health and Aging. In M. Gatz (Ed.), *Emerging issues in mental health and aging* (pp. 329–364). Washington DC: American Psychological Association.
Williams, J. B. (1988). A structured interview guide for the Hamilton Depression Rating Scale. *Archives of General Psychiatry, 45,* 742–747.
Williamson, G. M., & Schulz, R. (1992a). Pain, activity restriction, and symptoms of depression among community-residing elderly adults. *Journal of Gerontology: Psychological Sciences, 47,* 367–372.
Williamson, G. M. & Schulz, R. (1992b). Physical illness and symptoms of depression among elderly outpatients. *Psychology and Aging, 7,* 343–351.
Wing, J. K., Birley, J. L. T., Cooper, J. E., Graham, P., & Isaacs, A. D. (1967). Reliability of procedure for measuring and classifying "Present Psychiatric State." *British Journal of Psychiatry, 113,* 499–515.
Wolfe, R., Morrow, J., & Fredrickson, B. L. (1995). Mood disorders in older adults. In L. L. Carstensen, B. A. Edelstein, & L. Dornbrand (Eds.), *The practical handbook of clinical gerontology.* Thousand Oaks, CA: Sage.
World Health Organization (1977). *Manual of the international statistical classification of diseases, injuries, and causes of death* (9th rev., Vol. 1). Geneva: Author.
World Health Organization (1992–1993). *International statistical classification of diseases and related health problems* (10th rev.). Geneva: Author.
Yesavage, J. A., Brink, T. L., Rose, T. L., Lum, O., Huang, V., Adey, M., Leirer, V. O. (1983). Development and validation of a geriatric depression screening scale: A preliminary report. *Journal of Psychiatric Research, 17,* 37–49.
Zemore, R., & Eames, N. (1979). Psychic and somatic symptoms of depression among young adults, institutionalized aged and noninstitutionalized aged. *Journal of Gerontology, 34,* 716–722.
Zimmerman, M., & Coryell, W. (1987). The inventory to diagnose depression, lifetime version. *Acta Psychiatrica Scandinavica, 75,* 495–499.
Zimmerman, M., Coryell, W., Corenthal, C., & Wilson, S. (1986). A self-report scale to diagnose major depressive disorder. *Archives of General Psychiatry, 43,* 1076–1081.
Zorumski, C.F., Rubin E. H., & Burke, W. J. (1988). Electroconvulsive therapy for the elderly: A review. *Hospital and Community Psychiatry, 39,* 643–647.
Zuckerman, M., & Lubin, B. (1965). *Manual for the Multiple Affect Adjective Checklist.* San Diego, CA: EdITS/Educational and Industrial Testing Service.
Zuckerman, M., & Lubin, B. (1985). Manual for the MAACL-R: The Multiple Affect Adjective Checklist Revised. San Diego, CA: Educational and Industrial Testing Service.
Zung, W. W. K. (1965). A self-rating depression scale. *Archives of General Psychiatry, 12,* 63–70.
Zung, W. W. K. (1967). Depression in the normal aged. *Psychosomatics, 13,* 287–292.

7.10
Cognitive Development in Alzheimer's Disease: Charting the Decline Process

BRENT J. SMALL
Stockholm Gerontology Research Center, Sweden and Karolinska Institute, Stockholm, Sweden
AGENTA HERLITZ
Stockholm Gerontology Research Center, Sweden and Stockholm University, Sweden
and
LARS BÄCKMAN
Stockholm Gerontology Research Center, Sweden and Göteborg University, Sweden

7.10.1 INTRODUCTION

Several reviews agree that Alzheimer's disease (AD) results in a global cognitive impairment that involves deficits in perception, attention, psychomotor speed, memory, visuospatial functioning, intelligence, and language (Bäckman, 1992; Morris, 1996; Nebes, 1992).

This extension of cognitive impairment in AD is to be expected, given that this disease is associated with marked lesions in limbic structures as well as in the neocortical association areas (Braak & Braak, 1991, 1995; Frackowiak et al., 1981; Grady et al., 1990; Haxby et al., 1990).

However, the view that AD affects our cognitive functions in a global manner does not necessarily imply that all functions decline at the same time and at the same rate. By contrast, some variability in the degree to which different cognitive functions are compromised should be expected, given that (i) the neuropathological trajectory in AD may begin with lesions in medial-temporal regions that gradually radiate into neocortical (e.g., temporal, parietal, and frontal) areas (Braak & Braak, 1991, 1995; Fewster, Griffin-Brooks, MacGregor, Ojalvo-Rose, & Ball, 1991); and (ii) different cognitive tasks vary with regard to the extent to which overlearned skills, procedures, and knowledge could be utilized. Conceivably, this variability is likely to decrease as a function of increasing severity of dementia. Knowledge regarding whether AD related cognitive deficits occur in a lawful manner across the pathogenesis would seem to be imperative not only for advancing our scientific understanding of the disease itself, but also to facilitate early clinical diagnosis and be useful in behavioral intervention.

The purpose of this chapter is to provide an overview of recent research addressing the aforementioned issues. The overview is organized so as to parallel the disease development. That is, we begin by reviewing the evidence pertaining to potential preclinical cognitive markers of AD. This is followed by an examination of the cognitive tasks that may or may not be useful in differentiating early AD patients from normal old adults. The next step is to determine whether the same cognitive tasks that are particularly effective at detecting AD are also most sensitive in discriminating between patients at different phases in the disease process.

Most of the work examining the efficacy of cognitive measures in detecting and staging AD is cross-sectional in nature; this is reflected in the present review. However, an increasing number of longitudinal studies charting the cognitive progression in AD are available. Examining the results from these studies not only allows for an interesting comparison with the cross-sectional research on detection and staging of AD but also it provides the necessary means by which different cognitive functions can be compared with regard to rate of pathological change.

Although a major goal of the chapter is to examine whether there is a predictable development of cognitive decline in AD, there may also be individual differences among patients with regard to both the magnitude and rate of change in various cognitive functions. Individual difference variables (e.g., demographic, psychometric, biological) have been found to be powerful mediators of cognitive performance in normal aging (e.g., Elias, Wolf, D́Agostino, Cobb, & White, 1993; Wahlin et al., 1993; West, Crook, & Barron, 1992). Thus, an additional objective of this chapter is to determine whether variability in cognitive performance among AD patients can systematically be linked to specific subject-related factors.

Before describing the changes in cognitive performance that accompany AD, it is important to address a number of practical problems associated with studying this population of individuals. The most basic problem concerns the uncertainty of the diagnosis itself. Although the diagnostic criteria in the last few years have become increasingly strict (American Psychiatric Association, 1980, 1987, 1994; McKhann et al., 1984), there are still no specific clinical diagnostic markers for AD. Presently, the clinical diagnostic criteria are descriptive and exclusive, and pathological confirmation remains the current "gold standard" for AD diagnosis (Galasko et al., 1994; Huppert, Brayne, & O'Connor, 1994). Unfortunately, in AD research most studies have relied on the clinical diagnosis as the gold standard, which means that the criterion variable is far from perfect. It is possible that the clinical diagnostic criteria are not sensitive enough to detect very old subjects in a very early phase of AD. For example, what defines normality (e.g., in terms of physical, sensory, and cognitive status) may be rather equivocal in very advanced age (Brody & Schneider, 1986; Fries & Crapo, 1981), making diagnostic decisions uncertain (e.g., Fratiglioni, Grut, Forsell, Viitanen, & Winblad, 1992). Nevertheless, because these clinical criteria are one of the only means, at the present time, for rendering dementia diagnoses we must utilize what is available to us.

In addition to problems associated with dementia diagnosis, there are a number of issues regarding sample composition, such as sample selection, sample size, and dementia etiology that require consideration. These three facets all have the potential to influence the results that are found from studies that have examined cognitive performance in demented persons. The following section addresses these aspects of sample composition.

7.10.2 SAMPLE COMPOSITION

The source from which researchers select their populations of demented and nondemented (control) subjects has important implications for the severity of impairment that is observed, as well as the extent to which the results that are produced are generalizable to the population of adults at large. Typically, samples of demented and nondemented subjects are selected from clinical or population settings. One of the advantages of selecting patients from a clinical setting is often that relatively large numbers of subjects are available for study. Further, the accuracy of the dementia diagnosis is likely to be more precise, because clinicians are allowed to spend more time interviewing the patient and relevant family members as compared to population-based studies (Brayne et al., 1995). In addition, various diagnosis-related assessment procedures, including radiological assessment (e.g., computerized tomography, magnetic resonance imaging) as well as other medical procedures (e.g., blood sampling) are easier to implement in a clinical setting, thus enhancing diagnostic accuracy. Alternatively, there are also several disadvantages in selecting subjects from clinical populations. For example, it is likely that these subjects are biased towards being more demented than subjects from the community. In addition, the controls used in a clinical setting are likely to be healthier and cognitively superior compared with a random sample from the community. Both of these factors may result in an overestimation of the differences between patients and controls. Moreover, the greater initial impairment of the clinical population may make investigating mild changes in dementia difficult, because these populations are dominated by persons with more obvious signs of cognitive deficiencies. This may have negative repercussions concerning the generalizability of the findings that are observed. That is, when individuals self-select themselves for assessment in a clinical setting, the composition of this group, both demographically and cognitively, may be very different from studies who use patients that are sampled in a more representative fashion.

One of the chief advantages of sampling adults from the community is the ability to make generalizations back to the larger population. In addition, more diversity in terms of cognitive performance and demographic characteristics may be present in the samples as compared to clinical populations. This diversity is represented not only as milder levels of impairment among the demented subjects, but also in terms of increased variability in performance among those who are nondemented. Although there are benefits in examining cognitive performance in community-based samples of adults, there are also several disadvantages. Chief among them is the small sample size of demented adults that is often available. The relatively small sample size of demented persons in population-based studies is largely a byproduct of prevalence and incidence rates of AD. Several studies have shown that between 1.3 and 11.2% of adults over the age of 65 have AD (see Ebly, Parhad, Hogan, & Fung, 1994, for a review). Although prevalence rates increase with age, it remains that the population that must be sampled to achieve sufficient numbers of AD patients needs to be relatively large. Similar problems of small sample sizes are evident in studies that have examined incidence of dementia (e.g., Katzman et al., 1989; Tierney et al., 1996).

To combat problems with small sample sizes of AD patients, some authors have resorted to combining different dementia etiologies, typically AD and vascular dementia (VaD), into one group (e.g., Almkvist & Bäckman, 1993a, Herlitz, Hill, Fratiglioni, & Bäckman, 1995; Small & Bäckman, 1996). Although this procedure does reduce problems associated with sample size, it can be criticized on the grounds of potentially obscuring relationships with cognitive performance because of the different dementia types. For example, Gottfries, Blennow, Wallin, and Gottfries (1995) found that AD and VaD patients significantly differed in a number of cognitive dimensions. Specifically, on the one hand, AD patients experienced more parietal symptoms (e.g., sensory aphasia, visuospatial dysfunction), whereas VaD patients experienced more symptoms related to confusion (e.g., clouded consciousness, attentional problems) and subcortical impairments (e.g., psychomotor retardation). However, there is a growing body of evidence indicating nearly identical patterns of cross-sectional performance in tasks assessing various aspects of episodic memory for those individuals with AD and those with VaD (e.g., Almkvist, 1994; Almkvist, Bäckman, Basun, & Wahlund, 1993; Erkinjuntti, Laaksonen, Sulkava, Syrjäläinen, & Palo, 1986). A reasonable recommendation is that studies utilizing more than one dementia type should incorporate a test of the differences between the groups in their analyses. Only after different dementia groups have been found to be indistinguishable in the measures of relevance, is collapsing across dementia etiology justifiable.

In this chapter, we review studies that have focused exclusively on subjects with AD, but also on studies that have combined different dementia etiologies. This has been done for purely pragmatic reasons; the pool of available studies is so much larger when accounts that have used both subject selection methods are employed. Nevertheless, we will orient the reader to the use of these different subject groups and, where possible, indicate whether between-group comparisons were made.

7.10.3 INCIDENCE OF DEMENTIA

A number of studies have examined potential preclinical cognitive markers of dementia. In these studies, subjects are followed longitudinally and incident cases of dementia are identified. Investigators then compare the baseline cognitive performance of these two groups of individuals to determine whether a certain profile of cognitive performance is predictive of who will develop dementia. Identifying certain patterns of performance that may be particularly diagnostic of future dementia status has important clinical implications. Persons may be identified relatively early in the disease process and appropriate behavioral or pharmacological therapies may be designed to best deal with the impending disease process. Further, supportive opportunities (e.g., support groups, day care arrangements) for family members can be developed in attempts to lessen the impact of the dementia on loved ones.

Several studies have investigated the relationship between baseline performance on global indices of cognitive functioning and dementia incidence (Aronson et al., 1990; Katzman et al., 1989; Yoshitake et al., 1995). These measures, such as the Mini-mental state examination (MMSE; Folstein, Folstein, & McHugh, 1975), the Mattis dementia rating scale (MDRS; Mattis, 1976), and the Blessed information-concentration test (BIMC; Blessed, Tomlinson, & Roth, 1968) are designed to index a person's global level of cognitive performance. In general, research indicates that individuals who initially score at low levels on these cognitive indices are more likely to develop dementia than the remaining study sample. For example, Aronson et al. (1990) examined this relationship with the BIMC and found baseline performance on this measure to be a strong predictor of dementia incidence (AD, VaD, and mixed dementia). Similar results were reported by Yoshitake et al. (1995), whereby baseline performance on a Japanese test of global cognitive functioning, Hasegawa's dementia scale, was predictive of subsequent development of AD.

Although some investigators have focused on measures of global cognitive functioning as predictors of dementia incidence, others have examined specific aspects of cognitive performance. In these studies, larger batteries of cognitive tests, comprised of indices assessing domains such as episodic memory, visuospatial functioning, and verbal ability were administered at baseline. Among the specific measures of performance that have been found to be related to dementia incidence, evidence has indicated that markers of verbal ability, including the Boston naming test and measures of category fluency (Jacobs et al., 1995; Masur, Sliwinski, Lipton, Blau, & Crystal, 1994) may predict dementia incidence. In addition, Masur et al. (1994) found the digit symbol subtest from the Wechsler adult intelligence scale-revised (WAIS-R; Wechsler, 1981) to be predictive of dementia incidence, whereas Jacobs et al. found another WAIS-R subtest, word similarities, to be significantly related to incidence of AD.

Although these indices of verbal ability (category fluency, Boston naming), speeded psychomotor skill (digit symbol), and abstract reasoning (word similarities) have been found to be predictive of dementia incidence, the most salient predictor of who will become afflicted with dementia is baseline episodic memory performance. Numerous studies have found that individuals who perform poorly on measures of recall and recognition are more likely to develop dementia after a follow-up interval than their superior-performing counterparts. For example, Masur and colleagues (Masur, Fuld, Blau, Crystal, & Aronson, 1990; Masur et al., 1994) have found the delayed recall measure from the Buschke selective reminding test to be an effective predictor of dementia incidence. Similar relationships have been reported with the Fuld object memory test (Fuld, Masur, Blau, Crystal, & Aronson, 1990; Masur et al., 1994), and the logical memory subtest of the Wechsler memory scale (Linn, et al., 1995).

Tierney et al. (1996) addressed the relative importance of different memory tasks in predicting incident cases of AD. They examined 123 memory-impaired patients and identified 29 probable AD patients after a two-year follow-up period. At baseline, all subjects completed a comprehensive neuropsychological battery including multiple indices of memory, verbal fluency, and psychomotor speed. The results of a logistic regression analysis, predicting AD status (yes/no), indicated that two tests (delayed recall from the Rey auditory verbal learning test and the mental control subtest of the WMS) were predictive of dementia incidence. Furthermore, these variables were fairly successful at correctly classifying the proportion of patients diagnosed with dementia (sensitivity 76%), as well as correctly identifying those who were free of dementia (specificity 94%). This resulted in an overall accuracy rate of the model of 89%. The additional measures of verbal fluency and psychomotor speed added little diagnostic accuracy in predicting which individuals would develop AD. Taken together, the results from this research indicate that episodic memory measures may be the most salient predictors of dementia incidence.

Although the relationship between episodic memory performance and dementia incidence is well established, it is also apparent that not all memory tasks are created equal. For example, tasks may differ in terms of the amount of cognitive support that is offered the individual (see Bäckman, Mäntylä, & Herlitz, 1990; Herlitz, Lipinska, & Bäckman, 1992, for reviews). Cognitive support refers to characteristics of memory tasks that make successful retrieval more or less likely. For example, free recall of unrelated words can be considered to be a task with relatively little cognitive support. This is due to the fact that the to-be-remembered items have little inherent organizability, and the recall condition offers no cues as to which items should be remembered. One can increase the level of cognitive support in this task by selecting words from several superordinate categories (e.g., articles of clothing, musical instruments). This change makes the task more supportive by supplying organizational structure to the materials. In this manner, the subject can arrange the words into their respective categories facilitating memory for these items (Bäckman & Wahlin, 1995). Cognitive support can also be manipulated at retrieval. Instead of the relatively impoverished retrieval conditions prevailing in free recall, a cued recall task may be given whereby the subject is prompted by word stems or category names in order to improve recall performance. In addition, a recognition task, in which subjects are asked to choose among target and distractor items, could be used to further increase the supportive nature of the retrieval task (Craik, 1983).

Several authors have suggested that the supportive nature of episodic memory tasks can influence the success of these tasks in detecting early cases of dementia. For example, Branconnier, Cole, Spera, and DeVitt (1982) found that tasks that are well supported (e.g., recognition) were the best discriminators between mild cases of dementia and normal aging. A possible reason for this finding is that many older adults, especially very old adults, may have deficits in cognitively demanding tasks such as free recall, whereas recognition and cued recall are relatively well preserved (Bäckman & Larsson, 1992; Craik & McDowd, 1987; Schonfield & Robertson, 1966). Thus, when deficits in the well-supported task are present, this may indicate conditions other than normal aging (e.g., dementia, depression).

The role of cognitive support in episodic memory tasks in predicting incidence of dementia has received less empirical attention. Although several studies have included multiple measures of episodic memory (e.g., Fuld et al., 1990; Masur et al., 1990), the lack of systematic variation among memory tasks has made firm conclusions regarding the relationship between cognitive support and dementia status difficult. Small, Herlitz, Fratiglioni, Almkvist, and Bäckman (1997) attempted to examine the issue of cognitive support in episodic memory and incidence of dementia by including multiple episodic memory tasks that varied in terms of a number of encoding and retrieval demands. Specifically, tasks were chosen that varied in terms of encoding demands (e.g., unrelated vs. organizable items), retrieval conditions (e.g., recall vs. recognition), as well as the nature of the materials that were examined (e.g., faces vs. words). In this study, 26 incident cases of AD were identified after a three-year follow-up interval, whereas 179 remained nondemented. In addition to the memory tasks, measures of visuospatial ability (block design, clock test, Poppelreuter's figures), verbal fluency (letter and category fluency), and primary memory (digit span) were included to examine the predictive relationship between these measures and incidence of AD.

Results from a logistic regression analysis indicated that three measures, recall of organizable words, face recognition, and letter fluency, were significant predictors of AD. Other less supported memory tasks (e.g., free recall of unrelated words), as well as other measures of visuospatial ability, category fluency, and primary memory were not predictive of dementia incidence. By examining the sensitivity and specificity of the model, it was determined that the two memory measures, organized word recall and face recognition, provided the greatest ability to detect who would become afflicted with AD (sensitivity 62%). On the other hand, although letter fluency added significantly to the logistic regression equation, its role was in improving the ability of the model to detect individuals who would remain nondemented (specificity 99%). Thus, among the predictors of dementia incidence, it was the two episodic memory tasks that were most effective at predicting incident cases of AD. In addition, the results of this study confirmed the hypothesis that more supported memory tasks (i.e., face recognition, recall of organizable words) rather than less supported tasks (e.g., recall of unrelated words) are most effective at predicting incident cases of AD.

In summary, the results from studies that have examined preclinical cognitive markers of dementia provide important information as to the changes that accompany the pathogenesis of AD. Specifically, tests of episodic memory performance appear to be the most powerful predictors of dementia incidence. On the one hand, recent research suggests that episodic memory tasks that are cognitively well supported are the best predictors of development of dementia. On the other hand, the results from all relevant studies have shown that markers of other abilities, including verbal and visuospatial skill, are less effective predictors of dementia incidence. Thus, it seems wise to include episodic memory tasks, and especially those that are well supported (e.g., recognition, recall of organizable words) when developing a predictive model for AD.

7.10.4 DETECTION OF DEMENTIA

In the previous section, we described the effectiveness of cognitive performance measures, especially those that index episodic memory functioning, in predicting who will become demented. In this section, we change our focus slightly in that it is not the development of dementia that we are interested in; rather, the issue of interest is the ability to differentiate between adults who are already mildly demented compared with nondemented adults. For the purpose of the present chapter, we are interested in whether those same measures of cognitive performance that are able to predict development of dementia would be effective at discriminating between nondemented adults and persons who are in an early phase of the disease.

Two main statistical methods have been used to differentiate normal old from AD individuals, namely the algorithm approach (e.g., Fuld, 1984) and the discriminant analysis approach (e.g., Storandt, Botwinick, Danziger, Berg, & Hughes, 1984). In the following, we will limit our review to the more commonly used discriminant analysis method. In this method, researchers have tried to determine the cognitive tasks or tests that best discriminate between normal old and mild AD patients. As is true with research attempting to delineate preclinical markers of AD, the uncertainties regarding dementia diagnoses are problematic for attempts to detect dementia. Thus, it may be that the differentiation between normal old adults and AD patients is based on a less than perfect "answer key," which also means that we do not get a fair evaluation of the discriminative power of the cognitive tests.

With this problem fresh in mind, we now turn to the results from studies investigating how well cognitive measures can discriminate between normal old adults and early AD patients. Most studies have found that tasks assessing episodic memory are particularly sensitive in detecting early dementia (e.g., Almkvist & Bäckman, 1993a; Herlitz et al., 1995; Storandt et al., 1984; Welsh, Butters, Hughes, Mohs, & Heyman, 1991, 1992). For example, in groups of AD patients and community volunteers, matched on age and education, Welsh et al. (1991) found that a measure of episodic memory, delayed word recall, correctly classified 96% of the control subjects and 86% of the patients. However, the authors of this study pointed out that the AD patients were compared with high-functioning control subjects, and that the results cannot be generalized to older adults in the community at large.

A study investigated the relative importance of episodic memory tasks and visuospatial tasks in the detection of dementia (Herlitz et al., 1995). Subjects were sampled from the general population in Stockholm, Sweden. Thus, all subjects were randomly sampled from the same population, and were generally older than subjects in other studies. In addition to standardized neuropsychological tests, the test battery included specialized measures derived from the experimental literature to examine various features of episodic memory. Three-hundred and ninety-eight normal older adults and 63 mildly demented individuals participated in this study. The group of mildly demented adults consisted of patients diagnosed with AD, VaD, mixed dementia (AD and VaD), Parkinson's disease, and alcohol dementia. Separate analysis was conducted for the AD group and the entire dementia group, but it was found that the results were similar irrespective of dementia etiology.

The results of this study demonstrated that it is possible to differentiate those with mild dementia from normal old adults using mainly measures of episodic memory. Of the five measures that contributed to the differentiation of dementia from normal aging, four were indicators of episodic memory and, specifically, measures of recognition and cued recall. Thus, in contrast to the Welsh et al. (1992) study, no free recall task was included in the function, but rather highly supportive measures of episodic memory. As with the research on dementia incidence, it was hypothesized that a possible reason for this result is that many nondemented older adults, especially those in advanced age, already have deficits in free recall (see Craik & Jennings, 1992, for a review), whereas recognition and cued recall may be relatively well preserved. In the Welsh et al. study (1992), subjects were recruited from a clinical population with healthy volunteers from the community. Thus, differences in cognitive ability between the nondemented subjects in Welsh et al. (1992) and those in Herlitz et al. (1995) may have contributed to the differences in results.

Although episodic memory tasks provide a good classification of normal old and mildly demented subjects, a number of subjects are misclassified by these measures. Correct classification rates, ranging from 92%–96% and 67%–89%, have been achieved for normal old and mildly demented subjects, respectively (Almkvist & Bäckman, 1993a; Herlitz et al., 1995; Welsh et al., 1991, 1992). Herlitz et al. (1995) found an overall classification rate of 90.7%, misclassifying 22 normal controls as demented and 21 demented subjects as normals. Further analysis showed that the misclassified normal controls were older and had lower MMSE scores than the correctly classified normal older adults. By contast, the group of mildly demented subjects that were misclassified as normal controls, were younger, had higher MMSE scores, and consisted of more males than the group of correctly classified mildly demented subjects.

In a later study, Herlitz, Small, Fratiglioni, Almkvist, and Bäckman (1997) were able to provide follow-up information regarding dementia incidence of the subjects that were incorrectly classified as demented, by reassessing all subjects three years after the initial examination. It was found that out of the 14 surviving subjects (eight subjects died from time 1 to time 2), 10 had developed AD. This suggests that the misclassification of normal old as demented, by the cognitive tests administered at time 1, was fairly accurate in selecting subjects who would eventually develop dementia. Hence, the majority of the misclassified subjects may not have been misclassified at the baseline assessment, but rather been in an early phase of dementia already at time 1.

The reasons for the classification of subjects, who had a clinical diagnosis of dementia at time 1 as nondemented, were different. At time 2, it was found, among the 15 surviving subjects, that two subjects had their diagnosis changed from demented to nondemented. Thus, these subjects had received, incorrectly, a clinical dementia diagnosis at time 1 that was later corrected. However, the majority of subjects in this group, of course, remained demented, and it is reasonable to assume that the cognitive tests were unable to discriminate between the group of correctly classified dementia patients and this group of subjects who, were younger, had a higher MMSE scores, and consisted of more males. Thus, it appears that the clinical diagnosis of dementia is easier in younger, male, and highly educated subjects than it is in older, female, and less educated persons. These results indicate that cognitive tests, and especially tests of episodic memory, are effective at detecting subjects in a very early stage of dementia who are easily missed in the clinical diagnosis due to confounding variables such as age, education, and gender. Yet, although cognitive tests may be useful in the preclinical detection of dementia, these tests may also miss a sizeable proportion of prevalent dementia cases due to insensitivity to the same demographic indices.

Taken together, the results on cognitive detection of dementia show that episodic memory measures are particularly effective at discriminating between normal old adults and AD patients. In addition, this line of research demonstrates that memory tasks may be effective in the detection of AD at a very early phase—a finding which is consistent with research conducted on the incidence of AD (e.g., Small et al., 1997; Tierney et al., 1996). In particular, results indicate that performance on highly supported tests of episodic memory performance are especially salient predictors of future cases of dementia, as well as good discriminators between normal elderly adults and those in mild stages of the disease process.

7.10.5 STAGING OF DEMENTIA

It is of considerable interest whether the same or different cognitive tasks are particularly useful in the detection and staging of AD, respectively. Similarities or differences with respect to this issue are relevant to the understanding of the progression of AD. On the one hand, if the same cognitive functions would be involved in both detection and staging of dementia, this would mean that decline in these functions would be linear across the pathogenesis and, ultimately, that some cognitive abilities are relatively well preserved throughout the disease. On the other hand, if different functions are involved in the detection and staging of dementia, it would imply that different cognitive abilities may decline at different times in the disease process and at different rates.

In studies investigating staging of AD, the most common method has been to use a global cognitive assessment instrument (e.g., the MMSE) as the criterion variable. There are, of course, problems related to this method, the most important being that the global assessment instrument used consists of a given set of cognitive tasks, which means that how well a certain set of cognitive test measures can stage dementia, by means of discriminant analysis, is dependent on how well they are correlated with the criterion measure. Only a few studies have investigated the ability of cognitive tests to stage dementia, that is, to separate mildly demented subjects from moderately demented subjects (Almkvist & Bäckman, 1993a; Herlitz et al., 1995; Hill, Storandt, & LaBarge, 1992; Welsh et al., 1992). These studies have found that, although episodic memory tasks are critical in detecting dementia, tasks drawing on verbal skills and visuospatial abilities are more effective at staging dementia. For example, Hill et al. (1992) used the clinical dementia rating scale (George et al., 1990) as the criterion variable, and found that tasks assessing verbal naming, visuospatial copying, and episodic recognition separated between mildly and moderately demented AD patients, with an overall correct classification rate of 86.2%. Almkvist and Bäckman (1993a) staged very mildly, mildly, and moderately demented patients, with the MMSE as the criterion variable. This study found that tasks assessing visuospatial ability, semantic memory, psychomotor speed, and episodic memory separated the three groups of patients with an overall correct classification rate of 64%.

Herlitz et al. (1995) also used the MMSE as the criterion variable and found an overall classification rate of 84.3% in the differentiation of mildly and moderately demented subjects. As in the corresponding analysis on detection of dementia, all analyses were done with the patient group consisting of either AD patients or a mixture of dementia subjects. However, such a division made little difference to the outcome. Four test measures were included in the discriminant function, a free recall task, backward digit span, block design (WAIS-R; Wechsler, 1981), and modified trail making A (Armitage, 1946). Thus, in contrast to the tasks involved in the detection of dementia, two of the tasks in the discriminant function were visuospatial in nature and one was a measure of primary memory. Only one of the tasks in the discriminant function was an episodic memory measure. These results suggest that visuospatial and primary memory abilities may deteriorate later and/or at a slower rate than episodic memory functions in the early stages of dementia (see also Almkvist & Bäckman, 1993b).

The results on staging of dementia are less consistent than are the studies on detection, probably because different criterion variables have been used across studies. In addition, comparatively little research has addressed the efficacy of cognitive measures in the staging of dementia, hence making firm conclusions difficult. However, the majority of studies addressing this issue indicate that episodic memory plays a less dominant role than other cognitive abilities in the differentiation between mildly and moderately demented patients. We contend that the most parsimonious interpretation of these results is that cognitive abilities such as visuospatial functioning, semantic memory, and primary memory deteriorate later and/or at a slower rate than episodic memory in the early stages of dementia.

7.10.6 PROGRESSION OF DEMENTIA

In addition to studies that have examined the cognitive performance of mildly to moderately demented adults through attempts to stage dementia severity, research has focused on longitudinal changes in cognitive performance in these patients. Ultimately, information regarding rates of change, and whether there is a differential nature of cognitive change at later stages of dementia severity can only be inferred from studies that have examined data from more than one time of measurement. Studies that have attempted to stage and detect dementia are hampered by the lack of longitudinal evidence when deriving cognitive profiles of disease progression. The studies that we review in this section are based on data from more than one measurement point.

Grady et al. (1988) examined changes in memory, attentional, verbal, and visuospatial functioning in a group of 11 AD patients. They noted that among all of the measures of cognitive performance, impaired episodic memory performance was the first sign of cognitive dysfunction in dementia. Further, these investigators reported that visuospatial functioning and verbal ability were among the last abilities to show deficits in their sample of AD patients. Similar results were reported by Almkvist and Bäckman (1993b). In this case, longitudinal changes in a range of cognitive functions in AD were examined over a two-year period. Almkvist and Bäckman found that episodic memory measures exhibited the least amount of decline over the retest interval, but when the estimated onset of decline was examined, these measures were the first to exhibit decline in AD. Moreover, visuospatial functioning, indexed by block design and object assembly from the WAIS-R, exhibited a moderate rate of decline over the retest interval but were among the last measures to decline in the sample of AD patients.

Additional evidence for verbal and visuospatial functioning declining at a later point in the disease process comes from a study by

Haxby et al. (1990). This study examined changes in cognitive functioning over a two-year follow-up period in a group of 11 mildly demented AD patients. Haxby and colleagues found that the impairment that dominated at the initial time of measurement were localized to tasks measuring memory and ability to sustain attention. However, "neuropsychological impairment in mildly impaired AD patients became more severe and widespread as the disease progressed" (Haxby et al., 1990, p. 757).

Small and Bäckman (1997) also examined longitudinal changes in episodic memory, visuospatial functioning, and verbal fluency in a group of 26 AD and 10 VaD patients. In this study, longitudinal changes were less pronounced in the episodic memory measures, whereas performance in the visuospatial and verbal domains exhibited dramatic negative changes. Further, the changes in performance varied minimally as a function of dementia type, indicating approximately equivalent declines in performance for both the AD and VaD patients.

Taken together, the results from longitudinal studies that have examined changes in cognitive performance of mildly demented persons suggest a differential pattern of change depending on what domain of cognitive functioning is being measured. Specifically, changes in episodic memory functioning of mildly demented adults are less pronounced, probably as a result of the bulk of the dementia-related declines having occurred already. Certainly, this hypothesis is supported by the fact that impairment of episodic memory may be seen in persons who will later develop dementia several years before a clinical diagnosis is possible (e.g., Jacobs et al., 1995; Linn et al., 1995; Tierney et al., 1996). On the other hand, visuospatial and verbal functioning exhibit stronger declines at later stages of the progression of the disease. The results from the longitudinal studies thus converge with those seen in cross-sectional research attempting to stage dementia severity through cognitive performance indices. In particular, measures of visuospatial and verbal abilities may be particularly effective in staging dementia, because these abilities tend to decline at a later stage of the dementing illness than episodic memory skills.

7.10.7 TRAJECTORY OF DECLINE

Although there is some evidence to suggest that not all cognitive abilities decline at the same time, there is additional evidence to suggest that the shape of the decline function may also vary as a function of dementia severity. Several authors have suggested that the cognitive changes accompanying dementia follow a nonlinear pattern. For example, Haxby et al. (1990) examined the cognitive performance of 16 AD patients. They noted that changes in the WAIS, MDRS, and MMSE followed a biphasic pattern of change, that is, there was an initial plateau of performance followed by a sharp linear decline in cognitive functioning.

Additional evidence for nonlinear changes in cognitive performance in dementia comes from research reported by Brooks and his colleagues (Brooks et al., 1993; Brooks & Yesavage, 1995). These investigators proposed a trilinear model of cognitive change in AD, in which the cognitive decline function in AD is conceptualized as a tripartite curve. According to this view, there is an initial period of stability before detectable decline, followed by a period of decline, and ending with a final period of relative stability. Longitudinal evidence from Helmes et al. (1995) demonstrates that performance on their scale of global cognitive functioning, the extended scale for dementia, follows a trilinear pattern of change in dementia patients much like Brooks et al. have postulated.

The possibility of a nonlinear pattern of cognitive change in dementia has several implications for the way in which we study progression of cognitive changes across the disease process. For example, the use of statistical methodologies that assume linear changes in performance (e.g., multiple regression, analysis of variance) may be inappropriate because of the nonlinear changes that are embedded in performance. Perhaps the greatest implication deals with the number of measurement occasions that we choose to follow our longitudinal samples for. Obviously, in order to describe nonlinear patterns of change, at least three measurement occasions are required. Brooks et al. (1993) suggested that in order to adequately describe the trilinear decline function in AD, five measurement occasions should be planned for. In addition, if we wish to examine the trilinear shape of changes in memory and other cognitive abilities, even more measurement points will need to be examined. Recall from our reviews of incidence, detection, staging, and longitudinal changes, that episodic memory functioning may be the first cognitive ability to decline in dementia, whereas other cognitive functions, such as verbal and visuospatial skill, appear to decline at a later stage. The differential onset of changes in individual cognitive measures implies that persons will be at different stages in the trilinear model depending on what domain of functioning is being indexed. For example, some individuals may be experiencing decline in episodic memory functioning, but be at the initial plateau stage of verbal ability because they are relatively early in the course of dementia. By contrast, other persons may be experiencing decline in verbal ability, but be at the later plateau stage in terms of episodic memory functioning. Furthermore, this argument assumes that performance in each domain of functioning follows a similar trilinear pattern of decline, with comparable duration in each part of the function. Because much of the work on non-linear change in dementia has focused on more global indices of cognitive functioning (e.g., Brooks et al., 1993; Helmes et al., 1995), rather than individual domains of performance, it is unclear whether every domain of cognitive function (e.g., verbal ability, visuospatial functioning) will follow a similar trajectory of decline. Clearly, although the results presented here are suggestive of nonlinear changes in the cognitive performance of demented adults, additional evidence is necessary before firm conclusions can be made regarding the onset, shape, and duration of the respective change functions.

7.10.8 PREDICTORS OF DEMENTIA-RELATED DIFFERENCES AND CHANGES

We have argued that the changes accompanying dementia are somewhat predictable. For example, on the one hand, we have marshalled evidence to indicate that declines in episodic memory performance are among the first signs of a dementing illness. Indices of verbal and visuospatial functioning, on the other hand, begin to deteriorate markedly only after the diagnosis of dementia has been made and proceed to decline with increasing severity of dementia. In this section, we look again at the ability to predict dementia-related differences and changes in cognitive performance. However, although our previous attempts to examine the cognitive transitions in dementia have focused on the temporal progression of the disease, we focus here on whether cognitive performance is predictable by different demographic, biological, and psychometric indices.

In research on normal aging, there is a great tradition of using individual-difference variables to predict age-related differences, and age-related changes, in cognitive functioning (see Hultsch & Dixon, 1990; Salthouse, 1991, for reviews). For example, a number of studies have found age-related differences being predicted by demographic characteristics such as age, gender, and education (e.g., Herlitz, Nilsson, & Bäckman, in press; Inouye, Albert, Mohs, Sun, & Berkman, 1993; Wiederholt et al., 1993). Similarly, other studies have focused on the ability of biological indices, such as general health or vitamin status, in predicting cognitive performance (e.g., Hultsch, Hammer, & Small, 1993; Wahlin, Hill, Winblad, & Bäckman, 1996). Finally, investigators have identified a number of basic information processing indices, including measures of processing speed (e.g., Salthouse, 1991) and working memory (e.g., Hultsch, Hertzog, & Dixon, 1990; Salthouse, 1991) as important predictors of cognitive performance among normal elderly adults.

Although the role of these types of individual-difference variables in predicting age-related differences and changes in performance is well documented in the normal aging literature, it is less clear whether these same classes of variables can predict dementia-related differences or dementia-related changes in cognitive performance. Using global performance indices as target variables, a number of factors have been found to be associated with a more rapid rate of progression, including early onset age (e.g., Burns, Jacoby, & Levy, 1991), language deficits (e.g., Boller, Becker, Holland, & Forbes, 1991), visuospatial deficits (e.g., Becker, Huff, Nebes, Holland, & Boller, 1988), and psychomotor slowing (e.g., Berg et al., 1984). However, other studies have found the relationship between these individual-difference predictors and cognitive progression to be equivocal (e.g., Almkvist & Bäckman, 1993b; Mortimer, Ebbit, Jun, & Finch, 1992).

Bäckman, Hill, Herlitz, Fratiglioni, and Winblad (1994) reported that the role of individual-difference variables in predicting performance on episodic memory tasks is substantially reduced in dementia. In this study, Bäckman et al.(1994) examined the relationship between a variety of subject-related variables corresponding to the demographic (e.g., age, education, onset age, activities of daily living), biological (ferritin, albumin, folic acid, fructoseamine/albumin, vitamin B12, and thyroid stimulating hormone), and psychometric (e.g., block design, digit span) domains and performance on two episodic memory factors, recall and recognition. They found that after controlling for differences in disease severity, only two predictors contributed to performance. In one case, a marker of fluid intelligence (block design) was positively related to performance on a factor of word recall, and in the other, age was negatively related to performance on a measure of word recognition. However, the relative paucity of individual-difference variables that could predict dementia-related differences in episodic memory functioning stands in contrast to the variety of such measures that were significant predictors of episodic memory performance in the sample that contained nondemented adults from the same study population (e.g., Bäckman & Wahlin, 1995; Hill, Wahlin, Winblad, & Backman, 1995; Wahlin et al., 1993). In a related study, Hill, Bäckman, Wahlin, and Winblad (1995) demonstrated evidence for a limited number of predictors being related to visuospatial performance in dementia, once severity of dementia was statistically controlled. Specifically, using Poppelreuter's figures, the clock test, and block design as criterion variables, only one relationship out of a total of 15 possible predictor variables was observed, namely that education was positively related to block design.

Using the study of Bäckman et al. (1994) as a guide, we recently investigated whether the relatively paucity of individual-difference predictors also held when changes in the cognitive performance of demented adults were examined (Small & Bäckman, 1997). In this study, using the same constellation of predictor variables, we sought to determine whether longitudinal changes in episodic memory, visuospatial functioning, and verbal fluency could be predicted by these indices. Results indicated that none of the demographic, biological, or psychometric indices of performance were significant predictors of change in any domain of cognitive functioning. We concluded that although the rate of cognitive deterioration in dementia is highly variable, this variability in change appears to generalize across a variety of demographic, psychometric, and biological characteristics. A possible reason for the lack of effects is that the role of individual-difference variables in cognitive functioning in dementia is overshadowed by the pathogenetic process itself. Specifically, much of the systematic variation in performance may be absorbed by the severity of the disease (as indexed by, for example, the MMSE), hence leaving little predictive power to other subject-related factors.

In summary, it appears that although the role of individual-difference variables in predicting cognitive performance of nondemented adults has a long and successful heritage, the importance of these same variables appears to be substantially reduced in dementia when contrasted against the severity of the disease itself.

7.10.9 CONCLUSIONS AND EXTENSIONS

In this chapter, we have seen that as individuals make the transition from normal aging to dementia, as well as the transition from milder to more severe stages of dementia, there is a relatively predictable pattern of cognitive changes. The results from studies that have examined incident cases of dementia (e.g., Small et al., 1997; Tierney et al., 1996) indicate that baseline measures of episodic memory performance are the best predictors of who will become demented. Similarly, results from studies that have attempted to discriminate between nondemented and mildly demented adults on the basis of cognitive performance measures suggest that episodic memory performance is an important factor in making these discriminations (e.g., Herlitz et al., 1995; Welsh et al., 1992). However, the predictive role of verbal ability, visuospatial functioning, and primary memory at these early stages of dementia is considerably smaller. It is only after the disease has progressed that visuospatial functioning, verbal ability, and primary memory begin to deteriorate markedly. This is evidenced in studies that have found these measures to be effective at staging disease progression (Herlitz et al., 1995; Hill et al., 1992; Welsh et al., 1992), as well as in studies that have assessed longitudinal changes directly (Almkvist & Bäckman, 1993b; Grady et al., 1988; Small & Bäckman, 1996).

Although we still lack a complete understanding of why the different domains of cognitive functioning follow such a pattern of deterioration, analyzing the trajectory of cognitive decline in light of the biological changes that accompany AD may provide useful information. Specifically, it may be argued that the differential change in cognitive functioning is consistent with models of the pathogenetic process in AD based on both neuropathological (Arrigada, Growdon, Hedley-White, & Hyman, 1992, Braak & Braak, 1991, 1995) and brain-imaging (Grady et al., 1988, 1990) data. For example, Braak and Braak contend that initial changes in the brain structures of AD patients occur in the medial temporal regions (e.g., the entorhinal cortex and the hippocampus) and, as the disease process advances, these changes radiate into neocortical structures. It is well known from research with amnesic patients that the hippocampal formation plays an important role in episodic remembering (e.g., Mayes, 1988; Squire, 1987). Recent brain activation research using positron emission tomography supports the view that episodic memory is heavily dependent on the integrity of the medial–temporal cortex (e.g., Grady et al., 1995; Nyberg, McIntosh, Houle, Nilaaon, & Tulving, 1996). It is also known that the neocortical association areas are particularly critical to performance across a variety of verbal and visuospatial tasks (e.g., Raichle et al., 1994; Ungerleider & Haxby, 1994). Thus, the pattern of dementia-related cognitive decline across the pathogenesis makes perfect sense in view of independent research addressing the biological basis of human cognition. From a somewhat different perspective, it may further be noted that episodic memory performance has been found to be an especially sensitive cognitive indicator of a variety of conditions, including herpes simplex encephalitis (Williams, Watts, Macleod, & Matthews, 1988), hypoxic damage (Hashtroudi, Parker, DeLisi, & Wyatt, 1983), toxic changes (Teitelbaum et al., 1990), depression (Bäckman & Forsell, 1994), alcohol intoxication (Nilsson, Bäckman, & Karlsson, 1989), and sleep deprivation (Polzella, 1975). Tulving (1993; see also Schacter & Moscovitch, 1984) has speculated that episodic memory evolved relatively late phylogenetically and develops relatively late ontogenetically relative to other forms of memory and cognitive functions. Thus, following Ribot's law (Ribot, 1882), it may perhaps be expected that episodic memory should be especially prone to brain insufficiencies such as dementia.

7.10.10 SUMMARY

In summary, although the evidence we have presented here was gathered from a variety of sources that often differed in terms of sample composition, dementia severity, and selection of the specific cognitive tests that were employed, a relatively predictable pattern of cognitive deterioration in dementia was identified. On the one hand, it appears that episodic memory is the first ability to deteriorate at or even before the dementia diagnosis is rendered. On the other hand, visuospatial and verbal functioning decline somewhat later in the disease process, and this is likely to reflect the fact that additional brain structures are being affected by the disease process. We hope that this chapter, with its insights into the pattern of cognitive deterioration in dementia, may generate some considerations in the clinical setting. For example, knowledge pertaining to which specific cognitive tasks that may be particularly sensitive in detecting very early dementia-related changes (e.g., highly supported episodic memory tasks) should be helpful in improving the accuracy of early clinical diagnoses. Although we currently lack effective pharmacological or behavioral intervention procedures for AD and related dementia disorders, such procedures may be developed in the years to come. If that were to be the case, it is conceivable that treatment efficacy would be greatest at the earliest possible phase in the disease process. In addition, even in the present situation, accurate diagnostic information early in the disease process may be useful for the patient, practitioners, and caregivers alike in order to adjust optimally to the impending disease process.

ACKNOWLEDGMENTS

Preparation of this chapter was supported by grants from the Swedish Council For Social Research, and the Swedish Council For Research in the Humanities and the Social Sciences.

7.10.11 REFERENCES

Almkvist, O. (1994). Neuropsychological deficits in vascular dementia in relation to Alzheimer's disease: Reviewing evidence for functional similarity or divergence. *Dementia, 5,* 203–209.

Almkvist, O., & Bäckman, L. (1993a). Detection and staging of early clinical dementia. *Acta Neurologica Scandinavica, 88,* 10-15.

Almkvist, O., & Bäckman, L. (1993b). Progression in Alzheimer's disease: Sequencing of neuropsychological decline. *International Journal of Geriatric Psychiatry, 8, 755–763.*

Almkvist, O., Bäckman, L., Basun, H., & Wahlund, L.-O. (1993). Patterns of neuropsychological performance in Alzheimer's disease and vascular dementia. *Cortex, 29,* 661–673.

American Psychiatric Association (1980). *Diagnostic and Statistical Manual of Mental Disorders* (3rd ed.). Washington, DC: Author.

American Psychiatric Association (1987). *Diagnostic and Statistical Manual of Mental Disorders* (3rd ed. rev.). Washington, DC: Author.

American Psychiatric Association (1994). *Diagnostic and Statistical Manual of Mental Disorders* (4th ed.). Washington, DC: Author.

Armitage, S. G. (1946). An analysis of certain psychological tests used for the evaluation of brain injury. *Psychological Monograph, 60, 1–48.*

Aronson, M. K., Ooi, W. L., Morgenstern, H., Hafner, A., Masur, D., Crystal, H., Frishman, W. H., Fisher, D., & Katzman, R. (1990). Women, myocardial infarction, and dementia in the very old. *Neurology, 40,* 1102–1106.

Arragada, P. V., Growdon, J. H., Hedley-White, E. T., & Hyman, B. T. (1992). Neurofibrillary tangles but not senile plaques parallel duration and severity of Alzheimer's disease. *Neurology, 42,* 631–639.

Bäckman, L. (Ed.) (1992). *Memory functioning in dementia.* Amsterdam: North-Holland.

Bäckman, L., & Forsell, Y. (1994). Episodic memory functioning in a community-based sample of old adults with major depression: Utilization of cognitive support. *Journal of Abnormal Psychology, 103,* 361–370.

Bäckman, L., Hill, R. D., Herlitz, A., Fratiglioni, L., & Winblad, B. (1994). Predicting episodic memory performance in dementia: Is severity all there is? *Psychology and Aging, 9,* 520–527.

Bäckman, L., & Larsson, M. (1992). Recall of organizable words and objects in adulthood: Influences of instructions, retention interval, and retrieval cues. *Journal of Gerontology: Psychological Sciences, 47,* P273–P278.

Bäckman, L., Mäntylä, T., & Herlitz, A. (1990). The optimization of episodic remembering in old age. In P. B. Baltes & M. M. Baltes (Eds.), *Successful aging: Perspectives from the behavioral sciences* (pp. 118–163). Cambridge, UK: Cambridge University Press.

Bäckman, L., & Wahlin, Å. (1995). Influences of item organizability and semantic retrieval cues on word recall in very old age. *Aging and Cognition, 2,* 312–325.

Becker, J. T., Huff, J. P., Nebes, R. D., Holland, A., & Boller, F. (1988). Neuropsychological function in Alzheimer's disease: Pattern of impariment and rates of progression. *Archives of Neurology, 45,* 263–268.

Berg, L., Danziger, W. L., Storandt, M., Coben, L. A., Gado, M., Hughes, C. P., Knesevich, J. W., & Botwinick, J. (1984). Predictive features in mild senile dementia of the Alzheimer type. *Neurology, 34,* 563–569.

Blessed, G., Tomlinson, B. E., & Roth, M. (1968). The association between quantitative measures of dementia and of senile changes in the cerebral grey matter of elderly subjects. *British Journal of Psychiatry, 114,* 797–811.

Braak, H., & Braak, E. (1991). Neuropathological staging of Alzheimer-related changes. *Acta Neuropathologica, 82, 239–259.*

Braak, H., & Braak, E. (1995). Staging of Alzheimer's disease-related neurofibrillary changes. *Neurobiology of Aging, 16, 271–284.*

Branconnier, R. J., Cole, J. O., Spera, K. F., & DeVitt, D. R. (1982). Recall and recognition as diagnostic indices of malignant memory loss in senile dementia: A Bayesian analysis. *Experimental Aging Research, 8,* 189–193.

Brayne, C., Gill, C., Huppert, F. A., Barkley, C., Gehlhaar, E., Girling, D. M., O'Connor, D. W., & Paykel, E. S. (1995). Incidence of clinically diagnosed subtypes of dementia in an elderly population: Cambridge Project for Later Life. *British Journal of Psychiatry, 167,* 255–262.

Brody, J. A., & Schneider, E. L. (1986). Disease and disorders of aging: A hypothesis. *Journal of Chronic Disorders, 39,* 871–876.

Brooks, J. O., Kraemer, H. C., Tanke, E. D., & Yesavage, J. A. (1993). The methodology of studying decline in Alzheimer's disease. *Journal of the American Geriatrics Society, 41,* 623–628.

Brooks, J. O., & Yesavage, J. A. (1995). Identification of fast and slow decliners in Alzheimer disease: A different approach. *Alzheimer Disease and Associated Disorders, 9*(Suppl. 1), S19–S25.

Burns, A., Jacoby, R., & Levy, R. (1991). Progression of cognitive impairment in Alzheimer's disease. *Journal of the American Geriatrics Society, 39,* 39–45.

Craik, F. I. M. (1983). On the transfer of information from temporary to permanent memory. *Philosophical Transactions of the Royal Society of London, B302,* 341–359.

Craik, F. I. M., & Jennings, J. M. (1992). Human memory. In F. I. M. Craik & T. A. Salthouse (Eds.), *The handbook of aging and cognition* (pp. 51–110). Hillsdale, NJ: Erlbaum.

Craik, F. I. M., & McDowd, J. (1987). Age differences in recall and recognition. *Journal of Experimental Psychology: Learning, Memory, and Cognition, 13,* 474–479.

Ebly, E. M., Parhad, I. M., Hogan, D. B., & Fung, T. S. (1994). Prevalence and types of dementia in the very old: Results from the Canadian Study of Health and Aging. *Neurology, 44,* 1593–1600.

Elias, M. F., Wolf, P. A., D'Agostino, R. B., Cobb, J., & White, L. R. (1993). Untreated blood pressure level is inversely related to cognitive functioning: The Framingham Study. *American Journal of Epidemiology, 138, 353–364.*

Erkinjuntti, T., Laaksonen, R., Sulkava, R., Syrjäläinen, R., & Palo, J. (1986). Neuropsychological differentiation between normal aging, Alzheimer's disease, and vascular dementia. *Acta Neurologica Scandinavica, 74,* 393–403.

Fewster, P. H., Griffin-Brooks, S., MacGregor, J., Ojalvo-Rose, E., & Ball, M. J. (1991). A topographical pathway by which histopathological lesions disseminate through the brain of patients with Alzheimer's disease. *Dementia, 2,* 121–132.

Folstein, M. F., Folstein, S. E., & McHugh, P. R. (1975). "Mini-mental state:" A practical method for grading the cognitive state of patients for the clinician. *Journal of Psychiatric Research, 12,* 189–198

Frackowiak, R. S. J., Pozzilli, C., Legg, N. J., Du Boulay, G. H., Marshall, J., Lenzi, G. L., & Jones, T. (1981). Regional cerebral oxygen supply and utilization in dementia: A clinical and physiological study with oxygen-15 and positron tomography. *Brain, 104,* 753–778.

Fratiglioni, L., Grut, M., Forsell, Y., Viitanen, M., & Winblad, B. (1992). Clinical diagnosis of Alzheimer's disease and other dementias in a population survey: Agreement and causes of disagreement in applying DSM-III-R criteria. *Archives of Neurology, 49,* 927–932.

Fries, J. F., & Crapo, L. M. (1981). *Vitality and aging: Implications of the rectangular curve.* New York: Freeman.

Fuld, P. A. (1984). Test profile of cholinergic dysfunction and of Alzheimer-type dementia. *Journal of Clinical Neuropsychology, 6,* 380–392.

Fuld, P. A., Masur, D. M., Blau, A. D., Crystal, H., & Aronson, M. K. (1990). Object-memory evaluation for prospective detection of dementia in normal functioning elderly: Predictive and normative data. *Journal of Clinical and Experimental Neuropsychology, 12,* 520–528.

Galasko, D., Hansen, L. A., Katzman, R., Wiederholt, W., Masliah, E., Terry, R., Hill, L. R., Lessin, P., & Thal, L. J. (1994). Clinical-neuropathological correlations in Alzheimer's disease and related dementias. *Archives of Neurology, 51,* 888–895.

George, A. E., deLeon, M. J., Stylopoulos, L. A., Miller, J., Kluger, A., Smith, G., & Miller, D. C. (1990). CT diagnostic features of Alzheimer disease: Importance of the choroidal/hippocampal fissure complex. *American Journal of Neuroradiology, 11,* 101–107.

Gottfries, J., Blennow, K., Wallin, A., & Gottfries, C. G. (1995). Diagnosis of dementias using partial least squares discriminant analysis. *Dementia, 6,* 83–88.

Grady, C. L., Haxby, J. V., Horwitz, B., Sundaram, M., Berg, G., Schapiro, M., Friedland, R. P., & Rapoport, S. I. (1988). Longitudinal study of the early neuropsychological and cerebral metabolic changes in dementia of the Alzheimer type. *Journal of Clinical and Experimental Neuropsychology, 10,* 576–596.

Grady, C. L., Haxby, J. V., Schapiro, M. B., Gonzales-Aviles, A., Kumar, A., Ball, M. J., Heston, L., & Rapaport, S. I. (1990). Subgroups in dementia of the Alzheimer type identified using positron emission tomography. *Journal of Neuropsychiatry and Clinical Neurosciences, 2,* 373–384.

Grady, C. L., McIntosh, A. R., Horwitz, B., Maisog, J. M., Ungerleider, L. G., Mentis, M. J., Pietrini, P., Schapiro, M. B., & Haxby, J. V. (1995). Age-related reductions in human recognition memory due to impaired encoding. *Science, 269,* 218–221.

Hashtroudi, S., Parker, E. S., DeLisi, L. E., & Wyatt, R. J. (1983). On elaboration and alcohol. *Journal of Verbal Learning and Verbal Behavior, 22,* 164–173.

Haxby, J. V., Grady, C. L., Koss, E., Horwitz, B., Heston, L., Schapiro, M., Friedland, R. P., & Rapoport, S. I. (1990). Longitudinal study of cerebral metabolic asymmetries and associated neuropsychological patterns in early dementia of the Alzheimer type. *Archives of Neurology, 47,* 753–760.

Helmes, E., Merskey, H., Fox, H., Fry, R. N., Bowler, J. V., & Hachinski, V. C. (1995). Patterns of deterioration in senile dementia of the Alzheimer type. *Archives of Neurology, 52,* 306–310.

Herlitz, A., Hill, R. D., Fratiglioni, L., & Bäckman, L. (1995). Episodic memory and visuospatial ability in detecting and staging dementia in a community-based sample of very old adults. *Journal of Gerontology: Medical Sciences, 50a,* M107–M113.

Herlitz, A., Lipinska, B., & Bäckman, L. (1992). Utilization of cognitive support for episodic remembering in Alzheimer's disease. In L. Bäckman (Ed.), *Memory functioning in dementia* (pp. 73–96). Amsterdam: North-Holland.

Herlitz, A., Nilsson, L.-G., & Bäckman, L. (in press). Gender differences in episodic memory. *Memory and Cognition*.

Herlitz, A., Small, B. J., Fratiglioni, L., Almkvist, O., & Bäckman, L. (1997). Detection of mild dementia in community surveys: Is it possible to increase the accuracy of our diagnostic instruments? *Archives of Neurology, 54,* 319–324

Hill, R. D., Bäckman, L., Wahlin, Å., & Winblad, B. (1995). Visuospatial performance in very old demented persons: An individual difference analysis. *Dementia, 6,* 49–54.

Hill, R. D., Storandt, M., & LaBarge, E. (1992). Psychometric discrimination of moderate senile dementia of the Alzheimer type. *Archives of Neurology, 49,* 377–380.

Hill, R. D., Wahlin, Å., Winblad, B., & Bäckman, L. (1995). The role of demographic and life style variables in utilizing cognitive support for episodic remembering among very old adults. *Journal of Gerontology: Psychological Sciences, 50b,* P219–P227.

Hultsch, D. F., & Dixon, R. A. (1990). Learning and memory in aging. In J. E. Birren & K. W. Schaie (Eds.), *Handbook of the psychology of aging* (3rd ed., pp. 258–274). San Diego, CA: Academic Press.

Hultsch, D. F., Hammer, M., & Small, B. J. (1993). Age differences in cognitive performance in later life: Relationships to self-reported health and activity life style. *Journal of Gerontology: Psychological Sciences, 48,* P1–P11.

Hultsch, D. F., Hertzog, C., & Dixon, R. A. (1990). Ability correlates of memory performance in adulthood and aging. *Psychology and Aging, 5,* 356–368.

Huppert, F. A., Brayne, C., & O'Connor, D. W. (1994). *Dementia and normal aging*. Cambridge, UK: Cambridge University Press.

Inouye, S. K., Albert, M. S., Mohs, R., Sun, K., & Berkman, L. F. (1993). Cognitive performance in a high-functioning community-dwelling elderly population. *Journal of Gerontology: Medical Sciences, 48,* 146–151.

Jacobs, D. M., Sano, M., Dooneief, G., Marder, K., Bell, K. L., & Stern, Y. (1995). Neuropsychological detection and characterization of preclinical Alzheimer's disease. *Neurology, 45,* 957–962.

Katzman, R., Aronson, M., Fuld, P., Kawas, C., Brown, T., Morgenstern, H., Frishman, W., Gidez, L., Eder, H., & Ooi, W. L. (1989). Development of dementing illnesses in an 80-year-old volunteer cohort. *Annals of Neurology, 25,* 317–324.

Linn, R. T., Wolf, P. A., Bachman, D. L., Knoefel, J. E., Cobb, J. L., Belanger, A. J., Kaplan, E. F., & D'Agostino, R. B. (1995). The 'preclinical phase' of probable Alzheimer's disease: A 13-year prospective study of the Framingham cohort. *Archives of Neurology, 52,* 485–490.

Masur, D. M., Fuld, P. A., Blau, A. D., Crystal, H., & Aronson, M. K. (1990). Predicting development of dementia in the elderly with the Selective Reminding test. *Journal of Clinical and Experimental Neuropsychology, 12,* 529–538.

Masur, D. M., Sliwinski, M., Lipton, R. B., Blau, A. D., & Crystal, H. A. (1994). Neuropsychological prediction of dementia and the absence of dementia in healthy elderly persons. *Neurology, 44,* 1427–1432.

Mattis, S. (1976). Mental status examination for organic mental syndromes in the elderly patient. In L. Bellack & T. B. Kanasu (Eds.), *Geriatric psychiatry*. New York: Grune & Strattan.

Mayes, A. R. (1988). *Human organic memory disorders*. New York: Cambridge University Press.

McKhann, G., Drachman, D., Folstein, M., Katzman, R., Price, D., & Stadlan, E. M. (1984). Clinical diagnosis of Alzheimer's disease: Report of the NINCDS-ADRDA Work Group under the auspices of the Department of Health and Human Service Task Force on Alzheimer's Disease. *Neurology, 34,* 939–944.

Morris, R. G. (Ed.) (1996). *The neuropsychology of Alzheimer's disease*. Oxford: Oxford University Press.

Mortimer, J. A., Ebbit, B., Jun, S. P., & Finch, M. D. (1992). Predictors of cognitive and functional progression in patients with probable Alzheimer's disease. *Neurology, 42,* 1689–1696.

Nebes, R. D. (1992). Cognitive dysfunction in Alzheimer's disease. In F. I. M. Craik & T. A. Salthouse (Eds.), *The Handbook of aging and cognition* (pp. 373–446). Hillsdale, NJ: Erlbaum.

Nilsson, L.-G., Bäckman, L., & Karlsson, T. (1989). Priming and cued recall in elderly, alcohol intoxicated and sleep deprived subjects: A case of functionally similar memory deficits. *Psychological Medicine, 19,* 423–433.

Nyberg, L., McIntosh, A. R., Houle, S., Nilsson, L. G., & Tulving, E. (1996). Activation of medial temporal structures during episodic memory retrieval. *Nature, 380,* 715–717.

Polzella, D. J. (1975). Effects of sleep deprivation on short-term recognition memory. *Journal of Experimental Psychology: Human Learning and Memory, 104,* 194–200.

Raichle, M. E., Fiez, J. A., Videen, T. O., MacLeod, A. M. K., Pardo, J. V., Fox, P. T., & Petersen, S. E. (1994). Practice-related changes in human brain functional anatomy during non-motor learning. *Cerebral Cortex, 4,* 8–26.

Ribot, T. (1882). *Diseases of memory*. New York: Appleton.

Salthouse, T. A. (1991). *Theoretical perspectives on cognitive aging*. Hillsdale, NJ: Lawrence Erlbaum.

Schacter, D. L., & Moscovitch, M. (1984). Infants, amnesics, and dissociable memory systems. In M. Moscovitch (Ed.), *Infant memory* (pp. 173–216). New York: Plenum.

Schonfield, D., & Robertson, B. A. (1966). Memory storage and aging. *Canadian Journal of Psychology, 20,* 228–236.

Small, B. J., & Bäckman, L. (1997). *Predictors of longitudinal changes in memory, visuospatial, and verbal functioning in very old demented adults*. Manuscript submitted for publication.

Small, B. J., Herlitz, A., Fratiglioni, L., Almkvist, O., & Bäckman, L. (1997). Cognitive predictors of incident Alzheimer's disease: A prospective longitudinal study. *Neuropsychology, 11,* 413–420.

Squire, L. R. (1987). *Memory and brain*. New York: Oxford University Press.

Storandt, M., Botwinick, J., Danziger, W. L., Berg, L., & Hughes, C. P. (1984). Psychometric differentiation of mild senile dementia of the Alzheimer type. *Archives of Neurology, 41,* 497–499.

Storandt, M., & Hill, R. D. (1989). Very mild senile dementia of the Alzheimer type: II. Psychometric test performance. *Archives of Neurology, 46,* 383–386.

Teitelbaum, J. S., Zatorre, R. J., Carpenter, S., Gendron, D., Evans, A. C., Gjedde, A., & Cashman, N. R. (1990). Neurologic sequelae of domoic acid intoxication due to the ingestion of contaminated mussels. *New England Journal of Medicine, 322,* 1781–1787.

Tierney, M. C., Szalai, J. P., Snow, W. G., Fisher, R. H., Nores, A., Nadon, G., Dunn, E., & St. George-Hyslop, P. H. (1996). Prediction of probable Alzheimer's disease in memory-impaired patients: A prospective

longitudinal study. *Neurology, 46,* 661–665.
Tulving, E. (1993). Human memory. In P. Anderson, O. Hvalby, O. Paulsen, & B. Hökfelt (Eds.), *Memory concepts: Basic and clinical aspects* (pp. 27–46). Amsterdam: Elsevier.
Ungerleider, L. G., & Haxby, J. V. (1994). 'What' and 'where' in the human brain. *Current Opinions in Neurobiology, 4,* 157–165.
Wahlin, Å., Bäckman, L., Mäntylä, T., Herlitz, A., Viitanen, M., & Winblad, B. (1993). Prior knowledge and face recognition in a community-based sample of healthy, very old adults. *Journal of Gerontology: Psychological Sciences, 48,* 54–61.
Wahlin, Å., Hill, R. D., Winblad, B., & Bäckman, L. (1996). Effects of serum vitamin B12 and folate status on episodic memory performance in very old age: A population-based study. *Psychology and Aging, 11,* 487–496
Wechsler, D. (1981). *Wechsler Adult Intelligence Scale Revised: Manual.* New York: The Psychological Corporation.
Welsh, K., Butters, N., Hughes, J., Mohs, R., & Heyman, A. (1991). Detection of abnormal memory decline in mild cases of Alzheimer's disease using CERAD neuropsychological measures. *Archives of Neurology, 48,* 278–81.
Welsh, K., Butters, N., Hughes, J., Mohs, R., & Heyman, A. (1992). Detection and staging of dementia in Alzheimer's disease: Use of the neuropsychological measures developed for the Consortium to Establish a Registry for Alzheimer's disease. *Archives of Neurology, 49,* 448–452.
West, R. L., Crook, T. H., & Barron, K. L. (1992). Everyday memory performance across the life span: Effects of age and noncognitive individual differences. *Psychology and Aging, 7,* 72–82.
Wiederholt, W. C., Cahn, D., Butters, N. M., Salmon, D. P., Krtiz-Silverstein, D., & Barrett-Connor, E. (1993). Effects of age, gender and education on selected neuropsychological tests in an elderly community cohort. *Journal of the American Geriatrics Society, 41,* 639–647.
Williams, J. M. G., Watts, F. N., MacLeod, C., & Matthews, A. (1988). *Cognitive psychology and emotional disorders.* New York: Wiley.
Yoshitake, T., Kiyohara, Y., Kato, I., Ohmura, T., Iwamoto, H., Nakayama, K., Ohmori, S., Nomiyama, K., Kawano, H., Ueda, K., Sueishi, K., Tsuneyoshi, M., & Fujishima, M. (1995). Incidence and risk factors of vascular dementia and Alzheimer's disease in a defined elderly Japanese population: The Hisayama Study. *Neurology, 45,* 1161–1168.

7.11
Suicidal Behavior in Late Life

JANE L. PEARSON
National Institute of Mental Health, Rockville, MD, USA

7.11.1 INTRODUCTION

The research and clinical treatment of suicidal persons among any age group presents enormous challenges. One aspect of those challenges is to consider the influence of how societies view and tolerate suicidal behavior among their members. Stillion and McDowell (1996) have provided an historical overview of how suicide has been viewed in the Western world. Views on suicidal acts have ranged from Socrates' description of "honorable exits" in 399 BC to the Council of Toledo's declaration that instituted excommunication for the deceased suicide victim or attempter in AD 693. The recent US public health perspective (*Healthy People 2000*, 1991), which began in the 1960s (Shneidman, Farberow, & Litman, 1961), views suicide as an outcome of intolerable psychological distress and inadequately treated mental disorders. This more recent perspective, however, is not unanimously held in the USA. The Hemlock Society (Humphry, 1991, 1992) and a recent ruling by the 9th US District Circuit Court of Appeals (Compassion in Dying vs. State of Washington, 1996) consider suicide a right of individuals. Moreover, many persons hold the view that some persons have more of a right to this act than others; suicide in youth is still considered a tragedy relative to suicides by older, disabled, and less healthy persons (Marks, 1988–1989).

This perception, along with the higher percentage of media coverage devoted to suicides among young and middle-aged persons relative to the elderly could be interpreted as higher rates among youthful groups. However, in 1993 the suicide rate in the USA for persons age 85 and older was twice the rate than persons age 15–19 (10.9 per 100 000 compared to 22.8 per 100 000). If we consider the rates for white males, the highest risk group in the USA, the ratio is more than tripled: adolescents age 15–19 have a rate of 18.5 per 100 000, and older adults age 85+ have a rate of 73.6 per 100 000. This latter rate is over six times the rate of all age-adjusted suicides (National Center for Health Statistics, 1996).

In addition to agist views that consider an older life less valued than a young life, psychological research and clinical interest in elderly suicide may have been limited due to the fact that psychologists (as well as other mental health professionals) rarely see older patients who are suicidal. Generally speaking, older persons with mental disorders rarely seek help from mental health professionals, preferring to visit their primary care physician instead (German, Shapiro, & Skinner, 1985). In addition, psychologists may be less likely to see suicidal patients than psychiatrists: psychologists have a one-in-five chance, and psychiatrists a one-in-two chance of losing a patient to suicide during their careers (Chemtob, Hamada, Bauer, Kinney, & Torigoe, 1988; Chemtob, Hamada, Bauer, Torigoe, & Kinney, 1988). However, as depression is better recognized and effective treatments for depression are increasingly applied to the elderly population (NIH Consensus Development Panel, 1992), as more older persons receive mental health treatment, and as more psychologists become specialists in treating elderly patients (Niederehe, Cooley, & Teri, 1995), the probability that psychologists will encounter suicidal older adults will inevitably increase.

It is hoped that this review will highlight the incompleteness of our current understanding of late life suicide, and make apparent the need for more psychological research on this tragedy. In particular, the epidemiology and putative "risk factors" for completed suicides, and suicide completers' interface with the health system, are surveyed. Also reviewed are studies on elderly attempters, and research on the bioethical issues involved in assisted suicides. Suggestions for further research, including the consideration of possible subgroups at risk, and recommended clinical resources, are also discussed.

7.11.2 SOURCES OF DATA FOR STUDIES OF SUICIDAL BEHAVIOR IN THE ELDERLY

7.11.2.1 Mortality Data

The US national data on gender, age, race, marital status, and method of death characteristics of completed suicides are based on vital statistics information gathered by the Center for Disease Control and Prevention's National Center for Health Statistics. The source of this information is derived from death certificates that come from each state, each state being responsible for its own vital registry system. In addition to the variation by state policies, the qualifications for the coroner, medical examiner, or others responsible for completing death certificates also varies widely. The person may be an elected or appointed layman, lawyer, sheriff, mortician, general practitioner, or forensic pathologist. It is generally agreed that what systematic error exists, it will be toward conservative estimates: there are more "missed" suicide deaths than deaths of other causes miscounted as suicides (see O'Carroll, 1989 for a review). Clark (1992) has suggested that these undercounts are probably around 5%. Despite these sources of variation, mortality data has been used in epidemiologic methods to measure the magnitude of suicide as a public health problem, and assess the effects of public health policies (Healthy People 2000, 1991).

7.11.2.2 Community Studies Using the Psychological Autopsy Method

Although determining the cause of death in suspected suicides usually requires forensic work, such as in-depth interviews with the victims' associates, these efforts are not routinely recorded and available for research use. Therefore, although information such as recent life events, history of hospitalizations, or mental state of the person prior to the suicide may have been assessed, it is not systematically recorded at a state or national level. The psychological autopsy (PA) method was developed to integrate such information in order to achieve a better understanding of the psychological circumstances contributing to a death, and has been applied to a number of communities and populations. Clark and Horton-Deutsch (1992) describe the evolution of this method since the 1930s. As used today, the PA constructs a detailed picture of the victim's psychological state prior to death, including psychiatric symptomatology, behavior, and life circumstances in the weeks or months before death. The gathering of this information includes interviewing knowledgeable informants, reviewing available clinical records, and comprehensive case formulation by one or more mental health professional with expertise in postmortem studies (Beskow, Runeson & Asgard, 1990; Clark & Horton-Deutch, 1992). Clark and Horton-Deutch outline 12 standards for using this method in suicide research.

The application of the PA to suicides among the elderly has been slow in coming, due to the belief that older suicide victims are socially isolated from both formal and informal contacts and therefore there would be few knowledgeable informants to obtain data from. To the contrary, Younger, Clark, Oehmig-Lindroth, and Stein, (1990) described ample numbers of informants available: In Cook County, Illinois, 70% of elderly suicides were married; 90% had one knowledgeable informant and 50% had two informants. Several studies have further demonstrated that the PA method can be applied to elderly suicides: Conwell and Brent (1995) have reviewed a number of PA studies that compare younger and older adults. It is important to note that few psychological autopsy studies in general, and none that are focused on elderly suicides, have yet included appropriate case-controls that would maximize the benefits of this methodology.

7.11.2.3 Clinical Follow-up Studies

As will be discussed below, the majority of suicide victims have some sort of mental disorder. Among the elderly, first episode, unipolar depression is the predominating disorder among completed suicides (Conwell, 1994). A relatively efficient approach to obtaining data on suicides is to follow-up persons most at risk; those with depressive disorders. This has been most frequently conducted through retrospective cohort studies. In addition to the challenge of tracking of persons after treatment, this method also relies on medical records that are notoriously variable in accuracy and completeness. Although this approach has been used to examine suicides among young adult and middle-aged persons, few studies have examined what characteristics, in addition to clinical treatment for depression, place the elderly at risk for suicide. Of the studies that have considered "elderly" persons (those 50 and older), some have suggested that delusional depression is a risk factor, where other have not found this type of depression to be related to increased risk for later suicide (Coryell & Tsuang, 1982; Robinson & Spiker, 1985; Roose, Glassman, Walsh, Woodring, & Vital-Herre, 1983). When specific age groups such as the elderly are examined in these retrospective studies, limited sample sizes and variable follow-up periods often limit both the power to reliably discern risk rates and generalizability to other clinic populations.

Since the elderly are less likely to seek or obtain mental health services:(German et al., 1985), the biases in this approach are likely to favor the documentation of those more likely to see mental health services: women (Kessler, Brown & Broman, 1981; Nathanson, 1977), those with more severe depression, comorbid personality disorder, and persons who have used an overdose method (Lindesay, 1986; Vieta, Nieto, Gastó, & Cirera, 1992). Although it is important to study these biased samples in order to understand what are safe and effective treatments in such service contexts, they minimally overlap with community samples described by epidemiologic and PA methods: Characteristics of the later life suicides in epidemiologic populations and community samples include men, those with late onset, unipolar depression, persons unlikely to have received mental health care, and those who have used a firearm as a suicide method.

7.11.2.4 Suicide Attempter Studies

The PA approach, although providing a wealth of information, is most vulnerable to the retrospective reports of informants who may be biased by knowledge of the type of death of the subject of the inquiry. The PA method is also limited with regard to providing information on the subject's private self-perceptions, coping, or cognitive distortions. Such data can be obtained by interviewing persons who have survived a suicide attempt. However, attempters and completers have been described as distinct but overlapping populations (Linehan, 1986). Among younger groups, the ratio of attempts to completions is high, indicating that many more persons attempt than complete suicide, with variability in the intention for completion (Meehan, Lamb, Saltzman, & O'Carroll, 1992). In addition, women outnumber men in suicide attempts, but men exceed women in suicide completions in the general population both in the USA and the UK (Barraclough, Bunch, Nelson, & Sainsbury, 1974; Mościcki et al.,1988).

Among the elderly, however, the ratio of attempts to completions is estimated to be around 4:1 (Stenback, 1980). This has been interpreted to suggest that the elderly who attempt are more intent on completing suicide, and therefore may be more similar to completers than younger populations (Frierson, 1991; Merrill & Owens, 1990). In addition, previous studies of elderly suicide attempters find higher rates of later suicide completions relative to younger groups (Gardner, Bahn, & Mack, 1964; Kreitman, 1976a; Mościcki, 1995; O'Neal, Robins, & Schmidt, 1956). Because elderly attempters may be very similar to completers, and because studying attempters may offer valuable insight into the risk factors for late life suicide, this method would seem to be among the more promising methods to pursue to increase our knowledge about risk factors for completed suicide. In addition, elderly suicide attempters are an important group to study due to the significant morbidity and mortality that follows an attempt.

7.11.3 EPIDEMIOLOGY OF SUICIDAL BEHAVIOR IN LATE LIFE

7.11.3.1 Suicide Completions

7.11.3.1.1 Age, gender, and race

In the USA, like most other industrialized nations, the most consistent demographic factors associated with risk for suicide are older age and male gender (McIntosh, Santos, Hubbard, & Overholser, 1994; Mościcki, 1995; Pearson & Conwell, 1995). In the USA, older white males have by far the highest rate, followed by African-American men of all adult years. White females have the third highest rate among older persons, and African-American women having the lowest rate. Figure 1 illustrates these differences in rates.

A US Center for Disease Control and Prevention report declared that elderly suicides rates were on the increase (Suicide Among Older Persons, 1996). Fluctuations in suicide rates, such as these, have been the subject of cohort and period effect studies since the mid 1970s. Manton, Blazer and Woodbury (1987) examined age, period, and cohort effects separately on middle age and later life suicides; they concluded that when age and period effects were controlled, cohorts born before World War I and persons born after World War II (baby boomers) were at most risk relative to cohorts born between the World Wars. Murphy and Wetzel (1980), examining US rates from 1949 to 1974 by birth cohort, concluded that with more recent cohorts, rates were rising, regardless of race or gender, and raised an alarm that suicide rates would continue to increase in the USA unless major public health efforts were employed. Furthermore, given that the absolute numbers of the elderly will be increasing as the baby boomers age, the absolute numbers of suicides have been predicted to increase (Conwell, 1994).

However, Newman and Dyck (1988) proposed that the many national trends for "cohort effects" of increasing suicide rates could also be explained by period effects that may or may not be long-lasting. More recently, Fombonne (1994), in considering the evidence for increasing rates of depression and suicide, raised several issues that make it difficult to clearly conclude when changes in rates reflect cohort, period or age effects. These include the interaction among cohort, age and period, and the instability of effects due to selected age groupings. In studies of suicide rates, "the elderly" are often those considered age 65 and older (e.g., Kaplan, Adamek, & Johnson, 1994; McCall, 1991), but within this large age span, some age groups have shown more fluctuation or steeper rises in rates. White males age 65–69 had a suicide rate in 1980 of 30 per 100 000, and a 1993 rate of 27.8 per 100 000, which is a very slight decrease. In contrast, white males age 85 and older had a rate of 52.8 in 1980 but a rate of 73.6 in 1993, a very significant increase (National Center for Health Statistics, 1996). McCall and Land (1994) attempted to account for the increases in older suicides with social structural factors such as social security, cohort size, and widowhood. Although there was some evidence

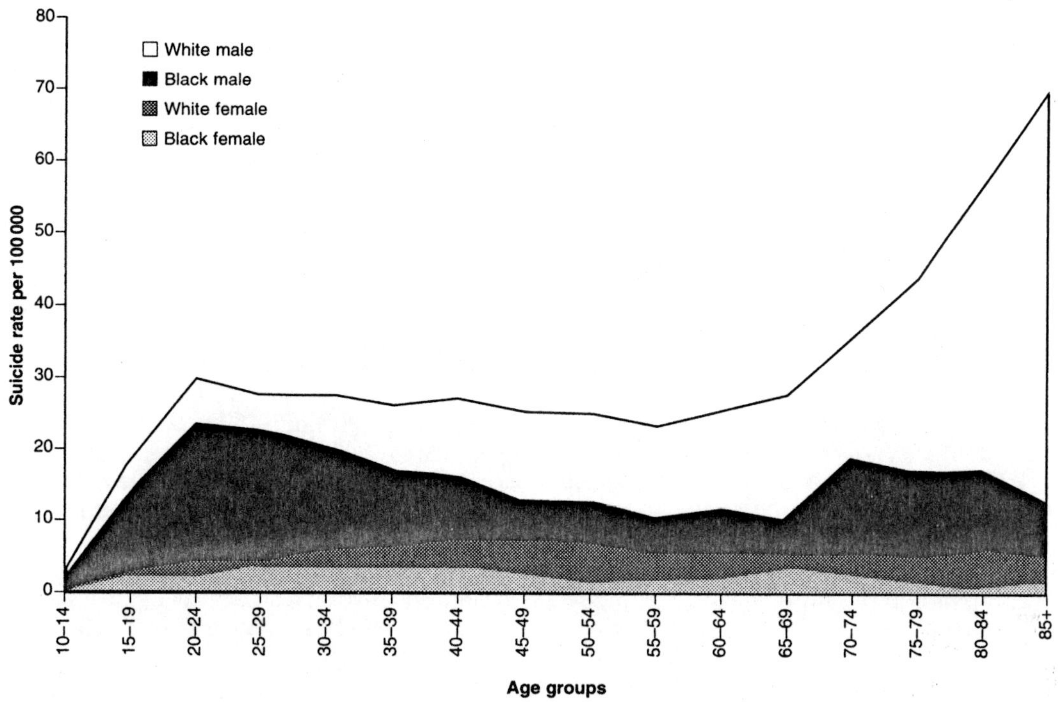

Figure 1 US suicide rates by age, gender, and racial groups, 1995. Source: National Institute of Mental Health, 1997. Data are from the Center for Disease Control and Prevention, National Center for Health Statistics.

for these factors being related to elderly suicides among the "young old" (ages 65–74), they found that none of the factors were related to suicides among the oldest old (ages 75 and older).

7.11.3.1.2 Marital status

In 1992, the rate for divorced and widowed men age 65 and older was 76.4 per 100 000. This was 2.7 times the rate for married men, and 1.4 times the rate for never-married men of this large age group (Suicide Among Older Persons, 1996). In a study comparing older widowed men and women, Li (1995) also reported that the risk of suicide for widowed men was three times greater than for widowed women over a 12 year period in a Maryland county sample. Buda and Tsuang (1990), using 1985 national statistics, reported age differences in specific rates for widowed and divorced males. Up to age 54, males who were widowed had higher rates than divorced males, but beginning with the age 55 group and higher, males who were divorced had higher rates of suicide compared to widowed males. Cohler and Jenuwine (1995) have considered the effects of age and marital status from a life course perspective. As an "off time" event, widowhood is less expected in earlier stages of life and therefore may be more stressful. This may be especially the case for men, where higher mortality rates occur during widowhood for younger men compared to younger women (Kaprio, Koskenvuo, & Rita, 1987), including suicide.

The higher rates of divorce among older men who suicided may reflect long-term family conflict or lack of supportive family interactions which increase risk for suicide. Indeed, family conflicts have been reported to play a role in elderly suicide attempts (Draper, 1994; Schmid, Manjee, & Shah, 1994; Zweig & Hinrichsen, 1993). These studies, along with the patterns of marital status and completed late life suicide rates highlight the need for more focused study on family process factors that may affect older persons' risk for suicidal behavior.

7.11.3.1.3 Methods of suicide

Death by firearms is the most common suicide method in the USA, and the elderly are more likely than any other age group to commit suicide with firearms (Kachur, Potter, James, & Powell, 1995; Kaplan et al., 1994; Meehan, Saltzman, & Sattin, 1991). Figure 2 illustrates the rate of suicides by method and by five-year age groups for 1992. Elderly males (those 65 and older) showed the most proportional increase in the use of firearms as a method of suicide from 1979 to 1992 (Kaplan et al., 1994; Meehan, et al., 1991; Suicide Among Older Persons, 1996).

Kaplan, Adamek, and Geling (1996) examined sociodemographic correlates of firearm use in white elderly male suicides from 1989 to 1991. Consistent with gun ownership patterns (Davis & Smith, 1989–1991), they found that nonmetropolitan residents and men with less than high school education were more likely to use firearms. With regard to marital status, single, never married, males were somewhat less likely than married, widowed, or divorced men to use firearms as a method.

Because efforts to reduce availability of methods of suicide have been reported to result in fewer deaths by suicide (Kreitman, 1976b; Nowers & Irish, 1988), it would seem logical that limiting access to firearms would reduce the rate of elderly suicide (Kaplan et al., 1996). For example, Dennis and Lindesay (1995) describe how a combination of limiting suicide methods on several fronts may have served to reduce elderly suicide rates in the UK. The detoxification of coal gas in the early 1960s was linked to a pronounced and prolonged drop in elderly suicides rates (Kreitman, 1976b), and restriction of prescribed barbiturates has also been associated with fewer deaths by self-poisoning in the elderly (Nowers & Irish). The introduction of exhaust emission laws led to a reduction of suicides by this method in the USA and abroad (Clarke & Lester, 1987).

Studies on the effects of reduced access to handguns and firearms have focused mainly on younger suicides. The degree to which such limitations have had significant effects remains controversial (Rich, Young, Fowler, Wagner, & Black, 1990), where rates of other methods (e.g., hanging) have been found to rise when guns (primarily handguns) are restricted. Sloan and his associates compared suicide rates between King County (Seattle) with the city of Vancouver BC, where the former has fewer restrictions on handgun ownership (Sloan, Rivara, Reay, Ferris, & Kellermann, 1990). Although persons aged 15 to 24 had higher rates of suicide by handguns in King County, the rate of death by firearms among middle-aged and elderly persons (age 45+) was virtually the same in these two communities. There has been no test of the limitations of firearms and its association with decreased suicides by firearms specifically among the elderly.

7.11.3.2 Suicide Attempts among the Elderly

Few epidemiologic studies have focused on the rates of suicide attempts in the elderly. Using data from the National Institute of

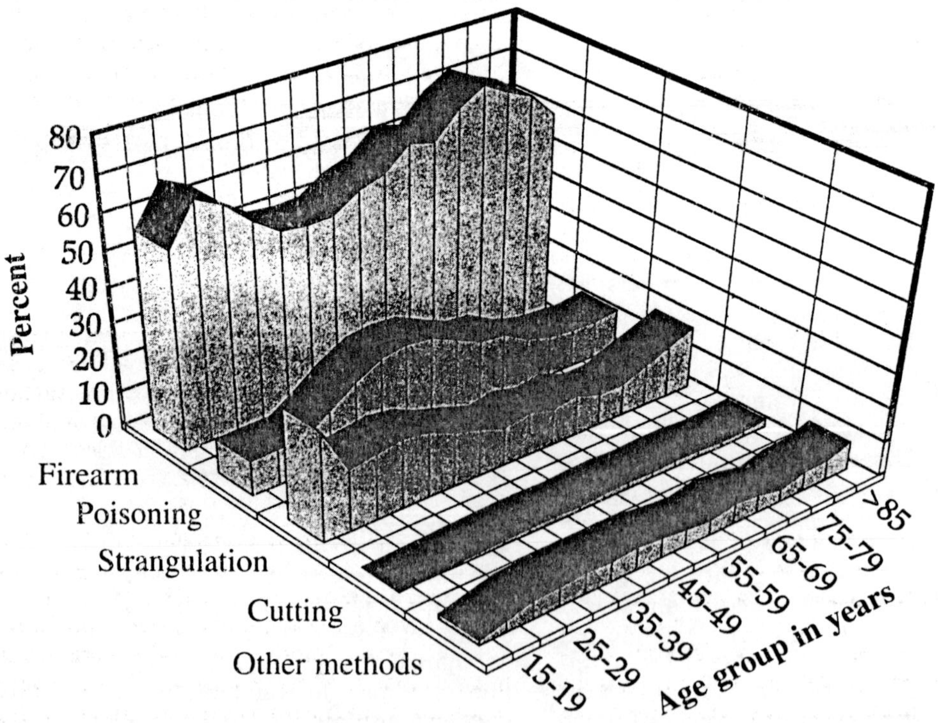

Figure 2 Percentage of suicides by age and method for 1992. From Kachur et al. (1995). Source: National Center for Health Statistics.

Mental Health Epidemiologic Catchment Area study (ECA; Regier et al., 1984), Mościcki et al. (1988) found a much lower prevalence of lifetime suicide attempts than younger populations. For persons age 65 and older, the lifetime prevalence for suicide attempt was 1.1%. In comparison, for persons age 25 to 44, the rate was 4%. There are no published ECA rates that examine older adults in smaller age groups, nor in combination with gender or race.

7.11.4 CORRELATES OF LATE LIFE SUICIDE COMPLETION

7.11.4.1 Psychopathology

The primary method for studying the psychopathology associated with suicide in late life is the PA. Structured diagnostic interviews with knowledgeable informants allow for comparisons of risk for various diagnoses. Various estimates indicate that psychiatric disorder and/or substance use were present in about 90% of suicides, with affective disorder the most common psychopathology, followed by substance use and schizophrenia (Conwell, 1994). The diagnostic profile of suicides, however, differs with age. Conwell and Brent (1995) reviewed 14 PA studies from the USA and Europe that examined psychiatric disorders across age groups. Schizophrenia, substance use, and conduct disorder are more common among younger persons, while affective disorder, primarily major depression of a late onset, is more characteristic of older suicides. In addition, the proportion of suicides associated with substance use disorders also declines with age. Although the disorders of dementia and delirium increase substantially in late life, few studies have found these diagnoses associated with risk for suicide (Conwell & Brent).

Conwell and his colleagues (Conwell, 1994; Conwell, Duberstein et al., 1996) make a strong case for late onset depression as the most powerful diagnostic risk factor for late life suicide. Conwell (1994) also cites a clinical follow-up study that illustrates this point. Gardner et al. (1964) linked psychiatric case register information with death certificates for Monroe County, New York. Age effects were considered among persons less than 55 compared to those 55 and older. Among persons with affective disorders, one year rates for suicide among the younger group were 207 per 100 000, while for the older group, the rate was 475 per 100 000.

7.11.4.2 Previous Suicide Attempts

Although elderly suicide victims are much less likely than younger victims to have a history of past suicide attempts (Conwell, 1994; Kreitman, 1976a; Merrill & Owens, 1990; Pierce, 1987), and as noted above, the elderly in general have low prevalence of lifetime suicide attempts compared to younger age groups (Mościcki et al., 1988), previous suicide attempts appears to be a potent risk factor for later completion. Although one could argue that competitive mortality and physical frailty may work to produce this effect, greater suicide intent and lethality among the elderly would suggest that these effects are not the major forces behind this pattern (Conwell). Moreover, in the clinical registry follow-up study by Gardner et al. (1964), of the persons age 54 or less who attempted suicide, 2% completed suicide within a year. In contrast, among the persons age 55 and older, 6% completed suicide in the same period. Nordentoft et al. (1993) reported more recently on a 10 year follow up of Danish patients admitted to a poison treatment center for suicide attempts, where greater age was among the significant risk factors for subsequent suicide.

7.11.4.3 Physical Illness

Several studies (Conwell, Rotenberg, & Caine, 1990; Sainsbury, 1955, Whitlock, 1978) have indicated that physical illness is a common diagnosis among elderly suicides. When making age comparisons with suicide rates, older persons are more likely to have experienced a physical illness as a "life event" relative to younger persons (Rich, Young, & Fowler, 1986). The British studies (Sainsbury and Whitlock) noted above, found that cancer, in particular, was a frequent correlate of suicide in late life. However, a case controlled study by Henriksson and his colleagues found depressive syndromes to be equally present (80% and 82%) among cancer patients who suicided (two-thirds were age 60 and older) and age- and sex-matched comparison suicides without cancer histories (Henriksson, Isometsä, Hietanen, Aro, & Lönnqvist, 1995).

Other studies have indicated that the actual rates of physical illness among elderly suicides are lower than expected. Clark (1992) reported that among 73 consecutive elderly suicides in Cook County, Illinois, only 14% were terminally ill and 23% were chronically or severely medically ill at the time of death. Given the high rate of physical illness (chronic, acute, terminal) among older persons, it is imperative to further pose this question in case controlled studies.

7.11.4.4 Personality Dimensions

Research on younger samples of completed suicides has indicated an association with personality disorders and certain personality characteristics (Angst & Clayton, 1986; Marttunen, Aro, Henriksson, & Lönnqvist, 1991; Paffenbarger, Lee, & Leung, 1994; Runeson & Beskow, 1991). Interest in personality characteristics and disorders in late life suicide may have been limited due to the challenge of assessing them through informants, as well as the belief that diagnosed personality disorders have less validity in the elderly (Sadavoy & Fogel, 1992).

Duberstein and his colleagues (Duberstein, 1995; Duberstein, Conwell, & Caine, 1994) have used an informant-based measure of the NEO-Personality Inventory (Costa & McCrae, 1985) to examine possible personality traits among older and younger suicides, relative to controls. The NEO inventory measures five general personality traits: neuroticism, extroversion, openness to experience, agreeableness, and conscientiousness. Suicides were found to have higher neuroticism scores, and older suicide victims had lower openness to experience scores than both younger suicides and normal controls. Clark (1993) has theorized that a "narcissistic" crisis, based on a personality predisposition, leaves the older person with increasingly rigid, inflexible thoughts under stressful life events.

Duberstein (1995) has theorized about the behavioral correlates of low openness to experience (OTE) with implications for clinical assessment, the possible gender differences in OTE and depression, biological correlates, and association between OTE and attempted suicide. Each of these offer important clinical implications and plausible research directions in suicidal behavior in late life.

Some reports suggest that it may be the confluence of personality, poor coping skills, fear of illness and the hopelessness of depression that influences the association between physical illness and suicide in the elderly. Conwell, Caine, and Olsen (1990) presented a series of eight cases where the victims' fears that they had cancer played a major role in committing suicide. Among these eight cases, only one was reported to have cancer upon autopsy, and five had diagnoses of major depression. Similarly, Horton-Deutsch, Clark, and Farran (1992), reporting on 14 cases from the study cited by Clark (1992) above, describe the co-occurrence of chronic dyspnea, increasing limitations in functional status, life events, and depression and anxiety among elderly men who suicided. Common to both of these studies is the description of the personality characteristics of the majority of elderly male suicides: appearance of being overtly strong and self-sufficient, yet covertly or overtly having difficulty in being dependent and accepting help, and having a rigid, inflexible coping style, not unlike a lack of OTE.

7.11.4.5 Life Events

7.11.4.5.1 Physical illness and loss

Significant age differences in recent life events among completed suicides have been reported in several studies (Rich et al., 1986; Heikkinen & Lönnqvist, 1995), where the proportion of victims with current somatic illness increases with age, and marital separations, family discord, and job problems are more common among younger suicides. When physical illness is excluded, few life events are found among elderly suicide victims. Outside physical illness, the most commonly cited life event associated with late life suicide is "loss." Loss in this context has referred to loss of spouse, family members, friends, job, physical autonomy, and impending nursing home placement (Conwell, 1994). Unfortunately, such losses are common in late life in general. Once again, without adequate control groups, it is not clear in what ways these events become risk enhancing for suicidal behavior.

7.11.4.5.2 Living alone

Another frequently cited risk factor is social isolation and living alone, which may or may not be linked to life events such as widowhood or family estrangement. Barraclough (1971) reported that among 30 suicides of persons age 65 and older, 50% lived alone, compared to 20% in the community from which they lived. More recent studies conducted in the USA have not found similar patterns. For example, Conwell et al. (1990) did not find an increase in living alone among complete suicides age 50 and older. Only 35% were found to be living alone; more than one-third of elderly suicide victims were married, and more than half lived with a spouse or family member.

Perhaps more important are the distinctions to be made among the constructs of living alone, social isolation, and loneliness. Living alone does not imply social isolation or loneliness. Younger et al. (1990) reported that among the nearly 50% of people living alone who had committed suicide, 60% had weekly visits with others outside the home and 98% had weekly contact with friends and family. The degree to which these suicide victims felt lonely, despite their contact with others, is not known and suggests the need for separating these constructs in both clinical assessment and future research.

7.11.4.6 Neurobiological Correlates

7.11.4.6.1 Serotonergic system

To date, there are still no specific biological markers for either depression or suicidal behavior. However, there are hopes that such biological information, in conjunction with psychologically assessed data, can improve detection of high risk persons, with prevention and treatment implications. If biological subtypes of suicidal behavior were to be discovered, for example, more targeted pharmacologic interventions might be developed. With regard to the elderly, it is conceivable that a "neurobiological vulnerability" to suicide might undergo modulation by age-related changes in neurobiological systems (Rifai, Reynolds, & Mann, 1992; Schneider, 1996). The consistency of suicide risk increasing with age and male gender across nations also suggests a possible neurobiological process (Conwell, Raby, & Caine, 1995). Decreased brain concentrations of serotonin, dopamine, norepinephrine and their metabolites (HVA, 5-HIAA); increased brain MAO-B activity; increased hypothalamic–pituitary–adrenal activity; and increased sympathetic nervous system activity are associated with both depression and normal aging (Schneider, 1996). Although it would seem that these correlates would have led to more neurobiological studies of elderly suicides, few have been conducted.

Several reviews have examined the evidence for neurobiologic abnormalities among elderly suicide victims relative to controls and have found too few studies that had included sufficient "elderly" subjects (older than 60 years) to draw any conclusions (Conwell & Brent, 1995; Rifai et al., 1992). This is particularly true of the subgroup of the elderly most at risk; those 85 and older. Conwell and Brent have also described the challenges to be met in obtaining sufficient cases to test various neurobiological hypotheses, and have outlined a protocol for standardization of data for postmortem research protocols.

7.11.4.6.2 Serum cholesterol

The association between serum cholesterol concentrations and late life comes from the heart disease outcomes literature. In clinical trial studies aimed at lowering serum cholesterol in persons either at risk for, or having heart disease, gains in lowered heart-related deaths have been off-set by increases in suicide and accidental deaths (e.g., Muldoon, Manuck, & Matthew, 1990). Among men age 70 and older, depression is also three times more common when plasma cholesterol concentrations are low (Morgan, Palinkas, Barrett-Connor, & Wingard, 1993). However, other studies have not found this association in free cholesterol levels, but have in the esterification of cholesterol (the reverse cholesterol transport; Maes et al.,1994). Clearly, further research in the cardiovascular and neurobiological correlates of suicidal behavior in later life are needed.

7.11.4.7 Health Service Use Patterns

Clark (1992) has noted that suicides in the USA are not higher for those with less access to health care. To the contrary, suicide rates are lower for African-Americans and Hispanics (groups who underuse health care) relative to their white counterparts. Indeed, a phenomenon common among elderly suicide completers and attempters is that the majority have recently visited a health care provider. Importantly, however, virtually none of these elderly had sought mental health services. This is in contrast to younger aged adults, where 25–30% were under the care of a mental health professional at the time of their death (Clark & Fawcett, 1992).

Instead, over 70% of older suicides have visited their primary care physician within the month of their suicide in the USA (Conwell, 1994) and the UK (Vassilas & Morgan, 1994). A similar pattern appears for elderly attempters in Japan (Takahashi et al., 1995), where more attempters relative to depressive controls sought out primary care physicians. This pattern may be in part due to physical concerns that reflect actual acute or chronic illness, as rates of comorbid physical illness among elderly suicides are also high compared to younger groups (Cattell, 1988; Conwell, 1994). This pattern may also be related to hypochondriacal concerns (Barraclough et al., 1974), and fear of pain, physical illness, and concomitant dependency as described above (Clark, 1993; Conwell et al., 1990; Duberstein, 1995; Horton-Deutsch et al., 1992).

The failure to recognize and adequately treat older adults with depression is probably due to several causes. First, the elderly themselves and their family members may incorrectly attribute depressive symptoms to the aging process, and see depression as a "normal" aspect of aging, and an expectable side effect of physical illness. Primary care physicians tend to spend less time with older patients and focus on physical problems to the exclusion of mental morbidity (German et al., 1985; Keeler, Solomon, Beck, Mendenhall & Kane, 1982). Second, there may be hesitancy or inability to report psychiatric symptoms even when specifically asked. Gallo, Anthony, and Muthén, (1994) have found that older depressed adults are less likely to endorse dysphoric mood as part of their symptom clusters. Older men, in particular, are less likely to report depressive symptoms (Allen-Burge, Storandt, Kinscherf, & Rubin, 1994; Lutsky & Knight, 1994). Third, primary care physicians, who are the most sought after health care providers among all persons with depression in the USA, typically do not recognize (e.g., Perez-Stable, Miranda, Munoz, & Ying, 1990) nor adequately treat depression among any age group (Sturm & Wells, 1995).

7.11.5 STUDIES OF ELDERLY SUICIDE ATTEMPTERS

Given the limited data on the epidemiology of late life suicide attempts, the bulk of this discussion focuses on studies of hospital based samples. In a review of attempted suicide in late life, Draper (1996) reviewed 12 studies published between 1985 and 1994. Despite variation in sampling contexts and approaches to measurement, and lack of adequate control groups, there were several consistent factors associated with attempted suicide in late life: depression, social isolation, and being unmarried. The degree to which physical health was a risk factor was unclear; in some studies it appeared to play a major role (Draper, 1994; Frierson, 1991; Nowers, 1993), while in another only about a third of the patients identified health as a factor (Pierce, 1987). Draper suggested that the interaction between psychosocial factors such as social isolation, loneliness, family conflict, and physical factors such as presence of pain and perceived limitations may be a more critical combination for risk of suicide attempt than physical illness alone. A gender difference by age pattern was also noted across the studies: the proportion of males attempting suicide increased with age, particularly among those age 75 and older. Without adequate control groups, however, these findings remain interesting leads rather than true advances in our understanding of risk factors for suicide attempts in late life.

Among the few studies with control groups, elderly depressives admitted for a suicide attempt have been more likely to have a later age of onset than elderly depressives who were not suicidal (Lyness, Conwell, & Nelson, 1992). In a German study an age by sex interaction in age of onset was noted, where men age 50 and older were more likely to have had an affective illness of late onset, and women had a younger age of onset and were more likely to have had previous suicide attempts (Bron, Strack, & Rudolph, 1991).

Psychosis and somatization have characterized the psychiatric symptoms of elderly suicide attempters. Lyness et al. (1992) and Roose et al., (1983) found psychotic depression to be more related to suicidal behavior than other affective disorders in retrospective cohort studies. Psychotic depression is interpreted by some to include delusions about physical symptoms. In a Japanese study of urban elderly attempters, Takahashi et al. (1995) examined the rates of somatization (defined as a separate entity from depression) among attempters and controls. Consistent with earlier descriptive studies of high rates of hypochondriasis among elderly attempters (Barraclough et al., 1974; De Alarcon, 1964), they found higher rates of somatization among attempters relative to controls. Although somatization can be defined as a type of psychosis, its unique role and cooccurrence with depression in late life appears worthy of further investigation.

7.11.6 SUBGROUPS OF ELDERLY AT RISK FOR SUICIDE

Suicide is a multidetermined, low base rate event. Despite the many correlates and posited risk factors identified, the prediction of suicidal behavior is next to impossible (Goldstein, Black, Nasrallah, & Winokur, 1991; Pokorny, 1983). However, since suicide risk in the elderly is strongly associated with certain demographic (white males) and psychological variables (depressive diagnoses and rigid coping), it follows that certain subgroups of the elderly are more or less likely to be at risk for suicidal behavior. The primary intent of proposing subgroups here is to stimulate research questions that consider the interaction of such demographic characteristics with other known risk or protective factors that may help the field move beyond studies that focus on main effects.

7.11.6.1 Intolerance for Physical Illness or Dependency

The discussions of somatization and findings pertaining to the role of physical illness in elderly suicide would suggest that there are persons, who, when faced with what they perceive to be an illness that may limit autonomy, become risks for suicide. White males, living in the community, who have taken pride in being independent and self-sufficient would be the prototype of this subgroup. Stated fears of losing what are considered markers of independence, such as driving or living independently, may reflect underlying intolerable anxiety and depression. These fears, in combination with suspicion of having an incurable illness with functional limitations, may create a lethal combination. In contrast, studies of patients with terminal illnesses, who have learned to readjust their expectations about life have a lower risk of suicidality (Marshall, Burnett, & Brasure, 1983). Measures of hopelessness (Beck, Brown, Berchick, Steward, & Steer, 1990; Beck, Steer, Kovacs, & Garrison, 1985; Hill, Gallagher, Thompson, & Ishida, 1988; Rifai, George, Stack, Mann, & Reynolds, 1994), limited openness to new experience (Duberstein, 1995), perfectionism (Hewitt, Flett, & Turnbull-Donovan, 1992), and willingness to adapt may help screen those elderly with physical illness who may be at risk for depression and suicidal ideation.

7.11.6.2 Older Alcoholics

Another group at risk for suicide are older male alcoholics with early onset who have survived to be among the "young old." Murphy and his associates described a number of factors associated with suicide among alcoholics. For the older male alcoholics, loss of the last social support has been found to be a pivotal event in suicide risk (Murphy, Wetzel, Robins, & McEvoy, 1992). Similarly, Duberstein et al. (1994) reported that interpersonal stressors and recent alcohol use combined to increase risk for suicide. In a Finnish sample, Heikkinen et al. (1994) compared nonalcoholic depressives and alcoholics who had committed suicide. Unlike depressives, alcoholics were likely to have recent interpersonal loss, unemployment, and financial trouble. Drinking patterns appeared to lead to these concurrent stressors. Assessment of depression as well as current social support among older alcoholics would seem to be essential in understanding risk for suicidal behavior in this subgroup.

7.11.6.3 Immigrants and Ethnic Minority Elderly

Studies conducted in Hong Kong (Yap, 1958), Singapore (Ko & Kua, 1995), Australia (Burvill, 1995); Burvill, Woodings, Stenhouse, & McCall, 1982), and Canada (Kliewer & Ward, 1988) indicate that suicide rates are higher among immigrants than natives of the host country. Such research is complicated as it must consider factors that may influence suicide risk in the country of origin (e.g., religion, the individuals' reason for leaving and mental health history); factors within the country of migration; and the society of settlement (e.g., similar or different in ethnicity, and degree of acculturation) (Murphy, 1977). With regard to elderly suicide, the study of these factors are even more challenging to consider as age of immigration can vary widely (e.g., the elderly migrant may have emigrated within the year of suicide, or 80 years prior), and familial networks will vary with the degree to which acculturation is desired or avoided. Despite these challenges, research on elderly suicide in countries and cities where immigration is high (e.g., USA, Hong Kong, Australia), comparing immigrant groups of varying rates of suicide, may help explicate the role of culture, religion, and family interactions in suicidal risk in the elderly (see Corin, 1995).

Very little empirical data exists about the risk or protective factors for suicidal behavior among African-American, non-white Hispanic, and Asian ethnic minority groups in the USA. However, theory development about risk and protective factors among ethnic minority Americans can be found (Griffith et al., 1989; Sorenson & Golding, 1988). Studies on the risk for depression in older ethnic minorities should provide clues as to risk for suicidal behavior in later life (e.g., Baker, 1996). As the number of American ethnic minority elderly are projected to increase substantially in numbers in the next few decades (US Bureau of the Census, 1996), much must be learned to best assess and treat suicidal behavior in these subpopulations in order to adequately provide care and service in the future.

7.11.6.4 Older Women

A fourth subgroup needing further study are elderly women. Canetto has discussed what is known about gender issues in suicide, including what little is known about older female suicides (Canetto, 1992, 1994, 1995). Of the many sociologic risk factors proposed to increase risk for suicide, including retirement, financial stress, widowhood, living alone, and poor physical health, older women suffer more than older men in each of these categories, yet have lower suicide rates (Canetto, 1995). Moreover, of the mental disorders thought to increase risk for late life suicide, depression is the most frequent disorder cited and older women have higher rates of depression than older men (Kennedy et al., 1989; Livingston, Hawkins,

Graham, Blizard, & Mann, 1990; Romanoski et al., 1992), as well as more functional impairment with depression (Kornstein, et al., 1995).

Because of these contradictions, Canetto has recommended that discussions of elderly suicide become more precise with regard to gender. Clearly, applying typical risk factors that reflect older male suicides in studies of older women will not yield great benefits. What may be of more utility is to examine gender differences in acceptability of completed suicide as a behavior (Canetto, 1995), as well as examining gender differences in coping and cognitive styles. Rumination, a cognitive style more common among women, may prolong depressive episodes and serve to increase prevalence rates (Nolen-Hoeksema, 1987; Nolen-Hoeksema, Morrow, & Fredrickson, 1993). Interpersonal sensitivity and a relational interactional style more common among women (Markus & Oyserman, 1989) makes them more sensitive and responsive to others' problems. Although this gender-typed style may contribute to prolonged depressive episodes among women, it may also protect them from acting on suicidal thoughts (Canetto, 1992). Little is known about how interpersonal sensitivity or a ruminative cognitive style are related to depression or suicidal ideation in older women, or what mediating factors such as social support influence these possible associations.

With regard to the older women who do complete suicide, one could hypothesize that older female suicides have had more previous attempts, based on epidemiologic data of middle-aged populations (Mościcki et al., 1988). Higher rates of previous attempts is also related to borderline personality disorder and less lethal attempts (Rich et al, 1986; Runeson & Beskow, 1991), which also are more common among women. Nolen-Hoeksema (1995) has articulated the biological and psychosocial theories of the evolution of gender differences in depression. There is evidence to suggest that some of the factors that increase rates for depression in women are similar to those for suicidal behavior, particularly histories of abuse in childhood and adulthood (Davidson, Hughes, George, & Blazer, 1996; Kaplan, Asnis, Lipschitz, & Chorney, 1995).

7.11.6.5 Nursing Home Patients

If nursing home settings are considered (where the vast majority of residents are female), less lethal and more passive attempts, such as refusal of food or adherence to medications may characterize suicidal behavior in this subgroup. Indeed, Osgood surveyed long-term care facilities and reported that most self-destructive behaviors in nursing homes were indirect, and that setting characteristics were related to rates of self-destructive behavior (Osgood, 1992; Osgood & Brant, 1990). Building on this work, Conwell, Pearson, and DeRenzo (1996) have summarized several research issues on self-destructive behaviors in nursing home patients. Included are patient-related factors (psychiatric illness, physical health, personality and coping styles, religious beliefs, and neurobiological beliefs), setting influences (nature and size of facility, quality of care provided) and their interactions, as well as ethical issues involved. Given the high prevalence rates of mental disorders in nursing homes that go undetected and untreated (Rovner, Kafonek, Filipp, Lucas, & Folstein, 1986; Strahan, 1991), the need for further study of self-destructive behavior, both direct and indirect, is clearly needed in these settings.

7.11.7 BIOETHICAL ISSUES

7.11.7.1 Physician Assisted Suicide

The question of risks for suicidal behavior in nursing homes brings to the surface the many complicated issues involved in passive and active euthanasia, advance directives, and physician-assisted suicide (see Chapter 6, this volume). Although there is consensus that decisions regarding the limitation of life-saving procedures are not "suicidal" in terminal illness, such as requesting do-not-resuscitate orders as a part of acute health care treatment, the role of the physician to hasten the process by active means remains controversial. The US public, health care guilds, and health care providers continue to debate patients' rights and physician-assisted suicide and in some cases, act on their beliefs (e.g., see Gibbs, 1993 on Kervorkian; Quill, 1991). In March 1996, the 9th US Circuit Court of Appeals (Compassion in Dying vs. State of Washington, 1996) ruled that *mentally-competent, terminally-ill* adults have a constitutionally protected liberty interest in hastening what might otherwise be a protracted, undignified and extremely painful death. The guiding principle here is that of patient autonomy. Patients have the right to control their own bodies and to decide for themselves the course of their own medical treatment.

The salience and complications of these issues vary with the health care context, perspective and health status of the patient, and age and perspective of the clinician (Marks, 1988–1989). Among adults with terminal illnesses who are cognitively intact, refusal of treatment or requests for physician-assisted suicide appears less controversial. With regard to the elderly, many of whom may not be competent to advocate for themselves, or may or may not have family members who can be trusted to represent their wishes, the issue is very controversial (Osgood, 1995). Competency is a pivotal issue, because cognitive impairment and depression often co-occur with terminal illness. Sullivan and Youngner (1994) highlight differences in clinicians' views on competency in the elderly by examining the refusal of life-sustaining treatment by patients with serious medical illness and comorbid depression. In medical settings, competence to refuse life-sustaining treatment is typically presumed unless the physician proves otherwise. In psychiatric settings, a desire to die is considered evidence of a mental disorder and proves justification of treatment.

7.11.7.2 Competency and Depression

Sullivan and Youngner (1994) recommended that depression in medical patients be treated to improve competency. If treatment is not successful, a residual diagnosis of depression is neither necessary nor sufficient for determining that the patients' medical decision is impaired. In their argument, depression and competency are separate issues. Yet others argue that depression can render limitations on consciousness, where alternatives other than suicide cannot be clearly considered by the patient (Clark, 1992; Koenig, 1993). Shneidman (1986) represents this same sentiment in his assessment of the cognitive narrowing and inflexibility of the suicidal patient: "It is not a thing to do while one is not in one's best mind. Never kill yourself when you are suicidal" (p. 8).

Studies on how depression affects decision making in late life are limited, but some evidence suggests that depression can affect the consistency in preferences for end of life decisions. Lee and Ganzini (1992) studied elderly persons seeking medical treatment, and found mild to moderate depression not to affect preference for life-sustaining medical therapy (intravenous fluids with medications, feeding tube, blood transfusions, intensive care, kidney dialysis, ventilatory support, and cardiopulmonary resuscitation). Among severely depressed elderly, however, there was less consistency in preferences over time. Lee and Ganzini (1994) have also documented little consistency among depressed older medical inpatients who recover from their depression. When depressed subjects who recovered changed their preferences, they were as likely to change from refusing to desiring a treatment as vice versa. Those who became depressed, and remained depressed, were likely to refuse an intervention they had initially asked for.

Sullivan and Youngner (1994) have argued that studies of nursing home residents provide equivocal evidence for the effects of depression on life-sustaining treatments, where depression in patients has been related to both decreased and increased desire for life-sustaining treatments (Garrett, Harris, Norburn, Patrick, & Davis, 1993) compared to preferences among nondepressed residents. What may contribute to inconsistencies in findings may be the mixing of research methods (hypothetical future illness versus current state of illness). Attempting to draw comparisons across diverse groups of elderly may be misleading due to the demographic and health differences among the elderly: community elderly seeking medical care are likely to differ significantly from nursing home residents with regard to age, gender, general health status, and perspectives on death.

Consistent with Lee and Ganzini's work, along with commonly found risk factors for late life suicide (male gender, white ethnicity), other evidence suggests that older persons' attitudes towards suicide may be related to their perceived social support and health and mental state (i.e., depression). Seidlitz, Duberstein, Cox, and Conwell (1995), using data from a Gallup Poll, found that nonreligious white men, especially those with strained family relationships and self-perceived failing health, were the most likely to endorse lenient attitudes toward suicide. Although owning such an attitude does not predict suicidal behavior, it does lower the threshold for tolerance of this option. Moreover, since lenient attitudes towards suicide may reflect hopelessness about family relations and self-perceived health—aspects that may be subject to change with intervention—treatment of depression or anxiety among patients holding such attitudes may affect lenient attitudes toward suicide.

7.11.7.3 Bioethical Research Needs

Future research that considers both patient-related and setting influences may help reconcile the seemingly contradictory evidence regarding depression, end-of-life decisions, and suicide. In considering these issues in the nursing home setting, Conwell, Pearson, and DeRenzo (1996) identified five patient-related factors relevant to self-harming behaviors: assessment of psychiatric symptomatology (dementia, depression, hopelessness, suicide intent, ideation); physical health (including somatic complaints and pain); personality and coping style (rigid coping style, openness to experience); religious beliefs; and neurobiological influences. Although setting influences described by Conwell, Pearson and DeRenzo (1996) were directed towards nursing homes, the context of access and willingness to seek health care, social supports, and attitudes of family members and health care providers can be assessed among the hospitalized and community dwelling elderly, and should be factored in the investigations of the individuals' decisions about end-of-life decisions.

An important implication of implementing right to refuse treatment policies or enacting physician-assisted suicide laws may be how such options affect older persons' attitudes about suicide. Increased availability and use of hospice care could conceivably affect older persons' attitudes towards suicide. If the end of life seems less likely to be characterized by pain, suffering, and dependence, dying by a "natural course" may seem more tolerable, and suicide a less preferred suicide option (Amenta & Shubert, 1995). For others, physician-assisted suicide may hasten death and reduce the time of enduring intolerable pain and suffering. Posner (1995) has argued that the perception that physician-assisted suicide can be available as needed, could be an effective means of suicide prevention in later life. These are researchable issues that can and should be addressed to best inform legislators and policy makers.

7.11.8 CLINICAL RESOURCES FOR TREATING SUICIDAL OLDER ADULTS

Suicide is an attempt to solve a problem of unbearable psychological pain, where few alternative solutions are seen or considered by the patient (Shneidman, 1992). The inability to consider that solutions, even though not obvious now, may be present in the future, reflects the serious hopelessness felt by suicidal patients (Beck et al.,1990; Beck et al., 1985; Rifai et al., 1994). Aspects of approaches to suicidal patients that appear particularly applicable to the elderly include the assessment of what Shneidman termed "cognitive constriction" (Shneidman, 1985). Constriction can be defined generally as dichotomous thinking, tunnel vision, or a narrowing of the range of options. As long as alternative solutions are not seen as plausible, suicide as a viable option remains and risk for acting on suicidal ideation is high. Clinical interventions for suicidal persons, whether they are individual, family, group, or pharmacologic in nature, must be effective in providing the alternative solutions to suicide.

As multiple psychological autopsy studies have shown, more than 90% of cases of adult suicides have had a recent major psychiatric disorder (Clark & Fawcett, 1992). Moreover, the lifetime probability of suicidal death is 15% for persons with a major affective disorder (Klerman, 1987). Therefore, the prevention of suicide in late life in both a crisis situation, and in the long run, will be best accomplished by the increased recognition and adequate treatment of depression (NIH Consensus Conference, 1992). As such, most of the clinical resources suggested below address treatment of depression primarily, with secondary benefits to reducing risk for suicide.

Unfortunately, there are few studies that address the effectiveness of various interventions with suicidal persons in general, and virtually none focusing on the elderly. Crisis hotlines are nearly impossible to evaluate (Lester, 1993), and little information exists on the elderly's use of such services in the USA (Conwell, 1994). Adamek and Kaplan (1996), in a survey of American Association of Suicidology listed crisis prevention centers, found that even though about a third had specialty programs for the elderly or specific outreach efforts, two-thirds of the staff did not know that older adults are the age group with the highest suicide rate. Although crisis lines may not be effective with the elderly, telephone outreach programs do show some promise of reducing psychological distress and suicidal ideation, if not completed suicide (see McIntosh, 1995, for a review).

With regard to comparative interventions with suicidal elderly, no studies exist, highlighting the need for this type of research. Therefore, the clinical resources described below are not proven to be effective treatments, but do reflect the state-of-the-art and limited science.

7.11.8.1 Psychotherapeutic Resources

There are a growing number of guidelines and descriptions of psychotherapeutic approaches to suicidal outpatients (e.g., Bongar, 1992; Leenaars, Maltsberger, & Neimeyer, 1994). Increasingly among these guidelines are articles, chapters, and even books, devoted solely to the suicidal elderly (e.g., Lester & Tallmer, 1994; McIntosh, et al., 1994; Richman, 1993). The most frequent author of chapters and papers on psychotherapeutic approaches to suicidal elderly is Joseph Richman, a family therapist who integrates research findings with nearly 30 years of clinical experience with suicidal elderly

(Richman, 1996). Richman's approach typically includes the family as well as the patient, as he considers the family an important context of the older person. The family can both contribute to the risk, and to the treatment of the suicidal elderly. His book, *Preventing elderly suicide,* reviews research that he has grounded his approach in, assessment, crisis intervention, and individual, family and group modalities (Richman, 1993).

Cognitive-behavior therapy has also been used successfully to treat suicidal persons (Beck, Rush, Shaw, & Emery, 1979; Beck & Weishaar, 1990), including the elderly. Generally described, cognitive behavior therapy, as applied to the suicidal individual, identifies the dysfunctional beliefs that are typically helpless and hopeless in character, the feelings associated with the beliefs, and then directs the client to problem solving methods. By forming a more precise description of the problem separate from depressed mood, breaking down the problem into components, and considering possible solutions, suicide as an only option begins to dissipate. DeVries and Gallagher-Thompson (1994) have described how this approach can be applied specifically to older adults in crisis, including suicidality.

Maltsberger (1991) applies a more psychoanalytic, "ego deficit" model of suicide in the elderly, where the suicidal person is narcissistically vulnerable, fearing loss of mental and physical capacity, as well as abandonment. If the older patient is unable to ask or obtain support for these functions and self-contempt and anxiety increase, the risk of suicide increases. In this approach, the therapist can play a critical role during this narcissistic crisis by providing resources through his or her warmth, encouragement, and availability.

7.11.8.2 Pharmacologic and Electroconvulsive Therapies

7.11.8.2.1 Pharmacologic therapies

Serotonergic abnormalities in patients who are suicidal would suggest that treatments using serotonin reuptake inhibitors (SSRIs, e.g., fluoxetine, paroxetine, sertraline) would be effective (Montgomery, 1993). Since the SSRIs are just as effective as the earlier tricyclic antidepressants but have lower side-effect profiles among the elderly (Schneider, 1996), acceptability and treatment compliance with SSRIs among the elderly may be improved. Furthermore, because fluoxetine has been shown to decrease suicidal ideation relatively early in treatment among adults ages 18–65 (Worthington et al., 1995), its use with older suicidal adults may be life saving. Although there is no research pointing to particularly effective pharmacologic treatments for suicidal elderly, there are several reviews that describe the many effective pharmacologic approaches to treating late life depression (Hay & Hay, 1996; Kennedy, 1996; Salzman, 1994). More studies that track the presence and change and continuity of suicidal ideation over time of treatment and follow-up are also needed (see Rifai et al., 1994 for one example).

7.11.8.2.2 Electroconvulsive therapy

Electroconvulsive therapy, although still controversial, can be an extremely effective treatment for elderly patients with depression who are not able to tolerate the side effects of pharmacotherapies. Moreover, it is often effective where patients have not responded to traditional pharmacologic interventions. The speed of onset of its action, which is typically more efficient than medication, also makes it an indicated treatment for suicidal persons and those with severe depressions in late life. The efficacy, applications, adverse effects, and contra-indications for use in the elderly have been reviewed elsewhere (Hay & Hay, 1996; Sackheim, 1994). Although there are no outcome studies specific to suicidal elderly, Avery and Winokur (1976, 1978) have demonstrated that electroconvulsive therapy does decrease the number of suicidal outcomes in depressed patients.

7.11.9 SUMMARY

Suicide among the elderly is one of the most critical public health problems facing us today. We have sufficient information on what appear to be strong correlates if not risk factors to address several levels of preventive interventions (Conwell & Duberstein, 1995; Rihmer, 1996). Although suicide in the elderly as a public health problem has probably been ignored due to agism, like other areas of psychopathology in late life, clinical, research, and policy interests in late life suicide (Suicide and the elderly: A population at risk, 1996) have grown with the increasing numbers of older persons in the USA, and other countries. Perhaps current older cohorts and younger cohorts will become more active in their interests in maintaining and increasing their own well-being (McIntosh, Pearson, & Lebowitz, 1997). As "baby boomers" age and demand more and better health care, the interest in the prevention and treatment of psychopathology of later life will certainly grow. It is hoped that this chapter has provided some useful groundwork, and has raised some potentially important research directions for the much needed information that will be required to meet the future needs and interests of the aging population and their family members.

ACKNOWLEDGMENTS

Dr. Paul Duberstein provided invaluable suggestions and comments on this chapter. His expert advice and criticism is greatly appreciated.

7.11.10 REFERENCES

Adamek, M. E., & Kaplan, M. S. (1996). Managing elder suicide: A profile of American and Canadian crisis prevention centers. *Suicide and Life-Threatening Behavior, 26,* 122–131.

Allen-Burge, R., Storandt, M., Kinscherf, D. A., & Rubin, E. H. (1994). Sex differences in the sensitivity of two self-report depression scales in older depressed inpatients. *Psychology and Aging, 9,* 443–445.

Amenta, M. O., & Shubert, V. (1995). Hospice care can obviate the need for suicide. *Home Healthcare Nurse, 13,* 72–74.

Angst, J. & Clayton, P. (1986). Premorbid personality of depressive, bipolar, and schizophrenic patients with special reference to suicidal issues. *Comprehensive Psychiatry, 27,* 511–531.

Avery, D., & Winokur, G. (1976). Mortality in depressed patients treated with electroconvulsive therapy and antidepressants. *Archives of General Psychiatry, 33,* 1029–1037.

Avery, D., & Winokur, G. (1978). Suicide, attempted suicide, and relapse rates in depression. *Archives of General Psychiatry, 35,* 749–753.

Baker, F. M. (1996). Suicide among ethnic elders. In G. J. Kennedy (Ed.), *Suicide and depression in late life: Critical issues in treatment, research and public policy* (pp. 51–79). New York: Wiley.

Barraclough, B. M. (1971). Suicide in the elderly: Recent developments in psychogeriatrics. *British Journal of Psychiatry, special supplement, 6,* 87–97.

Barraclough, B. M., Bunch, J., Nelson, B., & Sainsbury, P. (1974). A hundred cases of suicide: Clinical aspects. *British Journal of Psychiatry, 125,* 355–373.

Beck, A. T., Brown, G., Berchick, R. J., Stewart, B. L., & Steer, R. A. (1990). Relationship between hopelessness and ultimate suicide: A replication with psychiatric outpatients. *American Journal of Psychiatry, 147,* 190–195.

Beck, A.T., Rush, A. J., Shaw, B. F., & Emery, G. (1979). *Cognitive therapy of depression.* New York: Guilford.

Beck, A. T., Steer, R. A., Kovacs, M., & Garrison, B. (1985). Hopelessness, depression, and attempted suicide. *American Journal of Psychiatry, 142,* 559–563.

Beck, A. T., & Weishaar, M. E. (1990). Suicide risk assessment and prediction. *Crisis, 11,* 22–30.

Beskow, J., Runeson, B., & Asgard, U. (1990). Psychological autopsies: Methods and ethics. *Suicide and Life-Threatening Behavior, 20,* 307–323.

Bongar, B. (1992). *Suicide: Guidelines for assessment, management and treatment.* New York: Oxford University Press.

Bron, B., Strack, M., & Rudolph, G. (1991). Childhood experiences and loss and suicide attempts: Significance in depressive states of major depressed and dysthymic or adjustment disordered patients. *Journal of Affective Disorders, 23,* 165–172.

Buda, M. & Tsuang, M. T. (1990). The epidemiology of suicide: Implications for clinical practice. In S. J. Blumenthal & D. J. Kupfer (Eds.), *Suicide over the life cycle: Risk factors, assessment, and treatment of suicidal patients* (pp. 17–37). Washington, DC: American Psychiatric Press.

Burvill, P. W. (1995). Suicide in the multiethnic elderly population of Australia, 1979–1990. *International Psychogeriatrics, 7,* 319–333.

Burvill, P. W., Woodings, T. L., Stenhouse, N. S. & McCall, M. G. (1982). Suicide during 1961–1970 of migrants in Australia. *Psychological Medicine, 12,* 295–308.

Canetto, S. S. (1992). Gender and suicide in the elderly. *Suicide and Life-Threatening Behavior, 22,* 80–97.

Canetto, S. S. (1994). Gender issues in the treatment of suicidal individuals. In A. A. Leenaars, J. T. Maltsberger, & R. A. Neimeyer (Eds.), *Treatment of suicidal people: A series in death education, aging, and healthcare.* (pp.115–126). Washington, DC: Taylor & Francis.

Canetto, S. S. (1995). Elderly women and suicidal behavior. In S. S. Canetto & D. Lester (Eds.), *Women and suicidal behavior* (pp. 215–233). New York: Springer.

Cattell, H. R. (1988). Elderly suicide in London: An analysis of coroners' inquests. *International Journal of Geriatric Psychiatry, 3,* 251–261.

Chemtob, C. M., Hamada, R. S., Bauer, GB., Kinney, B., & Torigoe, R. Y. (1988). Patients' suicides: Frequency and impact on psychiatrists. *American Journal of Psychiatry, 145,* 224–228.

Chemtob, C. M., Hamada, R. S., Bauer, GB., Torigoe, R. Y. & Kinney, B. (1988). Patient suicides: Frequency and impact on psychologists. *Professional Psychology: Research and Practice, 19,* 421–425.

Clark, D. C. (1992). "Rational" suicide and people with terminal conditions or disabilities. *Issues in Law & Medicine, 8*(2), 147–166.

Clark, D. C. (1993). Narcissistic crises of aging and suicidal despair. *Suicide and Life-Threatening Behavior, 23,* 21–26.

Clark, D. C., & Fawcett, J. (1992). Review of empirical risk factors for evaluation of the suicidal patient. In B. Bongar (Ed.), *Suicide: Guidelines for assessment, management, and treatment* (pp.16–48). New York: Oxford University Press.

Clark, D. C., & Horton-Deutsch, S. L. (1992). Assessment *in Absentia:* The value of the psychological autopsy method for studying antecedents of suicide and predicting future suicides. In R. W. Maris, A. L. Berman, J. T. Maltsberger, & R. I. Yufit (Eds.), *Assessment and prediction of suicide* (pp. 145–181). New York: Guilford.

Clarke, R. V., & Lester, D. (1987). Toxicity of car exhausts and opportunity for suicide: Comparison between Britain and the United States. *Journal of Epidemiology and Community Health, 41,* 114–120.

Cohler, B. J. & Jenuwine, M. J. (1995). Suicide, life course, and life story. *International Psychogeriatrics, 7,* 199–219.

Compassion in Dying v. State of Washington. (1996). 96 C.D.O.S. 1507. [On-line]. Available: http://www.law.vill.edu/fed-ct/circuit/9th/opinions.

Conwell, Y. (1994). Suicide in elderly patients. In L. S. Schneider, C. F. Reynolds, B. D. Lebowitz, & A. J. Friedhoff (Eds.), *Diagnosis and treatment of depression in late life: Results of the NIH consensus development conference* (pp. 397–418). Washington, DC: American Psychiatric Press.

Conwell, Y. & Brent, D. (1995). Suicide and aging I: Patterns of psychiatric diagnosis. *International Psychogeriatrics, 7,* 149–164.

Conwell, Y., Caine, E. D., & Olsen, K. (1990). Suicide and

cancer in late life. *Hospital and Community Psychiatry, 41,* 1334–1339.
Conwell, Y., & Duberstein, P. R. (1995). Prevention of late life suicide: When, where, why and how. *Psychiatry and Clinical Neurosciences, 49*(Suppl), S79–S83.
Conwell, Y., Duberstein, P. R., Cox, C., Herrmann, J. H., Forbes, N. T., & Caine, E. D. (1996). Relationships of age and Axis I diagnoses in victims of completed suicide: A psychological autopsy study. *American Journal of Psychiatry, 153,* 1001–1008.
Conwell, Y., Pearson, J., & DeRenzo, E. G. (1996). Indirect self-destructive behavior among elderly patients in nursing homes. *American Journal of Geriatric Psychiatry, 4,* 152–163.
Conwell, Y., Raby, W. N., & Caine, E. D. (1995). Suicide and aging II: The psychobiological interface. *International Psychogeriatrics, 7,* 165–181.
Conwell, Y., Rotenberg, M., & Caine, E. D. (1990). Completed suicide at age 50 and over. *Journal of the American Geriatrics Society, 38,* 640–644.
Corin, E. (1995). From a cultural stance: Suicide and aging in a changing world. *International Psychogeriatrics, 7,* 335–355.
Coryell, W., & Tsuang, M. T. (1982). Primary unipolar depression and the prognostic importance of delusions. *Archives of General Psychiatry, 39,* 1181–1184.
Costa, P. T., & McCrae, R. R. (1985). *The NEO Personality Inventory: Manual.* Odessa, Fl: Psychological Assessment Resources.
Davidson, J. R. T., Hughes, D. C., George, L. K., & Blazer, D. G. (1996). The association of sexual assault and attempted suicide within the community. *Archives of General Psychiatry, 53,* 550–555.
Davis, J. A. & Smith, T. W. (1989-1991). *General social surveys, 1989–1991.* Chicago: National Opinion Research Center.
De Alarcon, R. (1964). Hypochondriasis and depression in the aged. *Gerontology Clinics, 6,* 266–277.
Dennis, M. S., & Lindesay, J. (1995). Suicide in the elderly—The United Kingdom perspective. *International Psychogeriatrics,* 7, 263–274.
DeVries, H. M., & Gallagher-Thompson, D. (1994). Managing psychological crises of older adults. In F. M. Dattilio & A. M. Freeman (Eds.), *Cognitive-behavior strategies in crisis intervention* (pp. 200–218). New York: Guilford.
Draper, B. (1994). Suicidal behaviour in the elderly. *International Journal of Geriatric Psychiatry, 9,* 655–661.
Draper, B. (1996). Attempted suicide in old age. *International Journal of Geriatric Psychiatry, 11,* 577–587.
Duberstein, P. R. (1995). Openness to experience and completed suicide across the second half of life. *International Psychogeriatrics, 7,* 183–198.
Duberstein, P. R., Conwell, Y., & Caine, E. D. (1994). Age differences in the personality characteristics of suicide completers: Preliminary findings from a psychological autopsy study. *Psychiatry: Interpersonal and Biological Processes, 57,* 213–224.
Fombonne, E. (1994). Increased rates of depression: Update of epidemiological findings and analytical problems. *Acta Psychiatrica Scandinavica, 90,* 145–156.
Frierson, R. L. (1991). Suicide attempts by the old and the very old. *Archives of Internal Medicine, 151,* 141–144.
Gallo, J. J., Anthony, J. C., & Muthén, B. G. (1994). Age differences in the symptoms of depression: A latent trait analysis. *Journal of Gerontology: Psychological Sciences, 49,* P251–P264.
Gardner, E. A., Bahn, A. K., & Mack, M. (1964). Suicide and psychiatric care in the aging. *Archives of General Psychiatry, 10,* 547–553.
Garrett, J. M., Harris, R. P., Norburn, J. K., Patrick, D. L., & Danis, M. (1993). Life-sustaining treatments during terminal illness: Who wants what? *Journal of General Internal Medicine, 8,* 361–368.
German, P. S., Shapiro, S., & Skinner, E. A. (1985). Mental health of the elderly: Use of health and mental health services. *Journal of the American Geriatric Society, 33,* 246–252.
Gibbs, N. (1993, May 31). R for death: The return of Dr. Death. *Time, 141*(22), 35–39.
Goldstein, R. B., Black, D. W., Nasrallah, A., & Winokur, G. (1991). The prediction of suicide: Sensitivity, specificity, and predictive value of a multivariate model applied to suicide among 1906 patients with effective disorders. *Archives of General Psychiatry, 48,* 418–422.
Griffith, E. E. H., Delgado, A. K., Foulks, E., Ruiz, P., Spiegel, J., Wintrob, R., & Yamamoto, J. (1989). *Group for the Advancement of Psychiatry: Report no. 128. Suicide and ethnicity in the United States.* New York: Brunner/Mazel.
Hay, D. P., & Hay, L. K. (1996). Biological treatment of severe late-life depression: Pharmacotherapy and electroconvulsive therapy. In G. J. Kennedy (Ed.), *Suicide and depression in late life: Critical issues in treatment, research, and public policy* (pp. 119–132). New York: Wiley.
Healthy People 2000 (1991). US Department of Health and Human Services, Public Health Service. DHHS Publication no. (PHS) 91-50212. Washington, DC: US Government Printing Office.
Heikkinen, M. E., Aro, H. M., Henriksson, M. M., Isometsä, E. T., Sarna, S. J., Kuoppasalmi, K. I., & Lönnqvist, J. K. (1994). Differences in recent life events between alcoholic and depressive nonalcoholic suicides. *Alcoholism: Clinical and Experimental Research, 18,* 1143–1149.
Heikkinen, M. E., & Lönnqvist, J. K. (1995). Recent life events in elderly suicide: A nationwide study in Finland. *International Psychogeriatrics, 7,* 287–300.
Henriksson, M. M., Isometsä, E. T., Hietanen, P. S., Aro, H.M. & Lönnqvist, J. K. (1995). Mental disorders in cancer suicides. *Journal of Affective Disorders, 36,* 11–20.
Hewitt, P. L., Flett, G. L., & Turnbull-Donovan, W. (1992). Perfectionism and suicide potential. *British Journal of Clinical Psychology, 31,* 181–190.
Hill, R. D., Gallagher, D., Thompson, L. W., & Ishida, T. (1988). Hopelessness as a measure of suicidal intent in the depressed elderly. *Psychology and Aging, 3,* 230–232.
Horton-Deutsch, S. L., Clark, D. C., & Farran, C. J. (1992). Chronic dyspnea and suicide in elderly men. *Hospital and Community Psychiatry, 43,* 1198–1203.
Humphry, D. (1991). *Final exit: The practicalities of self-deliverance and assisted suicide for the dying.* New York: Dell.
Humphry, D. (1992). Rational suicide among the elderly. *Suicide and Life Threatening Behavior, 22,* 125–129.
Kachur, S. P., Potter, L. B., James, S. P., Powell, K. E. (1995). *Suicide in the United States, 1980–1992. Violence Surveillance Summary Series, No. 1.* Atlanta, GA: Centers for Disease Control and Prevention, National Center for Injury Prevention and Control.
Kaplan, M. L., Asnis, G. M., Lipschitz, D. S., & Chorney, P. (1995). Suicidal behavior and abuse in psychiatric outpatients. *Comprehensive Psychiatry, 36,* 229–235.
Kaplan, M. S., Adamek, M. E., & Geling, O. (1996). Sociodemographic predictors of firearm suicide among older white males. *The Gerontologist, 36,* 530–533.
Kaplan, M. S., Adamek, M. E., & Johnson, S. (1994). Trends in firearm suicide among older American males: 1979–1988. *The Gerontologist, 34,* 59–65.
Kaprio, J., Koskenvuo, M., & Rita, H. (1987). Mortality after bereavement: A prospective study of 95 647 widowed persons. *American Journal of Public Health, 77,* 283–287.
Keeler, E. B., Solomon, D. H., Beck, J. C., Mendenhall, R. C., & Kane, R. L. (1982). Effect of patient age on

duration of medical encounters with physicians. *Medical Care, 20,* 1101–1108.
Kennedy, G. J. (1996). A brief antidepressant prescribing guide for the generalist. In G. J. Kennedy (Ed.), *Suicide and depression in late life: Critical issues in treatment, research and public policy* (pp. 133–138). New York: Wiley.
Kennedy, G. J., Kelman, H. R., Thomas, C., Wisniewski, W., Metz, H. & Bijur, P. E. (1989). Hierarchy of characteristics associated with depressive symptoms in an urban elderly sample. *American Journal of Psychiatry, 146,* 220–225.
Kessler, R. C., Brown, R. L., & Broman, C. L. (1981). Sex differences in psychiatric help-seeking: Evidence from four large-scale surveys. *Journal of Health and Social Behavior, 22,* 49–64.
Klerman, G. L. (1987). Clinical epidemiology of suicide. *Journal of Clinical Psychiatry, 48*(suppl.), 33–38.
Kliewer, E. V., & Ward, R. H. (1988). Convergence of immigrant suicide rates to those in the destination country. *American Journal of Epidemiology, 127,* 640–653.
Ko, S. M., & Kua, E. H. (1995). Ethnicity and elderly suicide in Singapore. *International Psychogeriatrics, 7,* 309–317.
Koenig, H. G. (1993). Legalizing physician-assisted suicide: Some thoughts and concerns. *The Journal of Family Practice, 37,* 171–179.
Kornstein, S. G., Schatzberg, A. F., Yonkers, K. A., Thase, M. E., Keitner, G. I., Ryan, C. E. & Schlager, D. (1995). Gender differences in presentation of chronic major depression. *Psychopharmacology Bulletin, 31,* 711–718.
Kreitman, N. (1976a). Age and parasuicide. *Psychological Medicine, 6,* 113–121.
Kreitman, N. (1976b). The coal gas story: United Kingdom suicide rates, 1960–1971. *British Journal of Preventive and Social Medicine, 30,* 86–93.
Lee, M., & Ganzini, L. (1992). Depression in the elderly: Effect on patient attitudes toward life-sustaining therapy. *Journal of the American Geriatrics Society, 40,* 983–988.
Lee, M., & Ganzini, L. (1994). The effect of recovery from depression on preferences for life-sustaining therapy in older patients. *Journal of Gerontology, 49,* M15–M21.
Leenaars, A. A., Maltsberger, J. T., & Neimeyer, R. A. (1994). *Treatment of suicidal people.* Washington, DC: Taylor & Francis.
Lester, D. (1993). The effectiveness of suicide prevention centers. *Suicide and Life-Threatening Behavior, 23,* 263–267.
Lester, D., & Tallmer, M. (Eds.) (1994). *Now I lay me down: Suicide in the elderly.* Philadelphia: Charles Press.
Li, G. (1995). The interaction effect of bereavement and sex on the risk of suicide in the elderly: An historical cohort study. *Social Science and Medicine, 40,* 825–828.
Lindesay, J. (1986). Trends in self-poisoning in the elderly 1974–1983. *International Journal of Geriatric Psychiatry, 1,* 37–43.
Linehan, M. M. (1986). Suicidal people: One population or two? *Annals of the New York Academy of Sciences, 487,* 16–33.
Livingston, G., Hawkins, A., Graham, N., Blizard, R., & Mann, A. H. (1990). The Gospel Oak study: Prevalence rates of dementia, depression and activity limitations among elderly residents in inner London. *Psychological Medicine, 20,* 137–146.
Lutzky, S. M., & Knight, B. G. (1994). Explaining gender differences in caregiver distress: The roles of emotional attentiveness and coping styles. *Psychology and Aging, 9,* 513–519.
Lyness, J. M., Conwell, Y., & Nelson, J. C. (1992). Suicide attempts in elderly psychiatric inpatients. *Journal of the American Geriatrics Society, 40,* 320–324.
Maes, M., Delange, J., Meltzer, H. Y., Scharpé, S., D'Hondt, P., & Cosyns, P. (1994). Lower degree of esterification of serum cholesterol in depression: Relevance for depression and suicide research. *Acta Psychiatrica Scandinavica, 90,* 252–258.
Maltsberger, J. T. (1991). Psychotherapy with older suicidal patients. *Journal of Geriatric Psychiatry, 24,* 217–234.
Manton, K. G., Blazer, D. G., & Woodbury, M. A. (1987). Suicide in middle age and later life: Sex and race specific life table and cohort analyses. *Journal of Gerontology, 42*(2) 219–227.
Marks, A. (1988–1989). Structural parameters of sex, race, age, and education and their influence on attitudes toward suicide. *Omega: Journal of Death and Dying, 19,* 327–336.
Markus, H., & Oyserman, D. (1989). Gender and thought: The role of the self-concept. In M. Crawford and M. Gentry (Eds.), *Gender and thought: Psychological* Perspectives (pp. 100–127). New York: Springer-Verlag.
Marshall, J. R., Burnett, W., & Brasure, J. (1983). On precipitating factors: Cancer as a cause of suicide. *Suicide and Life-Threatening Behavior, 13,* 15–27.
Marttunen, M. J., Aro, H. M., Henriksson, M. M., & Lönnqvist, J. K. (1991). Mental disorders in adolescent suicide: DSM-III-R Axes I and II diagnoses in suicides among 13- to 19-year olds in Finland. *Archives of General Psychiatry, 48,* 834–839.
McCall, P. L. (1991). Adolescent and elderly white male suicide trends: Evidence of changing well-being? *Journal of Gerontology: Social Sciences, 46,* S42–S51.
McCall, P. L. & Land, K. C. (1994). Trends in white male adolescent, young-adult, and elderly suicide: Are there common underlying structural factors? *Social Science Research, 23,* 57–81.
McIntosh, J. L. (1995). Suicide prevention in the elderly (Age 65–99). *Suicide and Life-Threatening Behavior, 25,* 180–192.
McIntosh, J. L., Pearson, J. L., & Lebowitz, B. D. (1997). Mental disorders of elderly men. In J. I. Kosberg & L. W. Kaye (Eds.), *Elderly men: Special problems and professional challenges* (pp. 193–215). New York: Springer
McIntosh, J. L., Santos, J. F., Hubbard, R. W., & Overholser, J. C. (1994). *Elder suicide: Research theory and treatment.* Washington, DC: American Psychological Association.
Meehan, P. J., Lamb, J. A., Saltzman, L. E., & O'Carroll, P. W. (1992). Attempted suicide among young adults: Progress toward a meaningful estimate of prevalence. *American Journal of Psychiatry, 149,* 41–44.
Meehan, P. J., Saltzman, L. E., & Sattin, R. W. (1991). Suicides among older United States residents: Epidemiologic characteristics and trends. *American Journal of Public Health, 81,* 1198–1200.
Merrill, J., & Owens, J. (1990). Age and attempted suicide. *Acta Psychiatrica Scandinavica, 82,* 385–388.
Montgomery, S. A. (1993). Suicide prevention and serotonergic drugs. *International Clinical Psychopharmacology, 8*(Suppl 2), 83–85.
Morgan, R. E., Palinkas, L. A., Barrett-Connor, E. L., & Wingard, D. L. (1993). Plasma cholesterol and depressive symptoms in older men. *Lancet, 341,* 75–79.
Mościcki, E. K. (1995). Epidemiology of suicide. *International Psychogeriatrics, 7,* 137–148.
Mościcki, E. K., O'Carroll, P., Rae, D. S., Roy, A., Locke, B. Z., & Regier, D. A. (1988). Suicide attempts in the Epidemiologic Catchment Area Study. *Yale Journal of Biology and Medicine, 61,* 259–268.
Muldoon, M. F., Manuck, S. B., & Matthews, K. A. (1990). Lowering cholesterol concentrations and mortality: A quantitative review of primary prevention trials. *British Medical Journal, 301,* 309–314.

Murphy, G. E., & Wetzel, R. D. (1980). Suicide risk by birth cohort in the United States, 1949 to 1974. *Archives of General Psychiatry, 37,* 519–523.

Murphy, G. E., Wetzel, R. D., Robins, E., & McEvoy, L. (1992). Multiple risk factors predict suicide in alcoholism. *Archives of General Psychiatry, 49,* 459–463.

Murphy, H. B. M. (1977). Migration, culture and mental health. *Psychological Medicine, 7,* 677–684.

Nathanson, C. A. (1977). Sex, illness and medical care: A review of data, theory and methods. *Social Science and Statistics, 11,* 13–25.

National Center for Health Statistics (January 18, 1996). Table 292A. Death rates for 282 selected causes, by 5-year age groups, color, and sex: United States, 1979–93.

Newman, S. C., & Dyck, R. J. (1988). On the age–period–cohort analysis of suicide rates. *Psychological Medicine, 18,* 677–681.

Niederehe, G., Cooley, S. G., & Teri, L. (1995). Research and training in clinical geropsychology: Advances and current opportunities. *The Clinical Psychologist, 48,* 37–44.

NIH Consensus Development Panel on Depression in Late Life. (1992). Diagnosis and treatment of depression in late life. *Journal of the American Medical Association, 268,* 1018–1024.

Nolen-Hoeksema, S. (1987). Sex differences in unipolar depression: Evidence and theory. *Psychological Bulletin, 101,* 259–282.

Nolen-Hoeksema, S. (1995). Epidemiology and theories of gender differences in unipolar depression, in M. V. Seeman (Ed.), *Gender and psychopathology* (pp. 63–87). Washington, DC: American Psychiatric Press.

Nolen-Hoeksema, S., Morrow, J., & Fredrickson, B. L. (1993). Response styles and the duration of episodes of depressed mood. *Journal of Abnormal Psychology, 102,* 20–28.

Nordentoft, M., Breum, L, Munck, L., Nordestgaard, A. G., Hunding, A., & Lawsen-Bjaeldager, P. A. (1993). High mortality by natural and unnatural causes: A 10 year follow up study of patients admitted to a poisoning treatment centre after suicide attempts. *British Medical Journal,* 306, 1637–1641.

Nowers, M. (1993). Deliberate self-harm in the elderly: A survey of one London borough. *International Journal of Geriatric Psychiatry, 8,* 609–614.

Nowers, M., & Irish, M. (1988). Trends in reported rates of suicide by self-poisoning in the elderly. *Journal of the Royal College of General Practitioners, 38,* 67–69.

O'Carroll, P. (1989). A consideration of the validity and reliability of suicide mortality data. *Suicide and Life Threatening Behavior, 19,* 1–16.

O'Neal, P., Robins, E., & Schmidt, E. H. (1956). A psychiatric study of attempted suicide in persons over sixty years of age. *Archives of Neurology and Psychiatry, 75,* 275–284.

Osgood, N. J. (1992). Environmental factors in suicide in long-term care facilities. *Suicide and Life-Threatening Behavior, 22,* 98–106.

Osgood, N. J. (1995). Assisted suicide and older people—A deadly combination: Ethical problems in permitting assisted suicide. *Issues in Law & Medicine, 10,* 415–435.

Osgood, N. J., & Brant, B. A. (1900). Suicidal behavior in long-term care facilities. *Suicide and Life-Threatening Behavior, 20,* 113–122.

Paffenbarger, R. S., Jr., Lee, I-M., & Leung, R. (1997). Physical activity and personal characteristics associated with depression and suicide in American college men. *Acta Psychiatrica Scandinavica, 377* (Suppl.), 16–22.

Pearson, J. L., & Conwell, Y. (1995). Suicide in late life: Challenges and opportunities for research. *International Psychogeriatrics, 7,* 131–136

Perez-Stable, E. J., Miranda, J., Muñoz, R., & Ying, Y. (1990). Depression in medical outpatients: Underrecognition and misdiagnosis. *Archives of Internal Medicine, 150,* 1083–1088.

Pierce, D. (1987). Deliberate self-harm in the elderly. *International Journal of Geriatric Psychiatry, 2,* 105–110.

Pokorny, A. D. (1983). Prediction of suicide in psychiatric patients: Report of a prospective study. *Archives of General Psychiatry, 40,* 249–257.

Posner, R. (1995). *Aging and old age.* Chicago: University of Chicago Press.

Quill, T. E. (1991). Death and dignity—a case of individualized decision making. *New England Journal of Medicine, 324,* 691–694.

Regier, D. A., Myers, J. K., Kramer, M., Robins, L. N., Blazer, D. G, Hough, R. L., Eaton, W. W., & Locke, B. Z. (1984). The NIMH Epidemiologic Catchment Area (ECA) Program: historical context, major objectives, and study population characteristics. *Archives of General Psychiatry, 41,* 934–941.

Rich, C. L., Young, D., & Fowler, R. C. (1986). San Diego suicide study: I. Young vs. old subjects. *Archives of General Psychiatry, 43,* 577–582.

Rich, C. L., Young, J. G., Fowler, R. C., Wagner, J., & Black, N. A. (1990). Guns and suicide: Possible effects of some specific legislation. *American Journal of Psychiatry, 147,* 342–346.

Richman, J. (1993). *Preventing elderly suicide: Overcoming personal despair, professional neglect, and social bias.* New York: Springer.

Richman, J. (1996). Psychotherapeutic approaches to the depressed and suicidal older person and family. In G. J. Kennedy (Ed.), *Suicide and depression in late life: Critical issues in treatment, research, and public policy* (pp. 103–117). New York: Wiley.

Rifai, A. H., George, C. J., Stack, J. A., Mann, J. J., & Reynolds, C. F. (1994). Hopelessness in suicide attempters after acute treatment of major depression in late life. *American Journal of Psychiatry, 151,* 1687–1690.

Rifai, A. H., Reynolds, C. F., & Mann, J. J. (1992). Biology of elderly suicide. *Suicide and life-threatening behavior, 22,* 48–61.

Rihmer, Z. (1996). Strategies of suicide prevention: Focus on health care. *Journal of Affective Disorders, 39,* 83–91.

Robinson, D. G., & Spiker, D. G. (1985). Delusional depression: A one year follow-up. *Journal of Affective Disorders, 9,* 79–83.

Romanoski, A. J., Folstein, M. F., Nestadt, G., Chahal, R., Merchant, A., Brown, C. H., Gruenberg, E. M., & McHugh, P. R. (1992). The epidemiology of psychiatrist-ascertained depression and DSM-III depressive disorders. *Psychological Medicine, 22,* 629–655.

Roose, S. P., Glassman, A. H., Walsh, B. T., Woodring, S., & Vital-Herre, J. (1983). Depression, delusions, and suicide. *American Journal of Psychiatry, 140,* 1159–1162.

Rovner, B. W., Kafonek, S., Filipp, L., Lucas, M. J., & Folstein, M. F. (1986). Prevalence of mental illness in a community nursing home. *American Journal of Psychiatry, 143,* 1446–1449.

Runeson, B., & Beskow, J. (1991). Borderline personality disorder in young Swedish suicides. *Journal of Nervous and Mental Disease, 179,* 153–156.

Sackeim, H. A. (1994). Use of electroconvulsive therapy in late-life depression. In L. S. Schneider, C. F. Reynolds, B. D. Lebowitz, & A. J. Friedhoff (Eds.), *Diagnosis and treatment of depression in late life* (pp. 259–277). Washington, DC: American Psychiatric Press.

Sadavoy, J., & Fogel, B. (1992). Personality disorders in old age. In J. E. Birren, R. B. Sloane, & G. D. Cohen (Eds.), *Handbook of mental health and aging* (pp. 433–463). New York: Academic Press.

Sainsbury, P. (1955). *Suicide in London.* Maudsley Monographs no. 1. London: Chapman & Hall.

Salzman, C. (1994). Pharmacological treatment of depression in elderly patients. In L. S. Schneider, C. F.

Reynolds, B. D. Lebowitz, & A. J. Friedhoff (Eds.), *Diagnosis and treatment of depression in late life* (pp. 181–244). Washington, DC: American Psychiatric Association.

Schmid, H., Manjee, K., & Shah, T. (1994). On the distinction of suicide ideation versus attempt in elderly psychiatric inpatients. *Gerontologist, 34,* 332–339.

Schneider, L. (1996). Pharmacological considerations in the treatment of late-life depression. *Americal Journal of Geriatric Psychiatry, 4*(suppl.), S51–S65.

Schneider, L. S. (1996). Biological commonalities among aging, depression, and suicidal behavior. In G. J. Kennedy (Ed.), *Suicide and depression in late life: Critical issues in treatment, research and public policy* (pp. 39–50). New York: Wiley.

Seidlitz, L., Duberstein, P. R., Cox, C., & Conwell, Y. (1995). Attitudes of older people toward suicide and assisted suicide: An analysis of Gallup Poll findings. *Journal of the American Geriatrics Society, 43,* 993–998.

Shneidman, E. (1985). *Definition of suicide.* New York: Wiley.

Shneidman, E. (1986). Some essentials of suicide and some implications for response. In A. Roy (ed.), *Suicide* (pp. 1–16). Baltimore: Williams & Wilkins.

Shneidman, E. (1992). What do suicides have in common? A summary of the psychological approach. In B. Bongar (Ed.), *Suicide: Guidelines for assessment, management and treatment.* New York: Oxford University Press.

Shneidman, E. S., & Farberow, N. L. (1961). Statistical comparisons between attempted and committed suicides. In N. L. Farberow, & E. S. Shneidman (Eds.), *The cry for help* (pp. 19–47). New York: McGraw-Hill.

Shneidman, E. S., Farberow, N., & Litman, R. (1961). The suicide prevention center. In N. Farberow, & E. S. Shneidman (Eds.), *The cry for help* (pp. 6–18). New York: McGraw-Hill.

Sloan, J. H., Rivara, F. P., Reay, D., Ferris, J. A. J., & Kellerman, A. L. (1990). Firearm regulations and rates of suicide. *New England Journal of Medicine, 322,* 369–373.

Sorenson, S. B., & Golding, J. M. (1988). Prevalence of suicide attempts in a Mexican–American population: Prevention implications of immigration and cultural issues. *Suicide and Life-threatening Behavior, 18,* 322–333.

Stenback, A. (1980). Depression and suicidal behavior in old age. In J. E. Birren & R. B. Sloane, (Eds.), *Handbook of mental health and aging* (pp. 616–652). Englewood Cliffs, NJ: Prentice-Hall.

Stillion, J. M., & McDowell, E. E. (1996). *Suicide across the life span: Premature exits* (2nd ed.). Washington, DC: Taylor & Francis.

Strahan, G. W.(1991). *Mental illness in nursing homes: United States, 1985.* Vital Health Statistics 13 (105). DHHS Publication No. (PHS) 91-1766. Hyattsville, MD: National Center for Health Statistics.

Sturm, R., & Wells, K. B. (1995). How can care for depression become more cost-effective. *Journal of the American Medical Association, 273,* 51–58.

Suicide Among Older Persons—United States, 1980n1992. (January 12, 1996). *Morbidity and Mortality Weekly Report, 45*(1), 3–6.

Suicide and the elderly: A population at risk, Senate Hearing, July 30, 1996.

Sullivan, M. D., & Youngner, S. J. (1994). Depression, competence, and the right to refuse lifesaving medical treatment. *American Journal of Psychiatry, 151,* 971–978.

Takahashi, Y., Hirasawa, H., Koyama, K., Asakawa, O., Kido, M., Onse, H., Udagawa, M., Ishikawa, Y., & Uno, M. (1995). Suicide and aging in Japan: An examination of treated elderly attempters. *International Psychogeriatrics, 7,* 239–251.

US Bureau of the Census (1996). *65+ in the United States.* Current Population Reports, Special Studies, P23-(No. 190). Washington, DC: US Government Printing Office.

Vassilas, C. A., & Morgan, H. G. (1994). Elderly suicides' contact with their general practitioner before death. (Letter to the editor) *International Journal of Geriatric Psychiatry, 9,* 1008–1009.

Vieta, E., Nieto, E., Gastó,C., & Cirera, E. (1992). Serious suicide attempts in affective patients. *Journal of Affective Disorders, 24,* 147–152.

Whitlock, F. A. (1978). Suicide, cancer and depression. *British Journal of Psychiatry, 132,* 269–274.

Worthington, J., Fava, M., Davidson, K., Alper, J., Nierenberg, A. A., & Rosenbaum, J. F. (1995). Patterns of improvement in depressive symptoms with fluoxetine treatment. *Psychopharmacology Bulletin, 31,* 223–226.

Yap, P. M. (1958). Suicide in Hong Kong. *Journal of Mental Science, 104,* 266–301.

Younger, S. C., Clark, D. C., Oehmig-Lindroth, R., & Stein, R. J. (1990). Availability of knowledgeable informants for a psychological autopsy study of suicides committed by elderly people. *Journal of the American Geriatrics Society, 38,* 1169–1175.

Zweig, R. A., & Hinrichsen, G. A. (1993). Factors associated with suicide attempts by depressed older adults: A prospective study. *American Journal of Psychiatry, 150,* 1687–1692.

7.12
Personality Disorders

DANIEL L. SEGAL and FREDERICK L. COOLIDGE
University of Colorado, Colorado Springs, CO, USA

7.12.1 INTRODUCTION

7.12.1.1 Evolution of the Diagnoses

Personality disorders (PDs) have been defined as long-standing and long-lasting maladaptive behaviors that seriously impair an individual's ability to perform adequately in a variety of settings including social, occupational, educational, and interpersonal. They have also been called character disorders, and one classic hallmark of the diagnosis has been that the patients are typically unaware or unperturbed about their disorder. Although anecdotal and literary descriptions of individuals who may have had PDs have been with us for thousands of years, the official diagnosis of PDs as a unique and separate diagnostic entity did not officially appear until 1952 with the publication by the American Psychiatric Association (APA) of the *Diagnostic and Statistical Manual of Mental Disorders (DSM)*.

7.12.1.1.1 Diagnostic and Statistical Manual of Mental Disorders

The *Diagnostic and Statistical Manual of Mental Disorders (DSM-I*; APA, 1952) contained seven major diagnostic categories including one named "Personality disorders." PDs were defined as developmental defects or pathological trends in the personality, with little or no sense of subjective distress. They were thought of as lifelong patterns of behavior and not likely to go into remission. Of the 12 PDs in *DSM-I,* four were "cardinal" types, (inadequate, schizoid, cyclothymic, and paranoid) indicating that individuals were rarely, if ever, altered by therapy; four were personality trait disturbances (emotionally unstable, passive–aggressive, compulsive personality, and an "other" personality trait disorder); and finally, four were types of sociopathic personality disturbance (antisocial, dyssocial, sexual deviation, and addiction).

The *DSM-I* descriptions for all 12 main types of PD consisted of, at most, two paragraphs and, most typically, four or five sentences. Although these types provided a major evolution in the diagnosis of PDs, psychological tests for the assessment of PDs lagged for more than 25 years. The *DSM* was widely used and no rival system existed in the USA. The international World Health Organization had produced the only worldwide alternative to the *DSM* and that was the *International Classification of Diseases (ICD),* which included a section on mental disorders. The eighth edition *(ICD-8)* was approved in 1966 and published in 1968. The second edition of the *DSM (DSM-II)* was published in 1968, and was then aligned with the *ICD-8.*

7.12.1.1.2 DSM-II

The *DSM-II* (APA, 1968) listed 10 specific types of PD. Their general description was very brief (two sentences only): "This group of disorders is characterized by deeply ingrained maladaptive patterns of behavior that are perceptibly different in quality from psychotic and neurotic symptoms. Generally, these are lifelong patterns, often recognizable by the time of adolescence or earlier." The 10 specific PDs were as follows: paranoid, cyclothymic, schizoid, explosive, obsessive compulsive, hysterical, asthenic, antisocial, passive–aggressive, and inadequate. One subtle change between *DSM-I* and *DSM-II* was the simple addition that PDs are recognizable by adolescence or earlier; *DSM-I* had mentioned that PDs tended to be lifelong, but there was no mention of when the onset occurred. Both the *DSM-I* and *DSM-II* noted the chronicity but neither noted any changes in PDs as a differential function of lifespan, or type of PD as a function of age.

7.12.1.1.3 DSM-III

The diagnosis of PDs took a quantum leap with the publication of *DSM-III* (APA, 1980). Its diagnostic, paradigmatic center shifted from a psychoanalytic to a more behavioral perspective. It also became multiaxial: major clinical syndromes and symptoms were to be coded on "Axis I" while PDs were to be coded on "Axis II." Also, a specific list of numbered criteria was presented for each PD, and patients had to meet a specified minimum number of criteria before receiving a diagnosis. *DSM-III* also mentioned aging as a factor. It stated "The manifestations of Personality Disorders are generally recognizable by adolescence or earlier and continue throughout most of adult life, though they often become less obvious in middle or old age" (p. 305). For the first time, in the history of the *DSM*, it was hypothesized that PDs may diminish with age.

Another interesting aspect of PD diagnosis in *DSM-III* was that they were grouped into three clusters. The odd or eccentric cluster comprised paranoid, schizoid, and schizotypal types. The dramatic, emotional, or erratic cluster contained histrionic, narcissistic, antisocial, and borderline types. The anxious or fearful cluster was composed of avoidant, dependent, compulsive, and passive–aggressive types.

Overall, *DSM-III* listed 11 specific PDs. Only four of these had remained essentially unchanged from the earlier editions. These were the paranoid, schizoid, antisocial, and passive–aggressive types. Two PDs had name changes (histrionic was formerly hysterical, and compulsive was formerly obsessive compulsive). Four specific disorders were eliminated: cyclothymic, inadequate, explosive, and asthenic. Five new PDs were also added since *DSM-II*: schizotypal, narcissistic, borderline, avoidant, and dependent.

7.12.1.1.4 DSM-III-R

A revised edition of *DSM-III* appeared only seven years later (APA, 1987). The 11 PDs remained, and again they were coded on axis II.

The odd or eccentric cluster of PDs from *DSM-III* officially became "Cluster A" in *DSM-III-R* and still comprised the paranoid, schizoid, and schizotypal types. There were also changes to the criteria for determining each type, although each PD diagnosis still consisted of a group of polythetic criteria. The dramatic, emotional, or erratic cluster became "Cluster B" and still consisted of the histrionic, narcissistic, antisocial, and borderline types. The anxious or fearful cluster became "Cluster C" and still consisted of the avoidant, dependent, and passive–aggressive types. The compulsive PD of *DSM-III* remained in Cluster C but was renamed the obsessive-compulsive PD. That change was highly ironic since in *DSM-I* it was the compulsive PD, in *DSM-II* it was the obsessive-compulsive PD, and in *DSM-III* it was again the compulsive PD. *DSM-III-R* also included two new and potentially controversial PDs that were placed in Appendix A for diagnostic categories needing further study. These were the sadistic and self-defeating types.

In terms of aging and developmental issues, *DSM-III-R* essentially repeated the same hypotheses as *DSM-III*, that is, PDs are generally recognizable by adolescence or earlier, continue through most of adult life, and become less prominent with age. These hypotheses were far too simplistic, however, and raised many more questions than they answered. For example, did all PDs diminish with increasing age? This certainly does not appear to be the case, at least intuitively, for the schizoid and avoidant PDs. Also, why do some PDs diminish with age? Is it simply an artifact of activity level or sociability, or is the phenomenon more complicated, that is, does the abnormal behavior diminishment associated with aging reflect underlying changes in neural substrate or chemical neurotransmitter functioning in the brain?

7.12.1.1.5 DSM-IV

The *DSM* was revised and published again after a further seven year interval (APA, 1994). This edition contained only 10 PDs on Axis II. The passive–aggressive PD was removed from Cluster C and was placed in Appendix B (for further study). An alternative name, negativistic PD, was given to the passive–aggressive PD. A new PD appeared in Appendix B, the depressive PD. The sadistic and self-defeating PDs were dropped completely from the diagnostic manual. The current list of PDs in *DSM-IV* is as follows: Cluster A—the odd or eccentric (paranoid, schizoid, schizotypal); Cluster B—the dramatic, emotional, or erratic (antisocial, borderline, histrionic, narcissistic); Cluster C—the anxious or fearful (avoidant, dependent, obsessive-compulsive); and Appendix B—criteria sets and axes provided for further study (depressive, passive–aggressive [negativistic]).

7.12.1.2 Age and the *DSM*

DSM-IV was the first version of the manual to include a specific section (along with cultural and gender topics) on the developmental issue of aging in the diagnosis of PDs. Again it recorded that a PD is usually recognized by adolescence or early adult life, and, by definition, the onset of a PD must occur before middle age for an official diagnosis to be made although, of course, an actual diagnosis might not be given until later adult life. Also noted in *DSM-IV* is that a PD may be exacerbated by social upheaval, such as the loss of a spouse or a job, although a clear change in personality in middle age or later adult life would more likely be due to a medical condition or substance-related disorder. Since, and again by definition, PDs are "enduring patterns of thinking, feeling and behaving" (APA, 1994, p. 632) they were also hypothesized to be consistent and stable throughout adulthood. However, the *DSM-IV* also noted that the antisocial and borderline PDs "tend to become less evident or to remit with age, whereas this appears to be less true for some other types (e.g., obsessive compulsive and schizotypal PDs)" (p. 632). Empirical research, however, in support or against these latter specific hypotheses has been scarce.

7.12.1.3 Dimensional vs. Categorical Classification

The diagnostic philosophy contained within *DSM-IV* is that PDs are distinct clinical categories or syndromes. Theoretically, these clinical syndromes form discrete entities of abnormal behavior patterns, and again, theoretically, they would be unrelated to normal personality dimensions, for example, the extraversion–introversion dimension. Currently, a more attractive and parsimonious theory is the dimensional diagnostic approach to PDs in which the PDs are viewed as maladaptive variations of normal personal traits. Thus, in the dimensional classification approach, normal and abnormal personality behaviors are simply points along a behavioral continuum. Typically, the extreme points at either end of a continuum might be reflective of a PD. For example, an extreme extrovert might be characteristic of the histrionic PD while an extreme introvert might be characteristic of a schizoid PD.

In the late twentieth century, dimensional trait research approaches have focused on finding the number of factors minimally required to describe an individual's personality, and whether those same dimensions can describe both normal and abnormal behavior. Eysenck (1978) originally proposed a two-factor model, extroversion and neuroticism, and then expanded his model to include a third factor, psychoticism. His model clearly covers the abnormal personality, although perhaps at the expense of normal personality constructs.

The most famous model of personality is that of Carl Jung from 1924 (1971). He conceptualized the personality as being fourfold: (i) one's preference to focus on the inner or outer world, (ii) how one perceives or acquires information, (iii) how one makes decisions, and (iv) how one orients one's self towards the outer world. This model was operationalized in a psychometric test, the Myers–Briggs Type Indicator (Myers, 1962), with four bipolar dimensions: (i) extraversion–introversion, (ii) sensing–intuiting, (iii) thinking–feeling, and (iv) judging–perceiving. This model, however, appears to be biased oppositely to Eysenck's model. The Myers–Briggs model appears to be more useful in explaining the normal personality rather than the abnormal one.

Norman (1963) developed and organized a pool of 2800 personality descriptors into sets such as states, traits, and roles. Based on his work, McCrae and Costa (1986, 1989) began a prodigious flow of research into a five-factor model describing both normal and abnormal personality; specifically, this included neuroticism, extraversion, openness, agreeableness, and conscientiousness. However, their model has been criticized for lacking diagnostic utility with regard to the *DSM-IV* PDs, for being unclear as to whether they were describing five, six, or even seven factors to account for PDs (Coolidge et al., 1994), for a lack of empirical research to support their claim that their model accounts for abnormal behavior, and the overgeneralization from statistical techniques (Millon & Davis, 1996). Furthermore, Kernberg (1996) wrote: "To develop factorial profiles for each personality disorder on the basis of those five factors has an eerie quality of unreality for the experienced clinician" (p. 107).

Cloninger (1987) originally proposed a three-factor model of personality based on three brain neurotransmitters: dopamine, serotonin, and norepinephrine. Later, he expanded his model to seven factors, operationalizing the measurement of his model with the Temperament and Character Inventory (TCI; Cloninger 1986, 1987; Cloninger, Przybeck, Svrakic, & Wetzel, 1994). This theory will be discussed further later in this chapter. By contrast, Cattell identified 16 source traits from data that he identified from surface traits, and he operationalized his theoretical personality structure into the Sixteen Personality Factor Questionnaire (16PF; Cattell, Saunders, & Stice, 1950). The 16PF has been a popular instrument in personality research, although more popular in nonclinical, rather than clinical, settings.

Thus, although *DSM-IV* approaches clinical diagnoses from a categorical perspective, most empirical personality research of abnormal behavior, particularly PDs, has entailed the use of dimensional models, typically ranging from 3 to 16 core factors or personality traits. However, little research has been devoted to how aging might affect these core traits and concomitant behaviors.

7.12.2 ETIOLOGY

Enduring, inflexible, and pervasive patterns of maladaptive behavior, coupled with an early onset, suggest that PDs may have an inheritable component. Thus, most conceptions about the etiology of PDs are based upon both biological and environmental contributions, although the theories vary in the emphasis placed upon these two components. Four major etiological theories, reflecting these ideas, will now be reviewed.

7.12.2.1 Rutter's Theory of Temperaments, Personality, and Personality Disorders

Rutter (1987) noted that temperaments are hypothesized to be biologically inherited predispositions for behaving in particular ways, and they emerge early in life. He specifically hypothesized, that temperaments were limited. According to Rutter, there are not a particularly large number of temperaments influencing behavior; such temperaments are nonmotivational and noncognitive. The search for the core number of temperaments may parallel the search for the core number of personality traits or factors, with the number varying from as few as three to as many as 16. There is a fairly substantial body of empirical research in support of heritability of temperaments and their enduring influence on behavior (e.g., McGue, Bacon, & Lykken, 1993; Plomin, Chipuer, & Loehlin, 1990; Thomas & Chess, 1977). Relatively undisputed is the hypothesis that the extraversion–introversion dimensional trait is reflective of a prominent temperament. Emotionality and activity levels have also received strong support as temperaments.

According to Rutter's theory, this limited number of temperaments helps to form what comes to be recognized as the individual's unique personality, although the personality is much broader than a simple collection of temperamental traits. Furthermore, Rutter proposes that as the individual interacts with family and society, these temperamental features may become reinforced by the social environment, thus producing the long-standing, enduring patterns of behavior that are characteristic of adult personalities. However, when particular temperamental features appear in the extreme or provoke unusual responses from the individual's environment, then PDs may result. The temperamental basis of a PD, along with its reinforcement history, therefore accounts for its enduring and inflexible nature.

Rutter's theory is confined to speculations about early childhood through adulthood, but there is little mention of issues related to later adulthood and the aged. Nevertheless, his theory can be used to generate a few hypotheses. Rutter argued that several longitudinal studies have shown "heterotypic" continuity, meaning that the phenotypic quality of the behavior changes over time while individual differences remain stable. Thus, early childhood passivity is predictive of noncompetitiveness in later adult life (Kagan & Moss, 1962). With respect to PDs, therefore, it is possible that the elderly should perhaps be evaluated according to different criteria or, at the least, the PD criteria should be examined for changes as a function of middle and later adulthood.

7.12.2.2 A Cognitive Theory of Personality Disorders

Pretzer and Beck (1996) have described difficulties in the psychotherapeutic treatment of patients with PDs, and they argue that even cognitive–behavioral treatments may prove counterproductive or ineffective if the therapist fails to recognize the specific nature of the PD and fails to modify treatment accordingly. In terms of the etiology of PDs from a cognitive perspective it is assumed that PDs develop phenomenologically, that is, through the person's view of their world. Thus, an individuals' perception of stimuli interacts with their prior beliefs and assumptions. An individual may react consciously and logically resulting in the observed emotional and behavioral responses to the perceived stimuli. However, prior misbeliefs (delusions) and false assumptions about the world may lead to inappropriate or maladaptive emotional responses and behavior. An individual may also commit "systematic errors in reasoning" which Pretzer and Beck labeled "cognitive distortions" that also result in inappropriate and maladaptive responses. They noted the prominence of at least 12 common cognitive distortions, such as viewing events in terms of mutually exclusive categories (dichotomous thinking) or focusing on one aspect of a complex situation to the exclusion of others (selective abstraction).

According to the theory, individuals are also likely to respond unconsciously or automatically to perceived stimuli. These ways of acting may have once been adaptive in an evolutionary sense. Beck (1992) has termed them "primeval strategies," and further, Pretzer and Beck (1996) have proposed that "human social change has outstripped physiological evolution [such that] we may well have also retained some biases in information processing that now tend to be maladaptive" (pp. 44–45). Thus, they argue that our inherited predispositions poorly fit some of the demands of modern society. For example, an earlier adaptive primeval strategy of predatory behavior may lead to the development of the antisocial PD, the earlier help-eliciting behavior may now result in the dependent PD, and earlier competitive behavior may now result in the narcissistic PD.

Nevertheless, Pretzer and Beck (1996) have argued that PD phenomena can be understood and treated without regard to inherited or inborn defects, and that inherited predispositions towards the development of PDs has not been clearly established. Moreover, their contribution appears neither simple nor straightforward. Overall, cognitive theory tends to emphasize that interactions between predispositions, the environment, and significant life events shape development rather than predispositions alone, and it is not external events that shape the personality but an individuals perception of those events that forms an individual's thinking and consequent behavior.

Although Pretzer and Beck's cognitive theory has a developmental perspective, it emphasizes early childhood influences upon the adult personality. Even though they hypothesize that traumatic experiences, either singular or recurrent, may alter an individual's personality over time, they do not address the influence of traumatic experiences upon the later adult personality. In fact, it could be easily hypothesized that 80 years of traumatic experiences should far outweigh a singular early traumatic experience. However, dramatic adult personality change is highly unlikely except for clear physiological reasons (e.g., brain disease, toxins, etc.). Thus, this aspect of their theory neglects personality issues of middle and late adulthood.

7.12.2.3 An Evolutionary Theory of Personality Disorders

Millon and Davis (1996) have proposed a highly complex and sophisticated evolutionary theory of PDs that attempts to link both normal and abnormal behavior to both phylogenetic and ontogenetic processes. Their theory explains why early experiences play a more profound role in the development of the personality than later experiences, drawing upon diverse sources of evidence such as Freud's writings about the influence of early childhood on the later adult personality and upon ethologists' observations of critical imprinting periods in maturational development.

Central to Millon and Davis' evolutionary theory are the hypotheses that four evolutionarily based "bipolarities" interact with four stages of early neuropsychological development to produce stable and consistent patterns of behavior that can either be adaptive or maladaptive. These bipolarities are pain–pleasure, active–passive, self–other, and thinking–feeling. The four bipolarities also reflect the parallel evolutionary processes of existence, adaptation, replication, and abstraction, respectively. The four parallel neuropsychological stages are sensory–attachment, sensorimotor–autonomy, pubertal–gender identity, and intracortical–initiative, respectively. Although their theory is comprehensive and far-reaching, they do not address PD issues of the elderly. Nor, despite the magnitude of their theory, does it offer much heuristically for the differential waxing or waning of PDs in the elderly.

7.12.2.4 Cloninger's Biosocial Theory and Personality Disorders

Cloninger (1987) has proposed a biosocial theory which asserts that phenotypic personality traits are the product of the interaction of genetically determined brain systems and environmental influences. He offered an operationalization of his theory in the TCI (Cloninger et al., 1994). This comprises seven major dimensions. There are four, purportedly genetically independent, trait dimensions: novelty seeking, harm avoidance, reward dependence, and persistence. The first three dimensions form the physiological component of the biosocial theory, and are identified with three primary monamine neurotransmitters: dopamine, serotonin, and norepinephrine. The first three traits are linked with these three neurotransmitters, respectively. Cloninger hypothesized that these three form neural temperaments which serve as discrete systems for the activation, inhibition, and maintenance of behavior in response to novelty, danger, and reward. The fourth character dimension, persistence, was not thought to be associated with a specific neurotransmitter. The decision to classify it as an autonomous factor in the model was based upon empirical statistical factor analyses.

The TCI also assesses three character dimensions: self-directedness, cooperativeness, and self-transcendence. These dimensions became later additions to the TCI to account for behavior not otherwise described by the initial three physiological dimensions and in order to determine whether a PD was present or not. The four temperament dimensions were designed to delineate clinical subtypes of personality but it appeared that they did not discriminate those individuals with PDs from those without PDs.

Another interesting feature of Cloninger's theory is that it attempts to link two primary components of human memory, procedural and declarative, to the formation of the seven trait and character dimensions. His theory postulates that the development of the four trait dimensions involves preconceptual responses to perceptual stimuli. Learned behavior patterns require the stimulus input of perceptual experience, but do not require conscious recall to replicate the behavior, which is the definition of procedural memory. The declarative memory system processes experience that is represented as words, images, or symbols. Once encoded, concept-based memories can be consciously retrieved, declared verbally, and willfully acted upon. Cloninger hypothesized that his three character dimensions reflected, in behaviorally expressed form, the information processed by the declarative memory system.

To account for PDs, Cloninger proposed that particular combinations of trait dimensions were predictive of various PDs. For example, he thought that the combination of high novelty seeking (high dopamine), low harm avoidance (low serotonin), and high reward dependence (high norepinephrine) was indicative of the histrionic PD, while the antisocial PD would be high on novelty seeking, and low on both harm avoidance and reward dependence. Presumably, all of the PDs would be low on the three character dimensions of self-directedness, cooperativeness, and selftranscendence.

Because the TCI is a relatively new test, there is a current lack of empirical evidence in support of Cloninger's biosocial theory. However, the previous version of the TCI (with only three trait dimensions) did receive modest but not overwhelming support in a few studies (e.g.,

Pfohl, Black, Noyes, Kelly, & Blum, 1990; Ruegg et al., 1993). Coolidge and Griego's (1996) study of the TCI with a new PD test (Coolidge Axis II Inventory; Coolidge & Merwin, 1992) provided moderate support for Cloninger's theory in a sample of 164 college students.

To date, Cloninger's biosocial theory makes no predictions about PDs as a function of the aging process. However, his biosocial theory is certainly fruitful for speculation. For example, there is substantial evidence (e.g., Morgan, May, & Finch, 1987) that there are normal age-related changes in the dopamine systems in humans and other mammals. There is an age-related, but not disease-related, loss in dopamine and its metabolites, a loss of dopaminergic neurons, and a decrease in particular types of dopamine receptors. Severe dopamine losses (greater than 75%) are characteristic of Parkinson's disease. Interestingly and anecdotally, these age-related losses of dopamine may, in part, account for the observation that some elderly persons do not typically engage in high novelty seeking behaviors. It appears that there are few or no age-related changes in the serotonin systems in humans. Although there appears to be a modest reduction in particular serotonin receptor sites, serotonin levels appear to be stable across the lifespan. Major serotonin level declines and serotonin receptor site losses are, however, indicative of Alzheimer's disease. Evidence regarding age-associated decreases in norepinephrine is scant.

In summary, it appears that Cloninger's biosocial theory is provocative and capable of generating a plethora of hypotheses concerning both pathological (PDs and brain syndromes) and nonpathological behaviors in the elderly. However, neurotransmitter systems in the brain are extremely complex and interactive, and it is doubtful whether singular descriptions of human behavior (e.g., novelty seeking) are based upon singular neurotransmitting systems. Furthermore, it is popularly suspected that many more neurotransmitters than have presently been discovered are yet to be discovered. Because of this, Cloninger's theory, at least in regard to PDs, may only be speciously complex and sophisticated.

7.12.2.5 Relevance of Personality Disorder Theories to the Elderly

It appears that many of the popular theories of PDs directly ignore issues related to aging and the elderly. Most of the theories, however, are useful in generating hypotheses about PDs in the elderly, regarding etiology, diagnosis, and treatment. For example, Rutter's hypothesis of heterotypic continuity in the lifespan is useful diagnostically, and it appears that comparisons of younger and older adults in terms of the *DSM* criteria for PDs may be useful. Pretzer and Beck's cognitive theory is provocative in that it appears to minimize the influences of traumatic experiences in the elderly. It appears that it would be fruitful to examine how, why, or if traumatic experiences vary from childhood to later adulthood. Also, it might be useful to determine whether and to what extent traumatic experiences differentially affect older people, that is, what characteristics do individuals possess that make them vulnerable or invulnerable to traumatic experience? Are there ways of inoculating the vulnerable? Are the elderly, as a group, more or less vulnerable? Also, Pretzer and Beck's primeval strategies are fascinating as a basis for the development of differences among the various PDs. Are there PDs unique to the elderly? If there are, do they have a primeval strategic basis?

Millon and Davis' evolutionary theory also does not address aging related issues. However, the four bipolarities (pain–pleasure, active–passive, self–other, and thinking–feeling) should be examined with respect to aging. Are there differences between younger and older persons? Also, evolutionary theories, in general, tend to ignore the latter end of the lifespan. After adaptation and replication, are humans simply devoid of evolutionary purpose? Do dramatic behaviors such as memory loss in the elderly have evolutionary meaning? What evolutionary purpose does personality stability possess?

Cloninger's biosocial theory can also be used to generate hypotheses about personality stability and change, and PDs in the elderly. To what extent do the chemical neurotransmitters in the brain affect behavior differentially in the elderly? How do declines in the neurotransmitter systems affect behavior in the elderly? Can classes of behaviors be directly linked to neurotransmitter systems in the elderly? If PDs are created by varying levels of neurotransmitters, can chemical interventions be developed to "cure" PDs?

This section on the etiology of PDs is far from an exhaustive review. However, a number of trends clearly emerge. The popular theories concerning PD attempt to integrate the biological and evolutionary factors with environmental influences. Most of these theories virtually, if not totally, ignore issues related to aging. It appears, however, that one can generate a host of provocative hypotheses from the theories with regard to aging issues, and psychologists should be encouraged to do so.

7.12.3 EPIDEMIOLOGY

Despite the growing body of literature about PDs in the elderly, there is a striking paucity of epidemiological and prevalence data for these interesting and challenging disorders in the older population. Moreover, reported rates for these conditions are far more inconsistent and controversial than estimates for more widely studied disorders, such as schizophrenia, cognitive impairment, or major depression. Such inconsistencies illustrate the difficulty clinicians and researchers have in accurately diagnosing PDs in the elderly.

Overall, surveys conducted in the 1980s show that prevalence rates for PDs in the older adult community range from as low as 2.8% to as high as 11% (Cohen, 1990). Prevalence figures are even more varied when mental health settings are considered. For example, Mezzich, Fabrega, Coffman, and Glavin (1987) conducted a retrospective chart review, and found that 5.1% of a sample of mixed inpatient and outpatient elders ($N=494$) manifested PDs. Casey and Schrodt (1989) reviewed charts of 100 consecutive admissions to a geriatric psychiatry unit and found that 7% received a diagnosis of PD as determined by psychiatrist rating. In the largest retrospective study to date, Fogel and Westlake (1990) ascertained prevalence of characterological disorder in 2332 older inpatients suffering from major depression. Again, diagnoses were assigned by attending psychiatrists, with results showing a 15.8% PD rate. In a related study, Kunik et al. (1993) evaluated depressed elderly inpatients and found that 37 of 154 (24%) met criteria for a PD based on consensus diagnosis among psychiatrists. Similarly, Thompson, Gallagher, and Czirr (1988) showed that 33% of depressed elderly clients participating in a psychotherapy outcome study were diagnosed with a PD. More recently, Molinari and Marmion (1995) used a structured PD scale to assess PDs in elderly patients with mood disorders, revealing a 63% prevalence rate.

Limitations of many older epidemiological studies include their use of retrospective chart assessments, reliance on clinical judgment in assigning diagnoses, and the absence of reliability or validity checks of PD diagnoses. Although the National Institute of Mental Health Epidemiological Catchment Area programs were successful at providing quality epidemiological data for many common mental disorders, the PDs (with the exception of antisocial PD) were neglected in these surveys. Clearly, large-scale cross-sectional and longitudinal studies that employ standardized, objective, and validated diagnostic instruments, such as structured interviews, are warranted to fully investigate the prevalence of PD in the aged.

Other factors have also hampered epidemiological studies of PDs. For example, estimates of PDs have fluctuated greatly depending on the type of sample (e.g., general population, medical patients, psychiatric patients), method of diagnosis (e.g., clinician diagnosis, self-report personality inventory, structured interview), and type of research design (e.g., retrospective chart review, crosssectional, longitudinal). Furthermore, different diagnostic criteria have been employed in different studies, including research diagnostic criteria (Spitzer, Endicott, & Robins, 1978) and various versions of the *DSM* system. Spar and LaRue (1990) suggest that "Few data have been gathered on Axis II disorders in elderly patients, in part because most of the personality disorders in *DSM-III-R* have not been defined long enough for thorough studies to take place" (p. 180). Indeed, diagnostic systems prior to *DSM-III* did not provide well-operationalized or specific criteria for each particular PD, and reliability of diagnosis was notoriously poor. Since early investigations of PDs in the elderly utilized classification systems that are dissimilar from contemporary *DSM-III-R* and *DSM-IV* conceptualizations (Kroessler, 1990), meaningful comparison of prior and more current data is difficult. Despite gaps in the epidemiological research base, it can be concluded that PDs in the elderly are not uncommon, and that many clients so disordered are presently on the caseloads of diverse mental health practitioners.

Another epidemiological issue concerns differential rates for PDs among older males and females. According to the *DSM-IV*, borderline, dependent, and histrionic PDs are diagnosed more frequently in females, while antisocial and obsessive-compulsive PDs, and, to a lesser extent paranoid PD, are more common in males. However, it is unclear to what extent these differences apply to older individuals who typically were not adequately represented in the research studies from which conclusions about sex differences were drawn. Hard data are also lacking about the stability or change in PD symptoms as one enters old age. As noted earlier, *DSM-IV* describes a PD as a lifelong, stable pattern of thinking, feeling, and behaving. However, it also suggests that some disorders (e.g., antisocial and borderline) tend to remit with age, while others may exacerbate (e.g., obsessive-compulsive and schizotypal). However, these hypotheses should be empirically tested.

Tyrer (1988) investigated empirically the relationship between PD and increasing age and suggested that "mature" forms of PD such as obsessive-compulsive, paranoid, schizoid, and schizotypal remain stable with age, while more "immature" or flamboyant disorders such as antisocial, borderline, histrionic, and narcissistic are likely to decrease with age. This observation certainly has some anecdotal support, culled from clinicians with vast experience in the diagnosis and assessment of older persons. For some elderly clients, their current personality and social functioning appears markedly improved compared to the interpersonal chaos and occupational disaster characteristic of their earlier years. On the other hand, some older clients show exacerbation in their personality styles. In an interesting study, Coolidge, Burns, Nathan, and Mull (1992) examined these questions about course of PDs by directly comparing PD rates in younger and older subjects. Their results showed that the elderly were significantly more obsessive-compulsive and schizoid than their younger counterparts (based on mean T-scores), and were equal on avoidant and dependent PD scales. Although this cross-sectional study is intriguing, definitive research about the long-term course of individual PDs is lacking. Longitudinal studies will provide the clearest evidence about this issue, but these studies are obviously time-consuming, expensive, and difficult to carry out. However, information is sorely needed about this important conceptual and clinical issue if we are to better understand our elderly clients.

7.12.4 DIAGNOSIS

7.12.4.1 General Issues

The awareness and importance of PDs as a diagnostic category took a major leap in 1980 with the publication of *DSM-III*, with its innovative multiaxial diagnostic system. Clinical syndromes (located on Axis I) were separated from long-standing PDs (located on Axis II). Since that time, PD diagnosis has been fraught with controversy and difficulty, with the psychiatric community expressing grave (and justified) concerns about the apparent lack of reliability for these disorders. In general, the reliability of measurement refers to consistency, replicability, or stability. In the context of psychiatric diagnosis, reliability often refers to the extent of agreement between two raters concerning presence or absence of a psychiatric diagnosis. If different diagnosticians cannot agree about particular diagnoses, then those diagnostic categories are, at best, of limited value and, at worst, virtually meaningless. A full discussion of reliability issues and procedures is provided by Segal (1997) and Segal, Hersen, and Van Hasselt (1994). In fact, classic investigations of inter-rater reliability for diagnosis of *DSM-III* PDs produced results that were unacceptably poor (see Mellsop, Varghese, Joshua, & Hicks, 1982; Spitzer, Forman, & Nee, 1979). Moreover, these values were considerably lower than values for major axis I disorders, such as depression and schizophrenia.

The pervasive lack of agreement between clinicians and researchers when diagnosing PDs is particularly troublesome, given that reliability is a necessary, but insufficient, prerequisite for validity (Grove, 1987). Fortunately, there recently has been much improvement in this area with the publication of *DSM-III-R* and *DSM-IV*. In an effort to enhance reliability (and validity) of diagnosis, these classification systems have provided more specific and behaviorally-operationalized trait criteria for each particular PD. Following the development of better diagnostic criteria, several structured diagnostic interviews (discussed later) were created and refined; this further enhanced the ability to diagnose PDs consistently.

Whereas reliability refers to reproducibility and stability, the validity of psychiatric diagnosis refers to the extent to which a diagnosis actually measures what it purports to measure. The issue here is one of diagnostic accuracy and meaningfulness. Unfortunately, the validity of PD diagnosis is much harder to gauge and document accurately; thus, it represents a formidable challenge for clinicians and researchers alike. A common strategy employed is to compare PD diagnoses generated by a structured interview with diagnoses from another source, such as a clinical interview, chart review, or other testing procedure. However, such practice is far from ideal, mainly because these other diagnostic measures often suffer from questionable reliability and validity in the first place. Indeed, a major problem encountered by clinical researchers interested in the validity of PDs concerns the lack of a solid criterion diagnosis, a sort of "gold standard," against which to compare an interview generated diagnosis. This inadequacy severely restricts conclusions drawn from many validity studies.

The reader should be aware that the current *DSM-IV* Axis II system, while considerably better than its predecessors, is far from ideal. PD diagnoses generally are still less reliable than those of the major Axis I conditions, and most Axis II disorders show extensive overlapping, with individuals typically meeting criteria for several PDs at one point in time (Oldham et al., 1992). This extensive pattern of comorbidity and the fact that "pure" types are rarely encountered has fueled debate and discussion among clinical researchers as to the validity of categorical diagnosis of PDs in the first place (Frances, 1982; Oldham et al.). As cogently noted by Oldham et al. most studies

> have found that at least 50% of patients have two or more coexisting PDs. It may be that a dimensional approach is better suited for Axis II disorders than a categorical one that results in an unwieldy list of presumably comorbid diagnoses to describe "character pathology" in a given patient. (p. 213)

Usefulness of the three clusters (odd–eccentric, dramatic–erratic, anxious–fearful) proposed by the *DSM* system has also been criticized (e.g., Morey, 1988). Unquestionably, accurate diagnosis of PDs in any age group is still widely viewed as a complex and challenging task.

7.12.4.2 Personality Disorder Diagnosis and the Elderly

In the elderly population, diagnosis of PDs is complicated by several additional factors. First, diagnosis is affected by the longtime, widely held (albeit erroneous) belief that personality dysfunction either was not present or was not a significant mental health problem for older people. With this diagnostic mindset, PD symptoms may be minimized or overlooked altogether by the clinician. In fact, some researchers have suggested that diverse service providers to older individuals are biased against diagnosing PDs or defining problems as characterological (Kroessler, 1990; Rose, Soares, & Joseph, 1993; Rosowsky & Gurian, 1992). According to Rose et al. (1993) the chronicity, rigidity, and resistance to intervention attributed to individuals carrying a PD diagnosis often make the client seem "hopeless" and service providers feel "helpless." Professionals may lack appropriate knowledge about the manifestations of PDs in older adults, and consequently may fail to address this component in their assessment procedures.

Second, misdiagnoses often occur because individuals with PDs often present clinically with comorbid symptoms of major axis I disorders, most notably depression and anxiety, which are more easily recognized by both clients and service providers. Typically, clients view such acute symptoms as distressing, while lacking insight into their maladaptive personality style. In some cases, the blatant psychiatric symptoms may be consequences of the chronic interpersonal and occupational difficulties experienced by those suffering from dysfunctional personalities, but this cause–effect relationship is difficult to evaluate. Moreover, many clinicians simply are more experienced with the diagnosis and treatment of major mental illnesses, not PDs.

A third obstacle to the accurate diagnosis of PDs in older adults is that some signs of personality disturbance (e.g., avoidance, dependency, social withdrawal, odd thinking, irritability, eccentric behavior, or emotional lability) are wrongly perceived by some young and old individuals as "normal" in the aged population, or they are dismissed as being attributed to "old age." Such faulty assumptions almost certainly preclude appropriate assessment and diagnosis.

A fourth impediment to diagnosis is that *DSM-IV* criteria for some PDs have limited relevance or applicability to aged clients given their unique physical, cognitive, and social circumstances. Just as somatic problems may confound diagnosis of Axis I disorders in older individuals (e.g., depression, or panic disorder), Kroessler (1990) notes similar difficulties with the diagnosis of PDs in the aged. For example, he points out that many symptoms of a dysfunctional personality (e.g., aggressiveness, impulsiveness, brawling, child-beating, recklessness, and promiscuity) require physical activity. These criteria may not be applicable to some older adults for purely biological reasons in terms of the expected declines in energy, strength, and mobility due to normal aging. Despite this, however, such symptoms do appear in some elderly persons. For borderline PD in particular, many classic symptoms of this condition in younger persons (e.g., impulsive acting-out, sexual promiscuity, self-mutilating behaviors, and substance abuse) are likely to decrease in intensity with increasing age and physical/social limitations, although the underlying psychodynamics remain present (Fogel & Westlake, 1990; Rosowsky & Gurian, 1991, 1992). Reflecting on the fact that older clients meet fewer criteria for borderline PD than they did as younger clients, Rosowsky and Gurian (1991) propose that this difference may actually be due to inadequate criteria for the elderly rather than the lack of the disorder. We suggest that these "age-biases" in diagnostic criteria also apply to other personality types. Alternatively, some symptoms of apparent personality dysfunction in older individuals may actually be due to age-related social and biological factors, rather than a disordered personality. For example: social withdrawal (characteristic of schizoid and avoidant PD) may increase due to physical disabilities and transportation problems experienced by some elderly people; perceptions of exploitation by others (characteristic of paranoid PD) may be attributable to realistic concerns about crimes and scams directed at the elderly; and impulsivity, emotional lability, poor social judgment, and uncontrollable rage (characteristic of borderline and histrionic PDs) may actually be due to frontal lobe damage caused by vascular accidents in some older persons.

Fifth, a major requirement for the diagnosis of any PD is the experience of clinically significant distress or impairment in social or occupational functioning (*DSM-IV*, criterion C). However, as individuals age, they work less frequently and have smaller social networks due to sensory and physical disabilities, as well as the cumulative loss of family and friends through death or relocation. Thus, the requirement of social/occupational impairment may preclude accurate PD diagnosis in older adults whose social world and work opportunities are much different from their younger counterparts upon whom many taxonomies are based. As age-related behavior changes may either mimic or mask PD symptoms we concur with Kroessler (1990) and also argue for inclusion of age-associated criteria in the diagnostic guidelines.

Several case reports have appeared in the literature documenting the unique diagnostic and intervention challenges faced by mental health professionals. Specifically, a vivid case description has been reported for borderline PD (Siegel & Small, 1986). More recently, case examples of antisocial (Howard, Bandyopadhyay, & Cook, 1992), histrionic, borderline, and avoidant PDs (Rose et al., 1993) in old age have been presented. It is obvious, however, that systematic research is necessary to clarify clinical manifestations and develop clearer profiles of each PD in the aged. As noted previously, longitudinal studies following personality-disordered individuals into later life are needed to assess changes over time in symptom patterns and personality characteristics of older individuals. It is probable that some symptoms are robust, some appear in muted format in the aged, and some are irrelevant. Given the diagnostic problems highlighted in this account, the need for elder-specific diagnostic criteria is underscored. For example, the number needed to assign a diagnosis (e.g., five out of eight for histrionic PD) may be modified (usually lowered) to improve diagnostic accuracy and application to the elderly. This issue can be determined empirically by validity studies assessing cut-off rates as the criteria requirements are adjusted. When evaluating and diagnosing PDs in the elderly, clinicians are also encouraged to recognize and be sensitive to potential age-biases in the *DSM-IV* system. In conclusion, a significant ramification of these diagnostic difficulties is that determination of the most appropriate form of intervention is often obfuscated. Treatment is often not indicated if the behavior is considered a "normal" concomitant of the aging process; or, when intervention is applied, it solely targets the blatant anxiety or depressive symptoms, while the etiologically significant underlying personality dysfunction is minimized, or even worse, completely ignored.

7.12.5 ASSESSMENT

Accurate assessment of PDs is a critical component of patient care given the fact that most clinicians working with older individuals will have some clients with PDs on their caseload. As diagnostic criteria for PDs has become more refined in recent years, the assessment of PDs has also flourished. Several instruments are available to the clinician, and these can be divided into two broad categories: self-report inventories and structured clinical interviews. Both assessment approaches are widely applied in clinical and research contexts, and both have their own advantages and disadvantages. On the one hand, structured interviews generally are more reliable and allow consideration of important observational data, but they require extensive training and experience on the part of the interviewer, and can be lengthy to conduct especially with severely disordered clients. On the other hand, self-report personality inventories are easy to administer and take less time, but in some cases tend to overpathologize and are prone to deviant test-taking response behaviors. This chapter now focuses on the description and development of several popular self-report inventories and structured interviews, as well as the application of these devices to older adults.

7.12.5.1 Self-report Personality Inventories

Instruments to be reviewed in this chapter include the *Millon Clinical Multiaxial Inventory-III (MCMI-III*; Millon, 1994), the *Personality Diagnostic Questionnaire-4 (PDQ-4*; Hyler, 1994), and the *Coolidge Axis II Inventory (CATI*; Coolidge, 1984; Coolidge & Merwin, 1992). These instruments are among the most commonly utilized tools for measuring *DSM-IV* PDs. Other self-report instruments have been developed to measure PDs, including the Wisconsin Personality Disorders Inventory (Klein et al., 1993). Also, Morey, Waugh, and

Blashfield (1985) have derived PD scales from the original Minnesota Multiphasic Personality Inventory (MMPI; Hathaway & McKinley, 1983). The MMPI, and its revision, the MMPI-II (Hathaway & McKinley, 1989), are not true measures of *DSM*-based PDs. Rather, they evaluate personality traits, symptom profiles, and axis I disorders. A full review of all measures is beyond the scope of this chapter. Therefore, we will restrict our reviews to *MCMI-III, PDQ-4,* and *CATI.*

7.12.5.1.1 Millon Clinical Multiaxial Inventory-III

The original *MCMI* (Millon, 1983) has undergone two revisions, that is, *MCMI-II* (Millon, 1987) and *MCMI-III* (Millon, 1994). *MCMI-III* is a 175-item, true-false, self-report inventory specifically designed to assess PDs. This instrument is widely used in research and clinical activities, and its taxonomy is "aligned" with *DSM-IV*. The *MCMI-III* includes 14 personality pattern scales (Axis-II related) including: schizoid, avoidant, depressive, dependent, histrionic, narcissistic, antisocial, aggressive (sadistic), compulsive, passive–aggressive (negativistic), self-defeating, schizotypal, borderline, and paranoid. Additionally, 10 symptom scales (Axis-I related) are provided, covering moderate clinical presentations (e.g., anxiety, dysthymia, alcohol dependence) and severe symptoms (e.g., thought disorder, major depression). It has three validity scales designed to detect random or confused response patterns and defensiveness. The *MCMI* is designed to be given only to those suspected of having a PD, and thus, should not be used for differential diagnosis in nonclinical populations. The *MCMI* has been the focus of numerous publications since its development in 1967, and earlier versions have been shown to have good psychometric properties, although it is said to be more reliable in diagnosing among PDs than in differentiating between clinical syndromes (Millon, 1992). Psychometric properties of the *MCMI-III* are currently being evaluated.

7.12.5.1.2 Personality Diagnostic Questionnaire-4

The original *PDQ* was revamped to match changes in the *DSM-III-R* system, and was renamed the *PDQ-R* (Hyler & Rieder, 1987). A newer version of *PDQ-R* has been created (*PDQ-4*; Hyler, 1994) and this is now consistent with *DSM-IV*. The *PDQ-4* assesses the 10 standard PDs in the *DSM-IV*. It contains 85 self-report, true-false items and takes about 30 minutes to complete. It has two validity scales: one detects underreporting of psychopathology and the other identifies those who are responding randomly or inconsistently. A supplementary clinical significance scale was designed for *PDQ-4*; to control for an excess of false positives. Also, a summed "total" score of all pathological items representing an overall level of personality dysfunction can be generated. Interestingly, an ancillary version, *PDQ-4+*, can be used to evaluate passive–aggressive and depressive PDs as listed in the appendix of *DSM-IV*. A computer-assisted version is available for administration and scoring. The *PDQ-R* has been demonstrated to be an efficient instrument for screening personality disorders according to *DSM-III-R* (Hyler, Skodol, Kellman, Oldham, & Rosnick, 1990; Hyler, Skodol, Oldham, Kellman, & Doidge, 1992), and has been found to have high sensitivity and moderate specificity for most axis II disorders (Hyler et al., 1990; Hyler et al., 1992). Most recently, Trull and Larson (1994) have conducted a validity study of the *PDQ-R*, comparing it to a structured clinical interview. They concluded that the *PDQ-R* was overly sensitive to psychopathology (false positives), although it was suggested that the *PDQ-R* might be helpful in ruling out PDs. The new clinical significance scale of the *PDQ-4* may help in this regard.

7.12.5.1.3 Coolidge Axis II Inventory

The *CATI* (Coolidge, 1984; Coolidge & Merwin, 1992) is a 225-item, self-report and significant-other report inventory developed and revised to assess PDs according to the diagnostic criteria of *DSM-IV*. The inventory currently contains 14 PD scales, retaining the *DSM-III-R* sadistic and self-defeating PDs, and offering the new *DSM-IV* depressive PD. The items on each PD scale were designed to cover all of the criteria listed in *DSM-IV* (or *DSM-III-R*). The *CATI* also provides assessment for 13 Axis I scales including depression, anxiety, schizophrenia, and post-traumatic stress disorder. The new *DSM-IV*, Personality Change Due to a General Medical Condition is also evaluated, with scores provided for each of the five subtypes: apathy, disinhibition, emotional lability, aggression, and paranoia. One unique feature of *CATI* is that it has an 18 item neuropsychological dysfunction scale for assessing symptoms of brain disease, trauma, and dysfunction, with three subscales assessing language dysfunction, memory and concentration difficulties, and somatic complaints related to brain dysfunction. The *CATI* also includes a 16 item executive functions scale with three subscales measuring poor planning, decision-making difficulty, and task incompletion. The test–retest reliability (one week intervening) for the *CATI* is good (mean r = 0.90; range = 0.78–0.97), and internal consistency is moderate (median r = 0.76; range = 0.66–0.87). With regard to validity, a 50% concordance rate with clinicians' diagnoses (based on *DSM-III-R* criteria) for 24 personality-disordered patients was found, and the *CATI* showed moderate concurrent validity with the *MCMI-II* (median r = 0.58; range = 0.10–0.87) with the same patients (Coolidge & Merwin, 1992).

7.12.5.1.4 Application to older adults

Application of the *MCMI* to older psychiatrically impaired adults has been explored in only one study. Hyer and Harrison (1986) administered the inventory to 60 elderly psychiatric inpatients. Results showed that rates of dependent and avoidant PDs were highest in this older group, a finding that mirrors results from younger age groups. In contrast, histrionic, narcissistic, and antisocial PDs had the lowest rates. These disorders were characterized as higher intensity personality styles. Notably, Hyer and Harrison suggested that these high energy personality types tend to become less prominent with increasing age.

Literature regarding the *CATI* and older adults is also limited. Coolidge and colleagues (1992) administered the *CATI* to normal younger (N=573; mean age 24.0 years) and older (N=36; mean age 69.4 years) individuals and compared results. They found that, for Axis I syndromes, older adults were significantly less anxious, but reported more signs of brain dysfunction. No group differences were reported on the depression scale. As for Axis II, the elderly scored significantly lower on antisocial, borderline, histrionic, narcissistic, paranoid, passive–aggressive, schizotypal, sadistic, and self-defeating scales than their younger counterparts. By contrast, the older adult sample was significantly more obsessive–compulsive and schizoid. No group differences were obtained for avoidant or dependent PD scales. Coolidge and colleagues (1992) noted that, in general, the older sample scored low on questions associated with impulsivity and endorsed items consistent with restricted emotional expressiveness. In this study, age differences on the *CATI* were assessed in nonclinical, normal subjects. To date, age comparisons have not been examined in psychiatric populations. We found no studies of the *PDQ* with older persons.

The dearth of studies applying the *PDQ*, *MCMI*, and *CATI* to older populations represents a major gap in the research literature. Recently, however, the concurrent validity of the *MCMI-II* and *CATI* has been evaluated in a pilot study (Silberman, Roth, Segal, & Burns, in press) targeting chronically mentally ill elderly inpatients (N=30; mean age 63.3 years). Patients were diagnosed by a psychiatrist as having a chronic mental illness (e.g., schizophrenia, bipolar disorder). The *MCMI-II* and *CATI* were concurrently administered in counterbalanced fashion and the data submitted to correlational analyses. The median correlation coefficient (raw score sums for the *CATI* and *MCMI-II*) for the 13 PD scales was 0.55 (range - 0.13 for schizoid to 0.88 for borderline), which was similar to the moderate results obtained by Coolidge and Merwin (1992) with a younger and less severe sample (24 psychiatric outpatients, mean age 38.0 years).

7.12.5.2 Structured Clinical Interviews

Since the 1960s, several structured diagnostic interviews have been developed for clinical, research, and training applications. Notably, structured interviews have been devised to assist in diagnosis of all standard Axis II PDs and all major Axis I clinical syndromes. Prominent interviews for Axis I conditions include the Schedule for Affective Disorders and Schizophrenia (Endicott & Spitzer, 1978), the *Diagnostic Interview Schedule* (original *DIS*; Robins, Helzer, Croughan, & Ratcliff, 1981; *DIS-IV*; Robins, Cottler, Bucholz, & Compton, 1996), and the Structured Clinical Interview for *DSM-IV* (First, Spitzer, Gibbon, & Williams, 1995a). (See recent review by Segal & Falk [in press] for further description of interviews for Axis I disorders.) Principal interviews for Axis II PDs include the Structured Interview for *DSM-IV* Personality (SIDP-IV), the International Personality Disorder Examination (IPDE), and the Structured Clinical Interview for *DSM-IV* Axis II Personality Disorders (SCID-II). Each PD interview is closely aligned to the *DSM* system, and subsequently has been revamped to match refinements in that classification scheme as it has evolved. Overall, structured interviews for PDs have improved clinical and research endeavors by providing a more standardized, scientific, and quantitative approach to the evaluation of these disorders. Indeed, these instruments have strongly contributed to the advancement in diagnostic clarity and precision for PDs. For each instrument, the purpose and construction will be briefly discussed, followed by some thoughts about the clinical applications of these instruments with older adults. PDs covered by the *DSM-IV* version of each instrument are presented in Table 1.

Table 1 *DSM-IV* personality disorders diagnoses covered by the SCID-II, IPDE, and SIDP-IV.

Personality disorders	*Structured interview* *SCID-II*	*IPDE*	*SIDP-IV*
Cluster A			
Paranoid	X	X	X
Schizoid	X	X	X
Schizotypal	X	X	X
Cluster B			
Antisocial	X	X	X
Borderline	X	X	X
Histrionic	X	X	X
Narcissistic	X	X	X
Cluster C			
Avoidant	X	X	X
Dependent	X	X	X
Obsessive-compulsive	X	X	X
Other personality disorders			
Mixed or PD NOS	X	X	X
Sadistic	no	no	no
Self-defeating	no	no	X
Depressive	X	no	X
Negativistic	X	no	X

7.12.5.2.1 Structured Interview for DSM-IV *Personality*

The SIDP-IV (Pfohl, Blum, & Zimmerman, 1995) is a comprehensive, semistructured diagnostic interview for *DSM-IV* PDs. The SIDP-IV covers 14 axis II diagnoses, including the 10 standard PDs, mixed PD, as well as self-defeating, depressive, and negativistic PDs which are proposed for "further study" in *DSM-IV*. The current edition of this popular instrument (SIDP-IV) has its roots in earlier versions that date back over a decade ago. In fact, the original Structured Interview for *DSM-III* Personality Disorders (SIDP; Stangl, Pfohl, Zimmerman, Bowers, & Corenthal, 1985) was the first structured interview designed to diagnose the full range of *DSM-III* PDs. Soon after, the Structured Interview for *DSM-III-R* Personality Disorders (SIDP-R; Pfohl, Blum, Zimmerman, & Stangl, 1989) was published to match changes in *DSM-III-R*.

Prior to the SIDP-IV structured interview, a full evaluation of current mental state or axis I conditions is required (Pfohl et al., 1995). This is not surprising given that self-report of enduring personality characteristics can be seriously compromised in a respondent experiencing acute distress. Indeed, the aim of all personality assessment measures is to rate the respondents typical, habitual, and lifelong personal functioning rather than acute or temporary states. For the most part, each SIDP-IV question corresponds to a unique *DSM-IV* axis II criterion. To help guide the interviewer, the specific *DSM* criterion associated with each question is provided on the form for easy reference. Items are not presented in a disorder-by-disorder fashion; rather, items are grouped according to 10 "topical sections" that reflect different dimension of personality functioning. Examples of these groupings include: interests and activities, close relationships, emotions, self-perception, and social conformity (Pfohl et al.). Questions typically are open-ended to encourage respondents to talk about their *usual* behaviors and long-term functioning. Based on patient responses, each criterion is rated on a scale with four anchor points, ranging from not present to strongly present and debilitating. The SIDP-IV requires that a trait be prominent for most of the last five years to be considered a part of the respondents' personality. This "five year rule" helps ensure that the particular personality characteristic is "stable and of long duration" as required by the "general diagnostic criteria" for a personality disorder described in *DSM-IV*.

Like the IPDE and SCID-II, significant clinical judgment is required to properly administer the SIDP-IV as interviewers are expected to ask additional questions to clarify patient responses when necessary. Also data are not limited to self-report; rather, chart records, and significant others such as relatives and friends who know the patient well should be consulted when available. Such collateral information is particularly prized when evaluating personality disordered individuals, who tend to lack insight into their own maladaptive personality traits and distort facts about their strengths and limitations. Moreover, informants can also provide diagnostic data that can help resolve the state/trait distinction about specific criterion behaviors. Overall, the SIDP typically requires 60 to 90 minutes for the patient interview, 20 minutes for interview of significant informants, and approximately 20 minutes to tabulate the responses and make diagnostic conclusions.

Reliability (inter-rater and internal consistency) of SIDP diagnoses has been evaluated in many studies (e.g., Stangl et al., 1985; Nazikian, Rudd, Edwards, & Jackson, 1990; Hogg, Jackson, Rudd, & Edwards, 1990; Jackson, Gazis, Rudd, & Edwards, 1991) with generally favorable results. Convergent validity has been assessed in several investigations in which SIDP diagnoses were compared to diagnoses from self-report Axis II instruments, such as the *MCMI*, and results typically have been modest at best (Hogg et al., 1990; Jackson et al., 1991; Miller, Streiner, & Parkinson, 1992; Nazikian et al., 1990; Turley, Bates, Edwards, & Jackson, 1992). It should be noted, however, that these studies may not be a fair test of the validity of the SIDP due to the differing assessment methods (interview vs. self-report) and the questionable validity of self-report PD measures.

7.12.5.2.2 International Personality Disorder Examination

The IPDE (Loranger et al., 1994) is an extensive, semistructured diagnostic interview for PDs. Although the 1994 version is compatible with the *DSM-III-R* and *ICD-10*, a version aligned with *DSM-IV* criteria has been produced by the World Health Organization (WHO; in press). The IPDE is an outgrowth of the Personality Disorder Examination (PDE) which was developed and refined over a five year period from 1983 to 1988 (Loranger, Hirschfeld, Sartorius, & Regier, 1991). Impetus for the development of the IPDE came from WHO and the US Alcohol, Drug Abuse, and Mental Health Administration (ADAMHA) in their joint effort aimed at producing standardized assessment instruments to measure mental disorders on an worldwide basis. The IPDE was selected by the WHO/ADAMHA for use as an instrument capable of assessing PDs in different languages, cultures, and countries. As such, the IPDE allows for diagnosis of PDs according to both the *DSM-IV* and *ICD-10* systems.

Items reflecting PD criteria according to the *DSM* and *ICD* are grouped into six thematic headings: work, self, interpersonal relationships, affects, reality testing, and impulse control (Loranger et al., 1991). Like the SIDP-IV, disorders are not covered on a one-by-one basis. IPDE sections typically begin with open-ended prompts to encourage respondents to elaborate about themselves in a less structured fashion. Then, specific questions are asked to evaluate each *DSM* and *ICD* criterion. There are separate modules for the *DSM-IV* and *ICD-10* classification systems. This division serves to reduce administration time, as interviewers typically follow one system or the other. Still, the IPDE typically requires 3–4 hours.

The IPDE requires that a trait be prominent during the last five years to be considered a part of the respondent's personality. Information about age of onset of particular behaviors is also explored to determine if a late-onset diagnosis is appropriate. When a respondent acknowledges a particular trait, interviewers follow-up by asking for examples and anecdotes to clarify the trait or behavior, gauge impact of the trait on the person's functioning, and fully substantiate the rating. Such probing requires significant clinical judgment and knowledge about each criterion on the part of interviewers. Moreover, some items are rated based on observation of the respondents behavior during the session, and this too requires a certain level of clinical expertise. To supplement self-report, interview of informants is encouraged. All items are rated on a three-point scale with the following definitions: "O" indicates that the behavior or trait is denied or within normal limits, "1" refers to present to an accentuated degree, and "2" signifies pathological/meets criterion (Loranger et al., 1994). The final output of the IPDE is extensive, including presence or absence of each criterion, number of criteria met for each disorder, a dimensional score (sum of individual scores for each criteria for each disorder), and a categorical diagnosis (definite, probable, or negative) (Loranger et al., 1994).

Like the SIDP-IV, inter-rater reliability of the IPDE (or PDE) generally is good, from report to report (Loranger et al., 1994; Loranger, Susman, Oldham, & Russakoff, 1987; Standage & Ladha, 1988). Not surprisingly, convergent validity coefficients typically have been weaker, ranging from 0.14 to 0.66 (Skodol, Oldham, Rosnick, Kellman, & Hyler, 1991; also see Hunt & Andrews, 1992; Pilkonis, Heape, Ruddy, & Serrao, 1991; Soldz, Budman, Demby, & Merry, 1993).

7.12.5.2.3 Structured Clinical Interview for DSM-IV *Axis II Personality Disorders*

To complement the Axis I version of the SCID, Spitzer and colleagues endeavored to develop a semistructured interview that would facilitate improved diagnosis of Axis II PDs. Their efforts resulted in publication of the SCID-II (version 1.0; Spitzer, Williams, Gibbon, & First, 1990), which targeted 11 PDs according to the then current *DSM-III-R* system. In 1994, the SCID-II was updated (SCID-II, version 2.0; First, Spitzer, Gibbon, Williams, & Benjamin, 1994) so that questions correspond to the new diagnostic criteria in *DSM-IV*. In this *DSM-IV* version, the 10 standard PDs are evaluated, along with the proposed depressive and negativistic PDs, while self-defeating and sadistic PDs have been deleted.

The SCID-II is usually employed in conjunction with the SCID-I, which typically is administered prior to personality assessment. This is encouraged so that the respondents present psychological state can be considered when judging accuracy of self-reported personality traits (First, Spitzer, Gibbon, & Williams, 1995b). A unique feature of the SCID-II is that it includes a 117 item, self-report, forced choice, yes/no screening component (called the Personality Questionnaire) that is completed prior to the interview portion and requires about 20 minutes to complete. The purpose of this screening measure is to reduce overall administration time. In the questionnaire, initial diagnostic items for each PD are presented, so that later sections of the structured assessment can be omitted if particular personality traits are denied.

During the structured interview component, only positively endorsed screening responses are further pursued to ascertain whether the symptom criteria is actually at clinically significant levels. Each SCID-II question taps a unique PD criterion, and the actual *DSM-IV* diagnostic criteria are printed on the interview page for easy review. Responses are coded on a three-point system (i.e., 1 = absent, 2 = subthreshold, 3 = threshold, ? = inadequate information). Each disorder is assessed completely and diagnoses are made before proceeding to the next disorder (First et al., 1995b). The modular format permits researchers and clinicians to tailor the SCID-II to their specific needs and reduce administration time. SCID-II administrators are expected to use their clinical judgment to clarify responses, gently challenge inconsistencies, and ask for additional information as required to accurately assess each disorder. Like the SIDP-IV and IPDE, collection of diagnostic information from ancillary sources is permitted. Complete administration of the SCID-II typically takes under 50 minutes (First et al., 1995b), which is substantially shorter than other structured measures. Training requirements and interviewer qualifications are similar to that of the other structured interviews for PDs.

With regard to psychometric properties of the SCID-II, an impressive large-scale multisite test–retest reliability project has recently been completed (First et al., 1995) with reasonably good results (overall weighted kappa = 0.53; range = 0.34–0.74). Other studies have reported even higher inter-rater reliability values for the SCID-II (Arntz et al.,1992; Brooks, Baltazar, McDowell, Munjack, & Bruns, 1991; Fogelson, Nuechterlein, Asarnow, Subotnik, & Talovic, 1991; Malow, West, Williams, & Sutker, 1989; O'Boyle & Self, 1990). Like the SIDP-IV and IPDE, less empirical attention has been devoted to validity of SCID-II diagnoses, and the studies that have been conducted generally produce only fair validity coefficients across different methodologies and criterion diagnoses used (O'Boyle & Self, 1990; Skodol et al., 1991; Skodol, Rosnick, Kellman, Oldham, & Hyler, 1988).

It is apparent that application of structured interviews for PDs over the last 15 years has greatly facilitated the task of psychiatric diagnosis for these conditions. Reliability values for the structured interviews generally indicate modest to excellent agreement with diverse patient populations and experimental designs. Most importantly, these values greatly surpass results from early investigations with unstructured interviews (Mellsop et al., 1982). Unfortunately, although reliability rates are now more acceptable for most PDs, it remains to firmly establish the validity. Most studies in this area have focused on basic reliability, differentiation of separate PDs from each other, and description of these conditions. Firm establishment of construct and predictive validity for the PDs is lacking in the literature. As such, investigation in this area should be the major focus of future research attention.

7.12.5.2.4 Application to older adults

As previously noted, each major structured interview has been subjected to extensive evaluation by clinical researchers. Unfortunately, the literature regarding specific application of these instruments with the elderly is sparse, although several clinical studies have been reported. For example, Abrams, Alexopoulos, and Young (1987) administered the

PDE to 21 older adults who had recovered from depression and 15 without a history of depression. The purpose of this study was to investigate the relationship between personality traits and late-life depression. Only two study participants met criteria for a PD and no reliability estimates were reported. In a more recent study also employing the PDE in a sample of 30 recovered depressed older adults, inter-rater reliability was high for all PDs, except histrionic (Abrams, Rosendahl, Card, & Alexopoulos, 1994). In a similar investigation, Schneider, Zemansky, Bender, and Sloane (1992) used the SCID-II to diagnose PDs in a group of older adults with history of major depression, although no reliability data were reported. Thompson et al. (1988) obtained Axis II formulations by using the SIDP in a sample of 79 depressed older adults, and found high inter-rater reliability. These clinical reports provide some evidence that the structured interviews can be successfully applied to older adults. However, larger reliability and validity studies are warranted especially with more diverse elder populations (e.g., medical patients, minorities, psychiatric inpatients).

Several additional concerns about the application of structured interviews with older adults should be noted. A common feature among all three structured interviews is that respondents are encouraged to describe their "typical or usual" functioning, rather than their often altered personality functioning during times of acute psychiatric illness. As such, during the course of the structured interview, respondents are sometimes asked to describe their behaviors at different points in time, possibly spanning several years. Unfortunately, such distinctions may be difficult for some elderly clients to make, as memory problems can preclude accurate self-report about behavior patterns many years ago. Another problem with the utilization of structured interviews with older clients is the considerable length of time required for completion. With young clients, administration time for the various interviews typically ranges from 1.5 to 3.5 hours. However, administration may take considerably longer with older persons. One reason for this is that older individuals simply have more extensive and complicated histories to review. Some older persons also require several "breaks" that may not be needed by younger individuals. Indeed, many older adults fatigue more quickly, and this must be monitored as responses will become less accurate if the client becomes inattentive or unmotivated. Older adults typically will perform their best when given frequent opportunities to stretch, take a brief walk, rest, or use the bathroom. Sometimes, it may be helpful to divide the structured interview into several shorter sessions.

Sensory impairments can also affect the evaluation. Older persons with hearing difficulties may misunderstand parts of the query or fail to answer the question entirely. It is often helpful to sit closer to the older client, face him or her directly, speak slowly and clearly, and reduce background noise in the evaluation room. The interested reader is referred to Edelstein, Staats, Kalish, and Northrop (1996) for full discussion of the effects of sensory deficits on the assessment of older adults. Finally, some older adults may respond negatively to the structure imposed by the interviews. In these cases, it is advisable to spend more time developing rapport, reflect more feelings during the interview, allow for more elaboration and venting from the client about troublesome symptoms, and explain the purpose and format of the structured interview. In all, flexibility and sensitivity are required when assessing and interviewing the personality-disordered older adult.

7.12.6 TREATMENT

The personality-disordered older adult is often ill-equipped to handle the challenges and changes associated with the normal aging process. A lifetime of social and occupational failures typically exacerbates the clinical picture, and increases the older adults sense of disappointment and hopelessness. As such, these individuals are often in need of counseling or supportive services to reduce their frustrations and difficulties. Unfortunately, little is currently known about the treatment of various PDs in the elderly. And, most of the literature is in the form of clinical case studies with a striking lack of group studies. Much of the literature we will discuss pertains to treatment models developed for younger individuals. The reader should be aware, however, that specific literature about treatment of PDs in the elderly is in short supply.

Evidence suggests that the majority of older adults with psychiatric problems do not seek or receive appropriate mental health services. Lazarus, Sadavoy, and Langsley (1991) have aptly described the many barriers to psychotherapy facing the current cohort of elderly persons: their attribution of psychiatric symptoms to physical rather than psychiatric causes, emphasis on medical treatment, stigmatization associated with psychiatric care, practical deterrents such as cost, transportation, and physical disabilities, and negative family and physician attitudes about geriatric mental health treatment. Unfamiliarity with current mental health treatment and a desire to remain independent also preclude intervention in some cases.

Two other factors specifically impede appropriate treatment of PDs in the elderly. The first concerns the lack of appropriate diagnosis. As we have discussed earlier, PDs are sometimes underdiagnosed by mental health professions due to their unfamiliarity with the disorders, the belief that PDs are rare in the elderly, an overemphasis on the Axis I symptoms that the client perceives as the problem, and a masking of Axis II diagnoses by the more flagrant or pressing Axis I symptoms. Although the underlying personality may not be taken into account, it certainly affects treatment outcome for these clients. Consider the treatment of an older male adult who is clinically depressed because he has recently retired and subsequently lost his wife to a fatal illness. Another elderly male may present with similar symptoms of depression, but his symptoms are not reflective of recent losses but rather are the effects of a lifetime of interpersonal chaos, self-destructive actions, and a poorly developed sense of self characteristic of borderline PD. Appropriate treatment for these two individuals most likely will take remarkably different forms. However, failure to recognize the moderating impact of personality dysfunction on psychiatric symptoms can result in poor treatment planning and therapeutic outcome. Indeed, in their classic report, Thompson et al. (1988) investigated whether presence of PDs affect outcome in treatment of 75 depressed older adults. They found that older adults with PDs did considerably worse in treatment than those without PDs, and these effects were still present at six month follow-up. Similar results have been reported in related studies with younger depressed clients with comorbid PD (Frank, Kupfer, & Jarret, 1987; Pilkonis & Frank, 1988).

The second factor hindering treatment of PD in older adults is that individuals (both older and younger) with a significant PD often fail to recognize their symptoms as signs of a psychiatric disturbance. In other words, they lack insight into the maladaptive nature of their behavior. Imagine an older adult suffering from narcissistic PD. This individual may have great difficulty maintaining adequate employment because of his sense of entitlement, condescending attitude, and difficulty following directions from his bosses whom the person regards as inferior. This older individual may blame his problems on his bosses who do not properly appreciate his talents or he may believe he is being discriminated against based on his age, when the real problem is the dysfunctional attitudes and behaviors characteristic of his personality type. Such individuals, who lack awareness of their own personality disturbance, typically see no need for personal change or psychiatric intervention. In general, individuals with a PD seek therapy when they begin to manifest troubling symptoms of an Axis I disorder, such as anxiety or depression. They see these symptoms as ego-dystonic and present at the clinician's office expecting relief. One tenet in treating older adults in this condition is to focus one's therapeutic attention initially on reduction of Axis I clinical symptoms until maximum therapeutic gain has been achieved (Abrams, 1991). At this early point, the therapeutic goal negotiated between therapist and client converge.

The early stage of treatment focusing on symptom relief is important for developing a therapeutic alliance and laying the foundation for later, more difficult, and more intensive treatment of the underlying character pathology. It is necessary to spend considerable time forming a therapeutic relationship with the older client. Indeed, a strong bond and safe environment is crucial to help older clients begin the process of viewing themselves and their behaviors more realistically (often more negatively). The older personality-disordered client may have few skills in this area and may have difficulty tolerating the negative feelings that often arise during this process. It is often helpful to proceed with caution and to be sensitive to increases in symptoms and distress. Typically, long-term psychotherapy is needed to address a lifetime of long-standing maladaptive behavior patterns. And, in some cases, treatment goals should be modest (Abrams, 1991).

Several models of treatment specific to PDs have appeared in the literature. For example, Young (1994) combines psychodynamic, object relations, and gestalt therapy concepts with standard cognitive therapy techniques in his schema-focused approach for treatment of PDs. Millon, one of the leaders in formulation and assessment of PDs, has developed a personologic and integrative treatment approach for PDs (Millon & Davis, in press), and Benjamin (1996) has presented her interpersonal approach to case conceptualization and treatment. These approaches have generated a great deal of anecdotal support, but little empirical validation has been reported. Other theorists have concentrated their attentions on one particular PD, with borderline PD receiving the most attention. For example, Paris (1994) describes a multidimensional treatment, while Horwitz et al. (1996) explicate a modified psychodynamic approach for borderlines. An innovative treatment for borderline PD, dialectical behavior therapy (DBT; Linehan, 1993) combines tenets from humanistic therapies and cognitive behavioral problem solving techniques. Several well-designed controlled outcome studies have been conducted to evaluate effectiveness of DBT with promising results (e.g., Linehan, Armstrong, Suarez, Allmon, & Heard, 1991; Linehan, Heard, & Armstrong, 1993), and DBT has recently been approved as an empirically validated treatment for borderline PD. The question remains whether this approach (as well as the others mentioned above) can be adapted for use with *older* individuals with severe personality dysfunction. In summary, although psychotherapy is generally considered the treatment of choice for PDs, few studies have actually tested various therapy models with older persons. The complexity of these disorders and well-established difficulty forming therapeutic relationships with personality-disordered individuals no doubt contribute to this lack of investigation.

Besides psychotherapeutic interventions, the psychopharmacological management of clients with PDs has been the focus of increasing attention in the past decade. Pharmacotherapy is sometimes used as an adjunctive strategy to ameliorate some acute depressive or anxiety symptoms and, in fact, can help some personality-disordered patients better engage in psychotherapy (Soloff, 1990). Such treatment is often welcomed by older clients who typically have been socialized to the medical model of intervention that requires little effort on their part. Unfortunately, the medication, while valuable in some instances in helping the patient regulate distressing affective, anxious, and cognitive symptoms, is not addressing the underlying pathology (i.e., the personality dysfunction) but is only providing symptom relief. Research on pharmacotherapy of PDs has mostly focused on Cluster B (dramatic, erratic, emotional) PDs, with generally promising, but preliminary results. For example, antidepressant medications have been found to show some positive effects for Cluster B patients (Ruegg & Frances, 1995), and antipsychotics have been found helpful for individuals with borderline PD, as they tend to reduce hostility, anxiety, and depression (Links & Steiner, 1988). The interested reader is referred to Soloff (1990) for an engaging and detailed review of pharmacological therapy for the PDs. Regrettably, pharmacotherapy studies typically have focused on younger and middle aged individuals. Despite encouraging findings, it remains to be seen how results with younger clients apply to geriatric clients. Indeed, older clients are particularly sensitive to interactive effects of medications and usually have greater side-effect profiles than younger persons. Pharmacotherapy studies with older clients are sorely needed.

7.12.7 SUMMARY

Initially in this chapter, we described the major evolution of the diagnosis of PDs from *DSM-I* to *DSM-IV*. By the placement of PDs on their own Axis in *DSM-III* and listing of specific and requisite criteria for each disorder in *DSM-III-R*, there was a tremendous growth in our knowledge of PDs and accompanying assessment tools and treatment techniques. Although there has been a parallel increasing interest in the psychology of older adults, clinical and investigative interest in PDs in this population is at the nascent stage. Many theories of the etiology of PDs have also been proposed, and we have reviewed several major biological, cognitive, evolutionary, and biosocial theories. It is clear from our review that most of these theories have ignored lifespan and aging issues, and, thus, there has been little or no attention to the nature or stability of PD symptomatology in the elderly.

Despite recent advances in the field, accurate diagnosis of PDs in the elderly is still a significant concern for clinicians and researchers. We have noted that some *DSM* diagnostic criteria may be inadequate for older individuals, given the unique physical, cognitive, and social complications encountered by the aged. We have suggested that the apparent decline in prevalence rates of some disorders (i.e., borderline, histrionic) may not be due to a maturation of the individual but rather the inability of the current diagnostic system to identify the age-related manifestations of these disorders. Some symptoms of PDs are erroneously attributed to old age and subsequently dismissed. Clients and professionals may also focus on Axis I symptoms and neglect to appreciate fully the role of the underlying personality dysfunction.

We have also reviewed the major self-report personality inventories and structured interviews employed to evaluate PDs. In clinical practice, all of the devices have been applied, no doubt, to older persons. However, formal reliability and validity studies of these instruments with the elderly are lacking in the literature. Recently, it has been demonstrated that the SCID for Axis I disorders can be reliably administered to older psychiatric populations (Segal, Hersen, Van Hasselt, Kabacoff, & Roth, 1993; Segal, Kabacoff, Hersen, Van Hasselt, & Ryan, 1995), and similar studies for Axis II instruments are needed. In the absence of empirical verification, it cannot be assumed that self-report devices and structured interviews for Axis II disorders have acceptable operating characteristics for this unique population. Definitive comparisons between instruments are also needed to advance the field. Our knowledge about the treatment of PDs in the elderly is presently limited, and much work remains to be conducted in this domain.

We hope that in this chapter we have delineated the problems and issues in the etiology, diagnosis, assessment, and treatment of PDs in the elderly. There have been some promising studies on these topics, and we feel confident that the growing general interest in aging and in PDs will lead to new contributions to this inchoate area.

7.12.8 REFERENCES

Abrams, R. (1991). Anxiety and personality disorders. In J. Sadavoy, L. W. Lazarus, & L. F. Jarvik,. (Eds.), *Comprehensive review of geriatric psychiatry* (pp. 369–386). Washington, DC: American Psychiatric Press.

Abrams, R. C., Alexopoulos, G. S., & Young, R. C. (1987). Geriatric depression and DSM-III-R personality disorder criteria. *Journal of the American Geriatrics Society, 35*, 383–386.

Abrams, R. C., Rosendahl, E., Card, C., & Alexopoulos, G. S. (1994). Personality disorder correlates of late and early onset depression. *Journal of the American Geriatrics Society, 42*, 727–731.

American Psychiatric Association. (1952). *Diagnostic and statistical manual of mental disorders*. Washington, DC: Author.

American Psychiatric Association. (1968). *Diagnostic and statistical manual of mental disorders* (2nd ed.). Washington, DC: Author.

American Psychiatric Association. (1980). *Diagnostic and statistical manual of mental disorders* (3rd ed.). Washington, DC: Author.

American Psychiatric Association (1987). *Diagnostic and statistical manual of mental disorders* (3rd ed. Rev.). Washington, DC: Author.

American Psychiatric Association (1994). *Diagnostic and statistical manual of mental disorders* (4th ed.). Washington, DC: Author.

Arntz, A., van Beijsterveldt, B., Hoekstra, R., Hofman, A., Eussen, M., & Sallaerts, S. (1992). The interrater reliability of a Dutch version of the Structured Clinical Interview for DSM-III-R Personality Disorders. *Acta Psychiatrica Scandinavica, 85*, 394–400.

Beck, A. T. (1992). Personality disorders (and their relationship to syndromal disorders). *Across-Species Comparisons and Psychiatry Newsletter, 5*, 3–13.

Benjamin, L. S. (1996). *Interpersonal diagnosis and treatment of personality disorders* (2nd ed.). New York: Guilford.

Brooks, R. B., Baltazar, P. L., McDowell, D. E., Munjack, D. J., & Bruns, J. R. (1991). Personality disorders co-occurring with panic disorder with agoraphobia. *Journal of Personality Disorders, 5*, 328–336.

Casey, D. A., & Schrodt, C. J. (1989). Axis II diagnoses in geriatric inpatients. *Journal of Geriatric Psychiatry and Neurology, 2*, 87–88.

Cattell, R. B., Saunders, D. R., & Stice, G. F. (1950). *The 16 Personality Factor Questionnaire*. Champaign, IL: Institute for Personality and Ability Testing.

Cloninger, C. R. (1986). A unified biosocial theory of personality and its role in the development of anxiety states. *Psychiatric Developments, 3*, 167–226.

Cloninger, C. R. (1987). A systematic method for clinical description and classification of personality variants: A proposal. *Archives of General Psychiatry, 44*, 573–588.

Cloninger, C. R., Przybeck, T. R., Svrakic, D. M., & Wetzel, R. D. (1994). *The Temperament and Character Inventory (TCI): A guide to its development and use*. St. Louis, MO: Center for the Psychobiology of Personality, Washington University.

Cohen, G. D. (1990). Psychopathology and mental health in the mature and elderly adult. In J. E. Birren & K. W. Schaie (Eds.) *Handbook of the psychology of aging* (3rd ed., pp. 359–371). San Diego, CA: Academic Press.

Coolidge, F. L. (1984). *Coolidge Axis II Inventory*. US Copyright TXU 182 026, Washington, DC.

Coolidge, F. L., Becker, L. A, DiRito, D. C., Durham, R. L., Kinlaw, M. W., & Philbrick, P. B. (1994). On the relationship of the five-factor personality model to personality disorders: Four reservations. *Psychological Reports, 75*, 11–21.

Coolidge, F. L., Burns, E. M., Nathan, J. H., & Mull C. E. (1992). Personality disorders in the elderly. *Clinical Gerontologist, 12*, 41–55.

Coolidge, F. L., & Griego, J. (1996). *A construct validity investigation between the Temperament and Character Inventory and the Coolidge Axis II Inventory*. Manuscript submitted for publication.

Coolidge, F. L., & Merwin, M. M. (1992). Reliability and validity of the Coolidge Axis II Inventory: A new inventory for the assessment of personality disorders. *Journal of Personality Assessment, 59*, 223–238.

Edelstein, B., Staats, N., Kalish, K. D., & Northrop, L. R. (1996). Assessment of older adults. In M. Hersen & V. B. Van Hasselt (Eds.), *Psychological treatment of older adults: An introductory text* (pp. 35–68). New York: Plenum.

Endicott, J. & Spitzer, R. L. (1978). A diagnostic interview: The schedule for affective disorders and schizophrenia. *Archives of General Psychiatry, 35*, 837–844.

Eysenck, H. J. (1978). Superfactors P, E, N in a comprehensive factor space. *Multivariate Behavioral Research, 13*, 475–481.

First, M. B., Spitzer, R. L., Gibbon, M., & Williams, J. B. W. (1995a). *Structured Clinical Interview for Axis I DSM-IV Disorders—Patient Edition (SCID-I/P, Version 2.0)*. New York: Biometrics Research Department, New York State Psychiatric Institute.

First, M. B., Spitzer, R. L., Gibbon, M., & Williams, J. B. W. (1995b). The Structured Clinical Interview for DSM-III-R Personality Disorders (SCID-II), Part I: Description. *Journal of Personality Disorders, 19*, 83–91.

First, M. B., Spitzer, R. L., Gibbon, M., Williams, J. B. W., & Benjamin, L. (1994). *Structured Clinical Interview for DSM-IV Axis II Personality Disorders (SCID-II, Version 2.0)*. New York: Biometrics Research Department, New York State Psychiatric Institute.

First, M. B., Spitzer, R. L., Gibbon, M., Williams, J. B. W., Davies, M., Borus, J., Howes, M. J., Kane, J., Pope, H. G., & Rounsaville, B. (1995). The Structured Clinical Interview for DSM-III-R Personality Disorders (SCID-II), Part II: Multisite test–retest reliability study. *Journal of Personality Disorders, 19*, 92–104.

Fogel, B. S., & Westlake, R. (1990). Personality disorder diagnoses and age in inpatients with major depression. *Journal of Clinical Psychiatry, 51*, 232–235.

Fogelson, D. L., Nuechterlein, K. H., Asarnow, R. F., Subotnik, K. L., & Talovic, S. A. (1991). Interrater reliability of the structured clinical interview for DSM-III-R, Axis II: Schizophrenia spectrum and affective spectrum disorders. *Psychiatry Research, 39*, 55–63.

Frances, A. (1982). Categorical and dimensional systems of

personality diagnosis: A comparison. *Comprehensive Psychiatry, 23,* 516–527.

Frank, E., Kupfer, D. J., & Jarret, D. (1987). Personality features and response to acute treatment in recurrent depression. *Journal of Personality Disorders, 1,* 14–26.

Grove, W. M. (1987). The reliability of psychiatric diagnosis. In C. G. Last & M. Hersen (Eds.), *Issues in diagnostic research* (pp. 99–119). New York: Plenum.

Hathaway, S. R., & McKinley, J. C. (1983). *The Minnesota Multiphasic Personality Inventory manual.* New York: Psychological Corporation.

Hathaway, S. R., & McKinley, J. C. (1989). *MMPI-2: Minnesota Multiphasic Personality Inventory-2: Manual for administration and scoring.* Minneapolis, MN: University of Minnesota Press.

Hogg, B., Jackson, H. J., Rudd, R. P., & Edwards, J. (1990). Diagnosing personality disorders in recent-onset schizophrenia. *Journal of Nervous and Mental Disease, 178,* 194–199.

Horwitz, L., Gabbard, G. O., Allen, J. G., Frieswyk, S. H., Colson, D. B., Newsom, G. E., & Coyne, L. (1996). *Borderline personality disorder: Tailoring the psychotherapy to the patient.* Washington, DC: American Psychiatric Press.

Howard, R., Bandyopadhyay, D., & Cook, M. (1992). Dissocial personality disorder in the elderly: A case history. *International Journal of Geriatric Psychiatry, 7,* 527–532.

Hunt, C., & Andrews, G. (1992). Measuring personality disorder: The use of self-report questionnaires. *Journal of Personality Disorders, 6,* 125–133.

Hyer, L., & Harrison, W. R. (1986). Later life personality model: Diagnosis and treatment. *Clinical Gerontologist, 5,* 399–416.

Hyler, S. E. (1994). *Personality Diagnostic Questionnaire, (PDQ-4)* (4th ed.). New York: New York State Psychiatric Institute.

Hyler, S. E., & Rieder, R. O. (1987). *PDQ-R: Personality Diagnostic Questionnaire—Revised.* New York: New York State Psychiatric Institute.

Hyler, S. E., Skodol, A. E., Kellman, H. D., Oldham, J. M., & Rosnick, L. (1990). Validity of the Personality Diagnostic Questionnaire-Revised: Comparison with two structured interviews. *American Journal of Psychiatry, 147,* 1043–1048.

Hyler, S. E., Skodol, A. E., Oldham, J. M., Kellman, H. D., & Doidge, N. (1992). Validity of the Personality Diagnostic Questionnaire-Revised: A replication in an outpatient sample. *Comprehensive Psychiatry, 33,* 73–77.

Jackson, H. J., Gazis, J., Rudd, R. P., & Edwards, J. (1991). Concordance between two personality disorder instruments with psychiatric inpatients. *Comprehensive Psychiatry, 32,* 252–260.

Jung, C. G. (1971). *Psychological types.* (A revision by R. F. C. Hull of H. G. Baynes, Trans.). Princeton, NJ: Princeton University Press. (Original work published in 1924).

Kagan, J. & Moss, H. A. (1962). *Birth to maturity.* New York: Wiley.

Kernberg, O. F. (1996). A psychoanalytic theory of personality disorders. In J. F. Clarkin & M. F. Lenzenweger (Eds.), *Major theories of personality disorder* (pp. 106–140). New York: Guilford.

Klein, M. H., Benjamin, L. S., Rosenfeld, R., Treece, C., Husted, J., & Griest, J. H. (1993). The Wisconsin Personality Disorders Inventory: Development, reliability, and validity. *Journal of Personality Disorders, 7,* 285–303.

Kroessler, D. (1990). Personality disorder in the elderly. *Hospital and Community Psychiatry, 41,* 1325–1329.

Kunik, M. E., Mulsant, B. H., Rifai, A. H., Sweet, R. A., Pasternak, R., Rosen, J., & Zubenko, G. S. (1993). Personality disorders in elderly inpatients with major depression. *American Journal of Geriatric Psychiatry, 1,* 38–45.

Lazarus, L.W., Sadavoy, J., & Langsley, P. R. (1991). Individual psychotherapy. In J. Sadavoy, L. W. Lazarus, & L. F. Jarvik, (Eds.), *Comprehensive review of geriatric psychiatry* (pp. 487–512). Washington, DC: American Psychiatric Press.

Linehan, M. M. (1993). *Cognitive-behavioral treatment of borderline personality disorder.* New York: Guilford.

Linehan, M. M., Armstrong, H. E., Suarez, A., Allmon, D., & Heard, H. L. (1991). Cognitive-behavioral treatment of chronically parasuicidal borderline patients. *Archives of General Psychiatry, 48,* 1060–1064.

Linehan, M. M., Heard, H. L., & Armstrong, H. E. (1993). Naturalistic follow-up of a behavioral treatment of chronically parasuicidal borderline patients. *Archives of General Psychiatry, 50,* 971–974.

Links, P. S., & Steiner, M. (1988). Psychopharmacologic management of patients with borderline personality disorder. *Canadian Journal of Psychiatry, 33,* 355–359.

Loranger, A. W., Hirschfeld, R. M., Sartorius, N., & Regier, D. A. (1991). The WHO/ADAMHA international pilot study of personality disorders: Background and purpose. *Journal of Personality Disorders, 5,* 296–306.

Loranger, A.W., Sartorius, N., Andreoli, A., Berger, P., Buchleim, P., Channabasavanna, S. M., Coid, B., Dahl, A., Diekstra, R. F. W., Feguson, B., Jacobsberg, L. B., Mombour, W., Pull, C., Ono, Y., & Regier, D. (1994). The International Personality Disorder Examination: The World Health Organization/Alcohol, Drug Abuse, and Mental Health Administration international pilot study of personality disorders. *Archives of General Psychiatry, 51,* 215–224.

Loranger, A. W., Susman, V. L., Oldham, J. M., & Russakoff, L. M. (1987). The Personality Disorder Examination: A preliminary report. *Journal of Personality Disorders, 1,* 1–13.

Malow, R. M., West, J. A., Williams, J. L., & Sutker, P. B. (1989). Personality disorders classification and symptoms in cocaine and opioid addicts. *Journal of Consulting and Clinical Psychology, 57,* 765–767.

McCrae, R. R., & Costa, P. T., Jr. (1986). Clinical assessment can benefit from recent advances in personality psychology. *American Psychologist, 41,* 1001–1003.

McCrae, R. R., & Costa, P. T., Jr. (1989). More reasons to adopt the five-factor model. *American Psychologist, 44,* 451–452.

McGue, M., Bacon, S., & Lykken, D. T. (1993). Personality stability and change in early adulthood: A behavioral genetic analysis. *Developmental Psychology, 29,* 96–109.

Mellsop, G., Varghese, F., Joshua, S., & Hicks, A. (1982). The reliability of Axis II of DSM-III. *American Journal of Psychiatry, 139,* 1360–1361.

Mezzich, J. E., Fabrega, H., Coffman, G. A., & Glavin, Y. (1987). Comprehensively diagnosing geriatric patients. *Comprehensive Psychiatry, 28,* 68–76.

Miller, H. R., Streiner, D. L., & Parkinson, A. (1992). Maximum likelihood estimates of the ability of the MMPI and MCMI personality disorder scales and the SIDP to identify personality disorders. *Journal of Personality Assessment, 59,* 1–13.

Millon, T. (1983). *Millon Clinical Multiaxial Inventory.* Minneapolis, MN: Interpretive Scoring Systems.

Millon, T. (1987). *Millon Clinical Multiaxial Inventory II (MCMI II) manual.* Minneapolis, MN: National Computer Systems.

Millon, T. (1992). Millon Clinical Multiaxial Inventory: I & II. *Journal of Counseling and Development, 70,* 421–426.

Millon, T. (1994). *Millon Clinical Multiaxial Inventory III*

(MCMI III) manual. Minneapolis, MN: National Computer Systems.

Millon, T., & Davis, R. D. (1996). An evolutionary theory of personality disorders. In J. F. Clarkin & M. F. Lenzenweger (Eds.), *Major theories of personality disorder* (pp. 221–346). New York: Guilford.

Millon, T., & Davis, R. D. (in press). *Synergistic psychotherapy: Integrative syndromic and personologic treatment*. New York: Wiley-Interscience.

Molinari, V., & Marmion, J. (1995). Relationship between affective disorders and Axis II diagnoses in geropsychiatric patients. *Journal of Geriatric Psychiatry and Neurology, 8*, 61–64.

Morey, L. C. (1988). The categorical representation of personality disorder: A cluster analysis of DSM-III-R personality features. *Journal of Abnormal Psychology, 97*, 314–321.

Morey, L. C., Waugh, M. H., & Blashfield, R. K. (1985). MMPI scales for DSM-III personality disorders: Their derivation and correlates. *Journal of Personality Assessment, 49*, 245–251.

Morgan, D. G., May, P. C., & Finch, C. E. (1987). Dopamine and serotonin systems in human and rodent brain: Effects of age and neurogenerative disease. *Journal of the American Geriatric Society, 35*, 334–345.

Myers, I. B. (1962). *Manual: Myers–Briggs Type Indicator*. Palo Alto, CA: Consulting Psychological Press.

Nazikian, H., Rudd, R. P., Edwards, J., & Jackson, H. J. (1990). Personality disorder assessment for psychiatric inpatients. *Australian and New Zealand Journal of Psychiatry, 24*, 37–46.

Norman, W. T. (1963). Toward an adequate taxonomy of personality attributes: Replicated factor structure in peer nomination personality ratings. *Journal of Abnormal and Social Psychology, 43*, 574–583.

O'Boyle, M., & Self, D. (1990). A comparison of two interviews for DSM-III-R personality disorders. *Psychiatry Research, 32*, 85–92.

Oldham, J. M., Skodol, A. E., Kellman, H. D., Hyler, S. E, Rosnick, L., & Davies, M. (1992). Diagnosis of DSM-III-R personality disorders by two structured interviews: Patterns of comorbidity. *American Journal of Psychiatry, 149*, 213–220.

Paris, J. (1994). *Borderline personality disorder: A multidimensional approach*. Washington, DC: American Psychiatric Press.

Pfohl, B., Black, D. W., Noyes, R., Kelly, M., & Blum, N. (1990). A test of the tridimensional personality theory: Association with diagnosis and platelet imiprimine binding in obsessive-compulsive disorder. *Biological Psychiatry, 28*, 41–46.

Pfohl, B., Blum, N., & Zimmerman, M. (1995). *Structured Interview for DSM-IV Personality SIDP-IV*. Iowa City, IA: University of Iowa.

Pfohl, B., Blum, N., Zimmerman, M., & Stangl, D. (1989). *Structured Interview for DSM-III-R Personality (revised) (SIDP-R)*. Iowa City, IA: University of Iowa.

Pilkonis, P. A., & Frank, E. (1988). Personality pathology in recurrent depression: Nature, prevalence, and relationship to treatment response. *American Journal of Psychiatry, 145*, 435–441.

Pilkonis, P. A., Heape, C. L., Ruddy, J. & Serrao, P. (1991). Validity in the diagnosis of personality disorders: The use of the LEAD standard. *Psychological Assessment, 3*, 46–54.

Plomin, R., Chipuer, H. M., & Loehlin, J. C. (1990). Behavioral genetics and personality. In L. A. Pervin (Ed.), *Handbook of personality: Theory and research* (pp. 225–243). New York: Guilford.

Pretzer, J. L., & Beck, A. T. (1996). A cognitive theory of personality disorders. In J. F. Clarkin & M. F. Lenzenweger (Eds.), *Major theories of personality disorder* (pp. 36–105). New York: Guilford.

Robins, L. N., Cottler, L. B., Bucholz, K., & Compton, W. (1996). *The Diagnostic Interview Schedule, (Version IV)*. St. Louis. MO: Washington University School of Medicine.

Robins, L. N., Helzer, J. E., Croughan, J., & Ratcliff, K. S. (1981). National Institute of Mental Health Diagnostic Interview Schedule: Its history, characteristics, and validity. *Archives of General Psychiatry, 38*, 381–389.

Rose, M. K., Soares, H. H., & Joseph, C. (1993). Frail elderly clients with personality disorders: A challenge for social work. *Journal of Gerontological Social Work, 19*, 153–165.

Rosowsky, E., & Gurian, B. (1991). Borderline personality disorder in late life. *International Psychogeriatrics, 3*, 39–52.

Rosowsky, E., & Gurian, B. (1992). Impact of borderline personality disorder in late life on systems of care. *Hospital and Community Psychiatry, 43*, 386–389.

Ruegg, R., & Frances, A. (1995). New research in personality disorders. *Journal of Personality Disorders, 9*, 1–48.

Ruegg, R. G., Gilmor, J., Ekstrom, R. D., Corrigan, M., Knight, B., Tancer, M., Leatherman, M. E., Carson, S. W., & Golden, R. N. (1993). A psychoneuroendocrine study of the unified biosocial theory of personality. *Biological Psychiatry, 34*, 885–888.

Rutter, M. (1987). Temperament, personality and personality disorder. *British Journal of Psychiatry, 150*, 443–458.

Schneider, L. S., Zemansky, M. F., Bender, M., & Sloane, R. B. (1992). Personality in recovered depressed elderly. *International Psychogeriatrics, 4*, 177–185.

Segal, D. L. (1997). Structured interviewing and DSM classification. In S. M. Turner & M. Hersen (Eds.), *Adult psychopathology and diagnosis* (3rd. ed., App. 24–57). New York: Wiley.

Segal, D. L., & Falk, S. B. (in press). Structured diagnostic interviews and rating scales. In M. Hersen & A. S. Bellack (Eds.), *Behavioral assessment: A practical handbook* (4th ed.). New York: Allyn & Bacon.

Segal, D. L., Hersen, M., & Van Hasselt, V. B. (1994). Reliability of the Structured Clinical Interview for DSM-III-R: An evaluative review. *Comprehensive Psychiatry, 35*, 316–327.

Segal, D. L., Hersen, M., Van Hasselt, V. B., Kabacoff, R. I., & Roth, L. (1993). Reliability of diagnoses in older psychiatric patients using the Structured Clinical Interview for DSM-III-R. *Journal of Psychopathology and Behavioral Assessment, 15*, 347–356.

Segal, D. L., Kabacoff, R. I., Hersen, M., Van Hasselt, V. B., & Ryan, C. F. (1995). Update on the reliability of diagnosis in older psychiatric outpatients using the Structured Clinical Interview for DSM-III-R. *Journal of Clinical Geropsychology, 1*, 313–321.

Siegel, D. J., & Small, G. W. (1986). Borderline personality disorder in the elderly: A case study. *Canadian Journal of Psychiatry, 31*, 859–860.

Silberman, C. S., Roth, L., Segal, D. L., & Burns, W. (in press). Relationship between the Millon Clinical Multiaxial Inventory-II and Coolidge Axis II Inventory in chronically mentally ill older adults: A pilot study. *Journal of Clinical Psychology*.

Skodol, A. E., Oldham, J. M., Rosnick, L., Kellman, H. D., & Hyler, S. E. (1991). Diagnosis of DSM-III-R personality disorders: A comparison of two structured interviews. *International Journal of Methods in Psychiatric Research, 1*, 13–26.

Skodol, A. E., Rosnick, L., Kellman, H. D., Oldham, J. M., & Hyler, S. E. (1988). Validating structured DSM-III-R personality disorder assessments with longitudinal data. *American Journal of Psychiatry, 145*, 1297–1299.

Soldz, S., Budman, S., Demby, A., & Merry, J. (1993). Diagnostic agreement between the Personality Disorder

Examination and the MCMI-II. *Journal of Personality Assessment, 60,* 486–499.
Soloff, P. H. (1990). What's new in personality disorders?: An update on pharmacological treatment. *Journal of Personality Disorders, 4,* 233–243.
Spar, J. E., & LaRue, A. (1990). *Concise guide to geriatric psychiatry.* Washington, DC: American Psychiatric Press.
Spitzer, R. L., Endicott, J., & Robins, E. (1978). Research diagnostic criteria: Rationale and reliability. *Archives of General Psychiatry, 35,* 773–782.
Spitzer, R. L., Forman, J. B. W., & Nee, J. (1979). DSM-III field trials: I. Initial interrater diagnostic reliability. *American Journal of Psychiatry, 136,* 815–817.
Spitzer, R. L., Williams, J. B. W., Gibbon, M., & First, M. B. (1990). *Structured Clinical Interview for DSM-III-R Personality Disorders (SCID-II, Version 1.0).* Washington, DC: American Psychiatric Press.
Standage, K., & Ladha, N. (1988). An examination of the reliability of the Personality Disorder Examination and a comparison with other methods of identifying personality disorders in a clinical sample. *Journal of Personality Disorders, 2,* 267–271.
Stangl, D., Pfohl, B., Zimmerman, M., Bowers, W., & Corenthal, C. (1985). A structured interview for the DSM-III personality disorders: A preliminary report. *Archives of General Psychiatry, 42,* 591–596.
Thomas, A. & Chess, S. (1977). *Temperament and development.* New York: Brunner/Mazel.
Thompson, L. W., Gallagher, D., Czirr, R. (1988). Personality disorder and outcome in the treatment of late-life depression. *Journal of Geriatric Psychiatry, 21,* 133–146.
Trull, T. J. & Larson, S. L. (1994). External validity of two personality disorder inventories. *Journal of Personality Disorders, 8,* 96–103.
Turley, B., Bates, G. W., Edwards, J., & Jackson, H. J. (1992). MCMI-II personality disorders in recent-onset bipolar disorders. *Journal of Clinical Psychology, 48,* 320–329.
Tyrer, P. (1988). *Personality disorders: Diagnosis, management, and course.* London: Wright/Butterworth.
World Health Organization. (1995). *The International Personality Disorder Examination (IPDE) DSM-IV module.* Washington, DC: American Psychiatric Press.
Young, J. E. (1994). *Cognitive therapy for personality disorders: A schema-focused approach* (Rev. ed.). Sarasota, FL: Professional Resources Press.

7.13
Schizophrenia and Related Conditions in Late Life

PHILIP D. HARVEY
Mount Sinai School of Medicine, New York, NY, USA

7.13.1 INTRODUCTION

Schizophrenia has been studied in detail from a psychological perspective. This research has focused on symptomatology, adaptive functioning, and cognitive impairments during the premorbid, early, and middle stages of the illness. In contrast to the huge volume of psychological research on schizophrenia in these earlier stages, there is considerably less research on schizophrenia and related conditions in late life. Understanding schizophrenia in late life is important for several reasons, including developing knowledge of the impact of aging on the illness, developing new treatments specifically targeted at older individuals, and understanding any differences between individuals with schizophrenia that has been chronic throughout the lifespan and individuals who develop schizophrenia late in life. With the aging of the population of the United States, the average age of psychiatric patients, including persons with schizophrenia, will increase as well. It is estimated that in 1997, there are 300 000 individuals over the age of 65 with a history of a schizophrenia diagnosis (Blazer, 1996), with many (20 000) still receiving institutional care of some sort (Hafner & Hambrecht, 1994). In addition, late-onset schizophrenia has been studied in considerably more detail in the early 1990s, with a number of interesting findings emerging regarding the similarities and differences between same-aged individuals with schizophrenia with early onset and those with a lifelong course of illness (Jeste et al., 1995).

This chapter focuses on the full range of psychological characteristics of schizophrenia, including clinical symptoms and phenomenology, cognitive functioning, adaptive skills, and treatments. Since schizophrenia has proven to be the most heterogeneous of all psychiatric conditions, the effects of aging on this condition would be expected to be very diverse and the developing research findings confirm this expectation. Symptoms, cognitive functions, and outcomes appear to vary greatly across elderly patients with a history of schizophrenia, ranging from complete disappearance of symptoms with stable residence in the community (Harding, Brooks, Ashikaga, Strauss, & Breier, 1987a, 1987b; Harding, Zubin & Strauss, 1992) to stays in chronic care hospitals of more than seven consecutive decades with complete dependence on others for all of their needs (Davidson et al., 1995). Thus, the extreme variability across individuals seen in schizophrenia in earlier life appears magnified in late life.

7.13.2 CONCEPTIONS OF SCHIZOPHRENIA AND IMPLICATIONS FOR RESEARCH ON SCHIZOPHRENIA IN LATE LIFE

Schizophrenia was initially described as a condition that developed in late adolescence and led to a deterioration in cognitive functions and behavior. The specifics of the deterioration have been in dispute since that time. Although Kraepelin (1919) referred to schizophrenia as "dementia praecox," it is not clear that he meant that schizophrenia was a condition which led to progressive deterioration in cognitive and behavioral functioning. It is clear, however, that his general perspective was that after the development of the illness, a full return to the previous level of functioning is almost never expected. In contrast, Bleuler's (1911/1950) conception of the illness allowed not only for a full remission of symptoms but also for considerable variation in symptom severity during the active illness itself. Thus, from the very first detailed descriptions of schizophrenia there has been controversy regarding the course of the illness and, by implication, the level of adaptive and cognitive impairment expected in older individuals with the illness.

Onset age has also been a controversial issue in the conceptions of the illness. Kraepelin delineated dementia praecox from paraphrenia, thus subdividing the illness on the dimension of age of onset. Paraphrenia was described as an illness of late onset, with predominantly persecutory (i.e., paranoid) delusions and minimal additional impairments. Hallucinations, if present, were not a central feature of the illness and delusions were nonbizarre. In the *Diagnostic and Statistical Manual of Mental Disorders (DSM-IV)* (American Psychiatric Association [APA], 1993), all hallucinations are required to be tactile or olfactory, not auditory, and must be related to the theme of the delusion. Patients with paraphrenia are classically described as lacking major changes in their affective response, and their level of motivation, and having preserved cognitive functions (Kraeplin, 1919). Their symptoms were seen as also remitting spontaneously with considerably more frequency than in dementia praecox. Bleuler disputed this conception, arguing instead that schizophrenia could develop in later life and that it was possible for a late onset of schizophrenia. Thus, the Bleulerian approach to the conception of the illness was that there was minimal difference in the characteristics of the illness seen as a function of onset age.

There has been controversy and evolution in diagnostic criteria for schizophrenia. Since the late 1970s, there has been considerable revision in diagnostic criteria for schizophrenia, with one of the major changes focusing on the issue of age at onset and the diagnosis for the disorder. The first of the new American diagnostic criteria, Research Diagnostic Criteria (RDC; Spitzer, Endicott, & Robins, 1978), required onset of symptoms between the ages of 16 and 45 for a diagnosis of schizophrenia. The rule-out for late onset was also present in *DSM-III* (APA, 1980), but was removed from the revision of these criteria in *DSM-IIIR* (APA, 1987). *DSM-IV* (APA, 1993) criteria also allow for schizophrenia to be diagnosed in individuals with an onset of symptoms at any age. No differences in symptomatology are required as a function of age of onset. One of the problems, of course, with diagnosing schizophrenia in later life is that many dementing conditions, including subcortical dementias such as Parkinson's disease and cortical dementias such as Alzheimer's disease, often have psychotic symptoms as a component of their symptom presentation (Jeste, Wragg, Salmon, Harris, & Thal, 1992). This situation can lead to complications in the initial diagnosis of schizophrenia.

7.13.3 DIAGNOSIS OF SCHIZOPHRENIA AND RELATED CONDITIONS IN LATE LIFE

Schizophrenia, as established by US and international criteria, is defined by the presence of characteristic symptoms, a clear decline in overall adaptive functioning, a minimum duration of illness, and the absence of other factors that could have caused the symptoms, such as affective disorder, substance abuse, brain dysfunction, or other general medical conditions (seizure disorders, etc.). Related conditions include schizophreniform disorder (illness meeting all criteria for schizophrenia other than the duration requirement), delusional disorder (a disorder with a single prominent, nonbizarre, delusion but not enough additional symptoms to meet criteria for schizophrenia), and schizoaffective disorder. As noted above, a major problem in diagnosing a new onset of any of these disorders in late life is the fact that degenerative dementing illnesses often have psychotic features as a symptom (Jeste et al., 1992). Thus, a careful cognitive assessment, including follow-up evaluation, is required at the time of diagnosis to rule out the presence of an alternative dementing condition. Neurological or neuroimaging assessment to rule out a cerebrovascular accident is also prudent.

One of the complexities of confirming a continued diagnosis of any of these disorders in individuals with a lifelong course of illness is that of ruling out alternative influences on symptoms. Aging-related physical illnesses and their consequences, including vascular disease, diabetes, and pulmonary problems, may cause cognitive impairments similar to those seen in schizophrenia. Thus, knowledge of current medical status is more important in generating a diagnosis of schizophrenia and related conditions in late life.

7.13.4 EPIDEMIOLOGY OF SCHIZOPHRENIA AND RELATED CONDITIONS IN LATE LIFE

Schizophrenia is well accepted to have a lifetime prevalence of around 1% of the population, across all cultures. Data suggest that there are slightly more male than female patients who meet diagnostic criteria for schizophrenia (Lewine, 1981), although onset age is quite important in determination of sex ratios of newly incident cases. Female patients are known to have a generally later age of onset for the illness (Faraone, Chen, Goldstein & Tsuang, 1994), although this finding may not hold true for patients who have a positive family history for schizophrenia in a first-degree relative (Albus & Maier, 1995). Prevalence of schizophrenia in late life is also a function of survival of early-onset cases, since schizophrenia has significant mortality associated with it. Most estimates of mortality associated with schizophrenia suggest that the first few years of illness are most dangerous, with accidents, suicide, and homicide accounting for mortality in these early periods. The large numbers of very old long-stay patients found in public psychiatric facilities in both the US and the UK suggest that long-stay patients as a group do not necessarily have an extremely abbreviated life expectancy. Two large-scale whole-hospital studies have found that female long-stay patients outnumber male patients (Davidson et al., 1995; Leff, Thornicroft, Coxhead, & Crawford, 1994), but differences in gender-related life expectancy might account for these findings.

There are an estimated 20 000 early-onset geriatric schizophrenic patients residing in chronic psychiatric hospitals in the US. In addition, there are another 200 000 living in nursing home care and an additional unknown number residing in community care (Meeks et al., 1990). It is not known how many former schizophrenic patients are living in relative remission in the community, but the results of some studies (Harding et al., 1987a, 1987b, 1992) suggest that this number may be substantial. Thus, the prevalence of diagnosable schizophrenia will be less than the sum of all cases still surviving who at one time carried a diagnosis of schizophrenia.

7.13.4.1 New Incidence of Schizophrenia in Late Life

Studies reviewed by Harris and Jeste (1988) suggested that approximately 15% of patients with a first episode of schizophrenia were over the age of 60 at the time of first psychiatric admission. In nearly every one of these studies, the proportion of females was greater than that of males in the new onset cases. These studies are often limited by virtue of being hospital admission studies and therefore fail to identify those cases who manifest the disorder but do not seek or otherwise obtain treatment. In a large-scale population-based prospective study, Castle and Murray (1993) examined the new-onset cases of schizophrenia in a London borough. They found that the average age of onset for males (31.2 years) was ten years younger than that of females (41.1 years) and that the prevalence and associated characteristics of the illness did not differ markedly as a function of the breadth of the schizophrenia criteria that were used. The male/female ratio changed as a function of age of onset, with the ratio at 1.6 to 1 for onset from ages 16 to 25 and 0.2 to 1 for onset age after 76. Patients with late onset were also much less likely to have a family history of schizophrenia, but some increase in familial prevalence of affective disorders was found in these patients. Previous studies of late-onset schizophrenia have suggested that late-onset schizophrenic patients typically have good adaptive functioning before the onset of illness, with some increase over normative expectations in the prevalence of schizoid or paranoid personality (Harris & Jeste, 1988).

7.13.4.2 New Incidence of Related Conditions in Late Life

A few studies have examined the characteristics of paraphrenia (i.e., late-onset delusional disorder) and compared it with schizophrenia. Parsons (1964) reported a prevalence of "late paraphrenia" of 0.17 to 0.24 cases per hundred community-dwelling elderly. Christenson and Blazer (1984) reported a 4% prevalence of paranoid delusions in community-dwelling elderly. Flint, Rifat, and Eastwood (1991) found a high incidence of "organicity" in the paraphrenia cases as compared with patients with late-onset schizophrenia. Yassa and Suranyi-Cadotte (1993) compared 20 patients with late-onset schizophrenia with 20 patients with late-onset paraphrenia. The incidence of paraphrenia was 4% of the total admissions over a 7-year period to a geriatric inpatient service, which was the same prevalence as for first-episode schizophrenia. Patients with paraphrenia were more likely to have had a concomitant physical illness and were less likely to have had a premorbid picture of personality abnormalities. These patients were also less likely to have a relapse after successful neuroleptic treatment.

Thus, many cases of schizophrenia apparently develop late in life, with several distinct epidemiological characteristics that separate them from early-onset cases and from related disorders with late-life onset. The prevalence of late-onset paraphrenia is more difficult to estimate, but is probably much less than that of schizophrenia. Since one-third of all cases of schizophrenia may have onset after age 50, the expected population prevalence of late-onset schizophrenia may be 0.33%, which is at least twice that of estimates of the prevalence of paraphrenia.

7.13.5 GENERAL OUTCOME OF SCHIZOPHRENIA IN LATE LIFE

Schizophrenia has long been noted for its variability in outcome, with a tendency toward negative outcomes dominating. Only about one-third of patients who meet diagnostic criteria for schizophrenia are able to resume adaptive functioning with any success and as many as one-third are chronically impaired and largely dependent on others for care on a lifelong basis (Wyatt, 1991). Comprehensive outcome studies suggest a wide variance in overall outcome (Ciompi, 1980). Although regional trends in mental health care may have as great an influence as the disorder itself on prevalence of patients with extremely long inpatient stay, a considerable number of schizophrenic patients have a very negative outcome with extended stays at high levels of care. Hospital-based studies have suggested that large numbers of geriatric patients with schizophrenia still reside in chronic psychiatric hospitals with low levels of functioning (Arnold et al., 1995; Davidson et al., 1995). These patients often have a relatively early age of onset, severe negative symptoms, poor adaptive functioning (both before and after the onset of initial symptoms), and severe cognitive impairments. Although some of these patients may be discharged from the hospital, many long-stay patients are simply referred to nursing home care (White et al., in press). Among the characteristics of patients who are difficult to discharge in late life are belligerent and hostile behaviors (White et al., in press), including both verbal and behavioral aggressiveness.

In contrast to hospital-based studies which tend to paint a fairly negative picture of outcome in the disorder, one comprehensive study has suggested that many individuals with an early diagnosis of schizophrenia go on to be discharged from the institution and to live in the community for decades with modest to no residual symptoms. The Vermont longitudinal study (Harding et al., 1987a, 1987b, 1992) suggested that many individuals with a diagnosis of schizophrenia in early adulthood are residing in the community, with modest to adequate adaptive, occupational, and interpersonal functions. Since this study was based in a rural state, which varies from urban areas in terms of levels of support and intactness of the community, the applicability of this study to patients from urban and suburban catchment areas is unclear. A study of community-dwelling geriatric schizophrenic patients (Bartels, Mueser, & Miles, 1997) based in the nearby state of New Hampshire found that there was considerably more impairment in adaptive functioning and clinical symptoms than reported in the Vermont study.

7.13.6 OUTCOME OF ACUTE PSYCHIATRIC ADMISSION IN LATE LIFE

While studies of chronic hospital populations may paint a gloomy picture of outcome in the disorder, there are some data from recent studies of acute care of geriatric patients with an acute admission for schizophrenia that also raise some questions about the outcome of even acute psychiatric care in the elderly patient with schizophrenia. Studies of nongeriatric first-admission patients (Loebel et al., 1992) suggest that over 90% of first-admission patients are in a state of remission within one year. Statistics for readmissions of patients with a previous history of schizophrenia are typically similar. While approximately 60% of acutely admitted nongeriatric psychiatric patients are discharged to the care of relatives, with another 30% being referred to some community residence, and only about 5% referred directly to chronic care (Keefe & Harvey, 1994), the two studies previously published on outcome of acute psychiatric admissions in geriatric patients suggested that only 50% at most of all acutely admitted patients who had been residing in the community returned to their former residence (Mulsant et al., 1993; Rockwood, Stolee, & Brahim, 1991). The geriatric schizophrenic patients in those two studies had a very high rate of referral to nursing home care (33% in Mulsant et al.) or long-term psychiatric hospitals (33% in Mulsant et al. and 20% in Rockwood et al.). These data suggest that there is a high risk for any single acute psychiatric treatment of a geriatric patient with schizophrenia to result in a referral to long-term care.

Explanations for this situation are complex. It is possible that acute psychiatric admissions in geriatric patients with schizophrenia are precipitated as much by medical or social crises as they are by exacerbation of symptoms of the illness. If there is an illness or other adverse event affecting a caregiver, a psychiatric admission may be precipitated, with the change in social environment precluding a return to the prior residence. An additional possibility is that what appears to be an admission for psychiatric reasons is actually precipitated by the onset of a degenerative dementia, such as Alzheimer's disease. The current set of short-term outcome studies do not allow for this possibility to be ruled out. Thus, it is not clear if schizophrenia alone, or if additional neurological or medical conditions are responsible for the relatively adverse outcome of geriatric acute psychiatric care.

7.13.7 CLINICAL SYMPTOMS IN LATE-LIFE SCHIZOPHRENIA

Clinical symptoms have been studied in both early- and late-onset cases of late-life schizophrenia. Symptoms of the illness are typically characterized in terms of three different dimensions: positive symptoms (i.e., florid), including delusions and hallucinations; negative symptoms (i.e., deficit symptoms), including reductions in affective response, language output, and motivated behaviors; and disorganized symptoms, including formal thought disorder, inappropriate affective, and bizarre behavior (Andreasen, Arndt, Alliger, Miller, & Flaum, 1995). For years, clinical lore held that positive and disorganized symptoms were "burned out" and that only negative or deficit symptoms would be detected in late life, even in long-stay institutionalized patients (Bridge, Cannon, & Wyatt, 1978). Several studies have suggested that this conception is partially to mostly incorrect.

In a large-scale study of chronically institutionalized schizophrenic patients ranging in age from 25 to 95 (Davidson et al., 1995), negative symptoms manifested an increase in severity over the age-range studied, while positive symptoms manifested a decrease. The severity scores for negative symptoms in this population were very elevated compared with those seen in younger patients. The decrease in severity of positive symptoms, however, was such that even the oldest of the patients studied manifested positive symptom severity scores at the 40th percentile for the standardization sample for the rating scale used (the Positive and Negative Syndrome Scale: PANSS; Kay, 1991). The severity of negative symptoms in the geriatric patients in this sample was found to increase slightly at a one-year follow-up of the sample, with no statistically significant decrease in positive symptoms (Putnam et al., 1996). This result is in contrast to studies of younger chronic schizophrenic patients (Mueser, Douglas, Bellack, & Morrison, 1991; Pogue-Geille & Harrow, 1984, 1985) where negative symptoms did not worsen in severity at similar follow-up intervals. In a study of formal thought disorder (Harvey, Lombardi et al., 1997), roughly parallel findings were seen. Geriatric chronically institutionalized patients manifested more severe poverty of speech and less severe "positive" thought disorders (e.g., derailment, tangentiality, loss of goal, and circumstantiality) than younger chronically institutionalized patients.

In a comparative study of late-onset, acutely ill patients with schizophrenia and early-onset chronic patients, paranoid symptoms were significantly more common on the late-onset cases (Jeste et al., 1995). In addition, late-onset patients were more likely to have better lifelong functioning, including marriage and a stable work history. A previous study (Harris, Jeste, Krull, Montague, & Heaton, 1991) had suggested that the deficit syndrome was present in approximately 30% of older patients with schizophrenia, with this prevalence probably not elevated from that seen in younger patients. When the stability of the deficit syndrome was examined in a large sample of geriatric chronic patients (Putnam et al., 1996), a high degree of cross-temporal stability was noted. Finally, White et al. (1994) used confirmatory factor analysis to compare the structure of symptoms in poor-outcome geriatric schizophrenic patients, divided on the basis of their level of cognitive dysfunction, with younger poor-outcome patients. No differences in the factor structure of clinical symptoms were found between older and younger patients or between the geriatric patients who varied in their level of cognitive impairment. The authors concluded that since schizophrenic cognitive impairment did not affect the structure of symptoms, it may be an instrinsic aspect of poor-outcome schizophrenia.

Any assessment of clinical symptoms in chronic schizophrenic patients, especially those with a long and often uninterrupted institutional stay, must seriously consider the role of iatrogenic factors. While life in a chronic care institution may not be likely to sustain the presence of positive symptoms, the level of impoverishment of the environment, years of treatment with antipsychotic medication, and the low staff-to-patient ratio could easily be argued to influence negative symptom severity. Although length of institutional stay had no relationship with the severity of negative symptoms in the Davidson et al. (1995) study, all patients had already been in the hospital for at least a decade. As in other discussions of cognitive functioning, chronic institutional care cannot be ruled out as a contributory factor to the severity of negative symptoms as measured in those studies. The results of longitudinal studies of early-stage patients with schizophrenia (Knight, Roff, Barrnet, & Moss, 1979) suggest that more severe negative symptoms early in the course of illness predict a more adverse outcome, and multiple cross-sectional studies of patients at approximately the same age suggest that negative symptoms are more severe in patients with a chronic course of illness and greater deficits in life skills. Positive symptom severity has been demonstrated to have no cross-sectional or longitudinal relationship with outcome (Green, 1996). More severe symptoms of disorganization, especially communication disorder, are associated cross-sectionally with poor outcome (Keefe et al., 1987). Thus, the most tempered interpretation of the data suggests that negative symptoms may start out worse in those patients with a lifelong stay in a chronic psychiatric hospital, with a late-life worsening where the institutional stay itself may affect symptom severity in certain patients.

7.13.8 COGNITIVE FUNCTIONING IN LATE-LIFE SCHIZOPHRENIA

Cognitive impairment is a very common symptom in schizophrenia, being present across the entire course of the illness (Kraeplin, 1919; Saykin et al., 1994). While a full discussion of the characteristics of cognitive impairment is beyond the scope of this chapter (see Gold & Harvey 1993 for a specific review of that symptom), it should be noted that deficits in academic functioning, relative to classmates, are identified in preschizophrenic individuals as early as the first grade (Crow, Done, & Sackler, 1995). Cognitive impairment appears to be stable within patients over time, across various follow-up intervals, and to predict outcome in the illness (Gold & Harvey, 1993). It should also be noted that there are many changes in cognitive functioning with aging in the normal population. While the domain of aging-related changes is enormous and beyond the scope of this chapter, several general points can be made. Major aging-related changes occur in motor speed and in memory functions, while the level of change in long-term memory and ability to access and utilize previously learned material is much more modest. As a consequence, baseline functioning can be estimated from performance on tests of old learning such as reading and vocabulary, because of the minimal aging-related changes in these areas. For a complete review of aging and neuropsychology, the reader is referred to Albert and Moss (1988). Since schizophrenic patients at their first episode often score 2 to 3 standard deviations below normal comparison groups (Saykin et al., 1994) or standardization samples, the possibility of detecting cognitive decline with aging is reduced because of floor effects. At the same time, it should be noted that the types of cognitive operations that change with normal aging (new learning and recall, concentration and attention, psychomotor and visuomotor speed) are the deficits most commonly noted in schizophrenic patients early in life. Thus, aging-related changes are likely to maximally impact those functions most impaired in schizophrenia earlier in life.

In younger schizophrenic patients, the typical assessment of cognitive functioning has either used assessment with clinical neuropsychological tests or with experimental measures of attention and memory. Across these studies, significant impairments have been found in learning and memory, attention, and executive functioning (see Gold & Harvey, 1993 for a review of these findings in younger patients), with lesser impairments noted in most other cognitive functions (Braff et al., 1991). In older schizophrenic patients, prominent cognitive impairments resembling dementia have also been reported. For example, in the Davidson et al. (1995) study, over 60% of the geriatric chronic schizophrenic patients would have met *DSM-IIIR* criteria for dementia in addition to schizophrenia. Similar findings were reported by Arnold, Franz, and Trojanowski (1994) in a separate sample. As demonstrated below, one of the issues that has been addressed in research on cognitive functioning is a comparison of the cognitive performance profiles of geriatric patients with schizophrenia, both early and late-onset, to the cognitive impairments seen in degenerative dementing conditions such as Alzheimer's disease (AD). Spurred by preliminary reports of an elevated prevalence of AD in postmortem brain specimens from patients who have a hospital chart diagnosis of schizophrenia (Prohovnik, Dwork, Kaufman, & Wilson, 1993), a number of studies have compared the cognitive profiles of patients with these two disorders.

One of the problems that develops in the assessment of geriatric patients is that of test selection. Patients who meet criteria for dementia may not be able to meaningfully complete many clinical neuropsychological tests, with their scores reflecting floor effects (Harvey, Mohs, & Davidson, 1993). One of the solutions that has been employed (Harvey et al., 1992) is the use of global screening measures, such as the Mini-Mental State Examination (MMSE; Folstein, Folstein, & McHugh, 1975 or a global assessment measure such as the Clinical Dementia Rating (CDR; Berg, 1988). These instruments have the advantage of being able to provide a global estimate of the level of cognitive functioning of the individual. They are limited by their focus on the cognitive impairments seen in degenerative dementia and their failure to include many of the content areas that are relevant to schizophrenia, such as executive functioning.

Studies of global estimates of cognitive functioning in patients with late-life schizophrenia have suggested that as many as 60% of geriatric chronically hospitalized patients have MMSE scores in the range suggestive of dementia. Davidson et al. (1995) used a cross-sectional design to compare MMSE scores in chronically hospitalized patients ranging in age from 25 to 95. There was a consistent linear relationship between MMSE scores and age, with the mean MMSE of patients who were aged 25 to 35 at 27 ("questionable impairment") and the mean MMSE of 85 to 95-year-olds only 9.6 ("severe dementia"). Even when low levels of premorbid education and age are considered (Crum, Anthony, Bassett, & Folstein, 1993), these scores are extremely low. There was a linear 3 MMSE points per decade reduction over the age-span of the patients studied. In contrast, in AD MMSE scores change an average of 3 points per year (Morris et al., 1993). When the geriatric patients who were still in the hospital were followed up 1 and 2 years later (Harvey, White et al., 1995) there was no measurable change in MMSE scores for the sample as a whole, the IntraClass Correlation Coefficient (ICC) was over 0.85 at each assessment, and one-month stability of the MMSE was found to be over 0.90 (ICC). When the sample of patients in the Davidson et al. sample was compared with similar-age, long-stay patients from the UK, there were no differences in their MMSE scores (Harvey, Leff, Trieman, Anderson, & Davidson, in press). In addition, MMSE scores of chronic schizophrenic patients in other US hospitals are strikingly similar across institutions (Gur et al., 1996).

These data suggest that globally estimated cognitive functions appear to manifest age-related differences, although these scores do not decline at a rate consistent with a degenerative dementia such as AD (Mohs, 1995). Further evidence for dissimilarity to AD was provided by Harvey, Lombardi et al.(1996), who used a battery of neuropsychological tests that was developed to assess the nature and progression of cognitive impairments in AD. At a one-year follow-up, none of these cognitive functions showed any evidence of decline. In addition, the profile of impairment was quite different from that seen in AD. A delayed recall memory deficit is the first reliable sign of mild AD (Welsh et al., 1991), with this deficit not progressing over time and being uncorrelated with overall MMSE scores (Morris et al., 1993). In the Harvey, Lombardi et al. study, delayed recall deficits were correlated with MMSE scores more strongly than any other measure. Further evidence of the dissimilarity of cognitive performance profiles in AD and geriatric schizophrenia is provided by the results of a cross-sectional study comparing late and early onset geriatric schizophrenic patients, nongeriatric schizophrenic patients, patients with AD, and normal controls on a expanded version of the Halstead—Reitan neuropsychological battery (Heaton et al., 1994). Patients with AD were found to perform worse than all schizophrenic patients on a measure of delayed recall, with the schizophrenic patients performing worse on several other summary measures. A very similar result was obtained by Davidson et al. (1996), who compared schizophrenic and AD patients who were matched on global cognitive impairment as measured by MMSE scores. Patients with AD were more impaired on delayed recall and less impaired on verbal and visuo-motor skills than schizophrenic patients who had similar MMSE scores. No differences in rate of learning were detected. Both of these studies suggest that schizophrenic patients are differentially impaired compared with patients with AD and both were careful to rule out alternative causes of cognitive impairment in their samples.

The results of these studies, combined with prospective studies of postmortem characteristics of geriatric schizophrenic patients failing to find evidence of AD-related neuropathology in the majority of cognitively impaired patients with schizophrenia (Arnold et al., 1995; Powchik et al., in press; Purohit et al., 1993), can be interpreted to conclusively demonstrate that the profound cognitive impairments seen in geriatric long-stay schizophrenic patients are not always due to degenerative dementia. What is considerably less clear, are the characteristics of cognitive impairment in geriatric schizophrenic patients and any possible differences between late- and early-onset cases, as well as the associations between outcome and cognitive impairments. In the Heaton et al. (1994) study, no differences in global neuropsychological summary scores were found between similar-aged early- and late-onset geriatric schizophrenic patients and no cognitive performance differences were found as a function of age in the schizophrenic sample. Similarly, Hyde et al. (1994) reported no age-related differences in cognitive functions in a cross-sectional study of schizophrenic patients ranging in age from the 20s to the late 60s. In contrast, several other studies of a large sample of extremely chronic institutionalized patients have found major age-related differences in both global indices of cognitive functions (Davidson et al., 1995) and in specific neuropsychological measures (Harvey, Leibman et al., in press; Harvey, Lombardi et al., 1995).

In terms of the specific characteristics of cognitive impairments seen in geriatric schizophrenic patients, Harvey, Powchik, Mohs, and Davidson (1995) compared geriatric chronic schizophrenic patients with either absent-mild or moderate cognitive impairments, defined by global ratings of a general clinical severity measure for dementia, on a battery of memory tests that have been demonstrated in brain-injured populations to be differentially sensitive to dysfunctions in the temporal and frontal lobes. They found that there were large differences in memory performance associated with global cognitive impairments and that patients, regardless of their level of cognitive impairment, tended to manifest patterns of performance consistent with either a temporal-lobe or frontal-lobe memory deficit. Paulsen, Heaton, Sadek, Perry, and Jeste (1995) also performed a comprehensive neuropsychological evaluation of profiles of memory impairment in schizophrenic patients, dividing their geriatric patients on the basis of cortical, subcortical, or unimpaired profiles. Cortical profiles include deficits in learning, recall, and recognition memory, while subcortical profiles include preserved recognition memory and increased benefits from cuing and encoding assistance. They found about one-third of the patients manifested an unimpaired profile, with 50% manifesting a subcortical profile. Only 15% of the patients manifested a cortical pattern of impairment. These results are quite consistent with the findings of Harvey, Powchik et al., who found that recognition memory performance did not vary across patients who differed considerably in their global level of cognitive impairment. In a study of verbal fluency performance, geriatric chronically hospitalized schizophrenic patients were found to be more impaired on phonemic fluency than younger chronic patients, with no age-related differences in category-based fluency when education differences between these two samples were considered (Harvey, Leibman et al., in press). Both groups of patients performed at least 2 to 3 standard deviations below age and education-corrected mean on category fluency and 1.5 to 2 standard deviations below the mean on phonemic fluency. An additional finding of some importance is that estimates of premorbid intellectual attainment (i.e., the Wide Range Achievement Test-Revised [WRAT-R; Jastak, 1984] reading subtest) were correlated with overall cognitive status in geriatric patients, but not nongeriatric patients. This suggests a possible bias effect that should be considered in later studies, as the WRAT-R or other similar tests are often employed as estimates of premorbid cognitive status in studies of cognitive functions in younger schizophrenic patients (O'Carroll, Walker, & Dunan, 1992).

In an examination of the long-term effects of psychosurgery in chronic schizophrenia, Harvey et al. (1993) studied 72 chronically hospitalized schizophrenic patients on a neuropsychological battery, comparing patients who had experienced a leukotomy with a sample matched for age, education, and overall cognitive status who had not. Consistent with earlier studies of leukotomized patients at younger ages (see Joschko, 1986 for a review), no major differences in cognitive functioning were found. These data suggest that a frontal lobe lesion that may disconnect the cortex and striatum does not interact with aging in chronic schizophrenia to produce even greater cognitive impairment, although there are some interpretive problems with the results. The geriatric chronic schizophrenic patients without leukotomy performed so poorly on tests sensitive to frontal lobe lesions, including the Wisconsin Card Sorting Test (WCST; Heaton, Chelune, Talley, Kay, & Curtiss, 1993), that it would be almost statistically impossible for the leukotomized patients to perform more poorly and reveal a differential performance deficit.

The results of these studies highlight the problem in studying cognitive performance in schizophrenic patients across wide ranges of age, chronicity, and severity of illness. Some of the inconsistent results may simply be the result of subject selection processes. The subjects in the studies conducted by Heaton and colleagues (Heaton et al., 1994; Paulsen et al., 1995) were largely outpatients residing in the community, in contrast to the subjects we studied, who had been continuously hospitalized for decades. Since more severe cognitive impairment is a powerful correlate of poor outcome in younger schizophrenic patients (Addington, Addington, & Maticka-Tyndale, 1991; Perlick, Mattis, Stastny, & Teresi, 1992), there is no reason to expect that extremely bad-outcome geriatric patients would not also have more severe impairments than those patients who are functioning adaptively in community. In the Hyde, Nawroz, Goldberg, Kleinman, and Weinberger (1994) study, relatively poor-outcome patients were studied, but younger and older patients were matched in WRAT-R scores in order to equalize premorbid intellectual functioning. As noted above, if WRAT-R scores are correlated with cognitive impairment in geriatric patients, matching on this variable would create a sample of geriatric patients who are preselected for reduced levels of cognitive impairment.

The previous research has revealed several important cohort effects when younger and older chronically hospitalized patients are compared. Geriatric chronic patients are consistently found to have a later age of first psychiatric admission and lower levels of formal education than younger patients (Arnold et al., 1995; Davidson et al., 1995). These differences have the potential of obscuring the interpretation of differences in cognitive functioning between the samples, because education and onset age have both been previously demonstrated to influence performance on cognitive tests. Performance differences between early and late-onset patients have the potential of being influenced by the correlates of chronic schizophrenia, including treatment and lifelong histories of social isolation, ostracism, and failure.

One area where age effects were not detected was in a set of studies examining the prevalence of age disorientation in chronic schizophrenia and affective disorder (Harvey, Lombardi et al., 1995; Lombardi et al., 1996). Age disorientation has been studied extensively by Crow and colleagues (Crow & Stevens, 1978; Liddle & Crow, 1984), with the consistent finding that approximately 25 to 33% chronic schizophrenic patients underestimate their age by 5 years or more. This finding has been demonstrated not to be caused by history of treatment, premorbid functioning, length of current hospital stay, age of onset, or age of the patients (Buhrich, Crow, Johnstone, & Owens 1988). Harvey, Lombardi et al. found that the prevalence of age disorientation was relatively stable, at approximately 40% from age 35 to age 75 in a sample of 393 chronically hospitalized schizophrenic patients. Age-related differences in cognitive functioning were found only in the patients who manifested age disorientation. Lombardi et al. found a similar rate of age disorientation (33%) in chronically hospitalized patients with affective disorders. These data suggest that one of the principal features of the cognitive impairment in schizophrenia may be orientation deficits. These deficits may be caused by impairments in episodic memory functions, which lead to faulty updating of personal information, in the same way that these memory impairments lead to poor performance on formal tests of memory functioning. Since only a portion of the patients manifest age disorientation, it cannot be due to some global factor associated with institutionalization. Furthermore, age disorientation was not associated, in either schizophrenic or affective patients, with history of premorbid functioning, including education, or history of somatic treatment, including leukotomy, insulin coma, or ECT, replicating previous findings (Buhrich et al., 1988). These data suggest that certain types of memory impairment may be correlated with poor outcome, regardless of diagnosis, and also clearly indicate that not all of the aspects of cognitive impairment in geriatric institutionalized schizophrenic patients could be attributed to aspects of institutional stay.

The main findings associated with the study of cognitive functioning in late-life schizophrenia is that there is very little evidence for the development of types of cognitive impairments that are qualitatively different from those seen in younger schizophrenic patients. While some studies find no age-related differences in cognitive performance, others do, with the principal variation between the studies being the nature of subject samples. The primary change appears to be a worsening of memory performance, in line with expected changes associated with normal aging, although this worsening still does not lead to performance as poor as seen in Alzheimer's disease. The association between extremely poor outcome and profound cognitive impairment leads to interpretive problems because of the very long length of stay and extensive treatment experienced by these patients. Since only a subset of these patients manifest age disorientation or other profound cognitive impairments, it is not possible that all aspects of their impairment are caused by institutional stay. Assuming that institutional stay and its correlates (e.g., medication treatment) have the potential to cause some of the cognitive impairments seen in geriatric chronically institutionalized patients, the variability across patients in level of impairment suggests that there may be individual difference factors that predict vulnerability to these effects. Identification of these factors is a useful target for further research.

7.13.9 ADAPTIVE IMPAIRMENT IN LATE LIFE SCHIZOPHRENIA

One of the principal sources of negative outcome in schizophrenia is a deficit in adaptive life functioning (Perlick, Stastny, Mattis, & Teresi, 1992; Serban & Gidynski, 1979; Tessler & Manderscheid, 1994). Many schizophrenic patients manifest severe and persistent disability because they are unable to care for themselves and become dependent on others for their care. Some of these impairments are more often present in patients with the negative symptoms (Mueser, Bellack, Douglas, & Wade, 1991) of schizophrenia as well as in patients with more severe cognitive impairment (Breier, Schreiber, Dyer, & Pickar, 1991). Patients who are dependent on others for their care are typically not more seriously affected by the positive symptoms of the disorder (Pogue-Geile & Harrow, 1985). Previous behavioral interventions in schizophrenia have often focused on remediation of these deficits in adaptive life functions (Hogg & Hall, 1992; Liberman, Mueser, & Wallace, 1986; Paul & Lenz, 1977), with some suggestions that pharmacological interventions should also be targeted at these types of deficits (Davidson & Keefe, 1995). As noted above, in younger chronic schizophrenic patients the presence of severe cognitive impairments is often correlated with the presence of these adaptive deficits (Green, 1996).

Limited information is available on adaptive functioning deficits in geriatric patients with schizophrenia. The available information suggests that the range of adaptive functioning is quite wide and that the level of care received by the patient is often correlated with their adaptive skill. Kincaid et al. (1995) studied 339 geriatric chronically hospitalized inpatients with schizophrenia, finding that clinical ratings of self-care and personal hygiene accounted for 9% of the variance in global ratings of severity of overall functional, cognitive, and behavioral impairment. Harvey, Davidson et al. (1997) developed the Social-Adaptive Functioning Evaluation (SAFE) scale, which was designed to evaluated overall adaptive dysfunction in geriatric institutionalized patients. They reported that total scores on the measure were strongly associated with the overall severity of cognitive impairment, as measured by the MMSE. In addition, the overall level of impairment was quite high in their population. For example, very severe impairments were found, on the average, for neatness and maintenance, money management, orientation and mobility, communication skills, and friendships, while impairments at a level that was considered "severe" were found on nine other measures of social, instrumental, and self-care skills. When a sample of 140 patients were followed prospectively for up to 3 years, it was found that deficits in the general areas of impulse control and self-care were quite predictive of discharge and placement. Patients with poor impulse control were likely to remain hospitalized, while patients with better self care were more likely to be discharged to a community setting. Social functioning did not discriminate between three different placement outcomes: remaining hospitalized, being referred to the community, or being transferred to a nursing home. In a study of over 800 geriatric psychiatric patients followed for 3 years during a period of downsizing of their psychiatric hospital, White et al. (in press) found that the presence of severe adaptive deficits was less strongly correlated with discharge from chronic care than the presence of hostile and belligerent behaviors. In patients who were discharged, however, severe deficits in adaptive functioning were more common in patients referred to a nursing home than in those discharged to the community.

In another study examining geriatric psychiatric patients residing outside of chronic hospitals and receiving community-based residential care, Bartels et al. (1997) evaluated patients with schizophrenia, major depression, and bipolar affective disorder. The severity of clinical symptoms was evaluated with the Brief Psychiatric Rating Scale-Expanded version (Lukoff, Liberman,& Nuechterlein, 1986) and with the Specific Levels of Functioning Scale (SLOF; Schneider & Streuening, 1983). The SLOF is a 43-item rating scale that comprehensively evaluates social, self-care, and community living skills, as well as disruptive behaviors. Schizophrenic patients, in addition to having more severe psychotic symptoms, were more impaired on all aspects of social and instrumental functioning than community-dwelling patients with affective disorders. These data suggest that the impairments in adaptive skills that characterize younger patients with schizophrenia are also present in late life, even in community-dwelling cases. Thus, severe adaptive deficits are present in many community-dwellers as well as in chronically hospitalized patients with schizophrenia.

In contrast, the results of the Vermont longitudinal study (Harding et al., 1987a, 1987b, 1992) suggest that some geriatric individuals with a history of schizophrenia are able to successfully adapt to life in the community and live there for extended periods without ever receiving any mental health services. Early identification of which patients are likely to have this type of adaptive success is not yet possible. When this constellation of characteristics predicting adaptive success is identified, early interventions for patients with a poor prognosis will be easier to target.

7.13.10 TREATMENT OF SCHIZOPHRENIA IN LATE LIFE

There is no specialized literature on the treatment of late-life schizophrenia with psychological interventions. At the same time, there is no information suggesting that current psychological treatments would be less effective in this type of population. Principal psychological interventions for schizophrenia with demonstrated efficacy are skills-based "rehabilitation" approaches and family intervention approaches designed to reduce expressed emotion (EE). Since EE approaches are applied to acutely ill patients, their applicability to geriatric schizophrenic patients with an early age of onset is limited. No specific EE research for late-life acute schizophrenia has been published up to 1997, although this may be a critical area for investigation. In particular, since many late-onset schizophrenic patients are referred to nursing home care directly from an acute psychiatric admission, assessment of EE characteristics at home may provide useful information in identifying those acutely ill late-onset patients who are at high risk to be referred to nursing home care because of negative aspects of their home life.

In contrast, skills-training approaches appear to be indicated for many of the geriatric patients (Bellack & Mueser, 1993). Since deficits in adaptive functioning are apparently extremely common in institutionalized and community-dwelling geriatric populations, this intervention would appear, at least superficially, to be likely to provide benefit to many of these patients. It is unclear how many of these geriatric patients have received such treatment earlier in their illness, without benefit, and how many have simply received "warehouse" institutional treatment or have been "dumped" into the community without follow-up plans. Previous studies suggest that even very severely ill younger patients may benefit from this treatment (Corrigan, Wallace, Schade, & Green, 1994), indicating that this population could be targeted for such an intervention.

A cautionary note is provided by the clear description by Green (1996) of cognitive barriers to such treatment. Since these interventions are essentially learning-based, deficits in the ability to learn with exposure, in performance on tests of vigilance, and in executive functioning have been demonstrated to markedly interfere with the success of these interventions in younger chronic schizophrenic patients. Since many geriatric patients with a chronic course of institutionalization manifest profound deficits in learning and memory, as described above, these patients would appear to be at high risk of failure in rehabilitation-type treatments (Mueser et al., 1991). Until techniques for cognitive enhancement are better supported with empirical research (see Vol. 18 (1992) of *Schizophrenia Bulletin* for a discussion of limitations in this regard), the application of social-instrumental skills-training approaches with geriatric patients with cognitive impairments appears to be quite likely to be unsuccessful.

Psychotropic medication for geriatric patients with schizophrenia is the most common treatment. While these interventions are not presently in the domain of clinical psychology, understanding of the issues involved in this type of treatment is important for any professional involved in the treatment of this population. As with many other drugs, dosing of geriatric patients is most useful at lower levels, a fact of which some treating physicians are apparently unaware. Geriatric patients are apparently more susceptible to the side effects of these medications as well. The reader is referred to a review paper by Jeste, Lacro, Gilbert, Kline, and Kline (1993) which addresses these issues, and others, in detail.

7.13.11 CONCLUSION

Schizophrenia is a lifelong illness that does not disappear with aging. Although some patients with schizophrenia have a good outcome in late life, the majority, both institutionalized and community dwelling, manifest severe deficits in adaptive functions. Clinical symptoms appear to be severe in most patients studied, with the level of symptoms seen across care settings arguing strongly against the idea that these symptoms burn out with age. Cognitive impairment appears to be a strong predictor of adaptive deficits and patients with a particularly poor outcome may actually show cognitive decline into the range of functioning commonly associated with dementia.

Schizophrenia appears to have a fairly high new case incidence in late life, with as many as 15% of all geriatric cases having had initial onset after age 65. These patients appear to resemble good-prognosis early-onset cases, other than for the high prevalence of females. Data on specific psychological treatments for late-life schizophrenic patients are completely lacking and are clearly necessary. As is clear from the data in this chapter, schizophrenia in late life is not benign and is associated with considerable disability in adaptive functioning and a clear burden on society or relatives. Development of effective treatments, psychological and pharmacological, for late-life schizophrenia is a clear goal for the future.

7.13.12 REFERENCES

Addington, J., Addington, D., & Maticka-Tyndale, E. (1991). Cognitive functioning and positive and negative symptoms in schizophrenia. *Schizophrenia Research,4*, 123–134.

Albert, M. S., & Moss, M. B. (1988). *Geriatric neuropsychology*. New York: Guilford.

Albus, M., & Maier, W. (1995). Lack of gender differences at age of onset in familial schizophrenia. *Schizophrenia Research. 18*, 51–57.

American Psychiatric Association (1980). *Diagnostic and statistical manual of mental disorders* (3rd. Ed.). Washington, DC: Author.

American Psychiatric Association (1987). *Diagnostic and statistical manual of mental disorders* (3rd Ed., revised). Washington, DC: Author.

American Psychiatric Association (1993). *Diagnostic and statistical manual of mental disorders* (4th. Ed.). Washington, DC: Author.

Andreasen, N. C., Arndt, S., Alliger, R., Miller, D., & Flaum, M. (1995). Symptoms of schizophrenia: Methods, meanings, and mechanisms. *Archives of General Psychiatry, 52*, 341–351

Arnold, S. E., Franz, B. R., & Trojanowski, J.Q. (1994). Elderly patients with schizophrenia exhibit infrequent neurodegenerative lesions. *Neurobiology of Aging, 15*, 299–303.

Arnold, S. E., Gur, R. E., Shapiro, R. M., Fisher, K. R., Moberg, P. J., Gibney, M. R., Gur, R. C., Blackwell, P., & Trojanowski, J. Q. (1995). Prospective clinicopathological studies of schizophrenia: Accrual and assessment of patients. *American Journal of Psychiatry, 152*, 731–737.

Bartels, S. J., Mueser, K. T., & Miles, K. M. (in press). Functional impairments in elderly patients with schizophrenia and major affective disorders living in the community: Social skills, living skills, and behavior problem. *Behavior Therapy*.

Bellack, A. S., & Mueser, K. T. (1993). Psychosocial treatment for schizophrenia. *Schizophrenia Bulletin,19*, 317–336.

Berg, L. (1988). Clinical dementia rating (CDR). *Psychopharmacology Bulletin,24*, 637–639.

Blazer, D. G. (1996). Epidemiology of psychiatric disorders in late life. In E. W. Busse & D. G. Blazer (Eds), *American Psychiatric Press handbook of geriatric psychiatry* (2nd ed., pp 155–171). Washington, DC: American Psychiatric Press.

Bleuler, E. (1911/1950). *Dementia praecox; or the group of schizophrenias*. New York: International Universities Press.

Braff, D. L., Heaton, R. K., Kuck, J., Cullum, M., Moranville, J., Grant, I., & Zisook, S. (1991). The generalized pattern of neuropsychological deficits in outpatients with chronic schizophrenia with heterogenous Wisconsin Card Sorting Test results. *Archives of General Psychiatry, 48*, 891–898.

Breier, A., Schreiber, J. L., Dyer, J., & Pickar, D. (1991). National Institute of Mental Health longitudinal study of chronic schizophrenia: Prognosis and predictors of outcome. *Archives of General Psychiatry,48*, 239–246.

Bridge, T. P., Cannon, E. H., & Wyatt, R. J. (1978). Burned-out schizophrenia: Evidence for age effects on schizophrenic symptomatology. *Journal of Gerontology, 33*, 835–839.

Buhrich, N., Crow, T. J, Johnstone, E. C., & Owens, D. G. (1988). Age disorientation in chronic schizophrenia is not associated with pre-morbid intellectual impairment or past physical treatment. *British Journal of Psychiatry, 152*, 466–469.

Castle, D. J., & Murray, R. M. (1993). The epidemiology of late-onset schizophrenia. *Schizophrenia Bulletin, 19*, 691–700.

Christenson, R., & Blazer, D. (1984). Epidemiology of persecutory ideation in an elderly population in the community. *American Journal of Psychiatry,141*, 1088–1091.

Ciompi, L. (1980). Catamnestic long-term study on the course of life and aging of schizophrenics. *Schizophrenia Bulletin, 6*, 606–618.

Corrigan, P. W., Wallace, C. J., Schade, M. L., & Green, M. F. (1994). Learning medication self-management skills in schizophrenia: Relationships with cognitive deficits and psychiatric symptoms. *Behavior Therapy, 25*, 5–15.

Crow, T. J., Done, D. J., & Sackler, A. (1995). Childhood precursors of psychosis as clues to its evolutionary origins. *European Archives of Psychiatry and Clinical Neuroscience, 245*, 61–69.

Crow, T. J., & Stevens, M. (1978). Age disorientation in chronic schizophrenia: The nature of the cognitive deficit. *British Journal of Psychiatry,133*, 137–142.

Crum, R. M., Anthony, J. C., Bassett, S. S., & Folstein, M. F. (1993). Population based norms for the mini-mental state examination by age and education level. *Journal of the American Medical Association, 269*, 2386–2391.

Davidson, M., Harvey, P. D., Powchik, P., Parrella, M.,

White, L., Knobler, H. Y., Losonczy, M., Keefe, R. S. E., Katz, S., & Frecksa, E. (1995). Severity of symptoms in chronically institutionalized geriatric schizophrenic patients. *American Journal of Psychiatry, 152,* 197–207.

Davidson, M., Harvey, P. D., Putnam, K., Welsh, K., & Mohs, R. C. (1996). Cognitive impairment in old-age schizophrenia: A comparative study of schizophrenia and Alzheimer's disease. *American Journal of Psychiatry, 153,* 1274–1279.

Davidson, M., & Keefe, R. S. E. (1995). Cognitive impairment as a target for pharmacological treatment in schizophrenia. *Schizophrenia Research, 17,* 123–129.

Faraone, S. V., Chen, W. J., Goldstein, J. M., & Tsuang, M. T. (1994). Gender differences in age at onset of schizophrenia. *British Journal of Psychiatry,164,* 625–629.

Flint, A. J., Rifat, S. L., & Eastwood, R. (1991). Late-onset paranoia: Distinct from paraphrenia. *International Journal of Geriatric Psychiatry, 6,* 103–109.

Folstein, M. F., Folstein, S. E., & McHugh, P. R. (1975). Mini-mental state: A practical method for grading the cognitive state of patients for the clinician. *Journal of Psychiatric Research, 12,* 189–198.

Green, M. F. (1996). What are the functional consequences of neurocognitive deficits in schizophrenia? *American Journal of Psychiatry, 153,* 321–330.

Gold, J. M., & Harvey, P. D. (1993). Cognitive deficits in schizophrenia. *Psychiatric Clinics of North America, 16,* 295–312.

Gur, R. E., Arnold, S. E., Moberg, P. J., Petty, R. G., Arnold, S., & Gur, R. C. (1996). The dementia of schizophrenia: Antemortem and postmortem studies. *Biological Psychiatry, 39,* 612.

Hafner, H. & Hambrecht, M. (1994). The elderly with schizophrenia. In E. Chiu & D. Ames (Eds.),*Functional psychiatric disorders of the elderly.* (pp. 287–302). Cambridge, UK: Cambridge University Press.

Harding, C. M., Brooks G. W., Ashikaga T., Strauss, J. S., & Breier, A. (1987a). The Vermont longitudinal study of persons with severe mental illness: I. Methodology, study sample, and overall current status 32 years later. *American Journal of Psychiatry,144,* 718-726.

Harding, C. M., Brooks, G. W., Ashikaga, T., Strauss, J. S., & Breier, A. (1987b). The Vermont longitudinal study of persons with severe mental illness: II. Long term outcome of subjects who retrospectively met *DSM-III* criteria for schizophrenia. *American Journal of Psychiatry, 144,* 727–735.

Harding, C. M., Zubin, J., & Strauss, J. S. (1992). Chronicity in schizophrenia: revisited. *British Journal of Psychiatry, 161* (Suppl.18), 27–37.

Harris, M. J., & Jeste, D. V. (1988). Late-onset schizophrenia: An overview. *Schizophrenia Bulletin, 14,* 39–55.

Harris, M. J., Jeste, D. V., Krull, A., Montague, J., & Heaton, R. K. (1991). Deficit syndrome in older schizophrenic patients. *Psychiatry Research, 39,* 285–292.

Harvey, P. D., Davidson, M., Mueser, K., Parrella, M., White, L., & Powchik, P. (1997). The social adaptive functioning evaluation: An assessment measure for geriatric psychiatric patients. *Schizophrenia Bulletin, 23,* 131–146.

Harvey, P. D., Davidson, M., Powchik, P., Parella, M., White, L., & Mohs, R. C. (1992). Assessment of dementia in elderly schizophrenics with structured rating scales. *Schizophrenia Research, 7,* 85–90.

Harvey, P. D., Leff, J., Trieman, N., Anderson, J., & Davidson, M. (in press). Cognitive impairment in geriatric chronic schizophrenic patients. A cross national study in New York and London. *International Journal of Geriatric Psychiatry.*

Harvey, P. D., Leibman, M., Lombardi, J., Parrella, M., White, L., Powchik, P., Mohs, R. C., & Davidson, M. (in press). Verbal fluency in geriatric and nongeriatric chronic schizophrenic patients. *Journal of Neuropsychiatry and Clinical Neurosciences.*

Harvey, P. D., Lombardi, J., Kincaid, M., Parrella, M., White, L., Powchik, P., & Davidson, M. (1995). Cognitive functioning in chronically hospitalized schizophrenic patients: Age-related changes and age disorientation as a predictor of impairment. *Schizophrenia Research, 17,* 15–24.

Harvey, P. D., Lombardi, J., Leibman, M., White, L., Parrella, M., Powchik, P., Mohs, R. C., & Davidson, M. (1996). Performance of geriatric chronic schizophrenic patients on cognitive neuropsychological measures sensitive to dementia. *International Journal of Geriatric Psychiatry, 11,* 621–627.

Harvey, P. D., Lombardi, J., Leibman, M., Parrella, M., White, L., Powchik, P., Mohs, R. C., Davidson, M., & Davis, K. L. (1997). Age-related changes in formal thought disorder in chronic schizophrenic patients: A cross-sectional study across 9 decades. *American Journal of Psychiatry, 154,* 205–210.

Harvey, P. D., Mohs, R. C., & Davidson, M. (1993). Leukotomy and aging in chronic schizophrenia: A followup study 40 years after psychosurgery. *Schizophrenia Bulletin, 19,* 723–732.

Harvey, P. D., Powchik, P., Mohs, R. C., & Davidson, M. (1995). Memory functions in geriatric chronic schizophrenic patients: A neuropsychological study. *Journal of Neuropsychiatry and Clinical Neurosciences, 7,* 207–212.

Harvey, P. D., White, L., Parrella, M., Putnam, K. M., Kinkaid, M. M., Powchik, P., Mohs, R. C., & Davidson, M. (1995). The longitudinal stability of cognitive impairment in schizophrenia: Mini-mental state scores at one and two year follow-ups in geriatric inpatients. *British Journal of Psychiatry, 166,* 630–633.

Heaton, R. K., Chelune, G. J., Talley, J. L., Kay, G. C., & Curtiss, G. (1993). Wisconsin Card Sorting Test (WCST) manual-revised and expanded. Odessa, FL: Psychological Assessment Resources.

Heaton, R., Paulsen, J. S., McAdams, L. A., Kuck J., Zisook, S., Braff, D., Harris, M. J., & Jeste, D. V. (1994). Neuropsychological deficits in schizophrenics. Relationship to age, chronicity, and dementia. *Archives of General Psychiatry, 5,* 469–476.

Hogg, L., & Hall, J. (1992). Management of long-term impairments and challenging behaviour. In M. J. Birchwood & N. Tarrier (Eds), *Innovations in the psychological management of schizophrenia: Assessment, treatment, and services* (pp. 171–203). Chichester, UK: Wiley.

Hyde, T. M., Nawroz, S., Goldberg, T. E., Kleinman, J. E., & Weinberger, D. R. (1994). Is there cognitive decline in schizophrenia? A cross-sectional study. *British Journal of Psychiatry, 164,* 494–500.

Jastak, S. (1984). The wide-range achievement test-revised. Wilmington DE: Jastak Associates.

Jeste, D. V., Harris, M. J., Krull, A., Kuck, J., McAdams, L. A., & Heaton, R. (1995). Late onset schizophrenia: Clinical and neuropsychological characteristics. *American Journal of Psychiatry, 152,* 722–730.

Jeste, D. V., Lacro, J. P., Gilbert, P. L., Kline, J., & Kline, N. (1993). Treatment of late-life schizophrenia with neuroleptics. *Schizophrenia Bulletin, 19,* 817–830.

Jeste, D. V., Wragg, R. E., Salmon, D. P., Harris, M. J., & Thal, L. J. (1992). Cognitive deficits of patients with Alzheimer's disease with and without delusions. *American Journal of Psychiatry, 149,* 184–189.

Joschko, M. (1986). Clinical and neuropsychological outcome following psychosurgery. In I. Grant & K. Adams (Eds), *Neuropsychological assessment in neuropsychiatric disorder* (pp. 300-320) New York: Oxford University Press.

Kay, S. R. (1991). *Positive and negative syndromes in schizophrenia.* New York: Brunner/Mazel.

Keefe, R. S. E., & Harvey, P. D. (1994). *Understanding schizophrenia.* New York: Free Press.

Keefe, R. S., Mohs, R. C., Losonczy, M. F., Davidson, M., Silverman, J. M., Kendler, K. S., Horvath, T. B., Nora, R., & Davis, K. L. (1987). Characteristics of very poor outcome schizophrenia. *American Journal of Psychiatry, 144,* 889–895.

Kincaid, M. M., Harvey, P. D., White, L., Parrella, M., Powchik, P., & Davidson, M. (1995). Validity and utility of the Alzheimer's Disease Assessment Scale-Late Version (ADAS-L) for the measurement of cognitive and functional impairment in geriatric chronic schizophrenic in patients. *Journal of Neuropsychiatry and Clinical Neuroscience, 7,* 76–81.

Knight, R. A., Roff, J. D., Barrnet, J., & Moss, L. (1979). Concurrent and predictive validity of thought disorder and affectivity: A 22 year followup of acute schizophrenics. *Journal of Abnormal Psychology, 88,* 1–12.

Kraepelin, E. (1919). *Dementia praecox and paraphrenia.* Edinburgh, UK: Livingstone.

Leff, J. P., Thornicroft, G., Coxhead, N., & Crawford, C. (1994). The TAPS Project. 22: A five-year follow-up of long stay psychiatric patients discharged to the community. *British Journal of Psychiatry, 165* (Suppl 25), 13–17.

Lewine, R. R. J. (1981). Sex differences in schizophrenia: Timing or subtypes? *Psychological Bulletin, 90,* 432–444.

Liberman, R. P., Mueser, K. T., & Wallace, C. J. (1986). Social skills training for schizophrenic individuals at risk for relapse. *American Journal of Psychiatry, 143,* 523–526.

Liddle, P. F., & Crow, T. J. (1984). Age disorientation in chronic schizophrenia is associated with global intellectual impairment. *British Journal of Psychiatry, 144,* 193–199.

Loebel, A. D., Lieberman, J. A., Alvir, J. M., Mayerhoff, D. I., Deisler, S. H., & Szymanski, S. R. (1992). Duration of psychosis and outcome in first episode schizophrenia. *American Journal of Psychiatry, 149,* 1183–1188.

Lombardi, J., Harvey, P. D., White, L., Parrella, M., Powchik, P., & Davidson, M. (1996). Age disorientation in chronically hospitalized patients with mood disorders. *Psychiatry Research, 60,* 87–90.

Lukoff, D., Liberman, R. P., & Nuechterlein, K. H. (1986). Symptom monitoring in the rehabilitation of schizophrenic patients. *Schizophrenia Bulletin, 12,* 549–602.

Meeks, S., Carstensen, L. L., Stafford, P. B., Brenner, L. L., Weathers, F., Welch, R., & Oltmanns, T. F. (1990). Mental health needs of the chronically mentally ill elderly. *Psychology and Aging, 5,* 163–171.

Mohs, R. C. (1995). Neuropsychological assessment of patients with Alzheimer's disease In F. E. Bloom & D. J. Kupfer (Eds.), *Psychopharmacology: The fourth generation of progress.* (pp. 1377–1388) New York: Raven Press.

Morris, J. C., Edland, S., Clark, C., Galasko, D., Koss, E., Mohs, R., van Belle, G., Fillenbaum, G., & Hayman, A. (1993). The Consortium to Establish a Registry for Alzheimer's Disease (CERAD). Part IV. Rates of cognitive change in the longitudinal assessment of probable Alzheimer's disease. *Neurology, 43,* 2457–2465.

Mueser, K. T., Bellack, A. S., Douglas, M. S., & Wade, J. H. (1991). Prediction of social skills acquisition in schizophrenic and major affective disorder patients from memory and symptomatology. *Psychiatry Research, 37,* 281–296.

Mueser, K. T., Douglas, M. S., Bellack, A. S., & Morrison, R. L. (1991). Assessment of enduring deficit and negative symptom subtypes in schizophrenia. *Schizophrenia Bulletin, 17,* 565–582.

Mulsant, B. H., Stergiou, A., Keshavan, M. S., et al. (1993). Schizophrenia in late life: Elderly patients admitted to an acute psychiatric care hospital. *Schizophrenia Bulletin, 19,* 709–722.

O'Carroll, R. E, Walker, M., & Dunan, J. (1992). Selecting controls for schizophrenia research studies: The use of the National Adult Reading Test (NART) as a measure of premorbid ability. *Schizophrenia Research, 8,* 137–141.

Parsons, P. L. (1964). Mental health of Swansea's old folk. *British Journal of Preventive and Social Medicine, 19,* 43–47.

Paul, G. T., & Lenz, R. J. (1977). *Psychosocial treatment of chronic mental patients: Milieu versus social-learning programs.* Cambridge, MA: Harvard University Press.

Paulsen, J. S., Heaton, R. K., Sadek, J. R., Perry, W., & Jeste, D. V. (1995). The nature of learning and memory impairments in schizophrenia. *Journal of the International Neuropsychologocal Society, 1,* 88–99.

Perlick, D., Mattis, S., Stastny, P., & Teresi, J. (1992). Neuropsychological discriminators of long-term inpatient or outpatient status in chronic schizophrenia. *Journal of Neuropsychiatry and Clinical Neurosciences, 4,* 428–434.

Perlick, D., Stastny, P., Mattis, S., & Teresi, J. (1992). Contribution of family, cognitive, and clinical dimensions to long-term outcome in schizophrenia. *Schizophrenia Research, 6,* 257–265.

Pogue-Geile, M. F., & Harrow, M. (1984). Negative and positive symptoms in schizophrenia and depression: A followup. *Schizophrenia Bulletin, 10,* 371–387.

Pogue-Geile, M. F., & Harrow, M. (1985). Negative symptoms in schizophrenia: Their longitudinal course and prognostic significance. *Schizophrenia Bulletin, 11,* 427–439.

Powchik, P., Haroutunian, V., Davidson, M., Gabriel, S., Harvey, P. D., & Davis, K. L. (in press). Postmortem studies in schizophrenia. *Schizophrenia Bulletin.*

Prohovnik, I., Dwork, A. J., Kaufman, M. A., & Wilson, N. (1993). Alzheimer-type neuropathology in elderly schizophrenia patients. *Schizophrenia Bulletin, 19,* 805–816.

Purohit, D. P., Davidson, M., Perl, D. P., Powchik, P., Haroutunian, V. H., Bierer, L. M., McCrystal, J., Losonczy, M., & Davis, K. L. (1993). Severe cognitive impairments in elderly schizophrenic patients: A clinicopathological study. *Biological Psychiatry, 33,* 255–260.

Putnam, K. M., Harvey, P. D., Parrella, M., White, L., Powchik, P., & Davidson, M. (1996). Symptom stability in geriatric chronic schizophrenic inpatients: A one-year follow-up study. *Biological Psychiatry, 39,* 92–99.

Rockwood, K., Stolee, P., & Brahim, A. (1991). Outcomes of admission to a psychogeriatric service. *Canadian Journal of Psychiatry, 36,* 275–279.

Saykin, A. J., Shtasel, D. L., Gur, R. E., Kester, D. B., Mozley, L. H., Stafiniak, P., & Gur, R. C. (1994). Neuropsychological deficits in neuroleptic naive patients with first episode schizophrenia. *Archives of General Psychiatry, 51,* 124–131.

Schneider, L. C., & Streuening, E. L. (1983). SLOF: A behavioral rating scale for assessing the mentally ill. *Social Work Research and Abstracts, 6,* 9–21.

Serban, G., & Gidynski, C. B. (1979). Relationship between cognitive defect, affect response, and community adjustment in chronic schizophrenics. *British Journal of Psychiatry, 134,* 602–608.

Spitzer, R., Endicott, J., & Robins, L. (1978). Research diagnostic criteria: Rationale and reliability. *Archives of General Psychiatry, 35,* 773–784.

Tessler, R. C., & Manderscheid, R. W. (1994) Factors affecting adjustment to community living. *Hospital and Community Psychiatry, 33,* 203–207.

Welsh, K. A., Butters, N., Hughes, J., Mohs, R. C., & Heyman, A. (1991). Detection of abnormal memory decline in mild cases of Alzheimer's disease using CERAD neuropsychological measures. *Archives of Neurology, 48,* 278–281.

White, L., Harvey, P. D., Parrella, M., Sevy, S., Knobler, H., Powchik, P., & Davidson, M. (1994). Empirical assessment of the factorial structure of clinical symptoms in schizophrenic patients: Symptom structure in geriatric and nongeriatric samples. *New Trends in Experimental and Clinical Psychiatry, 10,* 75–83.

White, L., Parrella, M., McCrystal-Simon, J., Masiar, S., Harvey, P. D., & Davidson, M. (1997). Characteristics of elderly psychiatric patients retained in a state hospital during downsizing: A prospective study with replication. *International Journal of Geriatric Psychiatry, 12,* 474–480.

Wyatt, R. J.(1991) Neuroleptics and the natural course of schizophrenia. *Schizophrenia Bulletin, 17,* 325–351.

Yassa, R., Suranyi-Cadotte, B. (1993). Clinical characteristics of late-onset schizophrenia and delusional disorder. *Schizophrenia Bulletin, 19,* 701–707.

7.14
Sleep Disorders

SONIA ANCOLI-ISRAEL, RUTH PAT-HORENCYZK, and
JENNIFER MARTIN
*University of California and Veterans Affairs Medical Center,
San Diego, CA, USA*

7.14.1 INTRODUCTION

Since the 1950s, increasing attention has focused on changes in sleep with advancing age. This chapter reviews what sleep is, how sleep is measured, and the major theories of sleep, and then focuses on the changes that occur in sleep with advancing age. Prevalent sleep disorders found in elderly populations are described, current methods of evaluation and treatments of these disorders discussed, and special emphasis is placed on adapting the interventions to the specific needs of elderly populations.

7.14.1.1 Measurement of Sleep

Sleep is an active process with changes occurring in physiological systems. Traditionally, sleep is studied by recording brain waves (EEG or electroencephalography), eye movement (EOG or electro-oculography), and muscle tension (EMG or electromyography). Information gained from these three channels of information allow the identification of the different stages of sleep. When additional clinical information is necessary, other systems such as heart rate, respiration, level of oxygen in the blood, limb movements, body position, and blood pressure may also be recorded. The recording of these variables is called a polysomnograph (PSG).

For diagnostic purposes, sleep is usually recorded for one full night. Since there may be some adaptation problems to the laboratory environment (referred to as "the first night effect"), for further assessment or for research purposes, sleep may be recorded for additional nights.

There have been many technical advances in the field of sleep with portable PSG now being available. Many of the same variables that are recorded in the laboratory can now be recorded in the patient's own home. Two major advantages of portable PSG are that the patient is more comfortable and relaxed at home and that it is less expensive than laboratory PSG. Much research is being conducted to determine the minimum number of channels of information necessary to screen for specific sleep disorders (Ferber et al., 1994).

An alternative approach for objectively measuring sleep/wake is the wrist actigraph. An actigraph measures wrist movement and significantly correlates with EEG for distinguishing wake from sleep (Sadeh, Hauri, Kripke, & Lavie, 1995). Wrist activity has been shown to provide valid and reliable measurements of the sleep/wake rhythm in elderly patients and has been used for elderly populations who might have difficulty with traditional EEG recordings such as elderly patients with insomnia (Hauri & Wisbey, 1994) and nursing home patients (Ancoli-Israel, Jones, et al., 1991). An additional advantage of wrist activity is the ability to record for consecutive 24-hour periods. The limitation of wrist actigraphy, however, is that it cannot distinguish between different sleep stages.

7.14.1.1.1 Sleep stages

Sleep is traditionally divided into two major states: rapid eye movement (REM) sleep and non-rapid eye movement (NREM) sleep. NREM sleep is further divided into four sleep stages. Each of the stages differs from one another in the amplitude and frequency of the brain waves, in the type of eye movements, and in the presence or absence of muscle tone. The four NREM stages roughly parallel a "depth of sleep" continuum, with arousal thresholds generally increasing from a low threshold in stage 1 to the highest threshold in stage 4. Stage 1 is the transitional phase between wakefulness and sleep and is characterized by low-voltage, mixed-frequency EEG and slow eye movements. Stage 1 sleep usually comprises about 2–5% of the night. Stage 2 sleep is considered the onset of sleep and is characterized by sleep spindles and k-complexes. Stage 2 usually comprises about 45–75% of the night. Stages 3 and 4 sleep are called deep sleep or slow-wave sleep and are characterized by high-amplitude, slow-frequency delta waves. Slow-wave sleep usually comprises 25% of the night in younger adults but almost 0% in the elderly. REM sleep is characterized by low-voltage, high-frequency EEG with minimal or no muscle tone and with rapid eye movements. REM sleep, which is also called dream sleep, comprises 20–25% of the night.

REM sleep is often called paradoxical sleep since it is characterized by high-frequency brain activity which resembles wakefulness. However, the arousal threshold is high (i.e., the subject is difficult to awaken) and there is motor paralysis or muscle atonia. This paralysis is believed to be a protective mechanism which keeps the dreamer from acting out dreams. REM sleep is also characterized by episodic bursts of rapid eye movements and irregular heart rate, respiration, and blood pressure.

7.14.1.1.2 Sleep cycles and architecture

NREM sleep and REM sleep alternate through the night in a cyclic fashion. The individual moves through the four NREM stages, then gradually returns to stage 2 sleep from which REM sleep is entered. NREM sleep generally comprises 75–80% of the sleep period, whereas REM sleep comprises 20–25% of the sleep period.

7.14.1.2 Theories on the Function of Sleep

Although we sleep for about one-third of our lives, the function of sleep remains enigmatic and controversial. The generally held assumption is that sleep is an essential and unavoidable condition. The strongest research evidence for the essential role of sleep comes from long-term sleep deprivation studies. For example, animal studies have shown that after 2–3 weeks of total sleep deprivation, rats die, suggesting that sleep is critical for survival (Glotzbach & Heller, 1996). These types of observable changes that occur during the process of sleep deprivation stimulated the development of several theories which have attempted to explain the underlying mechanisms of sleep.

There are four major theories on the function of sleep. The thermoregulatory theories of sleep suggest that sleep serves as a time for the organism to produce or to dissipate heat in order to maintain optimal body temperature (Nakao, McGinty, Szymusiak, & Yamamoto, 1995). The homeostatic drive hypothesizes that the sleep/wake system is driven by a homeostatic process (Borbely, 1994), i.e., as the duration of wakefulness (and therefore the length of time since the last sleep period) increases, the propensity for sleep increases. While the organism sleeps, this drive gradually decreases. The model suggests, however, that independent of the duration of the wake period, sleep is more likely at some circadian times than others. A third theory, that of memory consolidation, suggests that during some periods of sleep (i.e., REM sleep), certain types of memories are consolidated for the purpose of long-term storage (Carskadon & Dement, 1994). The fourth theory is that of the restorative function of sleep. This theory suggests that the physiological and biochemical degradation that occurs during the day is restored during deep sleep (Rechtschaffen, 1994). Each theory has data supporting it as well as data contradicting the models. The only conclusion that can be drawn at this time is that, although the full function is not yet known, sleep is crucial for survival.

7.14.1.3 Changes in Sleep Associated with Aging

Various epidemiological studies and population-based surveys have consistently indicated that up to 50% of people over age 65 experience some disruption of sleep (Foley et al., 1995). However, studies have indicated that these sleep disturbances were associated with poor physical health and depression (Monjan & Foley, 1996). Studies of healthy older people have shown that sleep complaints were infrequent, notwithstanding the presence of increased night-time wakefulness and decreased time in deeper stages of sleep (Prinz, Vitiello, Raskind, & Thorpy, 1990).

7.14.1.3.1 Objective sleep studies

The general findings, based on objective PSG measurements, are that in contrast to younger people, older people spend more time in bed but sleep less, and are more easily aroused from sleep. The most prominent finding is the profound decrease in slow-wave sleep (stages 3 and 4).

As people age, sleep becomes increasingly fragmented, resulting from both a rise in the number of transient arousals and an increase in the total amount of time awake throughout the night. Increased night-time wakefulness may cause increased daytime fatigue, daytime napping, and increased likelihood of falling asleep during the day. The question of whether daytime naps are the cause or the consequence of disturbed night-time sleep needs to be further explored.

Daytime napping is common among elderly populations. While surveys vary in their estimations of the frequency of napping in elderly populations, there is consensus that the amount of napping increases with age. Prinz (1977) reported that 25% of elderly people studied took a daytime nap, while Wauquier and colleagues reported that 80% of healthy elderly subjects napped on average for 30 minutes a day (Wauquier, Van Sweden, Lagaay, Kemp, & Kamphuisen, 1992).

Results obtained from objective studies which focused on daytime sleepiness also showed an increase in daytime sleepiness as measured by the multiple sleep latency test (MSLT). The MSLT consists of 4–5 opportunities to go to sleep at 2 hour intervals and is considered to be the standard for evaluating daytime sleepiness. Older people fell asleep faster than younger adults on all nap opportunities (Dement, Seidel, & Carskadon, 1982).

7.14.1.3.2 Subjective reports

Subjective complaints of the elderly tend to be consistent with PSG findings. Older people report taking longer to fall asleep, sleeping less at night, waking more often during the night, waking up early in the morning, and napping more during the day (McGhie & Russel, 1962).

Using a sample of over 9000 community-dwelling individuals over the age of 65, Foley et al. (1995) found that over half of the sample reported at least one of five of the most common complaints: trouble falling asleep, waking up during the night, waking up too early, needing a nap, and not feeling rested. Sleep complaints have also been found to relate to measures of depression (Benca, Obermeyer, Thisted, & Gillin, 1992).

7.14.1.3.3 Gender differences

Gender-related differences have been noted in sleep of the healthy elderly. A meta-analysis of PSG data conducted by Benca et al. (1992) showed that older women may sleep better than older men. Women also appeared to maintain sleep better than men (Rediehs, Reis, & Creason, 1990). It is noteworthy that older women were more likely than older men to complain of sleeping difficulties and thus receive hypnotics more often (Ohayon & Caulet, 1995).

Hormonal changes associated with menopause impact sleep. Menopause has been associated with both subjective complaints of insomnia, and objective changes including increased sleep latency, decreased REM sleep, and decreased total sleep time. Treatment with supplemental estrogens may help to alleviate some of these sleep disturbances (Wooten, 1994).

7.14.2 DISORDERS OF SLEEP

Sleep disturbances in elderly people may be due to primary sleep disorders (e.g., sleep-related respiratory disturbances or periodic movements in sleep)—the frequency and severity of which tend to increase with age—or they may be secondary to a variety of medical, psychiatric, pharmacologic, and psychosocial factors. Chronic sleep disturbances may also exacerbate illness, cause discomfort and frustration, and may be related to depression. The daytime effects of chronic sleep disturbances include impaired cognition, confusion, slowed psychomotor functioning, and increased risks of injuries due to falls, thus impairing the quality of life of the patients and their families.

7.14.2.1 Sleep-disordered Breathing

Sleep-disordered breathing (SDB), also called sleep apnea, is a repetitive process of respiratory cessation during sleep, often resulting in arousals during which respiration resumes. There are three types of SDB: (i) obstructive sleep apnea involves a collapse of the airway which partially or completely blocks the air flow, (ii) central sleep apnea results from failure of the respiratory neurons to stimulate the motor neurons that mediate respiration, (iii) mixed sleep apnea involves both a central and an obstructive component. Respiratory events involve either a complete cessation of breathing (apnea), or a partial obstruction of the airway resulting in a reduction in breathing (hypopnea). The number of apneas per hour of sleep (apnea index; AI) plus the number of hypopneas per hour of sleep (hypopnea index; HI) determine the respiratory disturbance index (RDI). SDB is generally diagnosed when a patient has 10 or more respiratory events per hour of sleep (i.e. $RDI \geqslant 10$) or five or more apneas per hour of sleep (i.e., $AI \geqslant 5$) (Kryger, 1989).

Several factors, acting alone or in concert, have been hypothesized to contribute to the presence and severity of SDB. These factors include age; obesity; micrognathia; jaw or nasal deformities; thyroid, pituitary, or neurologic impairments; and alterations of respiratory reflexes during sleep (Shepard, 1989). It has been demonstrated that the effect of weight on SDB is at least as great as chronological age, even above age 70 (Bliwise et al., 1987).

7.14.2.1.1 Symptoms

Snoring and daytime sleepiness are the two most common symptoms of SDB. Snoring itself is a partial obstruction of the airway, and is associated with a number of health problems including hypertension and cardiovascular disease (Fairbanks, Fujita, Ikematsu, & Simmons, 1987). The snoring of sleep apnea patients, especially those with OSA, is often so loud that it disrupts the sleep of the bed partner. Therefore, the bed partner is often the first to suspect a breathing disturbance.

Another common symptom of SDB is excessive daytime sleepiness which likely results from the frequent nocturnal awakenings caused by the apnea episodes as well as from the hypoxia experienced at night. The resulting daytime sleepiness can have serious implications as patients with SDB may have difficulty sustaining wakefulness while working, conversing with others, or driving a car.

With repeated decreases in respiration, patients with SDB often experience hypoxemia which may lead to other health problems such as hypertension, cardiac arrhythmias, myocardial infarction, and stroke, which have long-term health implications (Shepard, 1992).

7.14.2.1.2 SDB and hypertension

Many studies have shown a relationship between snoring and hypertension with those reporting frequent snoring reporting a higher prevalence of diagnosed hypertension (Hoffstein, 1990). In fact, research has shown that about one-third of all hypertensives have SDB (Ancoli-Israel, Bliwise, & Mant, 1993). Apneas are accompanied by a transient elevation of blood pressure suggesting that SDB may contribute to sustained systemic hypertension.

7.14.2.1.3 SDB and cognitive impairment

In addition to excessive daytime sleepiness, sleep apnea is also associated with problems in concentration, attention, and memory during the day (Bliwise, 1993). Numerous researchers have demonstrated a relationship between oxygen desaturations in patients with sleep apnea and cognitive functioning (Ancoli-Israel & Coy, 1994). Bliwise (1991) demonstrated that SDB has an effect on cognitive function independent of age and other risk factors; however, some researchers have not successfully replicated these findings (Findley, Presty, Barth, & Suratt, 1991). In elderly sleep apnea patients with no other health problems, this relationship may not be as strong (Hayward et al. 1992). It is important to note that extremely healthy elderly are not representative of the older population in general who typically suffer from one or more health problems in addition to sleep apnea. Although controlled studies have not been done, it appears that treatment of SDB may result in some improvement in cognitive functioning (Derderian, Bridenbaugh, & Rajagopal, 1988).

7.14.2.1.4 Mortality

Many investigators have studied the relationship between SDB and mortality (He, Kryger, Zorick, Conway, & Roth, 1988; Lavie et al., 1995), but few have studied the relationship in elderly. Ancoli-Israel, Kripke et al. (1996) reported that, in a population of community-dwelling elderly men and women, those with severe SDB had a significantly shorter survival time on follow-up than those with mild–moderate SDB or those with minimal or no SDB. Further, over 50% of the patients with SDB were more likely to die from cardiovascular disease, while only 35% of the subjects with minimal SDB died of the same cause. However, SDB was not predictive of death, while cardiovascular disease and pulmonary disease were. The relationship between SDB, cardiovascular disease, pulmonary disease, and mortality needs further exploration.

7.14.2.1.5 Prevalence

SDB is a common sleep disorder in elderly men and women, with most studies confirming that sleep apnea is more common in the elderly than in younger populations (Ancoli-Israel & Coy, 1994). In middle-aged adults (ages 30–60), the prevalence of SDB is estimated at 4% in men and 2% in women (Young et al., 1993). Ancoli-Israel and her colleagues have shown that 81% of those over 65 years had 10 or more respiratory events per hour of sleep, and 24% had five or more apneas per hour of sleep (Ancoli-Israel et al., 1991a). They also demonstrated that 33% of comparably aged inpatient populations, and 42% of an elderly nursing home population had at least five apneas per hour of sleep (Ancoli-Israel, 1989).

Few studies have been done examining the relationship between SDB and race. In a sample of older adults, it was found that although the prevalence of SDB was not different between Caucasians and African–Americans, the older African–Americans had more severe SDB (Ancoli-Israel et al., 1995).

7.14.2.1.6 Treatments

Some suggest that an RDI$\geqslant$20 should be aggressively treated since significant mortality risks have been demonstrated at this level. Until about the late 1980s, tracheostomy was the only available treatment for sleep apnea. Since that time, a variety of therapeutic options have become available. The appropriateness and efficacy of each treatment varies from one patient to another, and should be assessed on an individual basis.

(i) Positive airway pressure

Nasal continuous positive airway pressure (CPAP) and bilevel positive airway pressure (BiPAP) are highly effective treatments of OSA, and these are the most commonly used non-surgical treatments. Nasal CPAP acts by providing continuous pressure to the upper airway which prevents airway collapse (Sullivan & Grunstein, 1989). The CPAP system involves a mask worn over the nose at night which is connected via a hose to the CPAP machine. The pressure is adjusted by the prescribing physician until no more or very few respiratory events are seen.

(ii) Surgery

Some patients may be unwilling or unable to comply with CPAP or other treatments to control OSA. For such patients a surgical intervention may be appropriate. One of these surgical treatments is uvulopalatopharyngoplasty (UPPP) which is intended to widen the airway passages by shortening the uvula, removing unnecessary tissue, and tightening the flabby muscles of the airway. This surgery may improve snoring, and has been shown to decrease the number of apneas during the night to the level achieved by CPAP in about 50% of patients (Powell, Guilleminault, & Riley, 1994). Since it is possible for snoring to decrease without improvement of SDB, follow-up evaluation of sleep is extremely important.

One of the advances in the surgical treatment of snoring is laser-assisted uvulopalatoplasty (LAUP) (Standards of Practice Committee of the American Sleep Disorders Association, 1994). A laser beam is used to shorten or remove the uvula and trim the soft palate which vibrates while breathing during sleep. This procedure may alleviate snoring without improving the severity of SDB, and sleep should be reassessed following treatment. LAUP is not recommended as a treatment for SDB.

(iii) Dental devices

Numerous dental devices have been developed to open the airway by holding the tongue or jaw forward in order to reduce snoring and OSA. These devices are quiet, cost-effective, simple to use, and may be particularly appropriate for patients who have difficulty using CPAP or are not appropriate for surgery. Although these devices successfully increase the size of the airway, the actual reduction in RDI varies greatly between patients (Lowe, 1994).

(iv) Medications

Tricyclic antidepressants such as protriptyline (Vivactil) and flouxetine (Prozac) are respiratory stimulants and may improve sleep apnea. The side effects of these medications and their interaction with other drugs a patient may be taking should be considered, especially in the elderly who may be taking multiple medications.

(v) Weight loss

Since obstructive sleep apnea results from a closing of the airway, excess fatty tissue in the neck area may be a contributing factor. Ancoli-Israel, Kripke et al. (1996b) reported that elderly men and women with sleep apnea had significantly higher body mass indices than those with minimal or no sleep apnea, supporting evidence that weight plays a significant role in the presence and severity of SDB.

(vi) Other treatment strategies

Several other factors which may exacerbate SDB should be addressed in the treatment of afflicted patients. Alcohol, which is sometimes used by men and women suffering from insomnia, has been shown to exacerbate sleep apnea (Taasan et al., 1981). Supine body position was found to increase SDB and snoring in some patients (Cartwright, Diaz, & Lloyd, 1991). Taking measures to avoid sleeping on the back may reduce the number of respiratory events. Some medications such as hypnotics, narcotics, and barbiturates may also exacerbate respiratory problems and reduce the patient's ability to wake up and breathe (Ancoli-Israel et al., 1993). These medications should be used with extreme care in the elderly who are more likely to suffer from SDB, and who also use sleeping pills more frequently than any other age group.

7.14.2.2 Periodic Limb Movements in Sleep

Periodic limb movements in sleep (PLMS), also called nocturnal myoclonus, is characterized by repetitive leg kicks during sleep, occurring every 20–40 seconds, lasting 0.5–5 seconds and causing brief arousals (Coleman, 1982). The precise mechanisms underlying PLMS are not well understood although numerous hypotheses have been proposed.

7.14.2.2.1 Symptoms

The primary symptom of PLMS is leg kicking during sleep. The kick may be as mild as a muscle twitch, or may be an involuntary jerk. An uncomfortable sensation builds up into a need to kick which relieves the sensations. Sometimes the patients themselves are not aware of the leg kicks, although bed partners usually are. Other symptoms of PLMS include insomnia, motor restlessness, excessive daytime sleepiness, and sometimes cold feet (Ancoli-Israel, Seifert, & Lemon, 1986; Coleman et al., 1982).

7.14.2.2.2 Clinical evaluation

Patients complaining of night-time awakenings or sleep-onset trouble may suffer from PLMS. Patients with PLMS may also report daytime sleepiness as a result of the night-time sleep fragmentation resulting from arousals associated with the leg jerks. Interviewing the bed partner along with the patient provides additional information.

The only way to make an accurate diagnosis of PLMS is to record leg movements as part of a complete PSG. The number of leg jerks recorded per hour of sleep is called the myoclonus index (MI). A diagnosis is made when there are five or more leg kicks per hour of sleep (MI$\geqslant$5) each with an accompanying arousal. In patients with PLMS, periods of normal sleep alternate with disrupted sleep. The presence and severity of PLMS may vary from night to night (Mosko, Dickel, & Ashurst, 1988).

A related disturbance, restless legs syndrome (RLS), occurs more during the relaxed waking state. As summarized by Walters et al. (1995), patients experience "creeping" sensations in their legs. Moving the legs relieves this uncomfortable sensation, but the sensations return when the movement stops. Patients with RLS report difficulty falling asleep and symptoms may recur throughout the day or night. RLS is associated with caffeine intake, fatigue, exceptionally warm environment, prolonged exposure to cold, anemia, rheumatoid arthritis, and the last trimester of pregnancy. Almost all patients with RLS have PLMS, although the converse is not true.

7.14.2.2.3 Prevalence

The prevalence of PLMS in adults is estimated at 5–6% in the general population (Bixler et al., 1982). The prevalence increases with age, up to 45% in older populations, with no difference between men and women (Ancoli-Israel et al., 1991b).

Patients with PLMS sleep less than those with no leg jerks, and there is evidence for some sleep disturbance being associated with the leg kicks (Ancoli-Israel et al., 1991b). There is also evidence that patients with PLMS often suffer from SDB or narcolepsy (Coleman, Pollak, & Weitzman, 1979).

7.14.2.2.4 Treatments

PLMS is treated with medications and each treatment regimen has its advantages and disadvantages. Common treatments of PLMS include the use of sedative-hypnotics such as clonazepam or temazepam (Mitler, Browman, Menn, Gujavarty, & Timms, 1986), opiates such as Tylenol with codeine (Kavey, Walters, Hening, & Gidro-Frank, 1988), or levidopa/carbidopa (e.g., Sinemet or Sinemet CR) (Kaplan, Allen, Buchholz, & Walters, 1993). The fact that dopamine precursors and opiate drugs may alleviate PLMS in some patients suggests that one or both of these systems play a role in the pathophysiology of this disorder; however, both of these treatments are ineffective in some patients. Since many patients with PLMS also suffer from sleep apnea, a careful assessment of the sleep complaints should be conducted to determine whether SDB coexists with the PLMS since treatment of the PLMS with sedative-hypnotic medications may exacerbate sleep apnea. Whether the beneficial effects of long-term treatment with medications outweighs the risks associated with chronic use is yet unresolved.

7.14.2.3 Insomnia

The term "insomnia" (lack of sleep) refers to the complaint of an inability to initiate and/or to maintain sleep. Insomnia can be further divided into three subtypes: sleep-onset insomnia (difficulty in initiating sleep), sleep-maintenance insomnia (difficulty remaining asleep), and early morning insomnia (waking early and being unable to fall back to sleep). Many individuals experience a combination of the insomnia complaints. Younger adults are more likely to complain of sleep-onset insomnia whereas older adults are more likely to have sleep-maintenance or early morning insomnia, (Lichstein & Reidel, 1994). Insomnia is also defined by the duration of the disorder: transient insomnia refers to a very short-term insomnia that usually occurs in response to a sudden stress, short-term insomnia refers to a state that occurs over weeks and is often associated with acute medical or psychosocial factors, and chronic insomnia is a disturbance lasting months or longer.

Insomnia is the most common sleep complaint reported by elderly people. All epidemiological surveys that have evaluated the effect of age on sleep patterns have shown a higher prevalence of insomnia in older persons than in younger persons (Ford & Kamerow, 1989). Estimates of complaints of difficulties in falling asleep, of frequent or prolonged wakening, and of generally light and disturbed sleep range up to 40% for those 60 years of age and older (Miles & Dement, 1980), and estimates of severe insomnia complaints are more than 20% (Mellinger, Balter, & Uhlenhuth, 1985).

In addition to advancing age, female gender and concomitant health problems have been identified as important risk factors for insomnia (Klink, Quan, Kaltenborn, & Lebowitz, 1992). Women also tend to use more sedative medications to treat their insomnia than men (Mellinger et al., 1985). Individuals with chronic insomnia experience more psychological distress, are more preoccupied with somatic complaints, and utilize health care resources more often than good sleepers (Morin, Culbert, & Schwartz, 1994).

7.14.2.3.1 Clinical evaluation

Clinical evaluation of insomnia should encompass the various facets of the complaint. Insomnia should never be evaluated strictly as a night-time problem; rather the daytime effects on cognition and behaviors and the daytime behaviors that may contribute to the insomnia should also be examined (Morin, 1993).

(i) Clinical interview

As with any sleep complaint, a comprehensive clinical assessment includes a detailed medical and sleep history. The sleep interview usually examines the nature and the severity of the complaint, the daytime consequences of the insomnia, the environmental factors, the medication use, the dietary and smoking habits, the medical history, and the possibility for other sleep disorders.

Following the interview, Morin (1993) suggested that a functional behavioral analysis be conducted. The purpose of the functional analysis is to examine the antecedents, consequences, and the other controlling variables of the insomnia, and to identify the perpetuating factors. This understanding is essential for tailoring an intervention that is adapted to the specific difficulties of the individual. The assessment needs to be carried out with support and empathy and should focus on the patient's prebedtime routine, sleep incompatible activities, secondary gains, and typical responses to sleeplessness. The clinician may use and integrate information obtained by subjective daily sleep reports and by objective measurements. Compliance issues need to be addressed directly in individual discussions with the patient and, when possible, should involve the bed partners as they are most helpful in providing additional information.

(ii) Sleep diaries

Self-report measures are frequently used for assessment of the disturbance and for the evaluations of the treatment outcomes. Sleep diaries, also called sleep logs, are usually employed daily to collect descriptive data on sleep. A typical sleep diary is shown in Table 1. From the reported data, the total time in bed, total sleep time, and sleep efficiency can be calculated. Sleep diaries are useful for tracking treatment progress. Another advantage is that they demand active participation of the client. Despite the subjective nature of the sleep diaries, they tend to correlate significantly with PSG measures (Carskadon et al., 1976). Since insomnia is a subjective complaint, the treatment success, as defined by the patient, is more dependent on the patient's favorable perception of sleep than on objective changes.

(iii) Objective measurements

The usefulness of PSG for diagnosis of insomnia has been questioned. First, insomnia may be setting specific, thus laboratory PSG might not adequately represent the patient's insomnia as experienced at home (Hauri, 1983). Second, a single PSG might not detect chronic insomnia, given the nature of the disorder, since insomnia does not necessarily present every night, and repeated recordings are very costly. Conversely, it has been argued that PSG may be valuable for older patients since the presenting symptoms of insomnia may be secondary to sleep apnea, PLMS, or other sleep disorders that may have a similar clinical presentation to insomnia (Edinger et al., 1989). Lichstein and Reidel (1994) also conclude that PSG is indicated not only when there is a suspicion that other sleep disorders are present but also when insomnia treatments fail.

Wrist activity is an alternative objective measurement of the sleep–wake schedule. However, the results of actigraphy with insomnia patients may exhibit substantial disagreement with PSG results (Hauri & Wisbey, 1992). Nevertheless, actigraphy can be used effectively as part of psychological treatment to measure changes in sleep within subjects and can provide the patient with some reflection on the changes occurring in his or her sleep patterns.

Table 1 Sample sleep diary.

1. What time did you get into bed last night?
2. What time did you fall asleep last night?
3. How long do you think it took you to fall asleep?
4. How many times did you wake up during the night?
5. How long did it take you to fall back to sleep?
6. What time did you wake up in the morning?
7. What time did you get out of bed?
8. How did you feel when you woke up in the morning?
9. How much caffeine did you have yesterday?
10. How much alcohol did you have yesterday?
11. Did you nap? If yes, how many times and for how long?

Note. This questionnaire should be completed in the morning.

7.14.2.3.2 Etiology of insomnia

It is widely accepted that insomnia is a multifactorial symptom resulting from medical, behavioral, psychosocial, and environmental factors. *DSM-IV* (American Psychiatric Association, 1994) provides three categories for insomnia: primary insomnia, insomnia related to another mental disorder, and sleep disorders due to a general medical condition, insomnia type. The diagnoses are made on the basis of interview data. Chronic insomnia can have debilitating daytime consequences on mood, fatigue, performance, and motivation, as well as an adverse affect on an elderly person's quality of life and therefore on the public health system.

(i) Medical factors

The discomfort of medical conditions may disturb sleep, and some disorders, such as neurological and respiratory diseases, will directly alter sleep structure. Medical problems that are commonly associated with insomnia include neurological disorders, chronic obstructive pulmonary disease (COPD), cerebrovascular disease, headache, asthma, and any conditions that produce persistent pain (Wooten, 1994).

(ii) Psychiatric conditions

Sleep is also influenced by psychiatric conditions which can alter sleep patterns and architecture. It has been estimated that approximately 90% of depressed individuals exhibit some abnormality in sleep architecture (Reynolds, 1989). Depression has been related to early morning insomnia, although the most common finding was decreased REM latency (Benca et al. 1992). When sleep variables of elderly depressed individuals were compared with those of younger counterparts, the elderly show decreased sleep efficiency, decreased REM latency, decreased total sleep time, increased intermittent wakefulness, and decreased slow-wave sleep (Gillin et al., 1981).

(iii) Alcohol, caffeine, and nicotine

Alcohol, caffeine, and nicotine are all substances that are widely used (and abused), yet each can have a negative effect on sleep. Alcohol is the most commonly used nonprescription sleep medication. While it may initially decrease sleep latency, later in the night it causes sleep fragmentation, REM deprivation, and REM rebound. Alcohol use decreases with age, however, the sedating effects of alcohol may be more pronounced in elderly due to their decreased metabolic rate (Dufour, Archer, & Gordis, 1992). Furthermore, the combination of alcohol and hypnotics can also play a role in exacerbating existing insomnia.

Stimulant substances such as caffeine and food or drugs that contain caffeine (such as coffee, tea, certain sodas, chocolate, analgesics, bronchodilators, steroids, some antihypertensives, decongestants, and appetite suppressants) may produce insomnia as a side effect (Espie, 1991). Caffeine has been associated with an increase in sleep latency, decrease in total sleep time, and increase in spontaneous awakenings. Discontinuation of these substances may be associated with withdrawal symptoms of sleepiness, irritability, and depression (Diagnostic Classification Steering Committee, 1990). Nicotine may also produce insomnia and is related to lighter and more fragmented sleep.

(iv) Psychosocial factors

Life events (such as bereavement) and lifestyle behavior can affect sleep and instigate insomnia. Retirement and the lack of scheduled activities may cause more daytime napping (Kronholm & Hyyppa, 1985). Evidence shows that adhering to an active and structured schedule may be an important factor in maintaining satisfactory sleep (Hoch, 1991).

Physical activity has been related to improvement of both sleep onset and sleep maintenance. PSG reports of older adults who participate in regular exercise revealed more sleep consolidation (e.g., less wake time, more continuous and deeper sleep) than sedentary subjects (Edinger et al., 1993).

A diverse group of behaviors, sleep habits, and environmental variables tend to promote or impair sleep. Poor sleep habits, irregular sleep schedule, noise, room temperature, and changes in the sleep environment are related to sleep disruptions. Sensitivity to environmental factors increases with age and is also subject to individual difference.

(v) Cognitive factors

Patients with insomnia are more prone to cognitive arousals and anxiety than those with no insomnia (Lichstein & Fanning, 1990). Cognitive factors were identified by patients with insomnia as a more frequent source of sleep disruption compared with somatic complaints (Espie, Brooks, & Lindsay, 1988).

7.14.2.3.3 Pharmacological treatments

Older patients frequently take multiple prescription medications, often prescribed by more than one physician, as well as over-the-counter medications. Some of these medications may cause insomnia, contribute to daytime sleepiness, or exacerbate sleep apnea. Alcohol, beta blockers, bronchodilators, corticosteroids, CNS stimulants, decongestants, gastrointestinal drugs, cardiovascular drugs, and neurological drugs can all cause insomnia. Analgesics and benzodiazepines are known to cause daytime sleepiness. Antidepressants also affect sleep. Amitriptyline, sinequan, and trazodone are known to cause sleepiness, while buproprion, fluoxetine, paroxetine, sertraline, and venlafaxine are known to cause insomnia. Many antidepressants, such as desipramine, imipramine, and nortriptyline, can cause both insomnia and/or daytime sleepiness (Ancoli-Israel, 1996).

Pharmacotherapy is still the most commonly used therapy for insomnia in the elderly (Prinz et al., 1990), although it is complicated by age-related changes in pharmacokinetics and pharmacodynamics (Hicks et al., 1981). Sleep medication usage is disproportionally higher among older people, particularly among women.

There may also be adverse daytime effects including performance deficits (e.g., poor motor coordination, visual-motor problems), increased daytime sleepiness, and accidental injury (Roth, Roehrs, & Zorick, 1988). In addition, some hypnotics may alter sleep architecture by reducing slow-wave sleep and REM sleep. With continued use, tolerance can develop after only a few weeks, resulting in the return of the insomnia symptoms or requiring an increase in dosage in order to achieve the previous efficacy. Sleeping pills, therefore, when used inappropriately, can play a role in preserving and exacerbating insomnia rather than improving it. Withdrawal from hypnotics (especially abrupt cessation from long-acting drugs) may produce rebound insomnia, which is characterized by marked worsening of sleep and heightened anxiety. In addition, elderly are more likely to have disorders that can be aggravated by hypnotics such as respiratory, hepatic, renal, or cardiac disorders. As mentioned, hypnotics prescribed to patients who suffer from sleep apnea could exacerbate their oxygen desaturation and create serious medical risks (Gillin & Ancoli-Israel, 1992).

Elderly patients who are prescribed hypnotics should be given the lowest possible dose of a shorter-acting hypnotic for a short time period. The patient should be closely followed to decide if a renewal of the prescription is warranted.

All hypnotics impair performance while active; therefore, those with shorter half-lives and shorter duration of action have less impairment. Anterograde amnesia is a potential side effect of all hypnotics; however, the dose and duration will determine how severe the memory loss is. Since sleep itself produces amnesia, the interaction of the hypnotic with sleep onset will determine how much amnesia is experienced.

Rebound insomnia can also be caused by hypnotics, particularly those with short or intermediate half-lives. When the hypnotic is suddenly withdrawn, insomnia returns for several nights and the patient is tempted to resume taking the drug. For all these reasons, hypnotics are not recommended to be used on a nightly basis and should only be used for short periods of time.

All hypnotics, if given in adequate doses, will improve insomnia. The more commonly prescribed hypnotics include estazolam, flurazepam, quazepam, temazepam, triazolam, and zolpidem. The task is to determine the lowest adequate dose that promotes sleep with the fewest side effects. In addition, drug therapy should always be in conjunction with a nonpharmacological plan directed toward the underlying disorder.

7.14.2.3.4 Psychological treatments

The recognition of the role of psychological factors in creating, precipitating, or enhancing insomnia combined with acknowledgment of the limitations and the risks associated with long-term use of hypnotics prompted the development of nonpharmacological approaches for the management of insomnia. These alternative approaches include educational, behavioral, and cognitive interventions aimed at changing the maladaptive behaviors and attitudes toward sleep and insomnia.

(i) Sleep hygiene

Sleep hygiene is an educational approach for treatment of insomnia that was developed by Hauri and Linde, (1990). The basic premise of sleep hygiene is that poor behavioral habits (i.e., inadequate sleep hygiene) interfere with the maintenance of good quality of sleep and daytime alertness. Several habits may lead to disturbed sleep, for example, taking daytime naps; spending extended time in bed awake; keeping irregular sleep/wake schedules; excessive use of caffeine, nicotine, or other stimulants; exercise at inappropriate times; poor sleep environment; and engaging in exciting or emotionally upsetting activities close to bedtime. Providing basic knowledge about the structure of sleep and the factors that affect sleep constitute the core component of sleep hygiene. Table 2 lists the major rules of good sleep hygiene for the elderly.

Sleep hygiene has been incorporated into most psychological interventions for insomnia. Clinically, these instructions provide a good start for treatment. Hauri (1991) cautioned against giving a complete written list of sleep hygiene rules as that might overwhelm the patient. Instead, he recommended targeting a few rules which are pertinent to the patients' specific problem.

(ii) Stimulus-control therapy

Stimulus-control therapy, developed by Bootzin and Nicassio (1978), is based on the premise that sleep disturbances are behaviorally conditioned and therefore need to be reconditioned. The purpose of the intervention is to establish a consistent sleep/wake pattern, recondition the bed and bedroom as cues for sleep, and extinguish the maladaptive associations. Table 3 lists instructions for stimulus-control therapy.

The focus of the instructions is primarily to shorten sleep onset. For sleep-maintenance difficulties, the instructions are to be followed after awakening when the patient has difficulty falling back to sleep. Compliance is enhanced when the instructions are discussed individually and a rationale is provided for each rule. Two modifications of the rules have been suggested for older patients. For rules 2 and 3, those over the age of 60 are instructed to get out of bed after about 20 minutes, instead of 15 minutes. This recognizes that older individuals usually take longer to fall asleep than do younger individuals. The goals of rule 8 are to keep patients with insomnia from disrupting their sleep patterns by irregular napping and to prevent them from losing the advantage of the sleep loss from the previous night which increases the likelihood of faster sleep onset the following night. However, a short daily nap at the same time would be permissible. For those elderly patients with insomnia who feel that they need to nap, a short daily nap (30 minutes or less) or relaxation period as a nap substitute may be recommended (Bootzin & Engle-Friedman, 1987).

Table 2 Rules of sleep hygiene for the elderly.

1. Limit naps to less than 30 minutes per day
2. Take a walk both to exercise and to increase light exposure
3. Check the effect of medications on sleep
4. Avoid caffeine, alcohol, and tobacco
5. Limit liquids in the evenings
6. Keep regular hours

Table 3 Instructions for stimulus-control therapy.

1. Patient goes to bed only when sleepy
2. If not asleep within 15 minutes, patient gets out of bed, and does not return to bed until sleepy
3. When patient returns to bed, if not asleep within 15 minutes, gets out of bed again
4. Pattern is repeated until patient can fall asleep within a few minutes
5. Must avoid looking at the clock
6. Must get up at the same time each morning (even if only slept 2 hours)
7. Bed is used only for sleeping (not for watching television, reading exciting books, etc.)
8. All naps during the day must be avoided

Stimulus-control techniques have been shown to be effective with a variety of insomnia patients. Comparisons of stimulus-control interventions with placebo interventions have demonstrated superior sleep-latency curtailment for stimulus-control (Lacks, Bertelson, Gans, & Kunkel, 1996). Several studies reported improvement in sleep-maintenance insomnia in older patients (Morin & Azrin, 1988).

(iii) Sleep-restriction therapy

The approach to restrict time in bed and sleep duration in order to increase sleep efficiency was developed as a technique for the treatment of insomnia by Spielman, Saskin, and Thorpy (1987). It is based on the observation that many patients with insomnia spend excessive time in bed in futile attempts to achieve more sleep. Over time, the frustration and worry produced by excess awake time in bed serve to perpetuate the insomnia. Sleep-restriction therapy consists of curtailing the time spent in bed to the actual amount of time slept. The effects of restricting time in bed are twofold: first, this excess worry time is eliminated, and second, restriction may create an initial state of sleep deprivation, which itself produces more consolidated and satisfying sleep. Prescribed sleep-period durations from bedtime to arising time are based on self-reported sleep durations that are obtained from sleep diaries of the previous week. At first, patients may experience some sleep deprivation since they usually underestimate their amount of sleep, but this sleep deprivation may eventually work to reduce the sleep latency and to consolidate sleep. For example, if a patient reported sleeping 5 hours per night (out of 8 hours spent in bed) then the initial prescribed "sleep window" would be 5 hours per night. After sleep efficiency increases and the patient is "using effectively" the 5 hours for sleep, the allowed time in bed is increased by about 20 minutes each week, and this gradual increase is contingent on improved sleep efficiency. Implementation of the technique requires flexibility and adjustment to the individual patient and obviously a high level of cooperation and compliance. Table 4 lists the rules for sleep-restriction therapy.

Further modifications were added by Glovinsky and Spielman (1991) in order to increase compliance and to adjust the instructions to specific problems. For example, they included some flexibility with regard to setting the time in bed for patients with subjective perception of little or no sleep. For elderly patients, the sleep-efficiency criteria is lower by 5%. Research on sleep-restriction therapy, focused on older adults, showed good results (Friedman, Bliwise, Yesavage, & Salom, 1991). It has also been reported that sleep restriction combined with sleep hygiene and stimulus-control instructions can be effective for the treatment of sleep-maintenance insomnia in older patients (Gillin & Byerley, 1990). Lichstein and Reidel (1994) concluded that sleep-restriction therapy is probably the treatment of choice for geriatric insomnia.

A study examined the effects of sleep compression (restricted time in bed) combined with sleep education for older patients with insomnia (Riedel, Lichstein, & Dwyer, 1995). The study also looked at the differences between self-help techniques (using a guiding video) and therapist guidance. They found that the self-help insomniac group exhibited improvement on multiple sleep variables, but the addition of therapist guidance appeared to enhance treatment outcome for sleep latency, wake time after sleep onset, and sleep satisfaction. Interestingly, the sleep knowledge was equivalent for older patients with insomnia and no insomnia, suggesting that knowledge of age-related sleep changes may have a weaker influence than actual sleep-pattern differences on whether individuals consider themselves as having insomnia or not.

Table 4 Instructions for sleep-restriction therapy.

1. Patient is only allowed to stay in bed for the amount of time they think they sleep each night, plus 15 minutes. For example, if patient reports sleeping only 5.75 hours, they are allowed to stay in bed for 6 hours
2. Patient must get up at the same time each day. If normal waking time is 6.30 a.m., patient is allowed to go to bed at 12.30 a.m
3. Napping is not allowed
4. When sleep efficiency has reached 85%, the patient can go to bed 15 minutes earlier
5. This procedure is repeated until the patient can sleep for the desired amount of time

(iv) Cognitive interventions

Cognitive interventions for the treatment of insomnia are applications of the general principles of the cognitive model to psychotherapy as developed by Beck, Rush, Shaw, and Emery (1979), and others and further adapted specifically to the treatment of insomnia. The general principle of cognitive interventions is to focus on clarification and change of the maladaptive expectations, beliefs, and attitudes that the individual holds toward his or her problems; in this case, toward his or her sleep and sleeplessness. The cognitive change is ensued by using cognitive restructuring, reframing of the problem, challenging misconceptions, and enhancing the sense of self-control.

Morin, Stone, Trinkle, Mercer, and Remsberg (1993) described cognitive behavioral therapy for insomnia as an integration of behavioral, educational, and cognitive components which target the different facets of insomnia. The cognitive component is based on the principle of cognitive restructuring, applied by Morin (1993) to the special needs of the treatment of insomnia. The purpose of the cognitive intervention is to focus on dysfunctional beliefs and attitudes toward sleep and insomnia and to alter maladaptive attitudes that lead to or exacerbate sleep difficulties. Common misconceptions are held about sleep requirements, the causes for sleep difficulties, the consequences of insomnia and about the ability to control, predict, and promote sleep. These attitudes and misconceptions about sleep and sleeplessness may perpetuate a vicious cycle of insomnia, and may lead to or exacerbate existing sleeping difficulties. The fear of sleeplessness may then cause increased emotional arousal and anxiety that may create more problems in initiating and maintaining sleep.

Cognitive-behavior therapy sessions, as described by Morin, Kowatch, Barry, and Walton (1993), follow a three-step process: identification of the patient's specific dysfunctional beliefs, confrontation and challenging of those thoughts, and implementation of methods for revising and altering these thoughts with more rational and adjusted beliefs. A study conducted on elderly patients with insomnia showed that they exhibited more unrealistic sleep expectations, misattributed the causes of their sleep disturbances, and engaged in catastrophic thinking about the consequences of their insomnia, compared with normal-sleeper controls (Morin, Stone et al., 1993). Thus with elderly patients, the cognitive restructuring techniques should address the issue of normal changes in sleep with age versus pathological changes.

(v) Relaxation and biofeedback

A basic assumption behind various techniques of relaxation, meditation, and biofeedback is that the patients with insomnia are overaroused and anxious, and this arousal interferes with their ability to fall asleep and to resume sleep after being awakened in the middle of the night (Hauri, 1981). The purpose of the relaxation procedure is to teach the patients to relax so that they can fall asleep faster. It has been argued that the benefit may extend beyond the sleep problem and will facilitate a more general improvement in coping skills.

(vi) Summary

Two meta-analyses, conducted to examine the efficacy of psychological treatments for insomnia, summarized 59 and 66 treatment outcome studies, respectively (Morin et al., 1994; Murtagh & Greenwood, 1995). Both analyses concluded that nonpharmacological interventions produce a reliable and durable change in both sleep patterns and the subjective experience of sleep, compared with control groups. The improvement obtained by the psychological interventions was also maintained at short- and long-term follow-ups. Whereas Morin et al. (1994) concluded that the most effective single-therapy procedure was stimulus control and sleep restriction, Murtagh and Greenwood (1995) concluded that psychological treatments did not differ greatly in efficacy. Greater therapeutic gains were available for participants who were clinically referred and were not regular users of sedative hypnotics. It is possible that the drug users, because of their psychological reliance on hypnotics, had low self-efficacy for falling asleep naturally, which may have reduced expectations for improvement and consequently undermined treatment (Murtagh & Greenwood, 1995).

Although only a small number of studies focused on the elderly, the results show that insomnia in old age responds to psychological techniques. However, in a review, only five of the intervention studies with older adults included a no-treatment control group and the role of placebo has not been tested in geriatric insomnia (Lichstein & Reidel, 1994).

Studies have compared the efficacy of psychological vs. pharmacological therapies (McClusky, Milby, Switzer, Williams, & Wooten, 1991). Frequently, psychological treatments are used in combination with hypnotic therapy. In fact, there is a growing advocacy for a package approach combining both pharmacologic and behavioral interventions (Lichstein & Reidel, 1994).

7.14.3 CIRCADIAN RHYTHM CHANGES WITH AGE

The sleep/wake cycle is controlled by the body's circadian rhythms. The circadian rhythms, in turn, are controlled by the suprachiasmatic nucleus (SCN) located in the anterior hypothalamus. Studies have shown that surgical removal of the SCN results in animals taking multiple brief naps during the day and night rather than having one long sleep period at night.

Circadian rhythms are synchronized by external cues, or zeitgebers, such as light. Light enters the retina of the eye through the retinohypothalamic tract to the SCN. As the light intensity varies, our sleep/wake cycle varies. The circadian core body temperature rhythm and the circadian melatonin rhythm also interact with the timing and quality of sleep (Myers & Badia, 1995).

Much of the increased napping, daily fatigue, and daytime sleepiness in the elderly can be partially attributed to the breakdown in the body's circadian rhythm, manifested in the advancement of the rhythm and the decline in the rhythm amplitude (Bliwise, 1993; Vitiello, 1996). Czeisler et al. (1989) confirmed a phase advance of about 90 minutes and reduced amplitude of about 30% in the body temperature rhythms of older subjects compared with younger adults.

Circadian rhythm disturbances occur when the body's rhythm no longer matches that of the environment. One such common problem in the elderly is advanced sleep phase syndrome (ASPS). People with ASPS get sleepy earlier in the evening, around 8.00 p.m. If they were to go to bed at that point, they would most likely sleep for about 8 hours, waking up at 4.00 a.m. Most older people, though, do not go to bed early even if they are tired. Instead, they stay up until 10–11.00 p.m. Their bodies however, are still waking up at 4.00 a.m. Figure 1 illustrates the ASPS. In this way, older people are essentially depriving themselves of sleep by not allowing enough time in bed during the body's correct circadian phase to get sufficient sleep.

7.14.3.1 Bright-light Treatment

Studies of light exposure have shown that elderly living in the community are only exposed to 60 minutes of bright light a day, i.e., of 2000 lux or more. Alzheimer's disease patients living at home are exposed to 30 minutes of bright light a day (Campbell, Kripke, Gillin, & Hrubovcak, 1988). Studies on nursing home patients have shown that no

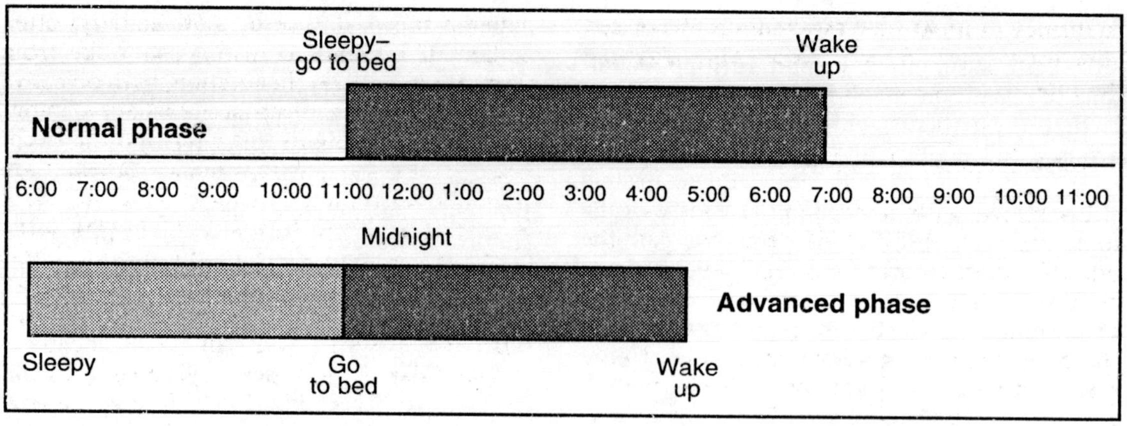

Figure 1 Advanced sleep phase syndrome. (Reprinted with permission of Mosby from Ancoli-Israel (1996).)

patient is ever exposed to over 2000 lux a day and on average, only 11 minutes are spent at levels over 1000 lux per day (Ancoli-Israel, Jones et al., 1991). Since light is such a strong zeitgeber, appropriately timed exposure to bright light can influence phase and amplitude of the circadian timing system (Czeisler et al., 1989). Specifically, bright-light exposure in the evening delays the circadian rhythm, i.e., pushes the rhythm forward so that the individual is no longer sleepy early in the evening. It has been shown that 2 hours of evening bright-light exposure (of at least 2500 lux) is beneficial for sleep maintenance insomnia in healthy older individuals (Campbell et al., 1995).

7.14.3.2 Melatonin

Melatonin, which is produced by the pineal gland at night, can reset sleep onset through its synchronizing effect on the internal biological clock (Dawson & Encel, 1993). With increasing age, the pineal gland secretes less melatonin (Reiter, 1995). The efficacy of administration of melatonin as a replacement therapy is a focus of growing interest. Haimov et al. (1995) reported a correlation between poor sleep and lower peak levels of melatonin in elderly patients with insomnia, suggesting that melatonin insufficiency may be a key variable in sleep disturbance of these older people. Garfinkel, Laudon, Nuf, and Zisapel (1995) conducted a follow-up study on 12 elderly patients with insomnia using a controlled-release formulation that provided effective concentrations of melatonin throughout the night. They found an improvement in sleep efficiency, and a reduction of the time awake after sleep onset during treatment, although total sleep time was not significantly different. The authors concluded that melatonin deficiency is a common cause of insomnia in the elderly and that replacement with controlled-release melatonin may effectively improve sleep quality in this population; however, patients should be screened for "melatonin deficiency" before administration of exogenous melatonin. These results were confirmed by Haimov et al. (1995).

Since the research on the efficacy of melatonin for improving sleep in general and for its specific efficacy on sleep consolidation in the elderly is in its first stages, more data are needed. Moreover, since melatonin is not regulated by the FDA and sufficient data are unavailable, caution should be taken with regard to the purity and dosage of the melatonin currently being sold over-the-counter and the time at which the melatonin is taken.

7.14.4 DEMENTIA AND SLEEP

Dementing illnesses include several nonreversible conditions (e.g., Alzheimer's disease, Parkinson's disease, Huntington's disease, multi-infarct dementia), and there is considerable evidence that dementia impacts sleep differently than the normal aging process (Bliwise, 1993). The sleep/wake rhythm in Alzheimer's disease (AD) patients has been found to be extremely disturbed (Ancoli-Israel, Klauber et al., 1996; Bliwise, Hughes, McMahon, & Kutner, 1995). As many as 70% of demented patients suffer from AD, and due to this high proportion of AD patients, most sleep studies include a majority of patients suffering from AD and often fail to distinguish between the specific type of dementia (Bliwise, 1993). Prinz et al. (1990) describe the sleep of AD patients as showing increased duration and frequency of night-time awakenings, decreased slow-wave and REM sleep, and daytime napping.

7.14.4.1 Laboratory Studies

Compared with nondemented control subjects, the waking EEG of dementia patients typically shows abundant diffuse slow activity, decreased alpha frequency, and other specific abnormalities associated with pathophysiological changes in the brain (Prinz & Vitiello, 1989). This slowing of EEG activity in dementia may cause distinguishing wake from sleep and differentiating between sleep stages to be very difficult. Temporal asymmetry frequently appears in both the waking and REM sleep EEG (Petit, Montplaisir, Lorrain, & Gauthier, 1992). Additionally, abnormalities in REM sleep measures (including REM percent and REM latency) are often found in AD patients, and may present only in the more severe stages of the disease (Reynolds, Kupfer et al., 1988).

7.14.4.2 Dementia and Depression

Demented patients presenting with depression may suffer from even more serious sleep disturbances than those with dementia in the absence of depression. This has been demonstrated with a PSG study comparing AD patients with age-matched depressives. This study showed that the depressed patients had even more disturbed sleep than the demented patients (Reynolds, Kupfer et al., 1988). In fact, elderly men and women with severe depression may appear to have symptoms of dementia (Reynolds, Hoch et al., 1988).

7.14.4.3 Nursing Home Patients

Sleep fragmentation has been shown to be extreme in institutionalized elderly (Ancoli-Israel, Parker, Sinaee, Fell, & Kripke, 1989). Disturbed sleep with frequent awakenings, night wandering, wakefulness, and confusion has been identified as one of the most common symptoms leading to the institutionalization of the elderly (Pollak & Perlick, 1991). Table 5 lists suggestions for dealing with sleep disturbances in this population.

Several attempts to objectively measure the sleep of nursing home patients with traditional EEG measures have had multiple problems. One drawback of EEG measurement is that the EEG wires themselves may exacerbate confusion and agitation in demented elderly (Cohen-Mansfield, Werner, & Freedman, 1995). A second problem is that the waking EEG in these patients shows diffuse or slow activity, often making it difficult to distinguish wake from sleep (Bliwise, 1993). In addition, both objective and observational sleep studies have demonstrated that the night-time sleep and the sleep/wake cycles of nursing home patients are extremely disrupted (Ancoli-Israel et al. 1989; Bliwise et al. 1995). Bliwise et al. (1995), using observational data collected by nursing home staff members, demonstrated that the level of night-time sleep fragmentation in AD patients was related to the severity of their dementia.

Ancoli-Israel and her colleagues (Ancoli-Israel, Klauber et al., 1996; Jacobs, Ancoli-Israel, Parker, & Kripke, 1989) conducted a series of studies using wrist actigraphy with nursing home patients. They computed the minutes of sleep and wake hour-by-hour, and found that, on average, over 24 hours, there was not a single hour that consisted of complete sleep or of complete wake; rather, a period of some sleep and some awakening occurred during each hour. Severely demented patients slept more in every hour of the 24-hour period than mild–moderately demented patients (Pat-Horenczyk & Ancoli-Israel, 1996). Times of most alertness were confirmed to be the meal times (Jacobs et al., 1989).

Previous results have shown great individual variation in sleep patterns and sleep pathology of cognitively impaired nursing home populations (Regestein & Morris, 1987). An exploration of the relationship between the severity of dementia and sleep found that overall, severely demented patients slept more both during the

Table 5 Dealing with sleep disturbances in nursing home patients.

1. Limit time in bed
2. Keep regular schedule of wake/sleep, meals, etc.
3. Avoid caffeine; make sure patients are not buying caffeinated snacks in the nursing home gift shop or getting gifts of chocolate from family and friends
4. Encourage time cues: serve meals at a table at the same time each day and avoid eating meals in bed; place large clocks and calendars around the home
5. Avoid frequent naps; limit to one daily nap
6. Keep night-time noise to a minimum
7. Keep resident rooms as dark as possible at night
8. Keep the nursing home as brightly lit as possible during the day
9. Match room-mates on basis of night-time as well as daytime behaviors and routines
10. Encourage exercise (appropriate to the patient's level of function)
11. Keep bedtime routines similar to prior routines at home whenever possible

day and during the night when compared with mild–moderately demented patients (Ancoli-Israel, Klauber et al., 1996). Systematic observations of sleep and wakefulness in a nursing home population also yielded similar results (Bliwise, Bevier, Bliwise, Edgar, & Dement, 1990).

A 1996 study explored the differences in profiles of alertness and sleepiness between severely and mild–moderately demented patients (Pat-Horenczyk, Jones, Martin, & Ancoli-Israel, 1996). Patients with mild–moderate dementia showed more alertness during the night, while patients with severe dementia showed more sleepiness during the day.

A multidimensional scaling analysis performed on the percentage sleep for each hour in severely demented patients and in mild–moderately demented patients suggested that in the mild–moderate dementia group, there was greater similarity in the level of sleep/wake between the daytime hours, whereas in the night-time hours the amount of sleep/wake varied greatly from hour to hour. In the severe dementia group, sleep/wake was equally disturbed during both the day and night. The authors concluded that sleep/wake patterns in severe dementia and in mild–moderate dementia were mainly different in the daytime hours. Mild–moderately demented patients had disturbed night-time sleep (sleep fragmentation), whereas the severely demented patients had both day and night disturbances (wake fragmentation during the day and sleep fragmentation during the night).

7.14.5 SUMMARY

In summary, sleep does change with age. Subjective complaints and objective measurements of sleep indicate an increase of sleep and wakefulness disturbances with old age. In general, elderly people sleep less deeply, have more fragmented sleep and tend to wake up earlier than younger adults. A central and controversial question is whether these changes constitute a decreased need for sleep with advanced age or whether it is the ability to sleep that diminishes with age.

Some of the changes in sleep are secondary to circadian rhythm changes. The circadian rhythm naturally advances a few hours with age, so older people may feel sleepy earlier in the evening and wake up earlier in the morning. There is also a high prevalence of sleep disorders, such as SDB and periodic limb movements in sleep, which contribute to sleep disruption. These disruptions in sleep lead to daytime sleepiness which has been objectively documented.

As mentioned, older people have a shorter sleep-onset latency on MSLT than younger adults, indicating more daytime drowsiness. Daytime drowsiness is caused by sleeplessness at night. This increase in daytime sleepiness seen in the elderly has been interpreted as support of the notion that it is the ability to sleep that changes with age and not the need for sleep. If the actual need for sleep decreased, there would be no daytime sleepiness. The fact that healthy elderly have normal sleep and that sleep complaints are associated with medical illness also supports the notion that it is the ability to sleep that decreases with age, rather than the need to sleep.

When evaluating an older person's sleep complaints, it is imperative to consider primary causes of sleep disturbances including medications, illness, depression, circadian rhythm changes, and sleep disorders. It is also important to remember that sleep of the elderly can be improved. Physical activity, natural light and sticking to a regular sleep/wake schedule may improve sleep and help to reset or stabilize the circadian clock. Not sleeping well at night and then napping during the day can cause a disturbed sleep/wake cycle.

Therefore, no matter what the age of the individual, a careful diagnosis needs to be made based on normal changes in sleep and on the complaints and history of that patient. Once the proper diagnosis is made, any sleep problem, regardless of the age of the individual, can be treated.

In conclusion, aging by itself does not cause sleep problems. Older adults do not need less sleep although sleep patterns do change with age. Rather, it is the ability to sleep that changes with age.

7.14.6 REFERENCES

American Psychiatric Association (1994). *Diagnostic and statistical manual of mental disorders (4th ed.)*. Washington, DC: APA.

Ancoli-Israel, S. (1989). Epidemiology of sleep disorders. In T. Roth & T. A. Roehrs (Eds.), *Clinics in geriatric medicine* (pp. 347–362). Philadelphia: Saunders.

Ancoli-Israel, S. (1996). *All I Want is a Good Night's Sleep*. Chicago: Mosby-Year Book.

Ancoli-Israel, S., Bliwise, D. L., & Mant, A. (1993). Sleep and breathing in the elderly. In N. A. Saunders & C. E. Sullivan (Eds.), *Sleep and breathing* (pp. 673–693). New York: Dekker.

Ancoli-Israel, S., & Coy, T. V. (1994). Are breathing disturbances in elderly equivalent to sleep apnea syndrome? *Sleep, 17*, 77–83.

Ancoli-Israel, S., Jones, D. W., Hanger, M. A., Parker, L., Klauber, M. R., & Kripke, D. F. (1991). Sleep in the nursing home. In S. T. Kuna, P. M. Suratt, & J. E.

Remmers (Eds.), *Sleep and respiration in aging adults* (pp. 77–84). New York: Elsevier.
Ancoli-Israel, S., Klauber, M. R., Jones, D. W., Kripke, D. F., Martin, J., Mason, W., Pat-Horenczyk, R., & Fell, R. (1997). Variations in circadian rhythms of activity, sleep and light exposure related to dementia in nursing-home patients. *Sleep, 20*(1) 18–23.
Ancoli-Israel, S., Klauber, M. R., Stepnowsky, C., Estline, E., Chinn, A., & Fell, R. (1995). Sleep-disordered breathing in African–American elderly. *American Journal of Respiratory and Critical Care Medicine, 152*(6). 1946–1949.
Ancoli-Israel, S., Kripke, D. F., Klauber, M. R., Fell, R., Stepnowsky, C., Estline, E., Khazeni, N., & Chinn, A. (1996). Morbidity, mortality and sleep disordered breathing in community dwelling elderly. *Sleep, 19* (4) 277–282.
Ancoli-Israel, S., Kripke, D. F., Klauber, M. R., Mason, W. J., Fell, R., & Kaplan, O. (1991a). Sleep disordered breathing in community-dwelling elderly. *Sleep, 14*(6), 486–495.
Ancoli-Israel, S., Kripke, D. F., Klauber, M. R., Mason, W. J., Fell, R., & Kaplan, O. (1991b). Periodic limb movements in sleep in community-dwelling elderly. *Sleep, 14(6)*, 496–500.
Ancoli-Israel, S., Parker, L., Sinaee, R., Fell, R., & Kripke, D. F. (1989). Sleep fragmentation in patients from a nursing home. *Journal of Gerontology, 44*(1), M18–M21.
Ancoli-Israel, S., Seifert, A. R., & Lemon, M. (1986). Thermal biofeedback and periodic movements in sleep: Patients' subjective reports and a case study. *Biofeedback and Self-Regulation, 11*, 177–188.
Beck, A. T., Rush, A. J., Shaw, B. F., & Emery, G. (1979). *Cognitive therapy of depression.* New York: Guilford Press.
Benca, R. M., Obermeyer, W. H., Thisted, R. A., & Gillin, J. C. (1992). Sleep and Psychiatric Disorders: A Meta-analysis. *Archives of General Psychiatry, 49*, 651–668.
Bixler, E. O., Kales, A., Vela-Bueno, A., Jacoby, J. A., Scarone, S., & Soldatos, C. R. (1982). Nocturnal myoclonus and nocturnal myoclonic activity in the normal population. *Research Communications in Chemical Pathology and Pharmacology, 36*, 129–140.
Bliwise, D. L. (1991). Cognitive function and sleep disordered breathing in aging adults. In S. T. Kuna, J. E. Remmers, & P. M. Suratt (Eds), *Sleep and respiration in aging adults* (pp. 237–244). New York: Elsevier.
Bliwise, D. L. (1993). Review: Sleep in normal aging and dementia. *Sleep, 16*, 40–81.
Bliwise, D. L., Bevier, W. C., Bliwise, N. G., Edgar, D. M., & Dement, W. C. (1990). Systemic 24-hr behavior observations of sleep and wakefulness in a skilled-care nursing facility. *Psychology and Aging, 15*, 16–24.
Bliwise, D. L., Feldman, D. E., Bliwise, N. G., Carskadon, M. A., Kraemer, H. C., North, C. S., Petta, D. E., Seidel, W. F., & Dement, W. C. (1987). Risk factors for sleep disordered breathing in heterogeneous geriatric populations. *Journal of the American Geriatrics Society, 35*, 132–141.
Bliwise, D. L., Hughes, M., McMahon, P. M., & Kutner, N. (1995). Observed sleep/wakefulness and severity of dementia in an alzheimer's disease special care unit. *Journal of Gerontology, 50A*(6), M303–M306.
Bootzin, R. R., & Engle-Friedman, M. (1987). Sleep disturbances. In B. A. Edelstein, & L. L. Carstensen (Eds), *Handbook of clinical gerontology.* New York: Pergamon.
Bootzin, R. R., & Nicassio, P. M. (1978). Behavioral treatments for insomnia. In M. Hersen, R. M. Eisler, & P. M. Miller (Eds), *Progress in behavior modification* (Vol. 6, pp. 1–45). New York: Academic Press.
Borbely, A. A. (1994). Sleep homeostasis and models of sleep regulation. In M. H. Kryger, T. Roth, & W. C. Dement (Eds), *Principles and practice of sleep medicine* (pp. 309–320). Philadelphia: Saunders.
Campbell, S. S., Kripke, D. F., Gillin, J. C., & Hrubovcak, J. C. (1988). Exposure to light in healthy elderly subjects and Alzheimer's patients. *Physiology and Behavior, 42*, 141–144.
Campbell, S. S., Terman, M., Lewy, A. J., Dijk, D. J., Eastman, C. I., & Boulos, Z. (1995). Light treatment for sleep disorders: Consensus report. V. Age-related disturbances. *Journal of Biological Rhythms, 10*(2), 151–154.
Carskadon, M. A., & Dement, W. C. (1994). Normal human sleep: An overview. In M. H. Kryger, T. Roth, & W. C. Dement (Eds), *Principles and practice of sleep medicine.* Philadelphia: Saunders.
Carskadon, M. A., Dement, W. C., Mitler, M. M., Guilleminault, C., Zarcone, V. P., & Spiegel, R. (1976). Self-reports versus sleep laboratory findings in 122 drug-free subjects with complaints of chronic insomnia. *American Journal of Psychiatry, 133*, 1382–1388.
Cartwright, R. O., Diaz, F., & Lloyd, S. (1991). The effects of sleep posture and sleep stage on apnea frequency. *Sleep, 14*(4), 351–353.
Cohen-Mansfield, J., Werner, P., & Freedman, L. (1995). Sleep and agitation in agitated nursing home residents: An observational study. *Sleep, 18*(8), 674–680.
Coleman, R. M. (1982). Periodic movements in sleep (nocturnal myoclonus) and restless legs syndrome. In C. Guilleminault (Ed.), *Sleeping and waking disorders: Indications and techniques* (pp. 265–296). Menlo Park, CA: Addison-Wesley.
Coleman, R. M., Bliwise, D. L., Sajben, N., Boomkamp, A., de Bruyn, L. M., & Dement, W. C. (1982). Daytime sleepiness in patients with periodic movements in sleep. *Sleep, 5*, S191-S202.
Coleman, R. M., Pollak, C. P., & Weitzman, E. D. (1979). Periodic nocturnal myoclonus in a wide variety of sleep-wake disorders. *Transactions of the American Neurological Association, 103*, 230–233.
Czeisler, C. A., Kronauer, R. E., Allan, J. S., Duffy, J. F., Jewett, M. E., Brown, E. N., & Ronda, J. M. (1989). Bright light induction of strong (type 0) resetting of the human circadian pacemaker. *Science, 244*, 1328–1333.
Dawson, D., & Encel, N. (1993). Melatonin and sleep in humans (Review). *Journal of Pineal Research, 15*, 1–12.
Dement, W. C., Seidel, W., & Carskadon, M. A. (1982). Daytime alertness, insomnia and benzodiazepines. *Sleep, 5*, S28-S45.
Derderian, S. S., Bridenbaugh, R. H., & Rajagopal, K. R. (1988). Neuropsychologic symptoms in obstructive sleep apnea improve after treatment with nasal continuous positive airway pressure. *Chest, 94*(5), 1023–1027.
Diagnostic Classification Steering Committee (1990). *International classification of sleep disorders: Diagnostic and coding manual.* Rochester, MN: American Sleep Disorders Association.
Dufour, M. C., Archer, L., & Gordis, E. (1992). Alcohol and the elderly. *Clinics in Geriatric Medicine, 8*(1), 127–141.
Edinger, J. D., Hoelscher, T. J., Webb, M. D., Marsh, G. R., Radtke, R. A., & Erwin, C. W. (1989). Polysomnographic assessment of DIMS: empirical evaluation of its diagnostic value. *Sleep, 12*(4), 315–322.
Edinger, J. D., Morey, M. C., Sullivan, R. J., Higginbotham, M. B., Marsh, G. R., Dailey, D. S., & McCall, W. (1993). Aerobic fitness, acute exercise and sleep in older men. *Sleep, 16*(4), 351–359.
Espie, C. A. (1991). *The psychological treatment of insomnia.* Chicester, UK: Wiley.
Espie, C. A., Brooks, D. N., & Lindsay, W. R. (1989). An evaluation of tailored psychological treatment of in-

somnia. *Journal of Behavior Therapy and Experimental Psychiatry, 19,* 51–56.

Fairbanks, D. N. F., Fujita, S., Ikematsu, T., & Simmons, F. B. (1987). *Snoring and obstructive sleep apnea.* New York: Raven Press.

Ferber, R., Millman, R., Coppola, M., Fleetham, J., Murray, C. F., Iber, C., McCall, V., Nino-Murcia, G., Pressman, M., Sanders, M., Strohl, K., Votteri, B., & Williams, A. (1994). Portable recording in the assessment of obstructive sleep apnea. *Sleep, 17*(4), 378–392.

Findley, L. J., Presty, S. K., Barth, J. T., & Suratt, P. M. (1991). Impaired cognition and vigilance in elderly subjects with sleep apnea. In S. T. Kuna, P. M. Suratt, & J. E. Remmers (Eds), *Sleep and respiration in aging adults* (pp. 259–265). New York: Elsevier.

Foley, D. J., Monjan, A. A., Brown, S. L., Simonsick, E. M., Wallace, R. B., & Blazer, D. G. (1995). Sleep complaints among elderly persons: an epidemiologic study of three communities. *Sleep, 18*(6), 425–432.

Ford, D. E., & Kamerow, D. B. (1989). Epidemiologic study of sleep disturbances and psychiatric disorders: An opportunity for prevention? *Journal of the American Medical Association, 262*(11), 1479–1484.

Friedman, L., Bliwise, D. L., Yesavage, J. A., & Salom, S. R. (1991). A preliminary study comparing sleep restriction and relaxation treatments for insomnia in older adults. *Journal of Gerontology, 46*(1), P1-P8.

Garfinkel, D., Laudon, M., Nuf, D., & Zisapel, N. (1995). Improvement of sleep quality in elderly people by controlled-release melatonin. *Lancet, 346,* 541–549.

Gillin, J. C., & Ancoli-Israel, S. (1992). The impact of age on sleep and sleep disorders. In C. Salzman (Ed.), *Clinical psychopharmacology* (pp. 213–234). Baltimore: Williams & Wilkins.

Gillin, J. C., & Byerley, W. F. (1990). The diagnosis and management of insomnia. *New England Journal of Medicine, 322,* 239–248.

Gillin, J. C., Duncan, W. C., Murphy, D. L., Post, R. M., Wehr, T. A., Goodwin, F. K., Wyatt, R. J., & Bunney, W. E. J. (1981). Age-related changes in sleep in depressed and normal subjects. *Psychiatry Research, 4,* 73–78.

Glotzbach, S. F., & Heller, H. C. (1996). Temperature regulation. In M. H. Kryger, T. Roth, & W. C. Dement (Eds), *Principles and practice of sleep medicine* (pp. 260–275). Philadelphia: Saunders

Glovinsky, P. B., & Spielman, A. J. (1991). Sleep restriction therapy. In P. J. Hauri (Ed.), *Case studies in insomnia* (pp. 49–63). New York: Plenum.

Haimov, I., Lavie, P., Laudon, M., Herer, P., Vigder, C., & Zisapel, N. (1995). Melatonin replacement therapy of elderly insomniacs. *Sleep, 18*(7), 598–603.

Hauri, P. J. (1981). Treating psychophysiologic insomnia with biofeedback. *Archives of General Psychiatry, 38,* 752–758.

Hauri, P. J. (1983). A cluster analysis of insomnia. *Sleep, 6*(4), 326–338.

Hauri, P. J. (1991). Sleep hygiene, relaxation therapy, and cognitive interventions. In P. J. Hauri (Ed.), *Case studies in insomnia* (pp. 65–84). New York: Plenum.

Hauri, P., & Linde, S. (1990). *No more sleepless nights.* New York: Wiley.

Hauri, P. J., & Wisbey, J. (1992). Wrist actigraphy in insomnia. *Sleep, 15*(4), 293–301.

Hauri, P. J., & Wisbey, J. (1994). Actigraphy and insomnia: A closer look, Part 2. *Sleep, 17*(5), 408–410.

Hayward, L., Mant, A., Eyland, A., Hewitt, H., Purcell, C., Turner, J., Goode, E., Le Count, A., Pond, D., & Saunders, N. (1992). Sleep disordered breathing and cognitive function in a retirement village population. *Age and Ageing, 21*(2), 121–128.

He, J., Kryger, M. H., Zorick, F. J., Conway, W., & Roth, T. (1988). Mortality and apnea index in obstructive sleep apnea: Experience in 385 male patients. *Chest, 94,* 9–14.

Hicks, R., Dysken, M. W., Davis, J. M., Lesser, J., Ripeckyj, A., & Lazarus, L. (1981). The pharmacokinetics of psychotropic medication in the elderly: A review. *Journal of Clinical Psychiatry, 42,* 374–385.

Hoch, C. C. (1991). Sleep in old age. In E. Murrow-Baines (Ed.), *Perspectives on gerontological nursing* (pp. 59–77). Newbury Park, CA: Sage.

Hoffstein, V. (1990). Snoring and hypertension. In F. G. Issa, P. M. Suratt, & J. E. Remmers (Eds), *Sleep and Respiration* (pp. 371–376). New York: Wiley-Liss.

Jacobs, D., Ancoli-Israel, S., Parker, L., & Kripke, D. F. (1989). Twenty-four-hour sleep-wake patterns in a nursing home population. *Psychology and Aging, 4*(3), 352–356.

Kaplan, P. W., Allen, R. P., Buchholz, D. W., & Walters, J. K. (1993). A double-blind, placebo-controlled study of the treatment of periodic limb movements in sleep using carbidopa/levidopa and propoxyphene. *Sleep, 16*(8), 717–723.

Kavey, N., Walters, A. S., Hening, W., & Gidro-Frank, S. (1988). Opioid treatment of periodic movements in sleep in patients without restless legs. *Neuropeptides, 11*(4), 181–184.

Klink, M. E., Quan, S. F., Kaltenborn, W. T., & Lebowitz, M. D. (1992). Risk factors associated with complaints of insomnia in a general adult population. Influence of previous complaints of insomnia. *Archives of Internal Medicine, 152*(8), 1634–1637.

Kronholm, E., & Hyyppa, M. T. (1985). Age-related sleep habits and retirement. *Annals of Clinical Research, 17,* 257–264.

Kryger, M. H. (1989). Management of obstructive sleep apnea: overview. In M. H. Kryger, T. Roth, & W. C. Dement (Eds), *Principles and practice of sleep medicine* (pp. 584–590). Philadelphia: Saunders.

Lacks, P., Bertelson, A. D., Gans, L., & Kunkel, J. (1983). The effectiveness of three behavioral treatments for different degrees of sleep onset insomnia. *Behavior Therapy, 14,* 593–605.

Lavie, P., Herer, P., Peled, R., Berger, I., Yoffe, N., Zomer, J., & Rubin, A. E. (1995). Mortality in sleep apnea patients: A multivariate analysis of risk factors. *Sleep, 18*(3), 149–157.

Lichstein, K. L., & Fanning, J. (1990). Cognitive anxiety in insomnia: An analogue test. *Stress Medicine, 6,* 47–51.

Lichstein, K. L., & Riedel, B. W. (1994). Behavioral assessment and treatment of insomnia: A review with an emphasis on clinical application. *Behavior Therapy,* 25, 659–688.

Lowe, A. A. (1994). Dental appliances for the treatment of snoring and obstructive sleep apnea. In M. H. Kryger, T. Roth, & W. C. Dement (Eds), *Principles and practice of sleep medicine* (pp. 722–735). Philadelphia: Saunders.

McClusky, H. Y., Milby, J. B., Switzer, P. K., Williams, V., & Wooten, V. (1991). Efficacy of behavioral versus triazolam treatment in persistent sleep-onset insomnia. *American Journal of Psychiatry, 148,* 121–126.

McGhie, A., & Russell, S. M. (1962). The subjective assessment of normal sleep patterns. *Journal of Mental Science, 108,* 642–654.

Mellinger, G. D., Balter, M. B., & Uhlenhuth, E. H. (1985). Insomnia and its treatment. Prevalence and correlates. *Archives of General Psychiatry, 42,* 225–232.

Miles, L., & Dement, W. C. (1980). Sleep and aging. *Sleep, 3,* 119–220.

Mitler, M. M., Browman, C. P., Menn, S. J., Gujavarty, K., & Timms, R. M. (1986). Nocturnal myoclonus: Treatment efficacy of clonazepam and temazepam. *Sleep, 9,* 385–392.

Monjan, A., & Foley, D. (1996). Incidence of chronic insomnia associated with medical and psychosocial factors: An epidemiologic study among older persons. *Sleep Research, 25,* 108.

Morin, C. M. (1993). *Insomnia: Psychological assessment and management*. New York: Guilford Press.

Morin, C. M., & Azrin, N. H. (1988). Behavioral and cognitive treatments of geriatric insomnia. *Journal of Consulting and Clinical Psychology, 56*(5), 748–753.

Morin, C. M., Culbert, J. P., & Schwartz, S. M. (1994). Nonpharmacological interventions for insomnia: A meta-analysis of treatment efficacy. *American Journal of Psychiatry, 151*(8), 1172–1180.

Morin, C. M., Kowatch, R. A., Barry, T., & Walton, E. (1993). Cognitive-behavior therapy for late-life insomnia. *Journal of Consulting and Clinical Psychology, 61*(1), 137–146.

Morin, C. M., Stone, J., Trinkle, D., Mercer, J., & Remsberg, S. (1993). Dysfunctional beliefs and attitudes about sleep among older adults with and without insomnia complaints. *Psychology and Aging, 8*(3), 463–467.

Mosko, S. S., Dickel, M. J., & Ashurst, J. (1988). Night-to-night variability in sleep apnea and sleep in sleep-related periodic leg movements in the elderly. *Sleep, 11*, 340–348.

Murtagh, D. R., & Greenwood, K. M. (1995). Identifying effective psychological treatments for insomnia: A meta-analysis. *Journal of Consulting Clinical Psychology, 63*(1), 79–89.

Myers, B. L., & Badia, P. (1995). Changes in circadian rhythms and sleep quality with aging—mechanisms and interventions. *Neuroscience and Biobehavioral Reviews, 19*(4), 553–571.

Nakao, M., McGinty, D., Szymusiak, R., & Yamamoto, M. (1995). Dynamical features of thermoregulatory model of sleep control. *Japanese Journal of Physiology, 45*, 311–326.

Ohayon, M. M., & Caulet, M. (1995). Insomnia and psychotropic drug consumption. *Progress in Neuro-Psycharmacology and Biological Psychiatry, 19*, 421–431.

Pat-Horenczyk, R., & Ancoli-Israel, S. (1996). 24 Hour sleep/wake in demented patients: A multidimensional scaling analysis. *Proceedings of Society for Research on Biological Rhythms*, 130.

Pat-Horenczyk, R., Jones, D. W., Martin, J., & Ancoli-Israel, S. (1996). Hour-by-hour sleep in demented nursing home residents. *Sleep Research, 25*, 130.

Petit, D., Montplaisir, J., Lorrain, D., & Gauthier, S. (1992). Temporal asymmetry in the awake and REM sleep EEG in mild to moderate Alzheimer's disease. *Sleep Research, 21*, 305.

Pollak, C. P., & Perlick, D. (1991). Sleep problems and institutionalization of the elderly. *Journal of Geriatric Psychiatry and Neurology, 4*, 204–210.

Powell, N. B., Guilleminault, C., & Riley, R. W. (1994). Surgical therapy for obstructive sleep apnea. In M. H. Kryger, T. Roth, & W. C. Dement (Eds), *Principles and practice of sleep medicine* (pp. 706–721). Philadelphia: Saunders.

Prinz, P. N. (1977). Sleep patterns in the healthy aged: Relationship with intellectual function. *Journal of Gerontology, 32*, 179–186.

Prinz, P. N., & Vitiello, M. V. (1989). Dominant occipital (alpha) rhythm frequency in early stage Alzheimer's disease and depression. *Electroencephalography and Clinical Neurophysiology, 73*, 427–432.

Prinz, P. N., Vitiello, M. V., Raskind, M. A., & Thorpy, M. J. (1990). Geriatrics: Sleep disorders and aging. *New England Journal of Medicine, 323*(8), 520–526.

Rechtschaffen, A. (1994). Mammalian sleep. In M. H. Kryger, T. Roth, & W. C. Dement (Eds), *Principles and practices of sleep medicine* (pp. 69–80). Philadelphia: Saunders.

Rediehs, M. H., Reis, J. S., & Creason, N. S. (1990). Sleep in old age: Focus on gender differences. *Sleep, 13*(5), 410–424.

Regestein, Q. R., & Morris, J. (1987). Daily sleep patterns observed among institutionalized elderly residents. *Journal of the American Geriatrics Society, 35*, 767–772.

Reiter, R. J. (1995). The pineal gland and melatonin in relation to aging: A summary of the theories and of the data. *Experimental Gerontologist, 30*, 199

Reynolds, C. F.I. (1989). Sleep in affective disorders. In M. H. Kryger, T. Roth, & W. C. Dement (Eds), *Principles and practice of sleep medicine* (pp. 413–415). Philadelphia: Saunders.

Reynolds, C. F., Hoch, C. C., Kupfer, D. J., Buysse, D. J., Houck, P. R., Stack, J. A., & Campbell, D. W. (1988). Bedside differentiation of depressive pseudodementia from dementia. *American Journal of Psychiatry, 145*, 1099–1103.

Reynolds, C. F., Kupfer, D. J., Houck, P. R., Hoch, C. C., Stack, J. A., Berman, S. R., & Zimmer, B. (1988). Reliable discrimination of elderly depressed and demented patients by electroencephalographic sleep data. *Archives of General Psychiatry, 45*, 258–264.

Riedel, B. W., Lichstein, K. L., & Dwyer, W. O. (1995). Sleep compression and sleep education for older insomniacs: Self-help versus therapist guidance. *Psychology and Aging, 10*(1), 54–63.

Roth, T., Roehrs, T., & Zorick, F. (1988). Pharmacological treatment of sleep disorders. In R. L. Williams, I. Karacan, & C. A. Moore (Eds), *Sleep disorders: Diagnosis and treatment* (pp. 373–395). New York: Wiley.

Sadeh, A., Hauri, P. J., Kripke, D. F., & Lavie, P. (1995). The role of actigraphy in the evaluation of sleep disorders. *Sleep, 18*, 288–302.

Shepard, J. W. J. (1989). Cardiorespiratory changes in obstructive sleep apnea. In M. H. Kryger, T. Roth, & W. C. Dement (Eds), *Principles and practice of sleep medicine* (pp. 537–551). Philadelphia: Saunders.

Shepard, J. W. J. (1992). Hypertension, cardiac arrhythmias, myocardial infarction, and stroke in relation to obstructive sleep apnea. *Clinics in Chest Medicine, 13*(3), 437–458.

Spielman, A. J., Saskin, P., & Thorpy, M. J. (1987). Treatment of chronic insomnia by restriction of time in bed. *Sleep, 10*, 45–56.

Standards of Practice Committee of the American Sleep Disorders Association. (1994). Practice parameters for the use of laser-assisted uvulopalatoplasty. *Sleep, 17*(8), 744–748.

Sullivan, C. E., & Grunstein, R. R. (1989). Continuous positive airway pressure in sleep-disordered breathing. In M. H. Kryger, T. Roth, & W. C. Dement (Eds), *Principles and practice of sleep medicine* (pp. 559–570). Philadelphia: Saunders.

Taasan, V. C., Block, A. J., Boysen, P. G., & Wynne, J. W. (1981). Alcohol increases sleep apnea and oxygen desaturation in asymptomatic men. *American Journal of Medicine, 71*, 240–245.

Vitiello, M. V. (1996). Sleep disorders and aging. *Current Opinion in Psychiatry, 9*(4), 284–289.

Walters, A. S., Aldrich, M. S., Allen, R., Ancoli-Israel, S., Buchholz, D. W., Chokroverty, S., Coccagna, G., Earley, C., Ehrenberg, B., Feest, T. G., Hening, W., Kavey, N., Lavigne, G., Lipinski, J., Lugaresi, E., Montagna, P., Montplaisir, J., Mosko, S. S., Oertel, W., Picchietti, D., Pollmacher, T., Shafor, R., Smith, R. C., Telstad, W., Trenkwalder, C., von Scheele, C., Ware, J. C., & Zucconi, M. (1995). Toward a better definition of the restless legs syndrome. *Movement Disorders, 10*(5), 634–642.

Wauquier, A., Van Sweden, B., Lagaay, A. M., Kemp, B., & Kamphuisen, H. A.C. (1992). Ambulatory monitoring of sleep-wakefulness patterns in healthy elderly males and females (>88 years): The "Senieur" protocol. *Journal of the American Geriatrics Society, 40*, 109–114.

Wooten, V. (1994). Medical causes of insomnia. In M. H. Kryger, T. Roth, & W. C. Dement (Eds), *Principles and Practice of sleep medicine*. (pp. 456–475). Philadelphia: Saunders.

Young, T., Palta, M., Dempsey, J., Skatrud, J., Weber, S., & Badr, S. (1993). Occurrence of sleep disordered breathing among middle-aged adults. *New England Journal of Medicine, 328*, 1230–1235.

7.15
Aging with Intellectual Disabilities and Later-life Family Caregiving

TAMAR HELLER
University of Illinois at Chicago, IL, USA

7.15.1 INTRODUCTION

7.15.1.1 Overview of Chapter

Adults with intellectual disabilities have needs for lifetime support and may require personal care, long-term health and mental health care, economic support, and social and housing services. The most consistent source of this care and support is the family. Nearly 80% of adults with intellectual disabilities live with their families (Fujiura, 1996). Although the likelihood of placement out of the home increases with age, family care still predominates for older adults with intellectual disabilities, at least while the parents are still alive (Meyers, Borthwick, & Eyman, 1985).

This chapter examines later-life caregiving for adults with intellectual disabilities from a life-course perspective that takes into account the social trends and changes in service patterns that effect these families. Older families have experienced pervasive changes in the context of caregiving. This life-course perspective aids in understanding their attitudes towards caregiving and their interface with the service system. The term "caregiving" includes both meeting socioemotional and instrumental needs. While we most often think of caregiving as unidirectional, in the case of older families caregiving can also be bidirectional encompassing support provided by the adult with intellectual disabilities to parents who are aging.

The introduction will present the sociodemographic trends affecting family caregiving. Subsequent sections will include: (i) description of life expectancy, demographic trends, and age-related changes for adults with intellectual disabilities; (ii) trends in services and supports and model of community inclusion; (iii) family caregiving across the life-course for mothers, fathers, and siblings and for various culturally diverse groups; (iv) support interventions that help adults with intellectual disabilities and their families cope with later-life transitions, including planning for the future; and (v) future research agenda.

7.15.1.2 Context of Family Caregiving

In the USA, the composition and structure of families have undergone major transformations since the 1950s that have changed families' abilities to provide care for dependent adults with disabilities. The traditional nuclear family consisting of a father who works out of the home and a mother at home providing care is in the minority. Rather, we see an increase in dual-income, single-parent, and step-families. We also see growing numbers of minority families and families living in poverty. At the same time increases in life expectancy extend the number of years for which families provide care for other members.

Increased life expectancy and lower fertility rates have contributed to the "aging" of the US population, with the median age rising from 28 years in 1970 to 33 in 1990. In 1950 the average life-course for persons born that year was 68 years. By 1990, average life expectancy had reached 78.8 years for women and 71.9 years for men. Projections are that average life expectancy will rise to 78 years by 2005 (US Bureau of the Census, 1992f). The percentage of adults aged 60 years and older is expected to increase from 17% of the US population in 1990 to 25% by the year 2030. The increase will be most dramatic for the oldest-old, with those over age 85 years projected to increase their numbers from 3.1 million in 1990 to 8 million by the year 2030 (US Bureau of the Census, 1992c). This growth of the elderly population will have a major impact on caregiving responsibilities within families across multiple generations as persons may need to provide care for parents, grandparents, and potentially, great-grandparents. This trend coupled with lower fertility rates, which have dropped from 3.6 children during the "Baby Boom Period" (1952–1964) to 1.8 in 1988, results in more demands for caregiving in later life and fewer siblings and children from which to draw support.

With an increasing number of single women bearing children, rising divorce rates, and higher life expectancy for women (Rossi, 1987), there has been a large increase in single parent households. Between 1970 and 1990 the percentage of US households with children under 18 years old headed by a single parent increased from 10% to 30%. This rise in single family households is most marked among African-American households, where by 1990 61% comprised single-parent households (US Bureau of the Census, 1992d).

Labor rate participation among women with children has increased in the last two decades. From 1975 to 1990 the percentage of married women with children under the age of 6 years who worked in paid employment increased from 37% to 59%. Across all ages 57% of married women and 68% of single women are in the workforce (US Bureau of the Census, 1992a). Hence, while the responsibilities of families across generations continue to increase, both the extent to which families can draw upon other family members for support and the time available for women caregivers has decreased. Furthermore, increased economic pressures on families have contributed to stress on caregivers. The economic situation has worsened for lower-income families, as the gap between the rich and poor has widened. As of 1990 13.5% of families in the USA were below the poverty level (US Bureau of the Census, 1992b).

There has been a rapid growth rate among racial/ethnic minority groups in the USA. Between 1980 and 1990 the growth rate was 108% for Asians, 53% for Hispanics, 38% for Native Americans, 13% for African-Americans, and only 6% for white non-Hispanics (Braddock, 1991). It is estimated that by the year 2050 the non-Hispanic white population will decline to only 53% of the US population (US Bureau of the Census, 1992e). Hence, any analysis of the caregiving experience for family members with intellectual disabilities needs to take into account differences among families attributed to cultural diversity and diverse family structures.

7.15.2 AGING IN ADULTS WITH INTELLECTUAL DISABILITIES

7.15.2.1 Life Expectancy and Demographic Trends

7.15.2.1.1 Growing numbers of older adults with intellectual disabilities

Intellectual disabilities (commonly referred to as mental retardation in the USA) is defined by the American Association on Mental Retardation as significant subaverage general intellectual functioning existing concurrently with deficits in adaptive behaviors which are first manifested before the age of 18 years (Luckasson et al., 1993). About 20% of adults with intellectual disabilities require assistance in performing basic activities of daily living such as dressing and bathing (Center for Vulnerable Populations, 1993). Generally, persons with intellectual disabilities show stability in their functional and cognitive levels in adulthood, at least prior to age-related changes in later life (Eyman & Widaman, 1987). Estimates of the prevalence of intellectual disabilities range from 1% to 3% of the population, depending on whether persons with mild forms of intellectual disabilities are included. The prevalence appears to be similar across ages, with some decrease at the oldest ages. However, the proportion of persons with intellectual disabilities who show up in the service system varies, with the greatest proportion served in the school age (McClaren & Bryson, 1987). It has been estimated that as many as 40% of adults with intellectual disabilities are not known to the service system (Krauss, 1986).

The number of older people with intellectual disabilities is not known. However, it is estimated that the age distribution will mirror that of the general population, with a large growth in the elderly population. Using the prevalence rate of 1.2% (which includes both persons known and not known to the service system) recommended by McClaren and Bryson (1987) it is estimated that the number of adults with intellectual disabilities aged 60 years and over in the US will increase from 503 000 in 1990 to 1 065 000 in 2030.

7.15.2.1.2 Increased life expectancy

Historically, persons with intellectual disabilities have had short life-spans, with many dying in childhood (Eyman & Borthwick-Duffy, 1994). With improved medical interventions, better social conditions, and technological advances, the life expectancy of adults with intellectual disabilities has improved substantially. From 1931 to 1980 the life expectancy increased from 15 years for males and 22 years for females to 58 years and 60 years, respectively, in 1976–1980 (Carter & Jancar, 1983). The increase had been most marked for persons with Down syndrome. Their life expectancy has risen from 9 years in 1929 to 55 years by 1995 (Adlin, 1993). Adults with milder forms of intellectual disabilities who do not have other physical disabilities, generally have the same life-span as the general population (Eyman & Borthwick-Duffy, 1994). Exceptions are people with Down syndrome, cerebral palsy, and more severe forms of intellectual disabilities (Heller, 1997).

With the longer life-spans of both adults with intellectual disabilities and their relatives, the period of family caregiving is much longer than in the past. Also, the likelihood that adult children with intellectual disabilities will outlive their parents has increased, with most expected to outlive their parents by several decades.

7.15.2.2 Age-related Changes

7.15.2.2.1 Biological and psychosocial changes

It is commonly assumed that persons with intellectual disabilities experience precocious aging. Yet, the research indicates that this phenomenon is only true for some subgroups, such as those with Down syndrome, severe levels of cognitive disability, cerebral palsy, or epilepsy (Heller, 1997). Persons with milder forms of intellectual disabilities experience age-related problems similar to those of the general population. In a large population study of adults with intellectual disabilities in Great Britain (Hogg & Moss, 1993) chronic diseases increased from age 50 years on, hearing loss from age 60 on, and mobility loss and incontinence from age 70 on. When compared with a general elderly group, older adults (age 50 years and over) with moderate to severe intellectual disabilities had a higher rate of incontinence and obesity, and a lower rate of angina (Wilkin, Durie, Wade, Jolley, & Stout, 1984). Cross-sectional analyses of age-related differences among adults with intellectual disabilities generally find a bias due to differential mortality, with those surviving to old age generally having better health and higher levels of cognitive ability.

Generally, studies that have examined adaptive behavior, maladaptive behavior, and cognitive changes among adults with intellectual disabilities have found few age-related changes, when persons with Down syndrome were not included. Researchers have noted some gradual decline in overall intellectual functioning after the age of 65 years (Fisher & Zeaman, 1970; Walz, Harper, & Wilson, 1986).

Losses in social support and in physical functioning can contribute to psychiatric disorders for older adults with intellectual disabilities. Often issues of death and bereavement are not adequately addressed in this population. Also, psychiatric problems tend to be underdiagnosed among adults with intellectual disabilities (Patel, Goldberg, & Moss, 1993). After thoroughly screening a community population of older adults with intellectual disabilities (age 50 and over) Patel et al. (1993) diagnosed 11.4% of the sample as having a psychiatric disorder (mostly depression and anxiety) other than dementia. Only one third of these cases had been identified and treated for their disorder.

7.15.2.2.2 Earlier aging for some conditions

Earlier aging occurs for persons with Down syndrome and to some extent for persons with cerebral palsy and epilepsy. Often, age-related changes can be due to secondary conditions related to the disability. For example, long-term use of antiseizure medication appears to be associated with an increased risk of osteoporosis and fractures (Adlin, 1993). For adults with Down syndrome there is a higher prevalence of Alzheimer's disease at a younger age (starting with age 50 years), which also is related to decrements in adaptive behaviors and increased maladaptive behavior (Janicki, Heller, Seltzer, & Hogg, 1996). Persons with Down syndrome also experience other age-related health problems, including hypothyroidism, depression, and sleep apnea, which can mimic the symptoms of dementia (Adlin, 1993).

For adults with cerebral palsy, aging-related changes have been noted starting in the 40s. These include decreased muscle strength and mobility, problems with choking and swallowing, increased pain, and incontinence (Turk, Overeynder, & Janicki, 1995). It is not uncommon for persons with cerebral palsy to begin using a wheelchair in middle age, as walking becomes more difficult and fatigue is greater.

7.15.3 TRENDS IN SERVICES AND SUPPORTS

7.15.3.1 Models of Care and Residential Services

7.15.3.1.1 Growth of community vs. institutional programs

Older adults with intellectual disabilities and their families have witnessed major changes in the service system and in ideologies concerning best models of care and support. For over 120 years from 1850 to the 1970s the dominant paradigm of care for persons with intellectual disabilities emphasized institutionalization and segregation. They often were sent to far-away institutions and special schools. Medical professionals dominated and made most of the decisions regarding the medical and educational needs of the children. Many older parents recall their early encounters with physicians who told them that their child had to be institutionalized because of the intellectual disabilities diagnosis. During this era there were no publicly funded schools or day/vocational programs for children with intellectual disabilities and few supports for families who chose to maintain their relative at home. At the height of this "institutional" era in 1967 there were 194 650 children and adults with intellectual disabilities and developmental disabilities in institutions (Braddock, Hemp, Bachelder, & Fujiura, 1995).

Beginning in the 1950s parents began to challenge the institutional and segregated model. They created the national Association for Retarded Children (renamed The Arc) which is the fourteenth-largest nonprofit organization in the USA. Largely through the efforts of the parent movement and class action lawsuits, legislation was passed that provided public education services to children with disabilities, including Public Law 194-142 in 1975, which guaranteed free and appropriate public education for all children with disabilities aged 3 to 21 years. Although older adults with disabilities were not able to benefit directly from this law as they already were adults by the time this law was passed, they have benefitted from its influence on families' expectations and advocacy for adult services.

The period 1976–1986 has been characterized as one of deinstitutionalization and community development (Bradley & Knoll, 1990). This phase emphasized a shift from the medical model to the developmental model, with specialized services that trained people for integration into more independent settings. During this era there were efforts to phase down or close large institutions and to develop other residential programs in the community, including large group homes and living centers. Concurrently, there was a major growth in schools, sheltered workshops, and activity centers located within the community. The model implied that there was a "continuum of services" and that persons needed to learn skills to advance to the less restrictive level of care. A major problem with this model was that without appropriate environmental supports most adults never "progressed" to the next level.

The 1990s model which is being promulgated is one of community membership. This approach emphasizes individualized functional supports to enhance community inclusion and quality of life. Services are being reconfigured to incorporate more emphasis on the role of informal family and community supports, consumer control, and individualized approaches. Rather than emphasizing skill development learned in specialized settings, its emphasis is on providing supports to individuals with disabilities in the natural setting, such as in supported employment, supported living arrangements, assistive technology and environmental accommodations, and family supports. There has also been an emphasis on civil rights for people with disabilities. This has been particularly evident with the passage of the Americans with Disabilities Act of 1990 (PL 101-336), which prohibits discrimination against individuals with disabilities in enjoyment of goods, services, privileges, and public accommodation.

Since the peak era of institutionalization there has been a steady decline in the institutional population and a concomitant increase in community-based services. By 1992 the majority of persons with intellectual disabilities living in out-of-home placements were living in small versus larger residences (170 077 vs. 165 119) (Braddock et al., 1995). However, older adults are much more likely than younger persons to be living in larger residential settings (Heller, 1997). Furthermore, there have also been federally mandated transfers of adults with developmental disabilities out of nursing homes and into other community-based settings. The Nursing Home Reform Act, part of the Omnibus Budget Reconciliation Act of 1987, required that all residents with a developmental disability who did not have skilled nursing medical needs move out, unless they had lived in the nursing home for over 30 months and chose to stay there. Between 1988 and 1992 their numbers decreased from 50 606 to 41 429 (Braddock et al., 1995).

7.15.3.1.2 *Waiting lists and unmet needs*

With the massive phase down of persons with intellectual disabilities from institutions and nursing homes and the lack of sufficient growth of alternative options to meet growing needs for residential supports, there has been a concomitant increase in the waiting list for residential services. A national survey indicated that in 1992, 60 876 people with developmental disabilities were on waiting lists for residential services in 37 states (Hayden, 1992). In addition, there is a big demand for day programs, with the same survey indicating that over 35 095 adults with developmental disabilities were on waiting lists for day habilitation or vocational services.

Services tend to go to persons already in the service system. Often, the older families who have chosen to rear their children at home and who have continued to care for them into adulthood face long waiting lists when they begin to look for placements. Furthermore, the actual demand is probably underestimated by waiting lists, as many families are unknown to the system (Krauss, 1986) and many other families, especially older ones, are wary of formal services. Some of this can be attributed to their earlier experiences with poor or nonexistent services when their children were younger. Other families may be unaware of the available options. Several outreach studies have identified numerous families who previously had not received any formal day or residential services for their relative with intellectual disabilities (e.g., Smith, Fullmer, & Tobin, 1994; Wood & Skiles, 1992). In a 1992 study of families age 55 and over caring for children with intellectual disabilities, only 33% had any involvement with any provider agencies (Wood & Skiles, 1992).

7.15.3.2 Community Inclusion Models for Older Adults

Paralleling the changing concepts of care for persons with intellectual disabilities, models for community inclusion of older adults with intellectual disabilities also have been rapidly changing. In the late 1970s through the 1980s there was a growing recognition that the population of older adults with intellectual disabilities was increasing and that they may require specialized services targeted to them. This segregated model focused on special senior programs within workshops or residential facilities. These programs were often modeled after seniors programs in the general population. The next phase emphasized community inclusion, either in terms of being integrated into the generic aging services programs or in terms of being included in the general community.

7.15.3.2.1 Integration into the aging service network

Integration into the aging service network has occurred on many levels: (i) federal and statewide legislation and memorandums of agreements in which the aging and disability networks agree to work together, (ii) integration of adults with intellectual disabilities into seniors residential and day programs, and (iii) combined outreach to families.

Amendments to the Developmental Disabilities Assistance and Bill of Rights Act (PL 100-142) and the Older American Act (PL 89-73) in the USA have fostered collaborative program planning and development across the aging and intellectual disabilities service systems. Examples of such programs include senior center/senior companion programs, nutrition programs, and senior adult day programs. The senior companion programs, in which staff, volunteers, or friends involve adults with intellectual disabilities in these various senior services and in other community activities has generally documented improvements in the social integration and self-esteem of participants (Roberts, 1990).

Outreach to older adults and their families has been successfully implemented through collaboration of both networks. For example, the Caregiver Resource Program in New York has outreached to numerous older family caregivers of adults with intellectual disabilities through the Area Agencies on Aging (Janicki, 1996). Many of the families who had never been linked to any formal services were more responsive to the aging network than to the intellectual disabilities service network. This could be attributed to lack of knowledge, previous negative experiences, or to feelings that their needs were primarily related to aging-related changes rather than to their child's intellectual disabilities.

7.15.3.2.2 Inclusion into the general community

Fitting in with the emerging model of community membership, other approaches to services and supports to older adults with intellectual disabilities focus on individualized programs that offer a wide variety of options. These can include making use of intellectual disabilities services, aging services, or services and activities offered to the general community. Examples of innovative programs using such an approach are the Community Entry Project (Blaney, 1995) and the Person-Centered Later Life Planning Project (Heller, Sterns, Sutton, & Factor, 1996). The Community Entry Project worked with older adults in creating a circle of support, which could include parents, guardians, staff members, friends, and service coordinators. This group then helped the individual connect with community activities in natural settings, such as YMCA programs, church groups, volunteer activities, and art classes. Another example, the Person-Centered Later Life Planning Project has developed a training program which helps older adults with intellectual disabilities become more informed about community options and better able to make choices and goals regarding their future. Also, it provides opportunities for greater choice-making through training of staff and families. Research examining the effectiveness of this program has indicated its success in increasing participants' knowledge of later-life options and increasing participation in leisure activities for participants living at home. Additionally, the training resulted in greater consideration of the preferences of older adults with intellectual disabilities in the actual goals developed in planning meetings with staff and families.

With the emerging models of community membership there is a greater emphasis on involving natural supports, including family and friends, than in previous segregated models that emphasized professional involvement. Hence, families are expected to be integrally involved in developing service plans, providing support, and in some cases directing services. This chapter more specifically discusses family support programs and new models of family consumer-direction in a later section.

In summary, the first three sections of this chapter provide a general overview of the historical changes that have effected the context of family caregiving for adults with intellectual disabilities. These have included changes in demographics and in service ideologies and trends. In addition, this chapter summarizes major biological and social psychological changes that adults with intellectual disabilities face as they age. These changes along with age-related changes of family caregivers affect their caregiving experience.

7.15.4 FAMILY CAREGIVING ACROSS THE LIFE-SPAN

7.15.4.1 Changes across the Life-span

7.15.4.1.1 Theories of family caregiving over the life-span

A life-span perspective on family caregiving recognizes that caregiving can span many decades and is usually a lifetime commitment for families of adults with intellectual disabilities. Unfortunately, the research examining caregiving across the life-span is sparse. Rather, most studies focus on particular ages, with the vast majority focusing on childhood. However, there have been studies focusing on older caregivers. In examining caregiving across the life-span, the terminology differs. Studies focusing on children typically refer to the "parenting" role; whereas studies focusing on adults refer to the "caregiving" role. A few studies have begun to examine caregiving reciprocity as adults with intellectual disabilities begin to serve caregiving roles for older parents (Heller & Factor, 1993a).

Over time, caregiving roles, stressors, and rewards are likely to have both stable and dynamic aspects. In examining the effects of caregiving over time, researchers need to take into account developmental transitions occurring for the person with a disability and the caregiver, changes in the availability of services and supports, and changes in societal attitudes towards the individual with a disability. Another important dimension could be the changing nature of societal expectations regarding caregiving and opportunities for fulfillment of other life roles. Several theories from the gerontological and intellectual disabilities literature address some of these dimensions in understanding the dynamic nature of caregiving over time.

Two contrasting theories emanating from the gerontological literature offer a framework for understanding family adaptation over the life-span. The "wear and tear" hypothesis predicts that the constant caregiving demands and accumulation of stressors will deplete the caregiver's physical and emotional resources (Johnson & Catalano, 1983). Several cross-sectional studies of caregivers of aging relatives have provided some support for this theory (e.g., Morycz, 1985; Zarit, Reever, & Bach-Peterson, 1980).

On the other hand, the "adaptational" hypothesis suggests that, with experience, caregiving becomes easier (Townsend, Noelker, Deimling, & Bass, 1989). The assumption is that when caregiving is a new role it is most stressful and that over time families learn to cope. Several longitudinal studies of caregiving for elderly relatives have reported less caregiving burden and depression over time despite deterioration in the condition of the elderly relative (Townsend et al., 1989; Zarit, Todd, & Zarit, 1986).

7.15.4.1.2 Findings on families of adults with intellectual disabilities

In the intellectual disabilities literature there has been support for both hypotheses, with reports of increases in both positive and negative adaptations over time and with much variability in family adaptations over time. The theories and research on intellectual disabilities also examine adaptation to caregiving from a developmental perspective that takes into account the normative life stage tasks faced by families at different life phases. Birenbaum (1971) and Farber (1975) have addressed the degree to which caregiving is normative vs. non-normative as the child with intellectual disabilities grows older. They suggest that as the child moves towards adulthood, caregiving becomes less normative, particularly if the child is still highly dependent on the parents. Birenbaum has noted that as the child gets older the rights and obligations of typical parenthood become more taxing and more divergent from normative roles. Similarly, Farber discusses the notion of "arrest in the life cycle," referring to the fact that as the child reaches adolescence and adulthood, the parents often are still involved in parenting tasks more typical in families with younger children. As children with intellectual disabilities become adults, most continue to live with parents, unlike what occurs in most families. Hence, parents of adults with intellectual disabilities are much less likely to experience an empty nest.

In addition to fulfilling roles that are less normative with age, parents of adults vs. children with intellectual disabilities are less likely to receive as much formal service support for their child. Suelzle and Keenan (1981) reported that families of adults were more stressed than families of children with intellectual disabilities. They attributed this greater stress to the lack of adult services. While there is US federal legislation mandating educational services for all children with disabilities, there are no mandates for educational, vocational, or residential services for adults with disabilities. Hence, in some families, the parents are the sole providers for their adult child with intellectual disabilities who may not be receiving any services or who may be on a waiting list for services. Furthermore, many of these adults lack friends and rely on their parents to meet their social recreational needs (Heller & Factor, 1988).

In discussing life-time accommodations to caregiving of a child with intellectual disabilities, Todd and Shearn (1996) discuss the meaning that parents give to the caregiving experience and its effect on their identity. They note that socialization into the parental role continues over the life course and entails a series of incremental changes and re-evaluations. They found different reactions of families depending on their interpretations of past experiences, anticipated futures, and personal aspirations. In their ethnographic study of 17 parents of adults with intellectual disabilities in Wales, Todd and Shearn describe how some of these older parents come to experience heightened stress as a consequence of their inability to end their parental responsibilities for their child with a disability. "In the beginning you know that you're going to be responsible for the rest of your life in one way or another, but you never really know in what way. It's like you just roll up your sleeves and get stuck in" (p. 8). Parents reported that adolescence was a turning point as their normalizing strategies were becoming less successful when the character of their own lives departed more from that of their peers. In the process of comparing themselves to others, caregivers (mothers in most cases) who had given up careers and other pursuits to care for their child with a disability, experienced greater discrepancy from the lives of their peers as their children got older.

On the other hand, there is also evidence supporting the adaptational hypothesis that, with time, caregiving for family members becomes less stressful and more rewarding. In a large study of 450 mothers aged 55 and over caring for an adult child with intellectual disabilities Seltzer and Krauss (1989) found, on average, favorable well-being. A higher proportion of these mothers rated their physical health as good or excellent (78%) than did a national probability sample of women their age (60%; Sweet & Bumpass, 1987) and they were less stressed than in other samples of caregivers of elderly relatives (e.g., Zarit et al., 1980) or relatives with intellectual disabilities (e.g., Friedrich, Greenberg, & Crnic, 1983).

In one of the few studies to examine family adjustment throughout the life-span Heller, Rowitz, and Farber (1992) compared 489 family caregivers grouped into five age phases based on the age of the person with intellectual disabilities: preschooler, young child, adolescent, young adult, and older adult. They found that perceived burden was lowest for caregivers of the youngest (under six years of age) and oldest (30 years and older) members with intellectual disabilities. They suggested that perhaps at this stage there is greater acceptance of the family member and greater reciprocity in caregiving as the child with intellectual disabilities takes on caregiving roles with aging parents. Seltzer and Ryff (1994) also suggest that for some mothers the experience of rasing a child with intellectual disabilities might lead to the development of new capacities and strengths that foster adaptational responses. Although the Heller et al. (1992) study was limited by its cross-sectional design and potential cohort effects, parents' retrospective reports further supported the notion of adaptational responses over the years. Families reported how over the years it became easier to adjust to the routines; they became more knowledgable about what was expected of them, and they understood their child better. Another frequent theme was that parents grew to love and appreciate their child more. These affectional bonds between the parent and child can nurture both the parent and the child (Seltzer & Ryff, 1994).

Todd and Shearn (1996) note that some parents make a career of parenting and redefine the centrality of parenting as the major line of activity open to them, beginning to interpret it more positively. Over time, parenting became a stronger source of self meaning and purpose.

While most of the research on adult children with intellectual disabilities has portrayed them as sources of burden to their primary caregiver, studies are beginning to document the positive contributions they can make to their families. Heller and Factor's (1988) study of 100 parents caring for adults with intellectual disabilities (aged 30 years and older) found that these children were an important source of support for them. In addition to providing meaning to their lives, many families reported that their child did chores for them, contributed financially through their Social Security Income, and kept them from feeling lonely. In a study of 85 family caregivers of adults (aged 30 years and over) that specifically addressed caregiving reciprocity, Heller and Factor (1993b) also found that adult children with intellectual disabilities provided considerable companionship support to their parents and help with household chores. Support from the child with intellectual disabilities was a key factor predicting parents' degree of perceived caregiving satisfaction and caregiving burden. Parents who received support from their adult child with intellectual disabilities experienced greater caregiving satisfaction and less caregiving burden. This reciprocal support may be particularly important as parents experience frailty due to aging or widowhood.

Both the "wear-and-tear" and "adaptational" hypotheses assume a linear relationship between time and caregiver well-being. Neither account for periodic variations in levels of stress as families experience major transitions, such as when the child enters or completes school or when the child moves out of the family home. Often the least stressful times are periods of stability in family roles (Wikler, 1986). These hypotheses also do not account for variability in characteristics of the child and in the family's coping and support resources.

7.15.4.1.3 Predictors of caregiver well-being in later life

Both characteristics of the child and of the family and coping and support resources can explain the wide variability in responses of families to caring for a child with intellectual disabilities over the lifespan. The major risk factors for stressful reactions in later life are having a child with more severe intellectual disabilities and more maladaptive behaviors (Heller & Factor, 1993b; Pruchno, Patrick, & Burant, in press).

The extent that formal services can reduce caregiver burden and increase families' ability to maintain caregiving in the home is unclear. However, in their two year longitudinal study of parents caring for adults with intellectual disabilities aged 30 years and over, increase in the number of perceived unmet formal needs was associated with increased caregiving burden and increased need for out-of-home placements (Heller & Factor, 1993b). However, greater use of services has not been associated with improved parental well-being. This chapter discusses the impact of family support services in greater detail in the section on "family support interventions and policies."

There is some evidence that informal support from family and friends can reduce burden (Heller & Factor, 1994; Seltzer & Krauss, 1989). In particular, a high level of sibling involvement with the adult child with retardation has been associated with positive maternal well-being. Seltzer, Begun, Seltzer, and Krauss (1991) found that when support was provided by the sibling to the adult child, mothers reported better health and life satisfaction than when mothers had no other children or received no such help from their other children. The critical variable was not the amount of support given to the mother, but the amount given to the adult child with a disability. They note that perhaps sibling involvement indicates potential continuity of family caregiving into the future.

7.15.4.2 Roles of Mother, Fathers, and Siblings

Much of the literature on family caregiving has focused on mothers, with little mention of the role of fathers or other siblings. Yet, each of the members' roles are interrelated and affect the ability of the family to cope with raising and caring for a child with intellectual disabilities.

7.15.4.2.1 Comparison of maternal and paternal caregiving

One of the most consistent findings in family research is that mothers are the primary caregivers across the lifespan (Hooyman & Gonyea, 1995). However, in the intellectual disabilities literature there have been only a few studies that compare the maternal and paternal roles and most of these studies have focused on families of young children. These studies have generally found that parental roles tend to be even more traditional in families that have a child with intellectual disabilities than in families that do not have a child with a disability. After the birth of a child with a disability, mothers are much less likely to return to work than are other mothers. In a study of two-parent families in which the mother worked prior to the birth of a child with a disability, Mardiros (1985) found that only 8% returned to work afterwards. Fathers of young children with a disability tend to assume less task involvement with the care of their child than do the other fathers. Willoughby and Glidden (1995) found that among parents of children with intellectual disabilities the only tasks in which fathers participated nearly equally with the mothers were those of play and helping with activities.

Several studies have found higher subjective caregiving burden among mothers than fathers of children (Beckman, 1991; Kazak, 1987) and of young adults with a disability (Hallum & Krumboltz, 1993), although some have found little differences in burden (Bruce & Schultz, 1994; Essex et al., 1992; Friedrich et al., 1983), or only in some dimensions of burden (e.g., pessimism) (Rousey, Best, & Blacher, 1992). In a cross-sectional study of 113 two-parent families of children and adults with intellectual disabilities, Heller, Hsieh, and Rowitz (in press) found that mothers spend more time in caregiving tasks for their child, offer more types of support, and perceive more caregiving burden than do fathers. These gender differences persist from childhood into adulthood and whether or not the child continues to reside in the family home.

In addition to the explanation that women have been socialized to play nurturant roles, another explanation for these gender differences in caregiving could be attributed to women having fewer competing roles and time demands, enabling more time to provide care. However, in a study of caregivers for elderly relatives (Stoller, 1983) employment has been shown to affect men's assistance to aging parents, but not women's care to parents. Among older fathers of children with intellectual disabilities, the father's retirement has not been related to increased involvement in the care of the child (Essex, Seltzer, & Krauss, 1992). Even when the mother is employed, men are not more likely to help with the household tasks or with care for the child with intellectual disabilities (Heller et al., in press; Marcenko & Meyers, 1991; Willoughby & Glidden, 1995). Also, women's employment does not seem to be related to the amount or type of help she provides her child with a disability. This could be one explanation for women reducing or giving up paid employment after the birth of a child with a disability. Both Heller et al. (in press) and Todd and Shearn (1996) have noted that many older mothers report that having a child with a disability hurt their job opportunities.

In examining predictors of maternal and paternal involvement and perceived burden, Heller et al. (in press) found that both mothers and fathers provided less support to the adult vs. the child with a disability and less to offspring who lived out of the home. Both mothers and fathers perceived less caregiving burden when children remained in the home and adult offspring with a disability were placed out of the home. Hence, placement out of the home seemed to be associated with reduced burden for parents of adults, but not for parents of children. One reason could be that launching out of the home is a normative function for adults, but not for children.

Given that mothers spend more time caring for the child having a disability than do the fathers, they appear to be more affected by the extent of the child's disability. Hence, in the Heller et al. (in press) study both the child's maladaptive behavior and physical health were related to higher perceived caregiving burden for the mother but not for the father. Also, mothers and fathers were differentially affected by their other role commitments and by the role commitments of their spouses. Mothers perceived the least burden when they were involved in organizational activities and when their husbands worked fewer hours. On the other hand, for fathers, neither their nor their wife's involvement in other roles had much effect on their perceived caregiving burden. However, given the correlational nature of the research it is also possible that fathers work more when their wives are more stressed either to provide better for the family or to avoid stressful family life (Farber, 1959).

Although family caregiving is predominantly a woman's task, fathers play a significant role in providing support. This support continues throughout the life-span, whether the offspring with a disability lives at home or out of the home. Often, fathers play an increasingly large role as their wife dies or becomes incapacitated, assuming the role of primary caregiver, previously held by the mother. Gordon, Seltzer, and Krauss (1996) found that upon the mother's death very few fathers sought out-of-home placement for their child with intellectual disabilities. These authors suggest that it is easier for fathers to move into the role of primary caregiver than to adjust to the empty nest after placement. Placement of their child also may remind fathers of their own mortality.

7.15.4.2.2 Sibling caregiver roles

Siblings provide the most durable relationships for adults with intellectual disabilities. They often share both common genes and the common experiences of growing up in the same family. Relationships among siblings without a disability are most typically egalitarian (Baskett & Johnson, 1982) and often intimate. The long-term impact of having a sibling with intellectual disabilities has been rarely studied.

There has been a large body of literature on the social and psychological effects of having a sibling with intellectual disabilities on children (Lobato, 1983). Generally, the research indicates that some siblings are at risk for greater emotional problems than other children. These siblings are more likely to have increased caregiving responsibilities, lower socioeconomic status, and anxiety or guilt surrounding the sibling with a disability (Begun, 1989). McHale and Gamble (1989) found that siblings of children with intellectual disabilities took on more household and caregiving responsibilities, but had similar well-being to that of siblings without a brother or sister with a disability. Other studies have noted the positive and valued aspects of having a sibling with a disability (Cleveland & Miller, 1977; Wilson, Blacher, & Baker, 1989). These studies have attributed the positive adjustment of siblings to parental attitudes and behaviors that fostered a family environment attentive to the needs of all members and that did not overly focus on the child with a disability.

There is some evidence that adult siblings of persons with intellectual disabilities continue to maintain involvement with their brother or sister with intellectual disabilities into adulthood and throughout the lifespan. Generally, these studies have found that these adult sibling relationships differ from those of other sibling dyads in that the relationships are less egalitarian and less intimate. Zetlin's (1986) study of sibling relationships of 35 adults with intellectual disabilities found that the relationship was hierarchical, with the disabled sibling being more emotionally dependent on the nondisabled sibling. Two larger studies of siblings of adolescents and adults (Heller, 1994; Seltzer et al., 1991) found that the nondisabled sibling performed nearly twice as many support functions for the other siblings than they received back from them. Heller (1994) also compared sibling involvement across ages. Among 175 siblings aged 11 years and older of siblings with moderate to profound intellectual disabilities, adults were more likely than adolescents to spend time helping their relative and to perform more support functions. This was despite the fact that adults were more likely than adolescents to be living out of the family home.

In examining the nature of supports provided by 326 siblings of adults with intellectual disabilities, Krauss (1993) found that these siblings were more likely to provide affective support (86%) than instrumental support (25%) to their sibling with a disability. The factors determining support functions provided differed for the two types of support. For affective support the key factor was past interpersonal climate of the family of origin, including greater cohesion and expressiveness; for instrumental support the key factor was the objective need for support, such as when the mother was older and widowed. The sibling was most likely to provide support when the sibling with a disability had less severe intellectual disabilities and the needs were seen as less demanding.

Several researchers have noted the positive but not intimate relationship between siblings with intellectual disabilities and their nondisabled siblings (Begun, 1989). Begun notes that these relationships were less intimate because it is more difficult to interact intimately with persons having limited language and social communication skills than it is to interact with nondisabled siblings. However, when the functioning level of the sibling with intellectual disabilities was higher the sibling relationship more closely resembled normative sibling relationships.

As parents can no longer care for their child with intellectual disabilities either due to frailty or death, other siblings begin to take on the role of primary caregiver. Griffiths and Unger (1994) reported that nearly 44% of 41 adult siblings interviewed were willing to take on future caregiving responsibilities if needed. Willingness to assume responsibility depended on the degree to which parents desired it and family communication was positive. In the Krauss, Seltzer, Gordon, and Friedman (1996) study of 140 adult siblings, 36% intended to coreside with their bother or sister with intellectual disabilities. These siblings were more likely to be sisters, as is typical of caregiving across disabilities (Hooyman & Gonyea, 1995). They also had siblings with less dependency needs and had engaged in more joint activities with their sibling. Hence, a sibling was more willing to take on the responsibility if the task did not seem too demanding. Furthermore, they were more likely to anticipate coresidence if their mother was already in poor health, making the transfer of responsibility more eminent.

Despite the fact that siblings are often expected to take on the primary caregiving role, often they are not consulted about future plans. For example, in the Krauss et al. (1996) study, only half of the siblings who expected to coreside with their sibling had discussions with their parents regarding future plans for their brother or sister. One explanation for families' reluctance to discuss these future plans is ambivalence about wanting another sibling to take on the responsibility. As a mother in one of our studies noted "I just do not want to burden our daughter." Another mother noted "My daughter has offered to care for her, but I know she works and it would be difficult for her." Hence, many siblings assume caregiving upon the death of their parents without sufficient planning and information about the needs and preferences of their siblings and the support services available to them.

In an examination of actual placements over a 3 year period following the death of parents, Gordon et al. (1996) found that in nearly one-quarter of the 21 families the adult with intellectual disabilities moved in with his or her sibling. They found that even when the adult with intellectual disabilities moved into an out-of-home placement, there was considerable sibling involvement, with many taking on the roles of guardian and advocate. In some cases they assumed these roles out of a sense of obligation to the deceased parents, and in others they did so out of personal desires to help their sibling.

7.15.4.3 Future Planning and Placement

As family caregivers age they increasingly face the prospect that their child with intellectual disabilities will outlive them. With increased frailty it may also be more difficult for parents to provide care. While planning for the future is a task faced by all persons as they age, the need to plan for their child is particularly salient and often stressful for these parents. Key aspects which usually need to be addressed include future living arrangements, guardianship, and financial planning. However, many of these older adults have great difficulty making future plans as do older adults in general (Heller & Factor, 1994).

7.15.4.3.1 Residential plans

Several studies have noted that only between one-third and one-half of aging parents make concrete plans for the their relative's future living arrangements (Freedman, Krauss, & Seltzer, 1997; Heller & Factor, 1994; Roberto, 1988; Smith, Fullmer, & Tobin, 1994). Residential planning is one of the most anxiety-provoking aspects of future planning as it reminds families of their mortality and it can invoke unspoken concerns regarding family responsibility, separation, and independence (Freedman et al., 1997). Furthermore, parents who have cared for their child at home for decades may be reluctant to relinquish their role. Older families often report that providing care for their relative within the family home provides meaning to their lives. The launching stage is a transition point which can result in considerable family accommodations, disequilibrium, and decreased well-being (Seltzer, Krauss, Choi, & Hong, in press).

While many families do not make concrete plans for living arrangements, most have preferences regarding the type of care they would like, and most would like to have plans in place in their lifetime (Heller & Factor, 1991; Roberto, 1988). About half of the families prefer continued care with another family member, usually a sibling of the adult with intellectual disabilities, and the other half would like an out-of-home placement. However, when families do begin to consider residential programs, they face long waiting lists (Hayden, 1992) and have significant concerns about the quality of housing options. A common sentiment of these families is that staff could not possibly provide the same degree of caring and understanding that a parent could. As one parent commented "It would break our heart to place her; there is no place like home and your parents; they know what their child is like" (Heller & Factor, 1988, p. 40). Wood and Skiles (1992) have noted that the caregiver's reluctance to plan may reflect both limited awareness of services and actual gaps in the service system. Apprehension about the residential service system may be particularly strong for older parents who may have had negative experiences when their children were young and when adequate community services were nonexistent.

Lack of planning by families can lead to emergency placements, difficulties for other family members who suddenly assume responsibility for their relative upon the death or frailty of a parent, pressures on the service system, and major disruptions in the daily life of the adult with intellectual disabilities. Also, without planning and discussions with other family members it is not possible to consider the views and preferences of various family members. Many parents do not discuss future plans with other family members or with their son or daughter with intellectual disabilities (Heller & Factor, 1994; Smith & Tobin, 1989). In a study that interviewed adults with intellectual disabilities (Heller & Factor, 1993a), we found that nearly half of the adults aged 30 years and older wanted to move out of the family home either to gain more independence or to live with friends. Those who wanted to remain with families stressed the desire for stability or the reciprocal supports they provided to and received from parents.

7.15.4.3.2 Predictors and outcomes of placement

Generally the parents who are most likely to make residential plans are those of higher socioeconomic status (Heller & Factor, 1991). Freedman et al. (1997) differentiate short-term (wanting a change in settings in less than two years) from long-term planners and note that the short-term planners are more likely to have health problems, worries about the future, and lower sense of purpose than longer-term planners or persons who had not made plans. The long-term planners had the most positive well-being of all the groups. A three-year follow-up indicated that the short-term planners were more likely to have achieved out-of-home placements.

The variables predicting preferences for future out-of-home placement versus actual placements differ. Heller and Factor's (1993b) longitudinal study indicated that over a two year period the major predictors of both outcomes were high perceived unmet need for formal services. High maladaptive behavior was associated with desire for placement, but not with actual placement. Actual placement was related to parents' perceptions that caring for their relative would become more difficult and to having placed their relative on a waiting list for residential services. In a study spanning three years, Seltzer, Greenberg, Krauss, and

Hong (1997) similarly found that placement was most likely to occur when the mother was in poor health and had placed her child on a waiting list. This pattern is similar to the factors predicting nursing home placement for elderly persons (Colerick & George, 1986; Pruchno, Michaels, & Potashnik, 1990) with characteristics of the caregiver playing a larger role than characteristics of the care recipient.

In examining outcomes of placement, Seltzer et al. (1997) found that parents' level of perceived caregiving burden was lower after placement. Although nearly 94% of the mothers maintained at least weekly contact with their child and at least one-third of the mothers continued providing them with some care, the mother's level of perceived burden was lower. With placement the daily caregiving responsibilities were reduced. In addition to reducing burden, out-of-home placement prior to the death of either or both parents can result in better outcomes for the adult with intellectual disabilities, in contrast with placements made after parental death. Gordon et al. (1996) found that the latter placements often result in more disruption in lifestyle, including not only a change in residence but also a change in day program and social life. These findings point to the importance of planning in advance of major parental declines in health.

7.15.4.3.3 Legal and financial planning

Legal and financial planning are other challenges for families who want to assure financial resources for their relative with intellectual disabilities without jeopardizing government benefits and who want to obtain guardianship if their relative is incompetent. In the Heller and Factor (1991) study nearly two-thirds of families of adults aged 30 years and over had made financial plans and nearly one-quarter had made guardianship plans. As with planning for living arrangements, the extent that families make plans is tied to their socioeconomic status. Certainly, families who are wealthier are more likely to make financial plans (Heller & Factor, 1991). However, lack of information and misinformation among families and professionals has often lead to inappropriate plans that do not protect government benefits or that deprive adults with intellectual disabilities of their rights. For example, some families will money or property to another child with the hope that the child with intellectual disabilities will be taken care of. There are many reasons why this approach is fraught with problems, including the high divorce rate and the encouragement of dependency of the adult child with a disability on another family member. Another example is the tendency of families to obtain full guardianship rather than partial guardianship where some of the rights of the adult with disability are retained. There has been very little research on advance directives: that is, plans regarding future health care needs.

7.15.4.4 Sociocultural Issues

The caregiving experience for families cannot be understood without taking into consideration their sociocultural context. We are just beginning to examine the commonalities and differences in the later-life experiences of families from different countries, ethnic backgrounds, racial heritage, and socioeconomic level.

7.15.4.4.1 Comparisons across countries

While this chapter primarily describes the service trends and research findings from the USA, many of the same trends are occurring in other countries, particularly in developed countries. For example in Germany, Adam (1992) has estimated that, from 1988 to 1998, the percentage of adults with intellectual disabilities receiving services in the Wilhlemshaven region will increase from 17% to 26% in the 50–64 year age group and from 3% to 4% in the over 60 years age group. The trend to close or phase down institutions and to develop community programs has been proceeding rapidly in Europe. For example, between 1980 and 1993 in Scandinavian countries and in the United Kingdom there has been a decrease in the institutional population at an average rate of 4.25% per year (Hatton, Emerson, & Kieman, 1995). As in the USA many countries have long waiting lists for residential services. Breitenbach (1995) has noted that in France there are few openings in residential programs for older adults who are living with families, as priority is given to persons already in the residential service system. Van Walleghem (1993) noted the long waiting lists awaiting older parents seeking residential services for their relative with intellectual disabilities in Belgium.

In a cross-national comparison Heller, Haveman, and Van Berkum (1996) report that in comparison with older caregivers in the USA, parents in the Netherlands are more likely to make future plans, have fewer unmet needs for supports, and perceive more caregiving burden. These results could be explained by differences in the two service systems. In the Netherlands the fact that families made more plans could be attributed to their greater use of case management services and less apprehension about the service system. The higher stipend given to persons with intellectual disabilities in the Netherlands than in the USA may explain the lower need for information about future financial planning. In both countries high unmet service needs and poor health of the adult with intellectual disabilities were related to higher caregiving burden.

In a study comparing older caregivers in the USA with caregivers in Ireland Seltzer et al. (1995) found that in Ireland caregivers were less likely to make future plans, had poorer health, a smaller support network, more parenting stress, and less life satisfaction. There were also differences between caregivers in the Republic of Ireland and in Northern Ireland, with caregivers from the Republic of Ireland reporting more social isolation. Both of these studies demonstrate the potential role that culture, society, and service availability and expectations play in shaping the caregiving experience for families.

7.15.4.4.2 Culturally diverse groups in the USA

Only in the 1990s have studies begun to examine caregiving issues among families of persons with intellectual disabilities from various minority groups. These studies have focused on residential placement and future planning, use of informal and formal supports, and perceived caregiving burden and satisfaction. Comparisons of African-American and white families have found that African-American families are less likely than other families to place their relative out of the family home (Markwardt, Heller, Rowitz, & Farber, 1993; Pruchno et al., in press). One reason could be attributed to difficulties minority families experience in accessing services, either due to lack of awareness or lack of available services in their communities (Vidal de Haymes, 1989). In a study of Hispanic families, Heller, Markwardt, Rowitz, and Farber (1994) found that in comparison with white non-Hispanic families these families reported significantly more problems with the service system, especially in finding information and finding support groups. Others have attributed low service participation to discrimination, lack of accessibility, and lack of bilingual services (Rosenthal & Carty, 1988).

Another explanation for the higher rate of coresidence with families for African-American adults with intellectual disabilities could be that African-American families tend to have more positive attitudes towards family responsibility and greater involvement with extended families. In one study of caregivers of adults with intellectual disabilities (Heller, Rowitz, & Farber, 1992) it was found that African-American families report a similar degree of caregiving burden to that of other families, but that they report less burden on the siblings of the adult with intellectual disabilities. On the other hand, Pruchno et al. (in press) found that African-American families of adults with intellectual disabilities or mental illness experienced less caregiving burden and greater caregiving satisfaction than did white caregivers, despite being poorer and in worse health.

Among African-American families, many express an interest in having a sibling take over responsibility when the parents can no longer provide care. In one focus group, many parents have stated that their other children have been more than willing to eventually take over the care. They noted that they did not need to ask the other siblings, as they came to them to offer their support: "My son has four sisters. All of them said that they would take over."

It has been noted that many older family caregivers of adults with intellectual disabilities do not make plans for the future care of their relative. When asked about reasons for not making future plans, two major themes have emerged: low socioeconomic status and religiosity contributed to a present-day rather than future focus. Examples of comments by African-American caregivers include: "We are close to God. God will lead us"; "We have no money with which to plan. I live from day to day. I can't afford big dreams; I just hope to stay healthy."

Given the changing structure and composition of the American family, and in particular the African-American family, with more single-parent households and females in the workforce, the reliance on the extended family may not be sufficient. Families will need increased help in providing support to their relative with intellectual disabilities and more information on residential services and financial planning so that they can secure a desirable future for their relative. A critical aspect for many minority families will be outreach to families not only through the aging or disability networks, but also through churches and other community resources.

7.15.5 FAMILY SUPPORT INTERVENTIONS AND POLICIES

As adults with intellectual disabilities and their parents age, they likely face some functional declines and greater difficulty in maintaining independence. Yet this group of families tends to make low use of services. Most of these families have been quite self-reliant in providing care for their child over the years. This section describes their service needs and use, the importance of formal services in sustaining their ability to provide care, and different models of service provision.

7.15.5.1 Family Needs and Service Use

As their children make the transition from childhood to adulthood, parents of adults with intellectual disabilities face the unique challenge of dealing with their own age-related declines in health and energy and the decreased formal services available for adults with a disability. Older parents have major unmet needs for information regarding residential programs, financial plans, and guardianship (Heller & Factor, 1994; Kelly & Kropf, 1995). Also, they have major needs for case management and advocacy (Kelly & Kropf, 1995) and financial assistance (Fujiura & Roccoforte, 1990). Fujiura and Roccoforte found that families spent an average of 20% of their pretax annual income on unreimbursed expenses for their adult relative with intellectual disabilities residing with them. In addition to needing services for their child, parents may also need services for themselves through the aging network.

Families often are unsure of appropriate goals and programs for their adult children and they may have reservations about using either the aging or intellectual disabilities formal services system. Many older caregivers have not had formal services available in the past and express fear that placement is the main aim of the formal service system (Janicki, 1996). Todd and Shearn (1996) note that for some families who have made a career of parenting, use of services reduces their roles and reduces their sense of purpose and identity. Other reasons why some families are reluctant to accept agency services are: (i) previous negative experiences, (ii) difficulties talking with providers who offer advice families do not agree with or who are not sensitive to their concerns, (iii) complex eligibility criteria for some services, and (iv) inflexibility of services. On the other hand, some families may have been long-term users of services. They may have been active in developing parent organizations, support groups, or provider agencies. The service families are most likely to use for their child is day programming. While many families desire respite, frequently the public financial resources for respite care are insufficient to meet demand.

The extent to which formal services improve the well-being of the caregiver is unclear. In our studies (Heller & Factor, 1991, 1993b) perceived unmet formal service needs was a key factor influencing the well-being of parents, with high unmet needs being related to caregiving burden. Use of services also has been related to parents' perceived current and future ability to provide care (Englehardt, Brubaker, & Lutzer, 1988).

7.15.5.2 Progam Models

Several models of support interventions help families in sustaining care and in coping with their relative. These include: (i) support and psycho-educational groups, (ii) outreach through the aging network, and (iii) family support programs.

7.15.5.2.1 Support and psycho-educational groups

At least one-quarter of the older family caregivers interviewed (Heller & Factor, 1991) expressed an unmet need for a support group. Support groups are one type of intervention that can provide aging families with information, skills, and support for helping the adult with intellectual disabilities, for helping themselves cope with the emotional aspects of caregiving, and for developing future plans. Smith, Majeski, and McClenny (1996) report that older families who participated in psycho-educational groups geared to caregivers of adults with intellectual disabilities most valued the information on future planning and formal services and the opportunity to interact with other parents having similar concerns. Parents who did not coreside with their adult child having intellectual disabilities reported benefitting the most from information on quality of residential programs. Although Smith et al. (1996) report family satisfaction with psycho-educational groups, few older family caregivers attend such events. Even when they would like to participate, older family members may have difficulty with transportation or scheduling. While these short-term interventions may ease stress on a short-term basis or provide some needed information, they do not tend to have long-lasting impacts. Also, Abel and Nelson (1990) caution that educational programs for caregivers can undermine the caregiver's own problem-solving capacity and sense of control over the situation.

Support groups for caregivers of elderly relatives have had modest benefits as measured by rating of participants' well-being and caregiving burden (Zarit & Toseland, 1989). Among families of persons with mental illness, they have been shown to help caregivers gain a sense of self-control and lower burden in some cases (Anthony & Blanch, 1989). No research has examined the effectiveness of support groups that are not psycho-educational groups on older caregivers of adults with intellectual disabilities.

7.15.5.2.2 Outreach through the aging network

Since US federal legislation was passed that targeted collaborative projects between the aging and developmental disabilities networks, there have been several model projects that targeted elderly caregivers of adults with intellectual disabilities. These projects entail coordination, network building, and internetwork coalition building (Factor, 1996; Janicki, 1996) between not only the aging and disabilities service agencies, but also other community agencies. One example of such a project is the Hispanic Coalition Network (Factor, 1996) that was developed in Chicago, which organized an Hispanic Fair that brought in 120 providers, elderly Hispanic family caregivers, and other community resources in a local community. In order to attract the families, health screenings and food were offered. Many families who had not previously received needed services became aware and linked up with a variety of services. Another example of a caregiver project is the New York Caregiver Assistance Project (Janicki, 1996), mentioned earlier in this chapter. That project operated from a mode which assigned outreach and assistance functions to a host agency. Major components included a needs assessment, targeting of special households, and a program of promoting community awareness. The project found that area agencies on aging could provide a safety valve for potential crises that would have resulted in immediate placement demands and referral to potentially more costly developmental disability programs. Another major finding was that working with cultural organizations within the local community resulted in greater willingness of families to accept services.

7.15.5.2.3 Family support public programs

In the 1980s and 1990s there has been a growing expansion of family support programs for families of persons with intellectual disabilities in the USA. Most of the earlier programs provided discrete types of services which were directed by agencies and by professionals. These included primarily respite, counseling, and parent training services. Later, cash subsidies were added in some states. However, with the emerging movement towards community empowerment and recognition of the need for persons with disabilities to remain in their communities and "natural" settings, new family-driven models have been promulgated. Generally, family support programs have been based on the goals of strengthening family functioning and enhancing growth and development of individuals and the family. Ultimately, most of these programs have the goals of maintaining persons with intellectual disabilities within the family home. As of 1995, 21 states had family support legislation (Bergman & Singer, 1996). Between 1988 and 1992 there has been an increase in intellectual disabilities state expenditures for family support services from 171 million to 277 million dollars allocated and from 163 330 to 198 827 families served (Braddock et al., 1995). While there has been an expansion of family support services, funding for them only represents 2% of expenditure for intellectual disabilities services (Braddock et al.) and many of these programs only target children.

Most of the innovative family support programs have developed models of consumer control in which families determine how resources are spent. These are based on the premise that families usually know best what it takes to maintain their relative with a disability in the family home. They also acknowledge the importance of using the informal network, including relatives, neighbors, and friends by allowing families to pay them for support services.

Most of the studies evaluating the impact of these family support programs have focused on families of children. These studies have documented their success in reducing stress and increasing life satisfaction for caregivers (Herman, 1991; Meyers & Marcenko, 1989). In a study of a family support program in Illinois geared to adults, it was found that family subsidies of about $1 300 combined with service facilitation and consumer control of services and expenditures resulted in many positive benefits over a 4 year period (Heller, Ruch-Ross, & Kopnick, 1995). In comparison with families who did not receive these services through a lottery selection process, the participant families reported greater caregiving satisfaction and greater feelings of competence and self-efficacy in helping their relative with intellectual disabilities. In addition, benefits included more community integration and improved interpersonal relations of the adult with intellectual disabilities, fewer unmet services needs, more satisfaction with services received, and less need for out-of-home placement. Also, families who participated were more likely to engage in legal and financial planning for their relative.

With the trend to community inclusion and consumer control of resources, and with pressures to cut costs by reducing residential services, there is likely to be an increase in family support programs. For older family caregivers this can result in added resources for maintaining caregiving within the family. However, with the advent of managed care approaches there is the danger that the funds will be too small or that sufficient residential options will not be in place for those families not able to provide care in the home setting. The Illinois family support program provides twice more funds per family than most of the other states' programs and is one of the few that targets adults.

7.15.6 RESEARCH DIRECTIONS

7.15.6.1 Summary of Research

The research on family caregiving for adults with intellectual disabilities is indicating tremendous variability in families' responses and the importance of understanding the life course and social context within which families operate. Some families devoted much of their lives to parenting a child with a disability through years when there were few services. Other families placed their relative out of the home and had various levels of continued involvement with their relative. With the advent of parent advocacy programs some families became active in promulgating new and expanded services in their communities. Certainly, during these eras there have been major demographic trends that have affected families' ability to provide care.

While expectations of family caregiving are higher, the resources within the family have often been diminished. This has been most acutely felt by women who most often are the primary caregivers. Yet, other members, such as fathers and siblings, also play crucial roles in supporting the adult with intellectual disabilities, not only during the parents' lifetime, but also afterwards.

Support programs and interventions have been one resource helping family caregivers. These have included support groups, counseling, parent training, respite, and cash subsidies. The effectiveness of these programs in helping families care for their relative and in enhancing the lives of the family members is being studied. Little is known about the best methods for providing supports to families. However, it is clear that, as they age, many families who have relied on their own resources will require some help from the formal service systems.

7.15.6.2 Research Agenda

To improve theoretical understanding of the caregiving experience and of ways to promote positive coping among families of adults with intellectual disabilities, comparative research across disability groups, across developmental periods, and across culturally diverse groups is needed. Most of the research up to 1997 focuses on one type of disability at one developmental period, usually that of parenting young children or of caregiving in later life. There are only a handful of studies that span different age phases, and these studies are hampered by their cross-sectional methodology.

With the exception of the research conducted by Seltzer and Krauss and their colleagues and by Heller and Factor there have been no longitudinal studies examining family caregiving among older family caregivers of adults with intellectual disabilities. With more longitudinal data it will be easier to delineate causal directions.

Another aspect that needs to be pursued further is the reciprocal nature of family caregiving and the impact of reciprocal supports on various family members. This line of research needs to take into account the perspectives of various family members—including the adult with intellectual disabilities, who may view the situation differently. Fathers and siblings also have been largely neglected in research; yet they play a critical role in supporting the adult with a disability and the mother.

There is little data on the impact of cultural, national and local differences on families' caregiving experience. There is a need for more studies that include various cultural groups and that examine the impact of differences in cultures and service networks in different communities, states, and countries. The challenge in this type of research is to disentangle the effects of socioeconomic status, culture, and service network differences on families.

Finally, more needs to be known about ways to help families cope. One way is to learn from families who have coped successfully, have nurtured a positive family climate, and have enhanced the development of the member with intellectual disabilities. These families have been able to successfully negotiate both the fulfillment of their own roles and the development of the adult with disabilities. In addition to quantitative data, there is a need for qualitative, ethnographic data to more richly elucidate this coping process .

Another way to learn more about ways to help families is to study the effectiveness of interventions and public programs. Most of the research is anecdotal or lacks empirically-sound comparison groups. In studying these interventions, a longer-term perspective needs to be taken. For example, to understand the impact on actual placement, a span of more than just 1 year must be looked at. As service models evolve examinations of both the mode in which services are delivered and the outcomes of these approaches are needed. Satisfaction of adults with disabilities and their families with the process and outcomes should be a major determinant of the program's success.

ACKNOWLEDGMENT

The preparation of this chapter was supported in part by funds provided by the National Institute on Disability and Rehabilitation Research and Training Center on Aging with Mental Retardation, Grant No. H133B30069.

7.15.7 REFERENCES

Abel, E. K., & Nelson, M. K. (1990). *Circles of care: Work and identity in women's lives* (pp. 65–91). Albany, NY: State University of New York Press.

Adam, G. A. (1992). German perspective. In S. Moss (Ed.), *Aging and developmental disabilities: Perspectives from nine countries* (pp. 37–44). Durham, NH: World Rehabilitation Fund University of New Hampshire.

Adlin, M. (1993). Health care issues. In E. Sutton, A. Factor, B. Hawkins, T. Heller, & G. Seltzer (Eds.), *Older adults with developmental disabilities: Optimizing choice and change* (pp. 49–60). Baltimore: Brookes.

Anthony, W., & Blanch, A. (1989). Research on community support services: What have we learned? *Psychosocial Rehabilitation Journal, 12,* 55–81.

Baskett, L. M., & Johnson, S. M. (1982). The young child's interactions with parents versus siblings: A behavioral analysis. *Child Development, 53,* 643–650.

Beckman, P. J. (1991). Comparison of mothers' and fathers' perceptions of the effect of young children with and without disabilities. *American Journal on Mental Retardation, 95,* 585–595.

Begun, A. L. (1989). Sibling relationships involving developmentally disabled people. *American Journal of Mental Retardation, 93,* 566–574.

Bergman, A., & Singer, G. H. S. (1996). The thinking behind new public policy. In G. H. S. Singer, L. Powers, & A. L. Olson (Eds.), *Redefining family support: Innovations in public–private partnerships* (pp. 435–464). Baltimore: Brookes.

Birenbaum, (1971). The mentally retarded in the home and the family cycle. *Journal of Health and Human Behavior, 12,* 55–65.

Blaney, B. (1995). *Aging with mental retardation.* Presentation at the Presidents Committee on Mental Retardation Collaborative Academy, Washington, DC.

Braddock, D. (1991). Technical note to census data. Chicago: Illinois University Affiliated Program, University of Illinois at Chicago.

Braddock, D., Hemp, R., Bachelder, L., & Fujiura, G. (1995). *The state of the states in developmental disabilities* (4th ed.) Washington, DC: American Association on Mental Retardation.

Bradley, V., & Knoll, J. (1990). *Shifting paradigms in services to people with developmental disabilities.* Cambridge, MA: Human Services Research Institute.

Breitenbach, N. (1995). *The lost generation.* Paris: Fondation De France.

Bruce, E. J., & Schultz, C. L. (1994). A cross-sectional study of parenting perceptions: Caring for children with intellectual disability. Special Issue: Family caregiving. *Australian Journal of Marriage and Family, 15,* 56–65.

Carter, G., & Jancar, J. (1983). Mortality in the mentally handicapped: A 50 year study at the Stokes Park group of hospitals. *Journal of Mental Deficiency Research, 27,* 143–156.

Center for Vulnerable Populations (1993). *Families focus: The status of America's vulnerable populations: A chartbook.* Waltham, MA: Brandeis University Press.

Cleveland, D.W., & Miller, N. (1977). Attitudes and life commitments of older siblings of mentally retarded adults: An exploratory study. *Mental Retardation, 15,* 38–41.

Colerick, E. J., & George, L. K. (1986). Predictors of institutionalization among caregivers of patients with Alzheimer's disease. *Journal of American Geriatrics Society, 34,* 493–498.

Englehardt, J., Brubacker, T. H., & Lutzer, V. (1988). Older caregivers of adults with mental retardation: Service utilization. *Mental Retardation, 26,* 191–195.

Essex, E. L., Seltzer, M. M., & Krauss, M. W. (1992). *Aging fathers as caregivers for adult children with developmental disabilities.* Paper presented at the National Institute on Aging Seminar on "Men's Caregiving Roles in an Aging Society," Washington, DC.

Eyman, R. K., & Borthwick-Duffy, S. A. (1994). Trends in mortality rates and predictors of mortality. In M. M. Seltzer, M. W. Krauss, & M. Janicki (Eds.), *Life-course perspectives on adulthood and old age* (pp. 93–105). Washington, DC: American Association on Mental Retardation Monograph Series.

Eyman, R. K., & Widaman, K. F. (1987). Life-span development of institutionalized and community-based mentally retarded persons, revisited. *American Journal of Mental Deficiency, 91,* 559–569.

Factor, A. R. (1996). *Final Report: Innovative internetwork service models serving older adults with developmental disablities and older family caregivers.* Chicago: Institute on Disability and Human Development, University of Illinois at Chicago.

Farber, B. (1959). Effects of a severely mentally retarded child on family integration. *Monographs of the Society for Research in Child Development, 24*(2, Serial No. 71).

Farber, B. (1975). Family adaptations to severely mentally retarded children. In M. J. Begab & S. A. Richardson (Eds.), *The mentally retarded and society.* Baltimore: University Park Press.

Fisher, M., & Zeaman, D. (1970). Growth and decline of retardate intelligence. In N. R. Ellis (Ed.), *International Review of Research in Mental Retardation* (Vol. 4, pp. 151–191). New York: Academic Press.

Freedman, R. I., Krauss, M. W., & Seltzer, M. M. (1997). Aging parents' residential plans for adult children with mental retardation. *Mental Retardation, 35,* 114–123.

Friedrich W. N., Greenberg, M. T., & Crnic, K. (1983). A short-form of the questionnaire on resources and stress. *American Journal of Mental Deficiency, 88,* 41–48.

Fujiura, G. (1996). *The demography of family care for adults with developmental disabilities.* Chicago: Institute on Disability and Human Development, University of Illinois at Chicago.

Fujiura, G., & Roccoforte, J.R. (1990, May). *Cost of disability to the American family.* Public Policy Forum, American Association on Mental Retardation, Washington, DC.

Gordon, R. M., Seltzer, M. M., & Krauss, M. W. (1996). The aftermath of parental death: Changes in the context and quality of life. In R. L. Schalock (Ed.), *Quality of life: Its applications to persons with disabilities* (pp. 23–40). Washington, DC: American Association on Mental Retardation.

Griffiths, D. L., & Unger, D. G. (1994). Views about

planning for the future among parents and siblings of adults with mental retardation. *Family Relations, 43*, 221–227.

Hallum, A., & Krumboltz, J. D. (1993). Parents caring for young adults with severe physical disabilities: Psychological issues. *Developmental Medicine and Child Neurology, 35*, 24–32.

Hatton, C., Emerson, E., & Kieman, C. (1995). Trends and milestones. *Mental Retardation, 33*, 132.

Hayden, M. F. (1992). Adults with mental retardation and other developmental disabilities waiting for community-based services in the United States. *Policy Research Brief, 4*, 1–18.

Heller. T. (1994). *Contemporary research on sibling issues.* Paper presented at the Brother and Sister: A Lifelong Connection conference of the New York Association for the Help of Retarded Children, New York.

Heller, T. (1997). Older adults with mental retardation and their families. In N. Bray (Ed.), *International review of research in mental retardation* (Vol. 20, pp. 99–136). San Diego, CA: Academic Press.

Heller, T., & Factor, A. (1988). *Development of a transition plan for older adults with developmental disabilities residing in the natural home.* Springfield, IL: Governor's Planning Council on Developmental Disabilities.

Heller, T., & Factor, A. (1991). Permanency planning for adults with mental retardation living with family caregivers. *American Journal of Mental Retardation, 96*, 163–176.

Heller, T., & Factor, A. (1993a). Support systems, well-being, and placement decision-making among older parents and their adult children with developmental disabilities. In E. Sutton, A. Factor, B. Hawkins, T. Heller, & G. Seltzer (Eds.), *Older adults with developmental disabilities: Optimizing choice and change* (pp. 107–122). Baltimore: Brookes.

Heller, T., & Factor, A. (1993b). Aging family caregivers: Changes in burden and placement desire. *American Journal on Mental Retardation, 98*, 417–426.

Heller, T., & Factor, A. (1994). Facilitating future planning and transitions out of the home. In M. M. Seltzer, M. W. Krauss, & M. Janicki (Eds.), *Life-course perspectives on adulthood and old age* (pp. 39–50). Washington, DC: American Association on Mental Retardation Monograph Series.

Heller, T., Sterns, H., Sutton, E., & Factor, A. (1996). Impact of person-centered later life planning training program. *Journal of Rehabilitation, 62*, 77–83.

Heller, T., Haveman, M., & Van Berkum, G. H.(1996). *Subjective and objective caregiving intensity and future planning among aging parents of adults with mental retardation: Comparison of United States and Dutch findings.* Annual Meeting of the International Association for the Scientific Study of Intellectual Disability, Helsinki, Finland.

Heller, T., Hsieh, K., & Rowitz, R. (in press). Maternal and paternal caregiving of persons with mental retardation across the lifespan. *Family Relations.*

Heller, T., Markwardt, R., Rowitz, L, & Farber, B. (1994). Adaptations of Hispanic families to a member with mental retardation. *American Journal on Mental Retardation, 99*, 289–300.

Heller, T., Rowitz, L., & Farber, B. (1992). *The domestic cycle of families of persons with mental retardation.* Chicago: University of Illinois Affiliated Program in Developmental Disabilities and School of Public Health, University of Ilinois at Chicago.

Heller, T., Ruch-Ross, H., & Kopnick, N. M. (1995). *The Illinois Home-Based Support Services Program evaluation report.* Chicago: Institute on Disability and Human Development, University of Illinois at Chicago.

Herman, S. (1991). Use and impact of a cash subsidy program. *Mental Retardation, 29*, 253–258.

Hogg, J., & Moss, S. (1993). Characteristics of older people with intellectual disabilities in England. In N. Bray (Ed.), *International review of research in mental retardation* (Vol. 19). New York: Academic Press.

Hooyman, N. R., & Gonyea, J. (1995). *Feminist perspectives on family care: Policies for gender justice.* Thousand Oaks, CA: Sage.

Janicki, M. P. (1996). *Help for caring—For older people caring for adults with a developmental disability.* Albany, NY: New York State Developmental Disablities Planning Council.

Janicki, M., Heller, T., Seltzer, G., & Hogg, J. (1996). Practice guidelines for the clinical assessment and care management of Alzheimer's disease and other dementias among adults with intellectual disability. *Journal of Intellectual Disability Research, 40*, 374–382.

Johnson, C., & Catalano, D. (1983). A longitudinal study of family supports to impaired elderly. *The Gerontologist, 23*, 612–618.

Kazak, A. E. (1987). Families with disabled children: Stress and social networks in three samples. *Journal of Abnormal Psychology, 15*, 137–146.

Kelly, T. B., & Kropf, N. P. (in press). Stigmatized and perpetual parents: Older parents caring for adult children with lifelong disabilities. *Journal of Gerontological Social Work, 23.*

Krauss, M. W. (1986). *Long-term care issues in mental retardation.* Paper presented at the National Institute of Child Health and Human Development and Kennedy Foundation Conference, Mental Retardation: Accomplishments and New Frontiers, Bethesda, MD.

Krauss, M. W. (1993). *Role variation among adult siblings of persons with mental retardation.* Paper presented at the Annual Meeting of the American Association on Mental Retardation. Washington, DC.

Krauss, M. W., Seltzer, M. M., Gordon, R., & Friedman, D. H. (1996). Binding ties: The roles of adult siblings of persons with mental retardation. *Mental Retardation, 34*, 83–93.

Lobato, D. (1983). Siblings of handicapped children: A review. *Journal of Autism and Developmental Disorders, 13*, 347–364.

Luckasson, R., Coulter, D. L., Polloway, E. A., Reiss, S., Schalock, R. L., Snell, M. E., Spitalnik, D. M., & Stark, J. A. (1993). *Mental retardation: Definition, classification, and systems of supports.* Washington, DC: American Association on Mental Retardation.

Marcenko, M. O., & Meyers, J. C. (1991). Mothers of children with developmental disabilities: Who shares the burden? *Family Relations, 40*, 186–190.

Mardiros, M. (1985). Role alterations of female parents having children with disabilities. *Canada's Mental Health, 33*(4), 24–26.

Markwardt, R., Heller, T., Rowitz, L., & Farber, B. (1993). *Adaptation of African-American families to a member with mental retardation.* Paper presented at the Annual Meeting of the American Association on Mental Retardation. Washington, DC.

McClaren, J., & Bryson, S. E. (1987). Review of recent epidemiological studies of mental retardation: Prevalence, associated disorders, and etiology. *American Journal of Mental Retardation, 92*, 243–254.

McHale. S. M., & Gamble, W. C. (1989). Sibling relationships of children with disabilities and nondisabled brothers and sister. *Developmental Psychology, 25*, 412–429.

Meyers, C. E., Borthwick, S. A., & Eyman, R. (1985). Place of residence by age, ethnicity, and level of retardation of the mentally retarded/developmental disabled population of California. *American Journal of Mental Deficiency, 90*, 266–270.

Meyers, J. C., & Marcenko, M. O. (1989). Impact of a cash subsidy program for families of children with severe developmental disabilities. *Mental Retardation, 27,* 383–386.

Morycz, R. K. (1985). Caregiving strain and the desire to institutionalize family members with Alzheimer's disease. *Research on Aging, 7,* 329–361.

Patel, P., Goldberg, D. P., & Moss, S. C. (1993). Psychiatric morbidity in older people with moderate and severe learning disability (mental retardation), Part II: The prevalence study. *British Journal of Psychiatry, 163,* 481–491.

Pruchno, R. A., Michaels, J. E., & Potashnik, S. L. (1990). Predictors of institutionalization among Alzheimer disease victims with caregiving spouses. *Journal of Gerontology: Social Sciences, 45,* S259–S266.

Pruchno, R. A., Patrick, J. H., & Burant, C. J. (in press). African-American and white mothers of adults with chronic disabilities: Caregiving burden and satisfaction. *Family Relations.*

Roberto, K. (1988). *Caring for aging developmentally disabled adults: Perspectives and needs of older parents.* (Final report presented to the Colorado Developmental Disabilities Planning Council). Greeley, CO: Department of Human Services, University of North Colorado.

Roberts, R.S. (1990). *Use of quality of life scales to measure outcomes of a project using volunteers with elderly* persons with mental retardation. Paper presented at the Growing Up and Growing Old symposium, Institute for Research on Mental Retardation and Brain Aging, Troina, Italy.

Rosenthal, E., & Carty, L. A. (1988). *Impediments to services and advocacy for black and Hispanic people with mental illness.* Mental Health Law Project, National Institute on Mental Health.

Rossi, A. (1987). Parenthood in transition: From lineage to child to self-orientation. In J. Lancaster, J. Altmann, A. Rossi, & L. Sherrod (Eds.), *Parenting across the life span: Biosocial dimensions.* New York: de Gruyter.

Rousey, A. M., Best, S., & Blacher, J. (1992). Mothers' and fathers' perceptions of stress and coping with children who have severe disabilities. *American Journal on Mental Retardation 97,* 99–110.

Seltzer, G., Begun, A. L., Seltzer, M. M., & Krauss, M. W. (1991). Adults with mental retardation and their aging mothers: Impact of siblings. *Family Relations, 40,* 310–317.

Seltzer, M. M., Greenberg, J. S., Krauss, M. W., & Hong, J. (1997). The end of co-resident caregiving: Predictive factors and changes in well-being in aging mothers of adults with disabilities. *Family Relations, 46,* 13–22

Seltzer, M. M., & Krauss, M. W. (1989). Aging parents with mentally retarded children: Family risk factors and sources of support. *American Journal on Mental Retardation, 94,* 303–312.

Seltzer, M. M., Krauss, M. W., Choi, S. C., & Hong, J. (in press). Midlife and later life parenting of adult children with mental retardtion. In C. D. Ryff & M. M. Seltzer (Eds.), *The parental experience at midlife.* Chicago: University of Chicago Press.

Seltzer, M. M., Krauss, M. W., Walsh, P., Conliffe, C., Larson, B., Birkbeck, G., Hong, J., & Choi, S.C. (1995). Cross-national comparisons of aging mothers of adults with intellectual disabilities. *Journal of Intellectual Disability Research, 39,* 408–418.

Seltzer, M. M., & Ryff, C. D. (1994). Parenting across the lifespan: The normative and nonnormative cases. In D. L. Featherman, R. Lerner, & M. Perlmutter (Eds.), *Life-span development and behavior* (Vol. 12, pp. 1–39). Hillsdale, NJ: Erlbaum.

Smith, G. S., Fullmer, E. M., & Tobin, S. S. (1994). Living outside the system: An exploration of older families who do not use day programs. In M. M. Seltzer, M. W. Krauss, & M. P. Janicki (Eds.), *Life-course perspectives on adulthood and old age* (pp. 19–37). Washington, DC: American Association on Mental Retardation Monograph Series.

Smith, G., Majeski, R., & McClenny, B. (1996). Psychoeducational support groups for aging parents: Development and preliminary outcomes. *Mental Retardation, 34,* 172–181.

Smith, G., & Tobin, S. (1989). Permanency planning among older parents of adults with lifelong disabilities. *Journal of Gerontological Social Work, 14,* 35–59.

Stoller, E. P. (1983). Parental caregiving by adult children. *Journal of Marriage and the Family, 45,* 851–858.

Suelzle, M., & Keenan, V. (1981). Changes in family support networks over the life of mentally retarded persons. *American Journal of Mental Deficiency, 86,* 267–274.

Sweet, J. A., & Bumpass, L. (1987). *American families and households.* New York: Russell Sage Foundation.

Todd, S., & Shearn, J. (1996). Time and the person: The impact of support services on the lives of parents of adults with intellectual disabilities. *Journal of Applied Research in Intellectual Disabilities, 9,* 40–60.

Townsend, A., Noelker, L., Deimling, G., & Bass, D. (1989). Longitudinal impact of interhousehold caregiving on adult children's mental health. *Psychology and Aging, 4,* 393–401.

Turk, M. A., Overeynder, J. C., & Janicki, M. P. (1995). *Uncertain future: Aging and cerebral palsy: Clinical concerns.* New York: New York State Developmental Disabilities Planning Council.

US. Bureau of the Census (1992a). *Households, families, and children: A 30-year perspective* (P-23, No. 181). Washington, DC: Government Printing Office.

US Bureau of the Census (1992b). How we're changing—demographic state of the nation: 1992. *Current Population Reports* (Special Studies, Series P-23, No. 177). Washington, DC: Government Printing Office.

US Bureau of the Census (1992c). Marital status and living arrangements: March 1992. *Current Population Reports* (Series P-20, No. 468). Washington, DC: Government Printing Office.

US Bureau of the Census (1992d). Marriage, divorce and remarriage in the 1990s. *Current Population Reports* (Series P-23, No. 180). Washington, DC: Government Printing Office.

US Bureau of the Census (1992e). Population projections on the United States, by age, sex, race and Hispanic origin: 1992 to 2050. *Current Population Reports* (Series P-25, No. 1092). Washington, DC: Government Printing Office.

US Bureau of the Census (1992f). Sixty-five plus in America. *Current Population Reports* (Series P-23, No. 178). Washington, DC: Government Printing Office.

Van Walleghem, M. (1993). Families with an elderly mentally handicapped child: Results of a qualitative study in Flanders Belgium. In M. K. Haveman & W. H. E. Buntinx (Eds.), *Family needs and family support in mental retardtion: An international perspective* (pp. 73–80). Nijmegen, The Netherlands: Kavanah Press.

Vidal de Haymes, M. (1989). *The Illinois Hispanic community living plan: Final report.* Springfield, IL: Illinois Hispanic Community Living Plan Advisory Board, Illinois Planning Council on Developmental Disabilities.

Walz, T., Harper, D., & Wilson, J. (1986). The aging developmentally disabled person: A review. *The Gerontologist, 26,* 622–629.

Wikler, L. M. (1986). Family stress theory and research on families of children with mental retardation. In J. Gallagher & P. Vietze (Eds.), *Families of handicapped persons: Research programs and policy issues* (pp. 167–196). Baltimore: Brookes.

Wilkin, D., Durie, A., Wade, G., Jolley, D., & Stout, I. (1984). *Specialist services for the elderly: A study of referrals to geriatric, psychiatric, and social services* (Research Rep. No. 5). Manchester, UK: University of Manchester.

Willoughby, J. C., & Glidden, L. M. (1995). Fathers helping out: Shared child care and marital satisfaction of parents of children with disabilities. *American Journal on Mental Retardation, 99,* 399–406.

Wilson, J., Blacher, J., & Baker, B. L. (1989). Siblings of children with severe handicap. *Mental Retardation, 27,* 167–173.

Wood, J. B., & Skiles, L. L. (1992). Planning for the transfer of care. *Generations, 16*(1), 61–62.

Zarit, S. H., Reever, K. E., & Bach-Peterson, J. (1980). Relatives of the impaired elderly: Correlates of feelings of burden. *The Gerontologist, 20,* 649–655.

Zarit, S. H., Todd, P. A., & Zarit, J. M. (1986). Subjective burden of husbands and wives as caregivers: A longitudinal study. *The Gerontologist, 26,* 260–266.

Zarit, S. H., & Toseland, R. W. (1989). Current and future directions in family caregiving research. *The Gerontologist, 29,* 481–483.

Zetlin, A. (1986). Mentally retarded adults and their siblings. *American Journal of Mental Deficiency, 91,* 217–225.

7.16
Falls Among Older Adults

BARRY A. EDELSTEIN and LISA W. DROZDICK
West Virginia University, Morgantown, WV, USA

7.16.1 INTRODUCTION

Falls are a common experience among older adults. Approximately one-third of community-dwelling older adults (Studenski et al., 1994; Tinetti, Speechley, & Ginter, 1988; Walker & Howland, 1991), 20% of older adults in acute care facilities (Kay & Tideiksaar, 1990), and half of older adults in long-term care facilities (Speechley and Tinetti, 1991; Tinetti, Baker, et al., 1994; Wright, Aizenstein, Volger, Rowe, & Miller, 1990) fall each year. Within a year, half of these fallers will have fallen again (Hernandez & Miller, 1986; Wolinsky, Johnson, & Fitzgerald, 1992). Studies suggest that these estimates may underestimate true fall rates. For example, Cummings, Nevitt, and Kidd (1988) found poor recall of past falls among community-dwelling older adults. Rates among institutionalized elderly may be higher as well, due to under reporting of noninjurious falls. This is a particular concern in studies utilizing chart reviews as their primary means of data collection (Kanten et al., 1993).

While the probability of falling is greater among nursing home residents, the vast majority of falls (85%) occur among community-dwelling older adults (Tideiksaar, 1993b). This is due to the greater number of older adults residing in the community; only 5–10% of older adults reside in long-term care facilities (Brock, Guralnik, & Brody, 1990). Nearly 50% of falls result in minor or soft tissue damage (Nevitt, Cummings, Kidd, & Black, 1989), while 10–20% result in more serious injury (Tinetti et al., 1988). Hospital admission follows 5–10% of falls (Gibson, Andres, Isaacs, Radebaugh, & Wore-Peterson, 1987) and falls account for 10–15% of emergency medical service (EMS) transports and trauma admissions among older adults (Mosenthal, Livingston, Elcavage, Herritt, & Stucker, 1995; Wofford, Heuser, Moran, Schwartz, & Mittelmark, 1994). Hip fractures result in tremendous physical and emotional consequences and an increased risk of death. Over 90% of the approximately 215 000 people who experience hip fractures each year in the USA (National Institutes of Health, 1991) occur as a result of a fall (cited in Graafmans et al., 1996). They are a leading cause of decreased independence and entrance into long-term care facilities (National Center for Health Statistics, cited in Greenhouse, 1994). Nearly half of older adult patients who enter a hospital due to a fall become long-term care patients following their injuries (Kay & Tideiksaar, 1990). Increased morbidity is also associated with falls (Rubenstein, Josephson, & Robbins, 1994). In 1987, 75% of all deaths due to falls in the USA occurred among older adults, even though they made up only 12% of the population at that time (Greenhouse, 1994).

The goal of this chapter is to provide an overview of the empirical literature on falls among older adults, beginning with a consideration of a few conceptual and methodological issues that plague this research area, and proceeding through the consequences of falls, factors associated with falls, and finally fall prevention. This is not intended to be an exhaustive review of the falls literature. Interested readers are referred to Tideiksaar (1997) for additional consideration of this literature.

7.16.2 CONCEPTUAL AND METHODOLOGICAL ISSUES

What constitutes a fall? The answer to this question varies according to who is being asked. One of the major problems with falls research is the failure to adopt a single definition of falls. Most definitions are consistent with the notion that a fall is an unintentional event that leads to an individual coming to rest on the ground or a lower level. However, specific aspects of a fall may be excluded from one study's definition while included in another. For example, Tinetti et al. (1988) defined a fall as "an event which results in a person coming to rest on the ground or other lower level, not as the result of a major intrinsic event (such as a stroke or syncope) or overwhelming hazard" (p. 1702). However, Hernandez and Miller (1986) included in their definition any abrupt accidental or purposeful change in position which could potentially result in an injury. While both definitions are acceptable, they make comparable results between the two studies difficult to interpret. In an effort to establish guidelines into research on falls, the Kellogg International Work Group (1987) proposed the following definition of a fall: "A fall is an event which results in a person coming to rest inadvertently on the ground or other lower level and other than as a consequence of the following: sustaining a violent blow, loss of consciousness, sudden onset of paralysis, as in a stroke, or an epileptic seizure" (Gibson et al., 1987, p. 4). Since this definition was proposed, it has been utilized in several studies. The use of such a single definition allows for comparisons across various studies, which has been difficult with the majority of published fall studies.

The definition of a fall is not the only problem found in the falls research literature. Diverse subject pools, different criteria for fallers, and disparate outcome measures also preclude comparisons among studies. Subjects in different studies vary along a variety of demographic variables (e.g., housing status, age, and health). Very few studies have included a wide age range of subjects (i.e., middle age and oldest-old adult subjects) and none have included samples across both community-dwelling older adults and nursing home residents. While studies have reported the populations investigated, sample differences may account for differences in the results rather than the experience of a fall. Studies have defined fallers both as individuals who have fallen at least once and individuals who have fallen two times or more. Since most results are based on differences between fallers and non fallers, discrepancies in criteria for group inclusion may account for variance in results. Finally, the use of a variety of outcome measures complicates the interpretation of results from various studies. Fall rates, total number of falls, and percentage of group experiencing a fall have all been used as outcome measures in studies of fall risk factors. These three outcome measures address different aspects of falls and are not always directly comparable. For example, a study showing a high total number of falls may have a low percentage of fallers and several repeat fallers may account for the large total number of falls. In contrast, a high total number of falls may be due to a relatively small number of falls among a large number of fallers. When interpreting or comparing the results of various studies, it is imperative that these fundamental methodological differences be considered.

7.16.3 CONSEQUENCES OF FALLS

7.16.3.1 Physical Consequences

Falls can result in a variety of physical consequences, ranging from minor injuries (e.g., abrasions, contusions, sprains, lacerations) to serious injuries (e.g., head trauma, spinal cord injuries, fractures, internal injuries). Thirty-one percent of falls result in minor injury and another 6% result in serious injury (Morse, Tylko, & Dixon, 1987). Though the percentage of falls resulting in fractures ranges from only 1–6% for the USA (Tinetti et al., 1988), France (Vellas, 1985, cited in Gibson et al., 1987) and Canada (Gryfe, Amies, & Ashley, 1977), "most deaths and long-term disability [related to falls] are ... due to the complications of fall-related fractures, especially hip fractures and other fractures among the elderly" (Melton & Riggs, 1985, p. 525). In view of the significance of fractures, falls related to fractures will be the focus of this section.

The most common fractures resulting from falls are to the wrist, upper arm, and pelvis (Melton & Riggs, 1985). The occurrence rate of fractures to the hip, wrist, pelvis and upper arm increases with age (Melton & Riggs, 1985), with such fractures among US, UK, and Scandinavian women outnumbering men between two and three to one (Evans, Prudham, & Wandless, 1979; Kreutzfeld, Haim, & Bach, 1984, cited in Gibson et al., 1987). The incidence of hip fractures increases after age 50 (Cummings, Kelsey, Nevitt, & Dowd, 1985), with a steep increase after age 70 (Gibson et al., 1987). Falls in the USA result in an estimated 215 000 hip fractures each year, resulting in 100 000 new cases of severe long-term disability (National Institutes of Health, 1991). On average, hip fractures result in a 21-day acute-care hospitalization (Baker & Harvey, 1985). The National Institutes of Health (1991) estimate that, by the year 2030, there will be 400 000 hip fractures incurred each year.

Of those individuals who are independently ambulatory prior to incurring a hip fracture, up to 75% will require ambulatory assistance for 6–12 months following the fracture (Tideiksaar, 1997). Of those hospitalized for a fall, only 50% survive one year (Tideiksaar & Kay, 1986). For those over the age of 85 residing in a nursing home, one fall out of five ends in death (Baker et al., 1984 as cited in Tideiksaar, 1989). Each year in the USA, 1800 falls are recorded as immediately fatal (Baker, O'Neill, & Karpf, 1984 as cited in Baker & Harvey, 1985).

Head trauma is a relatively common consequence of falls. Most head injuries resulting in acute hospitalization are from falls (Saywell, Woods, Rappaport, & Allen, 1989). Curtis, Wofford, and Branch (1995), cited in Tideiksaar, (1997), found that 54% of older adults hospitalized for subdural hematomas had fallen shortly before they were hospitalized.

Falls sometimes result in the faller remaining immobile for a period of time. Immobility secondary to a fall can result in hypothermia, broncho pneumonia, pulmonary emboli, and dehydration, all of which may lead to death (Mitchell, 1984; Tideiksaar, 1993c; Tideiksaar & Kay, 1986). The amount of time a person remains immobile immediately following a fall is termed "lie time" and is a marker for weakness, illness, and social isolation (Gibson et al., 1987). Moreover, lie time is a mortality risk factor. British studies indicate that lie times of at least 60 min are associated with death within six months (Wild, Nayak, & Isaacs, 1981, cited in Gibson et al., 1987). Unfortunately, data from France suggest that long lies are not uncommon. In Toulouse, 10 of 48 elderly patients hospitalized for falls had laid on the ground for an hour or more, and one for three days (Vellas, 1985, cited in Gibson et al., 1987).

7.16.3.2 Psychological Consequences

Older adults experiencing a fall also face potential emotional consequences. However, the psychological consequences following a fall are often ignored in falls research. Psychological consequences may lead to further physical decline. For example, an individual who experiences a fall may lose confidence in his/her ability to perform activities without falling again. Therefore, in an effort to avoid further falls, he/she restricts his/her activities. The decline in activities leads to a decline in physical health and muscle tone. If an individual remains inactive, he/she can become weak to the point of becoming unable to perform activities. Thus, psychological factors may result in decreased physical abilities and increased physical dependence.

Psychological factors have been examined as both risk factors and consequences of falls. Due to the retrospective nature of most falls research, it is difficult to determine if psychological problems related to a fall were present prior to, or appeared as a consequence of, a fall. This issue is further complicated by the fact that psychological factors can be both consequences and risk factors of falls. Many older adults experience a loss of confidence, depression, or fear of falling after a fall (Downton & Andrews, 1990; Tinetti, Richman, & Powell, 1990; Tinetti et al., 1988). The presence of any of these psychological problems may lead to decreased mobility and further physical decline as described previously.

The failure of many falls researchers to collect information on psychological consequences of falls reveals an emphasis on medical factors rather than psychological factors within falls researchers. Psychological factors are related to the occurrence and outcome of falls. Simpson and Mandelstam (1995) found that about 23% of hospital patients who had experienced a fall refused to participate in physical therapy training even though it was determined that they were capable of participation. Given that the patients were physically capable of participation, psychological factors likely account for the patient's refusals. This finding and others discussed below suggest that confidence in abiding abilities, self-perceived health status, depression, and fear of falling can have detrimental effects on health, activity level, and life satisfaction. It is important that research into psychological factors be conducted and prevention and treatment programs be developed.

Tinetti, Richman, and Powell (1990) developed the Falls Efficacy Scale (FES) to measure an individual's confidence in his/her ability to avoid a fall while performing specific activities. This scale was developed initially as a measure of fear of falling. Fear was defined as "low perceived self-efficacy or confidence at avoiding falls" (p. P239). Therefore, it is utilized more accurately as a measure of confidence. Decreased confidence has been shown to be related to a history of falls (Tinetti, Mendes deLeon, Doucette, & Baker, 1994). Poor ability to estimate mobility was a significant predictor of falls in a study conducted by Morse, Morse, and Tylko (1989). Poorer ability to accurately predict overall physical abilities appears to place one at risk of experiencing a fall.

Falls influence health ratings in otherwise healthy individuals (Cwikel, Kaplan, & Barell, 1990). People who have experienced a fall rate their health as being poorer after a fall than nonfallers (Cwikel et al.). Subjective health ratings are also related to severity of injury due to a fall. People requiring emergency room visits after a fall rate their health as poorer than fallers with less severe physical consequences (Cwikel et al.). Further, longitudinal studies demonstrate that subjective health rating is a predictor of morbidity and mortality (Kaplan, Barell, & Lutzky, 1988 cited in Cwikel et al.). Intuitively, it makes sense that people who report poor health and ability would fall more frequently, especially if their self-report is accurate. However, individuals who are actually in poor health but report good health (i.e., high confidence in a poor ability) may be more at risk. It is difficult to determine if subjective health ratings reflect actual health status. A complex interplay among reported health, actual health, and falls may be involved and warrants further investigation.

Depression has been found to be associated with falls (Tinetti et al., 1988), recurrent falls (Luukinen, Koski, Laippala, & Kivela, 1995), and to distinguish between groups of fallers and nonfallers (Tinetti, Liu, & Claus, 1993). The presence of depression significantly and independently predicted falls in community-dwelling psychogeriatric patients (Asada, Kariva, Kitarjima, Kakuma, & Yoshioka, 1994) and hospital patients (Soja, Kippenbrock, Hendrick, & Nyhius, 1992). Furthermore, antidepressant medications have been found to be associated with decreased risk of falling (Asada et al.), possibly due to the alleviation of depressive symptoms. These findings suggest that depression is a risk factor for falls. However, the majority of studies are retrospective in nature and should be interpreted with caution. Depression is a common diagnosis applied to older adults; therefore, it is difficult to determine from cross-sectional data whether depression is related to the occurrence of a fall or was a premorbid condition. Depression is often measured within fallers and nonfallers and then the two groups are compared. Researchers then conclude from these comparisons that the presence of depression is predictive of falls. However, a study which finds depression as a risk factor for falls by utilizing data collected after a fall may not be accurate. Findings may indicate that falls are predictive of depression. Prospective studies of depression and falls are needed to clarify the impact falls have on the expression of depression.

Fear of falling is reported by both older adults who have and have not fallen. Between 20 and 33% of nonfallers (Downton & Andrews, 1990; Howland, Peterson, Levin, & Fried, 1993) and 48 to 56% of fallers (Downton & Andrews, 1990; Tinetti et al., 1988) reported being afraid of falling. Walker and Howland (1991) found fear of falling to be the most prevalent fear reported by older adults living in a housing community for the elderly. Studies investigating the fear of falling are hindered greatly by the lack of a single definition or measure of fear of falling. Every study utilizes a different measure and differences in definition influence the results. For example, the FES discussed earlier is often used as a measure of fear of falling when it actually measures confidence in the ability to avoid a fall. Results from studies utilizing this scale cannot be compared with studies utilizing a direct measure of fear of falling. Using an open-ended question on fears, Null-Kogan (1996) found fear of falling to be the second most frequently reported fear among community-dwelling older adults. Of the 50 participants in this study, 68% reported at least a little fear of falling. Howland et al. (1993) demonstrated that injurious falls may create higher rates of fear of falling. Forty-one percent of people who experienced injurious falls reported a fear of falling as opposed to 29% of those who experienced noninjurious falls. Fear of falling is associated with higher dependency, greater physical symptomatology (Downton & Andrews, 1990), greater drug consumption (Downton & Andrews, 1990), higher reported depression and anxiety (Arfken, Lach, Birge, & Miller, 1994; Downton & Andrews, 1990; Howland et al.), restriction of movement and activities (Howland et al.), and increased morbidity. People with a severe fear of falling after a fall are more likely to have long hospital stays and die (Murphy & Isaacs, 1982).

One of the most serious consequences of falling is the subsequent restriction in movement accompanying the fear of future falls. In a study of nursing home residents using wheelchairs, 76% reported they used wheelchairs voluntarily because they were afraid of falling if they tried to walk (Pawlson, Goodwin, & Keith, 1986). Between one quarter and one half of fallers stated that they restricted or avoided activities due to fear of falling (Howland et al., 1993; Nevitt et al., 1989; Tideiksaar, 1993c; Tinetti, Mendes de Leon, et al., 1994). Restriction in movement can lead to social isolation and withdrawal as well as an increased risk of falling due to decreased muscle strength and mobility. Prolonged bed rest can lead to bone demineralization, lung and peripheral circulation stasis, skin and soft tissue damage, and altered supply of oxygen to the brain resulting in confusion and cognitive problems (Commodore, 1995). It can also lead to joint contractions, balance loss, pneumonia, pulmonary emboli, and death. Fear of falling and restriction of movement appear to be more common in people with a history of past falls.

7.16.3.3 Economic Consequences

It is estimated that the direct and indirect costs of accidental injury in the USA is between 75 and 100 billion dollars annually (Committee on Trauma Research, Commission on Life Sciences, National Research Council, & Institution on Medicine as cited in Urton, 1991). Falls are the leading cause of accidental injury. The direct costs include medical treatment, rehabilitation, nursing home care, medical equipment, and loss of productivity by the faller and their caregivers. A study conducted in Seattle in 1983 found that 1740 fall-related injuries cost US $500 000 for emergency room services alone (Hongladarom, 1983 cited in Commodore, 1995). The estimated cost of acute care for fractures is roughly 10 billion dollars each year (Sattin, 1992 cited in Tinetti, Baker et al., 1994). Hip fractures are the most serious fractures in terms of cost. In 1987–1988, a study conducted in the UK reported expenses of 160 million pounds for the medical treatment of hip fractures (Gibson et al., 1987). The annual cost of hospitalization and long-term care related to fall injuries is 2.5 billion dollars in the USA (Tideiksaar, 1997). Each year billions of dollars are spent to care for people after they experience a fall.

The economic cost of falls can also be indirect. For example, the additional costs of staff time and allotted hospital days for inpatient falls can mount quickly following a fall. Moreover, the additional care required of a fall victim is time taken away from other residents in the facility. Since falls are the leading cause of accidental traumatic injury in individuals over the age of 65, emergency medical costs are also affected by falls and fall-related injuries (Tinetti & Speechley, 1989). Campbell, Reinken, Allan, and Martinez (1981) found that patients admitted to a hospital for traumatic injury experienced longer stays than patients admitted for a nontrauma-related reason (43 days vs. 25 days). Individuals experiencing numerous falls are more likely to have longer stays and be placed in nursing homes (Wolinsky et al., 1992). In the UK and France, one of the leading causes of admission to geriatric hospitals, residential homes, and nursing homes is falls not resulting in fractures (Gibson et al., 1987). The demands of frequent fall-related trauma influence the allocation of resources.

Falls also impact psychological, familial, and societal resources. Loss of independence, depression, and fear of falling require emotional and psychological resources of health care providers, fallers, and families. For example, pain resulting from a fall can have far-reaching effects on an individual's functioning. Families may experience disruption in routines as family members adjust to living and interacting with a physically diminished individual. Once-independent members may require assistance from family members who must rearrange schedules or living situations to accommodate the new demands of caregiving. Finally, community resources may be allotted differently to meet the needs of physically limited older adults. For example, more funds may be designated for use in senior centers or elder care programs rather than building a new school. Falls can have far reaching effects on many diverse areas.

7.16.4 RISK FACTORS AND THE CONTEXT OF FALLS

A substantial number of extrinsic and intrinsic factors associated with falls have been identified. It is important to note that when considering these individual factors, the reader should be aware of the general finding that multiple risk factors are involved with any particular fall.

7.16.4.1 Extrinsic Factors

Every fall occurs within an environment. However, external or extrinsic factors are rarely the sole cause of individual falls. In a study conducted by Rubenstein et al. (1988), no fall could be completely explained by environmental factors. Most falls occur as a result of both intrinsic and extrinsic factors. For example, an older adult experiencing depression may trip over the edge of a rug overlooked due to inattentiveness. This might not have occurred had the individual been mentally healthy and attentive. Environmental factors are associated with approximately one-third of falls occurring within the home and two-thirds of falls occurring outside of the home (Nevitt et al., 1989). This may be an underestimation of the role of environmental factors due to the retrospective nature of research into falls. A faller's memory of factors involved in a fall may be faulty due to injuries, personal beliefs about the cause of the fall, or the passage of time. Moreover, a fall can alter the appearance of the physical environment (e.g., an obstacle may be moved following a fall), thereby influencing the recall of relevant environmental information. In a study investigating the prevention of falls, 53.8% of residents in a skilled nursing care facility and 35.1% of residents in a board and care facility were given recommendations regarding changes to their environment (Rubenstein et al.). The high rate of environmental hazards led the investigators to project that environmental factors may be involved in as many as 50% of falls. Some of the extrinsic factors considered in previous research are considered below.

7.16.4.1.1 Time of fall

Research into time-related factors has produced conflicting results. Several studies have found peak times for the occurrence or nonoccurrence of falls (Brown & Edelstein, 1995; Graffmans et al., 1996). Several studies suggest higher occurrences of falls in institutions during the morning and evening shifts (Marx, Cohen-Mansfield, & Werner, 1990; Walker & Howland, 1991), but no consensus exists across studies. Quail (1994) and Walker and Howland (1991) reported that increased fall rates occurred at times of increased activity. In their studies, falls were more likely to occur during toileting at night and while performing activities during the day. In addition, Heslin et al. (1992) found that falls from beds were more likely to occur at night. Thus, the location of specific activities influenced where falls occurred. It appears that falls are more likely to occur at periods of increased activity, and time of day influences which activities are being performed. The activities most frequently reported at the time of a fall were ambulation and transfer of position (Heslin et al.). These studies suggest that the differential effects of time of day reported in individual studies may be indicative of increased periods of activity.

Seasonal influences also impact fall rates. Commodore (1995) reported an increased number of falls during the winter months. This was likely due to increased numbers of slippery surfaces (e.g., ice) and outdoor environmental hazards (e.g., snow covering holes). Mobility is also restricted by bulky clothing during the colder winter months. Although it has not been examined in the literature, increased physical activity during the summer months may lead to a similar increase in falls during the summer months. More information is needed on seasonal fall rates to investigate seasonal contributions.

7.16.4.1.2 Location of fall

Previously mentioned fall rates differ across residential status. For example, nursing home residents are more likely to experience falls than community-dwelling older adults. In addition, recently admitted patients to a nursing home are more likely to fall than long-term residents (Quail, 1994), with over 60% of nursing home residents experiencing a fall during their first year (Tinetti, 1987). The unfamiliar environment of the nursing home is likely to contribute to many falls occurring with newly admitted residents.

Rubenstein et al. (1988) reported that 80% of falls occurring in a multilevel care facility occurred indoors. Similar results were found in a prospective study in residents of homes and apartments for the elderly in Amsterdam (Graffmans et al., 1996). Among acute care patients, 65% of falls occur in the bedroom, half of these occurring from the bed (Heslin et al., 1992). It is unclear if fall rates coincide with length of time spent in a specific location. For example, Brown and Edelstein (1995) found falls among psychogeriatric inpatients to occur more frequently in the bedroom, hallway, dining room, dayhall, bathroom, and outside. However, no overall percentage of time spent in these locations was reported. If an individual spends 75% of the day in bed, the chances of a fall occurring in his/her bedroom is higher than one occurring in another location. Lipsitz, Jonsson, Kelley, and Koestner (1991) found that older adults frequently fell when they ambulated or transferred position (e.g., stood up from a chair). It is likely that the frequency of activities occurring in specific locations influence fall rates in those locations.

Stairs are hazardous for many older adults. In one study, 10% of falls among community-dwelling adults occurred around stairs (Tinetti et al., 1988). Decreased visual perception may lead to miscalculation of the length or height of individual steps. Archea (1985), cited in Gibson et al. (1987), found that most accidents involving stairs occurred while the individual was descending the stairs and were often related to poor architectural design. Stair-related accidents occur more frequently among young-old adults (65–75 years) (Abrams, 1984 cited in Gibson et al.). This may be due to decreased use of stairs by old-old adults or increased caution while using them. However, old (75–85 years) and oldest-old (85 + years) adults experience more serious consequences from falls on stairs than young-old adults (Gibson et al.). Where a fall occurs can be influenced by the amount of time spent in a location, activities that occur in a location, and particular environmental characteristics of the location.

7.16.4.1.3 Walking aids

Improper use of a walking aid (e.g., cane, walker) is a common contributory factor to a fall. Fallers are more likely to use an ambulatory aid (Mahoney, Sager, Dunham, & Johnson, 1994; Morse et al., 1989; Robbins et al., 1989a, 1989b). It is unclear whether this is a direct result of previous falls or unrelated conditions. Tinetti (1987) found the use of a walking aid to be the most common external factor associated with falls in a nursing home population. Improper use of walking aids is also associated with the inability to get up following a fall (Tinetti et al., 1993). As previously discussed, individuals who are unable to get up after a fall are more likely to experience serious physical consequences than individuals who are able to get up after a fall. The increased risk of falling due to use of walking aids may be due to reasons related to the use of the walking aid. Campbell, Borrie, and Spears (1989) stated that the increased risk due to the use of walking aids was a reflection of frailty or poor mobility requiring the use of such aids. If this is found to be true, it is unknown if improper use of these aids would be an additional risk factor for experiencing a fall.

7.16.4.1.4 Restraints

Restraints have been used to prevent frail or confused older adults from falling and incurring injury. In a study conducted by Heslin et al. (1992), 98% of acute care patients who fell from a bed had restrictive devices and 2% had restraints on them at the time of the fall. This suggests that many falls may occur as a result of failed attempts to remove or escape from restraints. Increasing evidence suggests that restraints do not prevent falls (Evans & Strumpf, 1990) and may be associated with injurious falls (Heslin et al.). A study investigating the impact of removing restraints found that removing them led to a significant increase in the overall fall rate but not in the rate of serious falls when compared with a nonrestrained control group (Ejaz, Jones, & Rose, 1994). Given these results, restraints should be used with caution in individuals at risk of falling.

7.16.4.1.5 Footwear

In humans, contact between the foot and the ground is necessary to provide balance and stability. Loose or poor fitting shoes contribute to instability among older adults (Quail, 1994) by reducing the stability normally provided by contact between the foot and ground. Several studies implicate loose or poor fitting footwear (e.g., slippers) as major contributors to falls (Kinsman, 1983, cited in Gibson et al., 1987). Shoes with limited traction or slippery soles may also increase the risk of falling. Research into footwear appropriate for older adults needs to be conducted.

7.16.4.1.6 Environmental hazards

Numerous articles have attempted to list hazards commonly encountered in the home. Table 1 lists many of these potential hazards. Tinetti et al. (1988) found that 25% of falls occurred as a result of tripping over an object. Environmental hazards may be more of a factor in falls by active older adults. However, with increasing age and infirmity, environmental factors may play a significant role. Few studies have investigated the impact of specific environmental hazards or the utility of making environmental changes in an attempt to decrease falls.

7.16.4.2 Intrinsic Risk Factors

An extensive array of intrinsic variables associated with falls among older adults has been examined in the literature. The factors discussed include: demographic characteristics (e.g., gender, age); physical impairment (e.g., muscle weakness, hearing loss, visual acuity loss); the results of various physical impairments (e.g., ambulation, gait, and balance problems); number, types, and amount of medications (e.g., antidepressants, sedatives), medical disorders (e.g., Parkinson's disease, cardiovascular disease); and psychological factors (e.g., denial of limitations, cognitive status). A comprehensive survey of the research addressing intrinsic factors is beyond the scope of this chapter. Therefore, representative research findings regarding the most commonly examined intrinsic variables will be discussed.

7.16.4.3 Demographic Factors

Demographic information assembled from numerous studies allows clinicians to identify populations at risk for falls. Identification of high-risk groups helps clinicians predict the risk levels of specific individual clients and can aid in the development of treatment and prevention programs.

7.16.4.3.1 Gender

The findings of research on gender as a risk factor for falling have been contradictory (Brown & Edelstein, 1995), with some studies revealing gender differences and others finding no significant differences. However, the majority of studies suggest that women fall more frequently than men (Cwikel et al., 1990; Nevitt, Cummings, & Hudes, 1991; Poster, Pelletier, & Kay, 1991) and have more risk factors associated with falls than men (Campbell et al., 1989). For example, two studies conducted in US nursing homes (Gross, Shimamoto, Rose,

Table 1 Environmental hazards.

Location	*Hazard*
Outdoors	Ice, water, holes, cracks, steps
Bedroom	Improper bed height, wheels on furniture, nonlocking bed wheels, poor lighting
Bathroom	Mats, slippery floors, low or high toilet, poor lighting, glare from floor, lack of grab bars, sliding carpets, inaccessible tub or shower stall
Kitchen	Unsturdy step stools, poor lighting, slippery linolium floors, slippery bathtubs, glare from floor, high cabinets
Living room	Low furniture, extension cords, wheels on furniture, loose rugs, poor lighting, inappropriate chair height, high steps, worn stair treads, lack of arm rests
Everywhere	Objects in pathway, sliding throw rugs, worn carpets, poor access to switches and lamps, raised door sills, lack of night lights, clutter, limited walking space, waxed or slippery floors

& Frank, 1990; Kalchthaler, Bascon, & Quintos, 1978) found a greater rate of falls among women than men. Similarly, Campbell et al. found that among community dwellers 70 years of age and older, women were at greater risk than men of falling. Moreover, a French longitudinal study of community dwellers (mean age 73) conducted by Ousset et al. (1996) found that 48% of the women and 29.8% of the men reported one or more falls during a two-year period. A Japanese longitudinal study of community dwellers conducted by Yasumura et al. (1996) found the same pattern of results as Ousset et al. However, they found a lower incidence of falls with 14.7% of men and 23.5% of women reporting at least one fall during a one-year period. The shorter time period used in the Yasumura et al. study may account for the smaller fall rate than that reported by Ousset et al.

Women incur injury as a result of falls more frequently than men (Hornbrook et al., 1994), with elderly women over the age of 75 years most likely to experience a serious injury as a result of a fall (Gibson et al., 1987). Further, Abrams (1984), cited in Gibson et al., noted that while women in the UK represent only 25% of the 65+ population, they account for over 50% of hospital-treated falls within this population. The incidence of hip fractures among women increases around age 40 and doubles every five to six years after that (Brody, Farmer, & White, 1984, cited in Gibson et al.). Differences in risks factors have also been related to gender. For example, in their prospective study, Campbell et al. (1989) found total number of drugs taken, use of drugs that can cause postural hypotension, use of psychotropic drugs, use of hypnotic drugs, mental status, and joint replacement were risk factors for women but not for men.

In contrast to the previous studies, Van Dijk, Meulenberg, van de Sande, & Habbema (1993) found a significantly higher rate of falling among male than female demented nursing home residents. Other studies have found no relation between gender and falling among patients in a general hospital (Poster et al., 1991), patients in a veteran's center and geriatric unit (Morse et al., 1987), and individuals discharged from an acute-care hospital (Mahoney et al., 1994). The different findings among these studies may be attributable to subject differences (Brown & Edelstein, 1995), with community dwelling women showing a relatively consistent higher rate of falling than community dwelling men. In the nursing home studies, higher fall rates were found among male residents with dementia (Van Dijk et al.). The two studies that found higher fall rates among women in nursing homes (Gross et al., 1990; Kalchthaler et al., 1978) appeared to include a more cognitively heterogeneous population. The confusion and disorientation that often accompanies dementia could place dementia sufferers at greater risk of falling.

Studies suggest that gender differences dissipate with age and fall rates become roughly equal after the age of 70 (Luukinen et al., 1995; Poster et al., 1991). Moreover, gender does not appear to differentially influence fall rates in elderly nursing home patients (Luukinen et al.).

7.16.4.3.2 Age

The relation between age and falls is also unclear, with numerous studies supporting and failing to support a relation. Campbell et al. (1989) found fallers to be older than nonfalling inpatients, and Kalchthaler et al. (1978) found higher frequencies of falling among older nursing home residents 40 years of age and older. Members of the Kellogg International Work Group on the Prevention of Falls by the Elderly report that most falls occur among older women (Gibson et al., 1987) even when the fall figures were adjusted for the proportion of women in the population (Prudham & Evans, 1981). Graafmans et al. (1996) found age to be related significantly to recurrent falls (two or more falls) but not to single falls among a group of community-dwelling adults in Amsterdam. The participants were 1.7 times more likely to fall for each 10-year increase in age. Wofford et al. (1994) found that adults over the age of 85 were seven times more likely to experience a fall than those aged 65–74. A study conducted by Studenski et al. (1994) found that while the probability of falling increased with age, the probability of incurring an injury as a result of a fall did not increase. This may be due to the decreased number of vigorous activities performed by older adults. For example, Speechley and Tinetti (1991) found that "vigorous" older adults were more likely to incur an injury as a result of a fall than "frail" older adults. Despite conflicting reports on risk, older adults appear more likely to experience a fall (Cwikel et al., 1990; Greenhouse, 1994; Poster et al., 1991) than younger adults.

In contrast, several studies have failed to support the relation between falling and age. Lipsitz et al. (1991) studied 70 fallers and 56 nonfallers in a nursing home and found no significant difference in age between fallers and nonfallers. Similarly, Morse et al. (1987) did not find age to be a risk factor for classifying fallers and nonfallers. Van Dijk et al. (1993) found no relationship between fall rates and age among older adults with dementia. In a study of 306 community-dwelling adults aged 70-years and older, Studenski et al. (1994) found no significant age difference between fallers and nonfallers. Moreover, Rosen, Campbell, Villanueva, and Morgan (1985) found the mean age between nonfalling and falling community-dwelling residents age 70 or greater not statistically different. Mahoney et al. (1994) compared fallers and nonfallers after discharge from a community hospital and found no significant differences in age. Again, differences in subject pools complicate the interpretation of these results.

While age appears to influence risk of falling, other variables (e.g., health and mental status) often associated with aging may be more pertinent as moderator variables. These variables will be discussed later in the chapter. Carefully conducted studies, controlling for the presence of moderator variables, need to be conducted to determine the direct influence of age on falls.

7.16.4.3.3 Race

Tentative findings suggest that race is also associated with the risk of falling. Specifically, Wofford et al. (1994) and Nevitt et al. (1989, 1991) found that Caucasians have a higher risk of falling and requiring EMS transport following a fall than African-Americans. Further studies of the relations between falls and ethnic and racial variables are needed. The falls literature has not addressed racial and ethnic group differences. The relations found between falling and these demographic variables should be interpreted with care because of possible differences in the reporting of falls by the different groups. Many variables may influence the reporting of falls and these issues need to be addressed.

7.16.4.4 Sensory Impairments

Impairments of vision, the vestibular system, and the somatosensory system can contribute directly and indirectly to falls. For example, visual impairments can preclude the detection of obstacles that may lead to a fall. Inaccurate or inadequate visual or proprioceptive information or a malfunctioning vestibular system can all lead to gait or balance problems. Attenuated sensations of touch and pressure on the bottom of the feet (sometimes due to peripheral neuropathy secondary to diabetes mellitus) can contribute to poor control of balance during stance and gait. The ability of the somatosensory system to function properly declines with age, as does the ability of the sensory-motor system after age 55 (Lord, 1996) and the ability to correctly register joint movement and position (Simoneau & Lebowitz, 1996). On a more positive note, good vision can sometimes compensate for other sensory deficits (Whipple, Wolfson, Derby, Singh, & Tobin, 1993).

The few studies that have examined the relationship between sensory impairment and falls have produced inconsistent findings. Mahoney et al. (1994) compared fallers and nonfallers with regard to visual impairments and found a significantly higher rate of visual impairment among fallers. Similarly, Granek et al. (1987) found a significantly higher rate of falls among blind than sighted individuals. Nevitt et al. (1989) found both decreased visual acuity and depth perception to place individuals at increased risk of multiple falls. Similarly, Felson et al. (1989) found a relationship between risk of hip fracture and poor visual acuity. Interestingly, they also found that older adults with good vision in one eye and moderately good vision in the other had an increased risk of hip fracture. Lord (1996) suggests that this could be due to poor stereoscopic vision that, in turn, reduces depth perception and increases fall risk. Lord (1996) concluded from his studies that contrast sensitivity, "detection of large visual stimuli under low contrast conditions," is more important than visual acuity in predicting falls. The significance of these findings is particularly important when one considers that contrast sensitivity is essential for detecting edges, such as steps and misalignments of walking surfaces.

In contrast to the foregoing findings, Morse et al. (1987) found no significant differences between fallers and nonfallers with regard to visual impairments or hearing deficits. Similarly, Brocklehurst, Robertson, and James-Groom (1982) and Robbins et al. (1989a, 1989b) found no relation between visual acuity and falls among older adults beyond the age of 65. Though a comparison of findings regarding vision and falls is precluded due to methodological differences among studies, it is clear that the majority of studies suggest a relationship between falls and various measures of vision. More comparative studies utilizing similar subject populations and methodologies are sorely needed.

7.16.4.5 Muscle Weakness

The musculoskeletal system is essential for maintaining postural control and movement through the environment. Declines in muscle mass begin at approximately 25 years of age.

Muscle strength losses of 10–20% occur between the ages of 40 and 70, with losses of 30–40% occurring between the ages of 70 and 80 (Whitbourne, in press). The greatest declines in muscle strength in later years occur in muscle groups of the lower extremities, including the muscle groups involved in ambulation, transferring to and from seated positions, and climbing stairs.

Several studies have found hip and lower extremity muscle weakness to be related to falls (e.g., Campbell et al.,1989; Lipsitz et al., 1991; Robbins et al., 1989a, 1989b; Whipple, Wolfson,& Amerman, 1987; Wolfson, Judge, Whipple, & King, 1995). For example, Campbell et al., in a one-year prospective study, examined multiple risk factors for falling among community-based older adults. Female fallers had significantly less leg strength than female nonfallers, with a relative risk factor of 1.6. No differences were found in muscle strength between male fallers and nonfallers. Robbins et al. (1989) also examined multiple risk factors using both community-dwelling and institutionalized older adults. Hip weakness was one of the three risk factors identified. This risk factor yielded a 68% chance of falling within a one-year period, those without this risk factor had a 19% chance of falling within the same time period. Knee and ankle weakness have been found significantly more prevalent among fallers than nonfallers (Whipple et al.). Similarly, Wolfson et al. found that residents of a nursing home with histories of falls had less than half of the knee and ankle strength of nonfallers.

In summary, muscle weakness in the lower extremities is consistently found to be a risk factor for falling. This relation, however, may not always be direct since muscle strength is associated with a variety of other risk factors (e.g., gait, balance, speed). Fortunately, as later noted, muscle strength training can contribute to a decrease in falls.

7.16.4.6 Gait

Gait reflects the characteristics of a person's walking, which is controlled and influenced by a multitude of factors. Moreover, gait is a multidimensional construct that is measured in a variety of ways (see Duncan & Studenski, 1994, for a review). Disorders of gait affect 20–50% of older adults (Sudarsky, 1990). Impaired gait is considered to be a major contributor to falls, which can also contribute to negative psychological consequences (e.g., fear of falling) and the concomitants of fear previously discussed (e.g., immobility, further functional decline).

Numerous studies have found a relation between gait problems and falls. Morse et al. (1987), for example, found a greater percentage of gait problems among fallers (88%) than nonfallers (43%). Tinetti et al. (1988) found community-dwelling adults with balance and gait abnormalities to be as much as 1.9 times as likely to fall as those without these problems. Whipple et al. (1987) found fallers to have significantly slower gait speed and shorter stride length than nonfallers in a nursing home population. Also, Guimaraes and Isaacs (1980) found that fallers displayed slower walking speeds, shorter step length, and greater variability in their step length than nonfallers. Similarly, Wolfson, Whipple, Amerman, and Tobin (1990) revealed that fallers in nursing homes differed from nonfallers with regard to stride length and walking speed. Overall, studies of gait have found a high prevalence of gait disorders among older adults, placing them at significant risk of falling.

7.16.4.7 Balance

A balanced position requires the coordination and muscular control of individual body parts. Walking has been characterized as successive loss of balance episodes in which a fall is averted with each step by repositioning each foot (Simoneau & Leibowitz, 1996). Such postural control results from the coordination of sensory and musculo-skeletal systems. The ability to transfer from bed to floor, walk, and be seated requires balance obtained through these systems and their coordination. Therefore, problems with these systems can result in a loss of righting reflexes and an increase in body sway (Kay & Tideiksaar, 1990), leading to falls.

Poor control of posture (postural dyscontrol), as evidenced by poor balance, has been associated with falls for both community-dwelling and institutionalized older adults. Wild et al. (1981), as cited in Funk, Tornquist, Champagne and Wiese (1992), found that postural dyscontrol among community-dwelling older adults contributed to at least 67% of falls. In a prospective study of falls, Tinetti, Williams, and Mayewski (1986) found that residents recently admitted to an intermediate care facility with balance impairment were 5.4 times as likely to fall as those without a balance impairment. Similarly, Lipsitz et al. (1991), in a retrospective study of 126 nursing home residents, found subjects with a balance impairment to be 3.9 times as likely to fall as those without such an impairment. Tinetti et al. (1988), in a prospective study of community-dwelling adults 75 years of age and older, found that individuals with abnormalities of balance were 1.9 times as likely to fall when compared with individuals without such abnormalities. In a study of institutionalized and noninstitutionalized older adults, Robbins et al. (1989a, 1989b) found that fallers were significantly more likely than nonfallers to have impaired gait and balance. Balance was one of three risk factors that significantly and independently predicted falling among both populations.

Older adults may not lose their balance more often than younger individuals, but are simply less capable of correcting the imbalance (Overstall, 1992). One of the principal indices of imbalance is body sway. With increasing age there is a slowing of the ability to detect changes in posture or sway, which is associated with greater risk of falling. Brocklehurst et al. (1982) found a relation between postural sway, decreased proprioception, and falls. Similarly, Wild et al. (1981) found a relation between responses to pressure applied to the sternum (balance response) and risk of future falls. Several other studies have reported differences between fallers and nonfallers with regard to postural sway or unsteadiness (e.g., Lichtenstein, Burager, Shields, & Shiari, 1990; Overstall, Exton-Smith, & Johnson, 1977; Wolfson, Whipple, Amerman, & Kleinberg, 1986). Balance and gait tests have also been found useful in discriminating between residents of intermediate care facilities who fell two or more times from those who fell once or never fell (Tinetti et al., 1986). The findings of Tinetti et al. are particularly interesting because the situations in which balance was measured were those for which balance is particularly important (e.g., when rising, sitting, and turning around). Overall, the results of numerous studies suggest that poor balance, which increases with age, is a potentially significant risk factor for falls.

7.16.4.8 Medications

Medications have often been examined as potential factors influencing falls. However, research into the effects of drugs on fall rates is equivocal. Many studies have found that drugs influence fall risk (Cooper, 1994; Lipsitz et al., 1991; Tinetti et al., 1986), while others have found no significant effect of drugs on fall risk (Lord, Clark, & Webster, 1991; Mahoney et al., 1994; Morris, Rubin, Morris, & Mandel, 1987; Tinetti, 1987). Total number of medications taken (Lipsitz et al.; Robbins et al., 1989a, 1989b; Studenski et al., 1994), addition of a new medication (Tinetti et al., 1986), and recency of drug administration (Aisen, Deluca, & Lawlor, 1992; Lipsitz et al.; Nevitt et al., 1989) have all been associated with falls. Further, the use of more than six medications was associated with the inability to get up following a fall (Tinetti et al., 1993). Methodological differences between studies may explain disparate results. Drug variables entered into data analysis differ greatly between studies. Many studies group all drug classes together within a single category while others examine specific classes of drugs. While many studies fail to find a relation between a global medication measure and falls, the influence of particular classes of drugs have been found to influence fall risk. For example, antidepressants have been identified as a risk factor for further falls (Lipsitz et al.). In addition, there may be gender differences in drug influences on falls. Cambell et al. (1989) found the total number of drugs taken to influence fall rates among women but not among men.

Specific classes of drugs influence the risk of falls. Drugs directly influencing cognitive states or alertness may increase the risk of falling. For example, Quail (1994) found alcohol to be related to the occurrence of falls. Side effects of drugs also influence the risk of falling. For example, Downton and Andrews (1990) found sedatives associated with subjective reports of dizziness, which is related to increased risk of falling. Drug classes which have been investigated in the literature include antidepressants, sedative/hypnotics, anti-inflammatories and analgesics, cardiovascular agents, neuroleptic/antipsychotics, antihistamines/anticholinergics, antidiabetics, diuretics, anticonvulsants, nitrates, and anti-Parkinsonian medications. Several of these will be discussed in detail below. As new medications are introduced and utilized in the older adult population, the influence of medications on fall risk needs to be reevaluated.

7.16.4.8.1 Antidepressants

Antidepressants are utilized for their ability to elevate mood and increase energy. As with all the drug classes, research on antidepressants has produced mixed results. Antidepressant use has been associated with increased risk of falling among nursing home residents (Lipsitz et al., 1991), recurrent falls in long-term care patients (Luukinen et al., 1995), and distinguished between fallers and nonfallers among community-dwelling males and nursing home residents (Studenski et al., 1994; Lipsitz et al.). Moreover, it has been associated with decreased risk of falls in community-dwelling psychogeriatric patients (Asada et al., 1994). In contrast, other researchers have not found antidepressant use to be associated with falls among residents of homes for the elderly (Graffmans et al., 1996) or community-dwelling older adults (Nevitt et al., 1989). Differences in results may be attributable to differing classes of antidepressants.

Three major types of antidepressant are prescribed: tricyclics, monoamine oxidase inhibitors (MAOI), and selective serotonin reuptake inhibitors (SSRI). Each class will be discussed separately due to their various effect and side effect profiles. While each drug produces numerous side effects, only those relevant to falling will be mentioned. The exact mechanism by which tricyclic antidepressants produce their antidepressant effect is unknown but it is assumed that they block the reuptake of norepinephrine, dopamine, and/or serotonin. Tricyclics may produce orthostatic hypotension, heart palpitations, tremor, sedation, and delirium. Research into tricyclic antidepressants and falling is equivocal. Quail (1994) reported that tricyclics increased the risk of falling in an outpatient population, especially when they were combined with other drugs. In contrast, Mahoney et al. (1994) found no significant effect of tricyclics among discharged hospital patients. While no research has been conducted on MAOIs and SSRIs, they are important to mention due to their possible relation to falls. Both produce anticholinergic side effects such as dizziness, blurred vision, or nausea which can influence the possibility of falls. More research into the exact types of antidepressants producing positive relations with falling is needed to determine the risk of prescribing these drugs to the elderly.

7.16.4.8.2 Sedatives/hypnotics/anxiolytics

Sedatives/hypnotics are typically prescribed as sleep aids or calming agents. They may also be prescribed as anticonvulsants. However, they can have serious side effects including disrupted sleep patterns, confusion, light-headedness, and drowsiness. Sedatives have also been associated with subjective dizziness in community-dwelling older adults (Downton & Andrews, 1990). Sedative use has been associated with falls in community-dwelling older adults (Tinetti et al., 1988, 1993), recurrent falls of these individuals (Nevitt et al., 1989), and the inability of these individuals to get up following a fall (Tinetti et al., 1993). While a relationship has been found between sedative/hypnotic use among women (Campbell et al., 1989), many studies have failed to find a relation between falls and sedative/hypnotic use in male community-dwelling older adults (Studenski et al., 1994), ambulatory nursing home residents (Lipsitz et al., 1991), or community-dwelling psychogeriatric patients (Asada et al., 1994). The relation between alcohol use and falls has been unclear in the literature. Campbell et al. and Nevitt et al. (1989) found no relation between alcohol and falls in community-dwelling older adults, while Quail (1994) found alcohol to be related to falls among outpatients. Similar to research findings regarding antidepressants, disparate results may be attributable to different specific drugs within the classes. However, it is also possible that drugs are exacting different effects on different subjects.

Anxiolytics, of which the most common class is benzodiazepines, are utilized to reduce anxiety symptoms. Unfortunately, they are also addictive and can be fatal in high doses. No relation between benzodiazepines and falls in community-dwelling males (Studenski et al., 1994), residents of homes for the elderly (Graafmans et al., 1996), or discharged hospital patients (Mahoney et al., 1994) has been found. However, Aisen et al. (1992) found that PRN administration of benzodiazepines was two times more frequent in fallers. Moreover, in 24 of 33 falls among inpatient geropsychiatric patients, benzodiazepines were administered within 24 hours of the occurrence of a fall.

7.16.4.8.3 Neuroleptics/antipsychotics

Neuroleptics are sometimes referred to as the major tranquilizers due to their heavy sedating effect in high doses. Typically, they are prescribed for the treatment of psychotic disorders or agitation in elderly patients. They can result in extrapyramidal effects and blurred vision, both of which can increase the risk of falling. Brown and Edelstein (1995) found that the use of antipsychotic medications significantly increased the risk of falls among psychogeriatric inpatients. Lord, McLean, and Stathers (1992) found similar results with antipsychotic use being a significant risk factor for falls among community-dwelling older adults. Quail (1994) found similar results among outpatients with the use of major tranquilizers increasing the risk of falling by 50%. In contrast, Lipsitz et al. (1991) found no relation between antipsychotics and falls in ambulatory nursing home residents. Moreover, no relation was found between antipsychotics and falls among community-dwelling psychogeriatric patients (Asada et al., 1994) or discharged hospital patients (Mahoney et al., 1994).

7.16.4.8.4 Cardiovascular medications

Although a large portion of older adults are prescribed cardiovascular medications, very little research has been conducted on their relation to fall among older adults. Graafmans et al. (1996) is the only study which has found a positive relation between a type of cardiac medication, peripheral vasodilator, and the recurrence of falls. Cardiac medications were not associated with falls in nursing home or community-dwelling older adults (Robbins et al., 1989a, 1989b), psychogeriatric patients (Brown & Edelstein, 1995), or ambulatory nursing home patients (Lipsitz et al., 1991). Moreover, although antihypertensives led to severe postural symptoms among outpatients, they were not associated with falls (Graafmans et al.; Quail, 1994). Finally, diuretics, digitalis, and vasodilator were not significantly related to falls among long-term care patients (Luukinen et al., 1995).

7.16.4.8.5 Analgesics and anti-inflammatory medications

Medicines prescribed for the alleviation of pain or inflammation are often prescribed to older adults. In a study of ambulatory nursing home residents, fallers were significantly more likely than nonfallers to be taking analgesics (Lipsitz et al., 1991). However, the taking of analgesics was not found to be significantly related to falls among psychogeriatric inpatients (Brown & Edelstein, 1995) or residents of homes for the elderly (Graafmans et al., 1996). Ingestion of anti-inflammatory medications has not been found to be significantly related to falls among nursing home residents (Graffmans et al.; Lipsitz et al.).

The previous discussions regarding drugs demonstrate the need for research examining the relation between drugs and falls. Although some classes of drugs have been identified as potentially increasing the risk of falling, drug interactions may also account for increased fall rates. The majority of research on drugs has involved retrospective reviews. Unfortunately, very few subjects are prescribed only one drug. Therefore, differing results may be due to drug interactions. For example, a person taking an antidepressant may not be at increased risk of falling but an individual taking an antidepressant and a cardiovascular medication may be at increased risk. Medications have multiple effects on many systems within the body. It is likely that individual differences account for differential drug effects. The complex interplay of drugs and physiological systems requires more knowledge.

7.16.4.9 Medical Disorders

The relationship between the type of medical disorder and fall risk is unclear, as studies have yielded mixed results. Numerous studies have found relations between falls and underlying medical diseases (e.g., Campbell et al., 1990; Nevitt et al., 1989; Rubenstein et al., 1990). Rubenstein et al., following their review of several falls studies, estimated that 55% of falls are related to medical disorders, with the greatest percentage of these being due to chronic diseases. Among the disorders related to falls are arthritis of the knee, stroke (Campbell et al.,1989), Parkinson's disease (Davie, Blumenthal, & Robinson-Hawkins, 1981; Studenski et al, 1994), osteoarthritis, unspecified arthritis (Davie et al.), diabetes, and hypotension (Davie et al.; Lipsitz et al., 1991). Though considerable support has been found for relations between medical disorders and falls, several studies have failed to find this relation for some of the same disorders (e.g.,Lipsitz et al.; Morse et al., 1987; Studenski et al.). Brown and Edelstein (1995) noted that the only apparently consistent finding in this literature is the strong relation between musculoskeletal disorders and falling.

The mostly mixed and contradictory findings noted above are likely attributable to differences in numerous factors across studies (e.g., subject population, physical and mental status, age, nature and number of diseases, research procedures, length or severity of disorder) that can directly or indirectly influence reported fall rates. For example, Lipsitz et al. (1991) based their fall rate on falls witnessed by staff or self-reported by nursing home residents. In contrast, Davie et al. (1981) and Studenski et al. (1994) obtained data via telephone calls and interviews of community-dwelling adults. Davie et al. may have obtained results different from Lipsitz et al. and Morse et al. (1987) regarding falls among individuals with diabetes or hypotension because of participant differences. Davie et al. studied community-dwelling residents, whereas Lipsitz et al. and Morse et al. studied inpatients. Hospitalized older adults are generally at a greater risk of falling than community-dwelling adults, as they tend to be more cognitively impaired and less ambulatory. In conclusion, it may be naive to believe that the effects of individual medical conditions can be isolated and that findings across studies can be compared. It is not uncommon for older adults to simultaneously experience multiple medical disorders. When considering the problems of matching participants across studies on the many factors believed to be related to falls, the prospect of obtaining reliable results appears improbable.

The relationship between the number of medical disorders and fall risk also remains unclear. Studies by Kalchthaler et al. (1978) and Morse et al. (1987) found a positive relationship between number of medical disorders and falls.

Kalchthaler et al. found the largest number of falls among nursing home residents with three to six medical disorders. Similarly, Morse et al. found fallers had significantly more medical disorders than nonfallers. Although the medical disorder in fall literature is fraught with inconsistencies in methodologies and results, there is certainly sufficient support for the contention that medical disorders, particularly those of a chronic nature, place older adults at risk of falls.

7.16.4.10 Psychiatric Disorders

The effects of psychiatric disorders are difficult to separate from their treatment (e.g., psychotropic medications), the overall mental status of the participants, and the setting in which falls are examined. Institutionalized individuals are generally more likely to suffer from psychiatric disorders, be receiving psychotropic medications, and have poorer mental status than individuals still living in the community. In addition, they are more likely to fall. A small number of researchers have examined the relationship between psychiatric disorders and falls, some of which have found support for such a relationship. Hernandez and Miller (1986), for example, examined fallers on a psychogeriatric unit and found fallers to have the following psychiatric diagnoses: dementia (77%), depression (43%), and agitation or paranoia (21%). Similarly, Poster et al. (1991) found older adults in a psychiatric hospital with psychotic disorders to be at greater risk of falling than those without psychotic disorders. Granek et al. (1987) found significantly more depressed fallers than nonfallers in a long-term care facility.

Similar findings have been revealed among community-dwelling adults. Davie et al. (1981) found the presence of a psychiatric diagnosis to be related to falling among community-dwelling older adults. Similarly, Asada et al. (1994) found depressed community-dwelling individuals at a significantly greater fall risk than nondepressed individuals.

In contrast to the foregoing results, several studies have failed to find positive relations between psychiatric disorders and falls. For example, Hernandez and Miller (1986) and Granek et al. (1987) found no significant differences in the incidences of Parkinson's disease between fallers and nonfallers. Brown and Edelstein (1995) also found no relation between psychiatric disorders and falling. Moreover, there have been a few studies suggesting a possible protective effect of psychiatric disorders. For example, Poster et al. (1991) found patients with Bipolar Disorder to be at lower risk of falling than other patients. The only apparently consistent finding across several studies is the positive relation between depression and falling. Unfortunately, it cannot be determined whether this is primarily due to the disorder, cognitive deficits resulting from the disorder, the medications used to treat the disorder, or some combination of these and other factors that could serve to moderate this relationship.

In conclusion, there appear to be few intrinsic factors that reliably predict falls. However, a few factors have emerged as predictors in a sufficient number of studies to certainly warrant further investigation and exploration in prevention programs, particularly with regard to the type of intervention that is most effective for each particular risk factor.

7.16.5 PREVENTION OF FALLS

While the prevention of all falls is virtually impossible, numerous authors have offered suggestions for the development of prevention programs and limited empirical support has been found for some prevention practices. Recommendations for fall prevention have typically been based upon "common sense" (Gibson et al., 1987) and identified risk factors. However, Rubenstein and Josephson (1993) have aptly noted that while the literature is replete with such recommendations for preventing falls, few of the recommendations are based upon sound, controlled research. Similarly, Tinetti (1994) argued that fall prevention "studies reported in the literature to date have shown either no or only marginal reduction in fall rate" (p. 758). However, there has been evidence of successful prevention programming. In the following section approaches to prevention will be discussed and a few of the more promising studies published will be reviewed.

Falls can have multiple causes that vary across individuals. Thus, effective fall prevention programs must take into consideration a myriad of potential risk factors for each individual. Prevention programs might include risk factor identification, assessment following falls, exercise programs, alarm systems, and protective devices (Rubenstein & Josephson, 1993). Because the prevention programs often contain multiple interventions, it is difficult to compare studies in any meaningful way. Nevertheless, an attempt will be made to consider elements of prevention programs by following Tideiksaar's (1993a) categorization of prevention strategies, which include medical, rehabilitative, and environmental interventions.

7.16.5.1 Medical Prevention Strategies

Medical prevention strategies typically address risk factors through an initial risk factor assessment that might include mental status examination (to assess for delirium, dementia, depression), postural blood pressure measurement (to test for orthostatic hypotension), cardiac evaluation (to check for arrhythmias, valvular disorders), neurological evaluation, mobility assessment (e.g., ambulation, transfer from chair, bed or toilet), visual acuity testing, lower extremity muscle testing, balance testing (e.g., postural stress test), gait testing (e.g., Gait Abnormality Rating Scale), functional status evaluations, and a review of medications (Rubenstein & Josephson, 1993; Tideiksaar, 1993a). While many of these "conditions" cannot be prevented, many can be treated successfully, thereby reducing fall risk. In some cases the impact of these factors can be attenuated. For example, improved prescription practices (e.g., appropriate medication use, limiting number of medications, attention to drug interaction effects) can reduce fall rate. Several researchers have explored the effects of improving prescription practices. Goals included the reduction in amount of medication taken, reduction in the use of sedatives (particularly long-acting sedatives), and reduction in the use of tranquilizers. Rane-Szostak (cited in Gibson et al., 1987) attempted to reduce the number of falls in a large rehabilitation-oriented nursing home by asking physicians to reduce the use of sedatives (particularly long-acting sedatives) and tranquilizers. Nurses offered alternatives to medication for sleep, including changes in bedtime routines, using mild analgesics for pain, and providing evening snacks. A 70% reduction in the number of fall-related fractures has been attributed to the decreased use of sedatives and tranquilizers.

Once a fall has occurred, a detailed description of the circumstances surrounding the fall is recommended. The medically-oriented questions address such factors as loss of balance, dizziness, and other medically-related symptoms that have preceded the fall. The results of these inquiries can then be used in the development of prevention programs.

Tideiksaar (1993a) also suggested that these same questions following near-falls be explored. A near-fall involves a loss of balance without the occurrence of a fall due to gaining support from the environment (e.g., grabbing a hand rail). Near-falls are important to explore as they appear to portend future falls and may involve many of the same risk factors. Knowledge of these factors can be incorporated into prevention programs that could preclude or at least reduce the likelihood of future falls.

7.16.5.2 Rehabilitative Strategies

Fall risk can potentially be reduced through a variety of rehabilitative strategies. These might include muscle strengthening exercises, balance and gait training, and training in the proper use of ambulatory assistive devices. As previously noted, the relationship between lower extremity muscular strength and falls is quite strong. Weakened muscular strength can affect gait and balance, all of which can contribute to falling and fear of falling. Numerous studies have focused on increasing muscle strength with the goal of improving joint flexibility, gait, and balance (e.g., Fiatarone et al., 1994; Province et al., 1995). Such programs can include resistance exercises, weight-lifting, and leg stretching exercises. Flexibility and balance training, and even Tai Chi exercises, have shown positive results through improved gait and balance (e.g., Province et al.). Fiatarone et al. increased muscle strength by 113%, yielding a 12% increase in walking speed and a 28% increase in stair climbing ability through progressive resistance training among frail nursing home residents with a mean age of 87 years. Promising results have also been reported by Wolf, Kutner, Green, and McNeely (1993), who conducted a prospective, randomized controlled clinical trial comparing the effects of Tai Chi and computerized balance training with community-dwelling older adults. By 15 weeks, participants in the Tai Chi course reduced their fall rates by 47%, although the risk of falling was actually higher for those Tai Chi participants that experienced falls within the previous year. Fear of falling also decreased in the Tai Chi group.

7.16.5.3 Environmental Strategies

Environmental approaches to reduce fall risk attempt to do so by modifying the physical environment. Falls occur when there is a mismatch between an individual's performance level and the performance demands of environmental tasks (Hogue, 1992). Although physically fit individuals can lose their balance and fall, very frail individuals are probably the most dependent upon the environment to support the performance of tasks (Hogue, 1982, 1991; Waller, 1978). Frail individuals "may be unable to maintain postural control (prevent a fall) with virtually no external provocation" (Hogue, 1992, p. 45). The physical environment can often be modified to accommodate individuals whose abilities do not match the current environment. For example, higher seated chairs and toilets can replace lower seated ones to reduce the demands of transfer. Lighting can be intensified to reduce the risk of falls resulting from poorly illuminated areas, nonskid floor surfaces can replace slippery surfaces, stairways can be equipped with handrails for support, grab bars can be placed near toilets, bathtubs, and showers for support during transfers, and objects situated around the living environment that block or obstruct walk areas can be moved.

Tideiksaar (1997) noted that there is no definitive evidence of the efficacy of these environmental modifications in reducing falls. However, a few studies have offered promising results. Tideiksaar (1990), as reported in Tideiksaar (1997), eliminated various environmental hazards in the homes of older adults with multiple slip and trip falls. Slippery and irregular ground surfaces in the home were modified resulting in a decrease in number of falls over the following year.

Taking a more comprehensive approach, Wolf-Klein et al. (1988) provided medical management, home visits, and a falls prevention educational program for the participants in their study and their families, yielding a significant decrease in falls over the following year. Such comprehensive approaches have also been successful in institutional settings (e.g., Heslin et al., 1992; Hollinger & Patterson, 1992). Heslin et al. identified fall risk factors in acute, long-term, and residential health care settings and developed prevention strategies for each setting. Participants included 581 acute, 138 long-term care, and 247 residential care patients in a 966-bed teaching hospital. Fall rates at the beginning of the study were 2.16% for acute care, 1.46% for long-term care, and 9.38% for residential care. All but 17% of the fallers were 60 years of age or older. Prevention interventions targeted specific care settings and types of falls. Prevention in the acute care setting was directed at falls related to beds. The program included a fall risk assessment, nursing care plan, spot-the-dot (color-coded markers placed in risk areas), and bed sensors to alert staff to movement from beds. The number of bed-based falls decreased significantly (85%) over a three-month period using the sensor system. The spot-the-dot procedure was completely successful, with no bed-based falls following initial adjustments to the program on a medical unit. The long-term care interventions yielded similarly successful outcomes, with bed falls and transfers being targeted for interventions. When Huntington's Chorea patients who had experienced falls from bed had their restraints removed, their bed rails padded with cushions, and the bed surrounded with mattresses, injuries were reduced to zero. Bed to chair transfers, which account for approximately 50% of bed-based falls in the long-term care setting, were reduced by 92% through changes in transfer procedures and transfer devices.

Hollinger and Patterson (1992) developed and evaluated a falls precaution assessment and prevention program in an acute care setting. All participants were evaluated initially with a Fall Assessment Tool that addressed patient and environmental factors known to be risk factors for falling. Individualized prevention programs were then developed for individual patients based upon the findings with the Fall Assessment Tool. These programs included such precautions as use of assistive devices, night lights, and nonskid footwear. The fall rate over a six-month period was reduced significantly from a preintervention mean of 4.06 to a postintervention mean of 2.63.

7.16.5.4 Combined Prevention Strategies

Many of the reported prevention studies have employed a variety of intervention methods that involved medical, environmental, and rehabilitative approaches or some combination of two or more of these. For example, Tinetti et al. (1994) examined the effects of three different interventions with 301 men and women living in the community. All participants were at least 70 years of age and had at least one of the following risk factors: "postural hypotension; use of sedatives; use of at least four prescription medications; and impairment in arm or leg strength or range of motion, balance, ability to move safely from bed to chair or to the bathtub or toilet (transfer skills), or gait" (Tinetti et al., 1994, p. 821). The interventions were either usual health care or the combination of medication adjustment, behavioral change recommendations, and home-based exercise programs. Participants were followed for one year, during which 35% of the intervention group and 47% of the control group fell. The authors also demonstrated significant reduction in risk factors among the intervention group.

Although a broad range of prevention programs have been implemented, they have yielded mixed results. As Tinetti (1994) noted, the handful of clinical trials conducted prior to 1994 had somewhat discouraging results (see Hornbrook et al., 1994; Mulrow et al., 1994; Reinsch, MacRae, Lachenbruch, & Tobis, 1992; Rubenstein et al., 1990; Rubenstein, Robbins, & Josephson, 1991; Vetter, Lewis, & Ford, 1992). The recent "Frailty and Injuries:

Cooperative Studies of Intervention Techniques" (FICSIT) trials, however, offer more promising data from a large series of clinical trials (e.g., Tinetti, Baker et al., 1994; Wolf et al., 1993). Moreover, if empirical studies that do not meet the criteria for "prospective, controlled trials" are considered, the evidence in support of prevention programs is even more encouraging.

Perhaps what is most discouraging about the prevention literature is the failure to identify interventions that reliably reduce fall frequency or severity. Researchers may be at the point in prevention research that they must match interventions to the participants, with the hope of establishing which interventions are most effective with participants with particular characteristics and risk factors. Similarly, more effective prevention programs may be developed by considering such factors as whether the potential fallers are at little or great risk of falling, with different preventive approaches being most effective with one or the other of these two groups (Gibson et al., 1987). Perhaps attention should be focused on the prevention of particular types of falls. Tinetti (1994) has raised the provocative question of whether the goal of prevention programs should be the reduction in risk of all falls or the reduction in risk of injurious falls.

In conclusion, there is reason for optimism about the prevention of falls. Researchers have identified factors that place older adults at risk, have demonstrated that some of these factors can be changed through a variety of interventions, and have begun to demonstrate that some prevention programs can be effective with some individuals. The optimal approach for individuals with particular characteristics experiencing particular types of falls remains to be determined.

7.16.6 SUMMARY

This chapter has provided an overview of the empirical literature on falls among older adults. It began with considerations of conceptual and methodological issues, including how falls are conceptualized and measured. The many consequences of falls, including physical, medical, psychological, and economic consequences, were then discussed. Numerous intrinsic and extrinsic risk factors for falls were then considered, followed by a discussion of prevention approaches based upon these risk factors. Finally, the chapter concluded with a cautiously optimistic view of the prevention literature, suggesting that future preventive efforts focus on optimal matches of prevention programs to individual faller characteristics.

7.16.7 REFERENCES

Aisen, P. S., Deluca, T., & Lawlor, B. A. (1992). Falls among geropsychiatry inpatients are associated with PRN medications for agitation. *International Journal of Geriatric Psychiatry, 7,* 709–712.

Arfken, C. L., Lach, H. W., Birge, S. J., & Miller, J. P. (1994). The prevalence and correlates of fear of falling in elderly persons living in the community. *American Journal of Public Health, 84,* 565–570.

Asada, T., Kariva, T., Kitajima, E., Kakuma, T., & Yoshioka, M. (1994). Falls among community-dwelling psychogeriatric patients. *International Journal of Geriatric Psychiatry, 9,* 17–23.

Baker, S. P., & Harvey, A. H. (1985). Fall injuries in the elderly. *Clinics in Geriatric Medicine, 1,* 501–512.

Brocklehurst, J. C., Robertson, D., & James-Groom, P. (1982). Clinical correlates of sway in old age-sensory modalities. *Age and Aging, 11,* 1–10.

Brown, S. A., & Edelstein, B. A. (1995, November). *Factors associated with falls among psychogeriatric patients.* Paper presented at meeting of the Association for the Advancement of Behavior Therapy.

Campbell, A. J., Reinken, J., Allan, B. C., & Martinez, G. S. (1981). Falls in old age: A study of frequency and related clinical features. *Age and Ageing, 10,* 264–270.

Campbell, A. J., Borrie, M. J., & Spears, G. F. (1989). Risk factors for falls in a community-based prospective study of people 70 years and older. *Journal of Gerontology: Medical Sciences, 44,* M112–117.

Campbell, A. J., Borrie, M. J., Spears, G. F., Jackson, S. L., Brown, J. S., & Fitzgerald, J. L. (1990). Circumstances and consequences of falls experienced by a community population 70 years and over during a prospective study. *Age and Ageing, 19* (2), 136–141.

Commodore, D. I. B. (1995). Falls in the elderly population: A look at incidence, risks, healthcare costs, and preventive strategies. *Rehabilitation Nursing, 20,* 84–89.

Cooper, J. W. (1994). Falls and fractures in nursing home patients receiving psychotropic drugs. *International Journal of Geriatric Psychiatry, 9,* 975–980.

Cummings, S. R., Kelsey, J., Nevitt, M., & Dowd, K. (1985). Epidemiology of osteoporosis and osteoporotic fractures. *Epidemiologic Reviews, 7,* 178–208.

Cummings, S. R., Nevitt, M. C., & Kidd, S. (1988). Forgetting falls: The limited accuracy of recall of falls in the elderly. *Journal of the American Geriatrics Society, 36,* 613–616.

Cwikel, J., Kaplan, G., & Barell, V. (1990). Falls and subjective health rating among the elderly: Evidence from two Israeli samples. *Social Science and Medicine, 31,* 485–490.

Davie, J. W., Blumenthal, M. D., & Robinson-Hawkins, S. (1981). A model of risk of falling for psychogeriatric patients. *Archives of General Psychiatry, 38,* 463–467.

Downton, J. H., & Andrews, K. (1990). Postural disturbance and psychological symptoms amongst elderly people living at home. *International Journal of Geriatric Psychiatry, 5,* 93–98.

Duncan, P. W., & Studenski, S. (1994). Balance and gait measures. In M. P. Lawton & J. A. Teresi (Eds.), *Annual review of gerontology and geriatrics: Focus on assessment techniques, 14* (pp. 76–92). New York: Springer.

Ejaz, F. K., Jones, J. A., & Rose, M. S. (1994). Falls among nursing home residents: An examination of incident reports before and after restraint reduction programs. *Journal of the American Geriatrics Society, 42,* 960–964.

Evans, J. G., Prudham, D. A., & Wandless, I. (1979). A prospective study of fractured proximal femur: Incidence and outcome. *Public Health, 93,* 235–241.

Evans, L. K. & Strumpf, N. E. (1990). Myths about elder restraint. *Image: Journal of Nursing Scholarship, 22,* 124–128.

Felson, D. T., Anderson, J. J., Hannan, M. T. , Milton, R. C., Wilson, P. W. F., & Keil, D. P. (1989). Impaired vision and hip fracture: The Framingham study. *Journal of the American Geriatrics Society, 37,* 495–500.

Fiatarone, M. A., O'Neill, E. F., Ryan, N. D., Clements, K. M., Solares, G. R., Nelson, M. E., Roberts, S. B., Kehayias, J. J., Lipsitz, L. A., & Evans, W. J. (1994). Exercise training and nutritional supplementation for physical frailty in very elderly people. *New England Journal of Medicine, 330,* 1769–1775.

Funk, S. G., Tornquist, E. M., Champagne, M. T., & Wiese, R. A. (1992). *Key aspects of elder care: Managing falls, incontinence, and cognitive impairment.* New York: Springer.

Gibson, M. J., Andres, R. O., Isaacs, B., Radebaugh, T., & Worm-Peterson, J. (1987). The prevention of falls in later life. *Danish Medical Bulletin, 34* (Suppl. 4), 1–22.

Graafmans, W. C., Ooms. M. E., Hofstee, H. M. A., Bezemer, P. D., Bouter, L. M., & Lips, P. (1996). Falls in the elderly: A prospective study of risk factors and risk profiles. *American Journal of Epidemiology, 143,* 1129–1136.

Granek, E., Baker, S. P., Abbey, H., Robinson, E., Myers, A. H., Samkoff, J. S., & Klein, L. E. (1987). Medications and diagnoses in relation to falls in a long-term care facility. *Journal of the American Geriatrics Society, 35,* 503–511.

Greenhouse, A. H. (1994). Falls among the elderly. In M. L. Albert & J. E. Knoefel (Eds.). *Clinical neurology of aging* (2nd ed., pp. 611–626). New York: Oxford University Press.

Gross, Y. T., Shimamoto, Y., Rose, C. L. & Frank, B. (1990). Why do they fall?: Monitoring risk factors in nursing homes. *Journal of Gerontological Nursing, 16,* 20–25.

Gryfe, C. I., Amies, A., & Ashley, M. J. (1977). A longitudinal study of falls in an elderly population: I. Incidence and morbidity. *Age and Ageing, 6,* 201–210.

Guimaraes, R.M., & Isaacs, B. (1980). Characteristics of the gait in old people who fall. *International Rehabilitation Medicine, 2,* 177–180.

Hernandez, M., & Miller, J. (1986). How to reduce falls. *Geriatric Nursing, 7,* 97–102.

Heslin, K., Towers, J., Leckie, C., Thornton-Lawrence, H., Perkin, K., Jacques, M., Mullin, J., & Wick, L. (1992). Managing falls: Identifying population-specific risk factors and prevention strategies. In S. G. Funk, E. M. Tornquist, M. T. Champagne, & R. A. Wiese (Eds.), *Key aspects of elder care: Managing falls, incontinence, and cognitive impairment* (pp. 70–88). New York: Springer.

Hogue, C. C. (1982). Injury in late life. Part II: Prevention. *Journal of the American Geriatrics Society, 30,* 276–280.

Hogue, C. C. (1991). A person-environment model for understanding fall risk. In R. Weindruch & M. Ory (Eds.), *Frailty reconsidered: Reducing frailty and fall-related injuries in the elderly* (pp. 96–105). Springfield, IL: Charles C. Thomas.

Hogue, C. C. (1992). Managing falls: The current bases for practice. In S. G. Funk, E. M. Tornquist, M. T. Champagne, & R. A. Wiese (Eds.), *Key aspects of elder care: Managing falls, incontinence, and cognitive impairment* (pp. 41–57). New York: Springer.

Hollinger, L. M., & Patterson, P. A. (1992). A falls prevention program for the acute care setting. In S. G. Funk, E. M. Tornquist, M. T. Champagne, & R. A. Wiese (Eds.), *Key aspects of elder care: Managing falls, incontinence, and cognitive impairment* (pp. 110–117). New York: Springer.

Hornbrook, M. C., Stevens, V. J., Wingfield, D. J., Hollis, J. F., Greenlick, M. R., & Ory, M. G. (1994). Preventing falls among community-dwelling older persons: Results from a randomized trial. *The Gerontologist, 34,* 16–23.

Howland, J., Peterson, E. W., Levin, W. C., & Fried, L. (1993). Fear of falling among the community dwelling elderly. *Journal of Aging and Health, 5,* 229–243.

Kalchthaler, T., Bascon, R. A., & Quintos, V. (1978). Falls in the institutionalized elderly. *Journal of the American Geriatrics Society, 26,* 424–428.

Kanten, D.N., Mulrow, C. D., Gerety, M. B., Lichtenstein, M. J., Aguilar, C., & Cornell, J. E. (1993). Falls: An examination of three reporting methods in nursing homes. *Journal of the American Geriatrics Society, 41,* 662–666.

Kay, A. D., & Tideiksaar, R. (1990). Falls and gait disorders. In W. B. Abrams & R. Berkow (Eds.). *Merck manual of geriatrics* (pp. 52–68). Rahway, NJ: Merck Sharp & Dohme Research Laboratories.

Kreutzfeldt, J., Haim, M., & Bach, E. (1984). Hip fracture among the elderly in a mixed urban and rural population. *Age and Ageing, 13,* 111–119.

Lichtenstein, M. J., Burger, M. C., Shields, S. L., & Shiavi, R. G. (1990). Comparison of biomechanics platform measures of balance and videotaped measures of gait with a clinical mobility scale in elderly women. *Journal of Gerontology, 45,* M49–M54.

Lipsitz, L. A., Jonsson, P. V., Kelley, M. M., & Koestner, J. S. (1991). Causes and correlates of recurrent falls in ambulatory frail elderly. *Journal of Gerontology, 46,* M1114–M1122.

Lord, S. R. (1996). Instability and falls in elderly people. In C. Lafont, A. Baroni, M. Allard, R. Tideiksaar, B.J. Vellas, P. J. Garry, & J. L. Albarede (Eds.). *Falls, gait, and balance disorders in the elderly: From successfull aging to frailty.* New York: Springer.

Lord, S. R., Clark, R. D., & Webster, I. W. (1991). Physiological factors associated with falls in an elderly population. *Journal of the American Geriatrics Society, 39,* 1194–1200.

Lord, S. R., McLean, D., & Stathers, G. (1992). Physiological factors associated with injurious falls in older people living in the community. *Gerontology, 38,* 338–346.

Luukinen, H., Koski, K., Laippala, P., & Kivela, S. L. (1995). Risk factors recurrent falls in the elderly in long-term institutional care. *Public Health, 109,* 57–65.

Mahoney, J., Sager, M., Dunham, N. C., & Johnson, J. (1994). Risk of falls after hospital discharge. *Journal of the American Geriatrics Society, 42,* 269–274.

Marx, M. S., Cohen-Mansfield, J., & Werner, P. (1990). Agitation and falls in institutionalized elderly persons. *Journal of Applied Gerontology, 9,* 106–117.

Melton, L. J., & Riggs, B. L. (1985). Risk factors for injury after a fall. *Clinics in Geriatric Medicine, 1,* 525–539.

Mitchell, R. G. (1984). Falls in the elderly. *Nursing Times, January 11–17,* 51–53.

Morris, J. C., Rubin, E. H., Morris, E. J., & Mandel, S. A. (1987). Senile dementia of the Alzheimer's type: An important risk factor for serious falls. *Journal of Gerontology, 42,* 412–417.

Morse, J. M., Morse, R. M., & Tylko, S. J. (1989). Development of a scale to identify the fall-prone patient. *Canadian Journal on Aging, 8,* 366–377.

Morse, J. M., Tylko, S. J., & Dixon, H. A. (1987). Characteristics of the fall-prone patient. *Gerontologist, 27,* 516–522.

Mosenthal, A. C., Livingston, D. H., Elcavage, J., Merritt, S., & Stucker, S. (1995). Falls: Epidemiology and strategies for prevention. *Journal of Trauma: Injury, Infection, and Critical Care, 38,* 753–756.

Mulrow, C. D., Gerety, M. B., Kanten, D., Cornell, J. E., DeNino, L. A., Chiodo, L., Aguilar, C., O'Neil, M. B., Rosenberg, J., & Solis, R. M. (1994). A randomized trial of physical rehabilitation for very frail nursing home residents. *Journal of the American Medical Association, 271,* 519–524.

Murphy, J., & Isaacs, B. (1982). The post-fall syndrome: A

study of 36 elderly patients. *Gerontology, 28,* 265–270.

National Institutes of Health (1991). *Physical frailty: a reducible barrier to independence for older Americans* (NIH Publication No. 91–37). Washington, DC: National Institutes of Health.

Nevitt, M. C., Cummings, S. R., & Hudes, E. S. (1991).Risk factors for injurious falls: A prospective study. *Journal of Gerontology: Medical Sciences, 46,* M164–M170.

Nevitt, M. C., Cummings, S. R., Kidd, S., & Black, D. (1989). Risk factors for recurrent nonsyncopal falls: A prospective study. *Journal of the American Medical Association, 261,* 2663–2668.

Null-Kogan, J. (1996). *Self-reported fear in middle-aged and older adults and its relation to daily functioning and satisfaction with life.* Unpublished master's thesis, West Virginia University, Morgantown, WV.

Ousset, P.J., Hennia, A. O., Faisant, C., Sedeuilh, M., Reyes, G., Guiterez, L., Allard, M., Lafont, C., Vellas, B., & Albarede, J. L. (1996). A two years longitudinal study of falls, gait, and balance disorders in 267 healthy elderly persons living in the community: The ICARE study. In C. Lafont, A. Baroni, M. Allard, R. Tideiksaar, B. J. Vellas, P. J. Garry, & J. L. Albarede (Eds.), *Falls, gait and balance disorders in the elderly: From successful aging to frailty.* Paris: Serdi Publishing Company.

Overstall, P. W. (1992). Falls. *Reviews in Clinical Gerontology, 2,* 31–38.

Overstall, P. W., Exton-Smith, F. J., & Johnson, A. L. (1977). Falls in the elderly related to postural imbalance. *British Medical Journal, 1,* 261–264.

Pawlson, L. G., Goodwin, M., & Keith, K. (1986). Wheelchair use by ambulatory nursing home residents. *Journal of the American Geriatrics Society, 34,* 860–864.

Poster, E. C., Pelletier, L. R., & Kay, K. (1991). A retrospective cohort study of falls in a psychiatric inpatient setting. *Hospital and Community Psychiatry, 42,* 714–720.

Province, M. A., Hadley, E. C., Hornbrook, M. C., Lipsitz, L. A., Miller, J. P., Mulrow, C. D., Ory, M. G., Sattin, P. W., Tinetti, M. E., Wolf, S. L., & FICSIT Group (1995). The effects of exercise on falls in elderly patients: A preplanned meta-analysis of the FICSIT trials. *Journal of the American Medical Association, 273,* 1341–1347.

Prudham, D., & Evans, J. (1981). Factors associated with falls in the elderly: A community study. *Age and Ageing, 10,* 141–146.

Quail, G. G. (1994). An Approach to the assessment of falls in the elderly. *Australian Family Physician, 23,* 873–882.

Reinsch, S., MacRae, P., Lachenbruch, P. A., & Tobis, J. S. (1992). Attempts to prevent falls and injury: A prospective community study. *The Gerontologist, 32,* 450–456.

Robbins, A. S., Rubenstein, L. Z., Josephson, K. R., Schulman, B. L., Osterwell, D., & Fine, G. (1989a). Predictors of falls among elderly people: Results of two population-based studies. *Archives of Internal Medicine, 149,* 1628–1633.

Robbins, A. S., Rubenstein, L. Z., Josephson, K. R., Schulman, B. L., Osterwell, D., & Fine, G. (1989b). Predictors of falls among elderly people. *American Journal of Psychiatry, 143,* 1446–1449.

Rosen, A. M., Campbell, R. J., Villanueva, J., & Morgan, K. (1985). Factors affecting falling by older psychiatric inpatients. *Psychosomatics, 26,* 117–123.

Rubenstein, L. Z., & Josephson, K. R. (1993). Clinical research on falls in the nursing home. In L. Z. Rubenstein & D. Wieland (Eds.), *Improving care in the nursing home: Comprehensive reviews of clinical research* (pp. 216–240). Newbury Park,CA: Sage.

Rubenstein, L. Z., Josephson, K. R., & Robbins, A. S. (1994). Falls in the nursing home. *Annals of Internal Medicine, 121,* 442–451.

Rubenstein, L., Robbins, A. S., & Josephson, K. (1991). Falls in the nursing-home setting: Causes and preventive approaches. In P. R. Katz, R. L. Kane, & M. D. Mezey (Eds.), *Advances in long-term care* (Vol. 1, pp. 28–42.). New York: Springer.

Rubenstein, L. Z., Robbins, A. S., Josephson, K. R., Schulman, B. L., & Osterweil, D. (1990). The value of assessing falls in an elderly population. *Annals of Internal Medicine, 113,* 308–316.

Rubenstein, L. Z., Robbins, A. S., Schulman, B. L., Rosado, J., Osterweil, D., & Josephson, K. R. (1988). Falls and instability in the elderly. *Journal of the American Geriatrics Society, 36,* 266–278.

Saywell, R. M., Woods, J. R., Rappaport, S. A., & Allen, T. L. (1989). The value of age and severity as predictors of costs in geriatric head trauma patients. *Journal of the American Geriatrics Society, 37,* 625–630.

Simoneau, G. G., & Leibowitz, H. W. (1996). Posture, gait, and falls. In J. E. Birren, K. Warner Schaie, R. P. Abeles, M. Gatz, & T. A. Salthouse (Eds.), *Handbook of the psychology of aging* (4th ed. pp. 204–217). New York: Academic Press.

Simpson, J. M., & Mandelstam, H. (1995). Elderly people at risk of falling: Do they want to be taught how to get up again? *Clinical Rehabilitation, 9,* 65–69.

Soja, M. E., Kippenbrock, T. A., Hendrich, A. L., & Nyhuis, A. (1992). A risk model for patient fall prevention. In S. G. Funk, E. M. Tornquist, M. T. Champagne, & R. A. Wiese (Eds.), *Key aspects of elder care: Managing falls, incontinence, and cognitive impairment.* New York: Springer.

Speechley, M., & Tinetti, M. E. (1991). Falls and injuries in frail and vigorous community elderly persons. *Journal of the American Geriatrics Society, 39,* 46–52.

Studenski, S., Duncan, P. W., Chandler, J., Samsa, G., Prescott, B., Hogue, C., & Bearon, L. B. (1994). Predicting falls: The role of mobility and nonphysical factors. *Journal of the American Geriatrics Society, 42,* 297–302.

Sudarsky, L. (1990). Geriatrics: Gait disorders in the elderly. *New England Journal of Medicine, 322,* 1441–1446.

Tideiksaar, R. (1989). *Falling in old age: Its prevention and treatment.* New York: Springer.

Tideiksaar, R. (1990). The biomechanical and environmental characteristics of slips, stumbles, and falls. In B. E. Gray (Ed.), *Slips, stumbles, and falls: Pedestrian footwear and surfaces* (pp. 17–27). Philadelphia: American Society for Testing and Materials.

Tideiksaar, R. (1993a). Falls in older persons. *The Mount Sinai Journal of Medicine, 60,* 515–521.

Tideiksaar, R. (1993b). Mechanisms of falls in community residing older persons. *Pride Institute Journal of Long Term Home Health Care, 12,* 3–11.

Tideiksaar, R. (1993c). *Falls in older persons: Prevention and management in hospitals and nursing homes.* Boulder, CO: Tactilitics, Inc.

Tideiksaar, R. (1997). *Falling in old age: Prevention and management* (2nd ed.). New York: Springer.

Tideiksaar, R., & Kay, A. (1986). What causes falls? A logical diagnostic procedure. *Geriatrics, 41,* 32–50.

Tinetti, M. E. (1987). Factors associated with serious injury during falls by ambulatory nursing home residents. *Journal of the American Geriatrics Society, 35,* 644–648.

Tinetti, M. E. (1994). Prevention of falls and fall injuries in elderly persons: A research agenda. *Preventive Medicine, 23,* 756–762.

Tinetti, M. E., Baker, D. I., McAvay, G., Claus, E. B., Garrett, P., Gottschalk, M., Koch, M. L., Trainor, K., & Horwitz, R. I. (1994). A multifactorial intervention to reduce the risk of falling among elderly people living in the community. *New England Journal of Medicine, 331*, 821–827.

Tinetti, M. E., Liu, W. L., & Claus, E. B. (1993). Predictors and prognosis of inability to get up after falls among elderly persons. *Journal of the American Medical Association, 269*, 65–70.

Tinetti, M. E., Mendes de Leon, C. F., Doucette, J. T., & Baker, D. I. (1994). Fear of falling and fall-related efficacy in relationship to functioning among community-living elders. *Journal of Gerontology: Medical Sciences. 49*, M140–M147.

Tinetti, M. E., Richman, D., & Powell, L. (1990). Falls efficacy as a measure of fear of falling. *Journal of Gerontology: Psychological Sciences, 45*(6), P239–P243.

Tinetti, M. E., & Speechley, M. (1989). Current concepts in geriatrics: Prevention of falls among the elderly. *New England Journal of Medicine, 320*, 1055–1059.

Tinetti, M. E., Speechley, M., & Ginter, S. F. (1988). Risk factors for falls among elderly persons living in the community. *The New England Journal of Medicine, 319*, 1701–1707.

Tinetti, M. E., Williams, T. F., & Mayewski, R. (1986). Fall risk index for elderly patients based on number of chronic disabilities. *American Journal of Medicine, 80*, 429–434.

Urton, M. M. (1991). A community home inspection approach to preventing falls among the elderly. *Public Health Reports, 106*, 192–195.

Van Dijk, P. T., Meulenberg, O. G., Van de Sande, H. J., & Habbema, J. D. (1993). Falls in dementia patients. *Gerontologist, 33*, 200–204.

Vetter, N. J., Lewis, P. A., & Ford, D. (1992). Can health visitors prevent fractures in elderly people? *British Medical Journal, 304*, 888–890.

Walker, J. E., & Howland, J. (1991). Falls and fear of falling among elderly persons living in the community: Occupational therapy interventions. *American Journal of Occupational Therapy, 45*, 119–122.

Waller, J. A. (1978). Falls among the elderly: Human and environmental factors. *Accident Analysis and Prevention, 10*, 21–23.

Whipple, R. H., Wolfson, L. I., & Amerman, P. M. (1987). The relationship of knee and ankle weakness to falls in nursing home residents: An isokinetic study. *Journal of the American Geriatrics Society, 35*, 13–20.

Whipple, R., Wolfson, L., Derby, C., Singh, D., & Tobin, J. (1993). Altered sensory functions and balance in older persons. *The Journals of Gerontology, 48* (Special Issue), 71–76.

Whitbourne, S. K. (in press). Physiological aspects of aging: Relation to identity and clinical implications. In B. Edelstein (Ed.), *Clinical geropsychology*. Oxford: Elsevier.

Wild, D., Nayak, U. S., & Isaacs, B. (1981). Prognosis of falls in old people at home. *Journal of Epidemiology and Community Health, 35*, 200–204.

Wofford, J. L., Heuser, M. D., Moran, W. P., Schwartz, E., & Mittelmark, M. B. (1994). Community surveillance of falls among the elderly using computerized EMS transport data. *American Journal of Emergency Medicine, 12*, 433–437.

Wolf, S. L., Barnhart, H. X., Kutner, N. G., McNeely, E., Coogler, C., & Xu, T. (1996). Reducing frailty and falls in older persons: An investigation of Tai Chi and computerized balance training. *Journal of the American Geriatrics Society, 44*, 489–497.

Wolf, S. L., Kutner, N. C., Green, R. C., & McNeely, E. (1993). The Atlanta FICSIT Study: Two exercise interventions to reduce frailty in elders. *Journal of the American Geriatrics Society, 41*, 329–332.

Wolf-Klein, G. P., Silverstone, F. A., Basavaraju, N., Foley, C. T., Pascaru, A., & Ma, P. H. (1988). Prevention of falls in the elderly population. *Archives of Physical Medicine and Rehabilitation, 69*, 689–691.

Wolfson, L., Judge, J., Whipple, R., & King, M. (1995). Strength is a major factor in balance, gait and the occurrence of falls. *The Journals of Gerontology, 50a* (Special Issue), 64–67.

Wolfson, L. I., Whipple, R., Amerman, P., & Kleinberg, A. (1986). Stressing the postural response: A quantitative method for testing balance. *Journal of the American Geriatrics Society, 34*, 845–850.

Wolfson, L. I., Whipple, R., Amerman, P., & Tobin, J. N. (1990).Gait assessment in the elderly: A gait abnormality rating scale and its relation to falls. *Journal of Gerontology, 45*, M12–M19.

Wolinsky, F. D., Johnson, R. J., & Fitzgerald, J. F. (1992). Falling, health status, and the use of health services by older adults: A prospective study. *Medical Care, 30*, 587–597.

Wright, B. A., Aizenstein, S., Vogler, G., Rowe, M., & Miller, C. (1990). Frequent fallers: Leading groups to identify psychological factors. *Journals of Gerontological Nursing, 16*, 15–19.

Yasumura, S., Arai, H., Haga, H., Niino, N., Nagai, H., Suzuki, T., Amano, H., & Shibata, H. (1996). Risk factors for falls among elderly people living in an urban community in Japan: A longitudinal study. In C. Lafont, A. Baroni, M. Allard, R. Tideiksaar, B. J. Vellas, P. J. Garry, & J. L. Albarede (Eds.), *Falls, gait and balance disorders in the elderly*. Paris: Serdi Publishing Company.

7.17
Wandering

DONNA L. ALGASE
University of Michigan, Ann Arbor, MI, USA

7.17.1 WANDERING: A MODEL CASE

Mrs. G. walks intently toward the dining hall of the nursing home, a purse draped over her arm and golf hat sitting slightly askew atop her graying hair. When asked of her destination, she talks pleasantly in partial sentences of a luncheon date at the club. Mrs. G. enters the dining area and paces back and forth in front of a windowed wall overlooking a grassy courtyard. Appearing upset at times, she repeatedly attempts to slide the glass panels open. Passersby can hear her express determination to meet her husband, now long deceased, and observe her distress about his "overdue" arrival.

Most clinicians providing long-term care to cognitively-impaired persons encounter behavior such as this and call it wandering. Compared to its frequency in the clinical setting, the number of articles and studies of this behavior is small. Wandering has generally been viewed as an accompaniment to dementia or, worse, is seen as a nuisance. Perhaps its very commonness has worked against serious investigation of the phenomenon until the past decade.

This chapter presents a comprehensive review of the research and clinical literature on wandering. Sections addressing definitions and typologies, epidemiological data, putative risk factors and outcomes, etiologic factors and theories, assessment, and intervention are offered. Throughout each section, findings are summarized, gaps identified, suggestions for further research offered, and implications for clinical practice identified.

7.17.2 DEFINITIONS AND TYPOLOGIES OF WANDERING

Despite increasing interest in this perplexing behavior, the term "wandering" lacks a consistent meaning. Multiple definitions have been proposed from the clinical, conceptual, and empirical viewpoints of several disciplines, most notably psychology, nursing, and social work. Some definitions aim for objectivity while others impute a basis or cause for the behavior. Similarly, some attempt to circumscribe or limit the meaning to a narrow range of behavior while others use it loosely to include behaviors that accompany wandering, such as requests to leave, or are consequences of it, such as eloping or absconding from an expected or authorized area. The only universals in various characterizations of wandering discussed in this chapter are the presence of cognitive impairment and movement through large-scale space.

The term "wanderer" has also been applied to sleepwalkers (nocturnal wanderers) (Guilleminault, Kushida, & Leger, 1995; Guilleminault, Moscovitch, & Leger, 1995; Kushida, Clerk, Kirsch, Hotsin, & Guilleminault, 1995; Plazzi, Tinuper, Montague, Provini, & Lugaresi, 1995), vagrants (Weller & Jauhar, 1987), and patients who switch repeatedly from one physician to another (Pankratz & Jackson, 1994). These meanings of wandering are excluded from this review.

7.17.2.1 Clinical Views

Wandering poses a quandary for clinicians, inducing a conflict between the goals of affording both maximum freedom and safety for the afflicted. Consequently, clinicians usually advocate for a humane and tolerant approach to the behavior within a protected area. However, their definitions of wandering are among the most broad and imprecise and, thus, may inadvertently result in restriction of those whose ambulation poses no threat of harm. Coons (1988) defined wandering simply as self-initiated ambulation occurring independently of environmental cues to move, such as a ringing dinner bell or an invitation to an activity by a caretaker. While objective in that it is observable and infers no specific cause, Coons' definition is not particularly useful since virtually all spontaneous ambulation of cognitively-impaired individuals is included. In an early effort to clarify the behavior, Rader, Doan, and Schwab (1985) identified wandering as one end of a continuum of behaviors reflecting some effort to fulfill a social, emotional, or physical agenda or need that may or may not be rooted in current reality. While useful for pointing to possible constructive avenues for intervention, this definition fails to differentiate harmless from worrisome wandering and, thus, offers no clear guide for when to intervene.

7.17.2.2 Conceptual Schemes and Typologies

In efforts to more clearly delineate the behavior and explicate possible explanations for it, a number of others have taken more analytical approaches to defining wandering and classifying possible subtypes. Although data are offered in support of some of these typologies, most are more anecdotally than empirically derived.

Snyder, Rupprecht, Pyrek, Brekhus, and Moss (1978) defined wandering "as a tendency to move about, either in a seemingly aimless or disoriented fashion, or in pursuit of an indefinable or unobtainable goal" (p. 272). They also proposed the earliest typology of wandering based on chart reviews of eight nurse-identified wanderers. Three types were reported: (i) overtly goal-directed/searching behavior, associated with calling out repeatedly or approaching others in pursuit of a goal; (ii) overtly goal-directed/industrious behavior, typified by keeping busy with work-like actions, such as dusting; and (iii) apparently nongoal-directed behavior, described as ambulation that is aimless or shifts direction abruptly in response to changing environmental stimuli.

"Getting lost" or the inability to return to one's point of origin has also been suggested as a definition for wandering (Hussian, 1981, 1982). Greene, Smith, Gardiner, and Timbury (1982), who also equated wandering with getting lost, expanded this view by differentiating wandering types according to time of day (day or night) and location (outside vs. inside the home). However, wandering also entails a change in activity level that does not necessarily correlate with getting lost (Fairburn & Hope, 1988).

Based on observations of 13 residents in the geriatric unit of a state mental institution, Hussian and Davis (1985) proposed four independent types of wanderers: (i) akathesiacs, associated with extended hospitalization and long-term neuroleptic use and characterized by episodes of higher frequency and duration and lower attempts to leave or self-stimulate; (ii) exit seekers, associated with recent admission and characterized by frequent requests to leave, a high number and proportion of attempts to open exit (rather than other internal) doors, and a varied frequency and duration of ambulation episodes; (iii) modelers, who join with another ambulating resident and display little contact with door knobs, a low degree of self-stimulating behavior, and varying frequency and duration of episodes; and (iv) self-stimulators, who show other perseverative and stereotypical behaviors and no clear preference for exit doors. Analysis to support these categories was lacking.

More recently, a classification was proposed to differentiate dangerous from harmless wandering and to better target intervention strategies (Butler & Barnett, 1991). Based on the person's whereabouts and the patient's and nurse's knowledge of the same, four classes were delineated: purposeful (person and nurse know), escapist (person knows, nurse doesn't), aimless (nurse knows, person doesn't), and critical (neither know). While aimless wandering may be most stressful to caregivers, escapist and critical types are most dangerous due to associated elopements and injuries.

A time-in-motion approach was suggested to delineate wandering categories (Thomas, 1995). Continuous wanderers were said to be "moving constantly." Characteristics offered to describe this category included a higher level of cognitive impairment and inefficient travel behavior, a dissociation from feelings of fatigue or lack of awareness of the need to rest, and minimal social activity. On the other hand, sporadic wanderers move about occasionally. In addition to higher levels of cognitive function than continuous wanderers, sporadic wanderers were described as having greater ability to communicate verbally. While this classification scheme does reflect some clinically observed variations among wanderers also reported by others, Thomas used the cut-off point of 50% of time-in-motion to distinguish the category types without affording a rationale for this criterion.

One typology of wandering is clearly derived from an empirical base, where the travel patterns of wanderers ($n = 24$) and nonwanderers in a sample of 40 nursing home residents were evaluated (Martino-Saltzman, Blasch, Morris, & McNeal, 1991). Subjects' ambulation episodes occurring over a four-week period in pre-set locations were captured on videotape; 5768 events initiated without assistance of staff, visitors, or other residents were recorded. Each was described and then categorized by coders and the first author. Four patterns evolved: direct, travel between two points without diversion; pacing, repetitive back and forth travel within a limited area; lapping, repetitive travel encircling large areas; and random, haphazard travel between several locations without repetition. Coders achieved an acceptable inter-rater reliability (kappa = 0.79, $z = 13.2$, $p < 0.0001$) in a subsample of 231 events.

7.17.2.3 Empirically-based Descriptions and Features

Serious effort to evolve empirical descriptions and characterizations of wandering is limited to only a few recent studies. Two independent lines of research, differentiated by target population and methodology, are emerging. Although each approach has its limitations, these investigations are beginning to clarify what constitutes wandering behavior and to elucidate differences among wandering types.

Investigators in the UK are using community-based samples to uncover the inherent structure of wandering. Using a portion of the Present Behavioural Examination (Hope & Fairburn, 1992), a semistructured guide, they interviewed 29 caregivers of wanderers who were referred from the caseload of three community psychiatric nurses. The proportion of subjects showing each of the nine discrete behaviors at anytime since the onset of dementia was determined along with their gender, duration of dementia, and score on the Mini-Mental Status Examination (MMSE) (Folstein, Folstein, & McHugh, 1975). The following frequencies were reported: increased walking activity (17), wandering away from home (16), aimless walking (15), walking for an inappropriate purpose (14), checking/trailing (11), attempting to leave home (10), overactivity at night (9), pottering (6), and walking with appropriate purpose but an inappropriate frequency (4). No association with concomitant physical illness, medications, or premorbid activity levels was found. From these behaviors, a typology of wandering that could point to potential underlying etiologies was posed. These were: (i) increased overall walking activity, (ii) avoidance of being alone, (iii) diurnal rhythm disturbance, (iv) navigational problem, and (v) faulty goal-directed behavior (Hope & Fairburn, 1990). Although each subject exhibited more than one behavior, the time order of behaviors or any concurrent expression of them were not discussed. In a secondary analysis of the same data using Guttman scaling, Albert (1992) demonstrated that these nine behaviors were not a typology, but reflected a unidimensional hierarchical structure. Although the coefficient of reproducibility (0.78) fell slightly short of the 0.90 suggested by Guttman (1974), Albert argues that it is notable given the small sample size.

To challenge Albert's conclusion, Hope et al. (1994) conducted a factor analysis upon data from 83 subjects who were rated for 11 behaviors, that is, those listed earlier with the separation of checking/trailing and the addition of reduced walking. Only nine behaviors were used in analyses as wandering away from home and attempting to leave home did not correlate well with other behaviors. A four-factor solution explained 54.5% of the variance. Checking and trailing composed Factor 1, more and aimless walking constituted Factor 2, pottering stood alone as Factor 3, and inappropriate and overappropriate walking constituted Factor 4. Less walking and night-time walking did not load on any factor. In a scaling analysis of this data, neither the coefficients of reproducibility nor scalability were sufficient to support the conclusion of a hierarchical structure.

Investigators in the USA are using nursing home samples to describe various patterns of wandering in rhythmic terms (Algase, Beattie, Kupferschmid, & Beel-Bates, 1997; Algase, Beattie, Kupferschmid, & Therrien, 1997; Algase & Cheng, 1992a; Algase & Tsai, 1991). In their first study, a descriptive survey design and cluster sampling were used to screen 31 wanderers from a larger sample of 198 ambulatory, cognitively-impaired persons from eight randomly selected nursing homes. Wandering was viewed as a nonlinear, ultradian, biphasic rhythm with locomoting and nonlocomoting phases. It was operationalized by counting and timing cycles and their locomoting phases; each cycle was coded for impetus (self- or other-directed), location, and activity at onset and cessation of the locomoting phase using stop-watches and paper–pencil coding techniques. Without a typology for differentiating wandering from other ambulating, self-initiated cycles with locomoting phases ending in activity other than self-care (e.g., toileting, eating) were considered wandering. In accord with then current views of wandering as being aimless activity, "purposeful" ambulation, such as going to the toilet, was not counted as wandering. Wanderers were observed 1:1 for two 24-hour periods one week apart by coders trained on videotapes to time cycles to within 10 seconds of each other (Algase & Cheng, 1992a; Algase & Tsai, 1991).

Subjects averaged 79.24 wandering cycles (range = 19.5–162; SD = 39.33) and 110.07 minutes of locomotion (range = 69.04–257.02; SD = 61.32) daily. A distinct 24-hour pattern for hourly cycle frequency and hourly sum of locomoting phase durations was also identified (Algase, 1992a; Algase & Cheng, 1992a; Algase & Tsai, 1991), with the period from 1400 to 1600 representing the period of greatest wandering by both parameters for the sample as a whole. Night-time wandering was minimal, averaging less than one cycle per hour per subject.

Repeated measures ANOVA demonstrated that cycle frequency, locomoting and nonlocomoting phase durations, and percent of cycle locomoting were stable over a one-week period with no day effect or day by hour interaction effects. However, there was a significant hour effect on all cycle variables (Algase & Cheng, 1992a; Algase & Struble, 1992; Algase & Tsai, 1991). Further analysis also demonstrated that, of four start and stop types, solitary/unfocused starts (52%) and stops (45%) were most common, while social/unfocused starts (5%) and stops (5%) were least likely. Though relatively rare, cycles with social/unfocused starts had longer locomoting phases ($F = 3.76$; $p = 0.01$) and a higher percent of cycle locomoting ($F = 3.25$; $p = 0.02$). Variability in cycle period and nonlocomoting phases by start type and in all cycle variables by stop type were not significant (Algase & Cheng, 1992b). Though measures for wandering were cutting edge at that time, distinctions between wandering and nonwandering were crude and no classification to distinguish among any subtypes was used.

In a subsequent study, Algase, Beattie, Kupferschmid, and Beel-Bates (1997) estimated daily distribution, stability of direct and wandering ambulation cycles, and whether wandering occurring in a two-hour epoch is representative of that occurring in a 24-hour day. A correlational design incorporating direct observation and repeated measures over selected time periods was employed. Twenty-five ambulatory, cognitively-impaired residents from two long-term care settings served as the nonprobability sample.

Measurement of wandering was refined using Martino-Saltzman et al.'s (1991) typology to code the locomoting phase of each independent ambulation cycle. Accordingly, "inefficient" patterns (random, lapping, and pacing) were considered wandering, while "efficient" travel episodes (direct pattern) were not. Further, stopwatch methods were replaced with a portable terminal programmed to time entries, prompt coders, and store and transmit data for analysis. One subject per day was observed 1:1 over an initial 24-hour period beginning at 0700. On the third day following observation the subject was observed again for two two-hour periods: one standard (1400–1600) for all subjects, based on outcome of the study presented above, and a second unique period based on each subject's own 24-hour distributions of hourly ambulation cycle frequency and locomoting phase sums.

Distinct from previous studies, where researchers had classified subjects as wanderers or nonwanderers, this study revealed that all cognitively-impaired ambulatory subjects displayed wandering behavior as operationalized in this study. Although three subjects did not wander at all during the 24-hour period, they did wander during subsequent observation periods. All subjects, regardless of level of cognitive impairment, also displayed direct (nonwandering) ambulation. Descriptive statistics for wandering and direct cycle parameters are summarized in Table 1. Random was the dominant wandering pattern across all subjects, accounting for 77.2% of all wandering cycles, with lapping and pacing constituting 13.2% and 9.6%, respectively. Examination of the hourly frequency distributions of all ambulating revealed that the two-hour period of highest activity, 1700–1900 hours, was also the two-hour period in which the total wandering cycle frequency was greatest at 62 cycles per hour for the group as a whole.

To examine stability of wandering over a three-day period, wandering and direct cycle variables were compared at standard and individual periods. Wandering cycle frequency and locomoting phase sums were moderately and similarly correlated at both individual and standard periods; no direct cycle variable had a significant correlation at either period. For the standard period, all variables were stable for wandering and direct cycles. However, in the individual period, only the locomoting phase sum for wandering cycles was stable and there were more significant differences and, thus, less stability, among direct cycle variables.

The universal expression of wandering among all cognitively-impaired, ambulatory subjects has only been demonstrated in this one sample. Although subjects were drawn from two settings, the sample was small and nonrandom. Thus, further research is needed to validate and generalize this finding. However, it suggests that wandering may be a marker for disease progression or staging and could possibly serve as a measure for the efficacy of dementia treatment strategies in the future.

Table 1 Descriptive statistics for wandering and direct cycle variables over 24 hours ($N = 25$).

	Cycle frequency			*Sum locomoting phase*			*Mean % cycle locomoting*		
	Mean	*Range*	*SD*	*Mean*	*Range*	*SD*	*Mean*	*Range*	*SD*
Wandering	19.7	120	27.3	42.9	199.1	53.2	36.1	88	22.8
Random	15.2	104	23.2	34.6	173.1	46.4	40.1	88	26.2
Lapping	2.6	18	4.3	5.2	37.4	9.1	19.3	81.7	25.7
Pacing	1.9	9	2.6	3.1	26.6	5.8	20.8	85.5	27.7
Direct	22.0	64	13.2	29.0	92.3	18.8	28.9	34.9	10.2

7.17.3 EPIDEMIOLOGICAL DATA

7.17.3.1 Prevalence

Several estimates of wandering prevalence have been published, but all are flawed by unclear and inconsistent criteria for wandering and by mostly nonrandom, small, and incomparable samples. The basis for dementia may also vary by sample, a few being limited solely to subjects meeting diagnostic criteria for Alzheimer's disease (AD). Estimates are also likely influenced by other unknown or uncontrolled factors such as physical restraints and medications.

Among institutionalized demented elderly, estimates of the number of wanderers range from 6 to 24% (Dawson & Reid, 1987; Hiatt, 1980; National Center for Health Statistics, 1979; Wilkinson & Graham-White, 1980). In a random sample of eight nursing homes (Algase, 1988), wherein 747 residents (84% of those eligible) consented to cognitive screening, 5% were classified as wanderers by the nursing staff. As a percentage of those with cognitive impairments, the estimate doubled to 10%. Further, as a proportion of residents who were both cognitively impaired and ambulatory, the ratio was 1:4. Although not intended as an estimate of prevalence *per se,* Algase, Beattie, Kupferschmid, and Beel-Bates (1997) later found that in two long-term care settings, all ambulatory, cognitively-impaired residents, who had not necessarily been labeled as wanderers, displayed the behavior when directly observed over an extended time period. They concluded that if a person's overall ambulation activity was low or the proportion of their ambulation that was wandering was small, nurses tended to *underidentify* the phenomenon. However, in comparing nurses' ratings to observation, nurses have also *overestimated* the behavior (Milke, 1989). Conflicting conclusions may be due to different operational definitions for wandering in these studies.

In community samples of demented elderly, usually based on caregiver informants, estimates of wandering range between 19 and 56% (Burns, Jacoby, & Levy, 1990; Rabins, Mace, & Lucas, 1982; Teri, Larson, & Reifler, 1988). Among 92 consecutive patients with suspected dementia who received a home visit, approximately 37% were reported to get lost when outside the home and 28% when inside the home. These were most often persons with AD, as compared to vascular dementia, and level of cognitive impairment did not affect prevalence (Ballard, Mohan, Bannister, Handy, & Patel, 1991). In a survey of county sheriff's departments, sheriffs were called to locate one missing wanderer per year for every 1000 persons over the age of 65 years (Butler, 1990). Of these, five deaths occurred in 450 incidents. The cost to search for a missing wanderer was US$1200 per incident in law officer time alone. These estimates are conservative, as local police and volunteer fire departments are often the first line of assistance in such searches and therefore a number of events were likely excluded from this survey.

7.17.3.2 Incidence

No estimates for the incidence of wandering, either for the dementias in general or for any single type of dementia, were located. However, in staging dementia, "getting lost" is a criterion for stages 3 and 4 of the Global Cognitive Deterioration Scale (Reisberg, Ferris, deLeon, & Crook, 1982). By these instruments, at least one definition of wandering is accepted as an inevitable part of dementia, to be expected in every instance of the disease. However, the empirical basis for viewing this behavior as representative of a stage of dementia within these systems is unspecified.

7.17.4 PUTATIVE RISK FACTORS FOR WANDERING

7.17.4.1 Personal Factors

Currently, among those with cognitive impairments, knowledge is insufficient to predict who might wander or to specify the nature of the wandering behavior that one is likely to display. Although newer work has cast doubt on whether wandering is confined to a subgroup of cognitively-impaired ambulatory persons (Algase, Beattie, Kupferschmid, & Beel-Bates, 1997), older studies which compare wanderers and other nursing home residents may begin to illuminate the profile of a "problematic" wanderer. Since most of these older studies used nurses' or caregivers' judgments to identify wanderers, they likely represent comparisons between those with the most obvious display of the behavior and those with a low level or more subtle form of wandering. Variables most often reported include demographics, cognitive deficits, mobility, and psychosocial characteristics. Data from 12 samples are summarized in Table 2.

Most of these samples were not randomly chosen and, when comparisons were made with nonwandering controls, controls were generally also cognitively impaired. Wandering was noted in a wide age range of demented persons who were not consistently older or younger than controls. As might be expected, except for the two studies conducted on subjects from the Veterans' Administration, samples were largely female, representing a ratio of approximately 3:1. This gender ratio was maintained among wanderers. Samples were primarily ambulatory, with a few subjects in wheelchairs. When mobility was a variable of interest, wanderers with freedom to walk had better overall mobility than controls. Although wanderers were found among persons with all levels of cognitive impairment, as a group, their performance on global measures of impairment were generally worse than controls. On discrete cognitive tasks, poorer performance was found in memory and recall, abstraction, orientation, and visuospatial skills. Wanderers also had poorer language skills and were less able to communicate even though their personalities were generally more agreeable and extroverted. While none of these studies were strictly aimed at identifying risk factors, their overall results reveal that advanced cognitive impairment, good mobility, and impaired ability to communicate, particularly among individuals with a history of sociability, may portend a tendency to wander.

While the question of whether medical diagnosis, as a basis for dementia, might help to identify wanderers is an interesting one, few studies cast light on this possibility. Several studies do report various types of dementia among wanderers with a range of pathologies including AD, multi-infarct dementia (MID), and mixed dementia (Algase, 1992a; Hope et al., 1994; Thomas, 1997). However, due largely to small sample sizes and the limited nature of medical documentation in long-term care settings (from which most subjects are drawn), little analysis of the relationship between medical diagnosis and wandering has been done. In a random sample of 163 cognitively-impaired nursing home residents, 10% of one sample ($n = 163$) had only an irreversible basis for their dementia, 31% had only a reversible basis, and 59% had a mixed basis (both reversible and irreversible etiologies) noted in their medical records (Algase, 1992a). Wanderers tended to have their dementia due to mixed or irreversible causes. In a sample of 68 nursing home residents, drawn from a 911-bed nursing facility, wanderers ($n = 31$) tended to have a diagnosis of AD while nonwanderers were more likely to have a vascular dementia (Thomas, 1997). However, studies to examine the relative frequency, overall output, and type of wandering associated with various medical bases of dementia have yet to be conducted.

7.17.4.2 Potential Environmental Contributors

Although behavior in general (Lewin, 1935; Murray, 1938), among the aged (Whedon & Shedd, 1989), and within wanderers (Algase, 1992b; Algase & Struble, 1992; Hussian, 1981), is understood to arise as a function of person–environment interaction, few studies have yet explicated physical or social factors in the environment that may precipitate or otherwise influence wandering.

In a case study, observation of the intrusions of one wanderer into the rooms of other residents revealed a consistent pattern: attraction to a limited number of rooms which shared a common view of the outdoors and dalliance at a particular dresser with a mirror (Donat, 1984). By reassigning the wanderer to the room most frequently entered and containing the dresser, intrusions into other rooms decreased from an average of 16 per hour to less than two. While manipulating the environment had an effective outcome for those intruded upon, it made no real change in, but rather accommodated to, the subject's behavior. Thus, both the theoretical and practical value of this study is limited as no attempt to analyze attracting environmental features from a conceptual standpoint was made.

In analyses of the nursing home environment for its impact on agitated behaviors, observations of pacing (including "aimless" wandering) under naturally occurring conditions were also reported (Cohen-Mansfield & Werner, 1985; Cohen-Mansfield, Werner, & Marx, 1989;

Table 2 Characteristics of 12 samples of wanderers.

Author	*N*	*Control group*	*%wan.*	*Age*	*%fe*	*Cognitive status of wanderers*	*Mobilty status of wanderers*	*Communication/sociability of wanderers*
Algase (1992)	163	CI NHR[a]	20.0	mean = 83.7	77.0	more global impairment; $p<0.001$ poorer abstract thinking; $p<0.01$ poorer judgment, $p<0.001$ poorer spatial skills; $p<0.001$	ambulatory	poorer language skills, $p<0.001$
Cornbleth (1977)	48	CI NHR	62.5	68.7	0.0[b]	global impairment, ns	better if free to walk; $p<0.05$	worse social skills; $p<0.05$
deLeon et al. (1984)	16	CI NHR	31.3	72–90	nr	global impairment, ns poor parietal signs, $p<0.001$	nr	nr
Henderson et al. (1989)	28	AD	39.0	54–89; ns	ns	worse recall; $p<0.002$ poor visuoconstruction; $p<0.05$	ambulatory	nr
Hope and Fairburn (1990)	29	CI	100.0	55–92	69.0	MMSE 0–21	59% excessive	21% avoided being alone
Jackson et al. (1989)	8983	G NHR[b]	6.0	older; $p<0.01$	ns	more global impairment; $p<0.01$	better, $p<0.001$	poor communic, $p<0.0001$
Martino-Saltzman et al. (1991)	40	CI NHR	60.0	56–104	63.0	more impairment correlated with poorer travel efficiency		
Mayer and Darby (1990)	9	na	100.0	mean = 77.8	nr	100% severely impaired	walk or wc	nr
Monsour and Robb (1982)	44	CI NHR	50.0[c]	53–89	0.0[b]	55% severely impaired	walk or wc	nr
Ryan et al. (1995)	18	CI	33.3	70–92; ns	72.2; ns	more perseveration; $p<0.05$ attention, concentration; ns	ambulatory	nr
Snyder et al. (1978)	8	CI NHR	50.0[c]	ns	ns	worse memory, $p=0.001$ worse orientation, $p<0.001$	nr	alone more, $p<0.002$ poor conversing, $p<0.005$
Thomas (1997)	40	CI NHR	50.0[c]	younger $p<0.01$	ns	global, ns primarily AD; $p<0.05$	ambulatory	more extroverted; $p<0.01$ more agreeable; $p<0.01$

[a] Cognitively impaired nusing home residents. [b] General nursing home residents. [c] Matched sample. [d] VA setting.
ns = not significantly different from controls.
nr = not reported.

Cohen-Mansfield, Werner, Marx, & Freedman, 1991). Features of the physical environment in which wandering increased included location (corridor, nurses' station, and another resident's room) and normal lighting, noise, and temperature conditions. With colder temperatures, wandering decreased. Wandering also decreased significantly under certain social conditions, namely during structured activities and activities at daily living (ADLs), but increased in the presence of a few people (2–5) or when housekeeping staff or residents from another unit were present. However, these researchers made no attempt to manipulate environmental factors to elucidate effects on wandering.

Work on wandering in controlled environments wherein aspects of the environment are specifically manipulated is just beginning. To test the premise that the low light conditions associated with sundown increase confusion and wandering, a study of 10 wanderers was conducted in a specially controlled nursing home lounge. Preliminary analysis revealed no impact of various lighting conditions (dim, bright, or average ambient lighting) on the frequency of wandering episodes or total time wandering in the lounge (Algase, 1997a). However, although subjects were observed during the time of day when each was normally most active, they displayed very little wandering in the highly simplified, controlled environment of this study, suggesting that other aspects of the environment may have a greater potential to reduce wandering than light.

7.17.5 PUTATIVE OUTCOMES OF WANDERING

Outcomes of wandering have not been extensively studied and most knowledge concerning them has been derived from clinical experience. Falls and elopements are the direct, more immediate, and, due to their association with high morbidity (e.g., hip fractures) and mortality, the most serious outcomes of wandering. Weight loss, sleep disturbances, and fatigue are more indirect outcomes thought to reflect wandering's cumulative effects (Algase & Struble, 1992). An outcome that is not well documented, but frequently observed in the course of my clinical practice and research, is the tendency of other nursing home residents to shun or berate wanderers, most likely in an effort to protect themselves, their space, and their possessions from unwelcomed intrusions. Although effects of such negative responses to wandering on morale of wanderers is unknown, logic suggests that it is not a pleasant experience. In fact, it is not uncommon for such interactions to be verbally hostile, and they can escalate into physical aggression on the part of either party.

7.17.5.1 Falls

While cognitive impairment is the most important and frequently documented risk factor for falls (Buchner & Larson, 1987; Janken, Reynolds, & Swiech, 1986; Morse, Tylko, & Dixon, 1987; Nevitt, Cummins, Kidd, & Black, 1989; Reinboth & Gleidenvand, 1982; Rubenstein, Josephson, & Robbins, 1994; Tinetti, Speechley, & Ginter, 1988; Walshe & Rosen, 1979), little empirical data exists to support the clinical contention that wandering compounds the risk of falling (Cancro, 1968; Soverini & Borghesi, 1968). However, any such effects are probably mediated by disturbances in gait and balance associated with cognitive impairment itself (Kippenbrock & Soja, 1993; Morse, Tylko, & Dixon 1985; Morse et al., 1987). Characteristics of wanderers or types of wandering most likely to result in falls are unknown.

The higher frequency of and time spent in ambulation among wanderers may simply increase opportunity to fall. Wanderers as a whole are thought to be more physically able than less active persons with cognitive impairments. However, as dementia progresses, wandering increases at the same time as physical vigor declines for a given individual. Thus, the ability to apprehend and interpret environmental hazards worsens in tandem with deterioration in one's physical stamina. Based on a study of 60 institutionalized women with AD, researcher's concluded that falls were related to a decline in overall vigor in those who had been active (Brody, Kleban, Moss, & Kleban, 1984). Together, these factors may interact to increase the incidence of falls among wanderers.

7.17.5.2 Elopements

The most potentially dangerous consequence of wandering is elopement (Henderson, 1993–4; Mulrooney, 1993–4). Elopement, the unattended leaving of the premises, has been linked to out-of-facility deaths (Foxwell, 1993; Morino, 1989). While reported elopements have declined, largely due to growth of dementia units equipped with sophisticated security systems, they remain a serious and costly problem (Henderson, 1993–4). Death or serious injury occurring during elopement accounts for an estimated 17% of malpractice suits directed toward long-term care facilities (Kapp, 1986).

Risk management programs and in-service education, while essential in training personnel, have not demonstrated a reduction in the incidence of elopement (Kapp, 1986). Due to nursing home reforms contained in the Omnibus Budget Reconciliation Act (OBRA), the use of restraints to ensure safety for persons who wander is increasingly challenged, legally and empirically, because of known undesirable side effects of restraint use (Evans & Strumpf, 1989; Miller, 1975). Thus, the need for alternative approaches to reduce or control elopements, based upon a clearer understanding of particular wandering behaviors and circumstances precipitating egress, remains.

7.17.5.3 Weight Loss

Weight loss is associated with progressive dementia. In one study of hospitalized patients who were no longer mobile, those with AD were an average 11.3 kg (21%) lighter than those who were not demented and 6.6 kg lighter than those with MID despite comparable nutritional indices and food intake for all three groups (Singh, Mulley, & Lusowsky, 1988). In a retrospective comparison of weights recorded in the medical records of these same patients, body weight fell significantly for those with AD but did not change appreciably for the others. Reasons for these differences are poorly understood.

No studies examining the effects of wandering on weight, food intake, or nutritional indices were located. However, whatever the basis for weight loss in dementia and particularly in AD, wanderers may be prone to even greater losses for two reasons. First, their activity level and, therefore, their energy expenditure is high. Second, due to their activity level, wanderers are often difficult to keep seated and focused during mealtimes. Although they are usually capable of feeding themselves, wanderers often walk away from the table before having consumed their entire meal and, thus, may be at greater risk for insufficient caloric intake to offset their high level of energy expenditure.

7.17.5.4 Sleep Disturbance and Fatigue

Sleep patterns in dementia are altered to a degree even greater than that attributable to aging (Prinz, Peskind et al., 1982). The sleep of persons with dementia is punctuated with frequent arousals and nearly devoid of the deep sleep and REM sleep needed for physical and mental restoration (Vitiello, Poceta, & Prinz, 1991). Brief daytime naps are also common.

While the effects of wandering on sleep have not been reported, an examination of the individual 24 hour distributions of wandering episodes in 58 nursing home residents with cognitive impairment does confirm that wandering occurs during the night (Algase, 1997b). However, by comparison to daytime wandering, the frequency of night-time episodes and their total duration is quite small (see Figures 1 and 2). Distributions vary widely among subjects and not all daytime wanderers display the behavior at night. In an analysis of six cases, three with severe levels of cognitive impairment displayed wandering behavior during more hours in a day (9–19) than three with moderate levels of impairment (6–8). The longest period of time without a wandering episode was shorter for those with severe impairment (5–10 hours) than it was for those whose impairment was moderate (14–16 hours) (Algase, Beel-Bates, & Kupferschmid, 1995). Thus, wanderers, particularly those with more advanced cognitive loss, receive little uninterrupted rest.

What is unknown is whether the propensity to wander interferes with sleep to a greater degree than dementia itself or whether the fractured sleep patterns accompanying dementia inadvertently provide greater opportunity to wander. Clearly, more studies are needed to explicate relationships among sleep, fatigue, and wandering, as rest periods may be a potentially useful intervention (Hall & Buckwalter, 1987).

7.17.5.5 Other Possible Outcomes

Longitudinal effects of unrestrained wandering have been the focus of only one study (Cornbleth, 1977). Physical, psychosocial, and cognitive outcomes were assessed in a sample of 48 veterans prior to and at 6 and 12 weeks following their transfers between an experimental and other wards. Controlling for baseline performance, wanderers *on* the experimental ward, where they were free to walk about at will, showed greater physical ability (range of motion) at both postmove time points as did nonwanderers *off* the experimental ward. However, regardless of ward assignment, wanderers showed lower psychosocial functioning over time, reflected primarily in terms of friendliness, self-control, and communication skill than nonwanderers. Neither ward nor group had an effect on measures of cognitive performance.

Thus, not all outcomes of wandering are negative. Although no measures of wandering behavior were employed to demonstrate an actual increase in ambulation on the experimental ward, the above study reveals that

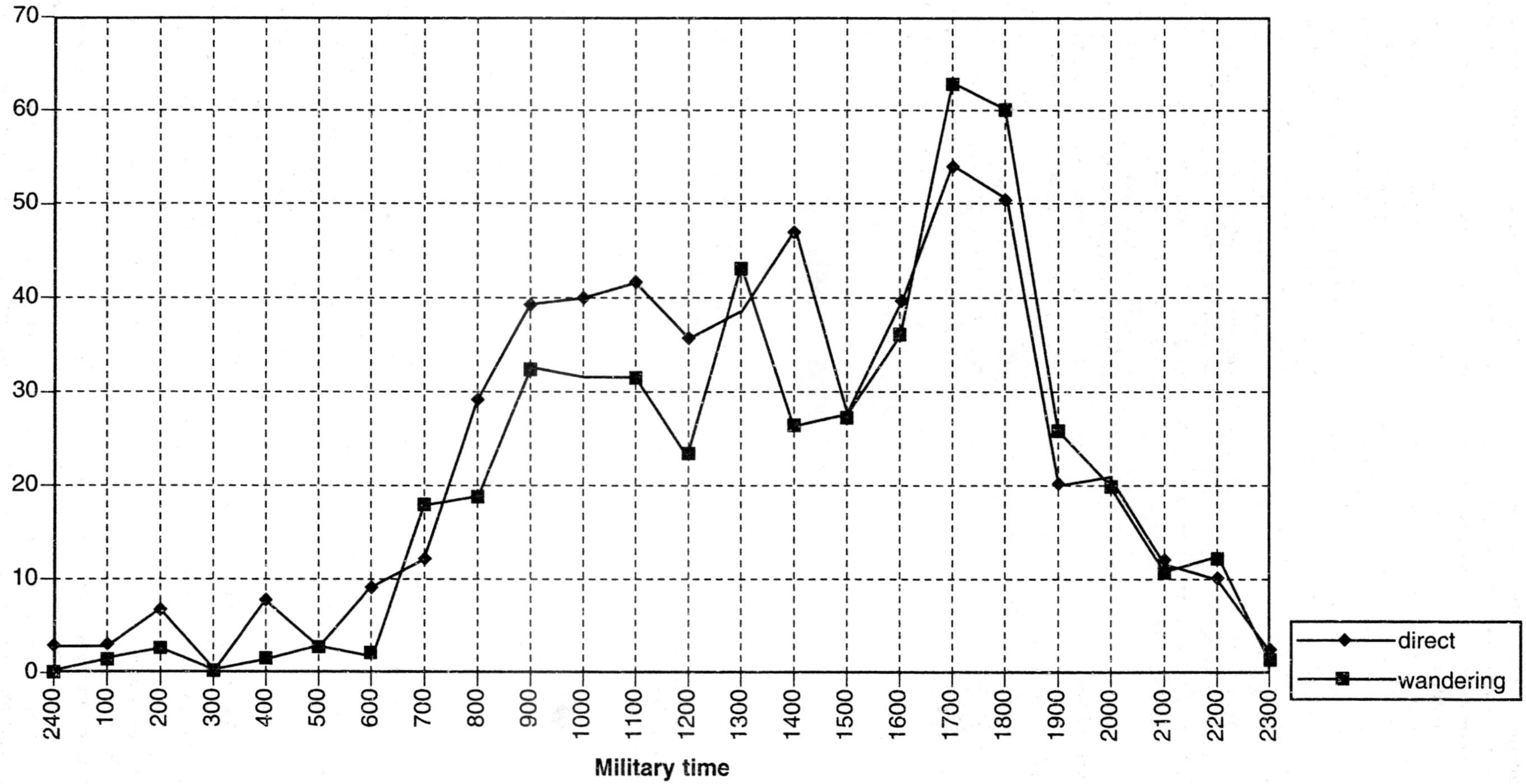

Figure 1 Sum of wandering and direct episode frequencies by hour ($N = 25$).

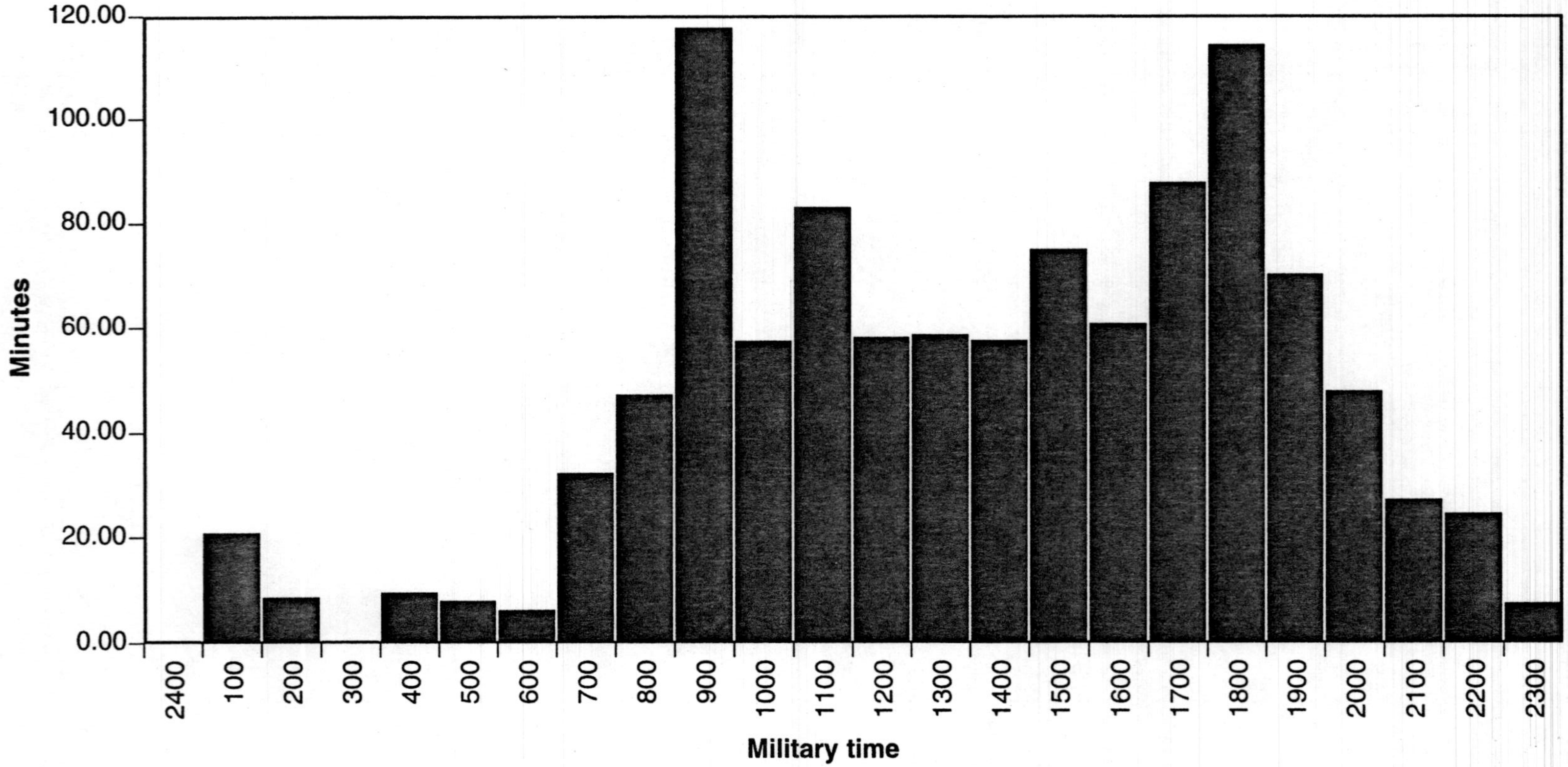

Figure 2 24-hour distribution of minutes spent wandering ($N = 25$).

physical functioning may be enhanced by freedom to wander. Unfortunately, on wards housing both wanderers and nonwanderers, such freedom for wanderers may adversely affect nonwanderers, who may inhibit their movements as a protective strategy. Further, wandering may have a negative impact on the psychosocial skills of those afflicted.

7.17.6 ETIOLOGIC THEORIES AND FACTORS

While several etiologies for wandering have been suggested, none as yet fully explain it. Most explanations are speculative, lacking adequate testing, yet all remain viable as hypotheses. The most glaring deficiency in efforts to test these "theories" is a reliance on proxy variables for wandering, rather than on any direct, valid, and reliable measure of the behavior itself. When eventually tied to observable features of wandering, each of these various theories may be able to explain some dimension or type of the behavior, thereby lending direction to more targeted intervention strategies for the most troubling aspects of wandering.

7.17.6.1 Wandering as Spatial Disorientation

Based on multiple findings from lesion and other studies on rats, the hippocampus (HPC), situated deep in the parietal lobe, is known to capture memories of spatial environments (Nadel, 1991). In humans, the right HPC has a special role in spatial learning (Goldsten, Canavan, & Polkey, 1989) and HPC damage is a classic neuroanatomical feature of dementia, particularly in AD. Further evidence supporting specific involvement of the right parietal lobe in wandering is drawn from a recent study of 18 subjects with vascular dementia, nine of whom were identified as wanderers on the basis of behaviors observed by staff in a long-term care setting (Meguro et al., 1996). Using positron emission tomography (PET), these researchers demonstrated that wanderers had significantly higher cerebral metabolic rate for glucose (CMR_{glc}) than nonwanderers in the left and right frontal lobe, left parietal lobe, temporo-parieto-occipital region, left occipital lobe, and cerebellum. Thus, while the CMR_{glc} of the right parietal lobe of wanderers was neither higher nor lower than nonwanderers, it was relatively lower than other brain regions for wanderers.

Impaired spatial memory is an expected feature of dementia and "getting lost" in familiar or unfamiliar surroundings has been used to characterize particular stages of cognitive decline (Reisberg et al., 1982). Several researchers have demonstrated the presence and nature of spatial disorientation in AD and other dementias. In tests of parietal lobe function, wanderers ($n = 5$) were shown to perform more poorly than similarly demented controls ($n = 16$) (deLeon, Potegal, & Gurland, 1984). Using neuropsychological measures of visuoconstructive (right parietal) performance, long-term declarative memory, attention, language performance, and dementia severity, Henderson, Mack, and Williams (1989) examined spatial disorientation, evaluated by caregiver ratings on four items (wandering, getting lost indoors, getting lost on familiar streets, unable to recognize familiar surroundings) from the Memory and Behavior Checklist (S. Zarit, Orr, & J. Zarit, 1985) in a sample of 28 ambulatory persons who met criteria for probable AD. Eleven subjects (39%) showed substantial spatial disorientation yet did not differ from remaining subjects by age, education, duration of symptoms, or gender. Correlations of neuropsychological measures to spatial disorientation ranged from 0.21 (attention) to 0.56 (long-term memory). Long-term memory and visuoconstructive performance together explained 41% of the variance in spatial disorientation with memory being the stronger predictor.

Visuospatial ability has also been examined in relation to right–left orientation (R/L-O) in AD and MID subjects with comparable dementia severity. Operationalized by putting geometric objects through holes of corresponding shape, visuospatial ability was significantly correlated to R/L-O (as applied both to self and external to self) in MID with focal lesions, but not in AD (Fischer, Marterer, & Danielczyk, 1990). In a study comparing AD and Parkinsons' dementia (PD), both groups, which were matched for dementia severity, age, and education, performed substantially worse on visuospatial tests than nondemented controls (Mohr, Litvan, Williams, Fedio, & Chase, 1990). Further, these PD subjects showed a selective deficit on the Object Assembly subscale of the WAIS-R, a task not principally associated with memory and thought to depend on frontal lobe functioning. However, the AD subjects performed more poorly on tasks with principal memory components, likely reflecting involvement of the HPC which, while always affected in AD, is not consistently so in PD (Chiu et al., 1986; Jellinger, 1987).

Still unknown from these works is the correspondence between these measures of visuospatial ability, which are done in grasping space, and performance of spatial tasks, such as way-finding, which occur in large-scale space. A study by Liu, L. Gauthier, and S. Gauthier (1991) lends support to linkages in performance at these two spatial levels. These researchers administered an array of tasks reflecting perceptual, cognitive, and functional spatial skills to 30 subjects, 15 with early AD and 15 age-matched normals. Perceptual spatial skills included figure-ground perception, visual and tactile shape recognition, visual and tactile size discrimination, position in space, spatial relations, and left–right orientation. Cognitive spatial skills were: spatial planning, decision-making, problem-solving, mental direction rotation, immediate spatial memory, spatial learning, and mental representation of both a familiar and a new environment. While all skills in the perceptual category and most in the cognitive category were performed within grasping space, one (problem solving) in the latter group did require walking in a large-scale space that afforded total visual accessibility. Orientation within a familiar and a new environment were the functional spatial skills examined. Both of these required walking to specified locations that were not immediately visible from one's point of origin.

Some perceptual skills were intact for AD subjects, namely visual shape discrimination, both visual and tactile size discrimination, and left–right discrimination. However, the measure of left–right discrimination favored application to self, as opposed to application external to self. AD subjects displayed gross disturbance of cognitive skills, performing significantly worse than normal controls on all tasks in this category. In finding their way about a highly familiar environment, AD subjects did as well as controls, but in a new setting they performed only half as well as controls.

While results of these studies indicate that spatial orientation is disturbed in dementia, the relationship of performance on various visuo-spatial tasks to observed travel patterns and ambulation efficiency and to the frequency, duration, distribution, and location of wandering remains unknown. Effective and efficient ambulation depends on spatial memories, also known as cognitive maps. In fact, building spatial memories requires some degree of exploration, which includes ambulation. As a kind of ambulation occurring concomitant with AD and other dementias, it seems reasonable to postulate that at least some aspects of wandering, most likely its geographic or spatial patterns, may reflect deterioration of such maps (i.e., difficulty remembering one's way around), or reduced capacity to form new maps (i.e., difficulty learning one's way around). Evidence for the link between spatial disorientation and the spatial patterns of wandering is found in the swim patterns of rats. Rats with unilateral and bilateral HPC damage swim in patterns resembling, respectively, the lapping and random travel patterns of demented elderly observed by Martino-Saltzman et al. (1991) (Holden & Therrien, 1993).

7.17.6.2 Wandering as a Movement Disorder

7.17.6.2.1 The HPC and locomotor output

Three presently unrelated views have been offered to explain the high level of movement in wanderers. The first again involves the HPC. In addition to its role in spatial orientation, researchers have demonstrated that the HPC also affects the amount of locomotion. Classical work (Ranck, 1973; Vanderwolf, 1969; Vanderwolf, Kramis, Gillespie, & Bland, 1975) first established that the electrical activity of cells in the HPC is correlated with locomotion. Work in 1994 by Whishaw, Cassel, Majchrzak, Cassel, and Will suggests that animals with damage to HPC shift towards more locomotion (i.e., shorter stop periods) on what is termed the mobility gradient. Specifically, theta units (groups of neurons, most likely HPC interneurons and/or dentate granule cells) produce a characteristic theta rhythm (7–10 Hz; also known as rhythmic slow wave activity). Rhythmical firing of theta units occurs when animals are walking, running, jumping, or moving the head. In contrast, predominantly irregular wave patterns and low rates of irregular firing or absence of theta is seen during motionless periods or with appetitive behaviors like grooming, chewing, etc. (Vanderwolf & Leung, 1983; Whishaw, 1991), suggesting that theta activity is involved in generating rhythmical locomotion and modulating movements and that intrinsic pacers of this rhythm basic to locomotion exist (Morgenson & Nielsen, 1984; Muller & Kubie, 1989; Traub, Miles, & Wong, 1989; Whishaw & Nikkel, 1975).

In humans, case reports of HPC theta exist from EEG recordings, although theta is difficult to record without invasive procedures and special electrode placements. However, Halgren (1991) has recorded action potentials related to movements requiring intention or high effort, indicating that human HPC neural activity strongly influences movement. Further he suggests (Halgren et al., 1980) that these are endogenous potentials or pacers. Thus, the well-established involvement of the HPC in AD and some other dementias may also explain the overall increase in locomotion observed among wanderers.

7.17.6.2.2 Perseveration

Perseveration, or difficulty in stopping or shifting behavior, is a second possible characterization for the overall high activity levels of wanderers. In other words, once walking is initiated, wanderers may have difficulty terminating an episode. Present with focal damage to the parietal and temporal lobes (Goldberg, 1986; Sandson & Albert, 1984) and with more diffuse central nervous system pathology (Goldberg, 1986), perseveration manifests as repetitive behavior, usually without a discernible stimulus. Perseveration is a documented feature in many cases of AD, MID, and PD (Fuld, Katzman, Davies, & Terry, 1982; Marley, 1982) and can involve repetitious speech patterns (e.g., echolalia, word intrusions) and motor behaviors.

This possible view of wandering was the basis of a study by Ryan et al. (1995). Eighteen community-residing subjects (72% female) with mild to moderate dementia were classified as wanderers ($n = 6$) or nonwanderers on the basis of caregiver ratings. Three types of perseverative motor behavior were quantified from subjects' drawings on the Bender Gestalt and clock drawing tests. The groups did not differ with regard to attention and concentration, spatial orientation, age, gender, or dementia severity. Wanderers demonstrated significantly greater perseveration than nonwanderers, although nonwanderers did perseverate. Wanderers were especially likely to have an ongoing, continuous, or repeated response to a singular stimulus, a form of perseveration associated with the right hemisphere and with attention or motor output deficits (Marley, 1982) or to carry over elements of one drawing into another, a form of perseveration associated with bilateral frontal or frontotemporal impairments (Sandson & Albert, 1987). Interestingly, authors of this study did not confirm spatial orientation deficits of wanderers reported above. They attributed this lack of difference to either their method for scoring the clock drawing test or to the earlier stage of dementia of their subjects.

7.17.6.2.3 Effect of neurotransmitters

A third hypothesis addressing the high degree of motor output of wanderers is not based on localization to particular brain structures or regions, but involves neurotransmitter systems. Weller (1987) suggested that the reduction of acetylcholine characteristic of AD may result in a relative excess of dopamine. Seeing wandering as indicative of restlessness, he further proposed that, analogous to its role in schizophrenia, this dopamine "excess" may account for wandering. However, no studies to evaluate this hypothesis could be located.

7.17.6.3 Wandering as a Circadian Rhythm Disruption

The suprachiasmatic nucleus (SCN) is thought the be the "biological clock" that governs daily fluctuations occurring in, at least, some physiological and behavioral phenomena in humans. Because the SCN is located atop and connected to major optic tracks in the brain, phenomena that naturally change in accord with the light–dark cycle, such as activity and rest, are more likely affected by it. The SCN decreases in size with aging and, to an even greater extent, in AD (Swaab, Fliers, & Partiman, 1985). Loss of neurons in the SCN accounts to a large degree for degradation in the normal sleep–wake cycle observed in both aging and AD (Prinz, Peskind et al., 1982; Prinz, Vitaliano et al., 1982; Witting, Kwa, Eikelenboom, Mirmiran, & Swaab, 1990). Further, if neuronal loss causes the SCN to fall below a certain critical mass, circadian periodicity may be completely obliterated (Brock, 1991).

Along with wandering, day–night reversal and "sundowning" are other clinical concerns observed in dementia that may coincide with shrinkage of the SCN. In fact, several authors have actually linked sundowning with wandering (Eisdorfer & Faan, 1982; Rindlisbacher & Hopkins, 1991). One group (Rindlisbacher & Hopkins, 1992; Rindlisbacher, Hopkins, & Grant, 1992) studying sundowning has used methodology (activity monitoring) similar to that used by researchers studying wandering (Algase, Beattie, Kupferschmid, & Beel-Bates, 1997; Satlin et al. 1991).

As sleep and physical activity are mutually exclusive, an inverse relationship between sleep and wandering would be expected. Thus, changes in overall circadian periodicity associated with AD and other dementias are likely to affect the daily distribution of wandering episodes. Figure 3 illustrates this likelihood as the data depicted for severely impaired cases, where SCN shrinkage would be advanced, show more night-time wandering and wandering occurring in more hours of the day than the data shown for moderately impaired cases. Further evidence supporting the role of the SCN in affecting wandering distribution is found in a comparison of AD subjects classified as "pacers" and "nonpacers" (Satlin et al., 1991). These researchers reported that relative amplitude in 24 hour activity patterns was lower for pacers, suggesting a weakening and loss of integrity in circadian periodicity that exceeds that of nonpacing AD victims.

7.17.6.4 Wandering as an Expression of Mood or Affect

Terming it "agenda behavior," clinicians have attributed wandering to affective states, such as anxiety or fear, underlying the here-and-now experience of a cognitively impaired person (Rader et al., 1985). However, while an appealing explanation because of its potential for intervention, little research yet exists to substantiate this claim. While Cohen-Mansfield and Marx (1990) demonstrated a connection between depression and screaming behaviors, no such relationship between depression and wandering was revealed. In a more recent work wherein agitation was viewed as a reflection of negative affective states such as anxiety or anger, researchers (Algase, Beattie, Kupferschmid, & Beel-Bates, 1997) used Cohen-Mansfield's Agitation Inventory (CMAI) to explain rhythmic parameters for various patterns of wandering. The physical aggression subscale (PA) of the CMAI, which contains behaviors suggestive of anger or frustration, accounted for 37% of the variance in cycle frequency and 43% of the variance in the sum of locomoting phases for all wandering patterns together (random, lapping, pacing) over a 24 hour day, with most of this attributable to the predominance of random-pattern wandering. The PA factor also accounted for 40% of the variance in the mean locomoting phase duration and 54% of the variance in the percentage of a cycle spent in locomotion for the pacing pattern. The physically nonaggressive subscale (PNA), which contains behaviors suggestive of anxiety or restlessness, accounted for 18% of the variance in cycle frequency, 19% of the variance in the 24-hour locomoting phase sum, 23% of the variance in the nonlocomoting phase mean, and 30% of the variance in the percentage of cycle locomoting for all wandering patterns together. Again, cycle frequency and locomoting phase sum results are largely attributable to the preponderance of random-pattern wandering displayed by subjects. However, nonlocomoting phase mean results were most influenced by lapping, for which the PNA predicted 39% of the variance. Results for the percentage of cycle spent in locomotion were largely influenced by pacing, for which the PNA predicted 61% of the variance. The verbal aggression subscale (VA), which contains behaviors suggestive of anger and general confusion, predicted only the nonlocomoting phase mean (19%) for random-pattern wandering. While promising, results should be viewed with caution as no controls for the effects of cognitive impairment were considered in these analyses. Although preliminary and based only on a convenience sample of 25 long-term care residents, these results do suggest that affect may be important in the expression of particular parameters of wandering and, with further study, these may be useful in identifying what kind and amount of wandering might be explained by affect and, thus, be potentially influenced by interventions targeted to change affect.

7.17.6.5 An Emerging Multifactorial Explanation for Wandering

A group of investigators devised a putative explanatory model for wandering and other dementia-related behaviors based on an extensive review of the literature (Algase et al., 1996). Potential etiologies were grouped and organized as either background factors (i.e., the relatively stable or slowly changing characteristics of persons with dementia) and proximal factors (i.e., the more fluid and dynamic features of the person or the environment). Background factors included dementia-compromised functions (e.g., memory, circadian rhythms), health state, demographics, and psychosocial variables (e.g., personality, response to stress); proximal factors included physiological need states (e.g., pain, hunger), psychological need states (e.g., affect), physical environment (e.g., light level), and social environment (e.g., staff stability). In addition to factors thought operative for any dementia-related behavior, a particular set of additional factors were also delineated for selected behaviors, including wandering. Additional variables posed as relevant to wandering were level of social engagement, complexity of environmental design, and crowding.

Figure 4 is a more recent schematic of the model as it pertains to wandering alone. Major propositions of the model are that: (i) background and proximal variables interact or combine in some way to produce wandering, (ii) proximal variables are perceived in the context of existing background variables, and (iii) some background variables may have a direct influence on wandering independent of any proximal variable. Accordingly, unless it is a direct result of an underlying neuropathology, wandering arises from some immediate perceived need and is expressed in a way that is compromised by dementia and mediated by environmental considerations.

The authors acknowledge that the model is tentative and requires empirical testing. How-

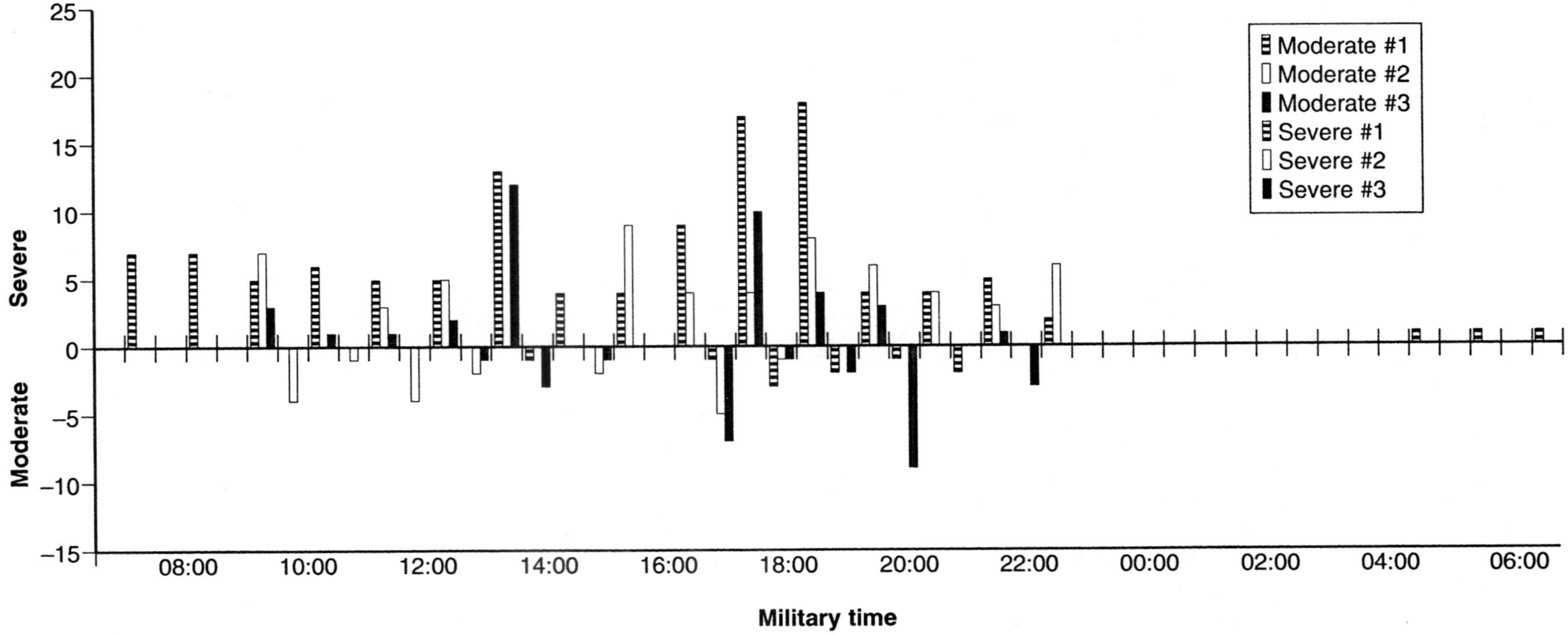

Figure 3 24-hour distribution of wandering episodes comparing moderate (n = 3) and severe (n = 3) cases.

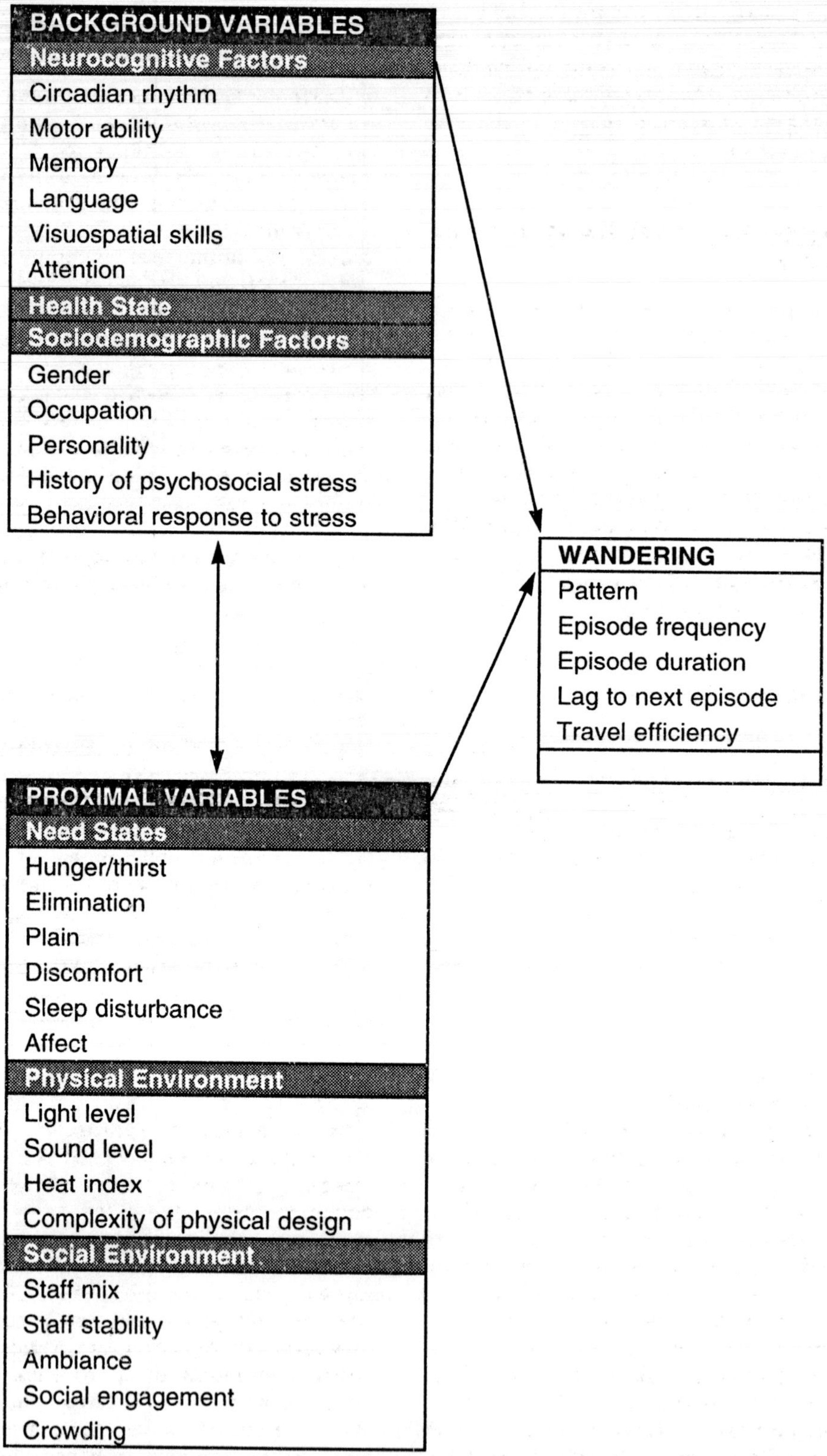

Figure 4 A tentative multifactorial model for wandering behavior.

ever, it is noteworthy in that it represents effort to advance a more comprehensive, integrated, and detailed view of this complex behavior. Further, it does so in a way that can lend support to development of specific intervention strategies for particular parameters or aspects of wandering that present problems or issues in particular contexts.

7.17.7 ASSESSMENT TECHNIQUES AND ISSUES

Most studies of wandering are actually studies of wanderers; few focus on the behavior itself and many of those actually target only exit behavior. Yet, research does provide some guidance for the clinical assessment of wandering behavior. Three measurement strategies used by researchers for quantifying wandering could be applied or adapted for the purposes of clinical assessment: mapping techniques, counting and timing strategies, and motion meters. Each is discussed in the sections that follow. In addition, sections addressing the assessment of clinical concerns and potential outcomes from wandering are offered.

7.17.7.1 Assessment Techniques for Wandering

7.17.7.1.1 Behavior mapping

The earliest study in which wandering behavior was quantified employed a behavior mapping strategy (Snyder et al., 1978). For designated time periods, episodes of locomotion were observed and traced on a floor plan of the unit where the wanderer resided. This approach captured approximate distance covered, areas of the unit where locomotion occurred, and number and heading of turns or direction changes. Robb (1987) extended this approach by adding recordings of time spent in each location and observation of several associated motor behaviors. Clinically, such data could be used to estimate relative amount of locomotion; to identify times of day when locomotion is greater or lesser than others; to document changes over time, including comparisons pre- and postintervention; and possibly to provide clues regarding both environmental stimuli that precipitate or repel wandering activity and personal factors that may influence the nature of one's wandering, such as lateral neglect. Supplemented by notes that capture other concurrent events or behaviors, mapping could reveal much about an individual's wandering to assist the selection or development of an individualized treatment program. However, this mapping approach does not differentiate wandering from nonwandering locomotion.

7.17.7.1.2 Counting and timing strategies

Researchers have also attempted to quantify wandering by counting and timing individual walking episodes (Algase & Cheng, 1992a; Algase & Tsai, 1991). Using a rhythm perspective, they cast each episode of wandering as a cycle with locomoting and nonlocomoting phases. By timing each phase, various parameters, such as cycle period (locomoting plus nonlocomoting phase) or percentage of cycle locomoting (locomoting phase divided by cycle period) can be calculated. By aggregating observations over specific time periods (e.g., hourly), additional parameters, such as cycle frequency or mean locomoting phase, can also be determined and graphed for a picture of variation over time. In later work, Algase combined her rhythm view with Martino-Saltzman and associates' typology of travel patterns to differentiate wandering from nonwandering locomotion and to compare cycle parameters for different wandering patterns (Algase, Beattie, Kupferschmid, & Beel-Bates, 1997). An example of a 24 hour graph of data resulting from this approach is shown in Figure 5. This strategy has also been combined with the recording of related behaviors, such as activity prior to and at the conclusion of the locomoting phase of each cycle (Algase & Cheng, 1992b).

The counting and timing of locomotion episodes, combined with the use of Martino-Saltzman's patterns and observation of antecedent and consequent activity or events, can provide powerful information, both scientifically and clinically. While researchers have observed continuously over time periods ranging from 2 to 24 hours and recorded data on portable terminals, a useful clinical picture can be obtained using less costly and technologically sophisticated approaches. By limiting observations to ten minutes per hour over a three-day period, a good baseline can still be documented for identifying times of relatively high and low activity and for comparing changes over time or in response to interventions (Algase & Struble, 1992). Low-tech stop watches and paper and pencil recording approaches can replace more sophisticated and costly computerized approaches. An individual's dominant wandering pattern, which may give cues to an underlying etiology, can also be determined. Further, by including observations of antecedents and consequences, assessment data can be used to inform the design of individualized behavior management strategies.

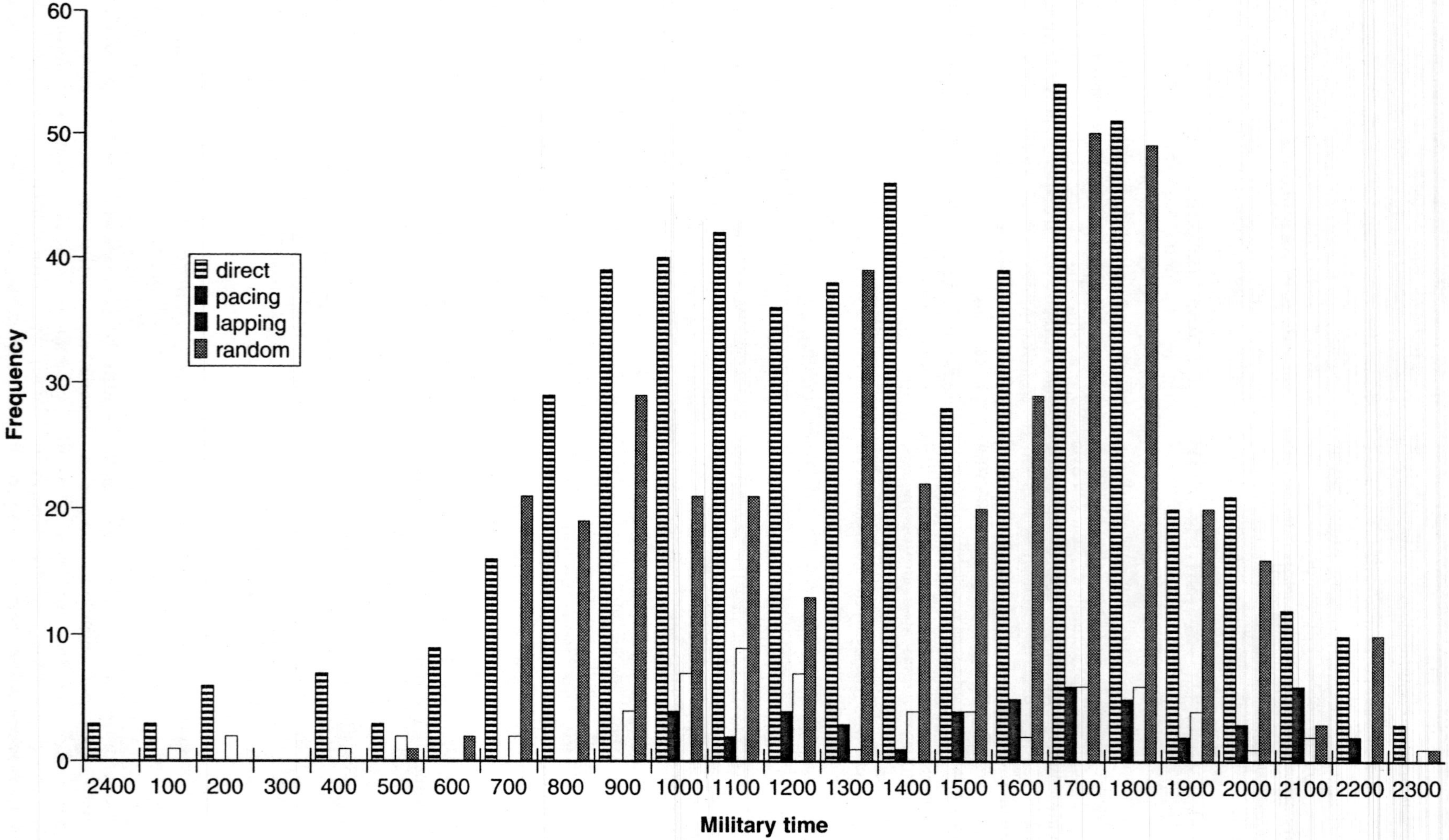

Figure 5 24-hour distribution of wandering episodes by pattern ($N = 25$).

7.17.7.1.3 *Activity monitors*

Cognizant of the expense and reliability issues associated with direct observation, researchers are beginning to test biomechanical motion detectors and pressure-sensitive counters for their ability to estimate wandering behavior (Algase, Beattie, Kupferschmid, & Beel-Bates, 1997; Algase & Cheng, 1992a; Madson, 1990). Although only in the preliminary stages of investigation, these devices hold promise for clinical as well as research purposes.

Large-scale integrated (LSI) monitors, watch-sized devices worn on the wrist, waist, or ankle, record changes in position by tripping an internal mercury switch. Movements are aggregated over time and registered in increments of 10 units or 160 movements. LSIs, originally developed for epidemiological research to quantify physical activity in the general population, are effective for aggregating frequency, but not intensity of movement (LaPorte et al., 1979). Because of their sensitivity, LSI monitors are considered well suited to assessing activity associated with skeletal muscle movement in elderly and/or disabled persons (LaPorte et al., 1983). Reliability estimates for LSIs (correlating day-to-total and evening-to-total readings) under laboratory and field conditions across a variety of populations, including postmenopausal women, are stable at values exceeding 0.70 (LaPorte et al., 1982).

In studies of wandering rhythm spanning 24 hours (Algase, Beattie, Kupferschmid, & Beel-Bates, 1997; Algase & Tsai, 1991), LSIs were used reliably; interunit reliability ranged from 0.76 to 0.93. They provided a relatively strong index of wandering over a 24-hour period but their ability to index wandering over a two-hour period was weaker; ankle applications were more valid than waist applications (Algase, Beattie, Kupferschmid, & Beel-Bates, 1997). LSIs were more effective for indexing parameters of wandering cycles alone than for approximating these for direct cycles alone. The use of LSIs as a proxy for direct observation over short time periods cannot be recommended confidently without further study using larger samples. Further, LSIs are not capable of detecting pattern.

Since 1990 new devices have been developed for the measurement of motor output. Examples are the Step-sensor (Madson, 1990) and Actillume (Ambulatory Monitoring Incorporated). Only the Step-sensor was developed specifically to quantify wandering. Composed of a heel pad, worn in the shoe, and a hardware component attached to the outer aspect of the shoe, the Step-sensor was highly reliable for recording actual number of steps taken when tested in a sample of elderly nursing home residents (Madson, 1990). These devices, alone or in combination, may estimate rhythmic aspects of wandering by demented persons more specifically and sensitively than LSI monitors. However, none yet posses the capacity to identify wandering patterns. The reliability, validity, and clinical acceptability of these devices for assessing wandering in a sample of demented elderly is unknown and is currently under investigation by Algase and associates in a nationally funded US study.

7.17.7.2 Assessment for Associated Clinical Concerns

A number of clinical concerns are associated with wandering and these deserve thorough assessment both for their contribution to and impact on this behavior. These are discussed below in relation to necessary foundational abilities, mediating factors, and antecedents and consequences.

7.17.7.2.1 *Foundational abilities*

Good gait, balance, and sensory capabilities undergird the ability of persons to walk safely. Regardless of deficiencies in these abilities, cognitively-impaired persons are known to move about their environment. Because of cognitive limitations, it is seldom effective to simply remind them to use special caution or assistive devices. Thus, good assessment and attention to these abilities is needed.

In contrast to declining intellectual abilities, systematic studies have established that motor function remains normal until the final stages of AD, the most prevalent dementia (Fayden & Townsend, 1976; Koller, Wilson, Glatt, & Fox, 1984; Molsa, Martilla, & Rinne, 1984). Progressive rigidity and limb flexion eventually lead to loss of balance, impaired ambulation and immobility, but psychomotor speed, posture, gait, and coordination are generally preserved. This has important clinical implications for the assessment and management of wandering behavior. Gait and balance are the fundamental physical skills which support independent mobility and thus wandering. Any patient with a history of wandering requires both gait and balance assessment. The purpose of assessment is to document the ability of the patient to ambulate safely. The extent of preserved safe ambulation behavior is the fundamental skill, second only to memory, underpinning "safe" wandering (i.e., the ability of the patient to negotiate the environment without harm to self or others).

With the exception of PD, normopressure hydrocephalus, and cerebral infarction with focal damage to relevant motor areas, abnormal gait or balance is not likely to be dementia-related until late in the course of the disease. Thus, examination for alternative explanations should be sought and resulting causes treated if such abnormalities are identified.

In the cognitively impaired patient gait and balance assessment may require modification to compensate for the inability of the individual to respond appropriately to verbal direction or gestures. In such a circumstance, discrete observation of the patient in a natural daily setting can substitute for specific testing of gait and balance. Since evidence suggests that wandering occurs in time-frames unique to each individual, gait and balance assessment timed to coincide with the patient's most active daily period will yield the most useful information.

Few gait and balance assessment tools with established reliability and validity exist for use with the elderly, and none have been specifically constructed for assessment of the cognitively impaired elder. In the absence of specific tools, those developed by Tinetti (1986) are widely used in clinical contexts and can be readily adapted to the needs of the cognitively impaired. While comprehensive gait and balance assessment will alert staff to specific mobility skills deficits, such testing cannot predict the success of preventative and adaptive safety measures for patients who wander. Anecdotal evidence suggests that many wanderers have superior mobility skills, can negotiate complex obstacles, and will persist in hazardous wandering despite safety measures. Recent empirical evidence suggests that, while a regular exercise program can increase muscle strength and stamina in AD, regular exercise has no significant effect on overall functional ability (Francese, Sorrell, & Butler, 1997).

The Tinetti gait assessment tool (Tinetti, 1986) covers nine areas of function basic to walking, including step height, length, symmetry and continuity, path deviation and turning while walking. The Tinetti balance assessment tool (Tinetti, 1986) covers sitting and standing balance, eyes closed balance, turning balance, rising, sitting, bending, and reaching. When testing gait and balance, observe the patient in an obstacle-free hallway and continue natural observation long enough for the severely cognitively impaired patient to demonstrate the required skills without verbal cueing. Less impaired patients may be able to respond to several of the simple commands required in both tools.

With a wandering patient it is critical to document as much of the data from formal assessment as possible, along with anecdotal accounts from staff and family of preserved mobility skills. For example, many wanderers, very late in their disease process, can climb and will be observed by staff climbing over chairs, up ladders, or onto ledges and tables. In addition, some patients had occupations in which climbing, balancing, and getting underneath or between structures was part of their daily work and remains part of their activity in institutions. Documented accounts of these preserved skills can help in the planning of individual environments free from known hazards.

With the cognitively impaired patient, balance and gait testing needs to be repeated at regular intervals or when cognitive status deteriorates from previous levels. While no standard time frame for re-evaluation has been established, periodic testing ensures the regular and systematic assessment of gait and balance as cognitive ability declines and provides a baseline against which to compare current function. Since the performance of motor skills is closely related to visuospatial ability, any deterioration in sensory capabilities or environmental change will also impact gait and balance, at least in the short term, and repeat testing should be considered.

In cognitively impaired wandering patients, pre-existing sensory loss of any type can complicate assessment. In addition, sensory loss interferes with communication and leaves fewer uncompromised options available to both subject and assessor. In those with cognitive impairment, even minimal assessment of sensory function is challenging and is based more on the subject's ability to function in the environment than on the results of objective testing. Wandering patients may not be able to remain still for long enough to complete formal testing of sensory function.

People with AD experience visual losses, specifically problems with color vision, depth perception, eye movements, contrast sensitivity, and higher-order visual perception (M. F. Mendez, M. A. Mendez, Martin, Smyth, & Whitehouse, 1990). In assessing vision, one looks for indications that the patient may be reading signs or books aloud, or that they appear clumsy and are bumping into furniture.

Hearing assessment in the wandering cognitively impaired patient relies heavily on knowledge of the patient's prediagnostic hearing ability. Wanderers frequently do not respond to voice instructions, even when their hearing appears to be intact. This seeming oblivion may have to do with lack of recognition of their name, the inability to distinguish individual sound amongst background noise, or a high level of preoccupation with their wandering behavior. None of these possibilities have been empirically tested. Clues about hearing ability can be obtained by watching for signs that the wanderer is hearing and responding to sound. For example, the patient may obviously enjoy music by tapping the feet or hands or singing along. Where there is existing hearing loss, three simple clinical tests using a tuning fork may help determine the type of hearing loss—the Rinne, Weber, and Schwabach tests, but each of these is highly dependent on the patient's ability to respond verbally to commands (Gallo, Reichel, & Andersen, 1995).

Cognitively impaired patient may experience deficits with taste and smell, but are often unable to report them. Wanderers will frequently appear with bruising related to bumping into things and have lost the ability to determine danger where there is hot water or electrical appliances. Some cognitively impaired persons also develop pica and many persons with late-stage AD will eat voraciously without regard for taste.

Crude assessment of kinesthetic sense in wanderers is possible during gait and balance testing by observing for ability to maintain sitting and standing balance and to recover from a gentle push against the shoulder. Fear of falling is apparent when a patient reaches out or braces, even when induced disequilibrium is slight. Wanderers are generally at less risk of kinesthetic deficits than less active or immobile patients because frequent walking stimulates proprioceptive and vestibular function.

Although assessment of sensory abilities in all modalities is important for safety considerations, anecdotal evidence gained from observations during our research suggests that some deficits may actually contribute to particular patterns or rhythmic parameters of wandering. However, the specific contribution of various sensory deficits to aspects of wandering behavior remains to be determined.

7.17.7.2.2 Mediating factors

Unlike foundational abilities, which are necessary for safe ambulation but may not actually affect the amount or type of wandering, mediating factors may play an active role in shaping this behavior. These factors include: cognitive strengths and deficits; mood, affect, agitation, physical discomfort; and personal patterns and preferences. As assessment of cognition, mood, affect, and agitation are the focus of other chapters, our discussion here is limited to personal patterns and preferences and physical discomfort.

To determine a wanderer's personal patterns and preferences, a personal interview and discussion with the patient and the primary informant is essential. Since patterns are laid down over time and stored in remote or procedural memory, many persist in the presence of recent memory loss and can be understood in the context of the patient's prediagnostic lifestyle and occupation. For example, a patient who once owned a chicken farm spent the early morning out in the yard making "shooshoo-ing" sounds and gesturing as if throwing seed down. Any attempt to interrupt the patient during this time resulted in an aggressive outburst. This type of habit behavior has been described as "agenda" behavior (Rader et al., 1985). Knowledge of such patterning can assist in understanding the origin and role of a behavior in a patient's life and bring new meaning to seemingly irrational actions.

Preferences, too, are long-standing and thus likely preserved late into a dementia. One of the most enduring preferences is that of food and many patients in advanced stages of the disease cannot choose between foods but will reject food they have always disliked. The role of personal patterns and preferences for daily routines, food, clothing, and any other aspect of the patient's environment is needed to understand their role in shaping wandering behavior. Such evaluation can greatly inform the design of effective targeted intervention strategies.

Although evaluations of efforts to preserve enduring life patterns and preferences for effects on parameters of wandering behavior are lacking, attention to such preferences has been used to reduce the problems arising from wandering. In a case study by Donat (1984), often repeated behavioral patterns were accommodated by reassigning a patient to the room most frequently entered and moving its then current occupant to new quarters. For the wanderer, this room reassignment eliminated exposure to the unhappy response her intrusive behavior precipitated from staff and the other resident; the gain for the other resident was exemption from unwanted intrusions into her private space.

Ability to accurately identify, personally address, or effectively communicate physical discomfort is hampered by cognitive impairment in wanderers. Increased restless or pacing behavior can signify such meaning. Common discomforts can be avoided or reduced in most cognitively impaired patients using systematic toileting, feeding and resting schedules. Food acceptance charting and routine weighing can aid in assessing hunger. Enforced daytime resting and napping, while offering respite from walking, may exacerbate circadian rhythm disturbance and create an artificial "need" for restraints. Observation and recording of the frequency and length of daytime napping and night sleep may assist in determining fatigue.

Although many wanderers are in better physical condition than nonwandering counterparts, they are not immune to arthritis, angina, and other acute and chronic conditions which cause pain. Additionally, wandering, by virtue of high activity levels, can aggravate certain conditions, such as arthritis, and precipitate others, such as foot blisters. Pain may account for noticeable changes in activity level.

Two instruments can assist in the assessment of discomfort in wanderers. (i) The Discomfort Scale-Dementia of the Alzheimer's type (DS-DAT), developed to assess for nonspecific discomfort (Hurley, B. Volicer, Hanrahan, Houde, & L. Volicer, 1992). The DS-DAT contains nine behaviors which reflect presence or absence of discomfort. Good construct validity (coefficient alpha = 0.77, $p < 0.001$) and test–retest reliability (0.60, $p < 0.001$) were reported on data from serial observations of 20 subjects with conditions known to cause discomfort. Inter-rater reliability ranges from 0.86 to 0.98 across four observations of five to nine subjects (Beck, personal communication, 1997). Again, this instrument was developed for the purpose of evaluating behavior captured in natural settings on videotape, but could be readily adapted for clinical use. (ii) An instrument for assessing pain that may be appropriate for use with wanderers is the Wong–Baker Faces Pain Rating Scale (FPRS). Useful for rating both presence and severity of pain, this series of six line-drawn faces was developed to evaluate pain in children who are at least three years old (Wong & Baker, 1988). In a sample of 97 adults (aged 21–65 years), Cason and Grissom (1994) report that the FPRS correlated with perceived pain intensity ($r = 0.79$) and a visual analog scale (0.67). Although reports of use with demented adults were not located, the fact that the FPRS is targeted to three-year olds suggests that it does not exceed the cognitive capacity of most demented elders (Thornbury, 1992).

7.17.7.3 Assessment of Wandering Outcomes

Outcomes most frequently associated with wandering are falls and elopement. Other outcomes of clinical interest include social functioning, weight loss and nutritional status, sleep and fatigue. Assessment concerns applicable to each are discussed in the following sections.

7.17.7.3.1 Falls

The management of highly mobile, wandering nursing home residents is a particular challenge because their increased mobility levels predispose them to increased extrinsic (e.g., tripping) and intrinsic (e.g., dehydration, fatigue) hazards (Berg & Cassels, 1990; Whall, Gillis, Yankou, Booth, & Beel-Bates, 1989). While mobility is crucial to functional ability and continued well-being during aging, associated falls are critical incidents for the elderly because of their serious immediate and long-term effects (Hogue, 1984; Rubenstein et al., 1994; Vallarino & Sherman, 1981). Falls by the elderly, "or events in which the patient came to rest on the floor from a lying, standing or sitting position" (Heslin et al., 1992) are widespread and well documented. Etiology, risk factors, and management are common research foci.

Limitations in mobility place cognitively intact individuals at higher risk of falls and fractures and the complications associated with them. A higher incidence of falls has been demonstrated among the institutionalized aged (25–61%) than among the community-based aged (Campbell, Reinken, Allan, & Martinez, 1981; Foerster, 1981; Hogue, Studenski, & Duncan,1990; Morris & Isaacs,1980; Overstall, 1978; Sehested & Severin-Nielsen, 1977; Tinetti, 1987; Tinetti et al., 1988; Wild, Nayak, & Isaacs, 1981). However, fall rates and fall-associated injuries vary greatly among and between hospitals and long-term care facilities and are highly dependent on fall reporting methods (Kanten et al., 1993). An epidemiological review of all large-scale published nursing home studies determined a mean incidence rate of 1.5 falls per bed per year (range 0.2–3.6 falls) (Rubenstein et al., 1994). Nursing home studies of the outcome of falls identified serious injuries such as hip fractures, cerebral contusions and hematomas as occurring in 3–6% of the subjects who fell (Morse et al., 1985, 1987; Tinetti, 1987).

The etiology of falls can be characterized as either extrinsic or intrinsic (Berg & Cassels, 1990). Extrinsic factors are general environmental factors, for example, lighting levels, time of day, placement of furniture, type of floor coverings, cleanliness of floors, and type of footwear worn. Critical intrinsic factors include the aging process itself, the presence of disease, increased general frailty, impaired postural control, limitations in mobility, poor vision, psychotropic medication intake, and gender (Barbieri, 1983; Cook, Exton-Smith, Brocklehurst, & Lampert-Barber, 1982; Louis, 1993; Tinetti, 1986; Wild et al., 1981). The relative contribution of each of these intrinsic factors to both fall risk and frequency has not been clearly elucidated.

Dementia can contribute to falls (Buchner & Larson, 1987; Janken et al., 1986; Morse et al., 1987; Nevitt et al., 1989). In a number of studies related to falls in nursing homes, cognitive impairment is the most important and frequently documented risk factor identified (Buchner & Larson, 1987; Reinboth & Gleidenvand, 1982; Rubenstein et al., 1994; Tinetti et al., 1988; Walshe & Rosen, 1979). In several studies, cognitive changes are associated with impaired gait, impaired balance, and wandering (Kippenbrock & Soja, 1993; Morse et al., 1985, 1987). Although thought to be an important factor in falls, the association between wandering and falls has not been well documented.

Conversely, elderly residents rated by nursing staff as alert had the greatest number of falls (Kalchthaler, Bascon, & Quintus, 1978) and a low incidence of mental confusion was found among residents involved in falls. Based on a study of 60 institutionalized women with Alzheimer's disease, researcher's concluded that falls were related to a decline in overall "vigor" in those who had been active (Brody et al., 1984).

While the relative contribution of critical intrinsic factors in the etiology of falls has not been clearly elucidated, the presence of a dementing process remains the most important and frequently documented intrinsic risk factor identified. Early work by Algase (1992b) examined antecedents and consequences as pacers for wandering cycles and determined that wandering is most likely to occur when the residents' activity is unfocused and solitary (52% of 2405 wandering episodes, $n=31$).

Retrospective chart auditing can establish incidence rates only for reported/recorded falls. While such data will provide a baseline, it is critical to determine actual rates more accurately by the systematic observation of at-risk patients. Examination of the at-risk patient for evidence of bruising and cuts caused by falling, and the comprehensive assessment of reports of pain-related behavior in cognitively impaired wandering patients, for example, wincing and limping, can reveal that a patient has had an unseen fall. The early identification of at-risk patients at the time of their admission to a facility, including previous fall history, drug history, and physical examination, is recommended (Brungardt, 1994).

*7.17.7.3.2 **Elopements***

Virtually all clinicians who work with wanderers are aware of elopement as a general hazard and have experienced the wiliness and persistence of some wanderers in successfully escaping the boundaries of their prescribed area. However, there are also those wanderers whose exits are accidental and whose spatial disorientation prevents them from recognizing that they are lost or disables retracing their steps for a safe return. While researchers have counted a variety of behaviors to signify elopement attempts (approaching exit doors, touching or manipulating door knobs, asking to leave, etc.) (Gaffney, 1986; Hussian, 1982; Namazi, Rosner, & Calkins, 1989), specific behavioral predictors for either "type" of elopement are unknown. Observing both antecedents and consequences of an individual's exit attempts can illuminate their unique pattern and thus inform the design of individualized interventions. Due to nursing home reforms contained in the Omnibus Budget Reconciliation Act (OBRA), the use of restraints to prevent elopement is increasingly challenged, legally and empirically (Evans & Strumpf, 1989). Strategies that are less restrictive and operate more passively, such as alarms, are preferred.

*7.17.7.3.3 **Social functioning***

While it has been suggested that wanderers were formally more sociable than nonwanderers (Monsour & Robb, 1982), the social functioning of wanderers is severely inhibited by their marked memory problems, impaired linguistic communication skills, and disinhibition. Assessing social behavior in the severely cognitively impaired is best accomplished by observation of the frequency and quality of interactions with staff, visitors, and other residents. The Minimal Social Behavior Scale (Dastoor et al., 1975) can be used to determine preserved aspects of 1:1 social interactive ability but does not address aspects of social behavior such as the ability to listen and respond appropriately to conversation, the ability to share an activity with others, and the ability to initiate social behavior.

As wanderers become more severely impaired, their ability to reach out and connect with others diminishes. Both staff and other patients frequently find wanderers irritating to deal with because they are forgetful, no longer adhere to social conventions, and unwittingly invade the personal space and privacy of others. Wanderers were the least favored patients in several surveys of caregivers (Lanceley, 1985; May, 1993). Surveys of caregivers and intimates of dementia sufferers indicate that visiting and spending time with a wanderer is a frustrating and difficult experience. The outcome of this potent combination of factors is the further isolation of the wanderer from others in the environment, which may impact the length of time a wanderer spends alone, which may in turn impact parameters of wandering behavior.

The comprehensive assessment of social functioning includes a detailed account of the patient's previous social network and family system and descriptions of the nature and purpose of current relationships (Zarit, Perlin, & Schaie, 1993). A wanderer is limited socially by several factors: (i) the inability to control or modulate their own activity levels and (ii) the loss of linguistic communication ability to the extent that others have difficulty listening to, interpreting, and responding to the wanderer's speech. Thus it is difficult for a wanderer to initiate and maintain social interaction unless another person is able to keep pace with them and tolerate a generally increased activity and a high level of impaired communication.

To date, most research on linguistic communication in dementia has focused on the identification and etiology of deficit rather than preserved functional skills. Several studies support the position that severely cognitively impaired nursing home residents may be capable of greater functional communication competence than has been thought previously (Murray, Marquardt, Richardson, & Nalty, 1984; Slauson, Bayles, & Tomoeda, 1987). Assessment of the preserved linguistic communication skills of the patient will assist in determining the type and nature of interaction the patient has the capacity to take part in. Several scales have been specifically developed for this purpose, including the Communication Observation Scale for the Cognitively Impaired (Tappen, 1988) which focuses on broad categories of impaired function such as the presence or absence of aphasia, blocking, perseveration, talkativeness, meaningless sentence production, and poverty of speech. Since problematic wandering appears to be associated with more severe levels of cognitive impairment, the majority of persistent wanderers will tend to have marked linguistic communication deficits.

A prime function of staff is to nurture the enduring relationships the patient has and to instruct others in ways to spend meaningful time with the patient. One simple way of doing this is to encourage others to walk with and accompany a wanderer, rather than expecting a wanderer to sit down and visit. Maintaining simple conversation focused in the here and now can assist in orientating the wanderer and increasing the interactive climate and expectations of the patient to remain social. However, little is known about the impact of expected social interaction and interactive pressure on levels of anxiety in wanderers, or on pattern and rhythm of wandering.

7.17.7.3.4 Weight loss and nutritional status

Patients with dementia have difficulty obtaining, preparing, and eating food. Patients who wander tend to have a higher lean muscle mass than less active patients, while requiring a higher calorie intake to support wandering activity. While overnutrition can be a problem early in the dementing process, the more likely scenario for a wanderer in the long term is a profile of undernutrition. Overnutrition may result from the inability of the patient to choose appropriate foods and uncontrolled eating. Undernutrition related to wandering is multifactorial resulting from the inevitable wasting related to dementia, the inability of the patient to sit still long enough to eat and drink adequately, changes in the condition of the mouth and teeth, increased activity levels occurring simultaneously with interrupted sleep patterns, and the inability of the patient to manipulate utensils. Severely cognitively impaired individuals may also spit, gag and stuff their mouths with food.

It is essential to calculate the weight and body mass index of the wandering patient and compare these measures to normative measures. The weight of a wanderer requires monitoring at regular intervals to prevent significant weight loss of going unreported. The nursing home standard of monthly weightings may be insufficient for wanderers. A dietary history including known allergies, food preferences, and usual eating times will assist in food selection and meal planning. Wanderers require increased calorie and fluid intake to balance the energy depleted in excessive motor output. A simple pedometer secured on the patient's clothing can give an estimate of miles traveled during waking hours and permit the calculation of calorie requirements for the patient in order to maintain current body weight. However, gait quality may affect the accuracy of pedometers as most work on impact and a more shuffling gait is common among wanderers. Assessment of the mouth and teeth, and correction, where possible, of mechanical problems associated with eating, will facilitate intake.

7.17.7.3.5 Fatigue and sleep disruption

Sleep disruption routinely occurring over extended time periods results in fatigue. In the wandering patient, fatigue levels may also be increased by persistent levels of physical overactivity. A characteristic anecdotal activity of wanderers is day-time napping but little empirical evidence exists to support this (Snyder et al., 1978). Sleep observation charting, at intervals of 30 minutes, will provide a reasonably accurate indication of the pattern of night waking, total uninterrupted sleep time, and daytime napping experienced by a wanderer (Bliwise, 1994), however, this method is staff intensive. Other methods of sleep assessment are both costly and cumbersome and therefore not yet clinically viable with this population.

7.17.8 INTERVENTION STRATEGIES

While the literature on wandering is certainly not vast, almost as many papers address interventions as discuss all other aspects of the behavior. Many suggested interventions have only clinical evidence to support their value. However, some have been tested empirically, but only a few of these have been refined through replication studies. Unfortunately, whether based on clinical experience or research, few interventions are theoretically driven or tied to putative etiologies for wandering. In the following sections, goals for treatment and intervention of wandering, as well as general health and safety considerations for wanderers, are outlined. Information on the range of tested and untested strategies and interventions are then summarized.

7.17.8.1 Goals for Treatment and Intervention

Overall goals for treatment and intervention with wanderers are: (i) assuring safety, (ii) preserving abilities, (iii) maximizing comfort, (iv) minimizing restriction, and (v) eliminating or reducing negative effects of wandering for the wanderer, other residents, and staff. Achieving these goals may entail efforts to reduce, redirect, contain, or redistribute wandering behavior itself. Further, strategies for achieving one goal can, at times, present challenges for attaining another. Prioritization of goals, which should include known personal preferences of the patient and involvement of both family and caregivers, can assist in resolving such conflicts. However, since knowledge of the etiology and purpose of the behavior remain limited at this time, measures designed to either restrict or facilitate the amount of wandering have little empirical basis and should be undertaken with extreme caution. A general rule of thumb is that such measures may be practiced if they do no harm, but careful monitoring to assure such is mandatory.

7.17.8.2 General Health and Safety Considerations

Sustained effort needs to be made to maintaining the physical condition and emotional well-being of the wandering patient. All possible measures for environmental safety need to be instituted to minimize or eliminate hazards associated with falling and elopement. In addition some simple environmental manipulation may assist the wanderer in way-finding and environmental interpretation.

Overall goals for maintaining the physical condition of wanderers are (i) ensuring adequate hydration, (ii) ensuring adequate nutrition, (iii) preventing exhaustion, (iv) minimizing circadian rhythm disturbance, (v) preserving skin integrity, and (vi) monitoring the dosage and undesirable effects of prescribed medications. Overall goals for promoting emotional well-being for the wanderer include (i) engaging the person in meaningful, supervised, and structured activity which provides sensory stimulation; (ii) creating regular opportunities for 1:1 purposeful communication at the person's level of comprehension; and (iii) preserving elements of previous meaningful life activities.

Overall goals for ensuring the physical safety of the wanderer are (i) removing safety hazards from the environment, (ii) enhancing lighting, (iii) preventing elopement, and (iv) balancing the level of stimulation in the environment. Since wanderers are cognitively impaired, aspects of the environment will grow increasingly unclear to them. Measures which may improve the functional ability of wanderers in negotiating their environment include (i) providing redundant cueing; (ii) decorating rooms with relevant personal items and photo identification; (iii) displaying orienting information in multiple, prominent places; and (iv) using rooms for a single, clear purpose.

7.17.8.3 Tested Techniques for Altering Wandering Behavior

7.17.8.3.1 Exercise

On the premise that directed energy expenditure could dissipate or reduce spontaneous wandering, Robb (1987) tested a program of exercise. In a quasiexperiment involving a multiple pre- and post-test design, the hypotheses that exercise would act to reduce the length of time spent in wandering, reduce overall energy expenditure, and improve night time sleep behavior in subjects with a medical diagnosis of dementia were tested. Twenty male subjects (aged 50–87 years) received 12 weeks of programmed outdoor exercise for two hours per day five days per week. Elements of wandering behavior, for example, change in location, time spent in each location, and limb and head movement, were measured during the day and at night prior to the intervention, at eight weeks into the intervention, and six weeks postintervention using behavioral mapping. All subjects received initial fitness and cognitive testing. Effort-induced physical harm was prevented with pulse checks and close observation.

Planned exercise had no significant effect on daytime wandering. However, reductions in night-time wandering were significant for number of locations visited and total time in motion. Serendipitous improvements in range of motion and energy expenditure were also reported. Despite its promise for reducing night-time wandering, no replication studies or clinical reports using exercise were found.

7.17.8.3.2 Cueing

The use of signs, whether composed of words, pictures, graphics, or familiar objects or pictures, has been widely advocated clinically to improve the spatial orientation of cognitively impaired persons. While this strategy has not been examined with regard to effect on overall amount or type of wandering behavior, it has been evaluated for its ability to enhance spatial orientation in the cognitively impaired.

In one experimental study, baseline route navigation and four location-to-location comparative trials were used to determine the effect of sign-post cueing on navigational ability in a sample of 20 spatially-disoriented long-term care residents (Cooke, Algase, & Terpenning, 1993). The sign-posting consisted of large, primary-colored, eye-level signs in simple shapes, such as circles, squares, and hexagons, or in shapes favored by or meaningful to the resident, such as cats or flowers, and labeled in large type. Sign-posts were strategically placed in doorways and corridors directing subjects to relevant locations, for example, the dining room, bathrooms, and their own rooms. Subjects navigated each of four routes sequentially without directional prompting but with occasional verbal reminders of the target location. Time to navigate the route, hesitancies, errors, and overall points scored were recorded for each route and all routes combined. Results of the study demonstrated that sign-posting, regardless of design, did not increase navigational ability.

7.17.8.3.3 Lighting

Several empirical studies have examined the effect of light on activity levels, defining wandering as one of a number of expressions of agitation in dementia. Early work by Evans (1987) identified the phenomenon of "sundowning" in which demented individuals become more agitated and restless with declining light levels in the late afternoon. Cohen-Mansfield et al. (1989) detected temporal patterns of activity disturbance over a 24-hour day in demented patients. Seasonal variation exists in agitated behavior (Bliwise, 1994; Bliwise, Carol, Lee, Nekich, & Dement, 1993), with agitation increasing in the darker winter months. In a Japanese study (Okawa et al., 1989), both morning and evening bright light treatment deceased agitation behavior. More recently, Lovell, Ancoli-Israel, and Gevirtz (1995) administered bright light at 2500 lux levels to six demented subjects (mean age = 82 years) for two hours in the morning for repeated 10-day periods in an ABABA design. Results indicated a significant difference in agitation levels on light-intervention days.

In the only known study of light directed at wandering, three light levels were specifically manipulated (baseline, bright light, and dim light simulating sundown) in a nursing home lounge outfitted for the study (Algase, 1997a). Ten cases were studied for three two-hour periods weekly over a six-week period in random assignment to either an ABAACA or ACAABA design; the second baseline week was intended as a washout period for any carryover effects. The time period was individually selected to match each case's most active period of the day. Although data analysis is incomplete at this time, preliminary results indicate that, regardless of lighting condition, wandering in the lounge was minimal. Logically, factors other than light account for the quite dramatic decrease in wandering observed. Simplicity of the lounge environment, which was completely accessible visually from any vantage point in the room and controlled most sources of stimulation, is the speculated explanation.

7.17.8.3.4 Social interaction

Interventions for wandering addressing aspects of social interaction are primarily related to restraint-reducing efforts. Many programs designed to increase and facilitate interactive social behaviors in the demented give anecdotal descriptions of the reduction in agitation and wandering produced by increased social opportunity and stimulation (Arno & Frank, 1994; Gerdner & Swanson, 1993; McGrowder-Lin & Bhatt, 1988; Mintzer et al., 1993). However, only one empirical study has so far explicitly sought to impact wandering.

Goldsmith, Hoeffer, and Rader (1995) report a test of Rader's (1987) "approach" to wandering (which includes steps to identify potential wanderers, programs and activities for safe ambulation, decreasing use of restraints and psychotropic medications, interaction strategies for managing exiting behavior, creating a safe and supportive physical and psychosocial environment) taught to nursing staff. The study used a single case design with a four-week preintervention phase, a four-week intervention phase, and a six-week postintervention phase. Use of medications and restraints decreased during the intervention phase, but medication use began to rise postintervention. Decreases were associated with increased Physical Self-maintenance scores. This approach had no demonstrable effect on problematic wandering (ambulating alone, exit-seeking while alone, alone in unsafe locations). During all phases of the study, 80% of observations documented a lack of social interaction between staff and subject, except during ADLs. The study was poorly controlled in that once staff were trained, it is theoretically possible, but unlikely, that they did not revert to their pretraining behavior during the postintervention phase of the study. The extent of reversion to pretraining habits and the amount of retraining required over time were not considered.

A recent study utilized a multiple case study design to examine the effect of a systematic, structured nurse–resident communication style on pattern and rhythm of wandering behavior in severely cognitively impaired nursing home residents (Beattie, 1996). An identical quasi-experiment was embedded within each case study as an interrupted time-series with multiple replications and nonequivalent dependent measures. The intervention was a modification of the Heron Six-category Intervention Analysis (Heron, 1976). Results were highly individual across cases, showing no consistent significant effect of the intervention.

7.17.8.3.5 Drug therapy

Older people have qualitative and quantitative differences from younger people in absorption, distribution, metabolism, and excretion of drugs. The wide use of drugs to control difficult behaviors associated with dementia has increased the potential for negative drug reactions. In the cognitively impaired patient, the management of drug therapy is a particular challenge because patients are frequently unable to report undesirable effects, and many patients have multiple pathology requiring concurrent medication.

The dangers of polypharmacy in the elderly are well known. In the cognitively impaired patient the general rule of "less is better" usually applies. A minimalist approach to medications is particularly important when trying to manage difficult behavioral symptoms and tease apart factors contributing to them. In addition, many cognitively impaired patients have difficulty accepting and swallowing medication and compliance must be carefully monitored. Regular and systematic review of medications can prevent some problems and minimize the impact of others. Wherever behavioral change occurs unexpectedly, or unusual behavior persists over a time period longer than a week, it is essential to consider the role of current drug therapy in the clinical presentation of the patient.

Two groups of drugs that are commonly prescribed in to patients with cognitive impairments may have a therapeutic effect on wandering: neuroleptics and benzodiazepines. The neuroleptics are most commonly prescribed for the treatment of agitation and hyperactivity, and are often differentiated on the basis of their undesirable effect profiles. The two major classes of neuroleptics are the phenothiazines (e.g., chlorpromazine and thioridazine) and the butyrophenones (e.g., haloperidol). In general the phenothiazines tend to be quite sedating and are associated with hypotension. Thus in the wandering patient the risk of circadian rhythm disruption, increased gait instability and fall risk, and hypothermia secondary to accidental elopement must be considered. The butyrophenones cause less sedation and few hypotension problems but are more frequently associated with neuroleptic-induced Parkinsonism, characterized by drooling, mask-like facial expression, muscular rigidity, and gait changes. Tardive dyskinesia (TD), an irreversible syndrome involving involuntary movements of the tongue, mouth, face, and neck, is usually associated with long-term neuroleptic use. In some cases, agitated behavior can be exacerbated by neuroleptic treatment so drug treatment should be conservative and time-limited. Over 90 studies of neuroleptic treatment of agitation in the elderly have been reported. Salzman (1987) and Sunderland and Silver (1988) report very similar levels of acceptance and behavioral control, with 70–80% of patients having none or minimal undesirable effects.

The benzodiazepines (e.g., diazepam, oxazepam, alprazolam, lorazepam) are frequently prescribed for symptoms of insomnia and anxiety in the elderly. To the extent that wandering is based on anxiety, they may be effective in its management. There are many age-related changes in response to this group of drugs, primarily due to pharmicokinetic alterations in drug metabolism which result in extended duration of action and lead to an accumulation of side effects (Greenblatt, Divoll, Abernethy, Harmatz, & Shader, 1982). Lorazepam has an uncomplicated metabolic pathway, but has been associated with specific memory impairments (Preston et al., 1988) and is thus a poor choice for the cognitively impaired patient.

7.17.8.4 Tested Techniques for Addressing Undesired Outcomes

Although several putative outcomes of wandering, discussed earlier, are thought hazardous, only one has received the attention of researchers. Reduction or control of egress has been the chief objective of such research. While not concerned with affecting the overall amount, distribution, or type of wandering, these studies focused mainly on reducing successful exits or exit attempts of known wanderers from their assigned unit or permitted range for free movement. The extent to which such exits or attempts occur during actual wandering, as compared to other self-directed locomotion, i.e., direct ambulation, remains unexamined. Three techniques have been tested: behavior modification, camouflage, and perimeter control devices.

7.17.8.4.1 Behavior modification

Principles of learning are frequently incorporated into planning wandering management, for example, rewarding constructive behavior and changing the consequences of the behavior (Hussian & Davis, 1985; Stokes, 1986). However, there are few examples in the literature of controlled, systematic behavior modification. Early work by Hussian (1982) investigated the effect of controlled stimuli and rewards on wandering patterns. The wandering behavior of three subjects (mean age = 73.4 years; mean length of hospitalization = 13 months) was conditioned using two sets of cardboard stimuli: orange rectangles and blue circles. Attention to the orange rectangles resulted in reinforcement with food; attention to the blue circles resulted in the aversive stimulant of an unpleasant noise. During conditioning, baseline data on ambulation behavior were obtained.

Following conditioning, the stimuli were affixed to walls where ambulation was either encouraged (orange) or discouraged (blue). Subjects were systematically observed for periods of 30 minutes. If no contact with the blue areas was made, subjects were rewarded with food. If contact with the blue areas occurred, subjects were returned to their point of origin without consequence. Over time the stimuli were faded by size reduction and eventually removed from the environment.

Mean number of entries into the designated blue trespass area was reduced across all subjects following conditioning by rates ranging from 13 to 100% per 30-minute period. However, booster sessions were required by all subjects at three months and the stimuli were replaced on the walls. Four booster conditionings were required over the 12-month period following initial conditioning. Eventually fading resulted in re-emergence of wandering to preintervention levels. While results of this study clearly demonstrate that wandering can be altered by environmental cueing, the effect on wandering will persist only as long as the cueing is maintained. Given the pattern of known decline in memory and visuospatial deficits in AD, the frequent reconditioning needed to maintain cueing effectiveness is not surprising. Using this method of behavioral control, cueing may need to be increased in intensity and frequency as cognitive functioning declined in order to achieve the same behavioral change. Further studies replicating Hussian's work would benefit from greater specification of level and stage of AD and finer gradation criteria for the fading of stimuli.

7.17.8.4.2 Camouflage

Problems with color vision, depth perception, eye movements, contrast sensitivity, and higher-order visual perception are known visual deficits associated with Alzheimer's disease (Mendez et al., 1990). Hussian and Brown (1987) proposed that these deficits might result in a misperception whereby a two-dimensional grid pattern, fixed to the floor with tape, would be seen as three-dimensional and, thus, unstable. If so, demented subjects may be hesitant to walk upon it and, if strategically placed in front of doorways, grids might reduce exits and exit attempts.

The effect of several different grid patterns made of low-contrast tape when applied to the floor in front of emergency doors were examined for effect on exiting behavior in a sample of eight male subjects with senile-onset, primary, degenerative dementia. Baseline data on attempted exits indicated that an attempt was associated with exit-door contact in 98% of observations. All grid patterns were effective in reducing exit attempts for all but one subject, who was never deterred by any pattern. Subjects did not cross the grid in 70% of their exit attempts.

Several researchers have attempted to replicate Hussian and Brown's results using a variety of color combinations and tape patterns and improvements in design of the original work (Chafetz, 1990; Hamilton; 1993; Hewawasam, 1996). Most were ineffective or results were equivocal. Inability to achieve success was attributed to factors such as confounding effects of medication or strength or "dose" effect of the grid intervention (i.e., grid insufficiently aversive to overcome enticing view through glass doors). However, grid patterns may be effective for patients diagnosed with AD due to associated problems in depth perception, but are not successful with other dementias (Hewawasam, 1996).

Based on the visual agnosia associated with dementia, visual barriers (i.e., door knob coverings or other disguising techniques that appear to create an obstruction, but do not actually impede egress through a door) have been suggested as an alternative camouflage strategy. Namazi et al. (1989) tested the effect of seven different visual barriers on resident exit behavior on an Alzheimer's unit. The subjects ($n = 9$; 55% female; mean time since diagnosis = 5.75 years) had similar cognitive abilities as measured by the MMSE (Folstein et al., 1975) and the Short Portable Mental Status Questionnaire (PMSQ) (Johnson & Grant, 1985). Barriers, which varied in color, material, width, angle of placement, and purpose, disguised both the exit and the door knob. Doorknob concealment was 100% effective in preventing exit behavior in all subjects. However, visual-spatial testing of subjects was not standardized and the exit behavior of subjects and their anxiety levels were not discussed.

In a replication of Namazi's work, the possible attraction of windowed doorways, which may have confounded efforts to replicate the original grid studies, was taken into account (Dickinson, McLain-Kark, & Marshall-Baker, 1995). A cloth panel matching the emergency door color and covering its panic bar was the visual barrier tested. In addition, a miniblind was used to control the view from a window in the door. A sample of seven ambulatory demented subjects (five male; two female; aged 70–87 years) with a history of exiting behavior were chosen from one dementia care unit; no other cognitive characteristics of the sample were reported. Three conditions were tested during a fixed time frame: closed miniblind alone, cloth panel alone, and both miniblind and cloth panel. After obtaining a one-week baseline count of exit attempts at the door, each test condition, which lasted for two hours per day over a one-week period, was followed by a one-week interval during which the blind was left open, no barrier was in place, and no counts were taken.

Overall, the miniblind alone reduced exit attempts by 44% from the baseline while the cloth panel reduced attempts by 96%. Together, the blind and panel were somewhat less effective (88%), suggesting a learning effect. When examining cases individually, four of the seven were found to have had five or fewer exits attempts during the baseline period. Of these, the blind alone was 100% effective for two cases while the panel alone was 100% effective in all cases. However, two of these four subjects returned to or exceeded their baseline count when the blind and panel were used together. The remaining three subjects accounted for 87% of the baseline exit attempts. The miniblind alone was 43% effective; however, the combined miniblind and panel remained nearly as effective (94%) as the panel alone (95%). Thus, the learning effect among these three cases was not as great. Only one of the three demonstrated an increase in exit attempts from the panel to the combined condition, but the increase was small (from 0 to 4) and still represented less than 10% of the subject's baseline count. Characteristics distinguishing those who made many exit attempts from those who made few were not reported. However, these characteristics may be important to delineate. Since these data suggest that those making fewer attempts may be more difficult to dissuade over time, such characteristics may help identify those whose exit attempts may persist and lead to harm.

7.17.8.4.3 Perimeter control devices

Reports of devices such as alarms, fences, and locks to control wandering began appearing in the literature in the 1970s (Miller, 1976). Many commercial electronic and computerized products now exist to provide perimeter control for wanderers, on the assumption that such devices will warn staff of an impending unsafe exit, or prevent such an exit. Devices generally operate in one of three ways: sounding an alarm when a patient crosses an electronic barrier, creating an electronic barrier by automatic closing of gates, doors, and windows, or tracking the patient via a unit worn on the body (Leach, 1985).

In tandem with the development of perimeter control devices, there has been an increase in sensitivity to issues in the humane and compassionate confinement of individuals with cognitive impairments, such as the right to the Least Restrictive Alternative (LRA), that is, to create a balance where individuals are confined at the lowest level considered appropriate to preserve their safety while retaining the highest possible levels of freedom, independence, and dignity (Ebersole & Hess, 1990). Many early perimeter control devices were large, cumbersome and conspicuous. Because these devices contradicted LRA principles, they were unpopular with relatives and staff. Further, they were likely to attract and be tampered with or removed by wanderers. In addition, concerns for the rights of patients have been expressed by ethicists and patient advocates who view electronic monitoring and alarms as violating the rights of privacy, dignity, confidentiality, and the right to give informed consent (Warrington & Eagles, 1995). Further, many practical problems have been associated with perimeter control devices over time, including inadvertent and purposeful triggering, multiple exiting, keeping devices comfortable and functional on patients, and the generally high costs of installation and maintenance.

Several studies have focused specifically on the effect of an alarm system designed to deter the wanderer and alert staff to a possible elopement, however, these studies did not employ definitions or criteria for the selection of wanderers and were uncontrolled (e.g., Gaffney, 1986). One study by Negley, Molla, and Obenchain (1990) focused on changes on resident behaviors when an alarm system is utilized to prevent elopement. Five ambulatory male subjects (mean age = 68.6 years), with various medical diagnoses and considered wanderers by the subjective assessment of senior medical and nursing staff, comprised the sample. Subjects wore wrist tags that activated an alarm concealed under a mat at the entrance to the ward. Observations totaling 120 hours were conducted at 30 hours per week for 4 weeks, with the test conditions varied each week as follows: (i) door unclosed and no sensor tags worn; (ii) door open, sensor tags worn, alarm off; (iii) door open, tags off, alarm on; and (iv) door open, tags off, alarm off. Results indicated a 67% decrease in attempted door exits between weeks 2 and 4.

7.17.8.5 Wandering Paths or Tracks

Many special care environments designed for dementia sufferers now incorporate specific paths or tracks, both indoor and outdoor, where patients can wander; see Zeisel, Hyde, and Levkoff (1994) for an example. By facilitating wandering in a safe environment, rather than restraining a wanderer, proponents suggest that wanderers would be more content and less aggressive, sleep better, and fall and elope less. While the shape of these walking paths varies from geometric to circular, the design is usually simple and the surrounds peaceful and interesting, with plants, pools, fountains, sculptures, and seats for resting. The pleasant atmosphere and accompanied walking which occurs within such environments are assumed to affect both mood and activity levels positively in wandering patients. Clearly, relatives and staff appreciate being able to visit in pleasant surrounds. However, the approach is atheoretical and disregards potential negative effects of encouraging or heightening wandering. Little research exists that tests the impact of tracks on level of wandering behavior or on wanderers, other residents, visitors, or staff.

An empirical study involving 14 subjects in a specially-designed dementia care unit (Kovach, Weisman, Chaudhury, & Calkins, 1997) explored the association of physical environment with behaviors and care of the demented. The study incorporated a "meaningful wandering path" in the facility design. The path circled a central area allowing continuous movement overlooking activities and involved small travel distances and landmarks, but the specific effect of this design element was not reported. To date, there is no evidence to suggest that such environmental manipulation alters parameters of wandering or benefits the wanderer.

7.17.8.6 Activities Programming

Most intervention studies using programmed activities have been global in intent and eclectic in content. Few have focused on a single systematic intervention targeting a single problem behavior such as wandering. These studies have assumed an unsubstantiated homogeneity among problematic behaviors associated with dementia and thus their clinical applicability and utility is limited (Cleary, Clamon, Price, & Shullaw, 1988).

Only one empirical study to date has explicitly sought to impact only wandering behavior (Goldsmith et al., 1995) with little success. The rationale for using activities to moderate wandering remains atheoretical. Anecdotal evidence suggests that it is difficult to find activities that are age-appropriate, span the abilities of a group of cognitively-impaired people, engage the interest of wanderers, and assure the success of wanderers with the activity.

7.17.8.6.1 Physical and chemical restraint

Physical restraint use by belts, wrist ties, vests, lap trays, and other mechanical devices remains common in wandering and agitation management (Werner, Cohen-Mansfield, Braun, & Marx, 1989), even though no published studies document the supposed reduction of wandering or agitation resulting from the use of physical restraints. Rather, a rebound effect in activity level may occur upon restraint release (Miller, 1975). Prevalence of restraint use is documented at between 18% and 85% in nursing homes (Folmar & Wilson, 1989;

Morrison, Crinklaw-Wianko, King, Thibeault, & Wells, 1987; Zimmer, Watson, & Treat, 1984). While these rates are from studies made before Federal criteria and restrictions for restraint use in long-term care settings were established to improve the quality of life and safety of the residents (OBRA, 1987), no more recent estimates were located. High levels of restraint use have also been found when residents are over age 75 years have a medical diagnosis of organic brain disease (Folmar & Wilson, 1989). Problems associated with restraints include: loss of dignity, urinary incontinence, constipation, muscle atrophy, limb ischemia, increased agitation, strangulation, and, in some cases, death (Beardsley et al., 1989; Werner et al., 1989).

In a post-OBRA implementation study, effects of physical restraints on psychotropic medication use in nursing homes were examined (Werner, Cohen-Mansfield, Karoknay, & Braun, 1994). A retrospective and prospective longitudinal design was used to obtain information about medication use and restraints over a two-year period at seven points in time: four, two, and one month prior to restraint removal; at the time of restraint removal and one, two, and four months after. Subjects (n = 88, 75% female, mean age = 86.3 years, mean length in residence = 5.2 years) were those physically restrained residents of a large nursing home and constituted 62% of the 140 residents who were restrained in the facility. Sixty-one subjects (69.3%) had a medical diagnosis of dementia and 18 had a specific diagnosis of AD.

Results indicated that the proportion of all residents receiving psychotropic drugs decreased from 83% to 70% during the study period, the most significant period of decrease being one month after restraint removal. Those with dementia evidenced the greatest decrease. In this group, medication use decreased from 87% four months prior to restraint removal to 57% four months after restraint removal. These results should be considered cautiously because they represent only one institution. However, adaptations to legal control of restraint use and medication withdrawal was clearly beneficial to those with dementia.

Neuroleptics and benzodiazepines are the most frequently used agents and psychotropic medications are often combined with other centrally acting agents. Zimmer et al. (1984) documented the frequency of interventions for agitation (often including wandering) used in skilled nursing facilities: psychoactive drugs (58% of patients), physical restraints (47%), reality orientation strategies (47%), and specialist psychiatric consultation (38%). In a survey of 1276 geriatric inpatients at 12 Veterans' Administration hospitals, 61% were receiving psychoactive drugs (Prien, Haber, & Caffey, 1985). Fifty-five percent of patients with organic brain syndrome were receiving psychotropics and the most frequently prescribed agents were neuroleptics (44%), antidepressants (11%), and antianxiolytics (10%). Another study of 101 demented inpatients reported that 38% received one psychotropic and 20% received two such medications, with neuroleptics being the agent of choice (Michel & Kolakowska, 1981).

An extensive body of literature, most of it descriptive and anecdotal, addresses the effectiveness of general pharmacological interventions for the control of wandering, agitation, and other behavioral symptoms. Barnes, Veith, Okimoto, Raskind, and Gumbrecht (1982) reported on the effectiveness of antipsychotic drugs for specific behavioral problems in a study of 60 demented subjects. In contrast, Druckenbrod, Rosen, and Cluxton (1993) advised limited use of psychoactive drugs because little data were available documenting the efficacy of their use in the elderly. Nevertheless, neuroleptics remain the mainstay treatment of behavioral disturbance in dementia (including wandering) and the intervention of choice in agitation management, although efficacy studies conclude that the effects are modest at best (Schneider, Pollock, & Lyness, 1990). Haloperidol is the most frequently chosen medication for agitation, restlessness, and wandering in older adults because of its reportedly benign cardiovascular and anticholinergic profile (Weiner, Bruhn, Svetlik, Tintner, & Hom, 1991). On the other hand, many elders are extremely sensitive to its extrapyramidal effects and are already at increased risk of drug-induced TD (Marsden, Milson, Parkes, Pycock, & Tarsy, 1975). For example, Prien et al. (1985) reported that in a small group of AD outpatients with psychotic symptoms, patients could not be maintained on more than 4 mg four times per day of haloperidol because of its extrapyramidal effects.

Neuroleptics have been more widely studied than any other class of pharmacological agent. Most controlled studies of neuroleptic use in dementia have suffered from major methodological flaws, for example, diagnostic heterogeneity was a common feature, methods of assessment were often global, and samples were comprised predominantly of severely demented subjects. In addition, the effects of neuroleptics on core psychotic features as well as behavioral disturbance (including wandering) were not assessed. Only a few published studies used a randomized, double-blind, placebo-controlled design.

Schneider et al. (1990) conducted a meta-analysis of placebo-controlled trials of neuroleptics in wandering, agitated patients with any form of organic brain syndrome. The methodological flaws mentioned previously compromised the utility of the meta-analytic approach to an extent. However, neuroleptics were found to be moderately more efficacious than the placebo (one-tailed $p = 0.004$), with effect size reduced by the high placebo response rate observed in some studies. These response rates may have been due to the inclusion of subjects with very mild behavior change only in order to increase sample size (Devanand & Levy, 1995).

To date no published randomized, double-blind, placebo-controlled study of neuroleptic use (without the concurrent use of other psychoactive agents) to treat wandering in a "pure" AD sample of either institutionalized or community-dwelling subjects have been published. A few reports of neuroleptic–benzodiazepine comparisons in the treatment of behavioral symptoms in demented samples are available.

Several other medications have been reported to be efficacious: trazodone (Pinner & Rich, 1988; Tingle, 1986); lithium (Schneider & Sobin, 1992); carbamazepine (Gleason & Schneider, 1990; Leibovici & Tariot, 1988); valproate (Mellow, Solano-Lozez, & Davis, 1993); propranolol (Pauszeck, 1991); and zolpidem, a nonbenzodiazepine hypnotic (Shelton & Hocking, 1997). Published data from randomized, double-blind, placebo-controlled study of all these medications are sparse. Szwabo, Woodward, Grossberg, and Shenn (1991) postulated that wandering is a response to anxiety and used Alprazolam, a short-acting antianxiolytic, in their 12-week study of 16 wanderers in a nursing home. Wanderers received cognitive testing pre- and postintervention and were placed on four weeks of 0.25 mg twice daily. Alprazolam, titrated to 0.5 mg if needed by a subject. A four-week period without Alprazolam followed the intervention. Behavioral change was monitored using daily ratings of total time spent dealing with wandering behavior and with the Nurse's Observation Scale for Inpatient Evaluation (Honigfeld, Gillis, & Klett, 1966). Results indicated statistically significant improvements in speech and irritability while on the drug, however, drowsiness increased.

Kamei, Oishi, and Takasu (1996) evaluated the use of fasudil hydrochloride, a novel cerebral vasodilator, for night wandering symptoms in two patients with a medical diagnosis of cerebrovascular dementia. Results indicated that wandering behavior disappeared in both patients during eight weeks of treatment, while memory function improved mildly. Wandering began again immediately after the cessation of treatment. Regional cerebral blood flow, measured by P-magnetic resonance spectroscopy and Xe-computed tomography, remained unaltered throughout.

7.17.9 RECOMMENDATIONS FOR FURTHER RESEARCH

7.17.9.1 Definition, Measurement, and Description

Lack of a standard, widely-accepted definition remains a primary challenge in research on wandering. While multiple authors have offered definitions of wandering, the scientific community has made little advance in the discussion and acceptance of a universal definition of the behavior. Reaching such a conceptual consensus would assist researchers in communicating effectively about the phenomenon and move them to issues of measurement and description which are required before interventions can be theoretically supported and rigorously tested. Fundamental questions such as: (i) Do all cognitively impaired individuals wander? (ii) What is the point at which an individual is classified "a wanderer"? (iii) Given that men and women are known to have different spatial abilities, are there gender differences in wandering behavior? and (iv) What are the natural limits to parameters of wandering, such as frequency and time in motion? will remain unanswered until consensus on a definition is reached.

In line with a need for a standard definition is that for valid and reliable measurement techniques for wandering. If there is any "gold standard" it is direct observation, the parameters of which are supported by some theoretical rationale and/or valid typology for wandering behaviors. An additional need, given the known costs and inter-rater reliability concerns with multiple raters in several settings, is for a biomechanical measure that reliably approximates at least some wandering parameters. One aim of our current study is to validate a range of mechanical devices for their utility in estimating frequency and total time in motion. However, there is yet no meter developed for capturing variations among any types or patterns of wandering. While our work has concentrated on the use of patterns (Martino-Salzman et al., 1991) as an organizer, there are other typologies which remain untested, for example, those developed by Hussian and Davis (1985) and Hope et al. (1994). The further testing and refining of mechanical measures, within a variety of typologies, would assist in moving us closer to understanding how best to quantify the phenomenon.

Studies of wandering tend to utilize small samples. While this issue relates to difficulties in the recruitment of aged subjects generally, and the frail elderly with dementia specifically, the result is that the overall pool of subjects about whom we have information remains small. The protocols for subject selection have tended to be loose, meaning that subject comparison across studies is limited and generalization is difficult, if not impossible. Refinement of protocols for subject selection using more sophisticated medical diagnosis parameters and neuropsychological testing, for example, the NINCDS-ADRDA (McKhann et al., 1984) for AD or for MID would result in more homogenous samples about which more robust generalizations could be made than those currently possible. Studies with larger and random samples will also facilitate breakdown of data into diagnostic groups.

To date we have few data describing the stability and normal variation for any parameter of wandering over time. Thus, studies incorporating baseline and repeated measures would assist in future methodological decision-making. In studies designed to evaluate episode frequency or time in motion, it is critical that both the period of intervention is in effect, as well as the distribution of wandering over the rest of a 24 hour period is determined. In other words, did the intervention change the volume or the distribution of wandering? Without such clarity, the overall utility of interventions cannot be meaningfully interpreted in terms of clinical management.

7.17.9.2 Etiologic Factors

Research to date has proffered multiple explanatory hypotheses and employed a wide variety of research paradigms, none of which adequately explain the phenomenon. Thus, there is a need for well-controlled studies to test competing hypotheses or to evaluate the relative contribution of various putative etiologies for explaining wandering. While a number of potential etiologies have been suggested, measurement poses a problem in evaluating some of these in persons with severe dementia. For example, while proxy measures of circadian rhythm disturbance such as sleep and body temperature are reasonable, it is not directly possible to measure the function of the suprachiasmatic nucleus given current technology. Further exploration of the role of previous personality in disturbing behaviors associated with dementia is indicated, as demonstrated by the results of research utilizing the NEO five-factor personality inventory (Kolanowski, Strand, & Whall, 1997; Thomas, 1997). If, as suggested, the basic features of an individual's personality are preserved predominantly intact in AD, patterns of motor activity integral to the expression of personality may also be preserved.

While a number of proximal factors thought to be associated with wandering have been proposed in the NDB model (Algase et al., 1996), the extent of the impact of individual and amalgamated proximal factors in either moderating or exacerbating wandering is not known. Likewise, the conditions under which wandering can be altered have not been elucidated as yet. A number of studies have recognized wandering as influenced by a variety of environmental factors, yet studies that link type and amount of wandering to particular outcomes are few. Studies that use a theoretical perspective to isolate and manipulate individual or conceptually-grouped environmental factors are needed.

Looking more broadly in relation to other or related behavioral issues in dementia, an overlap and lack of clarity persists in current understandings of restlessness, agitation, wandering, and confusion. Initial concept clarification, followed by further development, testing, and refinement of measures for each concept in a severely impaired population is necessary. Existing measures for agitation, for example, do not adequately capture the frequency and intensity of the behavior in many wanderers. Likewise, measures for evaluating physiological need states such as thirst, hunger, fatigue, and elimination in the cognitively impaired require development.

Few tests for assessing areas of specific cognitive deficits in individuals with severe impairments have been developed and most are quite dependent on language skills. The results of such testing, especially in combination with neuroimaging and behavioral measures, may prove invaluable in further understanding the nature and origin of intellectual deficits and the impact of specific deficits on wandering. In studies that have attempted to examine specific aspects of cognitive function in relation to wandering, such as by Liu et al. (1991), most testing was done in grasping space (space within one's reach). Yet we do not know how tests of visual-spatial ability done in grasping space correspond with actual functioning in large-scale space.

7.17.9.3 Intervention Studies

While the clinical need for such studies is appreciated, the majority of intervention studies designed to impact wandering behavior are both premature and atheoretical. It is unclear in many studies what dimension of wandering the researcher is trying to manipulate. In many studies, wandering is only one of multiple behaviors examined and is not the single dependent variable of interest. Wandering is considered in an homogenous cluster with other behaviors such as agitation and elopement. Focusing research specifically on the phenomenon of wandering isolates the behavior and assists in clarity of definition. Intervention studies would also be more useful if derived from theory or based on putative etiologies for wandering.

Case study designs are an underutilized strategy in wandering research. Case study research has the advantage of small sample size, a particular advantage when working with a fragile and difficult-to-recruit population. Case studies can yield rich and complex descriptive data. Those designs using multiple cases with theoretically-structured embedded experiments afford generalization to theoretical propositions based on replication logic (Yin, 1989). Such replication offers compelling support for the initial set of propositions and the observations for each case are considered independent, that is, the intervention for one case does not affect the intervention for the other cases. More systematic use of case studies to accomplish descriptive and explanatory work and to provide a preliminary test of interventions is recommended.

In addition, certain institutional level studies would also be useful to answer questions such as these: (i) Are there characteristics of social environments that affect wandering? (ii) Does a match between the personality of the wanderer and that of the staff impact the behavior? (iii) Do certain institutional policies or physical design elements actually induce or exacerbate wandering?

The relative risk of undesirable outcomes associated with specific aspects or parameters of wandering behavior requires exploration. Which kinds and amounts of wandering predict falls? Or elopements? Is there a threshold at which wandering escalates weight loss? While not exhaustive, answers to these questions and response to issues raised above will do much to advance our understanding of wandering and the development of rational, humane, and effective care for the afflicted.

7.17.10 SUMMARY

This chapter has aimed to present a comprehensive overview of the state of the science on wandering behavior and its implications for research and clinical practice. Review of definitions and typologies revealed a lack of standardization and few attempts of researchers to build on the work of others. Thus, knowledge is disjointed and the ability to interpret results and generalize findings is hampered. Although some estimates of prevalence and incidence have been reported, their value is questionable for the same reasons.

A profile of the cognitively impaired person who may be prone to wandering was derived from a summary of the characteristics of wanderers across a number of studies. In short, neither age, gender, nor medical basis for dementia appears to differentiate wanderers from other cognitively impaired persons. However, differences in the characteristics of wandering behavior among these subgroups is unknown. In general, wanderers have better mobility and worse cognitive impairment on global measures than nonwandering counterparts. Language and visual-spatial skills are particularly affected. Long-standing active behavior patterns and an outgoing personality may also characterize the wanderer.

In an effort to clarify and advance conceptualizations of wandering, the behavior was differentiated from its outcomes. The following putative outcomes were isolated: falls, elopements, weight loss, sleep disturbance and fatigue, improved physical stamina, and worsened social and cognitive skills.

Several possible etiologies for wandering were proposed and the evidence in support of each were summarized. Disturbances in visual-spatial ability and evidence of parietal lobe damage (particularly, the right parietal lobe, which is associated with spatial learning) were offered to support the hypothesis that wandering is a reflection of spatial disorientation. Hippocampal damage, perseveration, and neurotransmitter imbalances involving acetylcholine and dopamine were suggested as the basis for wandering characterized as increased movement. Deterioration of the suprachiasmatic nucleus and the fractured sleep and activity patterns that accompany it provided the rationale for viewing night-time wandering as a reflection of circadian rhythm disruption. While less evidence exists to support the roles of affect and needs in explaining wandering, they cannot be eliminated as etiologies based on existing knowledge.

Behavior mapping, counting and timing strategies, and activity monitoring devices were reviewed for their value in assessing wandering behavior. Multiple assessment techniques for related factors, such as sensory abilities, personal patterns and preferences, and physical discomfort, and for outcomes were discussed.

A range of tested and untested approaches to intervention were evaluated. Few proven and effective techniques were found. Exercise may mitigate night-time wandering, but further study is needed. The effectiveness of cueing and lighting have not been demonstrated. Social interaction approaches are promising, but also require further study before specific protocols can be advocated. Drug therapy is the mainstay of treatment, but effects are global rather than specifically targeted to wandering and multiple issues can arise with the use of medications.

Techniques for managing the elopement attempts were also reviewed. Behavior modification can be effective if conditioned stimuli are continuously applied. However, replication and further evaluation of useful protocols is needed. Two types of camouflage have been evaluated for reducing exit attempts. Results are conflicting, but approaches based on visual agnosia may prove effective if strategies to overcome learning effects are incorporated. A range of perimeter control devices was also discussed but lack of data prevents development of clear recommendations at this time. Several additional strategies such as wandering paths and tracks, activities programming, and use of restraints (both physical and chemical) were also considered. While they are popular in clinical settings, their efficacy and value are unsubstantiated.

Finally, suggestions for further research were offered in the areas of definition and measurement, explanation, and intervention.

ACKNOWLEDGMENTS

The author is grateful for the assistance of Elizabeth R. A. Beattie, Ph.D., Senior Lecturer at James Cook University, Queensland, Australia, for her assistance in the initial draft of sections on assessment and intervention.

7.17.11 REFERENCES

Albert, S. M. (1992). The nature of wandering in dementia: A Guttman scaling analysis of an empirical classification scheme. *International Journal of Geriatric Psychiatry, 7,* 783–787.

Algase, D. (1988). Cognitive and social discriminants of wandering among cognitively-impaired nursing home residents. Unpublished doctoral dissertation, Case Western Reserve University, Cleveland.

Algase, D. (1992a). Cognitive discriminants of wandering among nursing home residents. *Nursing Research, 41,* 78–81.

Algase, D. (1992b). A century of progress: Today's strategies for responding to wandering behavior. *Journal of Gerontological Nursing, 18,* 28–34.

Algase, D. (1997a). Impact of light levels on wandering. Unpublished data.

Algase, D. (1997b). Daily distributions of wandering. Unpublished data.

Algase, D., Beattie, E., Kupferschmid, B., & Beel-Bates, C. (1997). Estimates of stability of daily wandering behavior among cognitively-impaired long-term care residents. *Nursing Research, 46,* 172–178.

Algase, D., Beattie, E., Kupferschmid, B., & Therrien, B. (1997). Cognitive impairment and agitation as predictors of rhythmic parameters and patterns of wandering: A pilot study, unpublished data.

Algase, D., Beck, C., Kolanowski, A., Whall, A., Berent, S., Richards, K., & Beattie, E. (1996). Need-driven dementia compromised behavior: An alternative view of disruptive behavior. *American Journal of Alzheimer's Disease, 11,* 10–19.

Algase, D., Beel-Bates, C., & Kupferschmid, B. (1995). Wandering rhythms and patterns of cognitively-impaired elderly. Unpublished manuscript.

Algase, D., & Cheng, J. (1992a). *Wandering as a rhythm* [abstract]. In Proceedings of the 16th Annual Midwest Nursing Research Society Conference. Indianapolis, IN: Midwest Nursing Research Society.

Algase, D., & Cheng, J. (1992b). Antecedent and consequent activity as pacers for wandering cycles. *The Gerontologist* (Program Abstracts), *31,* 144.

Algase, D., & Struble, L. (1992). Wandering: What, why, and how? In K. Buckwalter (Ed.), *Geriatric mental health nursing: Current and future challenges* (pp. 61–74). Thorofare, NJ: Slack.

Algase, D., & Tsai, J. (1991). Wandering as rhythm. *The Gerontologist* (Program Abstracts), *30,* 140.

Arno, S., & Frank, D. (1994). A group for "wandering" institutionalized clients with primary degenerative dementia. *Perspectives in Psychiatric Care, 30,* 13–16.

Ballard, C. G., Mohan, R. N. C., Bannister, C., Handy, S., & Patel, A. (1991). Wandering in dementia sufferers. *International Journal of Geriatric Psychiatry, 6,* 611–614.

Barbieri, E. (1983). Patient falls are not patient accidents. *Journal of Gerontological Nursing, 9,* 165–173.

Barnes, R., Veith, R., Okimoto, J., Raskind, M., & Gumbrecht, G. (1982). Efficacy of antipsychotic medications in behaviorally disturbed dementia patients. *American Journal of Psychiatry, 139,* 1170–1174.

Beardsley, R. S., Larson, D. B., Lyons, J. S., Gottlieb, G. L., Rabins, R., & Rovner, B. W. (1989). Health services research in nursing homes: A systematic review of three clinical geriatric journals. *Journal of Gerontology, 44,* M30–M35.

Beattie, E. R. A. (1996). *Wandering and agitation behavior in severely cognitively-impaired nursing home residents: The impact of nurse–resident communication style.* Townsville, Australia: James Cook University.

Berg, R., & Cassels, J. (Eds.) (1990). Falls in older persons. Risk factors and prevention. In *The second fifty years: promoting health and preventing disability* (pp. 263–298). Washington, DC: National Academy Press.

Bliwise, D. L. (1994). What is sundowning? *Journal of the American Geriatrics Society, 42,* 1009-1011.

Bliwise, D. L., Carol, J. S., Lee, K. A., Nekich, J. C., & Dement, W. C. (1993). Sleep and "sundowning" in nursing home patients with dementia. *Psychiatry Research, 48,* 277–292.

Brock, M. A. (1991). Chronobiology and aging. *Journal of the American Geriatrics Society, 39,* 74–91.

Brody, E., Kleban, M. & Moss, M., & Kleban, F. (1984). Predictors of falls among institutionalized females with Alzheimer's disease. *Journal of the American Geriatrics Society, 32,* 877–882.

Brungardt, G. S. (1994). Patient restraints: New guidelines for a less restrictive approach. *Geriatrics, 49,* 43–50.

Buchner, D., & Larson, E. (1987). Falls and fractures in patients with Alzheimers type dementia. *Journal of the American Medical Association, 257,* 1492–1495.

Burns, A., Jacoby, R., & Levy, R. (1990). Psychiatric phenomena in Alzheimer's disease. IV: Disorders of behavior. *British Journal of Psychiatry, 157,* 86–94.

Butler, J. (1990). *The anatomy of a critical wandering episode.* Paper presented at the Arkansas Gerontological Society, Little Rock, AK.

Butler, J. P., & Barnett, C. A. (1991). Window of wandering. *Geriatric Nursing, 12,* 226–227.

Campbell, A., Rienken, J., Allan, B., & Martinez, G. (1981). Falls in old age: A study of frequency and related clinical factors. *Age and Ageing, 10,* 264–270.

Cancro, R. (1968). Elopements from the C. F. Menninger Memorial Hospital. *Bulletin Menninger Clinic, 32,* 228–238.

Cason, C. L., & Grissom, N. (1994). *Distraction as an intervention for short-term pain.* Intramural Grant Final Report. University of Arkansas for Medical Sciences, College of Nursing, Little Rock, AK.

Chafetz, P. K. (1990). Two dimensional grid is ineffective against demented patients' exiting through glass doors. *Psychology and Aging, 5,* 146–147.

Chui, H. C., Mortimer, J. A., Slager, U., Zarow, C., Bondareff, W., & Webster, D. D. (1986). Pathologic correlates of dementia in Parkinson's disease. *Archives of Neurology, 43,* 991–995.

Cleary, T. A., Clamon, C., Price, M., & Shullaw, G. (1988). A reduced stimulation unit: Effects in patients with Alzheimer's disease and related disorders. *The Gerontologist, 28,* 511–514.

Cohen-Mansfield, J., & Marx, M. S. (1990). Do past experiences predict agitation in nursing home residents? *International Journal of Aging and Human Development, 28,* 285–294.

Cohen-Mansfield, J., & Werner, P. (1985). Environmental influences on agitation: An integrative summary of an observational study. *The American Journal of Alzheimer's Care and Related Disorders and Research, 10,* 32–39.

Cohen-Mansfield, J., Werner, P., & Marx, M. S. (1989). An observational study of agitation in agitated nursing home residents. *International Psychogeriatrics, 1,* 153–165.

Cohen-Mansfield, J., Werner, P., Marx, M. S., & Freedman, L. (1991). Two studies of pacing in the nursing home. *Journal of Gerontology: Medical Sciences, 46,* M77–M83.

Cook, P., Exton-Smith, A., Brocklehurst, J., & Lampert-Barber, S. (1982). Fractured femurs, falls and bone disorders. *Journal of the Royal College of Physicians London, 16,* 45–49.

Cooke, D. A., Algase, D. A., & Terpenning, M. (1993). *Signposts and the institutionalized elderly: Effectiveness and principles of design.* Unpublished paper.

Coons, D. H. (1988). Wandering. *The American Journal of Alzheimer's Care and Related Disorders & Research, 3,* 31–36.

Cornbleth, T. (1977). Effects of a protected hospital ward area on wandering and non-wandering geriatric patients. *Journal of Gerontology, 32,* 573–577.

Dastoor, D. P., Norton, S., Boillat, J., Minty, J., Papadoupoulou, F., & Mullzur, H. F. (1975). A psychogeriatric assessment program. 1. Social functioning and ward behavior. *Journal of the American Geriatrics Society, 23,* 465–471.

Dawson, P., & Reid, D. W. (1987). Behavioral dimensions of patients at risk of wandering. *The Gerontologist, 27,* 104–107.

deLeon, M. J., Potegal, M., & Gurland, B. (1984). Wandering and parietal lobe signs in senile dementia of Alzheimer's type. *Neuropsychobiology, 11,* 155–157.

Devanand, D. P., & Levy, S. R. (1995). Neuroleptic treatment of agitation and psychosis in dementia. *Journal of Geriatric Psychiatry and Neurology, 8,* S518–S524.

Dickinson, J. I., McLain-Kark, J., & Marshall-Baker, A. (1995). The effects of visual barriers on exiting behavior in a dementia care unit. *The Gerontologist, 35,* 127–130.

Donat, D. C. (1984). Modifying wandering behavior: A case study. *Clinical Gerontologist, 3,* 41–43.

Druckenbrod, R. W., Rosen, J. & Cluxton, R. J. Jr. (1993). As-needed dosing of antipsychotic drugs: Limitations and guidelines for use in the elderly agitated patient. *Annals of Pharmacotherapy, 27,* 645–648.

Ebersole, P., & Hess, P. (1990). *Toward healthy aging: Human needs and nurses response.* St. Louis, MO: Mosby.

Eisdorfer, C., & Faan, W. (1982). Psychotropic drug side effects in the elderly. In *Treatment of psychopathology in the aging* (p. 211). New York: Springer.

Evans, L. (1987). Sundown syndrome in institutionalized elderly. *Journal of the American Geriatrics Society, 35,* 101–108.

Evans, L., & Strumpf, N. (1989). Tying down the elderly: A review of the literature on physical restraints. *Journal of the American Geriatrics Society, 37,* 65–74.

Fayden, A. I., & Townsend, J. J. (1976). Myoclonus in Alzheimer's disease. A confusing sign. *Archives of Neurology, 33,* 278–280.

Fairburn, C. G., & Hope, R. A. (1988). Changes in behaviour in dementia: A neglected research area, *British Journal of Psychiatry, 152,* 406–407.

Fischer, P., Marterer, A., & Danielczyk, W. (1990). Right–left disorientation in dementia of the Alzheimer's type. *Neurology, 40,* 1619–1620.

Foerster, J. (1981). A study of falls: The elderly nursing home resident. *Journal of New York State Nurses Association, 12,* 9–17.

Folmar, S., & Wilson, H. (1989). Social behavior and physical restraints. *The Gerontologist, 29,* 650–653.

Folstein, J., Folstein, S., & McHugh, P. R. (1975). " Mini-mental state". A practical method for grading the cognitive state of patients for the clinician. *Journal of Psychiatric Research, 12,* 189–198.

Foxwell, L. (1993). Risk management decreases incidence of falls, wandering. *Provider, 14,* 51.

Francese, T., Sorrell, J., & Butler, F. R. (1997). The effects of regular exercise on muscle strength and functional abilities of late stage Alzheimer's residents. *American Journal of Alzheimer's Disease, 12,* 122–127.

Fuld, P. A., Katzman, R., Davies, P., & Terry, R. D. (1982). Intrusions as a sign of Alzheimer's dementia: Chemical and pathological verification. *Annals of Neurology, 11,* 155–159.

Gaffney, J. (1986). Toward a less restrictive environment. *Geriatric Nursing, 7,* 94–95.

Gallo, J., Reichel, W., & Andersen, L. M. (1995). *Handbook of geriatric assessment* (2nd ed.). Gaisthersburg, MD: Aspen.

Gerdner, L., & Swanson, E. (1993). Effects of individualized music on confused and agitated elderly patients. *Archives of Psychiatric Nursing, 7,* 284–291.

Gleason, R. P., & Schneider, L. S. (1990). Carbamazepine treatment of agitation in Alzheimer's outpatients refractory to neuroleptics. *Journal of Clinical Psychiatry, 51,* 115–118.

Goldberg, E. (1986). Varieties of perseveration: A comparison of two taxonomies. *Journal of Clinical and Experimental Neuropsychology, 8,* 710–726.

Goldsmith, S. M., Hoeffer, B., & Rader, J. (1995). Problematic wandering behavior in the cognitively-impaired elderly: A single-subjected case study. *Journal of Psychosocial Nursing and Mental Health Services, 33,* 6–12.

Goldsten, L., Canavan, A., & Polkey, C. (1989). Cognitive mapping after unilateral temporal lobectomy. *Neuropsychologia, 27,* 167–177.

Greenblatt, D. J., Divoll, M., Abernethy, D. R., Harmatz,

J. S., & Shader, R. I. (1982). Antipyrine kinetics in the elderly: Prediction of age-related changes in benzodiazepine oxidizing capacity. *Journal of Pharmacol Expimental Therapeutics, 220*, 120–126.

Greene, J., Smith, R., Gardiner, M., & Timbury, G. C. (1982). Measuring behavioural disturbance of elderly demented patients in the community and its effects on relatives: A factor analytic study. *Age & Ageing, 11*, 121–126.

Guilleminault, C., Kushida, C., & Leger, D. (1995). Forensic sleep medicine and nocturnal wandering. *Sleep, 18*, 721–723.

Guilleminault, C., Moscovitch, A., & Leger, D. (1995). Forensic sleep medicine: Nocturnal wandering and violence. *Sleep, 18*, 740–748.

Guttman, L. L. (1974). The basis for scalogram analysis. In G. M. Maranell (Ed.), *Scaling: A sourcebook for behavioral scientists* (pp. 43–45). Chicago: Aldine.

Halgren, E. (1991). Firing of human hippocampal units in relation to voluntary movements. *Hippocampus, 1*, 153–162.

Halgren, E., Squires, N. K., Wilson, C. L., Rohrbaugh, J. W., Babb, T. L., & Crandall, P.H. (1980). Endogenous potentials generated in the human hippocampal formation and amygdala by infrequent events. *Science, 210*, 803–805.

Hall, G. R., & Buckwalter, K. C. (1987). Progressively lowered stress threshold: A conceptual model for care of adults with Alzheimer's Disease. *Archives of Psychiatric Nursing, 1*, 399–406.

Hamilton, C. (1993). *The use of tape patterns as an alternative method for controlling wanderers' exiting behavior in a dementia care unit.* Unpublished master's thesis, Virginia Polytechnic Institute and State University.

Henderson, J. N. (1993–4). Protecting the "frustrated eloper". *Journal of Long Term Care Administration, 21*, 13–15.

Henderson, V., Mack, W., & Williams, B. W. (1989). Spatial disorientation in Alzheimer's Disease. *Archives of Neurology, 46*, 391–394.

Heron, J. (1976). *Six-category intervention analysis.* London: Croom-Helm.

Heslin, K., Towers, J., Leckie, C., Thornton-Lawrence, H., Perkin, K., Jaques, M., Mullin, J., & Wick, L. (1992). Managing falls: Identifying population-specific risk factors and prevention strategies. In S. Funk, E. Tornquist, M. Champagne, L. Copp, & R. Wiese (Eds.), *Key aspects of elder care: managing falls, incontinence and cognitive impairment* (pp. 70–88). New York: Springer.

Hewawasam, L. (1996). Floor patterns limit wandering of people with Alzheimer's. *Nursing Times, 92*, 41–44

Hiatt, L. G. (1980). The happy wanderer. *Nursing Homes, 29*, 27–31.

Hogue, C. (1984). Falls and mobility in later life: An ecological model. *Journal of the American Geriatrics Society, 32*, 858–861.

Hogue, C., Studenski, S., & Duncan, P. (1990). The first step in preventing falls. In S. Funk, E. Tornquist, M. Champagne, L. Copp, & R. Wiese (Eds.), *Key aspects of recovery: Improving nutrition, rest and mobility* (pp. 275–280). New York: Springer.

Holden, J., & Therrien, B. (1993). Cue familiarity reduces spatial disorientation following hippocampal damage. *Nursing Research, 42*, 338–343.

Honigfeld, G., Gillis, R. D., & Klett, C. J. (1966). NOSIE-30: A treatment sensitive ward behavior scale. *Psychological Reports, 19*, 180–182.

Hope, T., & Fairburn, C. G. (1990). The nature of wandering dementia: A community based study. *International Journal of Geriatric Psychiatry, 5*, 239–245.

Hope, T., & Fairburn, C. G. (1992). The Present Behavioral Examination (PBE): The development of an interview to measure current behavioral abnormalities. *Psychological Medicine, 22*, 223–230.

Hope, T., Tilling, K. M., Gedling, K., Keene, J. M., Cooper, S. A., & Fairburn, C. G. (1994). The structure of wandering in dementia. *International Journal of Geriatric Psychiatry, 9*, 149–155.

Hurley, A. C., Volicer, B., Hanrahan, P. A., Houde, S., & Volicer, L. (1992). Assessment of discomfort in advanced Alzheimer's patients. *Research in Nursing and Health, 15*, 369–377.

Hussian, R.A. (1981). Psychotherapeutic intervention: Organic mental disorders. *In geriatric psychology: A behavioral perspective* (chap. 7, pp. 123–151). New York: Van Nostrand Reinhold.

Hussian, R. A. (1982). Stimulus control in the modification of problematic behavior in elderly institutionalized patients. *International Journal of Behavioral Geriatrics, 1*, 33–40.

Hussian, R. A., & Brown, D. C. (1987). Use of two dimensional grid patterns to limit hazardous ambulation in demented patients. *Journal of Gerontology, 42*, 558–560.

Hussian, R. A., & Davis, R. L. (1985). *Responsive care behavioral interventions with elderly persons.* Champaign, IL: Research Press.

Jackson, M. E., Drugovich, M. L., Fretwell, M. D., Spector, W. D., Sternberg, J., & Rosenstein, R. B. (1989). Pervalence and correlates of disruptive behavior in the nursing home. *Journal of Aging and Health, 1*, 349–369.

Janken, J., Reynolds, B., & Swiech, K. (1986). Patient falls in the acute care setting: Identifying risk factors. *Nursing Research, 35*, 215–219.

Jellinger, K. (1987). Neuropathological substrates of Alzheimer's disease and Parkinson's disease. *Journal of Neural Transmittors Supplement, 24*, 109–129.

Johnson, C. L., & Grant, L. A. (1985). *The nursing home in American society.* Baltimore: Johns Hopkins University Press.

Kalchthaler, T., Bascon, R., & Quintos, V. (1978). Falls in the institutionalized elderly. *Journal of the American Geriatrics Society, 26*, 424–428.

Kamei, S., Oishi, M., & Takasu, T. (1996). Evaluation of fasudil hydrochloride treatment for wandering symptoms in cerebrovascular dementia with 31P-magnetic resonance spectroscopy and Xe-computed tomography. *Clinical Neuropharmocology, 19*, 428–438.

Kanten, D., Mulrow, C., Gerety, M., Lichenstein, M., Aguilar, C., & Cornell, J. (1993). Falls: An examination of three reporting methods in nursing homes. *Journal of the American Geriatrics Society, 41*, 662–666.

Kapp, M. (1986). Preventing malpractice suits in long-term care facilities. *Quality Review Bulletin, 12*, 109–113.

Kippenbrock, T., & Soja, M. (1993). Preventing falls in the elderly: Interviewing patients who have fallen. *Geriatric Nursing, 14*, 205–209.

Kolanowski, A. M., Strand, G., & Whall, A. (1997). A pilot study of the relation of premorbid characteristics to behavior in dementia. *Journal of Gerontological Nursing, 23*, 21–30.

Koller, W. C., Wilson, R. S. , Glatt, S. L., & Fox, J. H. (1984). Motor signs are infrequent in dementia of the Alzheimer type. *Annals of Neurology, 16*, 514–516.

Kovach, C., Weisman, G., Chaudhury, H., & Calkins, M. (1997). Impacts of a therapeutic environment for dementia care. *American Journal of Alzheimer's Disease, 12*, 99–110.

Kushida, C. A., Clerk, A. A., Kirsch, C. M., Hotson, J. R., & Guilleminault, C. (1995). Prolonged confusion and nocturnal wandering arising from NREM and REM sleep: A case report. *Sleep, 18*, 757–764.

Lanceley, A. (1985). Use of controlling language in the

rehabilitation of the elderly. *Journal of Advanced Nursing, 10,* 125–135.

LaPorte, R. E., Black-Sandler, R., Cauley, J. A., Link, M., Bayles, C., & Marks, B. (1983). The assessment of physical activity in older women: Analysis of the interrelationship of activity monitoring, activity surveys, and caloric intake. *Journal of Gerontology, 38,* 394–397.

LaPorte, R. E., Cauley, B., Kinsey, C., Corbett, W., Robertson, R., Black-Sandler, R., Kuller. L., & Falkel, J. (1982). The epidemiology of physical activity in children, college students, middle-aged men, menopausal females and monkeys. *Journal of Chronic Diseases, 35,* 787–795.

LaPorte, R. E., Kuller, L. H., Kupfer, D. J., McPartland, R. J., Matthews, G., & Caspersen, C. (1979). An objective measure of physical activity for epidemiological research, *American Journal of Epidemiology, 109,* 158–167.

Leach, E. (1985). Safeguarding wandering patients. *Health Law Canada, 6,* 37–44.

Leibovici, A., & Tariot, P. N. (1988). Agitation associated with dementia: A systematic pproach to treatment. *Psychopharmacological Bulletin, 24,* 49–53.

Lewin, K. (1935). *A dynamic theory of personality: Selected papers by Kurt Lewin.* New York: McGraw-Hill.

Liu, L., Gauthier, L., & Gauthier, S. (1991). Spatial disorientation in persons with early senile dementia of the Alzheimer type. *American Journal of Occupational Therapy, 45,* 67–74.

Louis, M (1993). Falls and causes. *Journal of Gerontological Nursing, 9,* 143–156.

Lovell, B. B., Ancoli-Israel, S., & Gevirtz, R. (1995). Effect of bright light treatment on agitated behavior in institutionalized elderly subjects. *Psychiatry Research, 57,* 7–12.

Madson, J. (1990). *The development of a device to measure wandering in persons with senile dementia.* Unpublished master's thesis. University of Dubuque, Iowa.

Mardsen, C. D., Milson, J., Parkes, J. D., Pycock, C., & Tarsy, D. (1975). Proceedings: The effect of cholinergic and anticholinergic drugs on rotational behaviour in mice with destruction of one nigrostriatal pathway. *Journal of Physiology (London), 249,* 64P–65P.

Marley, M. L. (1982). *Organic brain pathology and Bender-Gestalt Test: A differential diagnostic scoring system.* New York: Grune & Stratton.

Martino-Saltzman, D., Blasch, B. B., Morris, R. D., & McNeal, L. W. (1991). Travel behavior of nursing home residents perceived as wanderers and nonwanderers. *The Gerontologist, 31,* 666–672.

May, C. (1993). Subjectivity and culpability in the constitution of nurse–patient relationships. *International Journal of Nursing Studies, 30,* 181–192.

Mayer, R., & Darby, S. (1991). Does a mirror deter wandering in demented older people? *International Journal of Geriatric Psychiatry, 6,* 607–609.

McGrowder-Lin, R., & Bhatt, A. (1988). A wanderer's lounge program for nursing home residents with Alzheimer's disease. *The Gerontologist, 28,* 607–609.

McKhann, G., Drachman, D., Folstein, M., Katz, R., Price, D., & Stadlan, E. M. (1984). Report of the NINCDS-ADRDA work group under the auspices of department of human and health services task force of Alzheimer's disease. *Neurology, 34,* 939–944.

Meguro, K., Yamaguchi, S., Yamazaki, H., Itoh, M., Yamaguchi, T., Matsui, H., & Sasaki, H. (1996). Cortical glucose metabolism in psychiatric wandering patients with vascular dementia. *Psychiatric Research Neuroimaging, 67,* 71–80.

Mellow, A. M., Solano-Lopez, C., & Davis, S. (1993). Sodium valproate in the treatment of behavioral disturbance in dementia. *Journal of Geriatric Psychiatry and Neurology, 6,* 205–209.

Mendez, M. F., Mendez, M. A., Martin, R., Smyth, K. A., & Whitehouse, P. J. (1990). Complex visual disturbances in Alzheimer's disease. *Neurology, 40,* 439–443.

Michel, K., & Kolakowska, T. (1981). A survey of prescribing psychotropic drugs in two psychiatric hospitals. *British Journal of Psychiatry, 138,* 217–221.

Milke, D. (1989). Comparisons of caregivers evaluations to systematic observations of wanderers. *The Gerontologist, 29,* 143A. Program for the 42nd Annual Scientific Meeting, Minneapolis, MN.

Miller, M. (1975). Iatrogenic and nurisgenic effects of prolonged immobilization of the ill aged. *Journal of the American Geriatrics Society, 23,* 360–369.

Miller, J. (1976). Control of the ambulatory senile. *Concern in Care of the Aging, 2,* 34–37.

Mintzer, J. E., Lewis, L., Pennypaker, L., Simpson, W., Bachman, D., Wohlreich, G., Meeks, A., Hunt, S., & Samson, W. (1993). Behavioral Intensive Care Unit (BICU): A new concept in the management of acute agitated behavior in elderly demented patients. *The Gerontologist, 33,* 801–806.

Mohr, E., Litvan, I., Williams, J., Fedio, P., & Chase, T. (1990). Selective deficits in Alzheimer and Parkinsonian dementia: Visuospatial function. *Canadian Journal of Neurological Sciences, 17,* 292–297.

Molsa, P. K., Martilla, R., J., & Rinne, U. K. (1984). Extrapyramidal signs in Alzheimer's disease. *Neurology, 34,* 1114–1116.

Monsour, N., & Robb, S. (1982). Wandering behavior in old age: A psychosocial study. *Social Work, 27,* 411–416.

Morgenson, G., & Nielsen, M. (1984). A study of the contribution of hippocampal- accumbens-subpallidal projections to locomotor activity. *Behavioral and Neural Biology, 42,* 38–51.

Morino, M. (1989). Preventing patient elopement at an outpatient Alzheimer's facility. *Contemporary Longterm Care, 12,* 84–86.

Morris, E., & Isaacs, B. (1980). The prevention of falls in a geriatric hospital. *Age and Ageing, 9,* 181–185.

Morrison, J., Crinklaw-Wiancko, D., King, D., Thibeault, S., & Wells, D. L. (1987). Formulating a restraint use policy. *Journal of Nursing Administration, 17,* 39–42.

Morse, J., Tylko, S., & Dixon, H. (1985). The patient who falls—and falls again: Defining the aged at risk. *Journal of Gerontological Nursing, 11,* 15–18.

Morse, J., Tylko, S., & Dixon, H. (1987). Characteristics of the fall-prone patient. *The Gerontologist, 27,* 516–522.

Muller, R. U., & Kubie, J. L. (1989). The firing of hippocampal place cells predicts the future position of freely moving rats. *Journal of Neuroscience, 9,* 4101–4110.

Mulrooney, C. (1993–4). Controlling exposure and exposing control. *Journal of Long Term Care Administration, 21,* 14–16.

Murray, H. A. (1938). *Explorations in personality.* New York: Oxford University Press.

Murray, J., Marquardt, T. P., Richardson, A., & Nalty, D. (1984). Differential diagnosis of aphasia and dementia from aphasia test battery scores. *Journal of Neurological Communication Disorders, 1,* 33–39.

Nadel, L. (1991). The hippocampus and space revisited. *Hippocampus, 1,* 221–229.

Namazi, K. H., Rosner, T. T., & Calkins, M. P. (1989). Visual barriers to prevent ambulatory Alzheimer's patients from exiting through an emergency doors. *The Gerontologist, 29,* 699–702.

National Center for Health Statistics (1979). *The national nursing home survey: 1977 summary for the United States: Vital and health statistics (1979).* Hyatsville, MD: Author.

Negley, E., Molla, P. M., & Obenchain, J. (1990). No exit: The effects of an electronic security system on confused patients. *Journal of Gerontological Nursing, 16,* 21–25.

Nevitt, M., Cummins, S., Kidd, S., & Black, D. (1989). Risk factors for recurrent nonsyncopal falls: A prospective study. *Journal of the American Medical Association, 261*, 2663–2668.

OBRA (Omnibus Budget Reconciliation Act) (1987). US Congress. Public Law 101–508.

Okawa, M., Mishima, K., Shimizu, T., Iijuma, S., Hishikawa, Y., Hozumi, S., & Hori, H. (1989). Sleep–waking rhythm disorders and their phototherapy in elderly patients with dementia. *Japanese Journal of Psychiatry and Neurology, 43*, 293–295.

Overstall, P. (1978). Falls in the elderly—epidemiology, aetiology and management. In B. Isaacs (Ed.), *Recent advances in geriatric medicine*. London: Churchill-Livingstone.

Pankratz, L., & Jackson, J. (1994). Habitually wandering patients. *New England Journal of Medicine, 331*, 1752–1755.

Pauszek, M. E. (1991). Propranolol for treatment of agitation in senile dementia. *Indiana Medicine, 84*, 16–17 .

Pinner, E., & Rich, C. L. (1988). Effects of trazodone on aggressive behavior in seven patients with organic mental disorders. *American Journal of Psychiatry, 145*, 1295–1296.

Plazzi, G., Tinuper, P., Montagna, P., Provini, F., & Lugaresi, E. (1995). Epileptic nocturnal wanderings. *Sleep, 18*, 749–756.

Preston, G. C., Broks, P., Traub, M., Ward, C., Poppleton, P., & Stahl, S. M. (1988). Effects of lorazepam on memory, attention, and sedation in man. *Psychoparmalogical Bulletin, 95*, 208–215.

Prien, R. F., Haber, E., & Caffey, D. (1985). Research overview of drug therapy in recurrent and chronic depression. *Advanced Biochemical Psychopharmacology, 40*, 121–130.

Prinz, P. N., Peskind, E. R., Vitaliano, P. P., Raskind, M. A., Eisdorfer, C., Zemcuznikov, N., & Gerber, C. J. (1982). Changes in the sleep and waking EEGS of nondemented and demented elderly subjects. *Journal of American Geriatric Society, 30*, 86–94.

Prinz, P. N., Vitaliano, P. P., Vitiello, M. V., Bokan, J., Raskind, M., Peskind, E., & Gerber, C. (1982). Sleep, EEG and mental function changes in senile dementia of the Alzheimer's type. *Neurobiology of Aging, 3*, 361–370.

Rabins, P. V., Mace, N. L., & Lucas, M. J. (1982). The impact of dementia on the family. *Journal of the American Medical Association, 248*, 333–335.

Rader, J. (1987). A comprehensive approach to problem wandering. *The Gerontologist 27*, 756–760.

Rader, J., Doan, J., & Schwab, M. (1985). How to decrease wandering, a form of agenda behavior. *Geriatric Nursing, 6*, 196–199.

Ranck, J. B. (1973). Studies on single neurons in dorsal hippocampal formation and septum in unrestrained rats, part I: Behavioral correlates and firing repertoires. *Experimental Neurology, 41*, 462–531.

Reinboth, J., & Gleidenvand, T. (1982). Pilot study of falls in an extended care setting. University of Iowa.

Reisberg, B., Ferris, S. H., deLeon, M. J., & Crook, T. (1982). The Global Deterioration Scale for assessment of primary degenerative dementia. *American Journal of Psychiatry, 139*, 1136–1139.

Rindlisbacher, P., & Hopkins, R. W. (1991). Sundowning syndrome: A conceptual analysis and review. *American Journal of Alzheimer Care and Related Disorders and Research, 6*, 2–9.

Rindlisbacher, P., & Hopkins, R. W. (1992). An investigation of the Sundowning syndrome. *International Journal of Geriatric Psychiatry, 7*, 15–23.

Rindlisbacher, P., Hopkins, R. W., & Grant, N. T. (1992). An investigation of the sundowning syndrome and ambient light. *American Journal of Alzheimer* Care and Research, 7, 22–27.

Robb, S. S. (1987). Exercise treatment for wandering. In H. J. Altman (Ed.), *Alzheimer's disease: Problems, prospects, and perspectives* (pp. 213–218). New York: Plenum.

Rubenstein, L., Josephson, K., & Robbins, A. (1994). Falls in the nursing home. *Annals of Internal Medicine, 121*, 442–451.

Ryan, J. P., McGowan, J., McCaffrey, N., Ryan, G. T., Zandi, T., & Brannigan, G. C. (1995). Graphomotor perseveration and wandering in Alzheimer's disease. *Journal of Geriatric Psychiatry and Neurology, 8*, 209–212.

Salzman, C. (1987). Treatment of the elderly agitated patient. *Journal of Clinical Psychiatry, 48*, S19–S22.

Sandson, J., & Albert, M. (1984). Varieties of perseveration. *Neuropsychologia, 22*, 715–732.

Sandson, J., & Albert, M. (1987). Perseveration in behavior neurology. *Neurology, 37*, 1736–1741.

Satlin, A., Teicher, M. H., Lieberman, H. R., Baldessarini, R. J., Volicer, L., & Rheaume, Y. (1991). Circadian locomotor activity rhythms in Alzheimer's Disease. *Neuropsychopharmocology, 5*, 115–126.

Schneider, L. S., Pollock, V. E., & Lyness, S. A. (1990). A meta-analysis of controlled trails of neuroleptic treatment in dementia. *Journal of American Geriatrics Society, 38*, 553–563.

Schneider, L. S., & Sobin, P. B. (1992). Non-neuroleptic treatment of behavioral symptoms and agitation in Alzheimer's disease and other dementia. *Psychopharmocology Bulletin, 28*, 71–79.

Sehested, P. & Severin-Nielsen, T. (1977). Falls by hospitalized elderly patients: causes, prevention. *Geriatrics, 32*, 101–108.

Shelton, P., & Hocking, L. B. (1997). Zolpidem for dementia-related insomnia and nighttime wandering. *Annals of Pharmacotherapy, 31*, 319–322.

Singh, S., Mulley, G., & Lusowsky, M. (1988). Why are Alzheimer's patients thin. *Age and Aging, 17*, 21–28.

Slauson, T. J., Bayles, K. A., & Tomeoda, C. K. (1987). *Communication disorders and late stage Alzheimer's disease*. Unpublished manuscript.

Snyder, L. H., Rupprecht, P., Pyrek, J., Brekhus, S., & Moss, T. (1978). Wandering. *The Gerontologist, 18*, 272–280.

Soverini, S., & Borghesi, E. (1968). On a strange case of wandering in an arteriosclerotic demented patient. *Gerontology, 16*, 846–851.

Stokes, G. (1986). *Wandering, common problems with the elderly confused*. Bicester, UK: Winslow Press.

Sunderland, T., & Silver, M. A. (1988). Neuroleptics in the treatment of dementia. *International Journal of Geriatric Psychiatry, 3*, 79–88.

Swaab, D. F., Fliers, E., & Partiman, T. S. (1985). The suprachiasmatic nucleus of the human brain in relation to sex, age and senile dementia. *Brain Research, 342*, 37–44.

Szwabo, P., Woodward, V., Grossberg, G., & Shenn, W. W. (1991). The use of Alprazolam for decreasing problem wandering in geriatric patients. *American Journal of Alzheimer's Care and Related Disorders and Research, 6*, 31–36.

Tappen, R. (1988). Revitalization: a developing approach to nursing care of the cognitively impaired. *Florida Nurse, 36*, 3.

Teri, L., Larson, E. B., & Reifler, B. V. (1988). Behavioral disturbance in dementia of the Alzheimer's type. *Journal of the American Geriatrics Society, 36*, 1–6.

Thomas, D. W. (1995). Wandering: A proposed definition. *Journal of Gerontological Nursing, 21*, 35–41.

Thomas, D. W. (1997). Understanding the wandering patient. *Journal of Gerontological Nursing, 23*, 16–24.

Thornbury, J. (1992). Cognitive performance on Piagetian tasks by Alzheimer's disease patients. *Research in Nursing and Health, 15,* 11–18.
Tingle, D. (1986). Trazodone in dementia [letter]. *Journal of Clinical Psychiatry, 47,* 482.
Tinetti, M. (1986). Performance-oriented assessment of mobility problems in elderly patients. *Journal of the American Geriatric Society, 34,* 119–126.
Tinetti, M. (1987). Factors associated with serious injury during falls by ambulatory nursing home residents. *Journal of the American Geriatrics Society, 35,* 644–648.
Tinetti, M., Speechley, M., & Ginter, S. (1988). Risk factors for falls among elderly persons living in the community. *New England Journal of Medicine, 319,* 1701–1707.
Traub, R. D., Miles, R., & Wong, R. (1989). Model of the origin of rhythmic population oscillations in the hippocampal slice. *Science, 243,* 1319–1326.
Vallarino, R., & Sherman, F. (1981). Stroke, fractured hip, amputation, pressure sores and incontinence: Principles of rehabilitation treatment. In L. Libow & F. Sherman (Eds.), *The core of geriatric medicine.* St. Louis, MO: Mosby.
Vanderwolf, C. H. (1969). Hippocampal electric activity and voluntary movement in the rat. *Electroencephalography and Clinical Neurophysiology, 26,* 407–418.
Vanderwolf, C. H., Kramis, R., Gillespie, L. A., & Bland, B. H., (1975). Hippocampal rhythmical slow activity and neocortical low voltage fast activity: Relation to behavior. In R. L. Isaacson & K. H. Pribram (Eds.), *The hippocampus: Neurophysiology* (pp. 101–128). New York: Plenum.
Vanderwolf, C. N., & Leung, L. (1983) Hippocampal rhythmic slow activity: A brief history and the effects of entorhinal lesions and phenycyclindine in neurobiology of the hippocampus. In W. Siefert (Ed.), *Neurobiology of the hippocampus* (pp. 275–302). London: Academic Press.
Vitiello, M. V., Poceta, J. S., & Prinz, P. M. (1991). Sleep in Alzheimer's disease and other dementing disorders. *Canadian Journal of Psychology, 45,* 221–239.
Walshe, A., & Rosen, H. (1979). A study of patient falls from bed. *Journal of Nursing Administration, 79,* 31–35.
Warrington, J., & Eagles, J. M. (1995). Day care for the elderly mentally ill: Diurnal confusion? *Health Bulletin, 53,* 99–104.
Weiner, M. F., Bruhn, M., Svetlik, D., Tintner, R., & Hom, J. (1991). Experiences with depression in a dementia clinic. *Journal of Clinical Psychiatry, 52,* 234–238.
Weller, M. P. I. (1987). A biochemical hypothesis of wandering. *Medicine, Science, and the Law, 27,* 40–41.
Weller, M. P. I., & Jauhar, P. (1987). Wandering at Heathrow airport by the mentally unwell. *Medicine, Science, and the Law, 27,* 37–39.
Werner, P., Cohen-Mansfield, J., Braun, J., & Marx, M. (1989). Physical restraints and agitation in nursing home residents. *Journal of the American Geriatrics Society, 37,* 1122–1126.
Werner, P., Cohen-Mansfield, J., Koroknay, V., & Braun, J. (1994). The impact of a restraint-reduction program on nursing home residents. *Geriatric Nursing, 15,* 142–146.
Whall, A., Gillis, G., Yankou, D., Booth, D., & Beel-Bates, C. (1989). *Journal of Gerontological Nursing, 18,* 13–17.
Whedon, M. B., & Shedd, P. (1989). Prediction and prevention of patient falls. *Image Journal of Nursing Scholarship, 21,* 108–114.
Whishaw, I.Q. (1991). Locale and taxon systems: no place for neophrenology. *Hippocampus, 1,* 272–274.
Whishaw, I. Q., Cassel, J. C., Majchrzak, M., Cassel, S., & Will, B. (1994). "Short stops" in rats with fimbria-fornix lesions: Evidence for change in the mobility gradient. *Hippocampus, 4,* 577–582.
Whishaw, I. Q., & Nikkel, R. W. (1975). Anterior hypothalamic electrical stimulation and hippocampal EEG in the rat: suppressed EEG, locomotion, self-stimulation, and inhibition of shock avoidance. *Behavioral Biology, 13,* 1–20.
Wild, D., Nayak, U., & Isaacs, B. (1981). How dangerous are falls in old people at home? *British Medical Journal, 282,* 226.
Wilkinson, I. M., & Graham-White, J. (1980). Psychogeriatric dependency rating scales (PGDRS): A method of assessment for use by nurses. *British Journal of Psychiatry, 137,* 558–565.
Witting, W., Kwa, I. H., Eikelenboom, P., Mirmiran, M., & Swaab, D. F. (1990). Alterations in the circadian rest activity rhythm in aging and Alzheimer's disease. *Biological Psychiatry, 27,* 563–572.
Wong, D., & Baker, C. (1988). Pain in children: Comparison of assessment scales. *Pediatric Nursing, 14,* 9–17.
Yin, R. K. (1989). *Case study research: Design and methods.* Newbury Park, CA: Sage.
Zarit, S., Orr, N., & Zarit, J. (1985). *The hidden victims of Alzheimer's Disease: Families under stress.* New York: New York University Press.
Zarit, S. H., Perlin, L. I., & Schaie, K. W. (Eds.) (1993). *Caregiving systems: Informal and formal helpers.* Hillsdale, NJ: Erlbaum.
Zeisel, J., Hyde, J., & Levkoff, S. (1994). Best practices : An environment behavior model (E-B) for Alzheimer special care units. *The American Journal of Alzheimer's Care and Related Disorders and Research, 9,* 4–21.
Zimmer, J. G., Watson, N., & Treat, A. (1984). Behavioral problems among patients in skilled nursing facilities. *American Journal of Public Health, 74,* 1118–1121.

7.18
Agitated and Aggressive Behavior

JANE E. FISHER, DIANE N. SWINGEN, and COLLEEN M. HARSIN

University of Nevada at Reno, NV, USA

7.18.1 INTRODUCTION

7.18.1.1 Agitated and Aggressive Behavior

Among the behavioral disturbances experienced by older adults with cognitive impairment, agitation and aggression present the most serious consequences for both patients and their caregivers. These behaviors increase the likelihood of an individual being institutionalized (Moak & Fisher, 1990) and experiencing physical or chemical restraint (Sloane, Mathew, & Scarborough, 1991). Numerous reports from studies of family and professional caregivers indicate that aggression in cognitively impaired individuals is the most stressful problem that caregivers confront (Fisher, Fink, & Loomis, 1993).

Within institutional settings physical and chemical restraints have historically been among the most common forms of managing aggression and agitated behaviors (Evans & Strumpf, 1989; Swearer, Drachman, O'Donnell, & Mitchell, 1988). Reliance on these intervention strategies with Alzheimer's disease (AD) patients is wrought with problems due to side effects such as increased risk of falls (Werner, Cohen-Mansfield, Braun, & Marx, 1989), concomitant reduction of desirable behaviors, and the risk of impairment in cognitive functions. Several of the medications commonly prescribed for the treatment of agitation and aggression are psychotropic drugs developed for problems quite different from those experienced by the cognitively impaired elderly. While medications such as haloperidol may be effective in reducing agitated and aggressive behavior they can also have undesirable effects on other behaviors. In addition, as an older adult's physiology changes due to normal (e.g., metabolism rate) or pathological processes (e.g., Alzheimer's disease, hypertension) the effects of medication may be altered. The etiology of the behavioral disturbances themselves may also change, and therefore they may not be responsive to formerly effective interventions.

While the use of physical and chemical restraints may decrease or temporarily eliminate agitation, it is becoming increasingly apparent that restraint-based interventions are not likely to lead to long-term alleviation of behavioral disturbances, and the risks involved in their use often outweigh the benefits.

Interest in the development of restraint-free alternatives for managing behavior problems has been prompted by US Federal legislation affecting nursing home care. In 1987 the US Congress passed the Omnibus Reconciliation Act of Nursing Home Reform (OBRA) requiring that facilities receiving Medicare or Medicaid funds adhere to a treatment program requiring psychotropic drug holidays and the implementation of behavioral programming in an effort to reduce reliance on psychotropic medication within nursing homes. While the essence of OBRA represents a commendable improvement in the care of the elderly within institutions, the requirements for alternative interventions were implemented prior to the development and empirical validation of such treatment alternatives.

Despite the obvious need for alternatives to physical and chemical restraints, and the increase in research addressing behavioral disturbances, there are still remarkably few established treatment alternatives. Three factors have hindered the development of alternative interventions. First, the study of behavioral disturbances in dementia patients has historically occurred within a medical model. The vast majority of studies on behavior problems in cognitively impaired older adults are pharmacological studies. Research on the environmental context of behavioral functioning in dementia has only emerged since the 1980s. Second, there is a lack of consensus within the field regarding basic issues of definition. This lack of consensus has impeded advances in explanation, prevention, and treatment of these problems, and limits comparison of findings across studies. Third, the large majority of nonmedical studies of aggression and agitation are descriptive accounts that have been conducted in an atheoretical context. Most research reports do not reference or employ any theoretical framework within which to consider findings. The atheoretical nature of the research has limited advances in the explanation, prediction, and treatment of behavioral disturbances in the elderly.

The development of restraint-free methods for managing behavioral disturbances in cognitively impaired older adults entails questions regarding the extent to which behavior continues to be influenced by environmental stimuli. Given the limited predictive validity of available classification systems of dementia, it is believed that answers to these questions will be found most effectively through idiographically based assessment and treatment planning methods.

This chapter describes a theoretical approach to the assessment and treatment of behavioral disturbances that considers the context in which behavioral disturbances occur, including physiological and environmental setting events, antecedent environmental stimuli, and the consequences of the behavior. Information on the epidemiology, etiology, assessment, and treatment of agitation and aggression in the elderly is reviewed. A discussion of definitional issues is presented first.

7.18.2 ISSUES OF DEFINITION

A requisite condition of efforts to explain, predict, and modify behavior is the reliable measurement of key elements of the behavior. The operationalization of a target behavior is a critical first step in progress toward reliable, consistent measurement (Johnston & Pennypacker, 1980). A difficulty in formulating an adequate definition of agitation or aggression involves addressing the multidimensional nature of these behaviors and the dynamic nature of the interaction between physiological functioning and response to environmental stimuli inherent in a degenerative disorder such as Alzheimer's disease. Selection of the relevant dimension depends upon the ultimate goal of a measurement or assessment process. Definitions of behavioral disturbances may be based on etiology, topographical features, natural history, environmental dependence, impact on others, or treatment response. Intra- and interindividual variation in these dimensions has been a consistent finding in the literature despite efforts to identify common elements associated with behavioral disturbance in older adults grouped on the basis of factors such as diagnosis, level of cognitive impairment or functional skill impairment, or duration of illness. Within individuals with degenerative forms of dementia, variation in the etiology, environmental dependence, and response to treatment of topographically similar behaviors may change over time, further complicating the reliable identification of agitated of aggressive behaviors.

Any definition of agitation or aggression must be evaluated on the basis of reliable measurement of the behavior as operationalized and the accumulation of evidence for criterion-related concurrent and predictive validity and ultimately construct validity. Despite difficulties inherent in identifying the dimensions relevant for reliable and valid definitions of behavior in dementia, it is evident that attention to this issue is mandated to facilitate advances in the field.

In defining agitation and aggression, researchers have proposed both molar definitions that represent broad inclusive categories and highly specific descriptions of behaviors that are accessible to direct observation. Molar definitions typically require higher inference judgements (Foster & Cone, 1986). The utility of a particular definition will be influenced by the population to which it is applied. This is due to the significant heterogeneity of the population characterized by the label "elderly."

Perhaps the most widely cited molar definition of agitation was proposed by Cohen-Mansfield and Billig (1986). Agitation was defined as "inappropriate verbal, vocal, or motor activity that is not explained by needs or confusion per se" (p. 712). The authors' statement that agitated behaviors are always inappropriate with regard to accepted social norms or the needs of the caregiver reflects the fact that this definition was developed for the general population of elderly. There are at least two problems with this definition of agitation when applied to dementia patients. First, applying the concept of "inappropriate" behavior to dementia patients may itself be inappropriate as it implies that the behavior is unsuitable or incompatible in a given context. When the behavior of dementia patients is considered within the context of a patient's declining competencies and, hence, an increasingly challenging environment, it can be argued that their behavior actually is adaptive rather than inappropriate. Second, when the concept of social norms is applied to dementia patients, agitation emerges as the norm, thus making the normative reference within this definition unsuitable for the population of cognitively impaired older adults.

Other authors have proposed molar definitions that incorporate reference to the motivation of agitation. Barnes and Raskind (1980) defined agitation as a behavioral term addressing excessive motor activity that is often nonpurposeful in nature and is commonly associated with feelings of internal tension, irritability, hostility, and belligerency on the part of the individual engaging in the behaviors. Other definitions of agitation incorporate reference to the *consequences* of behavior. Rosen, et al. (1994), for example, defined agitation as consisting of vocal or motor behavior that is disruptive, unsafe, or interferes with the delivery of care in a particular environment. When treatment outcome is a primary concern, measures which incorporate the consequences of a particular behavior for patients and caregivers may be particularly useful.

A limitation of molar definitions is that the higher-inference judgments required can result in reduced reliability. Two approaches have been employed in attempting to increase the specificity of the definitions of "agitation" and "aggression." First, some researchers have focused on the frequency, duration, and intensity of discrete behaviors that are accessible to direct observation (e.g., Yudofsky,

Silver, Jackson, & Endicott, 1986). Other researchers have provided lists specifying which behaviors are encompassed by the larger class of "agitation," and have grouped behaviors into various categories based on characteristics such as response modality (e.g., motoric vs. vocal) or dangerousness. For example, Rosen et al. (1994) described four behavioral classifications of agitation: (i) aberrant vocalizations (repetitious requests or complaints, and nonverbal vocalizations); (ii) motor agitation (pacing and wandering); (iii) aggressiveness (verbal or physical threats, harm to self or others, and physical behavior toward property); and (iv) resisting care (not taking medications or not cooperating with activities of daily living). Another example of a categorical approach to agitated behaviors is found in a study by Cohen-Mansfield (1986). Cohen-Mansfield included pacing, aimless wandering, inappropriate dressing or undressing, spitting, hitting, kicking, throwing things, screaming or making strange noises, biting, complaining, harming self or others, cursing, verbal aggression, constant unwarranted requests or statements, and general restlessness within the class of "agitated behaviors." A factor analysis produced three factors that have since been repeatedly cited as general forms of agitation and have been used to classify and study various aspects of agitation. The first factor is described as physically aggressive behavior, including spitting, biting, hitting, and throwing objects. The second factor includes verbal aggressive behavior such as cursing, threats, and verbal aggression. The third factor is described as nonaggressive behavior, including pacing, wandering, inappropriately dressing or undressing, and constant requests for attention.

Factor analytic methods of studying agitation and aggression may prove useful for understanding the etiology, natural history, or response to treatment of agitated or aggressive behavior. It is possible that behaviors associated with the various factors may emerge as having a similar etiology or response to treatment. Identifying behaviors that are functionally related will ultimately be the most effective for treatment development.

The difficulties inherent in defining agitated behaviors have had important implications for several areas of research, including epidemiological research.

7.18.3 PREVALENCE

Reports of prevalence rates of behavioral disturbances vary widely, depending upon the definition of agitated behavior used (e.g., summary terms such as "agitation" or "aggression" vs. specific behaviors such as screaming or hitting), the research methodology employed (e.g., caregiver report vs. direct observation), and characteristics of the population studied (e.g., nursing home residents vs. Alzheimer's disease patients). Prevalence rates of agitated behaviors also vary depending on whether the behavior is perceived to be a problem by others (Deutsch & Rovner, 1991). The following discussion of prevalence rates should be interpreted in light of these issues.

In a study of 408 residents in a large suburban nursing home, 93% of the residents were found to exhibit one or more of 29 agitated behaviors at least once a week as reported by caregivers using the Cohen-Mansfield Agitation Inventory (CMAI) (Cohen-Mansfield, 1986; Cohen-Mansfield, Marx, & Rosenthal, 1989). Participants in this study were identified as having various levels of cognitive impairment and physical limitations. General restlessness was the most commonly manifested behavior. Other high-frequency behaviors included pacing, repetitious sentences, constant requests for attention, complaining, negativism, and cursing. Physically nonaggressive behavior and verbally agitated behaviors were considerably more common than aggressive behaviors. In general, the frequency of agitated behaviors decreased throughout the day as the evening approached, and occurred least frequently at night when the majority of residents were sleeping. In contrast, a study by Teri, Larson, and Reifler (1988) reported that 26% of the total sample of 127 individuals with Alzheimer's disease exhibited agitation. Participants in this study were outpatients referred to a geriatric and family services clinic for a comprehensive geriatric evaluation. "Agitation" was considered separately from "wandering" and "restlessness." Levels of agitation varied with level of cognitive impairment as assessed with the Folstein Mini-Mental State Exam (MMSE; Folstein, Folstein, & McHugh 1975). Behavior problems were rated as present or not present by a physician based on observations or information provided by family of the participants. Ten percent of individuals with mild, 27% of those with moderate, and 38% of those with severe, cognitive impairment were identified as exhibiting agitation. Wandering and restlessness were evidenced in 26% and 45% of the entire sample, respectively.

7.18.4 ETIOLOGICAL FACTORS

Several factors have been proposed to contribute to the development of agitation and aggression in older adults. These factors include medication (Addonizio, 1987), illness such as infection (Yoshikawa & Norman, 1996), cognitive impairment (Cooper, Mungas, & Weiler, 1990), functional status (Cohen-Mansfield & Billig, 1986), environmental stimuli (Burgio et al., 1994; Cohen-Mansfield, Werner, & Marx, 1992; Fisher, Goy, Swingen, & Szymanski, 1994) and emotional states (Swearer, et al., 1988).

Based on the large variation in the physical and psychological functioning of older adults, the following guidelines may be useful for generating hypotheses regarding antecedent or etiological factors contributing to agitation or aggression in an older adult: (i) Given the significant variation in the health and cognitive status of older adults, identification of the etiology of aggression and agitation is best considered within an interactional model that includes physiological, psychological, and environmental factors; (ii) While an individual may exhibit topographically similar behaviors at different points in time, it should not be assumed that the same factors that contributed to the behavioral disturbance in the past are causing the current problem. Variation in etiology is a particularly salient issue when an individual has a degenerative condition such as Alzheimer's disease, in that topographically similar behaviors may have different etiologies over the course of the disease. Physiological and psychological factors that have been found to be associated with agitation and aggression in older adults are reviewed.

7.18.4.1 Physiological Factors

Physiological factors contributing to agitation and aggression can be conceptualized as falling into two categories: (i) direct precipitants of; or (ii) setting events for agitation or aggression. The term "setting events" refers to conditions of the individual or the environment in which the individual functions that affect the function of the antecedent or consequent stimuli associated with a particular response (Bijou & Baer, 1966; Kantor, 1959). Physiologically based setting events that may increase the risk of agitation or an aggressive response include patient fatigue, hunger, mood, health status, cognitive impairment, and sensory functioning. The categories of physiological factors described below may serve as a guide for generating hypotheses regarding factors influencing aggression or agitation in older adults.

Physiological conditions that have been identified as predisposing patients to become agitated or to behave aggressively include pain, physical discomfort, and sensory impairment. Evidence for their role in the etiology of agitation and aggression will be reviewed.

7.18.4.1.1 Pain

There are several painful physical conditions that may influence the occurrence of agitation and aggression. Infectious processes (Gerdner & Buckwalter, 1994), such as urinary tract infection, may produce pain in a cognitively impaired patient and may go undetected because of the inability of the patient to verbally express discomfort. Other sources of pain, such as heartburn, sinus congestion, arthritis, neuropathy from diabetes, or injury (e.g., stress fracture), may lead to agitation (Ferrell, Ferrell, & Rivera, 1995) or function as setting events in that they increase the likelihood of agitation or aggression occurring when stress is placed on the patient (e.g., when environmental stimulation is high or demands are placed on the patient in the context of caregiving).

7.18.4.1.2 Medication

Due to age-associated decreases in metabolism, older adults are at increased risk for iatrogenic effects associated with drug toxicity, drug interactions, and drug withdrawal (Gerdner & Buckwalter, 1994). Problems associated with polypharmacy have received extensive attention in the geriatrics literature for several years (Buck, 1988; Ray, Federspiel, & Schaffner, 1980; Williams & Betley, 1995). Surveys indicate that both psychotropic and nonpsychotropic medications continue to be widely over prescribed for older adults in nursing homes (Williams & Betley, 1995) and board and care homes (Spore, Mor, Hiris, Larrat, & Hawes, 1995). While polypharmacy often plays an important role in treatment of older adults, with increased numbers of medications, the risk of one medication negating, potentiating, or in some way altering the effects of another medication increases. Medications with side effects that may contribute to agitation in an elderly individual include but are not limited to neuroleptics (Addonizio, 1987), benzodiazapines (Wolf, Grohmann, Beiber, Brenner, & Luther, 1989) and nonprescription medication with anticholinergic properties (Hall, Beresford, Stickney, Nasdahl, & Coleman, 1985; see Callahan, 1993 for a review).

7.18.4.1.3 Sensory and perceptual deficits

Visual and hearing impairments may contribute to the occurrence of agitation and aggression in that they may produce or increase confusion and alter perception of the dangerousness of a situation. Perceptual impairments such as visual neglect due to stroke may also contribute to violent behavior.

7.18.4.2 Psychological Factors

7.18.4.2.1 Cognitive factors

The relationship between cognitive functioning and behavioral disturbance has received the largest amount of attention by researchers attempting to determine the cause of behavioral disturbance. Studies have examined the relationship between the number and/or types of behavioral disturbance and either cognitive status as measured by neuropsychological test performance and/or functional/adaptive skill level as measured by behavioral checklists. The results have varied. Some studies have reported a positive correlation (Cooper et al., 1990) while other researchers have found no relationship (Bolger & Dougherty, 1992; Teri, Borson, Kiyak, & Yamagishi, 1989) or a nonlinear relationship (Cohen-Mansfield, Marx, & Rosenthal, 1990) between overall number of behavior problems and cognitive status. Studies that have found a statistically significant relationship between cognitive status and behavioral disturbance have reported relatively low correlations accounting for little of the variance (e.g., Cooper et al., 1990).

In a study of Alzheimer's disease patients residing in a nursing home, Teri et al. (1988) found that the number of behavioral problems was positively correlated with cognitive impairment. The types of behavior problems manifested varied with the level of cognitive impairment. Wandering, agitation, and incontinence were found to be most heavily associated with level of cognitive impairment.

In a related study designed to further clarify the relationship between behavioral problems and level of cognitive and functional impairment in 56 moderately impaired Alzheimer's disease patients, Teri et al. (1989) found that the problems most strongly associated with level of cognitive functioning were confusion, disorientation, and memory loss. These problems constituted at least 50% of the total for problems that occurred more than twice per week as recorded by caregivers using the Behavioral Problems Checklist (BPC). The next most common problems were underactivity, loss of interest in activities, tension, depression, and apathy. No caregiver reported an absence of problems for an individual patient, and an average of seven of the 48 problems on the BPC were reported to have occurred more than twice per week. This study also identified gender differences in problem behaviors, as men were found to have significantly higher rates of the following problems: preoccupation with bodily functioning, loss of interest in activities, verbal aggression towards others, loss of interest in others, and poor personal hygiene. Perhaps the most important finding to emerge from this study is that no specific behavioral problem or pattern of behavior problems was associated with overall level of cognitive impairment.

7.18.4.2.2 Environmental factors

Research provides compelling evidence for the role of environmental influence on behavior in even very severely cognitively impaired older adults (Bourgeois, Burgio, & Schulz, 1995; Burgio et al., 1994; Vitaliano, Young, Russo, Romano, & Magana-Amato, 1993). Findings from observational research have been particularly informative in describing the influence of environmental factors on the occurrence of agitation and aggressive behavior (Anderson, 1970; Colenda & Hamer, 1991; Hamel et al., 1990; Vitaliano et al., 1993). Lindsley (1964) delineated four components for the functional analysis of behavior that can be applied to the behavior of dementia patients. These include (i) the antecedent stimulus or stimulus setting in which the behavior occurs, (ii) the behavior of interest (e.g., aggression or agitation), (iii) the contingencies of reinforcement, and (iv) the environmental events that follow the behavior. To this list others have added the concept of "setting events" (Kantor, 1959) which are conditions of the individual or the environment that affect the function of antecedent and consequent events.

(i) Setting events

Environmentally based setting events may include factors such as noise level, the presence of others, or a change in caregiver that affects the function of antecedent or consequent stimuli associated with agitation or aggression. Variation in the occurrence or intensity of aggression or agitation when the antecedent stimuli (e.g., caregiver's behavior) appear constant, may be associated with a change in environmental setting events (see Carr, Levin, McConnachie, Carlson, Kemp, & Smith, 1994). Time of day may also function as a setting event in that it has been shown that the frequency of aggressive acts decreased from day to evening to night (Cohen-Mansfield et al., 1989). Using the Cohen-Mansfield Agitation Inventory as a measure of agitated behaviors in 408 nursing home residents with varying degrees of physical and cognitive impairment, Cohen-Mansfield et al.

(1989) reported that the majority of behaviors occurred at significantly different rates across day, evening, and night shifts with frequency decreasing from day to evening to night. There are at least three possible explanations for this finding. First, patients may become increasingly fatigued as the day progresses, and therefore the decrease in agitated behaviors is a function of energy level. Second, the administration of medications and/or the application of physical restraints may decrease or preclude a patient's ability to engage in agitated or aggressive behaviors. Or third, the environment within the nursing homes changes across the day (e.g., due to changes in the caregiving or activity schedules). In short, the finding may reflect changes in environmental setting events (e.g., activities in the nursing home) or physiological setting events (e.g., fatigue or the use of medications).

The role of emotion as a setting event associated with agitation and aggression has been receiving increasing empirical attention. Research suggests that a patient's emotional state, such as level of anxiety or depression (Swearer et al., 1988) may be predictive of agitation and aggression. In a 1996 study Lawton, Van Haitsma, and Klapper (1996) reported that AD patients who were rated as "less content" were also considered more agitated by staff members. Swearer et al. (1988) found that 63% of caregivers reported that the patient for whom they provided care exhibited one or more symptoms of anxiety, including general fearfulness, a fear of specific objects or events, restlessness, pacing, and appearing to worry over insignificant matters and that these behavioral symptoms of anxiety tended to be significantly associated with angry outbursts

In a rare investigation of the association of premorbid history and agitation in nursing home residents, Cohen-Mansfield and Marx (1989) found that residents who experienced a major stressful event during their lives tended to exhibit a greater number of agitated behaviors—in particular, physically nonaggressive behavior. Residents who had not experienced relocation prior to being admitted to the nursing home exhibited more aggressive behavior and a greater number of agitated behaviors than did residents who had relocated at least once. The results of this study suggest that exposure to stressful events earlier in life may result in the development of coping skills or an increase in the threshold for perceiving events as stressful in later life. The changes produced by exposure to stress earlier in life may continue to influence behavior after the onset of a dementing process.

(ii) Antecedent stimuli

Several studies have reported that antecedent environmental stimuli such as task demands influence the occurrence of agitation and aggression. The finding of an association between environmental stimulation or caregiver demands and behavioral disturbance in cognitively impaired elderly indicates that these behaviors are not random or purposeless but instead may be functionally related to environmental stimuli.

Attempting to engage patients in activities of daily living, including being bathed, changed, or fed, has been described by nursing home staff as a primary cause of agitation (Cohen-Mansfield, 1986). These findings are consistent with those of Fisher et al. (1994) that aggressive behavior in Alzheimer's disease patients was consistently associated with a nurse's request to perform a task. In a study of 42 institutionalized dementia patients, Fisher et al. (1994) found that nurses described all physically assaultive AD patients as appearing distressed during episodes of aggressive behavior. For 80% of these patients, physically aggressive behaviors were described as being associated with an effort to escape from a stimulus, such as a nurse's request.

The concept of a "catastrophic reaction" (Goldstein, 1952) is frequently mentioned within the context of efforts to account for aggressive outbursts in dementia patients (e.g., Hall, Gerdner, Zwygart-Stuffacher, & Buckwalter, 1995). A "catastrophic reaction" occurs when demands presented by the environment exceed the patient's ability to cope. The individual becomes increasingly anxious and may attempt to terminate the anxiety-provoking stimulus by expressing a desire to be alone, screaming, or asking to go home. Continued stimulation may result in the individuals becoming extremely agitated or violent. The reports that aggression is often associated with an effort to escape from an aversive situation, described above, are consistent with the concept of catastrophic reaction.

The presence of other people has also been shown to be associated with agitation (Ryden, 1988; Cohen-Mansfield, Werner, & Marx, 1992). In a study involving 24 dementia patients described as highly agitated on the basis of CMAI scores, Cohen-Mansfield, Werner, and Marx (1992) reported that the agitated behaviors of pacing, strange noises, requests for attention, strange movements, aggressive behaviors, picking at things, and repetitious mannerisms were differentially affected by the presence of others. For example, strange noises were shown to increase when the patient was left alone while pacing decreased in the same situation.

Other environmental stimuli reported to influence behavioral disturbances include the caregiver's emotional expression (Vitaliano et al., 1993), lack of structure, and lack of attention (Cohen-Mansfield, 1986).

These findings support the hypothesis that certain behaviors that emerge during the course of dementia may serve a function for dementia patients in that they may be an adaptive (and the only available) means of increasing or decreasing stimulation. As a patient's behavioral repertoire diminishes over the course of a dementing process, behaviors characterized as "agitated" or "disturbances" may emerge to serve the function of previously available behaviors (e.g., those associated with language, leisure activities, or social interaction).

(iii) Environmental consequences

The consequences of agitated behaviors and aggression have received the least amount of attention by researchers. Little is known regarding how caregiver behavior following aggression functions to maintain or reduce aggression. Several possible relationships between behavior and consequences may be relevant. Aggressive behavior may be influenced by positive reinforcement if the former's occurrence is associated with the presentation of a consequent stimulus (e.g., caregiver attention) that increases the probability of the behavior occurring in the future. Alternatively, negative reinforcement may serve to strengthen aggressive tendencies through the contingent removal of an aversive stimulus (e.g., task demand). A few case studies (e.g., Bakke et al., 1994) discussed in detail in the intervention section, have described functional relationships between agitated behavior and environmental consequences.

(a) Social consequences. Aggression associated with positive reinforcement in the form of attention appears to be rare in dementia patients, although a few case reports have described an association between agitation and social contact (e.g., Rosberger & MacLean, 1983). When social contact is implicated in an aggressive episode, it is more often associated with an effort to terminate social contact (Fisher, 1995).

(b) Tangible consequences. Aggressive behaviors exhibited by cognitively impaired older adults may be associated with an effort to gain a tangible consequence such as food or an object. The role of tangible consequences in the development and maintenance of aggression within community settings has not been explored. Within institutional settings such as nursing homes, access to tangible objects is limited for safety purposes. The most frequent type of tangible consequence for a behavior that appears aggressive involves obtaining food from another resident (e.g., grabbing food from another resident) (Fisher et al., 1994).

In another scenario, a patient may grab onto or pinch the caregiver in a painful fashion during caregiving tasks. While the behavior may appear aggressive in that it causes pain for the caregiver, it may function to provide security or stimulation. Identifying an alternative response that is incompatible with the seemingly aggressive one, such as placing an object (e.g., a towel or small pillow) in the patient's hand prior to initiating the caregiving activity may prevent this form of aggression (Lundervold & Lewin, 1992).

7.18.5 ASSESSMENT

Interest in the assessment of behavioral disturbances in AD has increased since the mid-1980s. However, there are several limitations to our understanding of agitation and aggression and the reliability and validity of assessment procedures. First, there is a lack of consensus in the field regarding the definitions of agitation and aggression. Second, as discussed earlier in this chapter, the majority of available assessment instruments focus on the topographical features of agitation and aggression and have limited utility for treatment planning. Third, few of the available instruments have been validated for use with dementia patients. Psychometric studies have focused primarily on the reliability of instruments. The predictive validity and treatment utility of the majority of instruments have not been empirically evaluated.

The physiological, topographical, and functional characteristics of agitation and aggression in cognitively impaired older adults and the significance of each of these areas in assessment and treatment planning are explored in the following sections.

7.18.5.1 Physiological Assessment of Agitation and Aggression

For the purposes of determination of etiology and treatment planning, assessment of agitation should begin at the physiological level. Assessing and treating physical symptoms contributing to agitated behavior may eliminate the need for the more time-consuming assessment of environmental causes of agitation. While there have been few empirical investigation regarding the physiological correlates of agitation in dementia patients, pain and sensory impairment have been implicated in the etiology of agitation and is reviewed.

7.18.5.1.1 Pain

A particularly difficult challenge in caring for cognitively impaired individuals involves their limited verbal abilities. As verbal abilities decline, caregivers must increasingly rely on observation to determine whether a patient is experiencing pain or distress. It is crucial for adequate treatment planning to rule out physical pain as a precipitant to aggression. Regular physical examinations are a necessary component of adequate care.

Although assessment of pain is complicated by the impaired verbal abilities of the dementia patients, Ferrell et al. (1995) reported that 83% of a sample of 217 cognitively impaired dementia patients was able to complete at least one of the five unidimensional measures used to assess pain. The unidimensional measures used included: (i) a verbally administered questionnaire in which subjects were asked to choose among descriptors of pain listed in one-inch letters on large index cards (McGill Pain Questionnaire; Melzack, 1975); (ii) a verbally administered 0–10 Likert scale; (iii) a 100 mm visual analog scale with word anchors of "no pain" and "worst possible pain" (p. 593); (iv) a subscale of the Memorial Pain Card (Fishman et al., 1987) involving the visual and verbal presentation of eight words describing various intensities of pain ranging from no pain to excruciating; and (v) the Rand Coop Chart for pain (Nelson et al., 1987) that requires subjects to choose one of five cartoon characters accompanied by descriptive words depicting various levels of pain, ranging from no pain to severe pain.

Ferrell et al. (1995) report that 62% of subjects who were able to complete the assessment reported the presence of pain and 40% of the sample reported pain in more than one location. Further, for 37% of patients who reported pain, no etiology for the described pain was documented in the medical records. These findings indicate the high prevalence or pain among dementia patients.

While Ferrell et al. (1995) indicate that this study provides support for the ability of cognitively impaired dementia patients to report pain, several factors may limit the generalizability of the findings to moderately and severely impaired patients. First, the authors did not report the reasons why 17% of the sample was unable to complete the interview. The inability of a significant subset of the sample to complete the interview suggests that the results may not be generalizable to more impaired patients. Second, it is unclear whether the discrepancy between subject reports and medical records reflects inaccurate reporting by the dementia patients or insufficient documentation in patient charts. Research indicates that while interviewing is a helpful assessment tool with mildly impaired individuals, it is not effective as cognitive decline progresses (Davis & Robins, 1989). The limited utility of interviews with dementia patients is reflected by the elimination of 70 subjects prior to selection of the final sample in the Ferrell et al. study. The authors report that these subjects were eliminated, because they were "essentially mute and unresponsive, and no meaningful information could be obtained from the patient interview" (p. 594). The omission of severely impaired patients reflects the difficulty in clarifying the relationship between pain and agitation or aggression in dementia patients, since these behaviors are generally more likely to appear when cognitive impairment is moderate to severe (Kurita, Blass, Nolan, Black, & Thaler, 1993; Swearer et al., 1988).

Given the limitations of the use of interviews for assessing pain in severely impaired AD patients, it is usually necessary to rely on direct observation methods. Hurley, Volcier, Hanrahan, Houde, and Volcier (1992) developed the Discomfort Scale for Dementia of the Alzheimer's type (DS-DAT) to assess discomfort in AD patients through direct observation of facial expressions and body posture. The authors defined discomfort as "a negative emotional and/or physical state subject to variation in magnitude in response to internal or environmental conditions" (p. 369). Behavioral signs of discomfort on the DS-DAT include noisy breathing; negative vocalization; having a frown; fidgeting; and looking sad, frightened, or tense.

The construct validity of the DS-DAT was evaluated by administering the scale monthly to AD patients who were highly dependent on the nursing staff for their activities of daily living. During the course of the study 20 subjects were identified as having an acute illness typically manifested by fever. It was hypothesized that discomfort would be higher during a fever episode than during baseline. The results indicated that the DS-DAT was sensitive to changes in discomfort associated with fever episodes. A limitation of this study is that the observers were not blind to the patients' fever episodes. While this knowledge may have biased observations, the results indicate that reliable, systematic observation of discomfort in AD patients is possible. Such observation may provide caregivers with information necessary to assist in assessment of physiological factors in the etiology of agitation.

While no studies, up to 1997, have directly assessed the relationship between pain and agitation, it is important to continue to explore this relationship. The promising developments in the assessment of pain in dementia patients described above, support the need to explore this venue. Reliable methods for assessing pain in the cognitively impaired individuals may help in the identification of physiological factors contributing to agitation and aggression and, hence, inform treatment.

7.18.5.1.2 Sensory impairment

Sensory impairment may also contribute to agitation (Gerdner & Buckwalter, 1994). Dementia patients, who are unable to correct for inadequacies in sensory perception by gathering more information or by altering their behavior (Fisher & Carstensen, 1990) may experience significant confusion and subsequent distress associated with sensory decrements.

Deficits in vision and hearing may contribute to a patient's inaccurate perception of situational demands. Patients with severe sensory impairment may overestimate the dangerousness of a situation and behave aggressively out of fear and a perceived need for self-defense. Assessing the status of a dementia patient's sensory functioning may provide information regarding how they perceive the environment and whether sensory deficits are contributing to a tendency toward agitation or aggression.

7.18.5.2 Topographical Assessment of Agitation and Aggression

The majority of research regarding the assessment of agitation and aggression has addressed the topographical features of the behaviors. Topographical assessment is informative for the identification of target behaviors and the frequency and intensity of these behaviors. Topographical information is also critical for assessment of baseline levels of aggressive or agitated behavior and for monitoring the effects of interventions. Four assessment instruments designed to record the frequency and intensity of agitation or aggression will be reviewed.

7.18.5.2.1 Cohen-Mansfield Agitation Inventory

The Cohen-Mansfield Agitation Inventory (CMAI; Cohen-Mansfield, 1986) is a 29-item questionnaire designed to measure the types and frequencies of agitated behaviors exhibited by elderly nursing home residents. Respondents rate the frequency on a seven-point scale ranging from "1—never engages in" to "7—manifests the behavior on the average of several times an hour." Examples of items include "pacing," "cursing or verbal aggression," and "repetitious sentences or questions." Cohen-Mansfield et al. (1989) reported adequate interrater agreement for each behavior on the CMAI (average $r = 0.92$). Studies of the reliability of the CMAI by other groups have produced varying levels of support for interrater reliability. Finkel, Lyons, & Anderson (1992) found evidence for high internal consistency but high variation in interrater reliability across items. In 1995, Miller, Snowdon, and Vaughan (1995) reported adequate interrater reliability for aggressive ($r = 0.85$) and physically nonaggressive behaviors ($r = 0.73$) but low interrater reliability for agitated verbal behaviors ($r = 0.47$).

7.18.5.2.2 Pittsburgh Agitation Scale

The Pittsburgh Agitation Scale (PAS; Rosen et al., 1994) is designed to assess four categories of agitated behavior in dementia patients, including aberrant vocalization, motor agitation, aggressiveness, and resisting care. Behaviors are rated using a five-point scale ranging from "0" indicating that the behavior was not observed during the specified observation period, to "4" indicating severe intensity, frequency, and/or resistance to redirection of the behavior. The authors report adequate intraclass correlations and concurrent validity based on findings from studies of dementia patients from an acute-care geropsychiatric unit and a chronic-care nursing facility.

7.18.5.2.3 Overt Aggression Scale

The Overt Aggression Scale (OAS; Yudofsky et al., 1986) is a checklist designed to document specific aspects of aggressive behavior based on observable criteria. It is designed to be completed immediately following each aggressive incident. In addition to indicating which of 16 behaviors occurred during an incident, raters also record the intervention strategies used and the time of onset and duration of the incident. The 16 behaviors on the OAS are divided into four categories: verbal aggression, physical aggression against objects, physical aggression against self, and physical aggression against others. Sample behavioral items include "Makes loud noise, shouts angrily," "Bangs head, hits fists into objects, throws self onto floor or into objects (hurts self without serious injury)," and "Slams doors, scatters clothing, makes a mess." Sample intervention items on the OAS include "Talking to patient," "Closer observation," and "Use of restraints." Silver and Yudofsky (1991) reported that the OAS captured 98% of aggressive incidents documented in medication books, hospital charts, and ward communication books combined, indicating adequate concurrent validity.

A limitation of the OAS is that it may be logistically difficult to complete the form for each incident of aggression when they occur at a high frequency (Ratey & Gutheil, 1991; Sorgi, Ratey, Knoedler, Markert, & Reichman, 1990). In an effort to eliminate this problem, Sorgi et al. (1990) developed the retrospective OAS using the original 16 items contained in the OAS, but with a modified scoring and temporal interval. The frequency of occurrence for each item is rated on a five-point Likert-type scale ranging from "0" to "greater than 10 times." The retrospective OAS is designed to reflect the patient's behavior over the previous week. The authors report adequate interrater reliability ($r = 0.96$) and internal consistency ($\alpha = 0.75$). Ratey and Gutheil (1991) also developed a modified version of the OAS to reduce respondent burden. However, they did not report information regarding its psychometric properties.

While empirical reports of the use of the OAS and the retrospective OAS with dementia patients have not emerged, given that the behaviors and interventions included on the OAS are observed in dementia patients, it is reasonable to assume that the instruments are appropriate for use with this population.

7.18.5.2.4 Blessed Dementia Scale

The Blessed Dementia Scale (BDS; Erkinjuntti, Hokkanen, Sulkava, & Palos 1988) is a 22-item scale that assesses cognitive functions, activities of daily living, instrumental activities of daily living, and personality characteristics. The BDS is administered within the context of interview with an informed respondent. Activities of daily living are rated on the basis of the frequency with which the client is able to perform the task (e.g., daily, occasional, always). Changes in personality, interests, and drive are rated as present or absent. Examples of items from the activities of daily living category include "Inability to perform household tasks" and "Inability to recall recent events." Personality items include "Increased egocentricity," "Impairment of emotional control," and "Sexual misdemeanor." The BDS has been shown to discriminate between institutionalized dementia patients and elderly community residents with no organic impairment.

7.18.5.3 Assessment of Functional/Contextual Features

Information regarding the frequency, duration, and intensity of agitation and aggression is necessary but insufficient for treatment planning. Research has consistently indicated that environmental factors influence behavioral disturbances in dementia patients, and therefore systematic identification of the environmental characteristics associated with agitation or aggression is essential for the determination of whether a behavior is environmentally dependent, and if it is, the features of the environment on which it is dependent. Specific factors that merit attention in the functional analysis of agitation include setting events, antecedent environmental stimuli, response characteristics, and response consequences.

7.18.5.3.1 Setting events

Setting events include, but are not limited to, factors such as patient mood, fatigue, level of cognitive impairment, physical status, or sensory functioning that affect the relationship between antecedent stimuli and consequences associated with aggression or agitation. A challenge in developing interventions for patients with a degenerative dementia is the inherently dynamic nature of the relationship between setting events and behavior as neuropathology progresses. An idiographic approach to assessment will be the most effective for addressing variation in the interaction between cognitive impairment, environmental stimuli, and behavior.

7.18.5.3.2 Antecedent environmental stimuli

Evidence for the importance of identifying antecedent stimuli associated with aggression and agitation has emerged from several studies that have documented a systematic relationship between the occurrence of these behaviors and various environmental stimuli (Cohen-Mansfield, Marx, Werner, 1992; Ryden, 1988). When, through repeated pairing of a stimulus and a particular reinforcement contingency, a stimulus comes to signal that reinforcement is available contingent on a particular response, the behavior is considered to be under stimulus control. The stimulus which signals that reinforcement is available contingent on a particular response is termed a discriminative stimulus.

Factors associated with the development and maintenance of the stimulus control of behavior in dementia patients have not be delineated. Idiographically based methods for determining whether a particular behavior exhibited by a dementia patient is under stimulus control are described below.

7.18.5.3.3 Response characteristics

In consideration of response characteristics, the topography of aggression and agitation in dementia patients has been the primary focus of empirical attention. Patients' emotional responses to environmental stimuli have not been systematically investigated. Cohen-Mansfield (1986) reported that lack of attention can be a precursor to agitation. It is possible that lack of attention leads to boredom, thus producing a functionally adaptive self-stimulatory behavior in dementia patients, such as stereotypic movement.

Another emotional response characteristic that may influence response to environmental stimuli and the subsequent occurrence of agitation or aggression is anxiety. Hall et al. (1995) suggested that AD patients may overestimate the dangerousness of a caregiver session, for example, as a result of confusion caused by cognitive impairment. Perceiving the environmental stimuli as dangerous may result in high levels of anxiety. Due to cognitive limitations the patient's repertoire of behaviors for coping with an anxiety-provoking stimulus is reduced (e.g., the patient is unable to verbalize a request to terminate the interaction), and the patient may strike the caregiver. The aggressive behavior may be negatively reinforced by termination of the caregiver's demands and subsequent reduction in the patient's anxiety. In this situation assessment of emotion as a response characteristic may suggest a proactive intervention such as presenting the patient with a distracting stimulus such as soothing music or a soft object to carry.

7.18.5.3.4 Environmental consequences

The consequences of agitation and aggression have received the least amount of attention by researchers. Little is known about how patient and caregiver behavior following behavioral disturbances function to maintain or reduce these behaviors. It is possible that termination of caregiver's demands or the reduction of an aversive emotional state may function to negatively reinforce agitated or aggressive behavior.

The instruments described below may be useful for formulating hypotheses regarding the functional context of agitated behaviors.

7.18.5.3.5 Motivation Assessment Scale

The Motivation Assessment Scale (MAS; Durrand & Crimmins, 1988) is a 16-item questionnaire designed to identify variables maintaining self-injurious behavior. It addresses four categories of situational determinants of self-injurious behavior including social attention, tangible consequences, escape from unpleasant situations, and sensory consequences. Respondents are asked to rate the likelihood of the specified target behaviors occurring in each of the situations listed using a seven-point Likert-type scale ranging from "0—never" to "6—always." Sample questions include, "Does this behavior occur repeatedly, over and over, in the same way?" and "Does this behavior occur when you are talking to other persons in the room?" The four categories on the MAS were supported by a factor analysis conducted by Bihm, Kienlen, Ness, and Poindexter (1991).

Durrand and Crimmins (1988) investigated the psychometric properties of the MAS on a sample of 50 developmentally disabled children. They found that the scale had adequate internal consistency, test–retest, and interrater reliability. The scale also demonstrated adequate concurrent validity. The reliability and validity of this scale for use with dementia patients have not been empirically investigated.

Subsequent studies on the interrater reliability of the MAS have produced varied results. Zarcone, Rodgers, Iwata, Rourke, and Dorsey (1991) applied the MAS to a population of subjects with severe disabilities using self-injurious behavior as the target behavior and reported interrater agreement ranging from -0.24 to 0.44. Sigafoos, Kerr, and Roberts (1994) also found low interrater reliability ($r = 0.03$) of the MAS when applied to subjects with profound intellectual disability and using aggressive behavior as targets. However, Kearney (1994) reported adequate interrater reliability ($r = 0.55$–0.79) when using the scale with a sample of mentally retarded adults and a variety of agitated behaviors (e.g., aggression, self-injury, screaming) as targets.

7.18.5.3.6 Behavior Environment Taxonomy of Agitation

The Behavior Environment Taxonomy of Agitation (BETA; Fisher, 1995) is a 16-item checklist that asks respondents to describe the likelihood of specific agitated behaviors occurring in any of four classes of situations. The BETA represents a modification of the MAS. A preliminary study of the utility of the MAS for use with AD patients, involving 17 AD patients, found that the category "tangible consequences" was ranked last (i.e., least relevant) for 58% of cases with a mean ranking of four out a possible five. Items associated with tangible consequences were endorsed as relevant almost exclusively for the behavior "Grabbing." This association was judged to be uninformative. Therefore, in an effort to reduce respondent burden associated with completing the BETA and to improve its utility, items pertaining to tangible consequences were eliminated. The situations described in the BETA have been identified in the literature (Anderson, 1970; Colenda & Hamer, 1991; Hamel et al., 1990) and by caregivers (Fisher et al., 1994) as being associated with the occurrence of agitation in dementia patients and in other clinical populations, including developmentally disabled persons and psychiatric patients (Durand & Crimmins, 1988; Paul & Lentz, 1977). The classes of situations on the BETA include: (i) social attention; (ii) escape from unpleasant situation; (iii) increase sensory consequences; and (iv) reduce sensory consequences Nurses and CNAs rate the likelihood of occurrence of four examples of each of these classes of situations on a seven-point Likert-type scale ranging from "0—never" to "6—always."

To evaluate the interrater reliability of the BETA, mean scores for the four BETA categories were ranked. The approach of ranking of category scores was used, because this approach is most consistent with how the categories are used clinically. The highest mean score was given a rank of one. The other mean scores were given ranks of two, three, and four, respectively. Tie ranks were averaged. Spearman rank-order correlation coefficients for the category scores indicated consistency in BETA ratings between respondents (median $r = 0.83$, $p < 0.01$). Test–retest reliability was evaluated using Spearman rank-order correlation coefficients for the category scores. Results indicated consistency in BETA ratings over time (two to three week interval) (median Spearman $r = 0.80$, $p < 0.01$).

Initial investigations regarding the factor structure of the BETA using a normalized varimax rotation factoring program revealed that the four factors that emerged are essentially equivalent to the subscales proposed in the revision of the BETA. The exceptions appear to be associated with the category "Reduce sensory stimulation." Items which include a reference to "stimulation" may load more heavily on a separate factor. This finding may also be associated with respondents' interpretation of the term "stimulation."

7.18.5.3.7 Functional Analysis of Behavior Recording and Tracking Forms

The Functional Analysis of Behavior (FAB; Lundervold and Lewin, 1992) is designed to assess the antecedents and consequences of verbal abuse and combativeness. It is divided into two parts each of which is completed when the target behavior occurs. Respondents record the date and time of each occurrence and place a checkmark next to the situation that immediately preceded the behavior. Examples of situations described on the form include "Meal time," "Bath time," "Dressing," and "Command." A brief description of the intervention that was implemented to address the behavior problem is also recorded.

The FAB Tracking Form (Lundervold & Lewin, 1992) is designed for monitoring the frequency with which several target behaviors occur and treatment progress. Respondents record (i) the type of behavior exhibited and (ii) the time interval within which the problem behavior occurred. Behavioral categories include aggression, property destruction, self-injurious behavior, and noncompliant behavior. No information is available on the reliability and validity of these instruments.

7.18.6 INTERVENTIONS

7.18.6.1 Pharmacological Interventions

A search of the medical, nursing, and psychological literature on treatment studies for aggression and agitation reveals that the vast majority of treatment studies on agitation and aggression are pharmacological. Several types of medication have been used in the treatment of agitated behaviors and aggression in older adults. These include neuroleptics, anticonvulsants, antidepressants, and antianxiety agents. A detailed consideration of the pharmacology of these agents is beyond the scope of this chapter. Studies of treatment efficacy are briefly reviewed.

7.18.6.1.1 Neuroleptics

Neuroleptics are the most commonly prescribed medications for reducing behavioral symptoms in older adults (Devenand & Levy, 1995). Their effects on agitation have been widely documented (e.g., Barnes, Veith, Okimoto, Raskind, & Gumbrecht, 1982; Coccaro et al., 1990; Schneider, 1990) although their mechanism of action has not been clearly established. In a meta-analytic review of 17 placebo-controlled studies of the use of neuroleptics with dementia patients, Schneider, Pollock, & Lyness (1990) reported that 18% of patients improved with neuroleptic treatment.

The use of neuroleptics for the management of aggression and agitation remains controversial because of the severity of associated side effects, including sedation, orthostatic hypotension, and akathesia (Finkel, 1993). Age-associated changes in metabolism increase the risk and severity of the side effects of neuroleptic use in older adults. Extrapyramidal reactions and tardive dyskinesia are also risk factors. Anticholinergic effects may exacerbate symptoms of dementia resulting in increased confusion, memory loss, and disorientation.

7.18.6.1.2 Benzodiazepines

Benzodiazepines are commonly used for the treatment of insomnia, anxiety, and agitation in older adults. In comparing the efficacy of benzodiazepines and neuroleptics in reducing agitation in cognitively impaired nursing home residents, Coccaro et al. (1990) reported a greater treatment response for neuroleptics. Side effects associated with benzodiazepines include sedation, cognitive impairment (Larson, Kukull, Buchner, & Reifler, 1987) and cerebellar ataxia resulting in an increased risk of falls (Ray, Griffin, Schaffner, Bough, & Milton, 1987). Paradoxically, when benzodiazepines are administered for agitation they may result in daytime sedation which, when coupled with the cognitive impairment associated with dementia, can result in increased irritability and agitation (Finkel, 1993). Further, withdrawal from benzodiazapines can result in serious disturbance, including insomnia, agitation, and psychosis (Wolf et al.,1989).

7.18.6.1.3 Beta blockers

Several studies describe the use of beta blockers for the treatment of agitation in elderly dementia patients (e.g., Greendyke, Kantor, & Schuster, 1986; Weiler & Goodman, 1987; Weiler, Mungas, & Burnick, 1988). Beta blockers such as propranolol affect agitation levels by blocking beta-adrenergic receptors and thereby decreasing sympathetic activity. Up to 1997, no well-controlled studies have evaluated the effects of beta blockers on agitation in cognitively impaired older adults. In a review of research on beta blockers for the treatment of agitation, Schneider and Sobin (1991) describe preliminary support for efficacy based on small samples of patients with various dementia diagnoses. Side effects involve both cardiovascular and central nervous systems. Propanolol is contraindicated in patients with sinus bradycardia, congestive heart failure, heart block greater than first degree, and bronchial asthma.

7.18.6.1.4 Other antianxiety agents

Anxiolytics such as buspirone are receiving increasing attention in the management of agitation and aggression in cognitively impaired older adults. Buspirone has fewer side effects than other antianxiety agents and the advantages of not producing memory impairment, psychomotor deficits, sedative, or addictive effects (Gelenberg, 1994). When side effects do occur they tend to be associated with higher initial doses (e.g. 10 mg t.i.d. rather than 5 mg t.i.d.). These include dizziness, nausea, and headache. Well-controlled treatment outcome studies of the effects of buspirone with dementia patients have not been conducted to date. However, the few studies that have been reported indicate that buspirone is effective in reducing aggression in dementia patients, with few side effects (Colenda, 1988; Herrmann & Eryavec, 1993; Jeanblanc & Davis, 1995).

7.18.6.1.5 Antidepressants

Several antidepressants have been used in efforts to reduce agitation in older adults. Serotonin uptake inhibitors have been receiving increased attention in the treatment of behavioral disturbance in dementia patients. Nyth and Gottfries (1990) evaluated the efficacy of citalopram for the treatment of emotional disturbance in 98 AD patients within a placebo-controlled group design. Significant improvement in agitation was reported for patients in the citalopram group.

7.18.6.1.6 Anticonvulsants

Evidence for the effectiveness of anticonvulsants for the treatment of agitation is limited to clinical case studies. A review of reports by Schneider and Sobin (1991) found 22 cases of agitated AD patients treated with anticonvulsants. Four patients were described as improved, with the remaining 18 not responding or developing toxicity. No well-controlled studies have evaluated the efficacy of these medications for the treatment of agitation in dementia patients. The most severe reactions associated with the use of carbamazine include dizziness, drowsiness, unsteadiness, nausea, and vomiting (Physician's desk reference, 1996).

7.18.6.2 Psychological Interventions

Empirical accounts of psychological interventions for managing behavior disturbances in older adults provide compelling support for preventative or proactive behavioral interventions (Lundervold & Lewin, 1992). Preventative approaches emphasize environmental design and the stimulus control of agitated behaviors and aggression. Given the paucity of information regarding the influence of the dementing disorders on response to consequences, interventions that attempt to *prevent* the occurrence of these behaviors may be the most judicious. Stimulus control interventions are described first.

7.18.6.2.1 Environmental stimuli

There are four components of the setting and sequence of events that warrant attention in determining whether agitated behavior or aggression are associated with environmental stimuli. The four components are: setting events, antecedent stimuli, patient response characteristics, and the consequences of the agitation or aggressive response.

(i) Setting events

When physiological or environmental setting events are identified as being reliably associated with aggressive responding, the context of the problem behavior can be modified to reduce the probability of the behaviors occurring. To illustrate, if aggression tends to occur during caregiving in the evening and not early in the day, then a reasonable intervention may be to reduce demands over the course of the day. Completing tasks early in the day will reduce the influence of fatigue and minimize the risk of a catastrophic reaction. If assessment reveals an association between specific environmental conditions and aggression (e.g., aggression occurs only when certain caregivers are providing care) the level of intervention will involve restructuring the physical or social context (e.g., altering the communication style of the caregiver).

In considering the role of antecedent stimuli associated with aggression and agitation the behavior of the caregiver clearly warrants attention. Specifically, the manner in which demands/requests are presented, even when quite benign in appearance, may provoke agitation or aggression. When verbal information or physical prompts are considered within the context of a patient's limited competencies it is clear that they should be presented individually and at a slower pace than normal. Instructions or requests should be made within the context of short sentences to accommodate impairment in language abilities and short-term memory. Caregiver eye contact and touch may also influence the likelihood of an undesirable response.

(ii) Response characteristics

A patient's emotional response before and during aggressive episodes may have implications for treatment planning. In a study of behavioral disturbance in dementia patients by Swearer et al. (1988), 63% of caregivers surveyed reported that the patient for whom they provided care exhibited one or more symptoms of anxiety, including general fearfulness, a fear of specific objects or events, restlessness, pacing, and appearing to worry over insignificant matters. Behavioral symptoms of anxiety were also found to be significantly associated with angry outbursts. Based on the observed association between aggression and anxiety, two treatment approaches warrant consideration. These involve the reduction of the anxiety-provoking characteristics of demand tasks and/or altering the consequences of the aggression.

The reduction of anxiety in cognitively impaired older adults can involve two strategies: (i) modifying the setting events or antecedent stimuli associated with the behavioral disturbance as described above, or (ii) implementing a distraction-based intervention to draw the patient's attention away from the distressing stimulus (e.g., instructing the caregiver to sing during caregiving episodes). Distraction-based techniques have been described for the reduction of anxiety in noncognitively impaired individuals (e.g., Beck, 1995; Barlow, 1988). The utility of such methods for dementia patients warrants further consideration by researchers.

If aggressive behavior tends to occur when demands to perform a task are placed on dementia patients, the aggressive response may be negatively reinforced by termination of demands. Further, if anxiety precipitates the aggression and the aggressive behavior results in a reduction of anxiety through termination of the anxiety-provoking stimulus (e.g. caregiver) the aggressive behavior can be viewed as adaptive since it may be the only readily accessed response in the patient's repertoire (Fisher & Swingen, 1996).

(iii) Social consequences

Assessment may reveal that the aggressive behavior of a dementia patient is contingently associated with social consequences (e.g., attention by caregivers). Differential reinforcement of incompatible behavior (DRI) may be a reasonable option to consider in this situation. To illustrate, Roseberger and MacLean (1983) described the implementation of this procedure in the treatment of a 79 year-old stroke patient residing in a nursing home. The patient was aphasic and partially paralyzed. Problem behaviors included physically aggressive behavior directed at staff, other residents, and visitors, throwing objects, smearing feces, and disrobing in front of visitors. Mechanical restraint and medication (e.g. Haldol and Mellaril) resulted in unacceptable side effects. Following assessment of the behaviors identified as the most disruptive, a DRI intervention was implemented wherein staff were instructed to greet the resident and praise her cooperation whenever she was observed to be behaving appropriately. In addition, problem behaviors resulted in a brief time-out from social attention. The intervention proved effective in that the resident's aggressiveness was reduced from 16 episodes per week to zero by the third week. Treatment effects were maintained at a 5 month follow-up.

A case study involving a 72 year-old man diagnosed with AD also demonstrates the effective contingent application of social consequences for reducing agitated behavior (Bakke et al., 1994). The patient had been prescribed buspirone for the agitation and had been expelled from two day treatment centers previously because of the agitation. On the basis of interview and observational data it was hypothesized that this man's frequent efforts to leave a work program and statements about going home were maintained by consistent attention from staff, while on-task, in-seat behavior resulted in social attention only 15% of the time. The intervention involved increasing the rate of tangible and social reinforcement contingent on working while incorporating efforts to reduce fatigue, discomfort, and boredom through restructuring of the work setting and schedule. Results indicated that this multicomponent program produced a significant decrease in agitated behavior while maintaining work productivity.

Understanding the contingencies of reinforcement associated with the behavior of dementia patients presents unique challenges for researchers and caregivers in that the progression in neuropathology limits the adequacy of traditional standards of treatment generalization and maintenance (Fisher & Carstensen, 1990). As is the case for physiologically based interventions, the effects of environmentally based interventions for dementia patients require continuous monitoring of changes in the reciprocal influence between behavior and the environment associated with deterioration in brain function. Stimulus control procedures, designed to prevent the occurrence of problem behaviors may be the most reasonable approaches to pursue until information regarding the efficacy of other environmentally based interventions is available (Fisher & Carstensen, 1990; Hussian, 1988).

ACKNOWLEDGMENT

Preparation of this chapter was supported by Grant R29 AG11241 from the National Institute on Aging.

7.18.7 REFERENCES

Addonizio, G. (1987). Neuroleptic malignant syndrome in elderly patients. *Journal of the American Geriatrics Society*, *35*, 1011–1012.

Anderson, J. F. (1970). A study of disturbed behavior in patients with dementia in two hospital populations. *Gerontology Clinics*, *12*, 49–64.

Bakke, B. L., Kvale, S., Burns, T., McCarten, J. R., Wilson, L., Maddox, M., & Cleary, J. (1994). Multiple component intervention for agitated behavior in a person with Alzheimer's disease. *Journal of Applied Behavior Analysis*, *27*, 175–176.

Barlow, D. H. (1988). *Anxiety and its disorders: The nature and treatment of anxiety and panic*. New York: Guilford Press.

Barnes, R., & Raskind, M. (1980). Strategies for diagnosing and treating agitation in the aging. *Geriatrics*, *35*(3), 111–119.

Barnes, R., Veith, R., Okimoto, J., Raskind, M., & Gumbrecht, G. (1982). Efficacy of antipsychotic medications in behaviorally disturbed dementia patients. *American Journal of Psychiatry*, *139*, 1170–1174.

Beck, J. S. (1995). *Cognitive therapy: Basics and beyond.* New York: Guilford Press.

Bihm, E. M., Kienlen, T. L., Ness, M. E., & Poindexter, A. R. (1991). Factor structure of the motivation assessment scale for persons with mental retardation. *Psychological Reports*, *68*, 1235–1238.

Bijou, S. W., & Baer, D. M. (1966). Methods in child behavior and development. In W. K. Honig (Ed.), *Operant behavior: Areas of research and application.* Englewood Cliffs, NJ: Prentice-Hall.

Bolger, J. P., & Dougherty, L. M. (1992). Psychological determinants of aggressive behavior in geriatric inpatients. *Behavior, Health, and Aging*, *2*(1), 3–11.

Bourgeois, M. S., Burgio, L. B., & Schulz, R. (1993). Teaching caregivers of spouses with Alzheimer's disease to modify problem behaviors in the home. *The Gerontologist*, *33*, 260.

Buck, J. A. (1988). Psychotropic drug practice in nursing homes. *Journal of the American Geriatrics Society*, *36*, 409–418.

Burgio, L. D., Scilley, K., Hardin, J. M., Janosky, J., Bonino, P., Slater, & Engberg, R. (1994). Studying disruptive vocalization and contextual factors in the nursing home using computer-assisted real-time observation. *Journal of Gerontology: Psychological Sciences*, *49*, P230–P239.

Callahan, C. M. (1993). Psychiatric symptoms in elderly

patients due to medications. In J. Rowe & J. C. Ahronheim (Eds.), *Annual review of gerontology and geriatrics: Focus on medications and the elderly* (Vol. 12). New York: Springer.

Carr, E. G., Levin, L., McConnachie, G., Carlson, J.I., Kemp, D. C., & Smith, C. E. (1994). *Communication-based interventions for problem behavior: A users guide for producing positive change.* Baltimore: Paul H. Brookes.

Coccaro, E. F., Kramer, E., Zemishlany, Z., Thorne, A. Rice, C.M., Giordani, B., Duvvis, K., Patel, B.M., Tores, J., & Nora, R. (1990). Pharmacologic treatment of noncognitive behavioral disturbances in elderly demented patients. *American Journal of Psychiatry, 147,* 1640–1645.

Cohen-Mansfield, J. (1986). Agitated behaviors in the elderly, II: Preliminary results in the cognitively deteriorated. *Journal of the American Geriatrics Society, 34,* 722–727.

Cohen-Mansfield, J., & Billig, N. (1986). Agitated behaviors in the elderly, I: A conceptual review. *Journal of the American Geriatrics Society, 34,* 711–721.

Cohen-Mansfield, J., & Marx, M. S. (1989). Do past experiences predict agitation in nursing home residents? *International Journal of Aging and Human Development, 28*(4), 285–294.

Cohen-Mansfield, J., Marx, M. S., & Rosenthal, A. S. (1989). A description of agitation in a nursing home. *Journal of Gerontology: Medical Sciences, 44*(3), M77–M84.

Cohen-Mansfield, J., Marx, M. S., & Rosenthal, A. S. (1990). Dementia and agitation in nursing home residents: How are they related? *Psychology of Aging, 5*(1), 3–8.

Cohen-Mansfield, J., Marx, M. S., & Werner, P. (1992). Agitation in elderly persons: An integrative report of findings in a nursing home. *International Psychogeriatrics, 4*(Suppl. 2), 221–240.

Cohen-Mansfield, J. Werner, P., & Marx, M. S. (1992). The social environment of the agitated nursing home resident. *International Journal of Geriatric Psychiatry, 7,* 789–798.

Colenda, C. C. (1988). Buspirone in treatment of agitated demented patient. *The Lancet, ii,* 510.

Colenda, C. C., & Hamer, R. M. (1991). Antecedents and intervention for aggressive behavior of patients at a geropsychiatric state hospital. *Hospital and Community Psychiatry, 42,* 287–292.

Cooper, J. K., Mungas, D., & Weiler, P. G. (1990). Relation of cognitive status and abnormal behaviors in Alzheimer's disease. *Journal of the American Geriatrics Society, 38,* 867–870.

Davis, P. B., & Robins, L. N. (1989). History-taking in the elderly with and without cognitive impairment: How useful is it? *Journal of the American Geriatrics Society, 37,* 249–255.

Deutsch, L. H., & Rovner, B. W. (1991). Agitation and other noncognitive abnormalities in Alzheimer's disease. *The Psychiatric Clinics of North America, 14*(2), 341–351.

Devanand, D. P., & Levy, S. R. (1995). Neuroleptic treatment of agitation and psychosis in dementia. *Journal of Geriatric Psychiatry and Neurology, 8,* S18–S27.

Durand, V. M. & Crimmins, D. B. (1988). Identifying the variables maintaining self-injurious behavior. *Journal of Autism and Developmental Disorders, 18*(1), 99–117.

Erkinjuntti, T., Hokkanen, L., Sulkava, R., & Palos, J. (1988). The Blessed Dementia Scale as a screening test for dementia. *International Journal of Geriatric Psychiatry, 3,* 267–273.

Evans, L. K., & Strumpf, N. E. (1989). Tying down the elderly: A review of the literature on physical restraint. *Journal of the American Geriatrics Society, 37,* 65–74.

Ferrell, B. A., Ferrell, B. R., & Rivera, L. (1995). Pain in cognitively impaired nursing home patients. *Journal of Pain and Symptom Management, 10*(8), 591–598.

Finkel, S. I. (1993). The pharmacological management of agitation in demented nursing home elderly. In M. Bergener, R. H. Belmaker, & M. S. Tropper (Eds.), *Psychopharmacotherapy for the elderly: Principles of research and clinical implications.* New York: Springer.

Finkel, S. I., Lyons, J. S., & Anderson, R. L. (1992). Reliability and validity of the Cohen-Mansfield Agitation Inventory in institutionalized elderly. *International Journal of Geriatric Psychiatry, 7,* 487–490.

Fisher, J. E. (1995, August). *Agitation and adaptation: Functional characteristics of the behavior of dementia patients.* Paper presented at the Annual Convention of the American Psychological Association, New York.

Fisher, J. E., & Carstensen, L. L. (1990). Behavior management of the dementias. *Clinical Psychology Review, 10,* 611–629.

Fisher, J. E., Fink, C. M., Loomis, C. C. (1993). Frequency and management difficulty of behavior problems among dementia patients in long-term care. *Clinical Gerontologist, 13,* 3–12.

Fisher, J. E., Goy, E. R., Swingen, D. N., & Szymanski, J. (1994, November). *Functional characteristics of behavioral disturbances in Alzheimer's disease patients.* Presented at the Annual Meeting for the Association for the Advancement of Behavior Therapy, San Diego, CA.

Fisher, J. E., & Swingen, D. N. (1996). *Contextual features of behavioral disturbance in Alzheimer's Disease.* Presented at the 30th annual meeting of the Association for Advancement of Behavior Therapy, New York.

Fishman, B., Pasternak, S., Wallenstein, S. L., Houde, R. W., Holland, J. C., & Foley, K. M. (1987). The Memorial Pain Assessment Card: A valid instrument for the evaluation of cancer pain. *Cancer, 60,* 1151–1158.

Folstein, M. F., Folstein, S.E., & McHugh, P. R. (1975). Mini-mental state: A practical method for grading the cognitive state of patients for the clinician. *Journal of Psychiatric Research, 12,* 189–198.

Foster, S. L., & Cone, J. D. (1986). Design and use of direct observation procedures. In A. R. Ciminero, K. S. Calhoun, & H. E. Adams (Eds.), *Handbook of behavioral assessment* (2nd ed.). New York: Wiley.

Gelenberg, A. J. (1994). Buspirone: Seven-year update. *Journal of Clinical Psychiatry, 55*(5), 222–229.

Gerdner, L. A., & Buckwalter, K. C. (1994). A nursing challenge: Assessment and management of agitation in Alzheimer's patients. *Journal of Gerontological Nursing, 20,* 11–20.

Gilley, D. W., & Wilson, R. S. (1991). Nuisance parameters in the assessment of noncognitive manifestations of dementia. *Psychology and Aging, 6*(4), 528–532.

Goldstein, K. (1952). The effect of brain damage on the personality. *Psychiatry, 15,* 245–260.

Greendyke, R. M., Kantor, D. R., & Schuster, D. B. (1986). Propranolol treatment of assaultive patients with organic brain disease: A double-blind crossover placebo controlled study. *Journal of Nervous and Mental Disorders, 174,* 290–294.

Hall, G. R., Gerdner, L., Zwygart-Stauffacher, M., & Buckwalter, K. C. (1995). Principles of nonpharmacological management: Caring for people with Alzheimer's disease using a conceptual model. *Psychiatric Annals, 25*(7), 432–440.

Hall, R. C. W., Beresford, T. P., Stickney, S. K., Nasdahl, C. S., & Coleman, J. H. (1985). Psychiatric reactions produced by respiratory drugs. *Psychosomatics, 26,* 605–608; 615–616.

Hamel, M., Gold, D. P., Andres, D., Reis, M., Dastoor, D., Grauer, H., & Bergman, H. (1990). Predictors and consequences of aggressive behavior by community-based dementia patients. *The Gerontologist, 30*(2), 206–211.

Herrmann, N. & Eryavec, G. (1993). Buspirone in the management of agitation and aggression associated with dementia. *American Journal of Geriatric Psychiatry, 1*(3), 249–253.

Hurley, A. C., Volcier, J., Hanrahan, P. A., Houde, S., and Volcier, L. (1992). Assessment of discomfort in advanced Alzheimer patients. *Research in Nursing and Health, 15*(5), 369–377.

Hussian, R. A. (1988). Modification of behaviors in dementia via stimulus manipulation. *Clinical Gerontologist, 8*, 37–43.

Jeanblanc, W., & Davis, Y. B. (1995). Risperidone for treating dementia associated aggression. *American Journal of Psychiatry, 152*(8), 1239.

Johnston, J. M., & Pennypacker, H. S. (1980). *Strategies and tactics of human behavioral research.* Hillsdale, NJ: Erlbaum.

Kantor, J. R. (1959). *Interbehavioral psychology: A sample of scientific system instruction.* Bloomington, IN: Principia Press.

Kearney, C. A. (1994). Interrater reliability of the Motivational Assessment Scale: Another, closer look. *Journal of the Association for Persons with Severe Handicaps, 19*(2), 139–142.

Kurita, A., Blass, J. P., Nolan, K. A., Black, R. S., & Thaler, H. T. (1993). Relationship between cognitive status and behavioral symptoms in Alzheimer's disease and mixed dementia. *Journal of the American Geriatrics Society, 41*, 732–736.

Larson, E. B., Kukull, W. A., Buchner, D., & Reifler, B. V. (1987). Adverse drug reactions associated with global cognitive impairment in elderly persons. *Annals of Internal Medicine, 107*, 169–173.

Lawton, M. P., Van Haitsma, K., & Klapper, J. (1996). Observed affect in nursing home residents with Alzheimer's disease. *Journal of Gerontology: Psychological Sciences, 51*(1), P3–P14.

Lindsley, O. R. (1964). Geriatric behavioral prosthetics. In R. Kastenbaum (Ed.), *New thoughts on old age.* New York: Springer.

Lundervold, D. A. & Lewin, L. M. (1992). *Behavior analysis and therapy in nursing homes.* Springfield, IL: Charles C. Thomas.

Melzack, R. (1975). The McGill Pain Questionnaire: Major properties and scoring methods. *Pain, 1*, 277–299.

Miller, R. J., Snowdon, J., & Vaughan, R. (1995). The use of the Cohen-Mansfield Agitation Inventory in the assessment of behavioral disorders in nursing homes. *Journal of the American Geriatrics Society, 43*, 546–549.

Moak, G. S. & Fisher, W. H. (1990). Alzheimer's disease and related disorders in state mental hospitals: Data from a nationwide survey. *The Gerontologist, 30*(6), 798–802.

Nelson, E., Wasson, J., Kirk, J., Keller, A., Clark, D., Dietrich, A., Stewart, A., & Zubkoff, M. (1987). Assessment of function in routine clinical practice: Description of the COOP chart method and preliminary findings. *Journal of Chronic Disease, 40*, 55S–63S.

Nyth, A. L., & Gottfries, C. G. (1990). The clinical efficacy of citalopram in the treatment of emotional disturbance in dementia disorders: A Nordic multicentre study. *British Journal of Psychiatry, 157*, 894–901.

Omnibus Reconciliation Act of 1987, Subtitle of nursing home reform, Part C. Washington, DC: US Government Printing Office.

Paul, G. L., & Lentz, R. J. (1975). *Psychosocial treatment of chronic mental patients.* Champaign, IL: Research Press.

Physician's desk reference. (1996). Oradell, NJ: Medical Economics Company.

Ray, W. A., Federspiel, C. F., & Schaffner, W. (1980). Antipsychotic drug use in nursing homes: Epidemiological evidence suggesting misuse. *American Journal of Public Health, 70*, 485–491.

Ray, W. A., Griffin, M. R., Schaffner, W., Baugh, G. H., & Milton, L. J. (1987). Psychotropic drug use and the risk of hip fracture. *New England Journal of Medicine, 316*, 363–369.

Ratey, J.J., & Gutheil, C. M. (1991). The measurement of aggressive behavior: Reflections on the use of the Overt Aggression Scale and the modified Overt Aggression Scale. *Journal of Neuropsychiatry and Clinical Neurosciences, 3*(2), S57-S60.

Roper, J. M., Shapira, J., & Chang, B. L. (1991). Agitation in the demented patient: A framework for management. *Journal of Gerontological Nursing, 17*(3), 17–21.

Rosberger, Z., & MacLean, J. (1983). Behavioral assessment and treatment of "organic" behaviors in an institutionalized geriatric patient. *International Journal of Behavioral Geriatrics, 1*, 33–46.

Rosen, J., Burgio, L., Kollar, M., Cain, M., Allison, M., Fogleman, M., Michael, M., & Zubendo, G. S. (1994). The Pittsburgh Agitation Scale: A user-friendly instrument for rating agitation in dementia patients. *American Journal of Geriatric Psychiatry, 2*(1), 52–59.

Ryden, M. B. (1988). Aggressive behaviors in persons with dementia who live in the community. *The Alzheimer Disease and Associated Disorders: International Journal, 2*(4), 342–355.

Schneider, L. S., Pollock, V. E., & Lyness, S. A. (1990). A metaanalysis of controlled trials of neuroleptic treatment in dementia. *Journal of the American Geriatrics Society, 38*, 553–563.

Schneider, L. S., & Sobin, P. B. (1991). Non-neuroleptic medications in the management of agitation in Alzheimer's disease and other dementia: A selective review. *International Journal of Geriatric Psychiatry, 6*, 691–708.

Sigafoos, J., Kerr, M., & Roberts, D. (1994). Interrater reliability of the Motivation Assessment Scale: Failure to replicate with aggressive behavior. *Research in Developmental Disabilities, 15*(5), 333–342.

Silver, J. M., & Yudofsky, S. C. (1991). The Overt Aggression Scale: Overview and guiding principles. *Journal of Neuropsychiatry and Clinical Neurosciences, 3*(2), S22–S29.

Sloane, P. D., Mathew, L. J., & Scarborough, N. (1991). Physical and pharmacologic restraint of nursing home patients with dementia: Impact of specialized units. *Journal of the American Medical Association, 265*, 1278–1282.

Sorgi, P., Ratey, J., Knoedler, D. W., Markert, R. J., & Reichman, M. (1990). Rating aggression in the clinical setting: A retrospective adaptation of the overt aggression scale: Preliminary results. *Journal of Neuropsychiatry and Clinical Neurosciences, 3*(2), S52–S56.

Spore, D., Mor, V., Hiris, J., Larrat, P., & Hawes, C. (1995). Psychotropic use among older residents of board and care facilities. *Journal of the American Geriatrics Society, 43*, 1403–1409.

Swearer, J. M., Drachman, D. A., O'Donnell, B. F., & Mitchell, A. L. (1988). Troublesome and disruptive behaviors in dementia: Relationships to diagnosis and disease severity. *Journal of the American Geriatrics Society, 36*, 784–790.

Teri, L., Larson, E. B., & Reifler, B. V. (1988). Behavioral disturbance in dementia of the Alzheimer's type. *Journal of the American Geriatrics Society, 36*(1), 1–6.

Teri, L., Borson, S., Kiyak, A., & Yamagishi, M. (1989). Behavioral disturbance, cognitive dysfunction, and functional skill: Prevalence and relationship in Alzheimer's disease. *Journal of the American Geriatrics Society, 37*, 109–116.

Vitaliano, P. P., Young, H. M., Russo, J., Romano, J., & Magana-Amato, A. (1993). Does expressed emotion in spouses predict subsequent problems among care

recipients with Alzheimer's disease. *Journal of Gerontology: Psychological Sciences, 48*, P202–P209.
Weiler, P. G., & Goodman, T. A. (1987). The use of propranolol in Alzheimer's's disease patients with disruptive behavior. *Current Therapeutic Research, 42*, 364–374.
Weiler, P. G., Mungas, D., & Bernick, C. (1988). Propranolol for the control of disruptive behavior and senile dementia. *Journal of Geriatric Psychiatry and Neurology, 1*, 226–230.
Werner, P., Cohen-Mansfield, J., Braun, J., & Marx, M. S. (1989). Physical restraints and agitation in nursing home residents. *Journal of the American Geriatrics Society, 37*, 1122–1126.
Williams, B., & Betley, C. (1995). Inappropriate use of nonpsychotropic medications in nursing homes. Journal of the American Geriatrics Society, 43, 513–519.
Wolf, B., Grohmann, R., Beiber, D., Brenner, P. M., & Luther, E. (1989). Benzodiazapine abuse and-dependence in psychiatric patients. *Pharmacopsychiatry, 22*, 54–60.
Yoshikawa, T. T., & Norman, D. C. (1996). Approach to fever and infection in the nursing home. *Journal of the American Geriatrics Society, 44*, 74–82.
Yudofsky, S. C., Silver, J. M., Jackson, W., & Endicott, J. (1986). The Overt Aggression Scale for the objective rating of verbal and physical aggression. *American Journal of Psychiatry, 143*, 35–39.
Zarcone, J. R., Rodgers, T. A., Iwata, B. A., Rourke, D.A., & Dorsey, M. F. (1991). Reliability analysis of the Motivational Assessment Scale: A failure to replicate. *Research in Developmental Disabilities, 12*, 349–360.

7.19
Incontinence

JOHN F. SCHNELLE
University of California, Los Angeles, CA, USA

7.19.1 INTRODUCTION

Urinary incontinence (UI) affects approximately 13 million Americans (National Kidney and Urologic Diseases Board, 1994). It is a common problem among 10–35% of all adults, affecting 30% of persons over age 60 years and more than 50% of nursing home residents (Diokno, Brock, Herzog, & Bromberg, 1990). Despite its high prevalence, urinary incontinence in the community often goes undiagnosed and underreported due to the stigma it holds (United States Agency for Health Care Policy and Research [USAHCPR], 1996). Outside and in the nursing home, incontinence is most often treated by physicians and nurses as a result of federal clinical practice guidelines that focus on medical assessment and treatment. Psychologists and behavioral therapists have played a role in treatment involving biofeedback strategies for use with cognitively intact persons suffering from incontinence. The purpose of the present chapter is to present how and why psychologists should play a broader role in the treatment and management of incontinence, particularly among cognitively and physically impaired frail people. Due to a number of associated conditions, this is particularly true for the large population of people who suffer from incontinence in nursing homes.

The primary role of physicians and nurses in incontinence care is dictated by the fact that best-practice guidelines specify that basic medical assessment of this condition is the first step to good clinical practice (USAHCPR, 1996). In the case of the community dwelling elderly, surgery and pharmacological treatment are often suggested by these assessments, and despite their invasiveness, are acceptable to relatively healthy people who suffer from incontinence. As noted above, historically, psychologists and other behavioral professionals have been responsible for developing and implementing incontinence interventions based on biofeedback strategies with people who are cognitively intact and capable of following the protocols that underlie biofeedback training. This work has been an important contribution to the management of incontinence in community dwelling populations. The present chapter will describe these traditional approaches to incontinence care.

The case will be presented in this chapter that, in addition to traditional roles, psychologists could and should play a broader role in the treatment and management of UI among cognitively and physically impaired persons. This point holds particularly true for the large population of people who suffer from UI in nursing homes, since behavioral deficits, depression, motivation, and a variety of other nonphysiological factors play a much larger role in the UI problems of these institutionalized elderly than for those who live in the community. Psychologists are specially trained to assess and manage these problems. Frail institutionalized elderly are not good candidates for many of the available invasive treatments, even if medical justification for these interventions are present. The most effective treatment of UI problems in the frail elderly has involved noninvasive behavioral interventions that have been directed towards both the patient and the caregiver. The skills of the behavioral scientist both for assessing the need for these interventions and for successfully implementing them is critical.

The present chapter first describes the prevalence and sequela of UI problems in both community dwelling and institutionalized populations. A simple classification scheme to describe the different kinds of incontinence symptoms is presented, along with a brief description of three major classes of treatment: pharmacological, surgical, and behavioral. Evidence describing the efficacy of these treatments is provided, with particular emphasis on the behavioral interventions. The final section of the chapter is devoted to the assessment and management of UI among institutionalized elderly. The potential role behavioral healthcare professionals could play in this assessment and treatment is also highlighted.

7.19.2 PREVALENCE, MORBIDITY, AND CONSEQUENCES

Urinary incontinence is most prevalent among the elderly in both community and institutional settings (National Kidney and Urologic Diseases Advisory Board, 1994). It affects 30% of persons over age 60 years who live in the community, about 35% of older patients in acute care hospitals, and over 50% of those living in institutions (Help for Incontinent People, 1994). Urinary incontinence has significant adverse physical, psychological, and financial effects. It is a leading cause of infection among frail older persons, is considered an embarrassing stigma by many of its sufferers, and has an estimated annual cost of over US$15 billion (National Kidney and Urologic Disease Advisory Board, 1994). Coupled with its role as a primary predictor of institutionalization, these negative outcomes clearly justify more aggressive efforts to identify, evaluate, and treat UI. These efforts are further justified by growing evidence that appropriate management can reduce the morbidity and cost of incontinence, particularly in institutionalized populations (Ouslander, Palmer, Rovner, & German, 1993).

Reported prevalence rates of UI vary considerably, depending on the population studied, how UI is defined, and how the prevalence information is obtained (Diokno et al., 1990). Among the population aged between 15 and 64 years the prevalence of UI in men is in the range 1.5–5% and in women is 10–30% (Burgio, Matthews, & Engel, 1991; Harrison & Memel, 1994).

Prevalence of UI ranges from 15% to 35% for noninstitutionalized adults above the age of 60 years, with women having twice the prevalence of men. Of these incontinent older adults, 25–30% have frequent (i.e., daily or weekly) incontinence episodes (Burgio et al., 1991;

Diokno, Brock, Brown, & Herzog, 1986). Approximately 53% of homebound elderly are incontinent (Noelker, 1987); this being similar to the prevalence rates reported for institutionalized elderly.

UI among nursing home residents is more severe and more commonly associated with fecal incontinence than in the community populations. Incontinent nursing home residents generally have multiple incontinence episodes throughout the day and night, and approximately 50% are also incontinent of stool (Ouslander & Fowler, 1985; Ouslander, Kane, & Abrass, 1982). The reported prevalence of UI in institutionalized populations ranges from 40% to 70%, and even higher, varying considerably between individual facilities depending on the case mix of functional impairment found within the resident population (Ouslander & Schnelle, 1995).

UI is associated with substantial morbidity and costs in the nursing home. It can predispose residents to skin irritation, exacerbating pressure ulcers and making them difficult to heal (USAHCPR, 1996); and can result in symptomatic urinary tract infections (Ouslander, Greengold, & Chen, 1987; Warren et al., 1987). It is also associated with falls among residents with nocturia and impaired balance or gait (Stewart, Moore, May, Marks, & Hale, 1992). The adverse psychological effects of UI among nursing home residents have been difficult to document due to issues of cognitive status and lack of willingness to report. However, incontinent residents who do not have severe dementia have reported being often embarrassed and frustrated by their condition (Ouslander, Morishita, et al., 1987).

Nursing home staff generally consider UI to be one of the most onerous and difficult conditions for which they provide care, and they perceive that a disproportionate amount of time is spent on the care of incontinent residents. The economic costs of UI in the nursing home have been estimated to be close to US$5 billion annually, including the cost of staff time, laundry, and supplies (Hu, 1994).

Thus, UI is a severe problem for large numbers of older people. Yet, this condition becomes even more devastating when it is considered that UI is often associated with a variety of more severe conditions. Among community dwelling older adults, UI is listed as a common geriatric syndrome associated with (i) a general decline in upper and lower body strength, (ii) sensory and emotional decline, and (iii) a high risk of institutionalization (Tinetti, Inouye, Gill, & Doucette, 1995).

Among nursing home residents, UI is associated with a high rate of hospitalization (Murtaugh & Freiman, 1995). Incontinent nursing home residents are susceptible to a high rate of infection requiring costly medical treatment both in the hospital and within the nursing home. Furthermore, the act of hospitalizing a nursing home resident is expensive from both quality of life and economic viewpoints. When older persons are hospitalized, they are at risk for experiencing a deluge of dependencies (Creditor, 1993).

Elderly nursing home residents often deteriorate in their functional status during hospital stays and develop problems unrelated to the cause of the admission (e.g., pressure sores). It seems clear that reducing hospitalization rates in nursing home residents will both improve the quality of life of residents and reduce the overall costs of healthcare. In view of these data, it has been argued that prevention programs targeting incontinent nursing home residents should be developed (Murtaugh & Freiman, 1995). The intent would be to reduce serious side effects connected with UI (e.g., urinary tract infections, skin infections), or prevent the condition from occurring. One example of such a prevention program is described in Section 7.19.6.6

To launch preventative programs and productive interventions effectively, it is essential first to distinguish among specific types of UI and to design efforts that are appropriately based on etiology and symptoms.

7.19.3 TYPES OF URINARY INCONTINENCE

7.19.3.1 Urge Incontinence

Urge incontinence is characterized by the involuntary loss of urine associated with a strong (or urgent) desire to void. Normally, as the bladder (detrusor) fills with urine, stretch receptors send signals to the spinal cord indicating the need for contraction. Under normal circumstances these contractions are inhibited through the central nervous system control. The person with urge incontinence has a reduced ability either to sense the urgency to empty the bladder or to inhibit contractions from the point that such signals are recognized.

This condition is usually associated with involuntary detrusor contractions referred to as detrusor instability (DI). This response is urodynamically confirmed by filling a person's bladder slowly with fluid via a catheter and measuring bladder contractions. In the case of urge incontinence, bladder contractions occur before the patient can report that they are unable to hold further fluid. DI is at times associated with neurologic disorders, but can also occur in individuals who appear to be neurologically intact.

In cases where neurological lesions are established, the DI is distinguished as detrusor hyperreflexia (DH). The most common neurological disorder associated with DH is stroke. A second neurodynamic diagnosis associated with the symptom of urge incontinence in frail elderly people is detrusor hyperactivity with impaired bladder contractility (DHIC) (Resnick & Yalla, 1985). DHIC results in involuntary bladder contractions. However, symptomatically, patients must strain actually to empty their bladders. Patients with DHIC generally have symptoms of urge incontinence and elevated postvoiding residual volumes (i.e., the amount of urine left in the bladder after a person voluntarily attempts to empty his or her bladder). Clinically, the amount left in the bladder can be determined either by ultrasound or by catheterizing the person after they void and draining what remains in the bladder.

7.19.3.2 Stress Incontinence

Stress incontinence is characterized by the involuntary loss of urine during physical movements that increase intra-abdominal pressure, such as coughing, sneezing, laughing, or other physical activities. Stress incontinence is established if the urine loss is coincident with an increase in intra-abdominal pressure, but occurs in the absence of a detrusor contraction or an overdistended bladder (USAHCPR, 1996). The most common cause of stress incontinence occurs in women as intra-abdominal pressure results in a significant displacement of the urethra and bladder during exertion.

Stress incontinence may also be caused by a deficiency in the sphincter muscle that closes off the bladder outlet. Normally, the sphincter is relaxed when voluntary bladder emptying begins, but closes off the bladder outlet during other times. In women, this incontinence is commonly a result of multiple surgical procedures, low estrogen levels due to age or other causes, or both. In these cases, the urethra sphincter is unable to generate enough resistance to retain urine in the bladder when bladder pressure is raised. Patients with stress incontinence can leak continuously or with minimal exertion.

It is not unusual for people to have a combination of urge and stress incontinence. When both symptoms are present, the incontinence is called mixed. Mixed incontinence is particularly common in older women.

7.19.3.3 Overflow Incontinence

Overflow incontinence is the involuntary loss of urine associated with overdistension of the bladder due to a high volume of urine. Overflow incontinence may manifest itself in a variety of symptoms similar to those of stress incontinence. It may be caused by an underactive bladder (unable to contract efficiently) or a bladder-outlet obstruction leading to overdistension and overflow. The bladder may be underactive due to drugs, neurologic conditions, spinal cord injury, or as a side effect of diabetes. In men, overflow incontinence is often associated with obstruction caused by the prostate; outlet obstructions are rare in women. Overflow incontinence is best diagnosed by measuring a patient's postvoid residual volume, as described in Section 7.19.3.1.

7.19.3.4 Functional Incontinence

Functional incontinence is characterized by involuntary urine loss due to factors outside the lower urinary tract. For example, if a patient has no stress or urge symptoms or a high postvoid residual, but is incontinent because he or she cannot reach the bathroom in a timely manner, it may be termed functional incontinence. Functional incontinence is typically diagnosed in people with physical or cognitive impairment. Caution is recommended in making this diagnosis, in that it should only be made after other causes have been excluded. Because mobility and cognitive impairment may occur in patients suffering from other types of UI, it is essential first to rule out those types that could respond to specific therapies.

The most typical treatment for functional incontinence involves improving the patient's functional status, modifying transient causes for the incontinence (e.g., fecal impaction), and reducing environmental barriers to toileting or providing sufficient toileting assistance to avoid incontinence episodes. These latter treatments are suggested for consideration even if a lower urinary tract abnormality is present, since incontinence may be exaggerated by immobility and cognitive factors. The assessment and treatment of incontinence is now discussed.

7.19.4 BASIC ASSESSMENT

Best-practice guidelines recommend that all incontinent residents should undergo a basic evaluation that includes a history, physical

Table 1 Potentially reversible conditions that may contribute to urinary incontinence in nursing home residents, and the management of these conditions.

Conditions	*Management*
Impaired ability or willingness to reach a toilet	
Delirium	Diagnosis and treatment of underlying cause(s)
Illness, injury or restraint interfering with mobility	Regular toileting assistance. Use of toilet substitutes Environmental alterations.
Depression	Appropriate pharmacological and/or non-pharmacological treatment
Irritation or inflammation in or around the lower urinary tract	
Urinary tract infection (symptomatic with frequency, urgency, sudden onset, or worsening of UI, unexplained fever or functional decline)	
Antimicrobial therapy[a]	
Atrophic vaginitis/urethritis	Oral or topical estrogen[b]
Stool impaction	Disimpaction Use of stool softeners and laxatives as appropriate Adequate mobility and fluid intake.
Increased urine production	
Metabolic (hyperglycemia, hypercalcemia	Improved control of diabetes Therapy for hypercalcemia if indicated by underlying cause
Excess fluid intake	Reduction in diuretic fluid intake (e.g., caffeinated beverages)
Volume overload	
Venous insufficiency with edema	Support stockings Leg elevation Sodium restriction Diuretic therapy
Congestive heart failure	Medical treatment
Drug side-effects	
Rapid-acting diuretics causing frequency and urgency	Discontinuation of offending medication as possible
Rapid-acting diuretics causing frequency and urgency	Dosage reduction or modification of scheduling
Anticholinergics, narcotics, calcium channel blockers, α adrenergic agonists (in men) causing urinary retention	
α Adrenergic antagonists causing urethral relaxation and stress incontinence	
Psychotropic drugs with sedative or extrapyramidal effects causing sedation and immobility that interfere with toileting	

[a] For nursing home residents with bacteriuria (with or without pyuria) who have chronic, stable symptoms of UI and no other symptoms of urinary tract infection, antimicrobial therapy is not indicated (see text). [b] See text for specific recommendations.

examination, measurement of postvoiding residual volume, and urine analysis. This basic evaluation has three objectives:

(i) to identify potentially reversible factors for incontinence (e.g., stool impaction, drug side effects, and other factors, as listed in Table 1);

(ii) to identify serious underlying conditions that may require further urologic, gynecologic, or urodynamic evaluation (see Table 2 for listed conditions); and

(iii) to determine the types of incontinence and the appropriate plan for their management.

Depending on the outcomes of this basic evaluation, three general classes of treatment and several combinations of treatments may be justified. The three primary classes of treatment are now discussed.

Table 2 Conditions that may require further urologic, gynecologic, or urodynamic evaluation.

Conditions	*Comments*
History	
Incontinence with recurrent symptomatic urinary tract infections	Must first exclude structural abnormality or pathologic condition in the urinary tract predisposing the patient to symptomatic infection
Physical examination	
Marked pelvic prolapse protruding through vaginal introitus	Consider surgical repair or pessary management to prevent discomfort and tissue erosion
Possible prostate cancer	Surgical intervention to cure cancer would not be appropriate for most nursing home residents; however, cancer diagnosis may be important in managing the incontinence and other complications
Urinalysis	
Hematuria (sterile)	Consider urologic evaluation to identify pathologic conditions of the urinary tract
Determination of postvoid residual volume	
Residual volumes > 200 ml	No precise cutoff point can be recommended; however, residual volumes > 200 ml are abnormal and should prompt consideration of further evaluation of the urinary tract to identify complications (e.g., hydronephrosis or renal function impairment) and determine the cause of the retention (e.g., obstruction, impaired bladder contractility)

7.19.5 TREATMENT OPTIONS

7.19.5.1 Pharmacological Interventions

The most common pharmacological interventions involve medications given for detrusor instability with urge symptoms and for stress incontinence. Evidence for the efficacy of these medications is most complete for anticholinergic drugs, which are designed to limit the contractility of the normal bladder and which probably also reduce instable contractions in the bladder.

7.19.5.1.1 Drug interventions for urge incontinence

The pharmacological agent which has been most often tested in trials to reduce urge incontinence symptoms is oxybutynin. Oxybutynin proved superior to placebos in six studies of middle-aged patients, reducing UI frequency by 15–58% more than did the placebo (Holmes, Montz, & Stanton, 1989; Moore, Hay, Imrie, Watson, & Goldstein, 1990; Riva & Casolati, 1984; Tapp, Cardozo, Versi, & Cooper, 1990; Thuroff et al., 1991; Zeegers, Kiesswetter, Kramer, & Jonas, 1987). In two of these studies, 43–67% of the subjects became subjectively continent with oxybutynin, a significantly larger proportion than found in those receiving placebo.

To test its efficacy with a nursing home population, in a randomized clinical trial of nursing home residents, oxybutynin was administered only to those residents who failed to respond to a noninvasive behavioral intervention (prompted voiding) (Ouslander et al., 1995a). Oxybutynin was given as a supplement to prompted voiding for those residents who failed to reduce their UI level with the prompted voiding intervention to less than one episode per day. Oxybutynin showed very modest effects in this target group of residents, and did not reduce UI to levels which were regarded as clinically significant. Thus, given the cost of the medication and its potential negative side effects (dry mouth, constipation, urine retention), it is not recommended for the general treatment of UI among nursing home residents.

An expert consensus panel convened by the USAHCPR summarized the research findings for the use of pharmacological agents to treat detrusor instability as follows:

> Pharmacotherapy, at least in short-term trials, appears to benefit some patients with UI due to detrusor instability. However, involuntary bladder contractions are usually not abolished, the warning time between the appreciation of the need to

void and the onset of bladder contraction is usually not affected, the degree of improvement is modest and cure is uncommon. In addition, many of these medications are costly and most have bladder side effects. These drugs should be used only in conjunction with a voiding schedule or behavioral intervention and only if other factors contributing to UI have been addressed. (USAHCPR 1996, p. 47)

7.19.5.1.2 Drug interventions for stress incontinence

Medications have also been used for stress incontinence, the purpose being to enhance muscle control in the bladder neck, bladder base, and proximal urethra. It is anticipated in these cases that the drug will stimulate muscle contraction in these areas and increase bladder outlet resistance. Increasing resistance should result in less urine loss when intra-abdominal pressure is raised. The data from controlled trials of medications that stimulate such muscle contraction are less clear than for drugs given for detrusor instability. The expert USAHCPR panel concluded that pharmacological therapy treatment for stress incontinence appears to result in few cures, but may cause subjective improvement in 20–60% of patients over placebo responses.

Estrogen replacement therapy is also considered a potential treatment for stress incontinence. Presumably estrogen replacement therapy will increase the vascularity, tone, and responsiveness of the urethra muscle. This, in turn, should increase bladder resistance and decrease stress incontinence. The exact mechanism of how estrogen may work, however, is unknown.

Fantl, Cardozo, & McClish, (1994), for The Hormones and Urogenital Therapy Committee, provided a meta-analysis of estrogen effects from six randomized controlled trials and 17 uncontrolled clinical series. Positive results were found for all subjects in the trials, representing a significant number of patients who presented with stress incontinence symptoms.

7.19.5.2 Surgery

Surgical intervention for UI is a consideration for a small but important subgroup of nursing home residents and a much larger group of community dwelling elderly. Since UI is not a life-threatening problem, elective surgery should be considered only if the patient reports strong quality-of-life concerns. It is also recommended that in most, if not all, cases surgery be considered only after less invasive pharmacological or behavioral treatments have proven ineffective.

Two major types of surgery are used to treat UI. First, women with stress incontinence associated with significant pelvic prolapse and urethral hypermobility may benefit from bladder-neck suspension and repair of the pelvic prolapse. Although studies have not been done in the nursing home population, the short-term (1–5 years) success of this type of surgery for properly selected older women is approximately 75%, success being defined as a significant reduction or elimination of wetness USAHCPR, 1996). Surgical placement of artificial urinary sphincters has been used for younger patients with stress incontinence associated with intrinsic urethral deficiency. This requires a relatively major surgical procedure and is probably not appropriate for nursing home residents or very frail older people. Periurethral injections of collagen have recently been approved for patients with intrinsic urethral deficiency. It is unknown what the mechanism of the effects are, but periurethral injection has reportedly been effective in younger patients.

The other type of surgical intervention for UI is the removal of anatomical obstruction, most commonly an enlarged prostate in men or a urethral stricture. Newer, less invasive techniques are now available for the surgical relief of obstruction in men and may be especially appropriate for consideration in frail, older nursing home residents. Detailed discussion of the evaluation and surgical treatment of lower urinary tract obstruction is beyond the scope of the present chapter. However, it is important to note that candidates for surgery who are suspected of having obstruction should be referred for complex urodynamic evaluation.

7.19.5.3 Behavioral Interventions

Behavior-based treatment strategies are a relatively noninvasive form of treatment for UI and can be effective in many cases. Behavioral therapies can be divided into (i) caregiver-dependent techniques for patients with cognitive and motor deficits, and (ii) those requiring active rehabilitation and education of the patient. These distinctions are arbitrary and require a careful analysis of how the patient's abilities match the performance requirements of a specific behavioral protocol. For example, most biofeedback interventions require that a patient follow multistep instructions, which may be beyond the ability of a cognitively impaired frail older adult. Therefore, in order to characterize the full array of available behavioral techniques for the large range of cognitive and functional abilities represented among incontinent people, this section of the present chapter describes techniques ranging from those that require the most active involvement on the part of the patient to those that require the least.

7.19.5.3.1 Bladder retraining

Bladder retraining is strongly recommended for the management of urge and mixed incontinence. The goal of this training is to build bladder capacity or to increase intervals between voiding. This, in turn, will reduce the probability of involuntary contractions. Bladder training has been used primarily to manage incontinence caused by DI. This form of training has few side effects, but is difficult to implement in cognitively impaired persons.

Bladder retraining (also termed "bladder training") has many variations, but generally consists of three primary components: (i) education, (ii) scheduled voiding with systematic delay of voiding, and (iii) positive reinforcement.

The education component usually involves a combination of written, visual, and verbal instructions that describe the physiology and pathophysiology of the lower urinary tract. This provides the background understanding considered useful in promoting adherence to the behavioral protocol.

Scheduled voiding and delay of voiding involves retraining the patient in resisting or inhibiting the sensation of urgency, to postpone voiding, and to urinate according to a timetable rather than according to urge (McCormick & Burgio, 1984). Behavioral approaches are often designed to distend the bladder by adjusting fluid loads and/or delaying voiding. The goal is to progressively increase the volumes retained in the bladder as well as the intervals between voids (Keating, Schulte, & Miller, 1988). If the patient is unable to meet the delay goal, the schedule is adjusted and the interval reset. Generally, the interval goal is initially set between two and three hours, with consideration given to the patient's baseline. This technique is not usually applied during sleeping hours. Once established, the goal interval is progressively increased and new goals accomplished through the use of distraction or relaxation techniques. The patient is thus "trained" to delay voiding when the urge to void occurs.

Several reports demonstrate that bladder training is effective in reducing UI (Fantl et al., 1991; Ferrie, Smith, Logan, Lyle, & Paterson, 1984; Pengelly & Booth, 1980). Fantl et al. (1991) conducted a controlled, randomized study of 131 women with sphincteric incompetence and unstable detrusor function. Subjects participated in a bladder-training program that included patient education, behavioral strategies to decrease urge, and scheduled voiding. Of the 60 women in the treatment group, 12% became dry and 75% had at least a 50% reduction in the number of UI episodes. Control subjects did not have significant changes in incontinent episodes. The magnitude of the effect was somewhat larger in cases of DI and the effect of bladder training was maintained after six months.

7.19.5.3.2 Pelvic muscle rehabilitation

Pelvic muscle rehabilitation is designed to strengthen the voluntary muscles that contribute to the closing force of the urethra and to support the pelvic structures. Underlying these technologies is a strategy directed toward stress symptoms; but there is some evidence that it can also be successful with DI and urge incontinence as well. When pelvic muscle rehabilitation exercises are done alone they often are called Kegel exercises. However, these exercises are also frequently supplemented by biofeedback training designed to increase awareness of pelvic muscle functioning.

The first step in pelvic muscle exercises (PMEs) is to help the patient develop a better awareness of pelvic muscle function and control. PMEs are performed by voluntarily contracting the perivaginal muscles and anal sphincter as if to control urination or defecation (Rose, Baigis-Smith, Smith, & Newman, 1990). The goal is to accomplish this with minimal contraction of abdominal, buttock, or inner thigh muscles. Patients are trained to sustain a contraction for at least 10 seconds, followed by an equal period of relaxation. It is a goal to progressively increase the contraction time. PMEs should be performed about 30–80 times a day for at least eight weeks, and may need to be continued indefinitely. Patients should be taught to contract the pelvic muscles both before and during an incident when leakage may occur.

The most effective use of PME to date has been reported in an uncontrolled study by Benvenuti et al. (1987). Patients were provided with 10 hours of training, including 20 sessions for practice of PMEs and other behavioral strategies, and an intensive home program. Subjects were 20 women aged 35–65 years (mean age 50.8 years). This protocol resulted in a 95% reduction in incontinence episodes. PME also has proven effective in the treatment of older adults in a study by Flynn, Cell, and Luisi (1994) that involved treatment for transient UI in 37 older adults receiving home nursing care (mean age 76 years).

The intensity of the PME program significantly affects physiological and functional outcomes. Bo, Hagen, Kvarstein, Jorgensen, and Larsen (1990) found significantly greater reductions in UI among a group of patients receiving ongoing training of increasing intensity over a period of six months as compared to a group that received only a single session of instruction and a home exercise program. The group receiving the ongoing instruction reported a 60.1% cure/improvement rate compared with 17.3% among the home exercise group. This study also found significant differences between these groups in physiological measurements of improved pelvic strength. This finding indicates a possible systematic relationship between symptom reduction and objective physical changes. Benvenuti et al. (1987), Elia and Bergman (1993), and Mouritsen, Frimodt, and Moller (1991) also report findings that PME has the potential to change muscle physiology.

In all cases of PME training, patients must show the capability of memorizing multistep instructions and be motivated to practice exercises when not with the therapist. These performance requirements limit the use of pelvic floor muscle rehabilitation for cognitively impaired individuals.

(i) Pelvic muscle rehabilitation: biofeedback

Biofeedback therapy generally uses electronic or mechanical instruments to sensitize patients to their physiological activity. This sensitization is generally accomplished through the use of auditory, visual, or other feedback. The goal is to train patients to identify and modify physiologic responses that mediate bladder control. Studies reporting various applications of biofeedback combined with behavioral treatment report a range of 54–87% improvement in UI across various patient groups (USAHCPR, 1996).

Biofeedback protocols differ in their use of reinforcement or feedback, as well as in the measurement system used to establish this feedback. The biofeedback protocol that has achieved the largest and most consistent reduction in UI episodes (75.9–82%) simultaneously reinforces pelvic muscle contraction, inhibition of abdominal contraction, and inhibition of detrusor contraction (Burgio, Robinson, & Engel, 1986; Burgio, Stutzman, & Engel, 1989; Burgio, Whitehead, & Engel, 1985; Burton, Pearce, Burgio, Engel, & Whitehead, 1988; McDowell, Burgio, Dombrowski, Locher, & Rodriguez, 1992). The presumed benefit of this approach, defined by a multimeasurement procedure, is that it reinforces pelvic floor contraction with moment-to-moment feedback, thus providing the patient with highly specific internal references to upgrade muscle contraction. Combining bladder and sphincter biofeedback also allows teaching pelvic muscle contraction in response to increasing bladder volume and observed detrusor activity.

In comparing biofeedback to PME, the approaches have been found to have comparable results. In a randomized controlled study, Burns et al. (1993) studied 135 women (age range 55–75 years) with primary stress incontinence. One treatment group received PME, and another group received single-measurement biofeedback for 20 minutes per week. The two treatment groups demonstrated a 54–61% reduction in incontinent episodes, compared with a 6% reduction of UI in a control group. No significant difference between the two treatment groups was found. This study demonstrated that both PME and biofeedback have the potential to reduce UI, and provided evidence that symptom severity has a role in response.

(ii) Pelvic muscle rehabilitation: weight training

Specially designed vaginal weights to strengthen the pelvic muscles have also been used to supplement PME. In this therapy, the patient receives a set of vaginal weights of identical shape and volume but of increasing mass. As part of a progressive resistance program, women insert a weight intravaginally and are instructed to attempt to retain it by contracting the pelvic muscle for up to 15 minutes at least twice daily. It is to be worn while the patient is ambulatory. The mechanism of action that the sustained contraction requires to retain the weight increases the strength of the pelvic muscles in a way that provides heightened feedback as to the desired pelvic muscle contraction. Available literature on this technique includes observations made in women with stress incontinence, but no controlled trials have been conducted. Initial observation from four anecdotal studies indicate a subjective cure rate or improved status in 68–80% of women after 4–6 weeks of treatment (Bridges, Denning, Olah, & Aorrar, 1988). The preliminary data from vaginal weight training, as well as the simplicity of the procedure, make it an attractive treatment option. However, the procedure is not yet well evaluated and further research is needed.

7.19.5.3.3 Toileting assistance protocols

Toileting assistance interventions are necessary for many physically impaired people who cannot independently toilet and for cognitively impaired people who cannot remember the behaviors necessary to maintaining continence (e.g., finding the bathroom). Most of the estimated one million nursing home residents who suffer from UI have both physical and cognitive problems that prevent independent toileting. Therefore, it is necessary that their caregivers provide some level of assistance to compensate for the resident's deficits. Unfortunately, many of these cognitive and physical problems are not reversible in the nursing home population, and it is necessary that caregivers continue to provide toileting assistance indefinitely. Thus, the goal for most cognitively impaired patients is to increase dryness under conditions where staff or other caregivers implement a routine protocol. This is in contrast to less impaired populations, in which the goal is to rehabilitate patients to the point where they are capable of maintaining dryness independently. Several toileting assistance protocols have been described for application in nursing homes.

(i) Routine or scheduled toileting

Routine or scheduled toileting is conceptually the most simple toileting assistance procedure, and involves the caregiver placing the patient on the toilet every 2–4 hours. No systematic effort is made to have the patient delay voiding or to have him or her initiate or ask for toileting assistance, and there are relatively few mobility requirements. There are no controlled trials of scheduled toileting procedures, even though there have been some reports that it has positive effects (Burgio et al., 1989).

(ii) Habit training

Habit training is a modification of the scheduled toileting protocol in which caregivers first attempt to identify a resident's voiding pattern. A toileting schedule is then set based on this voiding pattern. Presuming predictable voiding habits can be identified, placing a patient on a toilet at the point that they are most likely to void should prevent UI episodes. One study has reported positive results with this procedure (Colling, Ouslander, Hadley, Eisch, & Campbell, 1992).

(iii) Prompted voiding

The toileting assistance protocol that has been most thoroughly evaluated is prompted voiding. The major objective for prompted voiding is to establish an awareness on the part of the patients as to their continence status (wet or dry) and to increase the probability that they will ask for toileting assistance. Residents are not placed on the toilet unless they respond to a prompt for assistance or self-initiate a request for toileting assistance. The major steps in prompted voiding are listed in Table 3. It should be noted that these steps are deceptively simple. Many nursing home residents show severe communication and attention problems, and therefore a high level of clinical skill is required to induce them to respond to prompts. A behavioral training program in which caregivers are taught to orient residents to questions with a series of verbal and manual prompts greatly increases the ability of caregivers to teach cognitively impaired residents to respond affirmatively to prompts.

Prompted voiding has been documented to be highly effective in nursing home residents when skilled staff implement the protocol, even with residents who have different types of urinary tract dysfunction (Schnelle, Newman, Abbey, et al., 1990). Data collected during three major clinical trials indicate that 25–45% of incontinent residents will respond to prompted voiding, with a reduction in their UI frequency from three to four episodes per day to one per day (Schnelle, 1991; Schnelle & Ouslander, 1996). Approximately 34–40% of these residents do not respond, either because of their refusal to respond to prompts, or their inability to initiate voiding once they are assisted to the toilet. Severe depression and cognitive impairment often characterize those residents who refuse to respond to prompts. Problems in the lower urinary tract characterize residents who cannot initiate toileting once on the toilet. Procedures to identify residents who are capable of responding to prompts, initiating bladder emptying when on the toilet, and maintaining dryness have been described, and responsive residents can be identified in a three-day run-in trial (Ouslander et al., 1995b). This run-in assessment procedure is described in more detail in Section 7.19.6.1.

Unfortunately, there is strong evidence that prompted voiding procedures are not consistently implemented by indigenous nursing home staff, even with residents who are highly responsive (Schnelle, Newman, & Fogarty, 1990a). The inconsistent application of the prompted voiding procedure invariably results, even with the most responsive residents, in an increase in UI frequency, since few nursing home residents are capable of independent toileting. The primary dynamic that causes staff to gradually withdraw toileting assistance and decrease implementation of prompted voiding relates to time

Table 3 Prompted voiding protocol.

1. Contact the residents every two hours from 7 a.m. to 7 p.m.
2. Focus residents' attention on voiding by asking them whether they are wet or dry
3. Check resident for wetness, record on bladder record, and give feedback on whether the resident's self-report was correct or incorrect
4. Whether wet or dry, ask the residents if they would like to use the toilet (or urinal).
   (a) If they say yes:
      (i) Assist them
      (ii) Record the results on the bladder record
      (iii) Give them positive reinforcement by spending an extra minute or two talking with them
   (b) If they say no:
      (i) In the event they have not attempted to void in the last four hours, repeat the request to use the toilet once or twice before leaving, and follow step 4(a) if an affirmative response is received
      (ii) Inform them that you will be back in two hours and request they try to delay voiding until then

efficiency (Schnelle, 1991; Schnelle, Sowell, Hu, & Traughber, 1988a). It has been documented many times that changing residents when they are wet is less time consuming for staff than is prompting them with sufficient frequency to maintain dryness (Schnelle, Sowell, Hu, & Traughber, 1988b). Furthermore, a resident is typically changed one to two times per eight-hour shift, despite best practice guidelines, and a successful prompted voiding program would require that a resident be prompted four times and provided toileting assistance approximately three of those times. It has been calculated that the time staff spend in managing incontinent patients is approximately seven minutes per eight-hour shift, whereas to implement the prompted voiding program so as to maintain dryness would take approximately 26 minutes per eight-hour shift (Schnelle et al., 1995).

Due to the time dynamic and other factors, behavioral management systems that reinforce nursing home staff to maintain prompted voiding protocols have proven necessary if the protocols are to be maintained. The most successful of these management systems is based on applied behavioral analysis strategies and work sampling systems that are used in the area of total quality management. This management system and issues relevant to implementing the system will be described later in this chapter (Schnelle, Newman, et al., 1993).

The successful implementation of the prompted voiding protocol in nursing homes within the framework of the best-practice guidelines, describing how UI should be assessed, generates major opportunities for the involvement of a behaviorally trained professional. An algorithm that describes how UI can be successfully assessed and treated within the nursing home setting is provided in Figure 1. This algorithm is described below, with particular emphasis on those points in the algorithm that require the expertise of behaviorally trained professionals.

The first section of the algorithm covers the basic UI evaluation that is recommended by best-practice guidelines for all patients. This basic assessment was summarized earlier in this chapter, and it is fully described in the USAHCPR incontinence guidelines. A trained nurse can complete this part of the algorithm, and we will not discuss these basic assessment procedures again at this point.

However, we should note that experience indicates that many nursing home residents will show transient causes for their incontinence at this stage, but also that the management of these conditions will not result in the elimination of incontinence. Immobility and dementia are such powerful causative factors for UI in the nursing home population that a program to compensate for these problems is almost always necessary if UI is to be improved. The term "compensate" is used in the above sentence as opposed to "rehabilitate" or "reverse" since there is strong evidence that the cognitive and physical impairments that exacerbate UI are not reversible in most cases, given the current treatment technologies and resource availability.

The most important section of the algorithm for the treatment and management of UI is the quality assurance monitoring system. This system requires that nursing supervisors and staff be trained in basic principles of behavior management and quality control, and is

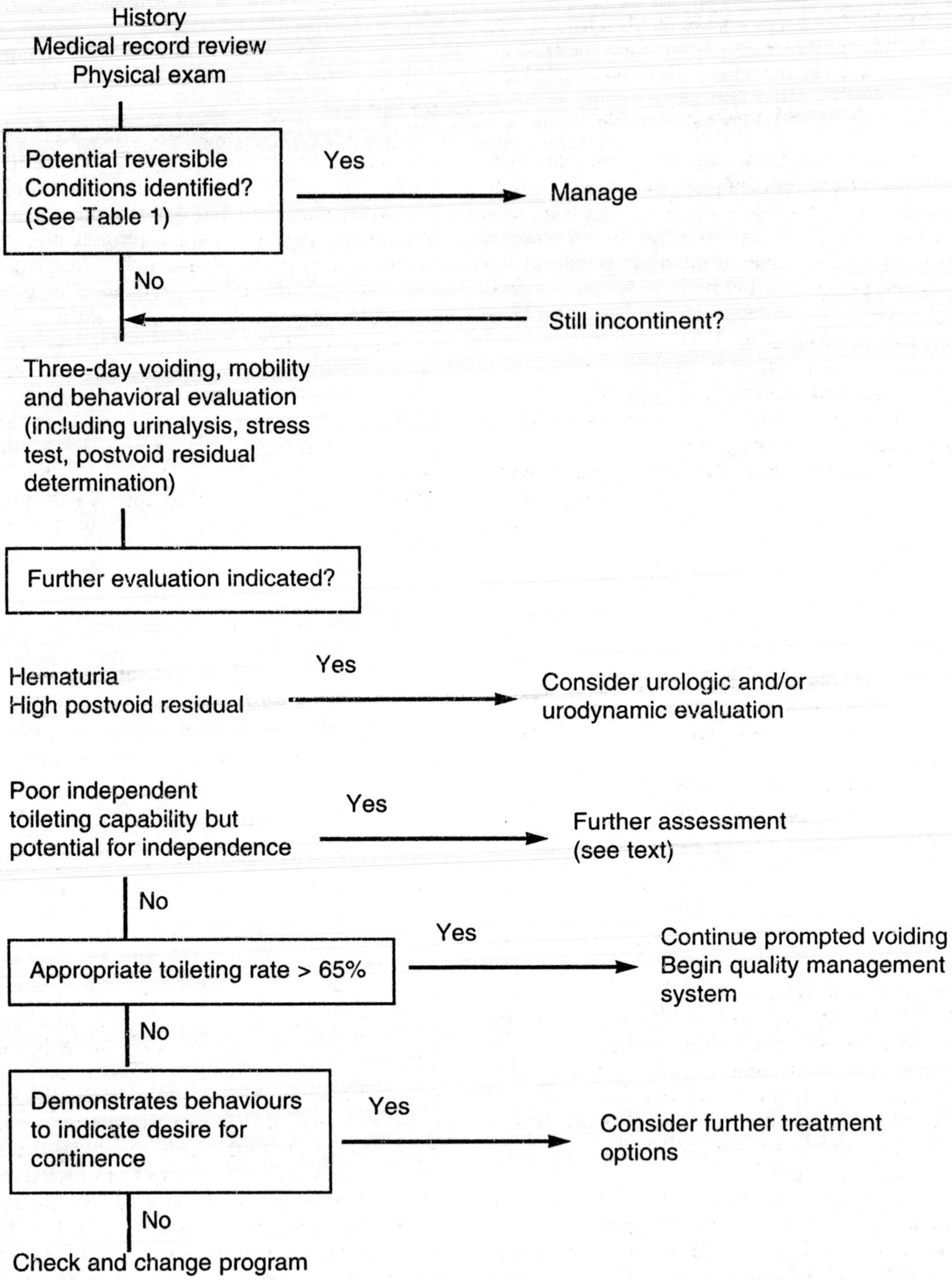

Figure 1 Assessment and treatment steps for urinary incontinence: basic evaluation.

described later in the present chapter. First, we discuss the critical assessment stage associated with prompted voiding.

7.19.6 IMPLEMENTATION OF AN INCONTINENCE MANAGEMENT PROGRAM IN NURSING HOMES

7.19.6.1 Prompted Voiding Assessment

The most important section of the algorithm for the assessment of UI in nursing home patients is a three-day voiding, mobility, and behavioral evaluation. This three-day evaluation can best be done by nurses in combination with the behavioral health professional who is expert in the assessment of behavioral competencies and motivation.

Critical information is collected during this stage regarding the following issues.

(i) Will a resident be responsive to a prompted voiding program?

(ii) Is the resident motivated to be continent, but not responsive to the prompted voiding protocol because of problems with the lower urinary tract?

(iii) Can the UI symptoms and problems with the lower urinary tract be identified and treated in the resident who is motivated to be continent, but who cannot maintain dryness?

(iv) Does a resident have mobility or cognitive problems which preclude safe independent toileting and can these problems be treated?

(v) What form of UI measurement is best for the resident who does not appear to be either a candidate for further treatment or who appears to not want further treatment?

The major activity during this three-day trial stage involves exposing the residents to a prompted voiding protocol every two hours between 8 a.m. and 4 p.m. (four times per day for three days = 12 prompts). Data are recorded at each prompt relevant to a resident's incontinent status (wet or dry); the resident's response to prompt (attempted to toilet successfully, attempted to toilet unsuccessfully, did not attempt to toilet), and the resident's behavioral response to prompt (shows resistance, agitation, or cooperation).

Prior to this three-day trial, the resident should be asked the following questions.

(i) Does it bother you to wet in your diaper?

(ii) Do staff help you to the toilet as much as you would like?

(iii) Do you want to be helped to the bathroom more often?

If the resident answers no to question (iii):

(iv) Do you want to be helped to the toilet less often?

(v) Do you want to be changed more often? If the answer is no, ask question (vi);

(vi) Do you want to be changed less often? Immediately after the three-day trial, the resident should be asked the same questions plus the question:

(vii) Do you like the amount of changing and toileting assistance you have received in the last three-days?

The most critical statistic calculated during this trial is the resident's appropriate toileting percentage. Appropriate toileting is calculated by dividing the total number of successful toilets by the total number of toilets plus the number of incontinence voids. Thus, a 50% appropriate toileting statistic will be derived if a resident appropriately toileted during six of the prompts on the three days and was wet on six of the prompts. Two separate major trials have determined that residents who have appropriate toileting percentages above 66% will very likely continue to be continent if exposed to prompted voiding over longer intervals (Schnelle, 1990; Schnelle, Ouslander, & Simmons, 1993); thus, it is recommended that all residents who show an appropriate toileting percentage of 65% or above be placed on a prompted voiding program. Residents who have appropriate toileting percentages of less than 65% seldom show responsiveness with longer term applications of prompted voiding. Based on previous studies in several major clinical trials, approximately 30–40% of residents will show a 66% appropriate toileting percentage or higher during this three-day trial.

The resident's response to the six questions asked prior to and after the three-day trial coupled with his or her behavioral responses to the prompts provided during the trial form the information base used to evaluate a resident's motivation to be continent. Approximately 80% of incontinent residents can provide answers to these questions. Surprisingly, however, approximately 10–20% of incontinent residents in nursing homes show no behavioral or verbal willingness to be either changed or toileted more frequently. Such residents respond to the questions with answers which indicate that they are not bothered by wetness and do not want to be changed or toileted more often. Moreover, when efforts are made to change or toilet such residents on a two-hour schedule during the three-day assessment period, there is often both behavioral and verbal evidence that this UI care is unwanted. For example, direct quotes taken during conduct of the protocol are as follows: "It hurts. I don't want to use the bedpan." "Leave me alone. I don't want changed." Similar comments are heard with noticeable frequency. Residents who express this type of resistance will typically not attempt to toilet even if consistently prompted by skilled and clinically sensitive staff. It is to be remembered that in prompted voiding, residents are not placed on the toilet unless they respond affirmatively to a prompt.

Even though a case can be made that the behavior of these resistive residents is not appropriate and may be caused by psychological conditions such as conditioned helplessness or depression, further treatment for these residents is not indicated at the present time due to three factors:

(i) there are no leads as to what types of behavioral, psychological, or medical interventions could be successful with these resistive patients;

(ii) there are so many incontinent nursing home residents that we currently strain resources to treat and manage UI with even those residents who are motivated to be continent; and

(iii) there is a distinct chance that some residents have such a high sickness burden that they do not care about staying dry and would prefer to not go through the activities involved with toileting, in which case prompted voiding would hinder rather than benefit quality of life.

Research investigating why some residents no longer care about their UI condition is highly appropriate, but treatment should not be considered until such research is completed.

Approximately 10–20% of residents will not attain a 66% appropriate toileting statistic but will show behavioral and verbal evidence that they are motivated to be continent and thatthey want further treatment. Further evaluation for these residents is indicated. The most important behavioral evidence to identify residents in potential need of further treatment is a statistic that reflects their positive response to prompts and their attempts to toilet during the three-day period. This statistic is different from the appropriate toileting statistic which requires not only an attempt to toilet, but also a successful void. If the resident attempts to toilet two times per day, even if they are not successful, it is an excellent sign that they are motivated to be continent. Many residents who attempt to toilet unsuccessfully cannot initiate the voiding process once they are placed on the toilet. Others will attempt to toilet frequently and void small amounts, but will continue to be wet between the checks and hence will not attain a 66% appropriate toilet ratio. These residents very often show stress incontinence, detrusor instability, or detrusor instability with impaired contractility, all of which were discussed in Section 7.19.3.1. Further information is collected during this three-day period which is highly relevant to determining which of these types of incontinence a resident may have. The purpose is to identify all problems appropriately treatable by other interventions. These procedures will be described next.

7.19.6.2 Postvoid Residual Determination and Urinalysis

During the three-day run-in evaluation for prompted voiding, an attempt is made to collect urine for analysis and also to measure a resident's postvoid residual, as is recommended for the basic assessment of people who suffer from incontinence. The basic prompted voiding protocol is temporarily modified in order to obtain this information efficiently. For further efficiency purposes, an attempt is made to collect these data the first time the resident successfully toilets during the three days of prompted voiding rounds. This toileting event offers the opportunity to collect urine for analysis with either a "clean catch" technology or by catheterization if the resident has to be catheterized to measure the amount of urine left in the bladder after urination (postvoid residual).

Clean urine may be difficult to obtain from incontinent, cognitively impaired, immobile nursing home residents. However, one can often noninvasively obtain a "clean catch" urine that accurately matches culture results from a catheterized specimen. For a woman, the technique involves careful cleaning of the perineum with a sterile preparation and then having her void into a disinfected collection device (Ouslander, Schapira, & Schnelle, 1995). For a man, after the penis has been cleaned with a sterile preparation such as betadine, a clean condom catheter can be applied (Ouslander, Schapira, Fingold, & Schnelle, 1995).

The primary purpose of the urinalysis is to exclude hematuria unless the purpose is to investigate symptoms other than UI which are suggestive of a urinary tract infection (e.g., dysuria, recent onset or worsening of UI, unexplained fever or functional decline). The urinalysis can also exclude sterile hematuria, which may be a sign of bladder or upper urinary tract pathology, and glucosuria resulting from poorly controlled diabetes. In nursing home residents it is important to note that bacteriuria should not be treated, because such treatment consistently has been found to have no effect on the severity of UI in this population (Ouslander, Schapira, Schnelle, Uman et al., 1995).

Although rapid urine screening methods are generally thought of as inaccurate for nursing home residents, they can be used to exclude bacteriuria with reasonable accuracy. The combination of negative dipstick tests for both nitrite and leukocyte esterase and a negative enzyme-based screen for bacteriuria (Uriscreen) has a negative predictive value of over 95% for significant bacteriuria among incontinent nursing home residents (Ouslander, Schapira, Fingold, & Schnelle, 1995).

Significant degrees of urinary retention can occur in the absence of symptoms or signs of obstruction or bladder contractility problems. In addition, physical examination (suprapubic palpation, bi-manual examination) is neither sensitive nor specific in detecting significant residual volumes.

Postvoid residual volume is usually determined by catheterization, but a portable ultrasound device is now available that can provide a noninvasive measurement with reasonable accuracy (Ouslander et al., 1994). It is important to note that postvoid residual volume demonstrates substantial intra-individual variability. The timing of the determination in relation to a void, the degree to which the void was natural, the nature of instructions provided to the patient, the amount of straining, and body position can all influence this measurement. Thus, when moderately elevated volumes are detected (e.g., 150–300 ml), repeated determinations may be appropriate. In these situations in particular, the use of ultrasound may be indicated, in order to avoid the need for repeated catheterization. Consistent residual volumes of more than 200 ml should prompt consideration of whether the patient should be referred for further evaluation.

7.19.6.3 Pad Test for Stress Incontinence

The second diagnostic modification of the prompted voiding run-in protocol is designed to evaluate signs of stress incontinence. Although the presence or absence of stress incontinence does not predict responsiveness to prompted voiding, this diagnostic measure is helpful in cases of residents who fail a trial of prompted voiding and who are candidates for other therapeutic interventions for stress incontinence. This test can be performed during the same toileting episodes in which a clean urine and postvoid residual are being obtained. It is performed by having the resident cough several times while standing. The test is positive if there is urine leakage simultaneous with the cough. If the test is negative and if the total bladder volume (voided volume plus residual) is less than 200 ml, the test should be repeated since a low bladder volume can cause a false negative result. In many cases, it is impossible to obtain an adequate stress test because of either low bladder volumes due to involuntary bladder contraction, low toileting frequency, or difficulty following instructions. Attempts to obtain a stress test should be terminated if it cannot be completed successfully during the first few toileting episodes.

7.19.6.4 Mobility Assessment

The third modification to the prompted voiding protocol evaluates the resident's mobility skills to toilet independently and to do so safely. Two critical questions are addressed by this assessment: (i) will a resident require ongoing prompted voiding management because of physical inability to safely toilet? and (ii) should a resident be placed on a rehabilitation program to improve mobility skills related to toileting?

The extent to which a resident can safely perform the mobility tasks involved in toileting can be evaluated most efficiently during the prompted voiding episodes, during which the resident must move for either changing or toileting assistance. This offers a time-efficient and natural opportunity to evaluate the resident's ability to perform three critical skills for independent toileting: standing, moving (either walking or wheeling a wheelchair) to the toilet, and transferring. A standardized behavioral assessment protocol has been designed to assess these skills (Schnelle, MacRae, Ouslander, Simmons, & Nitta, 1995). The instructions and prompting provided to the resident during this protocol are specifically designed to elicit the maximum possible independent effort. A resident is determined to be capable of independent toileting if he or she performs all three of the tasks either when instructed to do so or with instructions plus gentle manual guidance. Research conducted by the present author has demonstrated that 30–40% of nursing home residents are capable of independently performing all three skills necessary for independent toileting. However, many of these otherwise independent residents can complete these tasks only with major effort, due to deconditioning, muscular weakness, and balance problems, which place them at higher risk for falls. Many of the residents are aware of their safety risk and are so afraid to fall that they do not attempt to toilet independently because of this fear (Schnelle et al., 1994). These residents are candidates for further treatment of mobility problems, and it is anticipated that an unknown percentage of these residents may become capable of independent toileting. Mobility interventions that have been found to have positive outcomes for this group are described in Section 7.19.6.6.

The many residents who are not capable of toileting independently and who cannot be taught to do so safely will have to be maintained on prompted voiding indefinitely so as to receive toileting assistance even if other treatments for UI are attempted and successful. For example, even if a resident is capable of maintaining dryness for several hours at a time due to an intervention such as drug therapy, this resident will only be continent to the extent that staff offer him or her an opportunity to toilet on a regular basis.

Similarly, even residents who are capable of performing all toileting tasks independently must be maintained on prompted voiding if they are either very slow or show poor strength and endurance. Findings indicate that the average time it takes an incontinent resident to stand is six seconds; the average time span during which incontinent residents can sustain walking in a standardized endurance test is 2.6 minutes (Schnelle et al., 1994). These mobility problems limit the ability to stay dry, and the muscle weakness associated with the slowness and poor endurance place the resident at risk for falling. Thus, many such residents will have to be maintained on prompted voiding so that toileting assistance can be provided for the purpose of getting the residents to the bathroom quickly and safely. The issues involved in the maintenance of prompted voiding are complex and require an effective quality assurance system (described in Section 7.19.6.7). However, a decision regarding whether further evaluation is to be done should be made prior to determining if residents are to be managed on an ongoing basis with prompted voiding. The issue of who are candidates for further evaluation is discussed next.

7.19.6.5 Who are Candidates for Further Evaluation?

Urologic and/or urodynamic evaluation should be considered for residents with sterile hematuria or high (> 200 ml) postvoid residual volumes. Only residents who are candidates for specific interventions based on the results of these evaluations should be referred. Further evaluation may also be indicated for those residents who show positive stress symptoms or high wetness frequencies (two or more times per day), despite attempts to toilet two or more times a day. In these cases, either a stress or urge diagnosis is suspected, and the treatment options available for these conditions (described in Section 7.19.3) could be attempted. Given their attempts to toilet, these residents clearly have demonstrated at least the minimal cognitive capacity and motivation necessary to be appropriate candidates for these types of treatment. Recommendations for treatment with alternative behavioral, surgical, or pharmacological interventions should be qualified by the fact that there is no strong evidence that such interventions are successful, even with carefully targeted nursing home residents.

Further evaluation by a physical therapist is recommended for residents who either cannot independently perform all three mobility skills related to toileting or who do so very poorly and who are felt to have some potential for improving these skills. Based on previous work, we estimate that most incontinent residents will be in need of either a physical therapist consultation or a rehabilitative nursing exercise program designed to improve mobility, endurance, and muscle strength. Moreover, as discussed in Section 7.19.2, we reviewed data which indicates that UI and immobility problems are jointly predictive of a high rate of infection and hospitalization to treat these infections. An intervention program that addresses both risk factors is needed, even if the resident cannot attain toileting independence because of reversible physical or cognitive problems, since such a program may also prevent infections. Mobility interventions that may be effective with incontinent nursing home residents are now described.

7.19.6.6 Treatment for Mobility Problems that Limit Independent Toileting

It is not known to what degree physical therapy assessment and treatment is appropriate for incontinent nursing home residents who are chronically ill, demented, and who require maximal assistance to perform the three mobility skills related to independent toileting. Two separate exercise rehabilitation trials, each lasting for nine-week periods, have not been successful in significantly improving the independence level of these very dependent residents (Schnelle, MacRae et al., 1995). However, improvements have been found in endurance, speed, and safety levels for all three mobility skills among residents capable of performing these skills independently or with minimal physical assistance (Schnelle et al., 1996; Schnelle, MacRae et al., 1995). These findings are a result of a mobility intervention utilizing a functional incidental training (FIT) technique.

FIT is implemented concurrently with prompted voiding and involves two primary additions. The two additional FIT steps are done each time prompted voiding occurs when the resident is out of bed. First, the resident is encouraged to perform the toileting-related activities with minimal staff assistance. This is in contrast to standard care since, as a result of staff time constraints, aides typically provide maximal assistance to the residents in completing the prompted voiding sequence. In the absence of functional considerations, it is more efficient to provide such maximal assistance and to minimize the resident's involvement; however, the FIT intervention promotes functional activity. In the second FIT step, the resident is given repeated practice in each functional activity (e.g., standing, moving, transferring) and works toward an individualized goal, which is increased progressively as the resident demonstrates improvement.

The application of the FIT protocol three times per day for nine weeks has been shown in a controlled trial to result in significant improvements in walking endurance, standing speed, wheelchair endurance, and safety measures for a group of 38 residents (Schnelle, MacRae et al., 1995). Unfortunately, only 10% of the residents showed improvement on these mobility tasks to the point where they were rated as being at a low risk for falls. A modification of the FIT protocol is currently being tested which includes resistance training designed to further improve muscle strength. There is strong evidence from several trials that even very old nursing home residents will show strength improvements with resistance training (Fiatarone et al., 1994; Mulrow, Gerety, Kanten, & Cornell, 1994). In addition, FIT is being implemented for longer time periods to explore further its potential for producing a higher level of mobility independence and a lower risk for injury and infections which may require hospitalization.

However, even if these mobility interventions are successful, most residents will require routine prompting and some physical assistance to maintain continence and to maintain their improved mobility performance. A quality assurance system to assure that staff continue to provide such assistance is critical; therefore, the behavioral management skills that staff must learn to successfully implement such a system are discussed next. This behavioral management involves a system of accurately monitoring the resident incontinence status. It is in this critical arena that the role of the behavioral psychologist is most needed.

7.19.6.7 Staff Management and Continence Maintenance

Three major issues must be addressed if toileting assistance and the continence maintenance aspects of the prompted voiding program are to be accomplished. These issues, although discussed here specifically with regard to prompted voiding, are essential to any intervention requiring caregiver assistance. First, procedures are needed to target those residents who will respond well if ongoing toileting assistance is provided. Second, an information system must be developed to monitor incontinence outcomes effectively so as to facilitate quality control. Third, supervisors and direct care staff who actually implement the prompted voiding protocol must be taught how to use the outcome data to identify and correct problems. A comprehensive description of how these issues must be addressed to facilitate the implementation of prompted voiding can be found in several places (Ouslander & Schnelle, 1993; Schnelle, Ouslander, Osterwell, & Blumenthal, 1993).

The methodology to target residents who can be responsive to the prompted voiding toileting program has been described earlier in this chapter; specifically a three-day run-in assessment is described for this purpose. This same three-day assessment also provides the outcome data needed to maintain the incontinence system effectively. In review, during this three-day period residents are checked for wetness and prompted every two hours. Those residents who have a 66% appropriate toileting ratio or better are designated as responsive and are recommended for ongoing maintenance. The wetness data from these responsive residents collected during the two-hour checks can now be used to generate a control chart, which is the basic information tool used to monitor the prompted voiding program, thereby addressing the need for effective quality control (Fogarty, Schnelle, & Newman, 1989; Schnelle, Newman, Fogarty, Wallston, & Ory, 1991).

A control chart is a graphic display that allows the viewer visually to ascertain expected versus actual outcomes (Figure 2). The control chart in this case is constructed by graphing wetness data collected during each two-hour block during the three-day run-in period and calculating the average and standard deviation of this wetness. A warning limit is set two standard deviations above the average. This warning limit signifies unexpected variability and indicates either a failure of the prompted voiding work process to be implemented consistently or, perhaps, a change in the resident's status. For example, the control chart shown in Figure 2 was generated for a group of 22 residents. This control chart shows that 12% of the residents who showed $\geqslant$66% appropriate toileting rate during the three-day assessment period were found wet on the two-hour checks. A warning limit was set above this 12% average at 40%. This warning limit is two standard deviations above the average. An upper warning limit is established three standard deviations above the average. Supervisory nurses and direct care staff can now effectively monitor the prompted voiding program by randomly checking at least 10 residents per week for wetness. If the findings of this check, termed a control check, are within the average and two standard deviations of the expected average, the prompted voiding system can be said to be in control. If the wetness rate for the 10 patients exceeds the warning limit, then an analysis should be done to identify the causes of this excessive variability. A failure of staff to implement the prompted voiding program consistently or a deterioration in a resident's status are two potential explanations for an unusually high wetness check.

Software has been developed to facilitate the analysis and interpretation of the control checks, and supervisory and direct care staff have been taught how to use the software to identify problems and to provide feedback to the staff who are implementing prompted voiding. The implementation of this computerized system has resulted in successful maintenance of high levels of resident dryness during six-month to one-year evaluation periods in eight nursing homes (Schnelle, McNees, Crooks, & Ouslander, 1995). The failure of more traditional employee training methods to sustain such improvements have been described in several places (Schnelle, Newman, & Fogarty, 1990a). Unfortunately, the staff training and management interventions that have been evaluated have only been successful as long as research staff were present to provide support and social incentives to both supervisory and direct care staff to maintain the system.

The fact that maintaining resident dryness with a toileting program is more time consuming than simply changing residents when they are wet produces strong natural pressures that reduce staff motivation to maintain the program. The development of incentives to increase the motivation of nursing home staff to implement the more labor intense toileting program is an important new area to be investigated, and this is discussed in the next section.

7.19.7 FUTURE DIRECTIONS

Numerous areas related to incontinence treatment that are in need of research can be identified for both community dwelling and nursing home populations. Furthermore, many of these areas have direct relevance to behavioral scientists. For example, in the case of community dwelling populations major questions remain as to why most people with incontinence symptoms do not seek treatment. Behavioral interventions to increase people's willingness to be treated could possibly be developed if such information were available. Furthermore, such interventions to increase people's awareness of treatment options are clearly justified by the evidence that urinary incontinence is predictive of general functional decline in the community dwelling elderly. The fact that urinary incontinence is associated with a decline in measures of emotional functioning in the community dwelling elderly is also an area of interest for future behavioral research (Tinetti et al., 1995).

In the case of nursing home residents, major improvements have been made with incontinence problems by utilizing the assessment, treatment, and staff management system described in this chapter. In addition, the work to date suggests future research directions that should lead to further improvements in how incontinence care might be done in nursing homes. Two of these most important future directions have direct implications for behavioral scientists.

The first issue relates to the development of incentives that will motivate staff to maintain the quality control and information feedback system that is so critical to the maintenance of the prompted voiding program. The reality that maintaining continence is more time consuming than simply changing residents when they are wet contributes to the maintenance problem. However, the fact that even residents who are responsive to the prompted voiding program are not good self-advocates because of high sickness burden, dementia, or other unknown factors has not been discussed, and makes the need for incentives even more imperative. Unfortunately, most residents do not provide sufficient positive verbal feedback to nursing home staff when they provide toileting assistance so as to maintain the more labor intense toileting activities, and many residents can be convinced that they should accept their incontinence condition and a changing schedule as opposed to a prompting and toileting schedule.

Several approaches could be taken in reaction to this problem. First, external incentives that link the maintenance of the prompted voiding protocol to job advancement or salary increases could be attempted. These reinforcement strategies have been used successfully with other institutional populations that are not good self-advocates or are incapable of socially reinforcing staff for better care. A description of this behavioral research is available (Burgio & Burgio, 1990; Burgio et al., 1990).

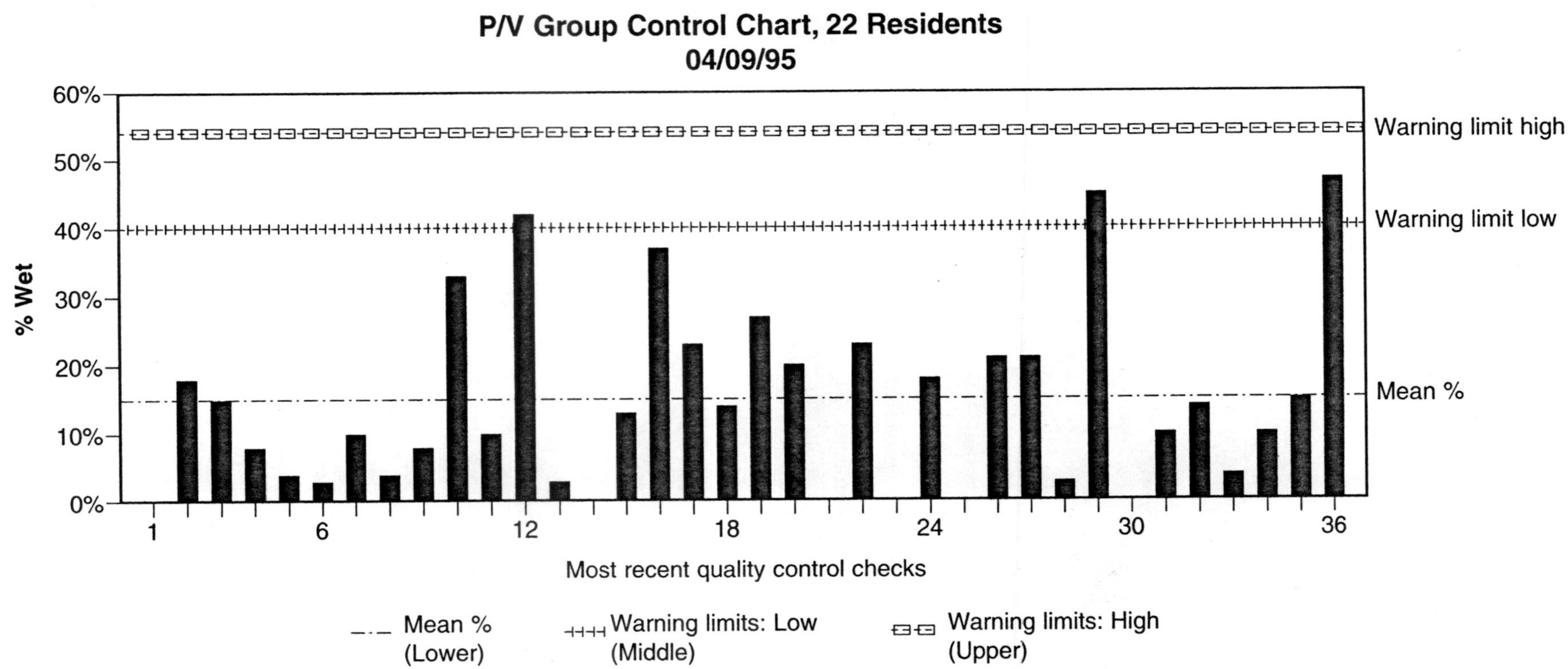

Figure 2 Sample control chart.

A second approach would be to develop interventions designed to make either residents or their families better advocates for their own care. With this approach, families and residents would have to be taught how to recognize good incontinence care and to interact with nursing staff in a manner so as to reinforce good care when it occurs. This form of patient/family involvement has been discussed by several consumer groups, but there have been no examples where this type of intervention has been done successfully.

A second direction for future behavioral research is related to the motivation of residents to be continent. The fact that many residents (estimated 15–30%) react negatively to the prompted voiding procedures and appear to prefer to be changed as opposed to toileted has been discussed previously in this chapter. These residents are not even carried into the staff management phase of the prompted voiding program because of their unresponsiveness to the prompting procedure during the run-in evaluation period. Research to measure residents' preferences for care and to determine the factors that contribute to these preferences would be important innovations that could guide how incontinence care should be delivered. For example, are preferences to urinate in pads and be changed as opposed to toileted influenced by the residents' reduced expectations of what is possible in the nursing home, or by true preferences for changing because it is less bothersome or painful than the toileting sequence? There are reasons to believe that both hypotheses may be plausible. The fact that many residents have experienced incontinence symptoms that were untreated before they entered the nursing home has been discussed in earlier sections in this chapter. It is thus plausible to predict that many residents may have adapted to the condition and sincerely are no longer bothered by wetness. Alternatively, it is also plausible to predict that some residents may have been convinced by nursing home staff that they should accept their incontinence condition because staff do not have time to help with toileting and thus have resigned themselves to the condition. Preferences based on the patient's acceptance and adaption to the condition versus preferences created by nursing home staff persuasion would require different interventions. In the first case it is arguable if anything should be done to convince residents of their need to be concerned about toileting, whereas in the second case an intervention to reverse the dependency and low expectations about care created by nursing staff is certainly necessary. Unfortunately, we know almost nothing about how to assess accurately the preferences of demented nursing home residents. The development of such a technology will allow us to begin the process of truly individualizing resident care according to their needs, not only in the case of incontinence care but also in other care areas.

7.19.8 REFERENCES

Benvenuti, F., Caputo, G. M., Bandinelli, S., Mayer, F., Biagini, C., & Sommavilla, A. (1987). Re-educative treatment of female genuine stress incontinence. *American Journal of Physical Therapy, 66*, 155–168.

Bo, K., Hagen, R. M., Kvarstein, B., Jorgensen, J., & Larsen, S. (1990). Pelvic floor muscle exercises for the treatment of female stress urinary incontinence. III. Effects of two different degrees of pelvic floor muscle exercises. *Neurourological Urodynamics, 9*(5), 489–502.

Bridges, N., Denning, J., Olah, K. S., & Aorrar, D. J. (1988). A prospective trial comparing interferential therapy and treatment using cones in patients with symptoms of stress incontinence. *Neurourological Urodynamics, 7*(3), 267–268.

Burgio, K., Whitehead, W. E., & Engel, B. T. (1985). Urinary incontinence in the elderly: Bladder–sphincter biofeedback and toileting skills training. *Annals of Internal Medicine, 103*, 507–515.

Burgio, K. L., Matthews, K. A., & Engel, B. T. (1991). Prevalence, incidence and correlates of urinary incontinence in healthy, middle-aged women. *Journal of Urology, 146*, 1255–1259.

Burgio, K. L., Robinson, J. C., & Engel, B. T. (1986). The role of biofeedback in Kegel exercise training for stress urinary incontinence. *American Journal of Obstetrical Gynecology, 154*(1), 58–64.

Burgio, K. L., Stutzman, R. E., & Engel, B. T. (1989). Behavioral training for post-prostatectomy urinary incontinence. *Journal of Urology, 141*, 303–306.

Burgio, L. D., & Burgio, K. L. (1990). Institutional staff training and management: a review of the literature and a model for geriatric long-term care facilities. *International Journal of Aging and Human Development, 30*(4), 287–302.

Burgio L. D., Engel, B. T., Hawkins, A., McCormick, K., Scheve, A., & Jones, L. T. (1990). A staff management system for maintaining improvements in continence with elderly nursing home residents. *Journal of Applied Behavior Analysis, 23*, 111–118.

Burns, P. A. Pranifoff, K., Nochajski, T. H., Hadly, E. C., Levy, K. J., & Ory, M. G. (1993, July). A comparison of effectiveness of biofeedback and pelvic muscle exercise treatment of stress-incontinence in older community-dwelling women. *Journal of Gerontology, 48*(4), 167–174.

Burton, J., Pearce, L., Burgio, K. L., Engel, B. T., & Whitehead, W. E. (1988). Behavioral training for urinary incontinence in elderly, ambulatory patients. *Journal of the American Geriatrics Society, 36*(8), 693–698.

Colling, J., Ouslander, J., Hadley, B. J., Eisch, J., & Campbell, E. (1992). The effects of patterned urge response toileting (PURT) on urinary incontinence among nursing home residents. *Journal of the American Geriatrics Society, 40*, 135–141.

Creditor, M. C. (1993). Hazards of hospitalization of the elderly. *Annals of Internal Medicine, 118*, 219–223.

Diokno, A. C., Brock, B. M., Brown, M. B., & Herzog, A. R. (1986). Prevalence of urinary incontinence and other urological symptoms in the non-institutionalized elderly. *Journal of Urology, 136*, 1022–1025.

Diokno, A. C., Brock, B. M., Herzog, A. R., & Bromberg, J. (1990). Medical correlates of urinary incontinence in the elderly. *Urology, 36*, 129–138.

Elia, G. & Bergman, A. (1993, February). Pelvic muscle exercises: When do they work? *Obstetrical Gynecology, 81*(2), 283–286.

Fantl, J. A., Cardozo, L., & McClish, D. K. (1994). Estrogen therapy in the management of urinary incontinence in postmenopausal women: A meta-analysis. First report of the hormones and urogenital therapy committee. *Obstetrical Gynecology, 83*, 12–18.

Fantl, J. A., Wyman, J. F., McClish, D. K., Harkins, S. W., Elswick, R. K., Taylor, J. R., & Hadley., E. C. (1991). Efficacy of bladder training in older women with urinary incontinence. *Journal of the American Medical Association, 265*(5), 609–613.

Ferrie, B. G., Smith, J. S., Logan, D., Lyle, R., & Paterson, P. J. (1984). Experience with bladder training in 65 patients. *British Journal of Urology, 56*, 482–484.

Fiatarone, M. A., O'Neill, E. F., Ryan, N. D., Clements, K. M., Solares, G. R., Nelson, M. E., Roberts, S. B., Kehayias, J. J., Lipsitz, L. A., & Evans, W. J. (1994). Exercise training and nutritional supplementation for physical frailty in very elderly people. *New England Journal of Medicine, 330*, 1769–1775.

Flynn, L., Cell, P., & Luisi, E. (1994). Effectiveness of pelvic exercises in reducing urge incontinence among community residing elders. *Journal of Gerontological Nursing, 20*(5), 23–27.

Fogarty, T. E., Schnelle, J. F., & Newman, D. R. (1989). Statistical quality control in nursing homes: A key indicator to evaluate patient incontinence care. *Quality Review Bulletin, 15*(9), 273–278.

Harrison, G. L. & Memel, D. S. (1994). Urinary incontinence in women: Its prevalence and its management in a health promotion clinic. *British Journal of General Practice, 44*(381), 149–152.

Help for Incontinent People (HIP) & the UCLA-JHA/Anna & Harry Borun Center for Gerontological Research (1994). *Managing incontinence in frail elderly dependent institutionalized and community dwelling persons: An agenda for research and care.* Monograph.

Holmes, D. M., Montz, F. J., & Stanton, S. L. (1989). Oxybutinin versus propantheline in the management of detrusor instability. A patient-regulated variable dose trial. *British Journal of Obstetrical Gynaecology, 96*(5), 607–612.

Hu, T. (1994). *The cost impact of urinary incontinence on health care services.* Paper presented at the National Multi-Specialty Nursing Conference on Urinary Continence, Phoenix AZ.

Keating, J. C., Jr., Schulte, E. A., & Miller, E. (1988). Conservative care of urinary incontinence in the elderly. *Journal of Manipulative Physiological Therapy, 11*(4), 300–308.

McCormick, K. A., & Burgio, K. (1984). Incontinence: An update on nursing care measures. *Journal of Gerontological Nursing, 10*(10), 16–23.

McDowell, B. J., Burgio, K. L., Dombrowski, M., Locher, J. L., & Rodriguez, E. (1992). An interdisciplinary approach to the assessment and behavioral treatment of urinary incontinence in geriatric outpatients. *Journal of the American Geriatrics Society, 40*, 370–374.

Moore, K. H., Hay, D. M., Imrie, A. E., Watson, A., & Goldstein, M. (1990, November). Oxybutyning hydrochloride (3 mg) in the treatment of women with idiopathic detrusor instability. *British Journal of Urology, 66*(5), 479–485.

Mouritsen, L., Frimodt, M. C., & Moller, M. (1991). Long-term effect on pelvic floor exercises on female urinary incontinence. *British Journal of Urology, 68*(1), 32–37.

Mulrow, C. D., Gerety, M. B., Kanten, D., & Cornell, J. E. (1994). A randomized trial of physical rehabilitation for very frail nursing home residents. *Journal of the American Medical Association, 271*, 519–524.

Murtaugh, C. M., & Freiman, M. P. (1995). Nursing home residents at risk of hospitalization and the characteristics of their hospital stays. *The Gerontologist, 35*(1), 35–43.

National Kidney and Urologic Diseases Advisory Board (1994, March). *Barriers to rehabilitation of persons with end-stage renal disease or chronic urinary incontinence.* Workshop summary report, Bethesda, MD.

Noelker, L. (1987). Incontinence in elderly cared for by family. *Gerontologist, 27*, 194–200.

Ouslander, J. G. & Fowler, E. (1985). Management of urinary incontinence in veterans administration nursing homes. *Journal of the American Geriatrics Society, 33*, 33–40.

Ouslander, J. G., Kane, R. L., & Abrass, I. B. (1982). Urinary incontinence in elderly nursing home patients. *Journal of the American Medical Association, 248*, 1194–1198.

Ouslander, J. G., Morishita, L., Blaustein, J., Orzeck, S., Dunn, S., & Sayre, J. (1987). Clinical, functional and psychosocial characteristics of an incontinent nursing home population. *Journal of Gerontology, 42*, 631–637.

Ouslander, J. G., Palmer, M. H., Rovner, B. W., & German, P. S. (1993). Urinary incontinence in nursing homes: Incidence remission and associated factors. *Journal of the American Geriatrics Society, 41*(10), 1083–1089.

Ouslander, J. G., Schapira, M., Fingold, S., & Schnelle, J. F. (1995). Accuracy of rapid urine screening tests among incontinent nursing home residents with asymptomatic bacteriuria. *Journal of the American Geriatrics Society, 43*, 772–775.

Ouslander, J. G., Schapira, M., & Schnelle, J. F. (1995). Urine specimen collection from incontinent female nursing home residents. *Journal of the American Geriatrics Society, 43*, 279–281.

Ouslander, J. G., Schapira, M., Schnelle, J. F., Uman, G., Fingold, S., Tuico, S., & Nigam, J. G. (1995). Does eradicating bacteriuria affect the severity of chronic urinary incontinence in nursing home residents? *Annals of Internal Medicine, 122*, 749–754.

Ouslander, J. G., & Schnelle, J. F. (1993). Assessment, treatment and management of urinary incontinence in the nursing home. In L. Rubenstein & D. Wieland (Eds.), *Improving care in the nursing homes: Comprehensive reviews of clinical research.* Newbury Park, CA: Sage.

Ouslander, J. G., & Schnelle, J. F. (1995). Incontinence in the nursing home. *Annals of Internal Medicine, 122*, 438–449.

Ouslander, J. G., Schnelle, J. F., Uman, G., Fingold, S., Nigam, J. G., Tuico, E., & Bates-Jensen, B. (1995a) Does oxybutynin add to the effectiveness of prompted voiding for urinary incontinence among nursing home residents? A placebo controlled trial. *Journal of the American Geriatrics Society, 43*, 610–617.

Ouslander, J. G., Schnelle, J. F., Uman, G., Fingold, S., Nigam, J. G., Tuico, E., & Bates-Jensen, B. (1995b). Predictors of successful prompted voiding among incontinent nursing home residents. *Journal of the American Medical Association, 273*(17), 1366–1370.

Ouslander, J. G., Simmons, S. F., Tuico, E., Nigam, J. G., Fingold, S., Bates-Jensen, B., & Schnelle, J. F. (1994). Use of a portable ultrasound device to measure post-void residual volume among incontinent nursing home residents. *Journal of the American Geriatrics society, 42*, 1189–1192.

Pengelly, A. W. & Booth, C. M. (1980). A prospective trial of bladder training as treatment for detrusor instability. *British Journal of Urology, 52*, 463–466.

Resnick, N. M. & Yalla, S. V. (1985). Management of urinary incontinence in the elderly. *New England Journal of Medicine, 313*, 800–805.

Riva, D. & Casolabi, E. (1984). Oxybutynin chloride in the treatment of female idiopathic bladder instability.

Clinical Experimental Obstetrics and cynecology, 11(1–2), 37–42.

Rose, M., Baigis-Smith, J., Smith, D., & Newman, D. (1990). Behavioral management of urinary incontinence in homebound older adults. *Home Healthcare Nurse, 8*, 10–15.

Schnelle, J. F. (1991). *Managing urinary incontinence in the elderly*. New York: Springer.

Schnelle, J. F., Keeler, E., Hays, R. D., Simmons, S. F., Ouslander, J. G., & Siu, A. L. (1995). A cost and value analysis of two interventions with incontinent nursing home residents. *Journal of the American Geriatrics Society, 43*(10), 1112–1117.

Schnelle, J. F., MacRae, P. G., Giacobassi, K., MacRae, H. S-H., Simmons, S. F., & Ouslander, J. G. (1996). Exercise with physically restrained nursing home residents: Maximizing benefits of restraint reduction. *Journal of the American Geriatrics Society, 44*, 507–512.

Schnelle, J. F., MacRae, P. G., Ouslander, J. G., Simmons, S. F., & Nitta, M. (1995). Functional incidental training, mobility performance, and incontinence care with nursing home residents. *Journal of the American Geriatrics Society, 43*(12), 1356–1362.

Schnelle, J. F., MacRae, P. G., Simmons, S. F., Uman, G., Ouslander, J. G., Rosenquist, L. L., & Chang, B. (1994). Safety assessment for the frail elderly: A comparison of restrained and unrestrained nursing home residents. *Journal of the American Geriatrics Society, 42*, 586–592.

Schnelle, J. F., McNees, P., Crooks, V., & Ouslander, J. G. (1995). The use of a computer-based model to implement an incontinence management program. *The Gerontologist, 35*(5), 656–665.

Schnelle, J. F., Newman, D. R., Abbey, J. C., Dray, R. J., Petrilli, C. O., & Hadley, E. C. (1990). Urodynamic and behavioral analysis of incontinence in nursing home patients. *Behavior, Health, and Aging, 1*(1), 43–49.

Schnelle, J. F., Newman, D. R., Fogarty, T. E., Wallston, K., & Ory, M. (1991). Assessment and quality control of incontinence care in long-term nursing facilities. *Journal of the American Geriatrics Society, 39*, 165–171.

Schnelle, J. F., Newman, D. R., & Fogarty, T. E. (1990a). Management of patient continence in long-term care nursing facilities. *The Gerontologist, 30*(3), 373–376.

Schnelle, J. F., Newman, D. R., & Fogarty, T. E. (1990b). Statistical quality control in nursing homes: Assessment and management of chronic urinary incontinence. *Health Services Research, 25*(4), 627–637.

Schnelle, J. F., Newman, D. R., White, M., Abbey, J., Wallston, K. A., Fogarty, T., & Ory, M. G. (1993). Maintaining continence in nursing home residents through the application of industrial quality control. *The Gerontologist, 33*, 114–121.

Schnelle, J. F., & Ouslander, J. G. (1996). Management of incontinence in long-term care. *Urinary incontinence*. St. Louis: MO: Mosby-Year Book.

Schnelle, J. F., Ouslander, J. G., Osterweil, D., & Blumenthal, S. (1993). Total quality management: Administrative and clinical applications in nursing homes. *Journal of American Geriatrics Society, 41*, 1259–1266.

Schnelle, J. F., Ouslander, J. G., & Simmons, S. F. (1993). Predicting nursing home residents' responsiveness to a urinary incontinence treatment protocol. *International Uro-Gynecology Journal, 4*, 89–94.

Schnelle, J. F., Sowell, V. A., Hu, T. W., & Traughber, B. T. (1988a). A behavioral analysis of the labor cost of managing continence and incontinence in nursing home patients. *Journal of Organizational Behavior Management, 9*(2), 137–153.

Schnelle, J. F., Sowell, V. A., Hu, T. W., & Traughber, B. T. (1988b). Reduction of urinary incontinence in nursing homes: Does it reduce or increase cost? *Journal of the American Geriatrics Society, 36*, 34–39.

Stewart, R. B., Moore, M. T., May, F. E., Marks, R. G., & Hale, W. E. (1992). Nocturia: a risk factor for falls in the elderly. *Journal of the American Geriatric Society, 40*, 1217–1220.

Tapp, A. J., Cardozo, L. D., Versi, E., & Cooper D. (1990, June). The treatment of detrusor instability in post-menopausal women with oxybutynin chloride: A double-blind placebo controlled study. *British Journal of Obstetrical Gynaecology, 97*(6), 521–526.

Thuroff, J. W., Bunke, B., Ebner, A., Faber, P., de Geeter, P., Hannappel, J., Heidler, H., Madersbacher, H., Melchior, H., Schafer, W., Schwenzer, T., & Stockle, M. (1991). Randomized, double-blind, multicenter trial on treatment of frequency, urgency and incontinence related to detrusor hyperactivity: Oxybutynin versus propantheline versus placebo. *Journal of Urology, 145*(4), 813–817.

Tinetti, M. E., Inouye, S. K., Gill, T. M., & Doucette, J. T. (1995). Shared risk factors for falls, incontinence, and functional dependence. Unifying the approach to geriatric syndromes. *Journal of the American Medical Association, 273*(17), 1348–1353.

United States Agency for Health Care Policy and Research (1996). *Urinary incontinence in adults: Acute and chronic management*. Rockville, MD: US Department of Health and Human Services, Public Health Services, Agency for Health Care Policy and Research.

Warren, J. W., Damron, D., Tenney, J. H., Hoopes, J. M., Deforge, B., & Muncie, H. L., Jr. (1987). Fever, bacteremia and death as complications of bacteriuria in women with long-term urethral catheters. *Journal of Infectious Diseases, 155*, 1151–1158.

Zeegers, A. G. M., Kiesswetter, H., Kramer, A. E. J. L., & Jonas, U. (1987). Conservative therapy of frequency, urgency and urge incontinence: A double-blind clinical trial of flavoxate hydrochloride, oxybutinin chloride, emepronium bromide and placebo. *World Journal of Urology, 5*(1), 57–61.

7.20
Community Mental Health Services in the United States and the United Kingdom: A Comparative Systems Approach

BOB G. KNIGHT and BRIAN KASKIE
University of Southern California, Los Angeles, CA, USA
BOB WOODS
University of Wales, Bangor, UK
and
EMILY PHIBBS
University College London, UK

7.20.1 INTRODUCTION

Community-based mental health services assist older adults with serious psychological disorders who have been moved out of institutional care facilities, as well as seeking to prevent older adults with such disorders from entering institutional care. In addition, community-based services assist older adults with acute psychological distress who are not at risk of placement in institutions. In this chapter, we describe community-based mental health services in the United Kingdom and the United States, we highlight similarities and differences, and we explore the historical and political–economic contexts that shaped these service systems.

7.20.2 MULTIPLE SYSTEMS OF MULTILEVEL CARE

The notion that community-based services for older adults with mental illness form one coordinated system is not a sufficient description. Knight (1991; Knight & Kaskie, 1995) argued that older adults with mental health problems are embedded in a variety of distinct care systems at both institutional and community-based levels: mental health systems, medical care services, long-term care for the elderly, and aging network services. Our understanding of community-based mental health services necessitates a systems level analysis where each system is considered independently and in relation to each other. This systems analysis departs from the more typical "coordination of services" and "gaps in the system" arguments in four distinct ways.

First, we contend that systems of care operate on different principles and create a legitimately confusing service world for both the older client and the professional service provider. Gaps in service provision exist because different systems were created for different purposes (mental health treatment, medical care, or social support). These systems have developed in response to different historical pressures rather than because someone overlooked elements while rationally laying out a system for older adults.

Second, failures to coordinate are more often dictated by economic pressures than by muddled planning or by providers' personal failings. Economic resources for mental health services are scarce and have become even more meager since the Reagan–Thatcher era of tax cuts and cost reductions to public services. Older people, especially those who need mental health services, continue to suffer from the "last-in, first-out" principle. In the UK, financial pressures and the increasing costs of acute medicine have drawn health services funding away from the chronic problems typical of those faced by older adults. In the US, support for older adults' mental health services by the Carter administration was rescinded by Reagan era cutbacks. Older adult services receive a minimal amount of funding, and continue to be subjected to further cutbacks. With such severely limited resources, the economic pressure is for systems to compete rather than to cooperate.

Third, service use is further complicated because older adults experience coexisting physical health and/or social difficulties, making it all too easy for each system to displace responsibility to another "more appropriate" system of care. A system may limit service delivery to existing clients and may not accept clients who "belong" to some other system. Further, limited financial support may cause a system to not provide adequate care even to those older adults who "belong" to the system. As noted by Gatz and Smyer (1992, p. 744), "everyone and no one is responsible for the clients." Indeed, the task of assuring appropriate community-based care for older adults with mental health problems becomes one of securing appropriate services from multiple competing systems, each of which has distinctive operating principles and incentives to provide services.

Fourth, the delivery of community-based services is further complicated by the fact that the different systems do not share the same definition of "community." For example, Knight and Lower-Walker (1985) noted that the mental health system moved older adults into nursing homes, which it defined as a transition from state hospital care to "the community." The aging network in the US has, in marked contrast, tended to define nursing homes as the prototypical institution from which older adults must be moved "to the community."

Our objective is to place the provision of mental health services for older adults in the context of the multilevel mental health services system as well as within other systems of care: long-term care, medical health care, and social services. In what follows, we begin with the long-term hospitals for older adults with mental disorders which are the historical antecedents of community care. The remainder of the chapter will consider community-based interventions.

7.20.3 THE STATUS QUO ANTE: LONG-TERM INSTITUTIONAL PSYCHIATRIC CARE

In the UK, county asylums emerged from the seventeenth and eighteenth century workhouses and institutions of confinement which were common throughout industrial–urban Europe (Foucault, 1965). The nineteenth century saw the development of psychiatry and the redefinition of these institutions as places for treatment of the insane (Foucault, 1965). Many county asylums became large institutions with several thousand inmates. Arie and Jolley (1982) commented that in the mid-1970s half of all asylums were occupied by people over 65, reflecting that:

> Mental hospitals which were built to provide asylum for the mentally ill before more active treatments were available, are nowadays increasingly occupied by old people whose numbers would grow even further were it not for enforced government rationing and not uncommon reluctance on the part of psychiatrists to admit them. (Arie & Jolley, 1982, p. 225)

Institutional psychiatric care developed in the US in the late nineteenth century as a humane alternative to imprisonment, to mistreatment in family homes, and to vagabond status for the mentally ill (Rosen, Pancake, & Rickards, 1995). The US had a shorter, less urban–industrial history, and so institutional care emerged as an alternative to no care rather than a redefining of existing institutions. Older adults were often over-represented in US inpatient psychiatric institutions in comparison to their representation in the general population. Between 1910 and 1950, for example, the state and county psychiatric hospital network expanded substantially in the US and admissions of older adults doubled (Grob, 1987; Rosen et al., 1995). Adults over the age of 65 represented 25% of the total patient population, and state and county psychiatric hospitals were the principal points of care for a population with an assortment of diagnostic, economic, and social attributes (American Psychiatric Association, 1993).

7.20.3.1 Deinstitutionalization of Mentally Ill

In the UK, the move to close large psychiatric institutions and replace them with local, community-based services began with the development of acute psychiatric units which were attached to local general hospitals during the 1960s and 1970s. The continued closure of mental hospitals was underpinned by rhetoric regarding the benefits of community-based care and driven by several Public Inquiry Reports of the scandalously poor conditions existing in such institutions. There were clear financial incentives also. The cost of maintaining and refurbishing the hospitals was growing and they became increasingly inefficient to operate with the falling number of patients. Also, there was an opportunity during the 1980s to transfer financial responsibility for patients from health budgets to the social security budget, through the transinstutionalization of patients from asylums to residential and nursing homes.

The movement of younger patients into the community led to older people forming an increasing proportion of the mental hospital population. Yet, the development of age-appropriate services varied greatly from area to area, often depending on the presence of a charismatic psychiatrist. By 1986, about 70% of the UK population had access to a specialist psychiatrist in old age mental health care (Ineichen, 1989) and developments have subsequently continued. This growth has helped to focus attention on the inadequacy of mental hospitals for older people with dementia or other mental health problems.

Beginning in 1955, older Americans were included in the mass "deinstitutionalization" of psychiatric patients from state hospitals to the community. Publicly supported psychiatric hospitals began an extended process of transferring older patients to the community (i.e., deinstitutionalization) or to other facilities such as nursing homes (i.e., transinstitutionalization). Moreover, state and county psychiatric hospitals applied more stringent admission criteria that reduced older adult admissions altogether (Kahn, 1975). This movement is generally attributed to the discovery of more effective psychopharmacological interventions and to a desire to provide more humane care in the least restrictive setting (Rosen et al., 1995), although cost control undoubtedly played a part. Hospitals were full and state legislatures were faced with the choice of building more or doing something else (Rounds, 1984). Moak and Fisher (1991) reported that 96% of the state hospitals had a floor, unit, or wing designated for geriatric patients. Yet, just 60% of the state hospitals retained a professional staff member who was trained in geriatric psychiatry and less than 20% of the hospitals provided any form of psychosocial treatment. These findings support the American Psychiatric Association's (1993) position that state and county hospitals rely on psychotropic medications and rarely use psychosocial interventions—even though well-designed, multidisciplinary treatment principles have been formulated.

7.20.3.2 Do The Old Institutions Still Exist?

The care of older adults who reside within institutional settings has changed. The image that county asylums and state hospitals provide only chronic, custodial care is contradicted by recent studies. In the areas of the UK where final closure has yet to occur, older patients are likely to be admitted to specialist inpatient assessment and rehabilitation units with a very few continuing care beds. Most of the long-term care admissions occur in areas where the independent sector has been slow to develop nursing home alternatives (Tomenson, Benbow, & Jolley, 1994; Wattis & Fairbairn, 1996).

In the US, Clark and Travis (1994) reported that just 20% of their older adult sample remained in the hospital for more than one year, while most of the rest were discharged. At least 15% of these older patients returned to the community while the remainder were released to another community-based facility such as a foster home, board and care facility, or nursing home (10% died in the hospital).

7.20.3.3 Who Was Discharged from Psychiatric Institutions?

In the UK, the older people affected by the closure of county asylums fit into two principal groups: (i) Chronic patients, usually with a long history of psychosis and having been hospitalized for many years. Arie and Jolley (1982) estimated they formed approximately 20% of the mental hospital population. They have often been discharged to hostels, residential and nursing homes (e.g., Dean, Briggs, & Lindesay, 1993). Anderson and Trieman (1995) suggested that over half this group may additionally have a moderate to severe degree of cognitive impairment. (ii) People with severe dementia—usually admitted because of behavioral problems and mainly discharged to nursing homes (e.g., Lyons, Cohen, Henderson, & Walker, 1995). In some cases, they are discharged to homes that are specially designed for people with dementia, for example, domus homes (Dean et al. 1993; Lindesay, Briggs, Lawes, MacDonald, & Herzberg, 1991; Skea & Lindesay 1996). These are small, "homely" living units, with specially trained staff and a philosophy encouraging attention to psychosocial aspects of care, to balance the traditional emphasis on physical care.

Based on the 1994 State and County Mental Hospital Inpatient Survey, Semke, Fisher, Goldman, and Hirad (1996) suggested that the US state hospital population could be sorted into three prominent groups: older adults with schizophrenia comprise 40.2% of the population, older adults with dementia total 30.0%, and those with depression and other late-onset disorders account for 13.1% of elderly patients. Another 10% were diagnosed with alcoholism, mental retardation, and other psychoses.

In summary, the image of county asylums and state hospitals as custodial warehouses where older patients are admitted and abandoned appears to be out of date. Rather, most hospitals provide limited inpatient services to older adults who are placed back to the community or another facility within a year of admission. In some places, the state or county hospital may be the only point of inpatient service. In considering policies surrounding community care, it is important to recognize that the county asylum and state hospital systems have changed dramatically. These hospitals have emerged as a form of community-based care, especially for older adults affected by psychoses, dementia, and severe affective disorders.

7.20.4 ACUTE PSYCHIATRIC INPATIENT SERVICES

In the UK, many districts have an inpatient old age psychiatry assessment unit on a general hospital site, with varying degrees of collaboration with geriatric medicine units (see Arie & Jolley, 1982; Ineichen, 1989). Typically, these are the central component of a community-based service for older people. Some of these inpatient units provide separately for those presumed to have dementia and those with an affective disorder. The advantages of having the inpatient unit on a general hospital site include increased access to the general hospital, access to specialists for coexisting physical health problems which might complicate the person's presenting state and course, and the opportunity to develop liaison services between mental health and general medical wards.

Over the last 20 years in the US, adult psychiatric inpatients have moved from state and county facilities, and now predominantly use general medical and private psychiatric inpatient hospitals (Kiesler, 1991). Narrow, Regier, Rae, Manderscheid, and Locke (1993) reported that 43.3% of all adult inpatients were admitted to either a general hospital psychiatric unit or scatter bed ("scatter bed" refers to individuals who are admitted to a hospital that does not have a special psychiatric unit or department), while 10.8% were admitted to a private psychiatric hospital. Atay, Whitkin, and Manderscheid (1995) examined the Inventory of Mental Health Organizations survey and, after excluding those older adults who resided in nursing homes, found that 21.6% of all elderly inpatients were treated in general hospitals, and 10.6% were treated in psychiatric hospitals. The remainder were treated in state or county hospitals, Veteran's Administration Hospitals, or by inpatient services affiliated with multiservice community mental health centers.

7.20.4.1 Who is Served in Geropsychiatric Inpatient Units?

Are these the psychotic and demented elderly who were the principal patient populations of state hospitals? Reports from individual hospital programs suggest that this may not be the case. In the UK, Domken, Bothwell, and McKeith (1995) analyzed discharge data from a well-established old age psychiatry unit. Comparison of the years 1985, 1988, and 1991 illustrated the growth in discharges to independent sector homes, together with increased admission rates and shorter lengths of stay. The proportion of patients having a functional disorder without organic impairment fell from 50% in 1985 to 25% in 1991, reflecting increasing reliance on day-hospital and community support for the functional disorders group.

In the US, Conwell, Nelson, Kim, and Mazure (1989) found that of 168 consecutively admitted patients to a geriatric inpatient unit in New Haven, 75% were diagnosed with an affective disorder and 25% with dementia. Knight and Carter (1990) reported that most geriatric admissions to a psychiatric inpatient unit in southern California were diagnosed with psychoses (47%) or with affective disorders (36%), with about 14% diagnosed with an "organic brain syndrome."

In summary, the role of acute psychiatric inpatient care has been overlooked when discussing community-based services, reflecting a tendency to equate inpatient care with custodial institutional care. However, impatient treatment of mentally disordered elderly appears successful using both psychopharmacologic (Schneider, 1995) and psychosocial (Gatz, Popkin, Pino, & VandenBos, 1985) interventions. Moreover, Knight (1983, 1986) reported that the utilization rates of inpatient and outpatient care by older adults in the counties of California were statistically independent of one another, suggesting that the systems serve different community-based populations. Short-term inpatient care close to home appears in fact, to be an important and distinct component of community-based care for older adults.

7.20.5 MENTALLY ILL OLDER ADULTS IN NURSING HOME CARE

In the UK, around 5% of older adults live in permanent institutional care. The majority (approximately 72%) of these older adults in 24 hour care live in residential or nursing homes which are not provided by the National Health Service (NHS), housing authority, or by local government. Many of these people are funded, at least in part, by a combination of Social Services and Social Security payments. The high prevalence of psychiatric morbidity in residential homes in the UK is well established. For example, Neville et al. (1995) assessed older people in four local authority residential homes. The great majority (82%) had some degree of dementia. Over half (53%) of the residents were assessed as having severe dementia. Of those (45%) able to complete a self-report depression scale, 17% scored in the depressed range. Of the whole sample, only 17% showed no evidence of dementia or depression. The rate of depression reported here is much lower than in previous studies (see Ames, 1991), where over a third of residents without severe dementia have been depressed.

The lower prevalence of depressed older adults in residential care may be due to improved assessment as well as more creative community treatment and support packages which enable older people with depression to remain in their own homes. An alternative hypothesis would be that the closure of hospital beds for severe dementia places pressure on local authority homes to accept a greater number of people with severe dementia, while independent sector nursing and residential homes—who have more choice over which residents to accept—absorb the less physically dependent and behaviorally disturbed group of depressed older adults. This illustrates the need to examine trends across the multiple systems (health, mental health, social) of institutional care. Examining one component in isolation gives an incomplete, and perhaps misleading, picture.

In the UK, the National Health Service and Community Care Act (1990) was motivated by the need to control the flow of resources into residential and nursing homes; previously, funding had been available without assessment of need. Although wrapped in rhetoric about providing better community support and services, assessments of need form the basis for targeting the provision of institutional care (see Gilleard, 1996a). "Need" for continuing hospital care is more likely to depend on availability than on any rational assessment; some districts have very few hospital beds, others retain a significant number (Tomenson et al. 1994).

Between 1963 and 1990, nursing homes expanded tremendously in the US from 445 000 to 1 772 000 individual beds as Medicare and Medicaid were initiated and included financial support for long-term care services (Darney, 1994; Schick & Schick, 1994). Moreover, the nursing home population grew as patients were supplied by the transinstitutionalization of older adults from state psychiatric hospitals (Kahn, 1975), a move which represented a cost-cutting strategy for state legislatures who moved the elderly mentally ill from totally state-funded psychiatric hospitals to partly federally-funded nursing homes (Estes, 1995).

In 1963, 48% of institutionalized mentally ill elderly were in state psychiatric hospitals with the remainder in nursing homes; in 1969, 75% were in nursing homes (Dorwart & Epstein, 1993). The nursing home setting would appear to be where many of the former psychiatric hospital population would now receive care: 50% of nursing home residents are demented, 30% have psychoses (Shadish, 1989).

More recently, the US Federal Government responded to the relocation of older mentally ill with the Nursing Home Act of 1987. This act recognized that older adults with psychiatric conditions were over-represented in nursing homes and stipulated that nursing homes must screen patients for psychiatric illness. If patients were diagnosed with a mental illness, then the nursing home was required to (i) provide appropriate psychiatric care, or (ii) deny admission to them and/or transfer them to a more appropriate facility (Smyer, 1989). Smyer, Shea, and Streit (1994) reported that at the time of the passage of this law, 65% of older adults in nursing homes who had mental health problems did not receive treatment for these problems. They also reported that for-profit homes tended to rely on bachelor's level counselors and government homes used psychiatrists, whereas private nonprofit homes used psychologists and social workers as well as psychiatrists. Early estimates suggested that between 2.4% and 18% of residents would be excluded from nursing home care by this act (Freiman, Arons, Goldman & Burns, 1990; Eichmann, Griffin, Lyons, Larson, & Finkel, 1992). However, later reports suggest sharp increases in mental health service provision in nursing homes after the passage of this law (Knight & Kaskie, 1995; Office of Inspector General, 1996), rather than discharges of patients with mental health problems. However, there are concerns about service standards and fraud: approximately 24% of Medicare billings in 1993 for mental health services to nursing home residents were estimated to be medically unnecessary (Office of Inspector General, 1996). Two-fifths of the insurance carriers for the Medicare program considered part of the problem to be "excessive entrepreneurialism" on the part of mental health professionals (Office of Inspector General, 1996, p. 13).

On the whole, the issue of providing adequate treatment to the transinstitutionalized older mentally ill resident of nursing homes in the US is still unresolved. For these individuals, "return to the community" has meant a shift from the mental health system to the long-term care system, reduced access to mental health treatment, a shift of care from the states to private sector institutions, and a shift of costs from states to a mix of federal-state (Medicaid) and private (patient and family) financing.

Lomranz and Bar-Tur (see Chapter 21, this volume) provide more comprehensive coverage of the nursing home population and service models for mental health treatment. Our point is that many, probably most, of those moved to "the community" were transferred to nursing homes from state hospitals, and that long-term psychiatric hospital treatment and care has been replaced by such homes in both the US and UK. In the remainder of this chapter, we explore community-based outpatient mental health services for older adults.

7.20.6 OLDER ADULTS IN COMMUNITY MENTAL HEALTH SERVICES

In this section, we cover the provision of mental health services to older adults outside of 24-hour care institutional environments. The range of services and settings described includes traditional and nontraditional outpatient services, partial hospitalization and related day care services, respite care, and support for caregivers.

7.20.6.1 Community-based Mental Health Outpatient Care in the UK

All community-based services in the UK operate in the context of Department of Social Services community care assessment and care management, intended to ensure that needs are properly assessed and that service provisions are targeted appropriately. Challis (1992) reviewed good models of providing community care through care management schemes. Some success is reported with mental health problems as well as with physical frailty. They have tended to include older people with dementia, rather than to focus specifically on them. Although apparently intended to be the basis of UK community care provision, important elements of the demonstration programs have often not been present in mainstream practice. The key elements included a high degree of flexibility, an available budget per person to "buy in" services, availability of paid volunteers, and a skilled assessment of need. There is widespread disappointment with the very basic packages of care being offered, and there is concern to ensure that specialist mental health services are involved more fully in assessment and care planning (Department of Health, 1996).

7.20.6.1.1 Multidisciplinary teams

The key element of such specialist community services in most areas of the UK would be a multidisciplinary team (MDT) usually seeing the older person in his/her own home. Most teams aim to respond quickly—within a few days—to referrals, more rapidly for urgent cases. The range of disciplines involved varies greatly; at a minimum, most members may be community psychiatric nurses, perhaps with an old age psychiatrist having a part-time input to the team. Elsewhere, occupational therapists, physiotherapists, social workers, speech therapists, clinical psychologists, and workers from voluntary agencies for older people may be team members. Typically the teams have been established by redirecting resources from mental health hospital provision; most teams liaise closely with inpatient old age psychiatry units and day hospitals. Often the team will share a hospital base with these services, although increasingly efforts are being made to locate such teams more accessibly, for example, in primary health care centers.

Most teams have a defined population to serve, and will usually see clients referred from residential and nursing homes within this area, as well as those living at home (Brown, Challis, & von Abendorff, 1996). Many teams will accept referrals from any agency, or from families or self-referrals; other teams maintain the traditional, less accessible, stance of only accepting referrals from the person's primary care physician. Some teams insist that all referrals are seen by a medical member of the team; others have a policy that a team member from any discipline may carry out the initial assessment meeting, where medical input would be available.

Coles, von Abendorff, and Herzberg (1991) evaluated the initial impact of a new community mental health team in an Inner London borough. This service replaced a traditional hospital-based system in which a consultant psychiatrist made domiciliary visits. The new community team was multidisciplinary, and used a keyworker scheme, where one member of the team would be allocated primary responsibility for the coordination and delivery of the service provided to each case. In a period of six months the team assessed over 90 more referrals than the consultant had seen in the equivalent period. The primary diagnosis for both the MDT and the consultant was dementia, which made up approximately 40% of all referrals. Depressive disorder accounted for 30.3% of diagnoses by the MDT and 18.3% of diagnoses by the consultant. The team was able to provide increased levels of input including treatment for depression, coordinating a range of services, and counseling and support for caregivers.

Junaid and Bruce (1994) investigated the effectiveness of community psychiatric nurse services for the elderly in a particular district. They found wide variation in the numbers employed per thousand people over 65 (from one per 2255 to one per 9200; The Royal College of Psychiatrists recommends one nurse per 5000 of the population over 65). They found large differences in the skill mix of the community teams. In some teams nurses would specialize in patients with specific diagnoses, for example, cognitive impairment, neurosis, or psychosis. Other teams would share case loads equally. In conclusion, Junaid and Bruce stated "Current provision appears to be based primarily on historical trends of resource allocation, and also on a varying commitment to community development which is evident in the philosophy or approach of the teams" (p. 718). It would seem that while the development of MDTs may have led to an improvement in services at a local level, the variation among teams' working practices and funding allocations has led to wide regional and inter-regional differences.

In the UK, some mental health teams (see Dening, 1992) specialize exclusively in working with people with dementia, whereas others cover all mental health problems of older people. Brown et al. (1996) provide details of referrals, caseloads, contact history, and outcomes of two well-established and pioneering teams which work with both organic and functional disorders. They took a random sample of 120 open cases on caseloads of two MDTs for elderly people, both with an open access policy, and followed up these cases over an 18-month follow-up. The teams' caseloads contained a greater proportion of patients with affective disorders, and less with dementia, in comparison with referrals to the team. The response to dementia appeared to be a briefer episode of contact, emphasizing assessment and diagnosis more than continuing support. A higher proportion of those with affective disorders remained at home at follow-up. This tendency for people with dementia and their caregivers to be rapidly discharged from the active caseload has led these teams to explore the use of specific long-term workers attached to the team to act as case managers for people with dementia and their families. Elsewhere, an innovative response has been the development of a specialist mental health nursing service to work specifically with family caregivers (see Woods, 1995), or teams working only with people with dementia, offering assessment, ongoing support, interventions to relieve caregiver strain, and facilitation of appropriate services.

Outcome studies of the work of such teams with people with dementia are yet to be completed. O'Connor, Pollitt, Brook, Reiss, and Roth (1991) have reported a controlled trial of the effect of an MDT on admission rates of people with dementia over the age of 75 over a two-year period. The team offered a wide range of help to people with dementia and their families identified in an ascertainment survey—including advice on and help in arranging services and benefits and respite admissions. No difference in admission rates, compared with control patients, was noted in those living with a caregiver. Those living alone were much more likely to enter residential care than controls. However, this study does not necessarily reflect outcomes in usual practice where the person or their family seeks help, rather than being identified as someone in need, as was the case here. More positive results are reported by Hinchliffe, Hyman, Blizard, and Livingston (1995) in a study where caregivers were offered an intervention devised by an MDT, which included components of behavioral, practical, and pharmacological input depending on the assessed needs of the situation. Caregiver mental health and the patient's behavioral difficulties improved compared with a waiting-list control group.

Although around 10% of the teams' caseload in Brown et al. (1996) had a diagnosis of schizophrenia, it is not clear what proportion of these had developed a psychotic illness such as paraphrenia in late life, as opposed to having a long-standing mental health problem. Generally, patients who have been receiving mental health services for many years are not transferred to old age services when 65, unless these services are more appropriate (e.g., because of the development of a dementia or physical health complications). Little has been documented regarding the effects of this approach.

In summary, community teams have developed widely, with very little in the way of evaluation, or even detailed descriptions of practice, since the early publications (Lindesay, 1991). Their service coordination role has, to an extent, been taken on formally by Social Services through the community care assessment and care planning process, and there are significant differences between areas in the extent to which the skills of the MDTs are utilized in carrying out specialist assessments and planning programs of care for older people with mental health problems. Some teams have very close links with social worker team members, and carry out many community care assessments; others find themselves much less involved, at best acting as an advocate for the patient's service needs. Although diversity of team functioning can be seen as flexibility to respond to local circumstances, the lack of consistency makes it difficult to know whether such teams do offer an effective way of organizing the response to mental health needs of older people in the community. Most teams attract high levels of referrals, and so appear to be meeting a demand, but this is of course an inadequate measure of efficacy. Two further developments—Memory Clinics and Family Therapy Clinics—in the UK are worthy of mention. Although their implementation is not yet as widespread as community teams, they promise to significantly shape the direction of future services.

7.20.6.1.2 Memory clinics

Early diagnosis of memory disorders is regarded as fundamentally important when treating and counseling individuals with dementia. The memory clinics have been developed to provide community-based services to older adults with dementia. All memory clinics provide an outpatient diagnostic assessment, and, in many centers, advice and counseling is offered to the person and their family, along with any appropriate treatment.

The first British memory clinic was established in 1983 at St. Pancras Hospital, London. A recent review of memory clinics in the British Isles (Wright & Lindesay, 1995) identified 20 clinics running in the UK and Ireland. Memory clinics provide diagnostic assessments for dementia and other memory disorders. Typically, patients receive a cognitive assessment involving standardized tests of cognitive functioning (including the Mini Mental State Examination, MMSE; Folstein, Folstein, & McHugh, 1975) and mood. A wide variety of physical investigations are used including full physical examination, computerized tomography scanning, magnetic resonance imaging, and blood tests. On average, around three-quarters of referrals to the clinics were diagnosed as having a dementing condition. Clinics vary in the cognitive tests and physical investigations used. The time taken to carry out full assessments was reported to vary from one to six hours. It is not clear whether the differences in practice have any clinical impact.

The number and type of staff running memory clinics vary. The professionals commonly involved are psychiatrists, geriatricians, neurologists, psychologists, and nurses, as well as speech therapists, social workers, and occupational therapists. Staffing levels vary as does the amount of any specific type of professional input to the service. Many of the memory clinics in the UK are actively involved in recruiting participants for research into dementia and specifically Alzheimer's disease. The research is both pharmaceutical and nondrug orientated.

Memory clinics provide an important service within the communities they serve. They are a useful point of referral for general practitioners, and may provide a starting point for many individuals to find help and information about memory impairment, as well as access to other community services. In a few areas, the follow-up from the clinic is extensive and caregivers receive considerable support over an extended time period (Bayer, Richards, & Phillips, 1990; Gilliard & Wilcock, 1993).

7.20.6.1.3 Family therapy clinics

Family therapy for older adults has only a brief history of implementation in the UK, although old age mental health service providers have long recognized the role of the family as being a significant factor in the psychological and physical well-being of older adults (Colwell & Post, 1959). UK research suggested that family-based work with older adults had useful clinical implications (Ratna & Davies, 1984). However, it is only in the last few years that family therapy for older families has begun to be implemented in practice. Traditionally, families with young children or adolescent members have been the prime focus for family therapy practice. In 1992, Gilleard, Lieberman, and Peeler set up a team for older adults in an established family therapy center in Inner London. The service was underutilized and referrals soon began to "dry up." Research revealed that professionals working with elderly people were unaware of the existence of the team, or had limited knowledge of family therapy with older people in general. Some professionals expressed doubts as to the usefulness of such a service, believing that there was little potential for change in the families of older people. Although misconceptions about older people did have some bearing on the lack of referrals to the new service, practical problems also played a large part. Professionals (especially community nurses and social workers) did not know that they were able to make referrals.

The overwhelming majority of professionals working with elderly people expressed positive attitudes towards family therapy. They suggested ways of making the service more accessible to their particular client groups, by limiting the amount of traveling and by holding all or some of the sessions in the client's home. Altering times of sessions to accommodate working hours was also suggested. By disseminating information regarding the service and by implementing changes suggested by health professionals, family therapy with older adults may become an important resource available to the community.

Research has highlighted the efficacy of family therapy to different elderly client groups (Gilleard, 1996b). Benbow, Marriott, Morley, and Walsh (1993) assessed the usefulness of family therapy with older adults suffering from dementia. The basic therapeutic techniques remained the same as for those older adults with other mental health problems, however, a few differences were found. Family therapy based treatment with dementia patients was often seen in terms of psychological management of the disorder and an increased focus on caregiver stress. Families were crisis-oriented and attended for fewer sessions. These difficulties present new challenges in providing family therapy for dementia sufferers. Continuing development indicates that family therapy with older adults will prove an important addition to older adult mental health services in the UK.

Curiously, family therapy for the elderly has grown slowly in the US. While there are services for caregivers (see Chapter 22, this volume) and well-known advocates for family therapy with the elderly (e.g., Qualls, 1996), there is no effort to establish family clinics as such.

In summary, for the foreseeable future, community MDTs seem likely to form the basis of specialist community mental health services for older people in the UK. Developments which reflect the importance of careful assessment and working with families, such as memory clinics and family therapy clinics, are likely to augment the basic service in some areas, and to influence practice within the teams more broadly.

7.20.6.2 Community Mental Health Outpatient Services in the US

In the US, the Community Mental Health Centers (CMHC) Act of 1963 financed the development of comprehensive community mental health centers. These centers were intended to provide services to the deinstitutionalized mentally ill and to provide services to persons who would have been institutionalized in the past. CMHC services target state hospital patients who do not require intensive supervision and CMHCs also serve community residents who need intermittent care (US Congress, Senate Committee on Labor and Welfare, 1973). CMHCs provide comprehensive mental health services including individual assessment, diagnosis, and treatment in acute inpatient, day treatment, or outpatient settings. Unlike the UK approach, the US CMHCs were newly created agencies rather than programs reaching out from existing hospital services.

As noted in Section 7.20.2, the focus on community-based services for the elderly did not begin in the mental health system until shortly before the national initiative was terminated and responsibility was returned to the states. Perhaps for this reason, the efforts at national planning of community mental health services for the elderly that are seen in the UK are lacking in the US. However, there are model programs that can provide guidance in conceptualizing what community mental health services could offer older adults.

Knight, Rickards, Rabins, Buckwalter, and Smith (1995) reviewed a variety of mental health programs for older adults with a range of mental health problems. The programs included community mental health services in Spokane, Washington, Cedar Rapids, Iowa, and Ventura County, California, as well as a multiservice program at Long Island Jewish Hospital in New York and a psychiatric consultation service to a federal housing program for the elderly in Baltimore. The services spanned urban and rural areas and used a variety of approaches to the coordination of care. These programs have shown that it is possible to provide high-quality, community-based mental health services to the mentally ill elderly. The programs also share some common features: (i) All emphasize accurate diagnosis of older adults. (ii) All are interdisciplinary and treatment focused. (iii) All use active case-finding methods and community education approaches to bring clients in. They also collaborate actively with other agencies that serve older adults and in three cases with postal carriers, meter readers, and other "community gatekeepers" (Raschko, 1990). (iv) All of them deliver mental health services to older adults at home. Mobile geriatric outreach teams, which use home delivered services and interdisciplinary teams (see Chapter 24, this volume) have proven effective in increasing service use by older adults in both urban (Knight, 1983) and rural areas (Buckwalter, Smith, Zevenbergen, & Russell, 1991). Mosher-Ashley (1994) also has highlighted the importance of home delivered services in reaching this population.

7.20.6.2.1 What types of clients are served?

In a survey of 349 older adult CMHC clients in Miami, Pruchno et al. (1983) reported that 54% were diagnosed with a unipolar or bipolar mood disorder, 21% had dementia, and 8.9% had schizophrenia or psychoses. Speer, Williams, West, and Dupree (1991) determined that 29% of their Tampa sample was diagnosed with dysthymia, 20% had mood disorder, and 10% had maritial problems. If these local samples are representative, it would appear that CMHCs serve high proportions of depressed older adults, but may be less successful in reaching the demented and psychotic populations that were a large part of the state hospital population.

7.20.6.2.2 Were CMHCs effective in outreach to elderly?

While the CMHCs did not develop sufficient services for older adults with mental illness (Lebowitz, 1988), they did not completely overlook older adults. In fact, the use of CMHC services by older adults grew steadily through the 1970s and 1980s. The Government Accounting Office (1982) reported that 4% of all CMHC clients were over the age of 65 in 1978, whereas by 1983 the elderly comprised 6% of the users of community mental health (Fleming, Rickards, Santos, & West 1986), with lower representation in other clinics and fewer still in private practices. In the 1990s, more of the elderly have begun to use mental health services. In 1990, the Inventory of Mental Health Organizations showed that 9.72% of all outpatient mental health clinic clients were older adults; 11.87% of clients in publicly supported clinics were older adults (Stiles, 1994).

Lebowitz, Light, and Bailey (1987) gathered information from 45% of the 624 CMHCs and found that 52% of those responding to the survey provided both professional mental health services to older adults and employed a geriatric staff specialist. However, 28% of their sample had neither age-targeted services nor a staff specialist. They concluded that older adults were offered more services by those CMHCs with trained staff or specific programs. In these centers, the older adult population represented 15.8% of the entire population; among the CMHCs with no staff or services, the older adult census averaged 8%. Also, Knight (1986) reported that for county mental health programs in California, service use by older adults was predicted by the number of specialist staff and was uncorrelated with percentage of elderly in the county population.

7.20.6.2.3 What comes next?

In the mid-1980s, Fox, Swan, and Estes (1986) reported that more than 60% of CMHCs were maintaining or increasing their services for older adult populations. More recently, they reported in a follow-up study that older adults services are more likely to be dropped than added to community-based mental health programs (Estes, Linkins, & Kane, 1994). Since the control of mental health programs was shifted back to the states, they have increasingly left individual CMHCs with a reduced budget, and without any stipulation concerning how the money should be spent (Christianson & Gray, 1994). In the mid-1990s, California continued the displacement of responsibility from federal to local governments by shifting control of mental health programs from states to counties, where these services compete with the medical care system for the indigent as well as with police and fire services for funding.

It seems unlikely that comprehensive CMHCs will be a major part of mental health services for older adults in the future. As mental health services in the US move to the private sector and to managed care organizations, active casefinding and other community mental health outreach strategies are likely to be inverted with probable negative impact on the accessibility of mental health services to older adults with depression, anxiety, substance abuse, and especially with long-term mental disorders like schizophrenia.

7.20.6.3 Summary: Community-based Outpatient Services

At this level, outpatient mental health services within the UK and US diverge most markedly. The UK's history of universal coverage has led to relatively systematic programming for the elderly, including MDTs, and more recently in some areas memory clinics and family therapy clinics. In the US, the federal role in mental health services has been more research-oriented than services-oriented with the individual states playing the major role in mental health services provision (Rosen et al., 1995). The history of federal–state relationships regarding mental health in the US has been characterized by shifting responsibility back and forth between the two with neither level of government taking clear responsibility at present. As noted by Liebig (1993) with regard to health and social policies for the aged, the federal system tends to lead to wide variation in policy among states, and in some cases the absence of policy. In the mental health sector, this is perhaps most clearly the case with dementia care, which some states would include in mental health services, while others would define it as in a different system, as its own system, or as not a state responsibility (Knight & Macofsky-Urban, 1990). The US has a few model programs for community-based outpatient services for the elderly, but lacks a system or a coherent national policy.

7.20.7 PARTIAL HOSPITAL SERVICES

7.20.7.1 British Models

In the 1970s and 1980s, day hospitals developed as the central component of many local older adults mental health services. By 1990, 20 000 older people were attending such day hospitals regularly, with over 1.7 million day places available per year (Fasey, 1994). Day hospitals have served a variety of functions: preventing admission to inpatient facilities, providing relief to caregivers of people with dementia, assessment, monitoring, and treatment of people with depression, facilitating discharge from an inpatient unit back to the community, and for observing the person's behavior and mental state for a longer period than is possible in the person's own home.

There is considerable debate concerning how effective the day hospital is in fulfilling these functions, and whether it represents the most effective use of resources (Fasey, 1994; Howard, 1994; Murphy, 1994). There is relatively little in the way of evidence to inform the debate. Day hospitals have not been effective in delaying admission to long-term care (Diesfeldt, 1992; Woods & Phanjoo, 1991), but do reduce strain for many (but not all) caregivers (Gilleard, 1987). However, some caregivers find the strain of getting the person ready for day care an additional burden, or find that most of their difficulties are at night and so they are not helped by day care. A few "night hospital" programs have been developed in response to this need. The role of day hospitals in the treatment of depression has not been evaluated in the UK context.

The UK also makes the distinction between "day hospitals" and "day centers," the former are health facilities, with a team including doctors, nurses, and therapists, and the latter are primarily "social care" resources but may have input from visiting health professionals. In reality, the distinction is not always clear, and those opposed to day hospitals argue that resources spent upon them are better used to provide more health input to day centers, many of which work well in providing relief for caregivers or as a social base for older people with depression needing to expand their social network.

Although Tester (1989) argued that day hospitals generally provide respite care for those older people whose behavioral problems or level of dementia proves "too severe" to be managed in a day center setting, Warrington and Eagles (1996) reported from a specific sample that the overall level of behavioral disturbance was no greater in cognitively impaired day hospital attenders than in those attending day centers.

7.20.7.2 American Models

Partial hospital programs have expanded significantly in the US in the last 10 years and have also become a more common form of mental health service for older adults. These partial hospital programs are organized under many different models that offer a range of social and medical services (Whitelaw & Perez, 1987).

Culhane and Culhane (1993) reported that 63% of day treatment programs in the US are located in CMHCs, 17% are affiliated with general hospitals, and 12% are found in private psychiatric hospitals. As fiscal incentives promote alternatives to inpatient care, partial psychiatric services seem to be expanding rapidly, especially in the private sector. For example, Stiles (1994) reported that partial hospital services increased by 50% between 1986 and 1990. Culhane and Culhane (1993) added that older adults represent between 4.8% and 7.9% of all partial hospital patients. The American Psychiatric Association (1993) noted that partial hospitals serve 18% of those older adults who actually use professional mental health services.

Since the history of partial hospitalization is directly related to substitution for hospital-based care, it is perhaps not surprising that the population served is more similar to the state hospital population. Eskew, Sexton, Tars, and Wilcox (1983) indicated that 34% of partial hospital patients were diagnosed with dementia, 32% had an affective disorder, and 24% were schizophrenic. The patient population appears to vary by program though; Plotkin and Wells (1993) reported that 60% of their partial hospital sample were depressed, 13% had a cognitive impairment, and 9% had an adjustment disorder. The majority of these patients received treatment subsequent to an inpatient hospital stay. In a program designed and implemented at the Florida Institute for Mental Health, Roger Patterson and associates designed a behaviorally-oriented social skills training approach to day treatment which assisted chronically mentally ill older adults to return to the community from state mental hospitals. As described and evaluated in Patterson et al. (1982), the program used applied behavioral analysis, behavioral intervention, and psychotropic medication to overcome effects of chronic psychosis and chronic institutionalization. Program attenders and graduates were more successful in community placements with lower recidivism rates.

7.20.7.3 Summary

The day program model has been used quite successfully for older adults in both the UK and the US and appears to be well suited to the needs of the older adults who formerly used long-term institutional care. However, this modality of treatment has neither been extensively reported in the clinical literature nor evaluated. We would hope that it would receive more attention in future research, clinical reports, and public policy consideration.

7.20.8 RESPITE CARE

As developed in the UK, respite care generally means a short stay in hospital or in another 24-hour care setting. In the US, respite has been used to refer to community-based social services such as social day care and in-home care workers. In the UK, respite can be considered as another partial hospitalization program. As noted above, this may be one of the functions of a day care program. Often a rationale will be made as to why a particular patient "requires" respite in a hospital rather than a residential or nursing home, in terms of severity of disturbance, or of need for nursing care. The availability of resources is of course an over-riding factor in these considerations, but the need to support caregivers in this way is widely recognized.

Residential respite care involves the patient staying in a residential/nursing home/hospital setting for a given period of time, thus allowing their caregiver to have a sustained period of time off from caring. Some beds are designated as "rota beds," in that a number of patients share the resource, taking turns to come into the facility. For example, four patients might each have two weeks in hospital and six weeks at home on a rotational basis, filling one bed continuously. Some relief schemes do not run on a rota system, but allow admission over a period when the caregiver may wish to go on holiday. Relief care may also include crisis admissions, say when a caregiver is taken ill.

Nolan and Grant (1992) carried out an extensive evaluation of such a hospital rota bed scheme, concluding that respite care fulfills a deeply felt need in caregivers, but also raises issues about caregivers' attitude towards institutional care. Caregivers possess unique knowledge of their relative, and often feel that the needs of the care recipient could not possibly be met by those working in an institution who have only limited knowledge of the care recipient (Worcester & Quayhagen, 1983). It is interesting to note that although this type of respite care is generally reported as being beneficial to caregivers, they also report feeling sad and lonely when their relative is away (Pearson, 1988). Guilt and worry may also be pervasive emotions felt by a caregiver who places a relative in residential respite care (Nolan & Grant, 1992).

Evaluations of respite care have shown that it has considerable benefit for caregivers. Levin, Moriarty, and Gorbach (1994) found respite was valued highly by caregivers. When respite services were introduced, they formed an ongoing source of support. Levin et al. emphasize the need for services to be targeted to the individual, noting that one "care package" may not suit all caregivers' needs. Flexibility of service is important, especially where disease progression is an element.

Some caregivers report that the person with dementia returns from respite more confused than when he/she was admitted. This may be understood in terms of the effects of a change in environment and routine on the person with dementia, and the difficulty of staff in ascertaining quickly the person's needs. Preadmission visits to a familiar place might reduce such effects, but an alternative strategy is to provide the respite care in the person's own home to minimize the disruption for them. This service is referred to as domiciliary respite where an outside agency will dispatch trained caregivers (i.e., a "sitter" or care attendant) to the home to take over the role of the caregiver for a given amount of time—a few hours or several days. Some care workers may even spend the night at the person's home, as this is often the most difficult time. There are some indications that caregivers find these services beneficial (Turvey & Toner, 1991).

In the US, day care and in-home respite services are not typically viewed as a part of mental health service systems but rather as a part of community-based long-term care or of home health services. Curiously, these services seem more effective at meeting mental health goals (i.e., improving the caregivers' life satisfaction or reducing emotional distress) than meeting community-based services goals of reducing care costs or preventing institutional care (Weissert, Cready, & Pawelak, 1988; Knight, Lutzky, & Macofsky-Urban, 1993). However, it has long been noted that respite may not be provided in sufficient quantity to meet these other objectives, and recent research tends to support the notion that longer respite may lead to reduced institutional care (Koslowski & Montgomery, 1995)

7.20.9 CAREGIVER SUPPORT

In the UK, caregiver support groups have been a popular development from the early 1980s. They take many different forms: some are organized as "training courses"; some are akin to therapy groups, being closed and having a facilitator; many are open-ended, self-help groups. Some are organized by voluntary agencies (especially the Alzheimer's Disease Society); others are based in day centers, day hospitals, residential homes, and primary health care centers. Few evaluations have been reported of their impact, although they are positively regarded by the caregivers attending. Morris, Woods, Davies, Berry, and Morris (1992) showed no differential impact of a coping skills-based group compared with a conventional course with invited speakers on strain and depression, although knowledge and use of coping skills did increase in both groups.

Services for caregivers in mental health settings have been a prominent feature of programs for older adults in the US since 1980. In a meta-analytic summary of program evaluation literature in the US, Knight et al. (1993) found that individual psychosocial interventions with caregivers appeared to be more effective than group interventions. Fully randomized evaluations of caregiver interventions have provided mixed results regarding the effectiveness of either individual or group interventions, a finding that is more curious given the effectiveness of psychological interventions with other groups of older adults (Scogin & McElreath, 1994).

7.20.10 MENTAL HEALTH SERVICES IN THE HEALTH CARE SYSTEM

In the UK, most mental health problems (including those of older people) are managed in primary care, without recourse to specialist mental health services. It is important to note that mental health problems are common in patients admitted to geriatric units (i.e., those designated for physical health care). Burn, Davies, McKenzie, Brothwell, and Wattis (1993) reported that 43% of such admissions who could be assessed had a diagnosable psychiatric condition (30% were depressed or anxious); many others could not be assessed because of a severe cognitive impairment. Conversely, significant physical health problems are also common in those admitted to old age psychiatry units (34% in one prospective study; Perry, Milner, & Krishnan, 1995).

In the UK, the problems center on the inaction of primary care physicians rather than the lack of recognition of mental disorders in older adults by physicians, which is more common among physicians in the US (Rapp, Parisi, Walsh, & Wallace, 1988). Jenkins and Macdonald (1994) indicated that general practitioners do recognize depression in their older patients, but rather rarely respond. A randomized controlled trial of depressed patients referred from primary care to a multidisciplinary team did not show any significant benefits—but the sample was small; the authors concluded that male patients might benefit from being referred more frequently, as their outcomes were slightly better.

Blanchard, Waterreus, and Mann (1995) achieved slightly more positive results. They identified older adults with depression from a community screening survey. The older patients were randomly allocated to intervention from a primary care nurse or to "usual care" from the general practitioner. Interventions were individually designed by a MDT, and included increasing the person's social network, antidepressant medication, counseling, and the involvement of relatives. Depression scores improved in this intervention group.

General practitioners in the UK refer people with dementia to specialist services at times of crisis, or when the dementia is well advanced—hence the need for open-access services described above. Wolff, Woods, and Reid (1995) have shown that GPs mainly saw dementia as a social rather than a health problem, and felt that early referral was unhelpful. They felt that they had little to offer patients with dementia, and this sense of helplessness may contribute to the failure to refer. Primary care teams are now encouraged to carry out an annual screening of individuals over the age of 75. This normally includes a rudimentary assessment of mental state. Consequently, the awareness of patients with dementia in the primary care context could grow.

In the US, there has been an increasing recognition that the health care system in general, and physicians' offices in particular, are a *de facto* part of the system of mental health care in the community. Analyses of service utilization data by George, Blazer, Winfield-Laird, Leaf, and Fischbach (1988) call attention to the fact that adults of all ages with a mental health problem are more likely to go to a health care provider than to a mental health professional. This tendency to seek mental health care from primary care physicians rather than from mental health professionals also appears to increase with age after the age of 55.

What happens during these visits is less clear. Physicians have been shown to be poor at detecting depression in medical impatients (Rapp et al., 1988) and outpatient service provision does not appear to be any better. Katz (1996) reported that primary care doctors often misdiagnose or overlook depression among older adults—one survey revealed that 26.4% of primary care physicians never evaluate the emotional status of individuals over the age of 75 (Mann, 1995). Further, primary care physicians tend to treat mental health problems only with psychotropic medications (Burns & Taube, 1990). These physicians are not likely to conduct clinical histories, involve family members with treatment, or to use psychosocial interventions.

Haley, Salzberg, and Barrett (1993) reported that geriatric specialists in medicine tend to be more open to psychological interventions and to working with psychologists as part of the care team than primary care physicians without geriatric training. Haley (1996) has also argued for the importance of staffing medical clinics with psychologists as part of the outreach effort to assure that older adults in need receive adequate services.

In short, it appears that on both sides of the Atlantic, mental health services for older adults are moving into the medical care system. While the move is conceptually unassailable and has the potential to improve access to mental health services and the coordination of mental health and medical services, short-term results suggest that the result may be decreased access to mental health services due to ineffective screening and intervention by primary care physicians. The multiple systems perspective would suggest that the medical system will, of course, recognize and treat medical disorders rather than mental health disorders and so the elimination of the separate mental health system may be undesirable.

7.20.11 DISCUSSION

7.20.11.1 Cross-national Systems Comparisons

The contrasting histories of mental health service systems in the UK and US are reflected in much of our previous discussion. While both systems have seen the demise of the large institutions, in the UK a long-term tradition of universal health care coverage and parity of coverage between mental health and health services created an environment in which old age psychiatry has developed as a new and influential speciality in psychiatry. New-style, community mental health services have been established with the resources released by hospital closure. However, as Murphy (1994) points out, not all the services that the asylums offered have been replaced. Extensive social support, health care, and social care resources have not been developed extensively. In the UK, institutional care still absorbs most of the available resources, despite preferences of families and older people and the stated aims of services.

In the US, community-based programs for older adults have never been well-funded and continue to face major threats to funding. Historically, federal policy in the US has placed restrictions on mental health services as supported by Medicare and Medicaid health insurance programs. These restrictions are beginning to be eliminated in the 1990s, but it is too early to assess the impact of increasing Medicare reimbursements to more providers or of recent moves toward parity in mental health insurance reimbursement. In summary, both nations have been more successful in closing down the institutions than in creating substitute systems in the community.

Research in both nations has focused on dementia and depression (rather than anxiety, alcohol abuse, or older schizophrenics) and on outpatient services rather than on inpatient or partial hospital services. These tendencies need correction to provide an empirical basis for comprehensive services in clinical geropsychology.

7.20.11.2 Dementia Services

The nature of services for older adults with dementia also differs. In the UK there is considerable focus on services to demented people themselves within the mental health sector with active concern for improving the well-being of the person with dementia. Kitwood (1996) provides a timely reminder of the "personhood" of the patient with dementia—psychological approaches to dementia must entail ensuring that the full human needs and potential of older people with severe cognitive impairments are recognized and nurtured. He contrasts his approach with the "neurological determinism" of the traditional model of working with the demented. The US, perhaps caught up in the "neurological determinism" viewpoint, has tended to conceptualize services for dementing elderly as services for the family caregiver and often places dementia services outside of the mental health sector: in social services, aging services, and so forth.

7.20.11.3 Mental Health and Primary Care

In the UK, mental health services for older people are likely to be provided in primary healthcare settings (see Mann, 1995) where most older people with mental health problems are actually found. A new relationship with the independent sector providing consultation outside the traditional NHS and Social Services settings needs to be established. This is a remarkably difficult change for clinicians brought up to feel that the NHS should provide care "from the cradle to the grave," at no cost at the point of service delivery.

In the US, the same change is likely to occur, driven in large part by the increasing organization of both health and mental health care into various types of managed care networks of providers. In the US, where the private sector is the traditional provider of health care and of much outpatient mental health care, resistance to these arrangements has more to do with the traditional independence of mental health providers and the differing organizational cultures of medical and mental health care. The latter reason has been offered as an explanation for the tendency to rely on separate managed care provider organizations for mental health services (Wholey, Christianson, & Peterson, 1996).

Indeed, as both nations move toward versions of managed care, primary care physicians will assume increased control over the provision of health and mental health services. For different reasons, this change may not bode well for access to required services since primary care physicians have not shown a great willingness to refer older adults for required mental health services (the UK) or even to recognize the need for such services (the US). In both cases, the problems may stem from the distinct world views of physical medicine and the mental health disciplines, a gap which must be bridged in order to effectively serve older adults. Creating the required levels of communication and collaboration will require orienting the two worlds to one another's languages, professional practices, and folkways (see Chapter 24, this volume; Qualls & Czirr, 1988).

However, as noted in the beginning of this chapter, older adults have a variety of medical, social service, and mental health needs which have traditionally been served by multiple systems of care, each with its own expertise, organizational structure, and economically driven imperatives. Mental health policy for the last few decades has tended to assume that people in general and older adults in particular would be better served by a single, formally organized system. Yet, participant observation would suggest that formal attempts to coordinate services have a tendency to serve the needs of the organization rather than those of the client; that is, groups of providers come together to discuss how to prevent clients from overusing services or to impose organizationally defined models of "appropriate" service use on the client. Myrtle and Wilber (1994) argued that a modern organizational theory, "loosely coupled systems," may better describe the functioning of services for the aged and also be a better model for assuring that the client gets the best services. Interlocking multiple systems can assure that specialized services are available for the client's multiple needs; restricted access systems (e.g., "single point of entry" and so forth) are likely to create barriers to some needs being met.

A salient example is the attempts in both the UK and the US to funnel older adults with mental health problems through primary care medicine, a gatekeeper strategy that seems likely (perhaps unintentionally) to deny care rather than assure it. An empirical test of an organized system of mental health care for children in the US (the Fort Bragg Demonstration) showed that the organized system provided better continuity of care but that clinical outcomes were no better and the cost was higher than in the business as usual fee-for-service system (Bickman, 1996).

Older adults often need a wide range of services from several different service systems and their needs may be met more effectively by an informed consumer who negotiates with the loosely coupled systems and interacts with those professionals who collaborate with other systems ("interpersonal coordination," Myrtle & Wilber, 1994). Their needs are less likely to be met within artificially constrained "megasystems" whose organizations make the individual systems less adaptable to specific, changing problems. Myrtle and Wilber (1994) argued that, over time, the informed consumer and gerospecialists would be expected to evolve their own norms for coordination of care and perhaps create a new aging-centered network of services in which current boundaries (e.g., between health and mental health or between mental health and social services) would have withered away.

7.20.11.4 Roles for Clinical Psychology in Community Care

There are many areas in community care where a key role could be assumed by a clinical psychologist. (i) In assessment, it is clear that individualized approaches are required to provide care in the community—in memory clinic contexts and elsewhere, neuropsychological assessment and professional consultation with other professionals is valued. The identification of neuropsychological problems underlying behavioral difficulties is important as is greater attention to differential assessment of emotional distress (anxiety versus depression) and personality disorders in older clients. (ii) Depression and anxiety are responsive to psychological treatment approaches (see Scogin & McElreath, 1994; Woods & Roth, 1996), and their adequate treatment would reduce a great deal of suffering. This treatment could be provided across a number of community-based systems. (iii) In support for family caregivers, there is evidence that psychological factors mediate strain and depression in family caregivers, and the development of more effective programs with psychological underpinning is desired (see Knight et al., 1993; Woods & Roth, 1996). (iv) In prevention and systems-level analysis and intervention, there is a strategic role in evaluating and developing more effective community services, and a need exists for a systemic approach to thinking, practice, and evaluation. For example, outcomes for caregivers and for their relatives with dementia cannot be viewed separately and in isolation. Also, the realities of elder abuse need to be considered alongside caregiver strain. The risk factors for institutionalization need to be understood more fully, along with better insight as to when entry to a nursing home is a good outcome for all concerned.

7.20.11.4.1 Development of clinical geropsychology

Clinical psychology with older people has had contrasting histories in the two countries. In the UK, in the 1960s and 1970s contact of clinical psychologists with older people concerned assessment, usually to attempt to answer the depression vs. dementia question. Very few psychologists specialized in aging. This changed during the 1970s when a small group developed a special interest in the field and explored a much broader range of roles, including treatment approaches to depression and dementia. By 1980, a formal interest group was formed and membership has continued to grow dramatically. The training of all clinical psychologists in the UK now requires experience in working with older adults, which includes working with people with depression and dementia and with family caregivers.

In the US, specialization in aging within clinical psychology developed later and more slowly. The first meeting on training psychologists to work with the elderly was held in 1981 (Santos & VandenBos, 1982). A follow-up conference in 1992 provided mixed impressions of the growth of the specialty during the 1980s (Knight, Santos, Teri, & Lawton, 1995); university-based training showed little expansion although internship training, especially in the Veterans Affairs hospital system, had expanded (Cooley, 1995). The national organization for clinical geropsychology in the US was formed in 1992 (Knight, Santos et al., 1995). Training for psychologists in aging is not widespread in the US and not a requirement for all psychologists as in the UK. The training models in the US emphasize university teaching and research, Veterans Affairs or university medical center employment, or independent practice as eventual employment opportunities in clinical psychology. Training and working within community-based mental health programs has been relatively ignored, except for the use of community practica in training geropsychologists (Qualls, Duffy, & Crose, 1995). Few psychologists with expertise in clinical geropsychology are found in community settings (Knight, Rickards et al., 1995; Qualls et al., 1995). Psychologists in the US are also facing increased competition from master's level providers not identified with psychology (e.g., clinical social work, marriage and family therapists). These other mental health professionals are employed as a less expensive provider of psychological services, especially under managed care approaches.

Training programs need to rethink their goals to train psychologists for the jobs of the twenty-first century. Clinical geropsychology tends to be progressive in its emphasis on the interface between medicine and mental health, between social services and mental health, and placing psychologists into nontraditional settings. The future of clinical geropsychology depends upon developments in public policy and in the management of health care services over the next several decades. Certainly, it would be helpful for clinical geropsychologists to study the successes and failures of colleagues in other countries.

7.20.12 SUMMARY

In both nations, clinical geropsychology can offer a great deal to the delivery of services to older adults. Clinical geropsychology focuses on the clinical psychology of medical illnesses, on services to demented older adults, and involves psychologists in services and research across a wide variety of hospital, partial hospital, clinic, and community settings. Training and practice in community-based clinical geropsychology is inherently multidisciplinary in focus. Clinical geropsychologists, like geriatricians and other specialists in aging services, are likely to be well-positioned on the mental health side for the kind of collaboration required to make the loosely coupled systems of services work for older adults.

7.20.13 REFERENCES

American Psychiatric Association (1993). *State mental hospitals and the elderly: A task force report of the American Psychiatric Association.* Washington, DC: Author.

Ames, D. (1991). Epidemiological studies of depression among the elderly in residential and nursing homes. Special Issue: Affective disorders in old age. *International Journal of Geriatric Psychiatry, 6.* 347–354.

Anderson, J., & Trieman, N. (1995). The TAPS Project. 21: Functional and organic comorbidity and the effect of cognitive and behavioural disability on the placement of elderly psychiatric inpatients: A whole hospital survey. *International Journal of Geriatric Psychiatry, 10,* 959–966.

Arie, T., & Jolley, D. (1982). Making services work: Organization and style of psychogeriatric services. In R. Levy & F. Post (Eds.), *The psychiatry of late life* (pp. 222–251). Oxford, UK: Blackwell.

Atay, J., Whitkin, M., & Manderscheid, R. (1995). *Data highlights on: Utilization of mental health organizations by elderly persons*. Rockville, MD: Center for Mental Health Services.

Bayer A. J., Richards V., & Phillips G. (1990). The Community Memory Project: A multidisciplinary approach to patients with forgetfulness and early dementia. *Care of the Elderly, 2*, 5–6.

Benbow, S. M., Marriott, A., Morley, M., & Walsh, S. (1993). Family therapy and dementia: Review and clinical experience. *International Journal of Geriatric Psychiatry, 8*, 717–725.

Bickman, L. (1996). A continuum of care: More is not always better. *American Psychologist, 51*, 689–701.

Blanchard, M. R., Waterreus, A., & Mann, A. H. (1995). The effect of primary care nurse intervention upon older people screened as depressed: *International Journal of Geriatric Psychiatry, 10*, 289–298.

Brown, P., Challis, D., & von Abendorff, R. (1996). The work of a community mental health team for the elderly: Referrals, caseloads, contact history, and outcomes. *International Journal of Geriatric Psychiatry, 11*, 29–39.

Buckwalter, K. C., Smith, M., Zevenbergen, P., & Russell, D. (1991). Mental health services of the rural elderly outreach program. *Gerontologist, 31*, 408–412.

Burn, W. K., Davies, K. N., McKenzie, F. R., Brothwell, J. A., & Wattis, J. P. (1993). The prevalence of psychiatric illness in acute geriatric admissions. *International Journal of Geriatric Psychiatry, 8*, 171–174.

Burns, B., & Taube, C. (1990). Mental health services in general medical care and in nursing homes. In B. Fogel, A. Furino, & G. Gottlieb (Eds.), *Mental health policy for older Americans: Protecting minds at risk* (pp. 63–84). Washington, DC: American Psychiatric Press.

Challis, D. (1992). Providing alternatives to long stay hospital care for frail elderly patients: Is it cost effective? *International Journal of Geriatric Psychiatry, 7*, 773–781.

Christianson, J., & Gray, D. (1994). What CMHCs can learn from two states' efforts to capitate Medicaid benefits. *Hospital and Community Psychiatry, 45*, 777–781.

Clark, W., & Travis, S. (1994) Elderly admissions to a state psychiatric hospital: Cohort characteristics, after care needs, and discharge destinations. *Journal of Gerontological Social Work, 21*, 101–115.

Coles, R. J., von Abendorff, R., & Herzberg, J. L. (1991). The impact of a new community mental health team on an inner city psychogeriatric service. *International Journal of Geriatric Psychiatry, 6*, 31–39.

Colwell, C., & Post, F. (1959). Community needs of elderly psychiatric patients. *British Medical Journal, 270*, 214–217.

Conwell, Y., Nelson, J. C., Kim, K., & Mazure, C. M. (1989). Elderly patients admitted to the psychiatric unit of a general hospital. *Journal of the American Geriatrics Society, 37*, 35–41.

Cooley, S. (1995). Geropsychology services and training in the US Department of Veterans Affairs. In B. Knight, L. Teri, P. Wohlford, & J. Santos (Eds.), *Mental health services for older adults: Implications for training and practice in geropsychology* (pp. 11–20). Washington, DC: American Psychological Association.

Culhane, D., & Culhane, J. (1993). The elderly's underutilization of partial hospitalization for mental disorders and the history of Medicare reimbursement policies. *Journal of Geriatric Psychiatry, 26*, 95–112.

Darney, A. J. (Ed.) (1994). *Statistical record for older Americans*. Detroit: Gale Research.

Dean, R., Briggs, K., & Lindesay, J. (1993). The domus philosophy: A prospective evaluation of two residential units for the elderly mentally ill. *International Journal of Geriatric Psychiatry, 8*, 807–817.

Dening, T. (1992). Community psychiatry of old age: A UK perspective. *International Journal of Geriatric Psychiatry, 7*, 757–766.

Department of Health (1996). *Assessing older people with dementia living in the community: Practice issues for social and health issues*. London: Social Services Inspectorate/Department of Health.

Diesfeldt, H. F. (1992). Psychogeriatric day care outcome: A five-year follow-up. *International Journal of Geriatric Psychiatry, 7*, 673–679.

Domken, M., Bothwell, R., & McKeith, I. (1995). Discharge patterns from a psychogeriatric inpatient unit. *International Journal of Geriatric Psychiatry, 10*, 41–46.

Dorwart, R. A., & Epstein, L. (1993). *The privatization of mental health care: A fragile balance*, Westport, CT: Auburn House.

Eichmann, M. A., Griffin, B. P., Lyons, J. S., Larson, D. B., & Finkel, S. (1992). An estimation of the impact of OBRA 1987 on nursing home care in the United States. *Hospital and Community Psychiatry, 43*, 781–789.

Eskew, R., Sexton, R., Tars, S., & Wilcox. F. (1983). Day treatment program evaluation. In M. Smyer & M. Gatz (Eds.), *Mental health and aging: Programs and Evaluations* (pp. 63–84). Beverly Hills, CA: Sage Publications.

Estes, C. L. (1995). Mental health services for the elderly: Key policy elements. In M. Gatz (Ed.), *Emerging issues in mental health and aging* (pp. 303–328). Washington, DC: American Psychological Association.

Estes, C. L., Linkins, K. W., & Kane, K. (1994, November). *Mental health services and the elderly: Organizations in transition*. Paper presented at the meeting of the Gerontological Society of America, Atlanta.

Fasey, C. (1994). The day hospital in old age psychiatry: The case against. *International Journal of Geriatric Psychiatry, 9*, 519–523.

Fleming A. S., Rickards, L. D., Santos, J. F., & West, P. R. (1986). *Mental health services for the elderly* (Vol. 3). Washington, DC: Retirement Research Foundation.

Folstein, M. F., Folstein, S. E., & McHugh, P. R. (1975). Mini-mental state: A practical method for grading the cognitive state of patients for the clinician. *Journal of Psychiatric Research, 12*, 189–198.

Foucault, M. (1965). *Madness and civilization: A history of insanity in the Age of Reason*. R. Howard (Trans.). New York: Random House (Original work published 1961).

Fox, P., Swan, J., & Estes, C. L., (1986). Trends in CMHC services to elderly populations. *Hospital and Community Psychiatry, 67*, 58–102.

Freiman, M. P., Arons, B. S., Goldman, H., & Burns, B. J. (1990). Nursing home reform and the mentally ill. *Health Affairs, 9*, 47–60.

Gatz, M., Popkin, S. J., Pino, C. D., & VandenBos, G. S. (1985). Psychological interventions with older adults. In J. E. Birren & K. W. Schaie (Eds.), *Handbook of the psychology of aging*. (2nd ed., pp. 455–488). New York: Van Nostrand.

Gatz M., & Smyer, M. A. (1992). The mental health system and older adults in the 1990's. *American Psychologist, 47*, 741–751.

General Accounting Office (1982). *The elderly remain in need of mental health services*. Pub. No. GAO/HRD 82–112. Washington, DC: Government Printing Office.

George, L., Blazer, D., Winfield-Laird, I., Leaf, P., & Fischbach, R. (1988). Psychiatric disorders and mental health service use in later life: Evidence from the epidemiological catchment area programs. In J. Brody & G. Maddox (Eds.), *Epidemiology and aging: An international perspective* (pp. 189–219). New York: Springer.

Gilleard, C. (1987). Influence of emotional distress among supporters on the outcome of psychogeriatric day care. *British Journal of Psychiatry, 150*, 219–223.

Gilleard, C. (1996a). Community care: psychological

perspectives. In R. T. Woods (Ed.), *Handbook of the Clinical Psychology of Ageing* (pp. 319–332). Chichester, UK: Wiley.

Gilleard, C. (1996b). Family therapy with older clients. In R. T. Woods (Ed.), *Handbook of the Clinical Psychology of Ageing* (pp. 561–573). Chichester, UK: Wiley.

Gilleard, C., Lieberman, S., & Peeler, R. (1992). Family therapy for older adults: A survey of professionals' attitudes. *Journal of Family Therapy, 14,* 413–422.

Gilliard, J., & Wilcock, G. (1993). Counseling for the carers. *Elderly Care, 5,* 24–26.

Grob, G. (1987). Mental health policy in post World War II America. *New Directions for Mental Health Services, 36,* 15–32.

Haley, W. E. (1996). The medical context of psychotherapy with the elderly. In S. H. Zarit & B. G. Knight (Eds.), *A guide to psychotherapy and aging: Effective interventions in a life stage context* (pp. 221–240). Washington, DC: American Psychological Association.

Haley, W. E., Salzberg, L. E., & Barrett, J. J. (1993). Psychologists in geriatric medicine: Results of a national survey. *Professional Psychology: Research and Practice, 24,* 491–495.

Hinchliffe, A. C., Hyman, I. L, Blizard, B., & Livingston, G. (1995). Behavioural complications of dementia: Can they be treated? *International Journal of Geriatric Psychiatry, 10,* 839–848.

HMSO (1990). *NHS and Community Care Act 1990.* London: HMSO.

Howard, R. (1994). Day hospitals: The case in favour. *International Journal of Geriatric Psychiatry, 9,* 525–529.

Ineichen, B. (1989). *Senile dementia: Policy and services.* London: Chapman & Hall.

Jenkins, D., & Macdonald, A. (1994). Should general practitioners refer more of their elderly depressed patients to psychiatric services? *International Journal of Geriatric Psychiatry, 9,* 461–466.

Junaid, O., & Bruce, J.M. (1994). Providing a community psychogeriatric service: Models of community psychiatric nursing provision in a single health district. *International Journal of Geriatric Psychiatry, 9,* 715–720.

Kahn, R. (1975). The mental health system and the future aged. *The Gerontologist, 15,* 24–31.

Katz, I. (1996). On the inseparability of mental and physical health in aged persons: Lessons from depression and comorbidity. *American Journal of Geriatric Psychiatry, 4,* 1–16.

Kiesler, C. A. (1991). Changes in general hospital psychiatric care, 1980–1985. *American Psychologist, 46,* 416–421.

Kitwood, T. (1996). A dialectical framework for dementia. In R. T. Woods (Ed.), *Handbook of the Clinical Psychology of Ageing* (pp. 267–282). Chichester, UK: Wiley.

Knight, B. G. (1983). Assessing a mobile outreach team. In M. Smyer & M. Gatz (Eds.), *Mental health and aging: Programs and evaluations* (pp. 23–40). Beverly Hills, CA: Sage Publications.

Knight, B. G. (1986). Management variables as predictors of service utilization by the elderly in mental health. *International Journal of Aging and Human Development, 23,* 141–148.

Knight, B. (1991). Outreach to older adults: Matching programs to specific needs. In N. Cohen (Ed.), *Psychiatric outreach to the mentally ill.* A monograph in the New Directions for Mental Health Services series. San Francisco: Jossey-Bass.

Knight, B., & Carter, P. M. (1990). Reduction of psychiatric inpatient stay for older adults by intensive case management. *The Gerontologist, 30,* 510–515.

Knight, B. G., & Kaskie, B. (1995). Models for mental health service delivery to other adults. In M. Gatz (Ed.), *Emerging issues in mental health and aging* (pp. 231–255). Washington, DC: American Psychological Association.

Knight, B. G., & Lower-Walker, D. (1985). Toward a definition of alternatives to institutionalization for the frail elderly. *The Gerontologist, 25,* 358–363.

Knight, B. G., Lutzky, S. M., & Macofsky-Urban, F. (1993). A meta-analytic review of interventions for caregiver distress: Recommendations for future research. *The Gerontologist, 33,* 240–249.

Knight, B., & Macofsky-Urban, F., (1990). Toward a policy for Alzheimer's disease in California. In P. Liebig & W. Lammers (Eds), *California policy choices for long term care* (pp. 145–170). Los Angeles: Andrus Gerontology Center.

Knight, B. G., Rickards, L., Rabins, P., Buckwalter, K., & Smith, M. (1995). Community-based services for mentally ill elderly. In B. Knight, L. Teri, P. Wohlford, & J. Santos (Eds.), *Mental health services for older adults: Implications for training and practice* (pp. 21–30). Washington, DC: American Psychological Association.

Knight, B. G., Santos, J., Teri, L., & Lawton, P. (1995). The development of training in clinical geropsychology. In B. Knight, L. Teri, P. Wohlford, & J. Santos (Eds.), *Mental health services for older adults: Implications for training and practice* (pp. 1–8). Washington, DC: American Psychological Association.

Kosloski, K., & Montgomery, R. (1995). The impact of respite use on nursing home placement. *The Gerontologist, 25,* 67–74.

Lebowitz, B. D. (1988). Mental health policy and aging. *Generations, 12,* 53–56.

Lebowitz, B. D., Light, E., & Bailey, F. (1987). Mental health center services for the elderly: The impact of coordination with area agencies on aging. *Gerontologist, 27,* 699–702.

Levin, E., Moriarty, J., & Gorbach, P. (1994). *Better for the break.* London: HMSO.

Liebig, P. S. (1993). The effects of federalism on policies for care of the aged in Canada and the United States. *Journal of Aging and Social Policy, 5,* 13–37.

Lindesay, J., Briggs, K., Lawes, M., MacDonald, A., & Herzberg. (1991). The domus philosophy comparative evaluation of a new approach to residential care for the demented elderly. *International Journal of Geriatric Psychiatry, 6,* 727–736.

Lindesay, J. (1991). *Working out: Setting up and running community psychogeriatric teams.* London: Research & Development in Psychiatry.

Lyons, D., Cohen, M., Henderson, T., & Walker, N. (1995). Partnership nursing home care for dementia: The Glasgow experience: The first twelve weeks. *International Journal of Geriatric Psychiatry, 10,* 557–560.

Mann, A. H. (1995). Future directions for the specialty of old age psychiatry: Some suggestions for debate. *International Journal of Geriatric Psychiatry, 10,* 87–92.

Moak, G., & Fisher, W. (1991). Geriatric patients and services in state hospitals: Data from a national survey. *Hospital and Community Psychiatry, 42,* 273–276.

Morris, R. G., Woods, R. T., Davies, K. S., Berry, J., & Morris, L. W. (1992). The use of a coping strategy focused support group for carers of dementia sufferers. *Counseling Psychology Quarterly, 5,* 337–348.

Mosher-Ashley, P. (1994). Therapy termination and persistence patterns of elderly clients in a community mental health center. *The Gerontologist, 34,* 180–189.

Murphy, E. (1994). A clinical role in service development: What should geriatric psychiatrists do? *International Journal of Geriatric Psychiatry, 9,* 947–955.

Myrtle, R., & Wilber, K. (1994). Designing service delivery systems: Lessons from the development of community based systems of care for the elderly. *Public Administration Review, 54,* 245–252.

Narrow, W. E., Regier, D. A., Rae, D. S., Manderscheid, R., & Locke, B. Z. (1993). Use of services by persons with mental illness and addictive disorders: Findings from the National Institute of Mental Health epidemiologic catchment area programs. *Archives of General Psychiatry, 50,* 95–107.

Neville, P. G., Boyle, A., Brooke, S., Baillon, S., Scothern, G., & Broome, C. (1995). Time for change: Psychiatric morbidity in residential homes for the elderly. *International Journal of Geriatric Psychiatry, 10,* 561–567.

Nolan, M. R., & Grant, G. (1992). *Regular respite: An evaluation of a hospital rota bed scheme for elderly people.* London: Age Concern England.

O'Connor, D. W., Pollitt, P. A., Brook, C. P. B., Reiss, B. B., & Roth, M. (1991). Does early intervention reduce the number of elderly people with dementia admitted to institutions for long-term care? *British Medical Journal, 302,* 871–875.

Office of Inspector General, Department of Health and Human Services. (1996). *Mental health services in nursing homes* (OEI–02–91–00860). New York: Author.

Patterson, R. L., Dupree, L. W., Eberly, D. A., Jackson, G. M., O'Sullivan, M. J., Penner, L. A., & Kelly, C. D. (1982). *Overcoming deficits of aging: A behavioral approach.* New York: Plenum.

Pearson, N. D. (1988). An assessment of relief hospital admissions for elderly patients with dementia. *Health Trends, 20,* 120–121.

Perry, D. W., Milner, E., & Krishnan, V. H. R. (1995). Physical morbidity in a group of patients referred to a psychogeriatric unit: A six month prospective study. *International Journal of Geriatric Psychiatry, 10,* 151–154.

Plotkin, D., & Wells, K. (1993). Partial hospitalization for psychiatrically ill elder patients. *American Journal of Psychiatry, 150,* 266–271.

Pruchno, R., Boswell, P., Wolff, D., & Faletti, M. (1983). A community mental health program: Evaluating outcomes. In M. Smyer & M. Gatz (Eds.), *Mental health and aging: Programs and evaluations* (pp. 41–62). Beverly Hills, CA: Sage Publications.

Qualls, S. H. (1996). Family therapy with aging families. In S. H. Zarit & B. G. Knight (Eds.), *A guide to psychotherapy and aging: Effective interventions in a life stage context* (pp. 121–138). Washington, DC: American Psychological Association.

Qualls, S. H., & Czirr, R. (1988). Geriatric health teams: Classifying models of professional and team functioning. *Gerontologist, 28,* 372–376.

Qualls, S., Duffy, M., & Crose, R. (1995). Clinical supervision and practicum placements in graduate training. In B. Knight, L. Teri, P. Wohlford, & J. Santos (Eds.), *Mental health services for older adults: Implications for training and practice in geropsychology* (pp. 119–128). Washington, DC: American Psychological Association.

Rapp, S. R., Parisi, S. P., Walsh, D. A., & Wallace, C. E. (1988). Detecting depression in medical inpatients. *Journal of Consulting and Clinical Psychology, 56,* 509–513.

Raschko, R. (1990). The gatekeeper model for the isolated, at-risk elderly. In N. Cohen (Ed.), *Psychiatry takes to the streets: Outreach and crisis intervention for the mentally ill.* New York: Guilford.

Ratna, L., & Davis, J. (1984). Family therapy with the elderly mentally ill: Some strategies and techniques. *British Journal of Psychiatry, 145,* 311–315.

Rosen, A. L., Pancake, J. A., & Rickards, L. (1995). Mental health policy and older Americans: Historical and current perspectives. In M. Gatz (Ed.), *Emerging issues in mental health and aging* (pp. 1–18). Washington, DC: American Psychological Association.

Rounds, J. (1984). Information and ambiguity in organizational change. In L. Sproull & P. Larkey, (Eds.), *Advances in information processing in organizations.* Greenwich, CT: JAI Press.

Santos, J. F., & VandenBos, G. R. (1982). *Psychology and the older adult: Challenges for training in the 1980s.* Washington, DC: American Psychological Association.

Scogin, F., & McElreath, L. (1994). Efficacy of psychosocial treatments for geriatric depression: A quantitative review. *Journal of Consulting and Clinical Psychology, 62,* 69–74.

Schick, F. L., & Schick, R. (Eds.) (1994). *Statistical handbook on aging Americans.* Phoenix, AZ: Oryx Press.

Schneider, L. S. (1995). Efficacy of clinical treatment for mental disorders among older persons. In M. Gatz (Ed.), *Emerging issues in mental health and aging* (pp. 19–71). Washington, DC: American Psychological Association.

Semke, J., Fisher, W., Goldman, H., & Hirad, A. (1996). The evolving role of the state hospital in care and treatment of older adults: Cross state trends, 1984–1993. *Psychiatric Services, 47,* 1082–1087.

Shadish, W. R. (1989). Private sector care for chronically mentally ill individuals: The more things change, the more they stay the same. *American Psychologist, 44,* 1142–1147.

Skea, D., & Lindesay, J. (1996). An evaluation of two models of long-term residential care for elderly people with dementia. *International Journal of Geriatric Psychiatry, 11,* 233–241.

Smyer, M. (1989). Nursing homes as a setting for psychological practice: Public policy perspectives. *American Psychologist, 44,* 1307–1314.

Smyer, M. A., Shea, D. G., & Streit, A. (1994). The provision and use of mental health services in nursing homes: Results from the National Medical Expenditure Survey. *American Journal of Public Health, 84,* 284–287.

Speer, D., Williams, J., West, H., & Dupree, L. (1991). Older adult users of outpatient mental health services. *Community Mental Health Journal, 27,* 69–76.

Stiles, P. G. (1994, November). *Utilization of ambulatory mental health services by the elderly: A preliminary report on the effects of recent Medicare reimbursement changes.* Paper presented at the meeting of the Gerontological Society of America, Atlanta.

Tester, S. (1989). *Caring by Day: A Study of Day Care Services for Older People.* Policy Studies in Ageing. London: Centre for Policy on Ageing.

Tomenson, B., Benbow S. M., & Jolley, D. J. (1994). Traffic Lights: Extracting order from the chaos of long-term care. *International Journal of Geriatric Psychiatry, 9,* 985–987.

Turvey, T., & Toner, H. (1991). The evaluation of a home based respite service for dementia sufferers and their carers. *Generations, 16,* 14–17.

United States Congress: Senate Committee on Labor and Public Welfare (1973). *Community Mental Health Center Act: History of the program and current problems and issues.* Washington DC: Government Printing Office.

Warrington, J., & Eagles, J. M. (1996). A comparison of cognitively impaired attenders and their coresident carers at day hospitals and day centres in Aberdeen. *International Journal of Geriatric Psychiatry, 11,* 251–256.

Wattis, J. P., & Fairbairn, A. (1996). Towards a consensus on continuing care for older adults with psychiatric disorder. *International Journal of Geriatric Psychiatry, 11,* 163–168.

Weissert, W. G., Cready, C. M., & Pawelak, J. (1988). The past and future of home and community based long term care. *The Milbank Quaterly, 66,* 309–388.

Whitelaw, C., & Perez, E. (1987). Partial hospitalization programs: A current perspective. *Administration in Mental Health, 15,* 62–72.

Wholey, D., Christianson, J., & Peterson, M. (1996). Organization of mental health care in HMOs. *Administration and Policy in Mental Health, 23,* 307–328.

Wolff, L. E., Woods, J. P., & Reid, J. (1995). Do general practitioners and old age psychiatrists differ in their attitudes to dementia? *International Journal of Geriatric Psychiatry, 10*, 63–70.

Woods, J. P., & Phanjoo, A. L. (1991). A follow-up study of psychogeriatric day hospital patients with dementia. *International Journal of Geriatric Psychiatry, 6*, 183–188.

Woods, R. (1995). Dementia care: Progress and prospects. *Journal of Mental Health, 4*, 115–124.

Woods, R. T., & Roth, A. (1996). Effectiveness of psychological interventions with older people. In A. Roth & P. Fonagy (Eds.), *What works for whom? A critical review of psychotherapy research* (pp. 321–340). New York: Guilford.

Worcester, M. I., & Quayhagen, M. P. (1983). Correlates of caregiving satisfaction: Prerequisites to elder home care. *Research Nursing Health, 6*, 61–67.

Wright, N., & Lindesay, J. (1995). A survey of memory clinics in the British Isles. *International Journal of Geriatric Psychiatry, 10*, 379–385.

7.21
Nursing Home Care and Interventions

JACOB LOMRANZ and LIORA BAR-TUR

The Herczeg Institute on Aging, Tel Aviv University, Israel

7.21.1 INTRODUCTION

Should a separate approach be taken to mental health for the aged in nursing homes? Could we not comprehend treatment of the aged in nursing homes as we comprehend the aged in the community? The answer is no. Furthermore, elaboration of this issue has been neglected, especially in light of the growing elderly population residing in nursing homes. This causes damage and reduces the quality of life for the elderly. While there certainly are similarities in the mental health approach to nursing home and community residents, there also are clear differences and unique demands of psychological treatment in nursing homes, based on specific knowledge of conceptualizations and clinical methodology. The absence of such knowledge hinders the function of the geropsychologist. The question whether elderly should age in organized and institutional frameworks of one kind or another has concerned modern society for many decades. But while debates continue as to the best, or necessary environment for the elderly to age, the fact is that in the postwar era organizational and institutional frameworks for the elderly have grown steadily. This growth parallels increased longevity and what is termed the "demographic revolution," that is, the colossal change in the population age structure, patterns of habitation, and the implications of these in all domains of life. Demographic projections suggest that the number of nursing home residents will triple in the 1990s (US Senate, 1987) since at least one person out of five will be institutionalized (Palmore, 1976). Keeping in mind that the needs of the elderly for mental health are extremely high, that psychiatric and medical institutionalization is unsatisfactory, and that the question of the appropriate residency in the later years is unsolved, there is a real danger that nursing homes will turn into centers inhabited by the most maladjusted elderly.

At the outset the reader was asked to bear in mind that many elderly do not suffer but enjoy their residency in nursing homes and experience well-being, development, and growth. Unfortunately, however, the problem of mental health in nursing homes is colossal. In this chapter, after defining the approach to mental health in the elderly, the issues of mental health as they appear in homes for the aged are addressed. The threats to adjustment of elderly people before, after, and during their relocation to homes for the aged are then delineated. To this end, the different nursing homes are noted as well as their inhabitants and then the utility of the nursing home is discussed, as well as the effects of institutionalization. This leads to an examination of the transitional process, the implication and effects of relocation, as well as the problems to overcome and the tasks to be achieved, in order for satisfactory adjustment to the new environment and for the preservation of mental health. While the initial focus is on the psychosocial process of adjustment, the prevailing psychopathology in these homes is discussed and then a psychological community-oriented clinical model is proposed, before a discussion of its organization and implementation as it applies to methods of treatment, including consultation, psychotherapy, and education, to staff and residents in nursing homes. The chapter ends with a future perspective on clinical geropsychology in nursing homes.

7.21.2 MENTAL HEALTH IN OLD AGE

7.21.2.1 Definition and Approach

The focus here is on the elderly person's ability to cope with personal aging processes in a specific, changing environment. Mental health is approached in the same way as those perceiving it beyond the absence of pathology. The modes of intervention and treatment are in line with such a broad perspective. The World Health Organization (1964) defines health as "a state of complete physical, mental and social well-being and not merely the absence of disease or infirmity" (p. 1). While many scholars are concerned with psychopathological aspects of mental health, the "positive mental health" approach (Jahoda, 1958) attempts to better understand the role of adaptive processes. Birren and Renner (1980) relate to four components in the concept of mental health: (i) the presence or absence of mental disease, (ii) the presence or absence of deficits or limitations in behavior, (iii) the satisfaction or contentment that is derived from one's life as it is being lived or has been lived, and (iv) some approximation of an ideal person. While the relevancy of (iii) and (iv) to the elderly could be understood in light of history, socialization processes, and life-review of the elderly, (i) raises problems since many elderly suffer from "social pathology," for example, loneliness (Pfeiffer, 1977) even in adjusted living, and (ii) is certainly complex since old age goes along with deficits and limitations in behavior. While mental health for the elderly may include many of the components applied to the young, such as adequate life satisfaction, self-acceptance, mastery of the self and environment, the ability to work, love, and play, the manner in which these criteria can be met changes in old age (Gatz, 1989).

While older adults experience the complete range of psychopathology seen in younger age groups (Knight, Santos, Teri, & Lawton, 1995), three points should be emphasized (Schaie & Willis, 1996). First, older people perform differently than younger on virtually all psychodiagnostic instruments, often resulting in inadequate assessment of their pathology. Second, in old age there is a high rate of physical or psychosocial loss which may constitute risk factors in mental illness. The third point concerns the major individual variability in old age. Some elderly may increase their psychological vulnerability through repeated inability to cope successfully with life stressors, while others may increase their sense of mastery as they improve resilience and become more resistant to mental illness. One should therefore be aware of the fact that applying various standards of mental health to the elderly in general, and to those residing in nursing homes in particular, is complex and requires clarification on the part of the clinical gerontologist.

A development-growth and not a depletion model is adopted to the elderly, in line with Gutmann (1994) who states that the second half of life should be viewed "neither catastrophically nor sentimentally; it is neither an exclusive tale of losses nor a golden age. Like any other sector in the life cycle, it has its own distinctive depletion, it has its own gains, and makes its own special contribution to individual development, social cohesion, and species continuity" (p. xviii). However, while adhering to this approach there is an awareness that due to, between others, lessened income, physical losses, poor health, enforced isolation, environmental relocation, retirement, interpersonal losses, widowhood, or the effects of drugs, many older persons cannot function according to the various standards of mental health. Elderly, especially in nursing homes, cannot always be autonomous and master their environments. They may lack the financial or personal and interpersonal resources to make decisions about their lives and, for certain individuals in specific situations, depression, hostility, apathy, or anxiety may be legitimate or even helpful (Gurland, 1973). Internal and environmental stress in the elderly may be more apt to produce mental disorder in the face of reduced physical and psychological reserves (Gatz, 1998). Therefore, when assessing the mental health of the elderly, it is more crucial to take into account the complete organism total life ecology, relocation being is a point in case. Exposition and explication of one's theory is crucial. Adherence to an adult developmental life-span approach is advocated (Baltes & Baltes, 1990), embedded in positive mental health as noted above and urge caution in defining and juxtaposing the different manifestation of "mental health" vs. "mental illness."

7.21.2.2 Mental Health In Nursing Homes

The problems in later life are singularly appropriate for psychological treatment. They include organic and cognitive loss, coping with stress, identity roles, interpersonal and family behavior, neurosis, psychosis and, indeed, every category to be found in any version of the *DSM* (Bienefeld, 1990). Although the magnitude and severity of the mental health problems in the elderly and their need for care are obvious, the extent of the treatment provided is severely limited and most needs are not met. The aged receive disproportionately less mental health services. It is estimated that only about 3% of all clinical services provided by psychologists go to the older adult population (Gatz, Popkin, Pino, & VandenBos, 1985). Given the higher rates of mental illness in homes for the aged, mental health care is proportionately even less then in the general population. Longevity may have increased, but not the quality of living.

Although many elderly persons enter long-term care institutions to improve their quality of life, unfortunately, the result is, at times, the opposite, with detrimental effects, often due to the inadequate quality of care (Kane & Kane, 1982). While mental disorders and symptoms are estimated between 15 and 25% (Schaie & Willis, 1996) for the population over age 65 years, in medical and institutional settings, such as nursing homes, the figure is dramatically higher, generally estimated to be in the range 60–90% (Cohen, 1991; Gatz & Smyer, 1992). A major criteria for mental health is a person's ability to cope with their environment. For many who are unable to live independently in the community, this criteria has to be met in adjusting to a nursing home. The absence of a caregiver or the lack of social support networks distinguishes most nursing home residents from equally impaired elders dwelling in the community. Twenty-five percent of nursing home placements are precipitated by the illness or death of the caregiver (Colerick & George, 1986). In the early 1980s, a national nursing home survey (Eisdorfer & Cohen, 1982) found that 30% of nursing home residents had "diagnosable" psychiatric disorders and that 61% had one or more mental impairments. While more older adults have dropped out of, or never entered, the mental health system, other organizational settings, notably nursing homes, have become the service destination for the mentally impaired elderly (Johnson &

Grant, 1985), especially since the Deinstitutionalization Act (Goplerud, 1979). Donahue (1978) estimated that 40% of the patients discharged from public mental hospitals eventually found their way into nursing homes. Despite the fact that a majority of nursing home residents are in need of mental health services (Newman, Griffin, Black, & Page, 1989), these settings are designed and staffed primarily for physical, rather than mental, health care (Smyer, 1989). In most nursing homes the staff is also untrained and too overburdened to deal with emotional problems, some of which are exacerbated or developed as a result of living in the home.

Psychotherapeutic mental health programs and provisions are rare. Psychiatric visits or consultations are the exception to the rule (Johnson & Grant, 1985). It has been noted that "the tragic irony about nursing homes is that they represent a major setting for the mentally ill, with grossly inadequate mental health attention" (Cohen, 1980, p. 983). There is a strong urgent need for interventions by mental health professionals such as psychiatrists, psychologists,or trained mental health social workers in order to handle the severe problems of mental health in homes for the aged.

7.21.3 NURSING HOMES: DIFFERENT SETTINGS OF LIVING AND CARE FOR DIFFERENT POPULATIONS

Although the generic term "nursing homes" has been adopted, the reader must realize the variability of these institutions. These habitats range from "sheltered homes" to "homes for the aged" to "convalescent homes." They differ in segregation (isolation from the outside world), policies, and control (the degree of autonomy permitted to patients). They range from "open" to "closed" institutions or floors, providing partial to total care, from secluded rural to urban community settings. They vary widely in quality, regulations, in the focus on instrumental and/or also social and affective needs, and offer various degrees of help in daily living. Some offer basic nursing and custodial care while others provide a variety of services to restore, or maintain, the residents' ability to function. Support in various homes may be related to the amenities and regulations of the facility and to the availability of more than minimal staff and care resources (Timko & Moos, 1990). Smaller facilities may, in certain instances, be more constructive since they resemble a home environment, better meet the resident's needs, and minimize the impact of institutionalization. As the size of the institution increases, the quality of communication, satisfaction, and active involvement of residents may decline (Schaie & Willis, 1996). It should be emphasized that the different structures and kinds of nursing homes bear different implications for their residents' behavior in terms of social life, humanistic or dehumanizing atmosphere, adequate health care, independence, control, well-being, and mental health.

Just as there are major difference between the various nursing homes, so do the residents differ in personality, coping abilities, mental health and cultural background. However, some generalities may be drawn. Generally, in contrast to the elderly dwelling in the community, most nursing home residents have the following in common: (i) their age is higher: 75% over 75 years of age and 35% of these are 85 or above (forecasts for the year 2003 suggest that 87% of nursing home residents would be over 75; National Center for Health Statistics, 1983); (ii) the majority are widowed; (iii) more have no surviving immediate family member living nearby; (iv) they are more functionally disabled; and (v) many more suffer from physical or mental problems as well as from chronic physical conditions involving pain, threat of hospitalization, and gradually increasing impairments.

7.21.3.1 Mental Health and the Role of Nursing Home

The function and utility of the nursing home in society is influenced by social forces, policy, economics, family structure, commitment, and social values. However, the climate and physical environment in which people live and work is related to life expectancy, stress, and various medical, physical, and mental disorders (Wantz & Gay, 1981). Nursing homes, therefore, determine to a great extent the well-being and mental health of their residents (Lawton, 1985).

For the elderly person with some deficit in self-care ability, the nursing home answers the major need for tending and care. It provides security, protection, and safety and assists in the activities of daily living. Usually nursing homes also attempt to satisfy the additional basic needs for shelter and human comfort. The family expects the nursing home to become a surrogate fulfilling the dual aspects inherent in the notion of care: providing concern, support and morale, as well as performing the direct work of tending. As illness, frailty, or loss in resources and support systems are often the background leading to nursing home admission (Hirschfeld & Fleishman, 1990), they highlight the fact that those admitted are vulnerable and in need of psychological support, in addition to tending. One task of the psychologist in nursing homes is to ensure that residents also receive mental support and care along with physical care.

Various studies indicated psychological and social improvements following the move to public housing facilities or retirement community centers (Lawton & Cohen, 1974), especially in homes which were designed specifically for the elderly and the residents themselves choose the home. However, disagreement exists with respect to effects of rehousing on health, and many studies found negative effects of relocation (e.g., Lieberman & Tobin, 1983). Butler (1975) claimed that most elderly people view the move to a nursing home with fear and hostility and believe that the move to an institution is a prelude to death. Farrari (1963) compared two groups moving from home to an institution, one voluntarily and the other with no option, and found that 10 weeks later mortality among the latter was to be extremely high. Lawton (1980) suggests that the differences in findings may be due to the variability in the quality of housing, sampling, economic status of inhabitants, and personality variables as well as to research design differences. Determining, in varying degrees, are also the detrimental effects of institutionalization.

7.21.3.2 The Effects of Institutionalization

Nursing homes are institutions and as such their inhabitants are subject to the effects of institutionalization. The very nature of an institution contradicts the nature of a "home," which implies intimacy, autonomy, privacy, and control. As Tobin and Lieberman (1976) state "it is difficult to avoid the implication that even the finest institutions cause the deleterious sequale commonly refered to as *institutional effects*" (p. 5). Basic factors leading to institutional effects include: physical and human ecology, territory and space constructions and limitations, the structuring of time, sharing of space and interaction with neighbors, regimes, inspections, routines, the burden of authority, use and abuse of dependency, ritualizations, stigmation, the impact of crowding, lack of privacy, group pressure, and engulfment (Goffman, 1961). Negative effects upon inmates of institutions include: changes in self-perception, feelings of inferiority, dependency, alienation, stress, depression, somatic and mental illness.

Such general factors have specific manifestations, impacts, and detrimental effects in nursing homes. The negative stereotyping of society incorporated by nursing home staff (Wright, 1988) may result in a negative atmosphere in the home and a lower self-concept of its residents. Insecurity and insufficient privacy (Firestone, Lichman, & Evans, 1980) may cause a sense of intrusion and fluidity of personal boundaries. Limitations in providing care may result in loss of self-esteem, estrangement, isolation, and deindividuation (Tobin & Lieberman, 1976). Low quality of care (Johnson & Grant, 1985; Kane & Kane, 1982), lack of sufficient personal attention, and respect may all induce depressive moods. Constricting freedom and control may be detrimental. Rodin and Langer (1977) have demonstrated how reducing restriction of choice and control in a home for the aged resulted in increased alertness, activity, and general well-being, while increasing restrictions have the opposite effect. They conclude that "some of the negative consequences of aging may be retarded, reversed, or possibly prevented by returning to the aged the right to make decisions and a feeling of competence" (pp. 897–902). Perlmuter and Monty (1979) suggest that the major problem for residents is the inability to exercise choice, control, and personal responsibility which then has a harmful effect on well-being and adaptation. Residents should be given greater control of their daily lives as well as participate in decisions affecting various aspects of the home's programs and policy (Moos & Lemke, 1985). Studies in social ecology of nursing homes show that reinforcing independence not only reduces dependence but also reduces the incidence of disease and death (Baltes, 1982).

Assembled in a common environment, the newcomer to the nursing home cannot escape the dreaded identification with their surroundings which include being sick, yearning for care, and feeling closer to death. In order to adapt, they have to participate with others in the cannons of the institution, but in doing so they may lose uniqueness, and become discontent, bitter, and hostile. The institutional structure and atmosphere may restrict or promote interpersonal and social contact (Hansson & Carpenter, 1994). It may decrease family visits leading to loss of contact with family members and friends. As family members recede into the background, the position of the institution as the last and "only" home for the elderly person is reinforced. The environment then signifies vulnerability, mutilation, and death, but at the same time protection and survival. Given all the above it should come as no surprise that individuals in nursing homes are significantly lower in psychological well-being than individuals with similar levels of physical and social function living in the community.

The impact of institutional processes, including staff burnout, may be so great as to undo and render useless the effects of professional therapeutic interventions (Lomranz, 1991).To counteract this impact, nursing homes should be viewed as communities whose subsystems mutually interact with the broader surrounding community and its social policy dimensions. At the same time, investment in nursing home staff should be aimed at active preventive programs to counteract institutionalization.

The chapter will now discuss the specific issues of the processes and mental health implications of moving to a nursing home and the factors involved in adjustment and adaptation.

7.21.4 MENTAL HEALTH IN LIGHT OF THE TRANSITION AND ADAPTATION TO A NURSING HOME: COGENT ISSUES

The transition to a nursing home involves significant change, including separation, loss, and readjustment. For many it means "closing" a 60+ year chapter of their lives. The new location encompasses a novel territory, neighborhood, social group, entire community, and access to the outside, larger world. The location chosen, its atmosphere and culture may be crucial. For most people a house is a meaningful life-space: "home is where the heart is." Home signifies stability, roots, a feeling of belonging, security, identity, intimacy, personal space, and generativity. Permanently relinquishing one's home can be a painful step. This surrender is especially hard for the elderly person who experiences many additional changes and may cling to the familiar for security and permanency. Thus, the need to adjust to a new framework involves the ability to separate emotionally from a previously meaningful stable world, that is, from habits and lifestyle held throughout many years, from defined identities, and from a familiar society and environment. Successful relocation, therefore, is a complex twofold process that requires reconciliation with loss as well as adaptation to a novel environment. The rationale to move to a nursing home, adjusting and maintaining well-being along time, all depend on a wide range of personal, interpersonal, and environmental resources. These include a complex range of factors, such as, individual characteristics and ego resources, past history, family structure, quality of relationships, economic status, social background, environment, and culture. Once in the nursing home, a variety of adaptational task are expected. Given the variability in nursing homes and in coping patterns of the individuals, it is almost impossible to predict adjustment patterns. Nevertheless, some basic factors are highlighted which are deemed critical to the adjustment process.

7.21.4.1 The Decision-making Process and its Impact

The decision to leave home and move to a nursing home is an emotionally-loaded process involving multiple aspects, phases, and actors (Groger, 1994). This major life decision often involves anxiety, stress, ambivalence, fears, doubts, hopes, and risk taking, feelings which may be unavoidable considering the life changes involved and the necessary uncertainty about the new habitat and the future. The family often plays a major role prior to admission and, thereafter, in the readjustment of the elderly. Overt and covert individual and family conflicts may often emerge. Family members frequently share the elderly person's ambivalence (Bar-Tur, 1993; Halpert, 1991). Institutionalization of an elderly parent may also create family crisis. Moreover, data suggests that above 50% of those entering homes for the aged do so without having taken a meaningful part in the decision-making process (Reinardy, 1992).

The decision-making process affects the person's adjustment to the nursing home. Elderly who exercised more control over the decision adjust better than those who have less control over the move. Often an elderly person may feel "dumped" by their family and consequently become alienated and depressed. Family structure has major impact. Having, for instance, one daughter or sibling reduces an older person's chances of admission by about one-fourth (Freedman, 1996). Sometimes family members act out conflicts in their relationships with the nursing home staff, further complicating the adjustment process. Children may seek professional help in the process of placing their parent in a nursing home. Guilt, anger, regret, and resentment are almost ubiquitous. Planning and implementing the decision with the family in a context of safety, nonthreatening, and open communication can minimize distortion and promote healing of the family (Bienenfeld, 1990). The psychological loaded milieu described here obviously indicates the possibilities for clinical geropsychologist to assist in conflict resolution and stress reduction for all those involved in this transition and relocation. At stake is not merely "adjustment" to the nursing home, but solving existential dilemmas to improve the quality of life.

Over one-half of the persons admitted to a nursing home are discharged within three months. This figure includes those who die as well those transferred to hospitals or to the community. Most of the hospitalized, as well as those discharged to the community, eventually return to the nursing home (Lewis, Cretin, & Kane, 1985). Cooperation between hospitals, the community, and nursing homes is crucial, especially when dealing with the chronically sick elderly.

7.21.4.2 Preadmission Screening

Elderly adults admitted to a nursing home usually present a combination of mental and physical health problems. Potential patterns of interaction between physical and mental health conditions among nursing home residents may be expressed in the four categories of (i) "classical" psychosomatic disorders; (ii) somatizing responses (e.g., conversion syndrome); (iii) physical illness causing psychiatric symptoms; and (iv) psychological responses to illness. Family and social issues are often embedded in all these. The preadmission screening procedure is therefore very important for certifying the type of care, mentally and physically, the new resident requires (Symer & Garfein, 1988). It may add clarification to the decision-making process as to the kind of home to seek and may lay the basis for the kinds of interventions needed to assist the individual's adaptation in the nursing home. It is recommended (Newman et al.,1989) that psychologists become more involved in the substance and process of preadmission screening, assessment being one of the applied psychologist's strengths. Depending on the results of the prescreening, the clinical psychologist may further refer the candidate to a medical, family, or consulting psychologist as well as to social workers.

7.21.4.3 Adaptational Tasks in Nursing Homes

The transition to a nursing home requires various adjustments. Some of the major tasks, in specific areas of daily living, that must be accomplished to promote an appropriate quality of life in the nursing home, are outlined in what follows.

7.21.4.3.1 Limited living space and seperation from personal effects

Exchanging a macro- for a microenvironment implies radical reorientation of spacial experience. Personal and interpersonal space has to be modified. Transition to diminished space, sometimes sharing one room with someone else, requires residents to limit drastically their living space and separate from many objects they have accumulated throughout many years. In such objects, a person's history, identity, and lifestyle are encapsulated. Separation from such meaningful objects, in addition to other losses experienced in old age, may create a painful sense of discontinuity. Relocation sometimes involves rapid renunciation, resignation, and separation, whereas mourning over the losses may be prolonged. For example, about one year after admission, Mrs. B. realized at her birthday party that she didn't have a single flower vase. She burst into tears at the memory of all the beautiful things she had been forced to leave behind, expressing a sense of deprivation. Mr. Z., a widower without relatives, negotiated for two years with a nursing home for them to accept him with his 200 books; he passed away, bitterly, in midst of negotiations. Neither had any contact with a mental health professional. Stripped of personal belongings and yearning for them may cause depressive mood. Attachment to familiar objects lends a sense of security and may serve as an adjustment mechanism. While the importance of transitional objects in young children (Winnicott, 1953) is recognized, they should be considered significant throughout the life-span. Just as the child therapist may utilize transitional objects to reinforce growth and development, the geropsychologist may do the same, but usually on the basis of the absence of such objects.

7.21.4.3.2 A novel geographic ecology

Adjustment to ecology includes the physical environment, the world of plants and animals, the human inhabitants, and the larger geographical surroundings. It also signifies the importance of environmental planning for older people (Moos & Lemke, 1985) and the behavioral and affective outcomes in the person-environment fit. Geographic experiences, defined as "the individual's involvement within the spaces and places of his life" (Rowles, 1979, p. 81), represent meaningful dynamics in the individual. Organization of a new living space is difficult. Residents must familiarize themselves with a whole new world. Mrs. B., a 90-year-old lady, said sadly "I lived in the same four-room apartment for 60 years, and everything had its place. Here, in one room, I have hardly anything and I still can't find nothing." The required adjustment not only concerns one's room, but also the facilities in the building and the surrounding area. Uncertainty as to what is usually posited firmly in our minds (e.g., rooms, buildings, streets, or bus schedules) may cause disorientation, especially for those who are confused, leading to anxieties and nightmares. Coping and adjusting to the ecological aspects consumes physical as well as mental energy but is crucial for enabling the residents to "feeling in place" and enhances belongingness.

7.21.4.3.3 Structured and leisure time

New residents face a transition from controlling and structuring their time, in the past, to a milieu in which almost all the time is structured for them and they also may be discontent about the way time is filled. Life in many nursing homes goes by a strict time schedule. There are specific hours for such things as eating, social activities, and receiving medication. Moreover, often these time-bound activities become the most significant events, the markers and content of existence and, as such, being after all very simple routines, may render the totality of life for the resident as boring and meaningless.

Transition to a nursing home frees time and energy that in the past were devoted to activities of independent daily living. Potentially individuals may enjoy, as many do, and use their time for a variety of creative and educational activities. However, although being released from burden and given freedom for pleasure and personal enrichment, many residents may find it difficult to shift from fulfilling duties to enjoying leisure time. Such an inability to shift relates to the difficulty in giving up roles, values, identities, and lifestyles, all molded during one's life-span. Neulinger (1981) postulated that the ability to enjoy leisure time depends on a certain mental state that includes a feeling of freedom together with basic motivation to experience and enjoy. Physically or emotionally frail residents may find it hard to learn new outlets for satisfaction and as a result experience low morale. The passage of time may also be experienced as monotonous, slow, and dispersonalized, features associated with the depressed elderly.

Further implications of temporality refer to the personal experience of time (Lomranz, Shmotkin, & Vardi, 1991) such as time perspective or the meaning of future time. Such aspects retain specific significance in the existence of nursing home residents and they present furtile ground for the work of the clinical geropsychologist.

7.21.4.3.4 Food and communal dining

Gutmann (1994) found, cross-culturally, food and oral preoccupation to be a major avenue of joy and pleasure and of highest significance for elderly people. Many nursing homes operate on the basis of communal dining and the issue of food becomes a major adaptational task for the resident. Coupled with changes in sense of taste, as well as the loss of familiar "home food," losing the role, especially for women, of "cook," and communal dining, can all be extremely frustrating and may become a major source of friction between residents as well as with staff. For an elderly resident, oral intake sometimes constitutes the only source of gratification and a main channel of communicating, interacting, and coping with the caretakers at the home and the world at large. Food, its quality and associated eating rituals, the conflicts as well as memories around it, all indicate personal and interpersonal significance. The psychological features associated with food: satisfying, receiving, giving, and caring, the ability to manipulate food as a means to interpersonal contact, are all severely restricted in communal dining and bear psychodynamic implications regarding mental health of residents, that the geropsychologist should be aware of.

7.21.4.3.5 Interpersonal and social adjustment

Adjustments in the interpersonal sphere and the social environment are perhaps the most crucial for the resident. The social circle, including residents as well as staff, is large, unknown, and unstable. Yet, new relationships have to be established. Many nursing homes are planned to have more than one resident per room. For some, the hardest tasks in adjusting to a nursing home are sharing personal space with a roommate, and forming a long-term intimate partnership. This requires a great deal of flexibility, compromise, and willingness to forego independence and freedom of choice regarding daily issues (e.g., when to turn out lights, cleaning and tidying, use of toilet, etc.) which take on increasing significance since they represent basic needs such as territory, belonging, or boundary intrusions, and become the ground for feelings of rejection, insult, or elicit aggressive behaviors.

Stripped of their previous acquaintances and social markers, the resident may feel insignificant and worthless. Loss of identity, together with the need to integrate into a new society, can cause insecurity, anxiety, and a sense of alienation. Mrs. B. said sadly, "for 60 years I lived in the same neighborhood and everyone knew me. When I came here, I suddenly lost my identity. I became anonymous, nobody knew who I am, what I have done all my life. I have become inferior in the world. I am just one old lady out of 300 old people." For many residents the absence of friends often renders the atmosphere in the home as distant and gloomy. Finding new friends and establishing personal relationships is a difficult task, especially in old age. Getting to know and be known requires motivation, risk-taking, confidence, learning, and adaptability, psychological qualities which the elderly resident may require professional help in utilizing for their well-being. The clinical geropsychologist may find here the appropriate ground upon which to help residents utilize their past experience, their social skills, and use ego strength to establish interpersonal and social relationships (Hansson & Carpenter, 1994). Since compatibility renders adjustment easier, the geropsychologist should be involved in decision-making about roommates. At times rearranging the environment may be useful. However, often they have to deal with already existing conflicts, in and between residents, and use them as analytic avenues towards adjustment and emotional security.

7.21.4.3.6 Reframing family relationships

Entering a nursing home necessitates the reformulation of relationships between the residents and their family. This sensitive process is emotionally loaded and may be the ground for deep conflict, as well reciprocal respect and love. The role of the family in the elderly's adjustment and their quality of life in the home is paramount. Relationships may become engulfed in ambivalence and stress, and past family dynamics may become the cornerstone for present conflicts or sound relationships. Although many families experience a heavy burden providing daily care for the older person at home, such stress often continues after the person's institutionalization (Stephens, Crowther, Hobfoll, & Tennenbaum, 1990). There is an ongoing launching process (Lomranz, 1995) in which, in contrast to the stage of adolescence, it is the parent who is being launched. Nevertheless, it bears similar launching characteristics, for example, guilt, ambivalence, letting go, holding on, transfer of responsibility, and mourning (Lomranz, Shmotkin, Eyal, & Zohar, 1996). Tobin (1987) describes children's mixed feelings, guilt and shame coupled with relief, in relocating a parent to a nursing home. Parents, however, may feel frustration stemming from their experience as they in the past shared lodgings with their own parents and grandparents. Although parents recognize the present difference in cohorts, housing arrangements, culture, and lifestyle, some may feel rejected and unwanted, believing that cohabitation would be possible if only desired by their children (Bar-Tur, 1993). Such beliefs may, in response, elicit guilt feelings and hostility in children. Zivoni (1993) found that positive intergenerational relationships had an indirect negative influence on application to a nursing home. Tobin (1987) described the importance of considering institutionalization as a family process. Tobin suggests that there will be a "good" figure (e.g., social worker or intern) satisfying the family's desire for individualized care for the resident, and a "bad" figure (e.g., administration) who could tolerate the family's anger. An elderly person's feeling of disconnection from their family may be detrimental to their mental health. Mutual ambivalence should be worked through. Intergenerational relations and the kind of daily involvement children have with the parent, family visits, and adequate contact with administration are extremely important for the well-being of the elderly and the family. In attending to their clients' problems, clinical geropsychologists sometimes have to involve the children (similar to the case of child therapy). Adult children should also be conceived as part of the social support network and in the role of caregivers, including the difficulties caregivers encounter (Stephens et al., 1990).

To summarize, nursing homes, the effects of institutionalization, and some core issues in a resident's adjustment to a nursing home, have been characterized from a mental health perspective. The elderly living in a nursing home should not be mainly preoccupied with coping and survival. Their quality of life should be the highest possible according to their potential. The nursing home should provide conditions which enhance physical and mental health and promote development and growth. This, however, is not always obtained and hence it is here that adaptational issues and the role and functions of the clinical geropsychologist are dealt with.

For growing numbers of aged people, especially (but not only) those who cannot live independently in the community, adjustment to a nursing home may be a major objective. The above explicated adaptational tasks actually refer to coping with aging processes and institutional effects. These tasks constitute the stage upon which the drama of life for the elderly resident is played out. They may continuously serve as "explosive potentials" as well as issues around which elderly may mask aggression, frustration, and depression. Thus, it is important for the clinical geropsychologist to be aware of them. Diminishment of these factors (e.g., spacial or geographical orientations, social circles) does not necessarily depend on length of residency, but may relate to lifestyle (e.g., a resident who is not mobile enough, or has no contact with the community), coping strategies, and quality of life in the home. For many elderly, life in nursing homes is dull and purposeless. Stripped of external responsibilities and social roles, the importance of the outlined existential components in the daily routine grows unproportionally, consuming physical and mental energy. Yet, at the same time, developmental processes fully operate, preoccupations with health, bodily concerns, life review, family issues, social surroundings, and processes relating to identity and the self. However, these processes may not find direct expression. Conflicts are expressed through the experience and events in daily life, be they tragedies or consumption of food. The clinical geropsychologist must be familiar with these ongoing adaptational tasks, their implications, and the personal meanings attached to them so as to be able to detect and utilize them as avenues to internal life.

If the foregoing may be comprehended in light of existential coping and "social pathology" (Pfeiffer, 1977), the chapter now focuses on more severe psychopathology.

7.21.5 MENTAL DISORDERS IN THE NURSING HOME

The extensive need for psychiatric treatment of nursing home residents has been noted above. Nursing homes report that they are admitting residents who are "sicker" and more frail than in the past. The prevalence of psychiatric behavioral disorders in nursing homes has been estimated to range from 68 to 94% (Grossberg, Hassan, & Szwabo, 1990). Burns et al. (1993) found mental illness among elderly nursing home residents at a rate of 64%; however, only about 4.5% received any mental health treatment in a given one-month period. When they did receive treatment, it was likely to be psychotropic medication only.

Manifestations of psychopathology in residents of long-term care facilities may include complaints of pain, anxieties, physical illness, impulse control problems, personality disorders, deliriums, thought disorders related to dementia, and chronic neurotic or psychotic behaviors. Evaluation of these behaviors and their differential diagnosis is complex and often not performed. Adequate treatment is prevented due to the lack of professional knowledge and facilities, limited resources, and staff. Norris, Snow-Turek, and Blankenship (1995) suggest that the environmental impact of institutionalization, as well as declining health, contributes to somatic and depressive symptomatology, as does frequent napping and use of psychotropic and sleeping medications prescribed (sometimes inappropriately) by general practitioners. The nursing home staff also suffer from such conditions. Everitt, Field, Soumerai, and Auron (1991) note that only minor attention has been focused on the effect on nursing home staff of agitating and disordered residents' behavior which might persist in spite of ongoing pharmacological therapy, although perhaps inappropriately managed. Staff, patients, physicians, and institutions are all leverage points for further intervention to improve the delicate balance between patient behavior, staff distress, and medication use.

7.21.5.1 Prevalence of Selected Syndromes and Interventions

The range of psychopatology in a nursing home is similar to that of the general population. Rovner and Rabins (1985) have divided psychiatric disorders seen in nursing home into three major groups: (i) cognitive disorders (e.g., delirium and dementias), (ii) depression, and (iii) behavioral disorders.

7.21.5.1.1 Dementia

Dementia is thoroughly presented in Chapter 10, this volume; here are highlighted some of their implications in homes for the aged. Estimates of incidence of the disease in individuals who are 80+ range from 10.8 to 47.2% (Gatz, Kasl-Godley, & Karel, 1996), hence its prevalence in many nursing homes is relatively high. As Chapter 10, this volume explicates, dementias appear in various patterns and modes of progression, a fact which carries many implications and difficulties in institutional management and care. Understanding emotions and moods of the older person suffering from dementia, correctly interpreting their behavior, and clarifying the impact of existing care practices are difficult tasks for the staff and pertain to the quality of care the institution is able to provide and the well-being of the demented (Cohen-Mansfield, 1996). Many of the demented elderly in nursing homes suffer from agitation reflected in a range of inappropriate behaviors: repetitive actions (e.g., pacing back and forth, repetition of words); socially inappropriate behavior (e.g., entering someone else's room and handling their belongings, or exposing themself nakedly); and aggressive behavior towards self or others. Often such patients walk out of the institution and cannot find their way back. Different agitating behaviors are associated with different individual characters, organicity, as well as situational characteristics. Such behavior is not only detrimental to the patient and their family, but creates fear and panic in the home where interaction is close and dense. "Healthy" and fearful residents express discontent of not being separated from persons even at early stages of Alzheimer. Each nursing home has its own covert norms and culture which are important for staff to be able to identify it in order to comprehend residents' behavior and reduce their own distress.

At various levels of dementia, aggressive behavior may be associated with poor-quality social interaction (e.g., responding to a roommate's minor invasion of personal space), or result from the patient's unsuccessful effort to interact verbally with their neighbor. Less aggressive behaviors tend to be manifested by persons who suffer from moderate to severe cognitive decline but are in relatively good physical health and under positive environmental conditions promoted by the institution. For some older persons, destructive behaviors may present a form of exercise or stimulation in the face of cognitive deterioration and reduced opportunities for other activities in the home. Various behavioral problems may occur frequently in a home inhabited by individuals suffering from a variety of illnesses, each at various levels of progression. It becomes an extremely difficult task for management to differentiate successfully and separate between such coexisting illnesses among residents.

A broad range of therapeutic functions and interventions are available to the geropsychologist. Proper neuropsychological assessment (see Chapter 7, this volume) is paramount to better understanding the cause of acute behavioral problems and in recommending appropriate treatment and case management. Delirium may be common in nursing homes and differentiation should be made whether or not it results from progressive demetia. The resident with multiple medical problems and receiving many medications may be particularly vulnerable to delirium. It takes special sensitivity to assess some deteriorated behaviors but also to reveal potential abilities and preserved areas. Some patients, for example, who do not respond otherwise, may respond to music even employing their memory. While often residents and staff avoid contact with a demented patient, it is important to provide them with social contact, a comfortable environment, and appropriate stimulation in order to maintain a proper quality of life. Psychotherapeutic interventions should address the different stages of dementia. Dynamic and primarily behavioral orientations ranging from personal to group interventions, including specified groups such as Reality Orientation, have all been used successfully. Other major avenues include working with the family and attending staff. Couples in the nursing home often have to be separated due to the deterioration of one of them, a traumatic event which often requires psychological intervention. The geropsychologist may advise staff regarding issues ranging from environmental safety of the wandering patient to impulse control problems, relevant neuropsychological presentations, and elevating staff distress. The various therapies should be promoted as important components of dignified management, in which the patient's entire life is respected and considered. This may also provide clues to the patient's resources that can to be drawn upon.

7.21.5.1.2 Depression

Depression has been considered the major mental health problem in aging. However, a more cautious approach is being seen. Differentiation in this category is related to issues such as prevalence, etiology, relation to physical illness, biology, and stress, as well as to methodology, screening, and diagnostic approaches (Blazer, Hughes, & George, 1987; Gatz, in press; Katz, in press; Teri, 1991). Affective disorders and depression are elaborated on in Chapter 9, this volume. This disorder in the nursing home setting should be emphasised. The prevalence of depression, its symptoms, or dysphoric mood rank high among residents of nursing homes. They may be subtle and often go unnoticed and untreated leading to excess disability, morbidity, and mortality. While the signs and symptoms are often ascribed to underlying medical problems and advanced age, in fact, some of depression's more prominent characteristics may be observed in many residents: loss of appetite and weight loss; severe fatigue; sleep disturbances; changes in bowel habits and somatization; sadness; feelings of loneliness; generalized lack of interest in life; apathy; increased time spent in bed; avoiding visits; nonparticipation in communal activity; low self-esteem; increased preoccupation with death; and a gloomy evaluation of one's present and future situation. More subtle signs in residents could include: memory problems (pseudodementia); difficulty in making even minor decisions; dreams of being lost and lonely in frightening, desolate places; and crying out for help with no one responding (Pachana, Gallagher-Thompson, & Thompson, 1994). Multiple losses appear in high concentration in nursing homes, perhaps rendering depressive symptoms as almost inevitable in some such institutions. Admission to a nursing home, especially involuntary, transition, and relocation, is often accompanied by an increase in depressive symptoms and lowlife satisfaction (Rovner et al., 1991), although confounding factors such as declining physical health, often the cause for the move, may be involved. Newmann, Engel, and Jensen (1991) have suggested the term depletion syndrome to describe a form of depression commonly observed in older adults, primarily involving lack of interest and feeling that everything is an effort. Blazer, Burchett, Service, & George (1991) term similar symptoms minor depression. These symptoms are often observed among residents and reinforce the search for more subtle signs of depression among nursing home residents. Etiology awaits further differentiation whether such symptoms constitute late-onset disorder, are secondary to residents' deteriorating health or reactive to being institutionalized.

Depressive disorders cause major distress to home and health care personnel. Residents at high risk would include those with a history of depression, poststroke individuals, new residents, those returning from hospitalization or admitted for rehabilitation, and those grieving or having severe adjustment problems. Differentiating between normal and pathological grief is critical. Also, several commonly prescribed medications can have mood-altering side effects, a significant factor when dealing with an institutionalized population which has, perhaps, the highest in intake of medical drugs. Often secondary depressions as manifestations of medical disorders are encountered. In order to provide treatment plans and direct the staff, the geropsychologist should administer diagnostic procedures, via clinical interview, symptom checklist, or more extensive testing. Although in most cases residents are referred to a psychiatrist for medication, the full range of causes for depression should be considered. These could include a variety of intrapsychic and psycho-social aspects, factors in which the geropsychologist's contribution is needed for evaluation and intervention. Effective therapies with depressive people, which also lend themselves well to the nursing setting, are behavior modification, cognitive, and psychodynamic therapies (Gallagher & Thompson, 1982).

7.21.5.1.3 Suicide

Suicide, its epidemiology, risks, and prevention, have been discussed in Chapter 11, this volume. This chapter emphasizes its special danger in the nursing home population. Many nursing homes constitute an assembly of suicide risk factors, as the discussion of depression indicates (Glass & Reed, 1993). Feeling helpless and hopeless, elderly candidates for suicide are less likely to make manipulative or suicidal gestures and they often signal their intentions, which are not always noticed. Some may, however, become unusually quiet and withdrawn. Recognizing the subtle signs of depression may require a high level of professional sensitivity. One clue is giving away valuable personal possessions. In either case, staff are often (it seems too often) "surprised" by the suicidal act.

The impact of suicide in an institutional perspective should be considered. Suicide in a nursing home can have an extreme impact on the residents and the staff. This may also be combated by defensive distancing. Usually it arouses anxiety, anger, and often a feeling of helplessness and inadequacy among those who were involved in the caregiving. Staff and management are often confused as death occurs (e.g., should obituaries be placed in the nursing home, should busing be arranged for funerals, etc.). There is always the threat of "contagion" as one suicide triggers suicidal thoughts or encourages other residents to attempt as well. This produces a threatening atmosphere in which fear of the "next" suicide prevails and is felt by most individuals in the home. At such times, interventions by staff may be crucial. In one nursing home six suicides were witnessed in a period of about two months. The atmosphere in the home became extremely tense. Both staff and residents were very anxious and many expressed guilt, helplessness, and desperation. Inspection revealed feelings of frustration, anger, and despair. A special intervention program was designed, including individual and group discussions in which residents were helped to deal with stressful life events and current obstacles, to ventilate, and were taught self-control and self-relaxation techniques. The psychologist's major task was to identify residents at risk and to provide immediate help for some residents, for example, those who had been friends of the suicidees or witnessed their death. A prevention program was also designed in which staff members were trained to identify signals of threat among residents, and certain security measures and technical devices (e.g., preventing accumulation of drugs, closing "risky" places such as roofs) were taken to prevent future suicidal events.

7.21.5.1.4 Psychotic symptoms and paraphrenia

A variety of delusions, often related to progressive dementia, are seen in patients in nursing homes. More frequent are the paranoid or accusatory behaviors. Late-onset schizophrenics, in contrast to early-onset schizophrenics, have an average life expectancy that seems to exceed that of the regular elderly population (Bienenfeld, 1990). Pharaphrenia, often regarded as late-onset schizophrenia, is usually described as having onset after the age of 60 and entailing paranoid delusions with or without auditory hallucinations, less thought disorder, and less flattening of affect.

Paraphrenia, which has a relatively high incidence among nursing home residents, can also be regarded as a delusional disorder characterized by an isolated delusion and no other symptoms, and with the delusion not necessarily signaling a neurological disorder (American Psychiatric Association, 1994). Delusions in older patients, according to Post (1987), take the form of "unshakable false belief" with remarkably "banal" content. Psychological diathesis for paraphrenia often include premorbid schizoid personality disorder (Pearlson et al., 1989). Traumas earlier in life, such as parental separation, being a refugee, and childlessness, may play a role in increasing vulnerability (Gurian, Wexler, & Baker, 1992), whereas recent stress may trigger the onset of the disorder. Residents who have immigrated from other countries seem susceptible to developing delusional disorders (Ruskin, 1990). Molinari and Chacko (1983) suggest that the development of paranoid symptoms in the elderly patient is usually the result of increased use of projection as a defense against grief or perceived loss of autonomy and control, typical occurrences in nursing homes. Many residents' ideation was often related to past experiences or unresolved conflictual relationships. Mr. G., aged 82, a frail elderly, blamed his wife of adultery since she became involved in the home's activities, while he remained in the room. In an other case, a widowed woman whose two daughters died in the last 10 years and who also suffered from hearing loss and eye sight deterioration, developed a paranoid ideation that her neighbor was stealing from her. These symptoms may defensively protect the resident from painful depression that some individuals experience as a reaction to loss and dependency. Some researchers have reported that hearing loss is associated with late-onset schizophrenia or paraphrenia and frequently among dementia patients with paranoid symptoms (Gurian et al., 1992). Paranoid symptoms may thus develop as a result of mental deterioration reflecting prethreshold organic brain change, sometimes in order to fill the gap created by impaired memory (Gatz, et al., 1996).

Late-onset psychotic symptoms often have an organic etiology. Therefore, a thorough medical and laboratory evaluation, together with a psychological one, should be obtained. A useful rule of thumb when dealing with psychotic symptoms in the nursing home is to ask to what degree these symptoms are disturbing to the patient or to the environment. Often such states are best treated nonchemically, late-onset schizophrenia does have more preservation of personality and less formal thought disorder then early-onset schizophrenia. If psychotic symptoms are disturbing, antipsychotic medication and ongoing psychiatric involvement is certainly called for. Case management interventions, such as encouraging the patient to remove from people or situations which stimulate the paranoid ideation, could be helpful. The role of the geropsychologist to could be to establish an alliance with the patient (Fried & Agassi, 1976), thus encouraging them to share thoughts about present and past experiences. When such communication can be established, the patient becomes less anxious and an ongoing treatment plan, with the consulting psychiatrist at the home, can be established.

7.21.5.1.5 *Personality disorders*

Personality disorders are discussed in Chapter 12, this volume, This discussion is limited to highlighting aspects relevant to nursing homes. Given the residents' advanced age, difficulties in diagnosis become apparent. Properly diagnosing personality disorders is further encumbered by the impact of the institutional environment, changes in cognitive processes, sorting out chronic from acute behaviors, and difficulties in obtaining history. A lifetime pattern of pathological interpersonal relationships, the present old-age experience of losses, and institutionalizational rules, all further promote regressive psychological functioning and may elicit primitive defenses such as splitting, all of which gain a special intense quality in an environment with multiple caregivers. Personality disorders are often seen in conjunction with other disorders, in particular major or masked depressions, frequent in nursing homes. Residents with personality disorders are especially ill-equipped to cope with the stress of institutionalization. Many of the "difficult" or "uncooperative" residents in a nursing home can be diagnosed as personality disorders, sometimes coupled with cognitive decline. Such residents may manifest inappropriate emotional responses or inconsistent control of impulse behavior, including aggression and violence. Sadavoy and Fogel (1992) suggest that these patients tend to represent a vulnerable personality that becomes increasingly less adaptive with new stressful events in old age due to eight critical age-specific stressors: interpersonal loss, physical disability, loss of external manifestations of the self (beauty, strength), loss of role, loss of defensive outlets; forced reliance on caretakers, confrontation with death; and conflict over the wish to live vs. the wish to die. Another major loss for such residents is the loss of resources of narcissistic gratification from others. These difficulties are often manifested in distorted ways such as self-perception oblivious to one's impact. This affects interaction with other residents and staff, and may lead to constant conflict with management. Difficulties in these individuals often result from the state in which they have to be dependent on others and to rely on them to supply their needs. They may fight for independence and autonomy in order to maintain their self-esteem by manipulating the staff, by refusing to obey rules, and acting out their anxieties and conflicts.

In spite of the difficulties with such patients, they may benefit from regular psychotherapeutic contact and are able to establish an alliance with the therapist. The relationship with the psychotherapist itself may gratify narcissistic needs which otherwise might have been expressed destructively. Work with the patient's family and staff caretakers is also indicated to introduce possible case management procedures shielding such a patient from stress or encouraging real and/or perceived autonomy and control (Perlmuter & Monty, 1979).

Although the major symtomatology has been outlined, it should be emphasized that the more "benign" disturbances and neurotic behaviors do not receive due attention, as if neuroticism disappears in old age and the elderly suffer only from cognitive difficulties, dementias, and psychosis. Reality is completely different; neurotic behavior and existential concerns are "there to stay," can be treated (including with psychotherapy), and present a major component in the mental health of the elderly in general and in nursing homes in particular. Other disturbances prevailing in nursing homes, and not discussed due to lack of space, include anxiety and somatoform disorders (Stanley and Beck, this vol.), drug abuse (Blow, this vol.), sleep disorders (Ancoli-Israel, this vol.), impulse control wandering, behavioral problems, family issues, further neurotic and psychotic disturbances, as well as surrogate decision-making for nursing home residents. Having emphasized that health problems do not receive adequate treatment, a comprehensive treatment model is presented to address all the explicated mental health issues discussed.

7.21.6 A CLINICAL GEROPSYCHOLOGICAL SERVICE IN NURSING HOMES: A PROPOSED MODEL

A geropsychological clinic operating in a nursing home in Isreal is described (Lomranz, 1991) and presented as a model clinic.

7.21.6.1 Setting and Clientele

The clinic operates within a nursing home housing a population of 750 residents. A psychiatrist serves as consultant. The elderly residents range from those functioning independently to those needing constant nursing care. The clinic is a recognized internship center for clinical psychology interns and is associated with the Tel Aviv University's Herczeg Institute on Aging. The target clientele consists of two main categories: the residents themselves and associated significant figures, mainly family, and the professional and paraprofessional staff. The clinic's framework includes regular staff meetings, case conferences, supervision, study groups, and seminars, as well as participation in many of the nursing home conferences, including referral conferences, admission committees, and meetings planning activities for residents.

7.21.6.2 Orientation and Philosophy

The philosophy constitutes the *zeitgeist* which prevails in the clinic and should be expressed in interaction with clientele, above and beyond the "professional approach." It is reflected in: (i) a dual focus on the image of a person, a Bo-psycho-social holistic view (Engel, 1977) embedded in a humanistic approach and respect for personal dignity, and a life-span developmental psychology orientation (P. Baltes & M. Baltes, 1993). The two orientations are eminently compatible. (ii) Comprehension of the environment and the significance of person/environment interaction; (iii) Aim: to improve mental health and upgrade the quality of life; (iv) Methods: The service adheres to a dynamic theoretical approach based on elaborations of clinical adult developmental theory (Nemiroff & Colarusso, 1990) and other eclectic clinical techniques of diagnosis and treatment. It has often been observed that mental health problems in nursing homes may go unnoticed for long periods of time. It is often only when a resident "becomes a nuisance" that they are dealt with. Early detection may improve the utility of treatment. It is therefore crucial that the service adheres to outreach, prevention, and community orientations.

7.21.6.3 Methods

The eclectic approach is tailored to the specific needs of the client. These approaches include dynamic, cognitive, and behavior modification, group methods, family and milieu systems, existential therapy, organizational, educational, and community approaches. Specific techniques found useful with the elderly are employed, including life review therapy, reminisence groups (Haight & Webster, 1995), family counseling (Brink, 1979), and educational programs and training (Garrison, 1978). These are applied to individuals, families, groups, community, staff, and interdisciplinary networks. Group work (e.g., psychotherapy, family, task groups, life review) is a major methodological component (MacLennan, Shura, & Weiner, 1988). Intervention are geared to eliminate psychopathology as well as preventive work to increase clients' sense of control and hopefulness about change. Reserve capacities are utilized, based on selection, optimization, and compensation (Baltes & Baltes, 1993; Ryff, 1989). Considerable attention is paid to assessment and diagnostics (Storandt, Siegler, & Elias, 1978). Existing diagnostic tools are adapted or modified, and specialized tools are developed in cooperation with the University Herczeg Institute on Aging. Thus, traditional and nontraditional approaches for intervention and assessment are employed. The psychologists work in cooperation with social workers, occupational, art- and physiotherapists. Special attention is given to psychosoma interaction, and ongoing communication is maintained with the medical and paramedical staff. Regular contact is held with the "Home mother," the caregivers, and technical departments (e.g., maintenance, cleaning, kitchen). Informal contact and interaction (discussions in the elevator, garden, etc.) are part of the approach and highly valued. All these activities also contribute to the integration of the clinic as an integral part of the nursing home.

7.21.6.4 Applications

Most referrals originate from interdisciplinary staff meetings, medical and social services, or individuals recommending neighbors. A minority are self-refered. Three principles of psychological interventions of a curative, preventive or palliative nature are categorized and for the sake of convenience, termed: (i) "treatment," basically consisting of a direct, short-term, or long-term systematic psychotherapeutic approach applied to different kinds of psychopathologies; (ii) "consultation," attending transitional, normative, or situational crises. This is mostly accomplished directly, but often indirectly (e.g., instructing a nurse, neighbor): short consultation or direction of other staff are central here; (iii) "prevention," consisting of two main activities of working with residents or staff on problematic issues or risk populations (e.g., groups work with isolated residents just before major holidays, or tackling staff problems of burnout) or of educational activities aimed at enriching the residents or furthering the professional development of the staff (e.g., lectures to residents on mental health or to staff on psycholpathology).

Thus, the psychological services in the nursing home comprises seven domains with their respective working goals of mental health.

7.21.6.4.1 Preadmission screening

Every applicant is interviewed and assessed to obtain information on cognitive as well as affective functioning and status. Thus, the service can be advise management in decisions to accept or reject an applicant. For those accepted, preadmission screening may be paramount in certifying the type of care and living facilities that the elderly requires (Smyer, 1989). While most people admitted to a nursing home have mental concerns and some physical problems, it is generally the latter which are documented and communicated to the staff, while mental or behavioral problems are rarely discussed professionally. At times, there is a tendency for the family and the older client to withhold information regarding deterioration of mental state. Such clients, once admitted, exhibit serious adjustment difficulty and, moreover, their cognitively impaired as well as affective state may deteriorate more rapidly. The psychologist can support the client and the family and can help reduce their initial anxiety, obtain their cooperation in assessing adequately the client and as a result prevent unnecessary misery and rapid decline in mental health.

7.21.6.4.2 Follow-up services

Working on the basis of data obtained in prescreening, the psychologist is later involved in assessing the follow-up of the new resident. Some residents need supportive sessions or crisis intervention, short-term therapy, focused on issues of separation and mourning over the losses they experience at the early phases of their transition to the nursing home. Others may be directed to task groups or activities in the home. The service conducts open-ended adjustment groups which focus on relocation effects during the first three to six months, a group in which every newcomer participates for at least several sessions.

7.21.6.4.3 Severe psychopathology

Here the clinic functions as any other psychiatric setting. Patients are refered and diagnosed, and treatment is planed and carried out. Often, combined psychopharmacological and psychological treatment is administered. Individual psychotherapy is increasingly being requested by residents.

7.21.6.4.4 Family interventions

A resident's family always occupies them in practice or in thought. The elderly person usually arrives at the nursing home accompanied by family members, with the adult children formally assuming "filial" responsibility, acting as "parents" as they relate to their parent and deal with staff and management. This role reversal is often likely to heighten the anxieties and difficulties of all parties concerned: children, parents, and staff. As some residents experience separation anxieties and relocation symptoms are manifested, the anxious, or guilt ridden, children may respond by engaging in acting-out behaviors. They may cause inconvenience, aggravate staff, and exhibit overdo concern. Parents, in turn, increase their fears and guilt by complaining, crying, expressing helplessness, and despair. This was the case with Mr. R., aged 88, who, prior to entering the home was functioning well, spending his time painting and sculpturing. He was forced to move to the nursing home after falling and became unable to take care of himself. He was the father of two devoted sons who encouraged him and helped him move to the home. Mr. R. seemed quiet and reserved in the admission interview. However, as soon as his sons left he became extremely anxious and restless. During his first week in the home he spent most of the day wandering around the phone box crying and calling his sons, asking them to visit. He nagged staff and other passers-by near the phone box to call his sons. His sons became concerned and paid visits a few times a day. Family sessions were held in which the children comprehended the father's separation anxieties and his intensive need for support. The sons were encouraged to talk about their own anxieties and work through their ambivalence at "launching" their father. The psychologist presented a treatment plan for the father with guidelines for the family and the nursing staff to help the father settle down and slowly shift towards self-control instead of enacting his need to control his sons. He gradually learned how to master his anxieties, his sadness declined, and his phone calls ceased.

Mr. G., 80-years old, lived in the nursing home for five years. His relationship with his only son was completely cut off, each accusing the other of ill-treating the mother/wife who passed away prior to Mr. G's move to the home. On memorial day each would come to the cemetery at a different hour. Mr. G. appeared to be well adjusted in the home until he developed a prostrate condition and feared he would die. At that point he began to long for his son who, stubbornly, refused to see him. The son had 20 hours of telephone discussions with one of the psychologists, during which he voiced his anger, discussed the role his mother played in his life, and his hate and ambivalence to his father. Only afterwards was a meeting arranged in which the two brought flowers to the mother's grave and joint treatment began.

7.21.6.4.5 From education to psychotherapy

Extending educational programs to residents and their families provides a channel leading residents to self-development. Psychological education is often a condition for various ethnic, economic, and less-educated residents to become utilizers of the psychological services.

Many elderly suffering in nursing homes may find it difficult to discuss personal issues and emotional problems with others, will not take the initiative to obtain psychological help, and may also refuse it when offered. One way to combat such difficulties is through offering relevant information, developing the proper atmosphere, and providing opportunities to meet therapists. Different psychologists and interns of the service provide a monthly lecture, open to residents, their families, and staff, on various aspects of the aging process, general psychology and adjustment issues in nursing homes. The psychologist then leads a discussion encouraging the audience to ask questions and to share ideas, thoughts, and feelings.

Mrs. J. approached the psychologist after a lecture on intergenerational relationships, seeking advice for problems her granddaugther has with her father. In the discussion she revealed her intense identification with the granddaughter voicing anger at her son. This became a basis for her visits to the service. She then focused on personal problems and remained in psychotherapy for eight months. Mrs. W., a highly educated 92-year-old, wished to continue the lecture on "successful aging" with the "young professor" (professional status being usually important, and overrated by elderly). This provided her with the opportunity to gain respect for her own knowledge and experience and eventually led to an extended and structured life review, after which she became more accepting of her present condition and learned new social skills. Obstacles in approaching the psychologist also reside in prejudice and stigmas about mental care, common in the older population. Public lectures, or special workshops (e.g., in communication skills, memory techniques) help the elderly, prospective client reduce anxieties and shame. Such activities, to most of which family members are also invited, may also serve as a vehicle of outreach to enhance constructive family involvement.

7.21.6.4.6 Working with nursing home staff

This is a primary goal in the work of the clinic. The clinic administers intervention programs aimed at reducing staff distress, professional upgrading, promoting team work (e.g., to eliminate stress between workers in the kitchen), assisting conflict resolution between various teams and between them and management, and preventing burnout.

Nursing homes often have high turnover rates and low staff morale, resulting from work pressures in dealing with threatening issues (aging, loss, illness, and death), distorted perceptions, and low intrinsic and extrinsic rewards. Psychologists in the service work with the interdisciplinary teams providing guidance, information, knowledge, and help in management of residents (e.g., how to address residents' hostile behaviors towards them), in coping with personal problems, and symptoms of burnout (increased fatigue, apathy, etc.). Workshops are conducted on improving interpersonal communication among the staff aiding managers to establish positive reinforcement techniques (Sbordone & Sterman, 1983), improving problem-solving on team building, and preventing burnout. Working educationally with different ranks of staff, the psychologist also conducts discussions, lectures, and case conferences with the various teams (e.g., medical, maintenance workers). Most interventions are based on short-term programs of two to six sessions.

The geropsychologist should project an independent, often "neutral," professional position in the home, thus promoting authority and the ability to work successfully with the various teams, management, and residents. The clinic has witnessed turnovers and shifts in staff roles as well as changes of management often resulting in unclarity and uncertainty as to structure and management. In one such instance staff had major difficulties adjusting to a transition period between managers. Discussions with the psychologist, working as an organizational consultant, revealed an accumulation of covert anger and coalitions between different team members detrimental to ongoing work. Often, in meetings, issues concerning complains about residents reveal conflicts between different teams of the staff. In another case, a nursing team became almost ineffective. It turned out that the team was understaffed, frustrated by hard work and lack of appreciation and recognition by management, and rapidly revealed burnout syptomatology. Group discussions combined with private sessions helped them release their feelings, work through some of the communication patterns with management, and address their complaints effectively. Some of the clinic's staff are also called for consultation to other nursing homes in the vicinity.

7.21.6.4.7 A university clinic

Coordinating links with the university's institute of aging and the nursing home, teaching and supervising students and interns, and cooperating in research are all part and parcel of the clinic. The staff includes postgraduate clinical psychologists who work as interns in the nursing homes, and provide supervision to undergraduate and graduate students of clinical psychology. Undergraduate students participate in a special practicum program involving them in activities which may range from friendly visits to more structured intervention, participation in group work, and providing lectures to the residents. Such liaisons with academic settings are beneficial to all parties involved and upgrade the quality of the home (Smyer & Garfein, 1988). They also encourage young students and interns to choose aging as their field of specialization (Kahana, 1986).

This section concludes with some general evaluative remarks. During two years of operation, residents have changed their attitudes to psychological services. They became less skeptic, have come to recognize the importance of the clinic, and make greater use of its services. Experience suggests the recommendation that as geropsychologists, even intermediately until clinics are set up, working as individuals in nursing homes, they should: (i) establish their position as consultants in a variety of roles; (ii) dwell on diagnostics and assessment; (iii) become major referal directors; (iv) operate as coordinators between teams; (v) be clinical-community oriented; (vi) advance milieu treatment; (vii) assert their impact on policy-making in the institute; (viii) plan and utilize interdisciplinary interventions; (ix) be liberal in using eclectic, traditional, as well as untraditional, intervention approaches, including psychotherapy; and (x) invest in educational programs and systematically accumulating knowledge through documentation and research.

The possibilities of psychotherapy in nursing homes should be emphasized as a challenge for every clinical psychologist. The goals of psychotherapy should be modified and theoretically they should consider gerontology, adult developmental processes, cognitive and medical losses and the effects of institutionalization, as well as clinical methodology. The dialectics between "case specificity" and "age specificity" have to be analyzed. Short-term treatment is often required (Brink, 1979; Gallagher & Thompson, 1982), and a relational approach to transference seems conducive (Frankel, 1995). In long-term therapy, sessions could be of short duration and may be conducted in the residents' personal environment (their room, or in the ward). Long-term psychotherapy often provides the resident with continuity assuring them of the therapist's availability as a secure base (Bowlby, 1980). Many problems of the aged person are fit for intrapsychic and interpersonal exploration and lend themselves to life review, development, and growth. While psychotherapy is always tailored to the specific case, its possible gains with the aged are (in the proper perspective) as unlimited as they are with younger populations. Psychotherapy should be considered as a viable option for the elderly (Shmotkin, Eyal, & Lomranz, 1989). The pleasure and growth in working with the suitable aged can be tremendously gratifying for all parties.

7.21.7 FUTURE PROSPECTS

There is undoubtedly an increasing need for mental health services in nursing homes. As the nursing home industry develops, this need intensively grows. Existing mental health facilities need to be expanded and improved, urgently, to answer neglected and increasing needs. Unfortunately, psychologists, not to mention geropsychological clinics, rarely are found in nursing homes. Also, the nursing home setting is ill-prepared to accept and employ psychologists. The absence of systematic assessment procedures, diagnosis and evaluation, consultations, therapy, and other appropriate interventions have a high cost. Unfortunately, there is a pronounced shortage of psychologists in gerontological clinical work in general (Gatz, 1995; Gatz et al., 1985). Clinical psychology as a discipline is still largely child-oriented and continues to reflect "professional ageism" (Butler & Lewis, 1982), especially with respect to nursing homes. The many misconceptions about the the older person (e.g., lack of energy, motivation, rigidity, and resistance to change) still remain after many decades and affect the "reluctant psychologist" who is unwilling to work with the elderly. Working with the elderly still seems to be rated by colleagues as having low professional status (Knight, Reinhart, & Field, 1982), all the more so in a nursing home. Psychologists may also tend to shrink from interdisciplinary collaboration and conflict (e.g., with psychiatrist, social workers, or other paraprofessionals). Working in a nursing home is often regarded as depressing and difficult since illness and death, helplessness, and hopelessness are confronted continuously. What then are the future prospects?

To meet the crucial challenge, a broader perspective should be adopted which associates geropsychology more strongly with clinical psychology at large and considers policy issues (Kane & Kane, 1990). Basic changes are recommended as stated in the following: (i) the discipline of clinical psychology has to further modify its developmental approach to include adulthood and aging; (ii) theory construction in clinical gerontology while thoroughly based on gerontology also needs to further integrate prevalent clinical theory (e.g., object relations); (iii) clinical methodology in geropsychology, on the aforementioned basis, should be eclectic and modified in goals and methods to fit the elderly population; (iv) policy should be further planned and policy makers have to present, perhaps more aggressively, the damage to nursing homes in cost-effective terms and develop reimbursement systems; (v) academic education and training has to be expanded intensively to include clinical geropsychology; (vi) governmental regulations should include the request for in-home psychological services in nursing homes as obligatory; and (vii) nursing homes should become academic-associated institutions, and clinics, as certified training placements and research units, should operate in each.

The major goal of the clinical gerontologist in nursing homes should be to contribute to a fundamental change which would render the various institutions as authentic "homes" in which residents could actualize their potentials for positive mental health, live with dignity, enhance their well-being, and live creatively. For that purpose, which to a certain extent will determine the kind of society that is built, the discipline of psychology, on its various domains, is expected to mobilize itself to change and meet that challenge.

7.21.8 REFERENCES

American Psychiatric Association (1994). *Diagnostic and statistical manual of mental disorders* (4th ed.). Washington, DC: Author.

Baltes, M. M. (1982). Environmental factors in dependency among nursing home residents: A social ecology analysis. In T. A. Wills (Ed.), *Basic processes in helping relationships*. New York: Academic Press.

Baltes, P. B., & Baltes, M. M. (Eds.) (1993). *Successful aging: Perspectives from the behavioral sciences*. Cambridge, UK: Cambridge University Press.

Bar-Tur, L. (1993). Adjustment to home for the aged as a developmental crisis in old age. *Gerontologia, 62*, 48–57.

Bienenfeld, D. (Ed.) (1990). *Verwoerdt's clinical geropsychiatry* (3rd ed.). Baltimore: Williams & Wilkins.

Birren, J. E., & Renner, V. J. (1980). Concepts and issues of mental health and aging. In J. E. Birren (Ed.), *Handbook of mental health and aging* (pp. 3–33). Englewood Cliffs, NJ: Prentice-Hall.

Blazer, D., Burchett, B., Service, C., & George, L. K. (1991). The association between age and depression among the elderly: An epidemiological exploration. *Journal of Gerontology: Medical Sciences, 46*, M210–215.

Blazer, D. G., Hughes, D. C., & George, L. K. (1987). The epidemiology of depression in an elderly community population. *Gerontologist, 27*, 281–287.

Bowlby, J. (1980). *Loss*. New York: Basic Books.

Brink, T. L. (1979). *Geriatric psychotherapy*. New York: Human Sciences Press.

Burns, B., Wagner, H. R., Taube, J. E., Magaziner, J., Permutt, T., & Landerman, L. R. (1993). Mental health service use by the elderly in nursing homes. *American Journal of Public Health, 83*, 331–337.

Butler, R. N. (1975). *Why survive? Being old in America*. New York: Harper & Row.

Butler, R. N., & Lewis, M. (1982). *Aging and mental health*. London: Merrill.

Cohen, G. D. (1980). Prospects for mental health and aging. In J. E. Birren & R. Sloane (Eds.), *Handbook of mental health and aging* (pp. 971-993). Englewood Cliffs, NJ: Prentice-Hall.

Cohen, C. (1991). The chronic mentally ill elderly: Service research issues. In E. Light & B. Lebowitz (Eds.), *The elderly with chronic mental illness* (pp. 194–219). New York: Springer.

Cohen-Mansfield, J. (1996). *Trends in the treatment of frail elderly persons*. Paper presented in the Herczeg Research Institute on Aging, Tel Aviv University, Israel.

Colerick, E. J., & George, L. K. (1986). Predictors of institutionalization among caregivers of patients with Alzheimer's disease. *Journal of the American Geriatrics Society, 34*, 493–498.

Donahue, W. (1978). What about our responsibility for the abandoned elderly? *The Gerontologist, 18*, 102–111.

Eisdorfer, C., & Cohen, D. (1982). *Mental health care of the aging: A multidisciplinary curriculum for professional training*. New York: Springer.

Engel, G. (1977). The need for a new medical model: A challenge for biomedicine. *Science, 196*, 129–136.

Everitt, D. E., Field, D. R., Soumerai, S. S., & Avron, J. (1991). Resident behavior and staff distress in the nursing home. *Journal of American Geriatrics Society, 39*, 792–798.

Farrari, N. (1963). Freedom of choice. *Social Work, 8*, 105–106.

Firestone, I. J., Lichman, C. M., & Evans, J. R. (1980). Privacy and solidarity: Effects of nursing home accommodation on environmental perception and sociability preferences. *International Journal of Aging and Human Development, 1*, 221–241.

Frankel, S. (1995). *Intricate engagements*. London: Jason Aronson.

Freedman, V. (1996). Family structure and the risk of nursing home admission. *Journal of Gerontology: Social Sciences. 51B*, S61–S69.

Fried, Y., & Agassi, J. (1976). *Paranoia: A study in diagnosis*. Dordrecht, The Netherlands: Reidel.

Gallagher, D. E., & Thompson, L. W. (1982). Treatment of major depressive disorders in older outpatients with brief psychotherapies. *Psychotherapy: Theory, Research and Practice, 19*, 482–490.

Garrison, J. (1978). Stress management training for the elderly: A psychoeducational approach. *Journal of the American Geriatrics Society, 26*, 397–403.

Gatz, M. (1989). Clinical psychology and aging. In M. Storandt & G. R. VandenBos (Eds.), *The adult years: Continuity and changes* (pp. 79-114). Washington, DC: American Psychological Association.

Gatz, M. (Ed.) (1995). *Emerging issues in mental health and aging*. Washington, DC: American Psychological Association.

Gatz, M. (1998). Towards a developmentally-informed theory of mental disorder in older adults. In J. Lomranz (Ed.), *Handbook of mental health and aging*. New York: Plenum.

Gatz, M., Kasl-Godley, J. E., & Karel, M. J. (1996). Aging and mental disorders. In J. E. Birren & K. W. Schaie (Eds.), *Handbook of the psychology of aging* (4th ed.). San Diego, CA: Academic Press.

Gatz, M., Popkin, S., Pino, C., & VandenBos, G. R. (1985). Psychological interventions with older adults. In J. E. Birren & K. W. Schaie (Eds.), *Handbook of the psychology of aging* (2nd ed., pp. 755–785). New York: Van Nostrand Reinhold.

Gatz, M., & Smyer, M. A. (1992). The mental health system and older adults in the 1990s. *American Psychologist, 47*, 741-751.

Glass, J. C., & Reed, S. E. (1993). To live or to die: A look at elderly suicide. *Educational Gerontology, 19* (8), 767–778.

Goffman, E. (1961). *Asylums: Essays on the social situation of mental patients and other inmates*. New York: Anchor.

Goplerud, E. (1979). Unexpected consequences of deinstitutionalization of the mentally disabled elderly. *Community Psychology, 7*, 315–328.

Groger, L. (1994). Decision as a process: A conceptual model of black elders nursing home placement. *Journal of Aging Studies, 8*, 77–94.

Grossberg, G. T., Hassan, R., & Szwabo, P. A. (1990). Psychiatric problems in the nursing home. St. Louis University geriatric grand rounds. *Journal of the American Geriatric Society, 38* (8), 907–917.

Gurland, B. J. (1973). Abroad clinical assessment of psychopathology in the aged. In C. Eisdorfer & M. P. Lawton (Eds.), *The psychology of adult development and aging* (pp. 343–377). Washington, DC: American Psychological Association.

Gurian, B. S., Wexler, D., & Baker, E. H. (1992). Late-life paranoia: Possible association with early trauma and infertility. *International Journal of Geriatric Psychiatry, 7*, 277–284.

Gutmann, D. (1994). *Reclaimed powers: Men and women in later life*. Evanston, IL: Northwestern University Press.

Haight, B., & Webster, J. (Eds.) (1995). *The art and science of reminiscing: Theory, research methods and applications*. London: Taylor & Francis.

Halpert, E. (1991). Aspects of a dilemma of middle age: Whether or not to place aged failing parents in nursing home. *Psychoanalytic Quarterly, 60*, 426–449.

Hansson, R., & Carpenter, B. (1994). *Relationships in old age. Coping with the challenge of transition*. New York: Guilford.

Hirschfeld, M., & Fleishman, R. (1990). Nursing home care for the elderly. In R. L. Kane, G. Evans, & D. Macfadyn (Eds.), *Improving the health of older people—A world view* (pp. 473–490). Oxford, UK: Oxford University Press.

Jahoda, M. (1958). *Current concepts of positive mental health.* New York: Basic Books.

Johnson, C. L., & Grant, L. A. (1985). *The nursing home in American society.* Baltimore: Johns Hopkins University Press.

Kahana, B. (1986). *A proposal to establish a Ph.D program in clinical-research gerontology.* Cleveland, OH: Cleveland State University.

Kane, R. L., & Kane, R. A. (Eds.) (1982). *Values and long term care.* Lexington, MA: Lexington.

Kane, R. L., & Kane, R. A. (1990). Health care for older people: Organizational and policy issues. In R. H. Binstock & L. K. George (Eds.) *Handbook of aging and social sciences* (3rd ed., pp. 415–437) San Diego, CA: Academic Press.

Katz, I. (in press). Depression as a pivotal component of secondary aging. In J. Lomranz (Ed.), *Handbook of mental health and aging.* New York: Plenum.

Knight, B., Resnhart, R., & Field, D. (1982). Senior outreach services: A treatment oriented outreach team in community mental health. *The Gerontologist, 22,* 544–547.

Knight, B. G., Santos, J., Teri, L., & Lawton, M. P. (1995). Introduction: The development of training in clinical geropsychology. In B. G. Knight, L. Teri, P. Wohlford, & J. Santos (Eds.), *Mental health services for older adults: Implications for training and practice in geropsychology.* (pp. 1–8). Washington, DC: American Psychological Association.

Lawton, M. P. (1980). Housing the elderly: Residential quality and residential satisfaction. *Research on Aging, 2,* 309–328.

Lawton, M. P. (1985). Housing and living environments of older people. In R. Binstock & E. Shanas (Eds.), *Handbook of aging and social sciences* (pp. 450–478). New York: Reinhold.

Lawton, M. P., & Cohen, J. (1974). The generality of housing impact on the well-being of older people. *Journal of Gerontology, 29,* 194–204.

Lewis, M. A., Cretin, S., & Kane, R. L. (1985). The natural history of nursing home patients. *Gerontologist, 25,* 382–388.

Lieberman, M., & Tobin, S. (1983). *The experience of old age. Stress, coping and survival.* New York: Basic Books.

Lomranz, J. (1991). Mental health in homes for the aged and the clinical psychology of aging: Implementation of a model service. *Clinical Gerontologist, 10,* 47–71.

Lomranz, J. (1995). Thus we live forever taking leave: The launching stage in the Israeli family. *Social Behavior and Personality,* 28, 287–302.

Lomranz, J., Shmotkin, D., Eyal, N., & Zohar, Y. (1996). Launching themes in Israeli fathers and mothers. *Journal of Adult Development, 3,* 159–170.

Lomranz, J., Shmotkin, D., & Vardi, R. (1991). The equivocal meanings of time. *Current Psychology: Research and Reviews,* 10 (1 & 2), 3–20.

MacLennan, B., Shura, S., & Weiner, M. (Eds.) (1988). *Group psychotherapies for the elderly.* Madison, WI: International Universities Press.

Molinari, V., & Chacko, R. (1983). The classification of paranoid disorders in the elderly: A clinical problem. *Clinical Gerontologist, 1,* 31–37.

Moos, R., & Lemke, S. (1985). Specialized living environments for the older people. In J. E. Birren & K. W. Schaie (Eds.), *Handbook of the psychology of aging* (pp. 864–889). New York: Reinhold.

National Center for Health Statistics (1983). *The national nursing home survey: 1977. Summary for the United States.* Washington, DC: Government Printing Office.

Nemiroff, R., & Colarusso, C. (Eds.) (1990). *New dimensions in adult development.* New York: Basic Books.

Neulinger, J. (1981). *To leisure: An introduction.* Boston, MA: Allyn and Bacon.

Newman, F. L., Griffin, B. P., Black, R. W., & Page, S. E. (1989). Linking level of care to level of need: Assessing the need for mental health care for nursing home residents. *American Psychologist, 44,* 1315–1324.

Newmann, J. P., Engel, R. J., & Jensen, J. E. (1991). Changes in depressive symptom experiences among older women. *Psychology and Aging, 6,* 212–222.

Norris, M. P., Snow-Turek, A. L., & Blankenship, L. (1995). Somatic depressive symptoms in the elderly: Contribution or confound? *Journal of Clinical Geropsychology, 1,* 5–17.

Pachana, N., Gallagher-Thompson, D., & Thompson, L. W. (1994). Assessment of depression. In M. P. Lawton & J. A. Teresi (Eds.), *Annual review of gerontology and geriatrics: Focus on assessment techniques* (vol. 14, pp. 234–256). New York: Springer.

Palmore, E. (1976). Total risk of institutionalization among the aged. *Gerontologist, 16,* 504–507

Pearlson, G. D., Kreger, L., Rabins, P. V., Chase, G. A., Cohen, B., Wirth, J. B., Sclaepfer, T. B., & Tune, L. E. (1989). A chart review study of late-onset and early-onset schizophrenia. *American Journal of Psychiatry, 146,* 1568–1574.

Perlmuter, L., & Monty, R. (Eds.) (1979). *Choice and perceived control.* Hillsdale, NJ: Erlbaum.

Pfeiffer, E. (1977). Psychopathology and social pathology. In J. E. Birren & K. W. Schaie (Eds.), *Handbook of the psychology of aging* (pp. 650–671). New York: Van Nostrand.

Post, F. (1987). Paranoid and schizophrenic disorders among the aging. In L. L. Carstensen & B. A. Edelstein (Eds.), *Handbook of clinical gerontology* (pp. 43–56). New York: Pergamon.

Reinardy, J. R. (1992). Decisional control in moving to a nursing home: Postadmission adjustment and well-being. *The Gerontologist, 32,* 96–103.

Rovner, B. W., German, P. S., Brant, L. J., Clark, R., Burton, L., & Folstein, M. F. (1991). Depression and mortality in nursing homes. *Journal of the American Medical Association, 265,* 993–996.

Rovner, B. W., & Rabins, P. V. (1985). Mental illness among nursing home patients. *Hospital Community Psychiatry, 36,* 119–120.

Rowles, G. D. (1979). The last new home. In S. M. Golant (Ed.), *Location and environment of elderly population.* Washington, DC: Winston

Rodin, J., & Langer, E. (1977). Long term effects of a control-relevant intervention with the institutional aged. *Journal of Personality and Social Psychology, 35,* 897–902.

Ruskin, P. (1990). Schizophrenia and delusional disorders. In D. Bienfeld (Ed.), *Verwoerdt's clinical geropsychiatry* (pp. 125–136). Baltimore: Williams & Wilkins.

Ryff, C. D. (1989). Beyond Ponc de Leon and life satisfaction: New directions in quest of successful aging. *International Journal of Behavioral Development, 12,* 35–55.

Sadavoy, J., & Fogel, B. (1992). Personality disorders in old age. In: J. E. Birren, R. B. Sloan, & G. D. Cohen (Eds.). *Handbook of mental health and aging* (2nd ed.) (pp. 433–462). New York: Academic Press.

Sbordone, R. J., & Sterman, L. T. (1983). The psychologist as a consultant in a nursing home: Effect on staff morale and turnover. *Professional Psychology: Research and Practice, 14,* 240–250.

Schaie, K. W., & Willis, S. L. (1996). *Adult development and aging* (4th ed). New York: HarperCollins.

Shmotkin, D., Eyal, N., & Lomranz, J. (1989). *Motivations and attitudes of clinical psychologist regarding treatment of the elderly.* Research report, The Sapir Foundation, Tel Aviv University, Israel.

Smyer, M. A. (1989). Nursing homes as a setting for psychological practice: Public policy perspectives. *American Psychologist, 44,* 1307–1314.

Smyer, M. A., & Garfein, A. (1988). Effective assessment approaches. In M. A. Smyer, M. Cohn, & D. Brannon (Eds.), *Mental health consultation in nursing homes* (pp. 64–81). New York: New York University Press.

Stephens, M. A., Crowther, J., Hobfoll, S., & Tennenbaum, D. (Eds.) (1990). *Stress and coping in later-life families.* New York: Hemisphere.

Storandt, M., Siegler, I., & Elias, M. (Eds.) (1978). *The clinical psychology of aging.* New York: Plenum.

Teri, L. (1991). Behavioral assessment and treatment of depression in older adults. In P. A. Wisocki (Ed.), *Handbook of clinical behavior therapy with the elderly client* (pp. 225–244). New York: Plenum.

Timko, C., & Moos, R. H. (1990). Determinants of interpersonal support and self-direction in group residential facilities. *Journal of Gerontology: Social Sciences, 45,* S184–S192.

Tobin, S. S. (1987). A structural approach to families. In T. H. Brubaker (Ed.), *Aging, health and the family: Long-term care* (pp. 42–55). Newbury Park, CA: Sage.

Tobin, S., & Lieberman, M. (1976). *Last home for the aged: Critical implications of institutionalization.* San Francisco: Jossey-Bass.

US Senate, Special Committee on Aging. (1987). *Developments in Aging, 1986* (Vols. 1–3). Washington, DC: US Government Printing Office.

Wantz, M. S., & Gay, J. E. (1981). *The aging process: A health perspective.* Cambridge, MA: Winthrop Publishers.

Winnicot, D. W. (1953). Transitional objects and transitional phenomena. *Collected papers: Through pediatrics to psychoanalysis, 1958,* (pp. 229–242). New York: Basic Books.

World Health Organization (1964). *Basic documents* (15th ed.). Geneva, Switzerland: Author.

Wright, L. K. (1988). A reconceptualization of the "negative staff attitudes and poor care in nursing homes" assumption. *The Gerontologist, 28,* 813–820.

Zivoni, M. (1993). Intergenerational relationships of the elderly and attitudes to residential facilities. *Gerontologia, 61,* 18–32.

7.22
Family Caregiving: Research Findings and Clinical Implications

STEVEN H. ZARIT, ADAM DAVEY, ANNE B. EDWARDS, ELIA E. FEMIA, and SHANNON E. JARROTT
Pennsylvania State University, University Park, PA, USA

7.22.1 INTRODUCTION

Family care of disabled older people has emerged as one of the most important clinical and social issues in an aging society. Historically the family has been the main source of help to the elderly, but in previous eras when most people did not survive to old age, families' involvement in providing care to parents or grandparents tended to be limited and brief. The demographic revolution of the late twentieth century has resulted in more people surviving to ages when rates of disability are high. As a result, increasing numbers of older people need at least some help to manage activities of daily living. The most frequent source of that help is the family. Providing care to a disabled elder poses considerable challenges to the family. Care needs may place physical strain on caregivers or may impinge on already full schedules of work and family responsibilities. The dependency of a spouse or parent can also intensify long-standing family problems, or overwhelm the psychological resources of caregivers. Formal social and health services can reduce the burden of care on families, but can also introduce new strains or problems. Clinicians can make timely and effective interventions to mobilize the family's resources, address family conflict, and maximize the ability of both the family and the disabled older person to meet the challenge of disability.

This chapter will present an overview of research on family caregiving and clinical interventions to relieve strain on the family. The chapter begins by introducing basic concepts to provide a foundation for examining research findings and clinical approaches. Three main areas of research on family caregiving are reviewed: how family relationships set the context for caregiving and in turn are affected by it, role conflict in caregiving, particularly, between employment and caregiving, and how the stresses of caregiving influence mental and physical health. The chapter concludes by examining clinical interventions and services designed to relieve stress on families and research on their effectiveness.

7.22.2 BASIC ISSUES IN FAMILY CAREGIVING

In this section the emergence of family caregiving as a major social issue is reviewed, and four issues are presented which guide understanding of this phenomenon: (i) caregiving as a career; (ii) stress proliferation and containment; (iii) the family context of caregiving; and (iv) the care recipient's perspective.

Caregiving has become an important concern because of the convergence of several social trends. The developed countries of the world are aging societies, that is, increasing proportions of their populations are 65 years of age and older. In fact, the fastest growing segment of the population is the "oldest old," people aged 80 years or over (Kinsella & Taeuber, 1993). Most older people live independently with few or no physical limitations, but the likelihood of disability increases with advancing age. By age 85 years, 60% of the population has at least some degree of disability which requires regular, ongoing assistance (Zarit, Johansson, & Berg, 1995). Among 85-year-olds with no disabilities, approximately 30% develop problems over the next two years, and another 30% do so in the following two years. Clearly, there is a growing risk of disability at very advanced ages.

How the aging of the population leads to increased risk of disability can be illustrated by the example of Alzheimer's disease. Although this disease can occur in people as young as 40 years of age, the greatest risk of incidence is after 75 (Johansson & Zarit, 1995; Jorm, Kortem, & Henderson, 1987; Kokman, Chandra, & Schoenberg, 1988). When most people in a society did not survive to 65, let alone 75 or 85, a disease such as Alzheimer's had a trivial impact. The dementia syndrome has been described since antiquity, but it has only assumed importance since the 1950s as large numbers of people have survived to the ages of greatest risk. For people surviving to their mid-80s, the cumulative risk of developing dementia due to any cause before death may be as high as 47% (Johansson & Zarit, 1995). The result is that many older people require considerable assistance for a period of time before their death.

Extension of the average life span has meant that people have, on average, a longer period of active life. They are able to live independently into their 70s, 80s, and even in some cases 90s. But the factors which have led to improved life expectancy, better medical care and improved public health, may also be contributing to a prolonging of the period of disability at the end of life. The Expansion of Morbidity Hypothesis (Cassel, Rudberg, & Olshansky, 1992) posits that people now survive longer with chronic diseases and with greater amounts of disability. While unequivocal data to support this hypothesis are not available, it is widely apparent that people with severe disabilities can survive for long periods of time. To cite one example, 50% of a sample of dementia patients (with varying diagnoses) were alive 11 years after the first onset of symptoms, and just under 40% survived more than 14 years (Aneshensel, Pearlin, Mullan, Zarit, & Whitlatch, 1995). This long duration of morbidity is an important factor in the heavy caregiver burden placed on families and society.

The net result of these trends is that more older people need help for longer periods of time than ever before. At the same time, families' resources for providing help have probably diminished somewhat. The most likely person to give assistance is a surviving husband or wife, but that person will also usually be elderly and may have disabilities which limit the amount or type of help that can be provided. Because of historic trends toward smaller family size, there are, on average, fewer children available to share the care of a disabled parent. Daughters and daughters-in-law have previously provided much of the assistance to elders, but with women's participation in the workforce, fewer full-time homemakers are available to take on caregiving responsibilities. Finally, historically high divorce rates in many Western countries weaken family ties and may diminish the amount of help available when a parent becomes disabled. Divorce in the parents' generation may have left strained or weakened ties with children, while divorce among children may result in their having fewer resources to commit to the care of an aging parent (Webster & Herzog, 1995).

These sociodemographic trends provide the context for caregiving. Four important concepts set the stage for discussion of research and clinical interventions: (i) caregiving as an ongoing, evolving process; (ii) stress proliferation and containment in caregiving; (iii) family systems theory; and (iv) the importance of addressing the needs of both caregiver and care recipient.

7.22.3 CAREGIVING AS AN ONGOING PROCESS: CAREERS OF CAREGIVERS

Caregiving involves an ongoing process, in which problems change and the caregiver's perceptions of problems also evolve. Just as the care recipient's disorder can span several years, caregiving also has a long duration. The tendency for studies to capture caregivers only at one point in time often obscures the temporal structure of what has come before and what lies ahead.

To describe this process, Pearlin (1993) has introduced the construct of caregiving careers, that is, that caregiving is a role involving certain predictable expectations and transitions. Using findings from a longitudinal study of caregivers of dementia patients (Aneshensel et al., 1995; Pearlin, 1993), Pearlin and his colleagues suggest three distinct phases in a caregiver's career. First is the period of role acquisition, during which caregivers recognize the growing disability in their relative and make the decision to take on the caregiving role. In progressive disorders such as dementia, this recognition develops gradually. Families frequently will ignore the growing signs of disability or hope that their relative will snap out of it and return to normal. A physician's diagnosis or a critical event, such as the patient getting lost or mishandling a sum of money, often changes how the family views the situation, although caregivers may still fluctuate in their acknowledgment of disability and their relative's need for assistance. The tendency in dementing illnesses for patients to deny their problems or disabilities, especially as the disease progresses (e.g., Kaszniak, 1996), undoubtedly contributes to families' ambivalence in recognizing the disorder and taking on care responsibilities.

The second phase in the caregiving career is role enactment, during which caregivers provide regular, ongoing assistance to their relative. Role enactment includes providing care to people in the home, and also in institutional settings. As we will see below, caregiving does not end at the institution's door. Families remain involved in care. While placement relieves some stresses, it introduces other problems and challenges for the family (Zarit & Whitlatch, 1992). The transition from home to institution may also be one of the most stressful times for families. Most of the available research addresses the period of role enactment, especially concerning caregivers providing care in the home.

The third phase in caregiving is disengagement, which is marked by the patient's death. Although psychological disengagement sometimes occurs sooner, death of the patient is a critical turning point that has complex effects on caregivers. Death of the patient is frequently welcomed when it brings release from a long, painful or deteriorated condition. Yet it also forces caregivers to re-examine and reorient their lives. Grief follows a predictable course, with symptoms greatest following the patient's death, and then gradually diminishing, although some caregivers remain distressed for a sustained period of time (Aneshensel et al., 1995).

Caregiving, then, should not be viewed as a static event that takes place for a limited duration of time. It is an ongoing process with some predictable demands and transitions. The pressures on the family depend to some extent on the phase of caregiving. Likewise, the type of clinical intervention will depend on whether caregivers are assuming the role, are in the midst of performing extensive caregiving activities, or are trying to reconstitute their lives following their relative's death. (For a description of varying clinical interventions over the full course of caregiving, see Zarit & Zarit, in press.)

7.22.4 CAREGIVING STRESS: PROCESSES OF PROLIFERATION AND CONTAINMENT

Caregiving has generally been viewed from the perspective of stress theory. Stressors represent all of the conditions, experiences, and activities that are problematic for people by thwarting their efforts, threatening their well-being, and disrupting otherwise stable systems (Aneshensel et al., 1995; Pearlin, Mullan, Semple, & Skaff, 1990). Chronic stress creates a state of perpetual arousal that taxes the individual's usual ability to adapt to the environment, and so compromises their ability to reach sought-after goals (Lazarus & Folkman, 1984).

A specific model is used to guide exploration of caregiving. The stress process model, developed by Pearlin and his colleagues (Aneshensel et al., 1995; Pearlin et al., 1990) has been used to guide a major longitudinal investigation of caregivers of dementia patients. This model identifies three major components in caregivers' experiences: primary stressors, secondary stressors and outcomes (see Figure 1). Primary stressors evolve directly from the needs of the patient and represent the actual tasks of caregiving. These stressors are called primary because they are intimately associated with the root of the stress, namely, the chronic disabilities of the care recipient (Pearlin et al., 1990). Examples of primary stressors are behavioral problems, memory problems, and difficulties carrying out activities of daily living (ADLs).

Coupled with the objective conditions of caregiving are the caregiver's subjective appraisals of the memory problems, behavioral disturbances, and ADL deficits. Some primary stressors are more problematic or challenging than others and so can affect coping skills and erode caregiver self-efficacy (Kinney & Stephens, 1989). Pearlin et al. (1990) specifically identify feelings of overload and role captivity, that is, a sense of being trapped in the caregiving role, as primary subjective stressors. They also propose that the caregiver's sense of loss of the relationship with the care recipient should be considered a primary stressor.

Evolving out of the primary stressors are the secondary stressors. Although termed secondary, these stressors are of no less importance. They represent the way in which primary stressors encroach upon and disrupt other areas of the caregiver's life, and thus are more variable and individual in their manifestation. Secondary stressors include family conflict, financial strain (e.g., reduced financial resources as a result of caregiving) and work conflict. They also involve psychological dimensions, such as diminished self-esteem and a feeling of loss of self, that the caregiver's identity has been absorbed totally in the caregiving role (Skaff & Pearlin, 1992).

Long-term exposure to stressors can produce a variety of physiological and psychological changes, or what are termed outcomes in the

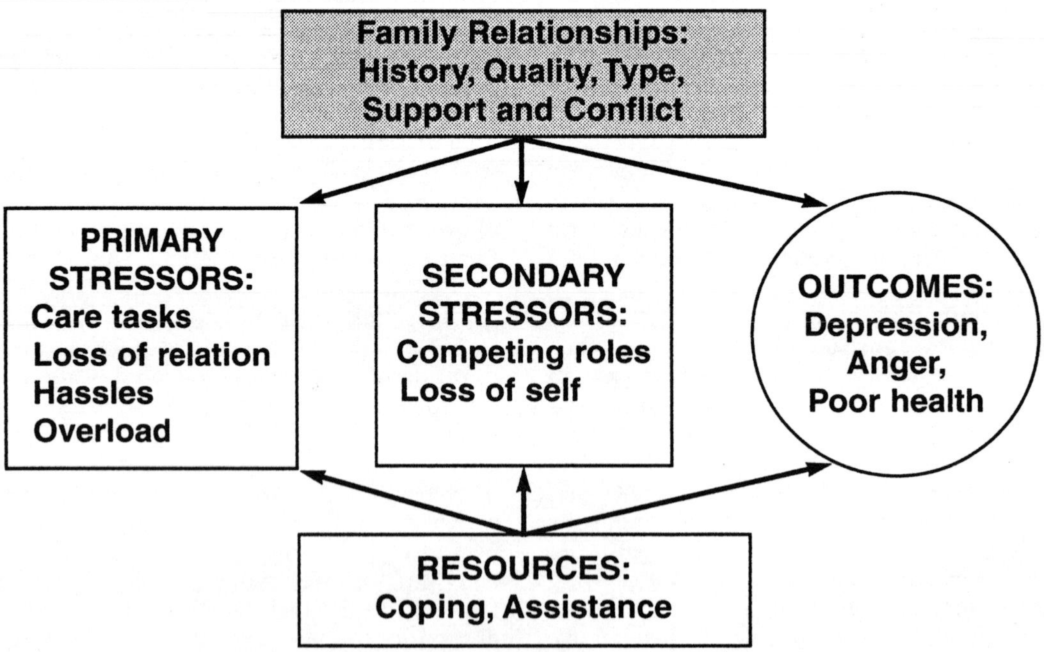

Figure 1 A model of caregiving stress and family relationships.

stress process model. Among the outcomes that have been studied are depression, anger, well-being and a variety of indicators of health. These outcomes occur as chronic stress which results in disruptions of people's homeostatic mechanisms that overwhelm their coping resources.

Stressors, however, do not have a fixed or constant effect on outcomes. The caregiving literature has documented considerable variability in how caregivers adapt to similar circumstances (e.g., Aneshensel et al., 1995; Haley, Levine, Brown, & Bartolucci, 1987; Wright, Clipp, & George, 1993; Zarit, Todd, & Zarit, 1986). The relation of stressors and outcomes is described in the stress process model in terms of two mechanisms: stress proliferation and stress containment (Aneshensel et al., 1995). Stress proliferation describes how the stressors involved in caregiving infiltrate and disrupt other areas of the caregiver's life. Primary stressors lead in varying degrees to secondary stressors, which in combination lead to negative outcomes. Stress proliferation is greatest when caregivers are assisting someone with higher levels of behavior problems and when there is a greater subjective effect of these stressors, for example, when caregivers feel overwhelmed or trapped in their role (Aneshensel et al., 1995; Haley et al., 1987; Zarit et al., 1986). Stress containment, in turn, describes how the caregiver's use of resources may limit or circumscribe the effects of stressors. How caregivers cope with specific problems as well as the amount of social and financial resources available to them can protect them from some of the adverse effects of stress.

The outcome of a particular configuration of caregiving stressors is variable. The amount of variance in caregiver outcomes, such as depression, that is accounted for by any particular stressor, for example, the patient's behavior problems or the amount of family conflict, is statistically significant but relatively modest (Aneshensel et al., 1995). Instead, outcomes depend on the extent of proliferation or containment.

The implications of this framework for clinical intervention are twofold. First, clinicians need to assess which primary and secondary stressors are present in a given situation. Caregiving and caregivers' resources are sufficiently varied so that the constellation of problems and stressors will differ considerably from one family to another. Rather than assuming that a constellation of stressors will be overwhelming or that a caregiver will necessarily experience work or family conflict, clinicians need to conduct an assessment to identify the specific proliferation of stress in the caregiver's life. Second, the goal of clinical interventions is to reduce sources of stress proliferation and enhance the caregiver's resources that lead to containment. Although it may not be possible to change the patient's underlying disability or to alter the primary stressors on caregivers, interventions can modify their impact on the caregiver's life (Whitlatch, Zarit, & von Eye, 1991). In the sections below, research is highlighted which suggests which factors are associated with greater or less stress for family caregivers and which may be amenable to clinical intervention.

7.22.5 CAREGIVING IN A FAMILY CONTEXT

Stress theory is useful for characterizing the problems and challenges faced by caregivers, but it does not take into account the specific family context in which caregiving occurs. The relationship between caregiver and care recipient and their relationships with other family members should be considered. A family systems perspective focuses on what roles and functions a person performed within the family as well as the quality of these relationships (Zarit, Orr, & Zarit, 1985). Because of illness and disability, the care recipient can no longer perform certain activities and functions for the family. A spouse caregiver, for example, may experience the loss of a confidant and sexual partner, and may have to take over activities that his/her spouse previously performed in the household. Besides these specific losses, care recipients and caregivers have varying amounts of prestige and influence in the family, which affects how much help and assistance other people will provide. Children who view a caregiving mother as extremely competent may not view her as needing help. Conversely, a mother who is viewed as needy or lacking competency may get too much help or a mixture of criticism and assistance. Caregiving can also reawaken or intensify long-standing conflicts in the family.

7.22.6 THE PERSPECTIVE OF THE CARE RECIPIENT

Lost in much of the caregiving literature is the perspective of the person receiving care. In part, this omission is due to the extensive focus on providing care to people with dementia, who lose the ability to report their experiences reliably as the disease progresses. This exclusion, however, means that the care recipient's perspective often is overlooked. Care recipients can continue to provide some types of help, assistance, or comfort to the caregiver, even in cases of moderate to severe dementia. The care recipient's well-being and needs should be considered along with the caregiver's, in decisions about living arrangements and care. It is important to consider whose interests are being represented when making a clinical intervention. What is good for the family may, in some circumstances, not be in the patient's best interest. The clearest example is nursing home placement, which relieves strain on families but puts the dementia patient at risk for a variety of adverse outcomes, including an increased risk of mortality (Aneshensel et al., 1995). Though often omitted from research, the patient's perspective needs to be incorporated consistently into clinical intervention.

7.22.7 RESEARCH ON FAMILY CAREGIVING

The following review of the research literature focuses on the stress process and family relationships. It starts by emphasizing caregiving in its family context, and the relationships of caregiver and care recipient to one another and to other family members. One of the main secondary stressors, is then considered, that is, when there is strain or conflict between caregiving and employment. Finally, consideration is given to what is known about the effects of caregiving on physical and mental health and some of the correlates of negative outcomes.

7.22.8 CAREGIVING AND FAMILY RELATIONSHIPS

In this section, attention is focused on caregivers and their family relationships. Two primary themes underlie the organization of this section. First, family caregiving arises within a long-standing, often life-long, relationship. As a result, the caregiving relationship can be seen as an extension of the prior relationship history and its associated pattern of interactions. Second, informal caregiving is best understood when considered as a system, rather than as the characteristics of a single individual or a single relationship. As suggested by the stress-process model outlined above, events within the caregiver–care recipient relationship can have consequences, both positive and negative, for other familial relationships and caregiver well-being.

Despite the vast literature on family caregiving, surprisingly little is known about its effects on family relationships. In this section, the effects of caregiving on the relationship between caregiver and care recipient are considered, as well as the effects of caregiving on relationships outside the primary caregiving dyad, particularly between the caregiver and his or her spouse and siblings. Most is known about caregivers who are the spouses or children of the care recipient. Siblings sometimes take care of a brother or sister, and other relatives and even nonkin may take on the caregiving role (e.g., Cicirelli, 1985, 1992), but little is known about how caregiving affects these relationships.

7.22.9 NORMATIVE FAMILY RELATIONSHIPS IN LATER LIFE

Recognition of the importance of family relationships in later life has spawned a large body of research examining normative patterns of intergenerational exchanges. Overwhelmingly, this literature has demonstrated that older adults typically remain both active donors and recipients of support until very late in life. In this intergenerational context, older adults generally give more to their adult offspring than they, in turn, receive (Eggebeen & Wilhelm, 1995; Zarit & Eggebeen, 1995).

Reciprocity and the balance of exchanges have received particular attention because of their potential influence on psychological well-being (e.g., Ingersoll-Dayton & Antonucci, 1988). Using a large, nationally representative Canadian sample, Hirdes and Strain (1995) found a curvilinear relationship between age and the balance of instrumental exchanges between generations with the greatest balance occurring at midlife. Morgan, Schuster, and Butler (1991) examined the balance of exchange between older parents and their adult offspring as a function of parents' age. They found that parental giving and receiving declined with increasing parent age, but that older adults typically continued to give more than they received beyond age 85. Unlike Hirdes and Strain (1995), who focused only on instrumental exchanges, Morgan et al. (1991) also considered emotional support, which partially accounts for these observed differences.

Related to intergenerational exchanges are norms of filial responsibility. Hamon and Blieszner (1990) report that older parents and their children strongly endorse expectations of filial responsibility in times of need. There is ample evidence that these norms are robust across a wide variety of cultures and family structures (e.g., Brody, Johnsen, & Fulcomer, 1984; Chow, 1983; Fadel-Girgis, 1983; Hanson, Sauer, & Seelbach, 1983; Kendig & Rowland, 1983; Kivett & Atkinson, 1984; Maeda, 1983; Weihl, 1983; Worach-Kardas, 1983).

It appears that these cultural norms are readily translated into action, with relationships with adult children assuming greater importance for older adults in later life. Field and Minkler (1988) report that frequency of contact with adult children remains high from early to late old age. Whereas interactions with friends and their perceived importance decreases, satisfaction with relationships with children increases across the same period.

7.22.9.1 Family Structure and Caregiving

Caregiving grows out of these normative patterns of intergenerational exchange and interaction. Strong social norms govern who is most likely to become a caregiver. By any estimation, gender is the single strongest predictor of who will become a caregiver, with women comprising approximately 70% of all caregivers (Aneshensel et al., 1995; Stone, Cafferata, & Sangl, 1987). Most research has suggested that caregivers assume their role hierarchically within the family structure. Married individuals will turn first to a spouse for assistance in times of need. In the absence of a spouse, adult children are the next choice, followed by siblings, more distant relatives, and finally neighbors and friends (e.g., Penning, 1990). Wives, daughters, and daughters-in-law are the most common female caregivers, and husbands the most common male caregivers, followed distantly by sons (Aneshensel et al., 1995; Stone et al., 1987), who are only likely to assume the caregiving role in the absence of a female sibling (Horowitz, 1985).

In most caregiving situations, one person takes over the primary responsibility, providing the most help or spending the most time with the care recipient. Other family members may also provide considerable assistance. Although sons do not frequently assume the role of primary caregiver, they often give considerable help to their sisters. Similarly, a parent caring for his or her spouse will typically receive help from children. The relationships between primary and secondary caregivers are an important source of support, but can also be a focal point for conflict and disagreement (Semple, 1992).

In studies of how siblings take responsibility for care tasks, Matthews (1987; Matthews & Rosner, 1988) found that family structure (birth order, number of siblings, gender composition), history of parent-child affectional ties, and extrafamilial roles (employment status, marital status, and geographic proximity) all influence which sibling provides parent care (see also Brody, 1990). In families with two or more adult daughters, shared care was the norm, whereas sons consistently appeared to play less central roles.

According to Matthews (1995), both adult daughters and sons draw upon cultural norms for gender-appropriate behavior in shaping their caregiving behavior. Adult daughters are viewed as being primarily responsible for caregiving activities regardless of the actual division of labor, and their brothers' contributions to caregiving are seen as peripheral and unimportant.

Another important distinction in the caregiving situation is whether or not the caregiver and care recipient share the same household (Chappell, 1990; Tennstedt, Crawford, & McKinley, 1993; Townsend, Noelker, Deimling, & Bass, 1989). Spouse caregivers usually live in the same household, but children may or may not live with a parent. An important source of cross-cultural differences is the extent to which aged parents and their adult children share a household (Sundström, 1992; Davey et al., 1996). In some countries such as the USA, rates of shared households have been relatively high, with children frequently taking in a disabled parent. In other countries, such as Sweden, two-generation households have been quite rare.

The implications of shared or separate households are considerable. A shared household probably places more continuous strain on family members and has been found to result in higher levels of stress (Townsend et al., 1989). In contrast, some different problems confront families who provide care to a parent in a different household, including needing to coordinate help that may be brought into the home, and worrying about the safety of the elder when no one is around. A special situation is trying to provide care at a long distance, which can be a source of considerable anxiety to children.

Marital status of parents and their children have emerged as important predictors of caregiving and intergenerational exchange. Specifically, parental divorce has been shown to affect the quality of relationships and frequency of contact between fathers and their adult children and the frequency of contact with mothers (Webster & Herzog, 1995). In general, the effects of divorce were much greater for fathers than for mothers (Cooney & Uhlenberg, 1990; White, 1992).

Disruption in adult children's marital status has also been found to relate to lower levels of help given to elderly parents, perceptions that parents need less assistance, and a lower sense of filial obligation to provide assistance (Cicirelli, 1983). A study by Brody and her colleagues (Brody, Litvin, Albert, & Hoffman, 1994) elaborates upon these findings, suggesting that daughters' marital status can have considerable effects on the amount of care they provide to an older parent. In particular, never-married and widowed daughters were found to provide the greatest proportion of care needed by a frail older parent by themselves. Never-married daughters, in particular, were most likely to be sole caregivers for their elderly parents. Conversely, married daughters were more likely to receive assistance with care tasks from informal sources, and divorced daughters were more likely to report using formal services.

7.22.9.2 Caregiver–Care Recipient Relationships

The relationship between caregiver and care recipient is an important and often overlooked aspect of these situations. Probably the most important distinction is between cognitively-intact people who can maintain some continuity in their relationships with caregivers, and those suffering from dementia.

Providing care to an elderly relative with dementia presents stressors which differ in fundamentally important ways from situations in which cognition is spared, or recovery is possible. When comparing caregivers of people with dementia but no physical limitations to caregivers of people with functional disabilities but no cognitive deficits, Birkel (1987) found that the former experienced much higher levels of care-related stress. In a comparison of caregivers of relatives with dementia and of relatives with cancer, Clipp and George (1993) found that dementia caregivers reported poorer self-rated health, greater substance use, poorer emotional health, reduced social functioning, and poorer financial status, even when the effects of employment status, age, and duration of illness were controlled.

Wright (1993) compared a small, nonrepresentative sample of Alzheimer's disease (AD) caregiving couples with well couples across a variety of dimensions. The study is unique in that she considered the perspective of both members having each report on specific aspects of their marriage. AD caregivers reported decreased companionship and difficulty dealing with changes in sexual intimacy. Wright also found that ratings of past marital happiness were associated with current valuing of the afflicted spouse as a unique individual, but not with future commitment, which was lower among caregiving spouses.

Majerovitz (1995) found a relationship between family adaptability and outcomes for caregivers of dementia patients. Caregivers who reported high adaptability in their families had lower depression, even when there were high levels of care-related stressors. She also reported that low-adaptability spouses were more likely to cling to an unrealistic role for their cognitively-impaired spouse, expecting their partner to continue to meet former expectations. While these data are cross-sectional, they suggest that caregivers with more realistic expectations of their demented spouse are likely to experience fewer negative consequences as a result of the care they provide.

In spousal relationships, relationship quality between the caregiver and care recipient may also play a role in the decision to institutionalize. Pruchno, Michaels, and Potashnik (1990b) found that spouses reporting a better quality of relationship with the care recipient reported less desire to institutionalize, but this finding did not extend to actual decisions regarding institutionalization. By the same token, however, desire to institutionalize was a strong predictor of actual institutionalization, suggesting that an indirect link may exist.

These findings offer support to the idea that there is something uniquely debilitating about losing a spouse to dementia as compared to another terminal illness in which cognitive functioning is typically spared. Because dementing illness results in deterioration in cognition and behavior, patients lose the ability to participate in the family or to have a say about the course of their own care. Caregiving becomes completely one-sided, with the patient unable to reciprocate in any way and, often, unable even to acknowledge the help that is provided. The progressive course of these disorders means that families face a somewhat predictable pattern of deterioration. Care of patients who are cognitively intact is not without its stresses; rather, care demands do not have the unrelenting pattern found in dementia and care recipients can acknowledge and show appreciation for the assistance they receive. Families caring for someone with another type of major psychiatric disorder may experience similar levels of distress as caregivers of dementia patients (Pearson, Verma, & Nellett, 1988). It may be that disorders which involve behavioral and emotional disturbances, and which are more disruptive of the usual family relationships, have the greatest impact on caregivers. The past relationship between children and their parents has considerable influence on caregiving experiences. Feelings of attachment and obligation have both been found to predict the amount of help daughters provided to their older parents (Cicirelli, 1993). Those who reported stronger feelings of attachment experienced lower levels of burden, whereas those who reported higher levels of obligation experienced higher levels of burden. Thus, children providing care out of a sense of obligation rather than affection may experience greater negative consequences as a result.

There are other important implications of the quality of prior relationships for the caregiving experience. Caregivers with a poor relationship with the care recipient are less likely to assume the caregiving role and, if they do, to experience more stress within it (Whitlatch & Noelker, in press). In an intriguing study by Uchino, Kiecolt-Glaser, and Cacioppo (1994), higher ratings of pre-illness affection for the care recipient were associated with lower heart rate reactivity, a physiological indicator of stress, measured two years later.

Walker, Martin, and Jones (1992) examined the role of intimacy in predicting adult daughters' and mothers' perceived costs and benefits of caregiving. Adult daughters' feelings of intimacy were associated with fewer feelings of having insufficient time for extra-caregiving activities, less frustration with caregiving, and less anxiety about providing care. For mothers receiving care, intimacy was related to less anger and resentment about the care they received. Other research has found conflict in the caregiver–care recipient relationship to be associated with greater caregiver strain and negative affect (Sheehan & Nuttall, 1988).

Townsend and Franks (1995) found that adult childrens' perceptions of relationship quality with their parent was an important mediator between the parent's cognitive impairment and the adult child's well-being. In their study of 90 adult–child caregivers, perceived closeness was associated with lower levels of reported caregiver burden and a greater sense of caregiving efficacy. Their study also underscores the importance of conflict in the relationship, which was associated with higher levels of stress, efficacy, and depression.

While most research has examined quality of the relationship, Aneshensel and her colleagues (1995) looked at the extent to which caregivers reported the loss of their relationship with a relative suffering from dementia. As their relative's disease progressed, caregivers reported a greater loss of the relationship. This sense of loss continued to play a role even after the patient's death. Caregivers who had previously reported a greater loss recovered more quickly than those who still held onto the relationship.

One extreme outcome of a poor relationship between caregiver and care recipient is violence directed toward the elderly care recipient. In a study of 236 caregivers to a relative with dementia, Pillemer and Suitor (1992) examined predictors of violence and violent feelings toward the care recipient. With regard to care recipient characteristics, they found that both violent behaviors and disruptive behaviors were associated with caregivers' greater fear of becoming violent with their relative. Violent behaviors by the care recipient were also associated with a greater likelihood of actual violence on the part of the caregiver. Caregivers who lived with their relative were more likely to report being afraid of acting violently toward their relative, and spouse caregivers were more likely to have acted violently toward their relative than adult children.

Thus, there is evidence to suggest that aspects of the past and present relationship quality between caregivers and care recipients play an important role in the caregiving experience, and that these characteristics have an effect, for both spouses and adult children, on the burden experienced as a result of caring.

7.22.9.3 Social Support from Family and Other Informal Sources

One of the most important sources of help to caregivers is the assistance and emotional support provided by other family members. Although actual estimates vary widely, there is general consensus that a majority of caregivers have support in their role from a secondary caregiver (e.g., Aneshensel et al., 1995; Stone et al., 1987; Tennstedt, McKinlay, & Sullivan, 1989). Social relationships can also involve conflict, and it has been suggested that negative social interactions can have greater impact on satisfaction with social support than measures of support received from others (e.g., Krause, 1995). In many instances, the same relationship can be a source of support and conflict.

Clipp and George (1990a) report considerable stability in the social support caregivers receive over a one-year period. They also report a lack of relationship between objective needs (dementia symptoms, duration of caregiving) and social support received. In other words, some families provide support whether the need for help is great or small, while other families do not help much at all, whatever the circumstances.

Thompson and colleagues (Thompson, Futterman, Gallagher-Thompson, & Lovett, 1993) examined potential differential effects of various types of social support in predicting measures of caregiver burden. Reduced social participation with friends and family was the most consistent social support predictor of the burden indicators they considered (see also, Haley et al., 1995). Specifically, higher levels of social participation were associated with lower levels of burden, having a less restricted social life, and a less negative relationship with the care recipient. That social support may also come with associated costs to caregivers was also indicated by their research. Caregivers who received material aid or financial assistance tended to report more negative interactions with family and friends.

Using longitudinal data, Aneshensel and her colleagues (1995) expanded on this theme that different types of support are related to different outcomes. Using the stress process model described earlier, they found that instrumental support from informal helpers (family and friends) can contain the experience of overload that results from primary stressors, whereas emotional support is not effective to this end. Similarly, instrumental support reduces proliferation of stress into other important roles held by the caregiver, such as work. Emotional support appears to be most effective in containing the effects of stress on outcomes such as depression.

For caregivers who are married, their relationship with a husband or wife can be both a source of support or a point of increased strain, as they experience conflicting demands on their time and energy. In an intriguing study, Creasey and his colleagues (Creasey, Meyers, Epperson, & Taylor, 1990) investigated how caring for a parent or parent-in-law with AD affected the relationship between husband and wife with each other and with their parents and children. Women caring for a parent (or parent-in-law) experienced a loss of support both from their husband and parent. Support from their own children, however, was not affected by caregiving, nor did their involvement lead to increases in negative interactions with their spouse or parent. Their husbands reported less support from parents, but not from wives or children.

Suitor and Pillemer (1992; see also Franks & Stephens, 1996) found, not surprisingly, that when husbands provided emotional support to caregiving wives, marital satisfaction was higher. Conversely, marital satisfaction was lower when husbands hindered their wives' caregiving in some way.

Caregiving grows out of a relationship with a long history and previously well-established expectations for interactions. There is evidence that this history has a substantial influence on the caregiving experience. As the nature of the caregiver–care recipient relationship changes, positive and negative interactions in other important family relationships can also be found. How much the support from others helps caregivers depends on how and what type of support are given, in a complex, but comprehensible fashion. Support from family and friends is a readily available resource for caregivers, which is not limited to the working hours of formal service agencies, nor bound by bureaucratic rules. Finding ways to increase support to caregivers while reducing conflict is an important goal for clinical intervention, as we shall discuss later.

7.22.10 SECONDARY STRESSORS: COMPETING ROLES AND STRESS PROLIFERATION

Caregivers have dimensions in their lives outside the demands of caregiving. These other roles can create additional stress on the caregiver, or they can help to alleviate the stress of caregiving, depending on the nature and quality of these outside roles. In the model guiding this chapter, these outside influences fall under the term secondary stressors.

Secondary stressors contain both role strains and intrapsychic strains. Role strains may arise from family, work or informal responsibilities outside of the caregiving situation, but are generated or aggravated by the demands of caregiving (Aneshensel, Pearlin, & Schuler, 1993). These stressors include family conflict, work-caregiving conflict, and economic strain. Intrapsychic strains involve dimensions of self-concept and psychological states.

There are two main hypotheses regarding the effect of different roles on the well-being of a person. The scarcity hypothesis proposes that additional roles create strain. Goode (1960) introduced the concept of role strain, or the difficulty in meeting expected role demands. In this view, role strain is seen as normal and even inevitable; therefore, the task for everyone is to discover ways to reduce this strain. This corresponds to the competing commitment perspective within the caregiving literature. This concept focuses on the time dimension of the conflicts among multiple roles, and assumes that the other roles of caregivers create further demands on the caregivers' time (Stoller & Pugliesi, 1989).

In contrast to the scarcity hypothesis, Sieber (1974) introduced the expansion hypothesis, that there are positive effects of accumulating additional roles. Even though the obligations of a role may be taxing, the rights gained within that role may negate any detrimental outcomes that might occur because of the acquisition of the role. One way in which multiple roles might compensate for role strain is by allowing people to fall back on successes in one role if they fail within another. A number of studies have found that occupying multiple roles is associated with better overall well-being (Thoits, 1983; Verbrugge, 1983).

One important focus of multiple roles is on daughters who balance caregiving with being a wife and mother. Studies by Stephens and her colleagues (Stephens, Franks, & Townsend, 1994; Stephens & Franks, 1995) have identified both positive and negative consequences of these multiple roles. An important feature of these studies is that they examine how each role has stresses and rewards, which affect how one role might affect the other. Both stress and rewards in the role of mother were associated, respectively, with positive and negative affect reported by caregivers. Stress and rewards in the role of wife were also associated with ratings of physical health.

Quality of the marital relationship can also have important consequences for the effects of caregiving on adult daughters, and vice versa. Stephens and Franks (1995) examined positive and negative perceptions that one role (either caregiving or spousal) had affected the other ("spillover"). Whereas positive spillover from the role of wife to caregiver was only related to higher levels of marital satisfaction, positive spillover from the caregiver to wife role was associated with lower levels of depression and greater positive affect. Conversely, negative spillover from wife to caregiver roles was associated with less positive affect and lower marital satisfaction; negative spillover from caregiver to wife roles was associated with significantly greater depression.

The main area in which these competing hypotheses about multiple roles have been explored is work and caregiving. Work has a central role in many people's lives and the difficulties that balancing work and caregiving responsibilities pose make it a particularly challenging issue. The rapid increase in the number of working women in first-world nations has made work and caregiving conflict an important social issue, as well as a consideration in clinical situations. An unusual longitudinal study of work and caregiving documents the increased rate at which women are combining both roles. This study examined a group of women who were originally interviewed in 1956 and then interviewed again 30 years later about caregiving histories (Moen, Robison, & Fields, 1994). Over 60% of the women in the study were caregivers to relatives with disabilities at some time in their lives. In this study, women were as likely to combine working and caregiving as they were to be only caregivers. Women seem to be adding to their roles rather than giving up a role when a new role must be acquired.

Working and caring for an elderly relative produces some special challenges and issues. When studying mothers and their daughter caregivers, Brody and Schoonover (1986) found that mothers received the same amount of help whether their daughters worked or not. But when employed women were compared with their nonemployed sisters, significant differences were found in the amount of help given when their parents' functional status was poor, with working women providing less assistance (Matthews, Werkner, & Delaney, 1989). Working women, then, are often providing extensive help in the caregiving role, but there are limits to their ability to help, which become evident in situations involving more extensive disabilities.

The question of whether an employed woman should make adjustments to her employment situation or quit her job is one that many caregivers face. A sizable number of caregivers leave their jobs within three months of becoming a caregiver (Franklin, Ames, & King, 1994). Leaving a job or reducing work hours is the most dramatic change that a caregiver can make in order to deal with the competing demands of work and caregiving. Workers generally try to rearrange their schedules or reduce their hours before leaving the job (Mutschler, 1994). There are many different factors that contribute to the decision or need to leave a job because of caregiving responsibilities. Caregivers who leave their jobs or reduce their work hours tend to have relatives who have more severe disabilities (Brody, Kleban, Johnsen, Hoffman, & Schoonover, 1987) and have faced work constraints for a longer period of time (Mutschler, 1994).

Reports of strain are common among working caregivers (Mutschler, 1994; Scharlach & Boyd, 1989). But there is the question of what contributes to that strain. The four main predictors of conflict between work and caregiving are: (i) the elderly family member's emotional health; (ii) the number of caregiving tasks performed by the caregiver; (iii) the presence of children in the caregiver's residence; and (iv) having caregiving responsibilities when beginning at the current job (Gibeau & Anastas, 1989). In addition, sociodemographic variables such as the employee's gender, marital status, household income, job status, occupation, and flexibility of work schedule are related to employees' levels of absenteeism and stress (Neal, Chapman, Ingersoll-Dayton, Emlen, & Boise, 1990). Other studies have found that the severity of disability of the elderly relative and the intensity of the caregiving responsibilities are related to work and caregiving conflict (Gibeau & Anastas, 1989).

Beyond the simple distinction between working and nonworking caregivers, the type of occupation has an effect on strain or burden. Mutschler (1994), for example, reports that production workers have less opportunity to adjust their work and care demands than workers in executive, sales, or clerical positions.

The relationship between experiences in the employment role and caregiving stress may be more complicated than originally thought. As was the case when balancing roles of caregiver, mother, and wife, the dual commitments of work and caregiving involve rewards as well as stress. High satisfaction with work seems to be associated with fewer depressive symptoms, except for those caregivers who experience high levels of caregiving stress (Martire, Stephens, & Atienza, 1997). The number of hours that a caregiver worked is associated with negative outcomes under conditions of high caregiver stress. Martire, et al. (1997) also found that women working part-time experienced poorer physical health and less positive affect than those women who were working full-time. One reason for this may be the increased amount of time that full-time workers are away from the impaired relative (Brody, 1990; Scharlach, 1994). Another reason may be that full-time work provides greater knowledge, benefits, and support (Matthews et al., 1989).

Workers tend to be interested in work benefits that are designed to make work and caregiving easier. The ideas for benefits that generated the most interest were respite care, flexible work hours, reduced hours without reduced benefits, adult day care, and job sharing. Caregivers using formal services understood that the availability of those services was critical if they were to maintain their employment and meet their family member's need for care (Gibeau & Anastas, 1989).

In summary, the findings from research on competing roles indicate that the additional roles that a caregiver occupies can result in both stress proliferation and containment. In order to get a complete understanding of the challenges that the caregiver faces, it is necessary to understand the quality of the roles and the rewards as well as stresses that the various responsibilities bring. Advising a caregiver, for example, to reduce her work responsibilities before having a clear picture of the entire caregiving situation would be ill advised. Rather, the challenge in clinical situations can be to find ways to balance competing roles more effectively and to minimize the spillover of stress from one activity to another.

7.22.11 OUTCOMES OF CAREGIVING: HEALTH AND MENTAL HEALTH EFFECTS

Caregiving is a uniquely stressful event. Being a long-term caregiver has been found to be associated with a variety of negative outcomes. The consensus among studies examining physical and mental health outcomes is that a majority of caregivers report feeling physically and emotionally distressed (Anthony-Bergstone, Zarit, & Gatz, 1988; Brodaty & Hadzi-Pavlovic, 1990; Clipp & George, 1990b; George & Gwyther, 1986; Haley, Levine, Brown, Berry, & Hughes, 1987; Kinney & Stephens, 1989). Several studies report higher levels of psychological morbidity among caregivers compared to noncaregiving samples of the population. Anthony-Bergstone and her colleagues (1988) noted the increased feelings of hostility, anger, and anxiety among caregivers as compared to the general population. An Australian study showed that mean scores on the General Health Questionnaire (GHQ), a measure of psychological morbidity, were higher in the caregiving sample and among caregiving spouses than the general population or other subsamples of caregivers (Brodaty & Hadzi-Pavolovic, 1990). Women caregivers generally report higher levels of psychological distress than men (Anthony-Bergstone et al., 1988; Zarit & Whitlatch, 1992).

Schulz, Visintainer, and Williamson (1990) reviewed several studies showing the psychiatric morbidity effects of caregiving. In studies using self-report measures such as the Beck Depression Inventory (BDI) or the Center for Epidemiological Studies Depression Scale (CES-D), three general conclusions emerged. First, greater severity of the care recipient's problems is linked to more depressive symptomatology. Second, women have higher rates of depression than men. Third, the more representative the caregiving population, the lower the rate of depression. Thus, caregivers drawn from specific subsamples such as daughters taking care of severely demented relatives or those seeking help from a service program show higher rates of depression symptoms.

A second group of studies has used clinical assessment tools (e.g., the Schedule for Affective Disorders and Schizophrenia Interview) which yield rates of clinical diagnoses of depression and other problems. These studies have found that caregivers frequently meet diagnostic criteria for depression or other diagnoses (e.g., Cohen & Eisdorfer, 1988; Drinka, Smith, & Drinka, 1987; Goldman & Luchins, 1984). In one of the most comprehensive studies of this kind, Gallagher and colleagues (Gallagher, Rose, Rivera, Lovett, & Thompson, 1989) found prevalence rates for depression ranging from 31% for men to 46% for women. These studies provide strong evidence that caregivers are at risk of increased psychiatric symptoms and clinical disorders.

The model of the stress process described earlier in the chapter illustrates how primary and secondary stressors can have a cumulative effect on caregiver mental well-being and physical health. Among the primary stressors, behavior problems are most likely to lead to adverse outcomes for family caregivers. The common behavior problems identified by caregivers as difficult or stressful for them are incontinence of the bowel and/or bladder, crying easily, hiding things, acting restlessly or agitated, and becoming irritable, angry, or accusatory (Haley & Pardo, 1989). These behavioral problems require vigilance, surveillance, and control on the part of the caregiver. Pruchno and Resch (1989) found that asocial and disoriented behaviors on the part of the care recipient are associated with greater burden, decreased social participation, and less satisfaction with caregiving. For forgetful behaviors, the consequences for caregiver's mental health increase at first, and then diminish as the severity of behavior problems increases, suggesting a curvilinear relationship between the two.

In a study of depression in dementia caregivers, Redinbaugh, MacCallum, and Kiecolt-Glaser (1995) found that caregivers who experienced chronic depression over a three-year period reported their relative's behavior as more problematic, and had higher levels of upsetting social support than non-depressed caregivers or caregivers who had experienced a transient depressive episode during the course of the study.

Vitaliano and colleagues (Vitaliano, Young, Russo, Romano, & Magana-Amato, 1993) were interested in examining the possibility that caregiver behaviors, specifically in the form of expressed emotion, were predictive of subsequent care recipient behaviors one and a half years later. Controlling for initial levels of problem behaviors, dementia patients who were cared for by an individual with high levels of expressed emotion displayed significantly more negative behaviors at follow-up. These findings are significant because caregiver expressed emotion is correlated with higher levels of depression, suppressed anger, and lower life satisfaction (Bledin, MacCarthy, Kiupers, & Woods, 1990; Vitaliano et al., 1993).

Burden, guilt, inadequacy, and negative perceptions of patient mood and functioning are words that describe the motivation to engage in caregiving activity (Hadjistavropoulos, Taylor, Tuokko, & Beattie, 1994). Lack of time, lack of help, and difficulty in managing patient behavior describe the caregiver's ability to engage in the caregiving process. These stressors have a cumulative impact on caregiver well-being.

Two broad domains have been investigated for the extent to which they buffer or contain the stressors of caregiving: social support and coping. The role of social support was reviewed earlier. Coping resources potentially represent an important way of containing stress. Research in this area has identified some promising leads on what type of coping strategies are more effective, but limitations in current research make it difficult to draw firm conclusions.

Pruchno and Kleban (1993) studied the relative effectiveness of emotion-focused vs. problem-focused coping strategies in mediating stress experienced by caregivers to an institutionalized relative. Their findings suggest that, contrary to coping research in other caregiving contexts (e.g., Stephens, Norris, Kinney, Ritchie, & Grots, 1988), emotion-focused coping was associated with better mental health than problem-focused coping. These findings highlight the importance of recognizing caregiving as a chronic stressor which is less amenable to change than many other situations. As a result, caregivers may be more successful if they focus on dealing with their responses to the situation than if they take a more traditional, instrumental approach.

Williamson and Schulz (1993) examined the relationship between a number of coping strategies and the burden experienced across three domains of the caregiving relationship: dealing with memory deficits, loss of communication, and the decline of a loved one. Their results suggest that different strategies are more and less successful, depending on the specific domain. Use of wishfulness as a coping strategy was related consistently to the experience of greater burden for all three stressors considered. Similarly, use of direct action strategies in response to memory deficits was associated with greater depression. Strategies which are more successful for caregivers included using relaxation as a way of coping with memory problems and seeking support to deal with loss of the relationship with the care recipient. Finally, acceptance of the situation was associated with lower depression related to loss of a loved one and loss of communication.

Gignac and Gottlieb (1996) considered caregivers' use of 12 kinds of coping strategies in dealing with specific behavior problems exhibited by the care recipient. They found considerable variation in the kinds of strategies caregivers used over a five-month period, suggesting that caregivers modify their approach to dealing with stressors over time. Caregivers who focused on gaining insights into how their coping strategies affected the relationship with the care recipient, both in attributing behavior problems to the disease process and in understanding the contingencies between caregiver and care recipient behaviors reported lower levels of stress at follow-up, even when initial levels of stress were controlled.

Thus, the effects of coping are complex. Strategies which attempt to change elements of the disease process are unsuccessful and perhaps even harmful. Conversely, strategies which focus on acceptance of changes in the caregiver–care recipient relationship appear much more helpful. Again, support seeking can be helpful in this regard.

One of the most comprehensive examinations of the determinants of mental health problems of caregivers was conducted by Aneshensel et al. (1995). Using a longitudinal panel of caregivers of dementia patients, they were able to examine how changes in stressors were related to increased or decreased mental health symptoms over a four-year period of time. Stress proliferation took place when primary stressors, such as behavior problems or ADL disabilities, led to feelings of overload or role captivity (see above). Thus, there needed to be both the occurrence of specific care-related problems and a subjective sense that those problems were overwhelming. In those instances, secondary stressors such as work or family conflict were more likely to emerge, as were mental health problems. In turn, receiving more informal social support from family and better coping, specifically higher feelings of mastery, resulted in some containment of stress. These results suggest that both objective indicators of the patient's disabilities and caregivers' subjective evaluation of their impact are needed to understand the processes leading to depression and other mental health problems.

Reports that caregiving is associated with high rates of psychiatric symptoms are probably not surprising, given the multiple pressures experienced. More intriguing are the results of studies which suggest that caregivers may be at risk of poorer health or even increased risk of mortality. There is less consistency across studies in reporting health effects, but sufficient evidence has been found to suggest there is at least some risk.

Studies of the effects of caregiving on health generally focus on self-reported problems, although a few investigations have used more objective indicators. Caregivers generally report they are in poorer health than age-matched controls (e.g., Pruchno & Potashnik, 1989; Schulz et al., 1990). In a nationally-representative sample from the USA, one-third of women caregivers reported fair or poor health compared to only one-fifth of age-matched peers (Stone et al., 1987). Other studies (e.g., Haley et al., 1987; Pruchno & Potashnik, 1989) have found that caregivers visit their physicians more often and use more prescription drugs compared to noncaregivers. These results, however, have not been confirmed in other studies of medical service use (e.g., George & Gwyther, 1986; Kiecolt-Glaser et al., 1987). Finally, several studies have found specific increases in health problems, such as respiratory illnesses, hypertension, and cardiovascular disease (Moritz, Kasl, & Ostfeld, 1992; Schulz et al., 1990; Wright et al., 1993).

Undoubtedly, the response of caregivers to chronic caregiving stress can follow the patterns of the general adaptation syndrome (Selye, 1976). Caregivers are exposed to a great deal of rage, grief, despair, and other intense emotions that can have effects on the blood and heart as well as clinical depression and anxiety. Caregivers may also exert a great deal of physical effort that can raise blood pressure and initiate atherosclerotic responses. The most common risk factors for health problems include being a spouse caregiver (Wright et al., 1993), living arrangements (Pratt, Wright, & Schmall, 1987), financial strain, and the intensity of primary stressors and secondary stressors. As stated before, these risk factors become detrimental to health when they are chronic.

One of the most intriguing findings linking chronic stress to health problems is that caregivers of dementia patients may experience changes in immune system functioning. In investigations which examined caregivers and a sample of matched controls, Kiecolt-Glaser and her colleagues (Keicolt-Glaser et al., 1987; Kiecolt-Glaser, Dura, Speicher, Trask, & Glaser, 1991) found that caregivers had poorer immune function, and these changes were linked to higher rates of illness in some subjects.

Caregivers' health problems may increase due to compromised self-care and health behavior (Brodaty & Hadzi-Pavlovic, 1990; Kwee, Zarit, Edwards, Davey, & Jarrott, 1995; Lieberman & Fisher, 1995). Caregivers may not go to the doctor when ill, or may not get enough rest or exercise. Nutritional intake can be affected, with some caregivers not getting adequate nutrition and others eating too much. Other caregivers may smoke more, use alcohol excessively, or even take tranquilizing medications prescribed for the patient. Consistent with the stress process model, compromised health behavior follows a model of competing demand whereby caregivers are faced with dwindling resources of energy, time, and money, and so must choose between self-care and care of their relative (Kwee et al., 1995). Often, caregivers feel no choice but to neglect their own health to continue to give care to their loved one (Bunting, 1989). Neglected self-care then acts as a mediating variable between stressors and the outcome of physical and mental health.

The process by which mental and physical health are affected as a result of caregiving stressors is admittedly complex. Uncertainties in causal directionality of independent and dependent variables and the possible existence of feedback loops due to the dynamic nature of an elder's disabilities add to the difficulty of making causal statements. Based on findings of the research, a theoretical model can be summarized as follows: the relative's illness creates the environment of primary stressors that proliferate or spillover to the creation of secondary stressors. Primary stressors, as represented by the mental and physical hardships of caregiving (e.g., motivation and ability), have both a main effect and a mediated effect (through secondary stressors) on caregiver mental and physical health. The secondary stressors that result are manifested through the caregiver's inability to take proper physical and mental care of him/herself because of a lack of energy or time. Prolonged exposure to primary and secondary stressors affects well-being. Research suggests a lagged relationship between depression and physical health, with depression leading to greater levels of physical illness (Pruchno, Kleban, Michaels, & Dempsey, 1990a).

In this framework, healthfulness is the result of continually achieving the best possible adaptation to the environment and involves interdependent physical, psychological, and social aspects (Capra, 1982). Illness occurs if stress pushes the system away from balance in response to environmental influences. To regain balance, the individual depends on his/her physical and mental response mechanisms. Because of the extensive demands that caregiving places on primary caregivers, it is not surprising that some fail to adapt to changing environmental situations and so experience severe disruption and breakdown. The challenge now is twofold: to identify the factors that protect good health in caregivers, and to design interventions that alleviate chronic stress at points in time before the body becomes ill.

Although the negative outcomes of caregiving have been emphasized, these adverse effects are sometimes balanced by positive experience. Feelings of gain, a growing sense of competency, or satisfaction with having met one's obligations or done a job well can offset the negative consequences (Aneshensel et al., 1995; Lawton, Brody, & Saperstein, 1989a). For some caregivers, fulfilling an obligation in the ways they define it is more important than putting themselves at risk of health problems or depression. Clinicians need to recognize that these commitments represent deeply-held beliefs, and not neurotic guilt (although that can be a motivator for some people). Successful clinical interventions involve helping caregivers explore and sometimes redefine their commitments, rather than confrontation over what the clinical decides is inappropriate or irrational. Solutions may also involve finding better ways of fulfilling a commitment, as described in the following sections.

7.22.12 CLINICAL RESEARCH AND SERVICES

The unprecedented stress associated with family caregiving warrants an organized response to help share a portion of the burden. At the broadest level, it is in the interest of society to encourage families to provide care, since that reduces the demand for more expensive institutional care. From the care recipient's perspective, being cared for at home for as long as possible is usually preferred. Families as well usually prefer to do as much as they can to help older family members.

Clinical interventions can be organized with two goals in mind. Interventions can be used to bring in new resources in ways that directly relieve families of a portion of their responsibilities. Respite services such as adult day care or home help serve this function. The most extensive new resource is an institutional setting, which takes over most of the care. Interventions can also build up the caregiver's own abilities for managing the situation more effectively. The review that follows, will look first at respite services, including institutional care, and the benefits and drawbacks for families. It will then consider clinical interventions for caregivers.

7.22.13 RESPITE SERVICES

Respite services for caregivers of elderly relatives with dementia are widely advocated by professionals and sought after by caregivers. While there is no clear definition of what services comprise respite, day care, in-home help, and short- and long-term institutionalization are some of the most frequently used services. Respite is designed to serve both caregiver and patient. With the growing awareness that institutional care is often not optimal for older people, respite services have been promoted as a means by which impaired elders could remain in the community longer while reducing the cost of care provision.

Despite reports of high satisfaction with respite services (e.g., Burdz, Eaton, & Bond, 1988; Kosloski, Montgomery, & Borgotta 1990;

Lawton et al., 1989a, 1989b; Montgomery & Berkeley-Caines, 1989; Montgomery & Borgatta, 1985), there has not been much evidence of the benefits for caregivers or patients. Some investigations have found little impact of respite services, leading to the suggestion that these programs may be of no value to the family (Callahan, 1989). These negative findings, however, may be the consequence of poor programing or low or inconsistent levels of service utilization. This section describes different respite services and considers outcomes of and obstacles to utilization.

7.22.13.1 Adult Day Care

Adult day care programs are designed for individuals with dementia or other mental or physical disabilities. They provide the patient with a few hours of supervised, structured activity, and give the family caregiver time to rest or perform other chores and responsibilities. Typically an individual will attend a day care program two to three days each week for about five hours each day (Weissert et al., 1990). Program activities include orientation exercises, socializing, and reminiscing. Programs frequently provide services such as health screening, podiatrist and eye doctor visits, and prescription administration. Out-of-home care allows the caregiver to stay at home and enjoy their privacy or have time with other family members (Montgomery, 1995). Day care gives the patient the opportunity to meet others and have a change of scenery and activities while remaining in a safe environment.

Despite reports that caregivers are very satisfied with day care (Burdz et al., 1988; Lawton et al., 1989a, 1989b; Miller, Gulle, & McCue, 1986; Sands & Suzuki, 1983), benefits for the caregiver are equivocal. Some research supports the idea that day care usage results in improved physical and mental health, better relationships, and increased confidence in caregiving abilities among family caregivers (Montgomery & Borgatta, 1985; Scharlach & Frenzel, 1986). Other studies, however, have found that day care has little or no effect on caregiver burden or well-being (Burdz et al., 1988; Lawton et al., 1989b; Montgomery & Borgatta, 1989).

The effects, or lack thereof, of day care programs on caregiver burden may depend on the characteristics of the individual in the caregiving situation (Montgomery, 1995). Caregivers' employment, health, or responsibility for another family member could affect utilization and mediate the benefits of a day care program. Failure to find benefits may also be due to low utilization of programs. For example, Lawton et al. (1989a) found no effects of program participation on caregiver burden, but the caregivers in the program utilized day care less than once a month. Inability to control how much families utilize day care prevents firm conclusions being drawn about the benefits of adult day care. Some caregivers find the programs too inaccessible (MaloneBeach, Zarit, & Spore, 1992), and some relatives would rather remain at home.

Preliminary results from a large-scale trial of adult day care for dementia are more promising (Zarit, Stephens, Townsend, & Greene, 1996). In this study, caregivers received adequate amounts of respite (at least two days per week) from well-developed programs with expertise in care of dementia patients. Measures were also developed to be specific to the strains likely to be addressed by this kind of respite care. Results showed that caregivers using day care experienced lower feelings of overload, decreased anger and depression, and increased well-being compared to a control sample not receiving day care or other respite services. These results suggest that well-designed day care programs may relieve stress on caregivers.

7.22.13.2 In-Home Respite

Respite services provided in the home include attendance to the patient's physical needs, such as bathing and feeding, and "sitting" with the patient, either for a short period or overnight. Providers may include a companion, homemaker, home health aide, or a nurse (Isett, Kraus, & Malone, 1984). Levels of in-home care can be low or high, for a short or an extended period of time. Home respite is intended for patients who still live alone and need assistance, and for the coresiding caregiver of a more dependent patient.

Reports on benefits of in-home respite for the caregiver are generally positive. In-home care eliminates the need for transportation and may be scheduled with some flexibility (Montgomery, 1995). Benefits of in-home respite for the caregiver include improved mood (Gwyther, 1989) and decreased time spent in caregiving activities (Berry, Zarit, & Rabatin, 1991). In addition to being satisfied with in-home help, caregivers usually want more of it. At the conclusion of a 12-month program during which respite services were available, Lawton et al. (1989b) found that all caregivers in the study wanted more respite than any other class of services. MaloneBeach et al. (1992) also reported that caregivers wanted more help in the home.

Caregivers using in-home help have also voiced concerns with the services provided. Complaints about in-home help have focused on the qualifications, reliability, and continuity of respite providers, and availability and flexibility of scheduling (MaloneBeach et al., 1992; Montgomery, 1995). Obstacles to use of in-home respite include bureaucracy and disengagement of the caregiver from the service system (MaloneBeach et al.). Caregivers report that the structure of the service system is too narrow as it often does not meet all of the patient's or caregiver's needs. Caregivers also report that the system is unaccommodating of changes in patients' conditions unless they fit into the service levels of a schedule fixed by the respite program. These studies, which were conducted in the USA, may not capture caregivers' experiences in countries that provide better access to and coordination of services.

Although many consider in-home respite a means by which family caregivers may keep their relative with dementia in the community longer, use of respite is sometimes associated with short or long-term institutionalization (Montgomery 1995; Montgomery & Borgatta, 1985; Montgomery & Kosloski, 1990). Lawton et al. (1989b) reported that caregivers who spent the most time and effort caregiving were most likely to use respite, particularly nursing home respite. As caregivers learn to be more comfortable sharing the burden of caregiving, it may become more acceptable to them to place their relative in an institution (Montgomery, 1995). An alternative explanation is that respite services are a stepping stone to institutionalization in the progression of the patient's illness.

7.22.13.3 Institutionalization and its Consequences

Short-term institutionalization offers overnight respite for family caregivers and provides skilled nursing for the patient. A short-term admission may be scheduled every couple of weeks for two to three nights or less frequently for one to two weeks (Montgomery, 1995). While short-term institutionalization offers the benefit of an extended period of respite, it tends to be less flexible than in-home care. Institutions cannot usually offer emergency respite because of the cost of keeping a bed free (Scharlach & Frenzel, 1986). Some patients have difficulty adjusting to a new environment (Mace & Rabins, 1981), and some will resist institutional respite for fear that it is a permanent placement (Montgomery, 1995). In a study of two weeks of institutional respite, Burdz et al. (1988) expected dementia patients to show increased problems due to the confusion of being in a new environment. The patients, however, demonstrated significant decreases in problem behaviors, and caregivers rated the program as highly beneficial, though few said their situation had improved after the program. Even with an extended break from caregiving, short-term institutionalization frequently precedes long-term placement (Montgomery & Borgatta, 1989).

Placement of a relative in a long-term care facility may be viewed as a final release of caregiver stress and responsibility, but it is accompanied by its own stressors (Townsend, 1990; Zarit & Whitlatch, 1992). Institutionalization may ease some of the strain of everyday care, but many caregivers continue to provide assistance even after transferring their relative to an institution. While primary stressors such as feelings of overload decrease following placement, feelings of depression and other mental health indicators are often unchanged (Zarit & Whitlatch, 1992). MaloneBeach et al. (1992) found that family caregivers with a relative in a nursing home reported that their relative still needed additional services not provided in the nursing home. Caregiving strains may persist for as long as four years after placement (Aneshensel et al., 1995).

The high levels of satisfaction which caregivers report with all respite services is encouraging. However, the results of empirical studies indicate that respite services do not reduce caregiver burden and stress consistently. A major problem in these studies has been low rates of use of services, which is often related to barriers to or problems in service delivery. Availability and accessibility is another obstacle to service utilization. For example, waiting lists at US day cares are more common than in Sweden where the municipality provides sufficient access to day programs (Jarrott, Zarit, Berg, & Johansson, 1996). Flexibility of scheduling and services are essential, along with personal contact with a case worker and regular care providers. Once caregivers are taken off a waiting list and admitted to a program, many patients attend sporadically because hours or transportation are inconvenient (Montgomery, 1995). Cost and clear guidelines on qualifications for different services need to be provided along with the support which permits all those in need of assistance to receive it.

Despite caregivers' concerns about respite programs and the inconsistent findings of benefits, families overwhelmingly say it is important to them and most would like more respite. Respite services may need to be considered for their long-term effects

(Fortinsky & Hathaway, 1990). Greene and Coleman (1990) suggest that available services may serve a preventive function, so that stress on the family does not reach an overwhelming level. Other families, however, consider caregiving a personal responsibility and only look for assistance when they have reached their own limits. More active recruitment of family members early in their caregiving career may result in greater long-term relief from burden and stress. Perhaps when caregivers feel more comfortable turning to respite services for assistance, utilization will be greater and effects will be evident.

7.22.14 CLINICAL SERVICES

Clinical protocols have been developed to lower stress on family caregivers by increasing their ability to manage care-related problems and improving their access to help from other family members and from formal services (e.g., Zarit, Orr, & Zarit, 1985; Zarit, 1996). These interventions build on existing research by identifying modifiable aspects of the stress process. As observed, behavior problems do not have a fixed or constant effect on caregiver outcomes. By improving how caregivers manage behavior disturbances, the impact of these problems will be reduced and caregivers will experience less stress. Similarly, increasing support from and reducing conflict with other family members should lead to improvements in the caregiver's situation.

A model for clinical interventions is shown in Figure 2. As with any intervention, the starting point is assessment. Assessment focuses on both care recipient and caregiver and serves several functions. First, it is important to confirm the care recipient's disabilities and to make sure that treatable components have not been overlooked. Symptoms of memory loss sometimes have treatable causes and should not be assumed to be due to dementia, unless an appropriate medical and neuropsychological examination has been conducted. Second, the clinician can assess the specific problems, disabilities, and strengths of the care recipient. Although the focus is often on decrements, care recipients may retain some abilities and resources, even when suffering from dementia or other progressive disorders. Strengths can include activities the person currently is able to perform, or past interests and activities that may be possible to enhance in the present situation. Third, the assessment should indicate which problems are stressful for the caregiver. As emphasized throughout this chapter, caregivers experience potential stressors in different ways. What is difficult for one person may not be so for another. That includes management of specific behaviors, such as incontinence or wandering, or handling potential conflicts between caregiving and work or other roles. Finally, the clinician should consider the extent to which the care recipient can participate in a clinical intervention, either jointly with the caregiver, or separately. There have been reports that short-term counseling and support groups are helpful for dementia patients in the earlier stages of their illness (Teri, 1994; Zarit & Zarit, in press). For cognitively intact people, a wide range of clinical interventions might be appropriate.

Following the initial assessment, clinicians can draw upon three treatment strategies when working with caregivers: increasing the caregiver's understanding of the patient's illness and disabilities; problem solving to manage daily care-related problems; and support. A starting point for interventions is often to increase caregiver's understanding of the care recipient's illness. Families often have questions that have not been answered by medical personnel, or they have trouble understanding the implications of a diagnosis. Often they will have questions about the possibilities for treatment.

An important facet of understanding the disorder is learning to view changes in the patient's behavior as part of the disease process. In disorders like dementia that have considerable impact on behavior, families often misunderstand or misinterpret common problems. They may, for example, believe that a patient asks the same question over and over to annoy the caregiver or to get attention, or because of laziness. Families should be encouraged to look at why someone with a memory-impairing disease would behave this way. They should also avoid reasoning or arguing with patients over factual issues. Patients may insist that they want to see their long-deceased mothers, or to go home, when they are already at home. Experience shows that caregivers cannot persuade patients they are mistaken. In fact, reminding patients that their mothers are dead is often upsetting, since they experience it as a new loss, and the result is more agitation. Instead, families are encouraged to think about why someone with memory loss would behave this way, and what they must be feeling at this time. Although families cannot respond effectively to the content of these types of communications, they can respond to the underlying emotions, for example, by providing comfort or reassurance, or by reminiscing about the patient's mother.

Increasing the caregiver's understanding of problem behaviors flows naturally into a more formal approach to problem solving. Problem

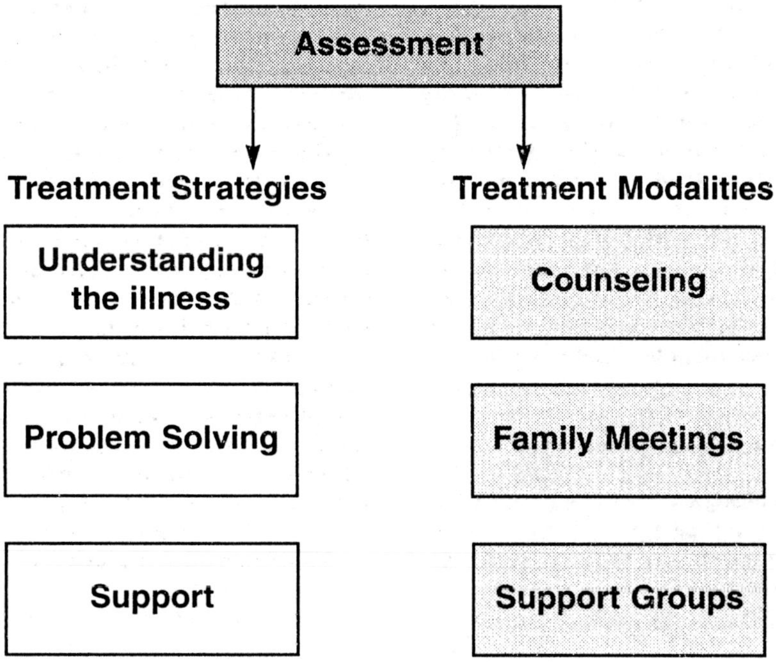

Figure 2 A model of intervention with caregivers.

solving can be used to address persistent troubling behaviors. Drawn from contemporary behavior therapy, problem solving involves a series of steps to identify causes and reinforcers of current problems and to generate and implement possible solutions (see Table 1). The starting point is to pinpoint a specific behavior or problem (e.g., agitation, depressed behaviors), and to have the caregiver observe it over a period of several days. Caregivers should note when the problem occurs, what went before it (antecedents), and what followed the behavior (reinforcers). This step provides a baseline of how often the problem occurs, against which interventions can be measured. It also identifies how the behavior may function. In dementia, for example, agitated behavior typically follows a period of inactivity or napping and is reinforced by attention.

Once a pattern is identified, the caregiver can be encouraged to think about strategies to change or head off the problem. Strategies need to be specific and practical and within the ability of the caregiver to manage. Caregivers may have difficulty selecting a solution. In that case, they can compare different strategies with the method of pros and cons, by which they write down advantages and drawbacks of each approach (including doing nothing). Planning and rehearsing the solutions before trying them out heads off problems if the plan is not realistic. After implementing a solution, caregivers should continue monitoring how often the problem occurs in order to evaluate how successful this strategy has been.

Although it is a behavior technique, problem solving is compatible with the use of medications. In fact, medications to control behavior or mood should be considered as one of the possible strategies for intervention. If the caregiver obtains a baseline of the frequency of the targeted problem before a medication is introduced, then it will be possible to get an accurate evaluation of the effectiveness of treatment. As clinicians know, medications often have uncertain and variable effects. Neuroleptics are widely used for control of behavior problems in the elderly, but they are not consistently effective or sometimes work for a while and then lose their effectiveness (Schneider, Pollock, & Lyness, 1990). By viewing medications as one of several possible

Table 1 The problem solving process.

	Stage
1	Pinpoint a behavior and assess when it occurs and how often
2	Identify antecedents and consequences
3	Identify possible strategies
4	Select a strategy (use pros and cons)
5	Plan and rehearse implementing the strategy
6	Try out strategy and evaluate

strategies and carefully monitoring their effectiveness, clinicians can develop more rational treatment approaches.

Problem solving can also be used to identify antecedents and consequences of caregiver stress. Rather than pinpointing a specific behavior problem, caregivers can note when they feel the most stress, and what has led up to that. Sometimes, it will be revealed that no one problem or behavior is overwhelming. Instead, the accumulation of small stressors without a break leads to difficulties. Solutions can then focus on how the caregiver can prevent the build up of stress, such as arranging for respite care.

The third treatment strategy is support. Clinicians can provide support directly with empathy for the caregiver and a nonjudgmental attitude. Interventions can also work to increase support and understanding from family and friends, and to gain more help from formal service providers. Clinicians can help families address the perceived and actual obstacles in respite services.

Three intervention modalities have been used with caregivers: one-to-one counseling; family meetings; and support groups. Each brings a different element to treatment. Short-term counseling can provide caregivers with the opportunity to explore their situation in depth and to consider the options and alternatives available to them in a supportive and nonjudgmental situation. Family meetings offer the opportunity to address directly areas of conflict and misunderstanding in the family and to build support and assistance for the primary caregiver. Support groups give caregivers the opportunity to discuss their situation with other people in similar situations. Groups may be an efficient means of sharing information and learning about new approaches and strategies.

Several studies document the effectiveness of these approaches. Whitlatch, Zarit, and von Eye (1991) found that caregivers receiving individual counseling and a family meeting had lower stress than people receiving only a support group or who were on a waiting list. In a series of studies, Toseland and his colleagues (Toseland, Rossiter, Peak, & Smith, 1990) have also found that counseling is more effective in the short run for relieving a caregiver's distress than support groups.

Mittelman and her colleagues (1993; 1995) developed a comprehensive intervention program that combines individual and family counseling during an initial four-month period, followed by sustained treatment in a support group. Caregivers in the treatment group had lower burden and distress and placed their relatives in nursing homes at a lower rate than people in a control group (see also, Whitlatch, Zarit, Goodwin, & von Eye, 1995).

These findings demonstrate the effectiveness of planned interventions designed to lower the stress of family caregivers. By increasing caregivers' skills in managing problems and stressors and bringing in new resources to support the caregiver whenever possible, clinicians can provide substantial assistance even in the face of a deteriorating condition. Through these interventions, caregivers can function as well as possible, while providing an optimal care environment for their relative. Timely use of these interventions may be cost-effective by preventing the breakdown of the family caregiving system, and encouraging a rational use of respite services, including institutional care when that is appropriate.

7.22.15 CONCLUSIONS

One of the major features of an aging society is that families are caring for disabled elders more often and for longer periods of time than ever before. There is considerable individual variability in how caregiving is handled and experienced, but it is typically stressful for the primary family helper and sometimes for the extended family network. The phenomenon of caregiving cannot be captured within a single measure of burden or stress. Rather, the many dimensions involved in the family's responses and the types of different stressors or problems caregivers experience have been observed. The stress of caregiving is an ongoing process, which evolves as the demands of care change and as caregivers develop new understanding, utilize different resources, or become overwhelmed by the unrelenting problems they face.

The challenge for the future is to find ways to support families so that they can provide high-quality, personalized care without excessive strain on themselves. The cost of care for social and health programs for the elderly has become an increasing problem for those countries with a significant proportion of their populations over age 65 years. As the number of elderly increase, cost-efficient means of providing care that do not sacrifice quality are needed. The responsibility for care cannot fall exclusively on families, because the burdens are too great, nor on society, since the cost will be too high. There need, instead, to be partnerships that find creative ways of sharing care, and which address the needs of both care recipient and caregiver. What shape those alliances will take, or the best models of working to support families, remain to be discovered. A small, but growing, clinical literature suggests that timely and well-conceived clinical interventions can be an important part of this partnership, helping families develop better strategies for managing a patient's disabilities and regulating the stress on themselves.

7.22.16 REFERENCES

Aneshensel, C. S., Pearlin, L. I., Mullan, J. T., Zarit, S. H., & Whitlatch, C. J. (1995). *Profiles in caregiving: The unexpected career.* New York: Academic Press.

Aneshensel, C. S., Pearlin, L. I., & Schuler, R. H. (1993). Stress, role captivity, and the cessation of caregiving. *Journal of Health and Social Behavior, 34,* 54–70.

Anthony-Bergstone, C. R., Zarit, S. H., & Gatz, M. (1988). Symptoms of psychological distress among caregivers of dementia patients. *Psychology and Aging, 3,* 245–248.

Berry, G. L., Zarit, S. H., & Rabatin, V. X. (1991). Caregiver activity on respite and nonrespite days: A comparison of two service approaches. *The Gerontologist, 31,* 830–835.

Birkel, R. C. (1987). Toward a social ecology of home-care households. *Psychology and Aging, 2*(3), 294-301.

Bledin, K. D., MacCarthy, B., Kuipers, L., & Woods, R. T. (1990). Daughters of people with dementia: Expressed emotion, strain, and coping. *British Journal of Psychiatry, 157,* 221-227.

Brodaty, H.,. & Hadzi-Pavlovic, D. H. (1990). Psychosocial effects on carers of living with persons with dementia. *Australian and New Zealand Journal of Psychiatry, 24,* 351–361.

Brody, E. M. (1990). *Women in the middle: Their parent-care years.* New York: Springer.

Brody, E. M., Johnsen, P. T., & Fulcomer, M. C. (1984). What should adult children do for elderly parents? Opinions and preferences of three generations of women. *Journal of Gerontology, 39,* 736–746.

Brody, E. M., Kleban, M. H., Johnsen, P. T., Hoffman, C., & Schoonover, C. B. (1987). Work status and parent care: A comparison of four groups of women. *The Gerontologist, 27,* 201–208.

Brody, E. M., Litvin, S. J., Albert, S. M., & Hoffman, C. J. (1994). Marital status of daughters and patterns of parent care. *Journals of Gerontology, 49,* S95-S103.

Brody, E. M., & Schoonover, C. B. (1986). Patterns of parent-care when adult daughters work and when they do not. *The Gerontologist, 26,* 372–381.

Bunting, S. M. (1989). Stress on caregivers of the elderly. *Advances in Nursing Science, 11,* 63-73.

Burdz, M. P., Eaton, W. O., & Bond, J. B., Jr. (1988). Effect of respite care on dementia and nondementia patients and their caregivers. *Psychology and Aging, 3,* 38–42.

Callahan, J.J., Jr. (1989). Play it again, Sam—There is no impact. *Gerontologist, 29,* 5–6.

Capra, F. (1982). Wholeness & health. In *The turning point: Science, society and the rising culture.* (pp. 305–330). New York: Bantam Books.

Cassel, C. K., Rudberg, M. A., & Olshansky, S. J. (1992). The price of success: Health care in an aging society. *Health Affairs, (Summer),* 87–99.

Chappell, N. L. (1991). Living arrangements and sources of caregiving. *Journals of Gerontology, 46,* S1–S8.

Chow, N. W. (1983). The Chinese family and support of the elderly in Hong Kong. *The Gerontologist, 23,* 584–588.

Cicirelli, V. G. (1983). A comparison of helping behavior to elderly parents of adult children with intact and disrupted marriages. *The Gerontologist, 23,* 619–625.

Cicirelli, V. G. (1985). The role of siblings as family caregivers. In W. J. Sauer & R. T. Coward (Eds.), *Social support networks and the care of the elderly: Theory, practice, and research* (pp. 93–107). New York: Springer.

Cicirelli, V. G. (1992). Siblings as caregivers in middle and old age. In J. W. Dwyer & R. T. Coward (Eds.), *Gender, families, and elder care* (pp. 84–104). Newbury Park, CA: Sage.

Cicirelli, V. G. (1993). Attachment and obligation as daughters' motives for caregiving behavior and subsequent effect on subjective burden. *Psychology and Aging, 8,* 144–155.

Clipp, E. C., & George, L. K. (1990a). Caregiver needs and patterns of social support. *Journals of Gerontology, 45,* S102–S111.

Clipp, E. C., & George, L. K. (1990b). Psychotropic drug use among caregivers of patients with dementia. *Journal of the American Geriatrics Society, 38,* 227–235.

Clipp, E. C., & George, L. K. (1993). Dementia and cancer: A comparison of spouse caregivers. *The Gerontologist, 33,* 534–541.

Cohen, D., & Eisdorfer, C. (1988). Depression in family members caring for a relative with Alzheimer's disease. *Journal of the American Geriatric Society,* 36, 885–889.

Cooney, T. M., & Uhlenberg, P. (1990). The role of divorce in men's relations with their adult children after midlife. *Journal of Marriage and the Family, 52,* 677–688.

Creasey, G. L., Myers, B. J., Epperson, M. J., & Taylor, J. (1990). Couples with an elderly parent with Alzheimer's disease: Perceptions of familial relationships. *Psychiatry, 53,* 44–51.

Davey, A., Kwee, E. E., Shea, D. G., Zarit, S. H., Sundström, G., Berg, S., & Smyer, M. A. (1996, November). *How much do families help? Cultural and policy perspectives.* Paper presented at the annual meeting of the Gerontological Society of America, Washington, DC.

Drinka, T. J., Smith, J., & Drinka, P. J. (1987). Correlates of depression and burden for informal caregivers of patients in a geriatrics referral clinic. *Journal of the American Geriatrics Society, 35,* 522–525.

Eggebeen, D. J., & Wilhelm, M. O. (1995). Patterns of support given by older Americans to their children. In S. A. Bass (Ed.), *Older and active: How Americans over 55 are contributing to society* (pp. 122–168). New Haven, CT: Yale University.

Fadel-Girgis, M. (1983). Family support for the elderly in Egypt (1983). *The Gerontologist, 23,* 589–592.

Field, D., & Minkler, M. (1988). Continuity and change in social support between young-old and old-old or very-old age. *Journals of Gerontology, 43,* P100–P106.

Fortinsky, R. & Hathaway, T. (1990). Information and service needs among active and former family caregivers of persons with Alzheimer's Disease. *The Gerontologist, 30,* 604–609.

Franklin, S. T., Ames, B. D., & King, S. (1994). Acquiring the family eldercare role: Influence on female employment adaptation. *Research on Aging, 16,* 27–42.

Franks, M. M., & Stephens, M. A. P. (1996). Social support in the context of caregiving: Husbands' provision of support to wives involved in parent care. *Journals of Gerontology, 51B,* P43–P52.

Gallagher, D., Rose, J., Rivera, P., Lovett, S., & Thompson, L. W. (1989). Prevalence of depression in family caregivers. *The Gerontologist, 29,* 449–456.

George, L. K., & Gwyther, L. P. (1986). Caregiver well-being: A multidimensional examination of family caregivers of demented adults. *The Gerontologist, 26,* 253–259.

Gibeau, J. L., & Anastas, J. W. (1989). Breadwinners and caregivers: Interviews with working women. *Journal of Gerontological Social Work, 14,* 19–40.

Gignac, M. A. M., & Gottlieb, B. H. (1996). Caregivers' appraisals of efficacy in coping with dementia. *Psychology and Aging, 11,* 214–225.

Goldman, L. S., & Luchins, D. J. (1984). Depression in the

spouses of demented patients. *American Journal of Psychiatry, 14,* 1467–1468.
Goode, W. J. (1960). A theory of strain. *American Sociological Review, 25,* 483–496.
Greene, V. L., & Coleman, P. D. (1995). Direct services for family caregivers: Next steps for public policy. In R. A. Kane & J. D. Penrod (Eds.) *Family are giving in an aging society: Policy perspectives* (pp. 46–63). Thousand Oaks, CA: Sage
Gwyther, L. P. (1990). *Barriers to service utilization among Alzheimer's patients and their families* (Report to the US Congress, Office of Technical Assessment, National Technical Information Service #PB89–225205. Durham, NC: Duke University Center on Aging.
Hadjistavropoulos, T., Taylor, S., Tuokko, H., & Beattie, B. L. (1994). Neuropsychological deficits, caregivers' perception of deficits, and caregiver burden. *Journal of the American Geriatrics Society, 42,* 308–314.
Haley, W. E., Levine, E. G., Brown, S. L., & Bartolucci, A. A. (1987). Stress, appraisal, coping and social support as predictors of adaptational outcome among dementia caregivers. *Psychology and Aging, 2*(4), 323–330.
Haley, W. E., Levine E. G., Brown, S. L., Berry, J. W., & Hughes, G. H. (1987). Psychological, social, and health consequences of caring for a relative with senile dementia. *Journal of the American Geriatrics Society, 35,* 405–411.
Haley, W. E., & Pardo, K. M. (1989). Relationship of severity of dementia to caregiving stressors. *Psychology and Aging, 4,* 389–392.
Haley, W. E., West, C. A. C., Wadley, V. G., Ford, G. R., White, F. A., Barrett, J. J., Harrell, L. E., & Roth, D. L. (1995). Psychological, social, and health impact of caregiving: A comparison of black and white dementia family caregivers and noncaregivers. *Psychology and Aging, 10,* 540–552.
Hamon, R. R., & Blieszner, R. (1990). Filial responsibility expectations among adult child-older parent pairs. *Journals of Gerontology, 45,* P110–P112.
Hanson, S. L., Sauer, W. J., & Seelbach, W. C. (1983). Racial and cohort variations in filial responsibility norms. *The Gerontologist, 23,* 626–631.
Hirdes, J. P., & Strain, L. A. (1995). The balance of exchange in instrumental support with network members outside the household. *Journals of Gerontology, 50B,* S134–S142.
Horowitz, A. (1985). Sons and daughters as caregivers to older parents: Differences in role performance and consequences. *The Gerontologist, 25,* 612–617.
Ingersoll-Dayton, B., & Antonucci, T. C. (1988). Reciprocal and nonreciprocal social support: Contrasting sides of intimate relationships. *Journals of Gerontology, 43,* S65–S73.
Isett, R. D. Krauss, C., & Malone, M. (1984). *A study of the Intercommunity Actions, Inc. In-home respite care project.* Unpublished manuscript. Mid-Atlantic Long Term Care Gerontology Center.
Jarrott, S. E., Zarit, S. H., Johansson, L., & Berg, S. (1996, June). *A comparison of day care in Sweden and the United States.* Paper presented at the Nordic Gerontology Congress, Helsinki, Finland.
Johansson, B., & Zarit, S. H. (1995). Prevalence and incidence of dementia in the oldest old: A longitudinal study of a population-based sample of 84-90 year-olds in Sweden. *International Journal of Geriatric Psychiatry, 10,* 359–366.
Jorm, A. F., Korten, A. E., & Henderson, A. S. (1987). The prevalence of dementia: A quantitative integration of the literature. *Acta Psychiatry Scandinavia, 76,* 465–479.
Kaszniak, A. W. (1996). Preparing for treatment of the elderly: Assessment. In S. H. Zarit & B. Knight (Eds.), *A guide to psychotherapy and aging: Clinical intervention in a life stage context.* Washington, DC: APA Books.
Kendig, H. L., Rowland, D. T. (1983). Family support of the Australian aged: A comparison with the United States. *The Gerontologist, 23,* 643–649.
Kiecolt-Glaser, J. K., Dura, J. R., Speicher, C. E., Trask, O. J., & Glaser, R. (1991). Spousal caregivers of dementia victims: Longitudinal changes in immunity and health. *Psychosomatic Medicine, 53,* 345–362.
Kiecolt-Glaser, J. K., Glaser, R., Shuttleworth, E. C., Dyer, C. S., Ogrocki, P., & Speicher, C. E. (1987). Chronic stress and immunity in family caregivers of Alzheimer's Disease victims. *Psychosomatic Medicine, 49,* 523–535.
Kinney, J. M., & Stephens, M. A. P. (1989). Hassles and uplifts of giving care to a family member with dementia. *Psychology and Aging, 4,* 402–408.
Kinsella, K., & Taeuber, C. M. (1993). *An aging world II. International Population.* Reports P95/92–3. US Department of Commerce, Economics, and Statistics Administration, Bureau of the Census, Government Printing Office, Washington, DC.
Kivett, V. R., & Atkinson, M. P. (1984). Filial expectations, association, and helping as a function of number of children among older rural-transitional parents. *Journal of Gerontology, 39,* 499–503.
Kokmen, E., Chandra, V., & Schoenberg, B. S. (1988). Trends in incidence of dementing illness in Rochester, Minnesota, in three quinquennial periods, 1960–1974. *Neurology, 38,* 975–980.
Koslowski, K. D., Montgomery, R. J. V., & Borgotta, E. F. (1990). Predicting nursing home utilization: Is this the best we can do? In S. M. Stahl (Ed.), *The legacy of longevity: Health and health care in later life.* Newbury Park, CA: Sage.
Krause, N. (1995). Negative interaction and satisfaction with social support among older adults. *Journals of Gerontology, 50B,* P59–P73.
Kwee, E. E., Zarit, S. H., Edwards, A. B., Davey, A., & Jarrott, S.E. (1995, November). *Caregiver's health-seeking behavior: Impact of the intensity of stressors.* Poster presented at the Fortyeighth Annual Meeting of the Gerontological Society of America, Los Angeles, CA.
Lawton, M. P., Brody, E. M., & Saperstein, A. R. (1989a). A controlled study of respite services for caregivers of Alzheimer's patients. *The Gerontologist, 29*(1), 8–16.
Lawton, M. P., Brody, E. M., Saperstein, A. R., & Grimes, M. (1989b). Respite services for caregivers: Research findings for service planning. *Home Health Care Services Quarterly, 10*(1/2), 5–32.
Lazarus, R. S., & Folkman, S. (1984). *Stress, appraisal, and coping.* New York: Springer.
Lerner, M. J., Somers, D. G., Reid, D., Chiriboga, D., & Tierney, M. (1991). Adult children as caregivers: egocentric biases in judgements of sibling contributions. *The Gerontologist, 31,* 746–755.
Lieberman, M. A., & Fisher, L. (1995). The impact of chronic illness on the health and well-being of family members. *The Gerontologist*, 35, 94–102.
Mace, N. L. & Rabins, P. V. (1981). *The 36-hour day: A family guide to caring for persons with Alzheimer's disease, related dementing illness and memory loss in later life.* Baltimore: Johns Hopkins University Press.
Maeda, D. (1983). Family care in Japan. *The Gerontologist, 23,* 579–583.
Majerovitz, S. D. (1995). Role of family adaptability in the psychological adjustment of spouse caregivers to patients with dementia. *Psychology and Aging, 10,* 447–457.
MaloneBeach, E. E., Zarit, S. H., & Spore, D. L. (1992). Caregivers' perceptions of case management and community-based services: Barriers to service use. *The Journal of Applied Gerontology, 11*(2), 146-159.
Martire, L. M., Stephens, M. A. P., & Atienza, A. A. (in

press). The Interplay of work and caregiving: Relationships between role satisfaction, role involvement and caregivers' well-being. *Journals of Gerontology: Social Sciences, 52B,* S279-S289.

Matthews, S. H. (1987). Provision of care to old parents: Division of responsibility among adult children. *Research on Aging, 9,* 45–60.

Matthews, S. H. (1995). Gender and the division of filial responsibility between lone sisters and their brothers. *Journals of Gerontology, 50B,* S312–S320.

Matthews, S. H., & Rosner, T. T. (1988). Shared filial responsibility: The family as the primary caregiver. *Journal of Marriage and the Family, 50,* 185–195.

Matthews, S. H., Werkner, J. E., & Delaney, P. J. (1989). Relative contributions of help by employed and nonemployed sisters to their elderly parents. *Journal of Gerontology: Social Sciences, 44,* S36–S44.

Miller, D. B., Gulle, N. & McCue, F. (1986). The realities of respite for families, clients and sponsors. *The Gerontologist, 26,* 467–470.

Mittelman, M. S., Ferris, S. H., Shulman, E., Steinberg, G., Ambinder, A., Mackell, J., & Cohen, J. (1995). A comprehensive support program: Effect on depression in spouse-caregivers of AD patients. *The Gerontologist, 35,* 792–802.

Mittelman, M. S., Ferris, S. H., Steinberg, G., Shulman, E., Mackell, J. A., Ambinder, A., & Cohen, J. (1993). An intervention that delays institutionalization of Alzheimer's disease patients: Treatment of spouse-caregivers. *Gerontologist, 33,* 730–740.

Moen, P., Robison, J., & Fields, V. (1994). Women's work and caregiving roles: A life course approach. *Journal of Gerontology, Social Sciences, 49,* S176–S185.

Monahan, D. J., & Hooker, K. (1995). Health of spouse caregivers of dementia patients: The role of personality and social support. *Social Work, 40,* 305–314.

Montgomery, R. J. V. (1995). Examining respite care: Promises and limitations. In D. E. Biegel, & R. Schulz (Series Eds.) & R. A. Kane & J. D. Penrod (Vol. Eds.), *Family Caregiver Applications Series: Vol. 5. Family caregiving in an aging society* (1st ed., pp. 29–45). Thousand Oaks, CA: Sage.

Montgomery, R. J., & Berkeley-Caines, L. (1989). Effects of in-home volunteer respite services on caregivers: A final report to Detroit Catholic Social Services. Detroit, IL: Wayne State University Institute of Gerontology.

Montgomery, R. J. V., & Borgatta, E. (1985). *Family support project: Final report to the administration on aging.* Seattle, WA: University of Washington

Montgomery, R. J. V., & Borgatta, E. (1989). The effects of alternative support strategies on family caregiving. *The Gerontologist, 29,* 457–464.

Montgomery, R. J. V., & Kosloski, K. (1990, November). *Adult children and the nursing home decision.* Paper presented at the Fifty-second Annual Meeting of the National Council on Family Relations, Seattle, WA.

Morgan, D. L., Schuster, T. L., & Butler, E. W. (1991). Role reversals in the exchange of social support. *Journals of Gerontology, 46,* S278–S287.

Moritz, D. J., Kasl, S. V., & Berkman, L. F. (1989). The health impact of living with a cognitively impaired elderly spouse: Depressive symptoms and social functioning. *Journals of Gerontology, 44,* S17–S27.

Moritz, D. J., Kasl, S. V., & Ostfeld, A. M. (1992). The health impact of living with a cognitively impaired elderly spouse: Blood pressure, self-rated health, and health behaviors. *Journal of Aging and Health, 4,* 244–267.

Mutschler, P. H. (1994). From executive suite to production line: How employees in different occupation manage elder care responsibilities. *Research on Aging, 16,* 7–26.

Neal, M. B., Chapman, N. J., Ingersoll-Dayton, B., Emlen, A. C., & Boise, L. (1990). Absenteeism and stress among employed caregivers of the elderly, disabled adults, and children. In D. E. Biegel & A. Blum (Eds.), *Aging and caregiving: Theory, practice, and research* (pp. 160–183). Newbury Park, CA: Sage.

Pearlin, L. I. (1993). The social contexts of stress. In L. Goldberger & S. Breznitz (Eds.), *Handbook of stress: Theoretical and clinical aspects* (2nd ed., pp. 303–315). New York: Free Press.

Pearlin, L., Mullan, J., Semple, S., & Skaff, M. (1990). Caregiving and the stress process: An overview of concepts and their measures. *The Gerontologist, 30,* 583–594.

Pearson, J., Verma, S., & Nellett, C. (1988). Elderly psychiatric patient status and caregiver perceptions as predictors of caregiver burden. *The Gerontologist, 28,* 79–83.

Penning, M. J. (1990). Receipt of assistance by elderly people: Hierarchical selection and task specificity. *The Gerontologist, 30,* 220–227.

Pillemer, K., & Suitor, J. J. (1992). Violence and violent feelings: What causes them among family caregivers? *Journals of Gerontology, 47,* S165–S172.

Pratt, C. P., Wright, S., & Schmall, V. (1987). Burden, coping, and health status: A comparison of family caregivers to community dwelling and institutionalized Alzheimer's patients. *Journals of Gerontological Social Work, 20,* 99–112.

Pruchno, R., & Kleban, M. H. (1993). Caring for an institutionalized parent: The role of coping strategies. *Psychology and Aging, 8,* 18–25.

Pruchno, R. A., Kleban, M. H., Michaels, E., & Dempsey, N. P. (1990a). Mental and physical health of caregiving spouses: Development of a causal model. *Journals of Gerontology: Psychological Sciences, 45,* P192–199.

Pruchno, R. A., Michaels, J. E., & Potashnik, S. L. (1990b). Predictors of institutionalization among Alzheimer disease victims with caregiving spouses. *Journals of Gerontology: Social Sciences, 45,* S259–S266.

Pruchno, R. A., Peters, N. D., Kleban, M. H., & Burant, C. J. (1994). Attachment among adult children and their institutionalized parents. *Journals of Gerontology: Social Sciences, 49,* S209–S218.

Pruchno, R. A., & Potashnik, S. L. (1989). Caregiving spouses physical and mental health in perspective. *Journal of the American Geriatrics Society, 37,* 697–705.

Pruchno, R. A., & Resch, N. L. (1989). Aberrant behaviors and Alzheimer's disease: Mental health effects on spouse caregivers. *Journals of Gerontology, 44,* S177–S182.

Redinbaugh, E. M., MacCallum, R. C., & Kiecolt-Glaser, J. K. (1995). Recurrent syndromal depression in caregivers. *Psychology and Aging, 10,* 358–368.

Reis, M. F., Gold, D. P., Gauthier, S., Andres, D., & Markiewicz, D. (1994). Personality traits as determinants of burden and health complaints in caregiving. *International Journal of Aging and Human Development, 39,* 257–271.

Sands, D., & Suzuki, T. (1983). Adult day care for Alzheimer's patients and their families. *The Gerontologist, 23*(1), 21–23.

Scharlach, A. E. (1994). Caregiving and employment: Competing or complementary roles? *The Gerontologist, 34,* 378–385.

Scharlach, A. E., & Boyd, S. L. (1989). Caregiving and employment: Results of an employee survey. *The Gerontologist, 29,* 382–387.

Scharlach, A. E., & Frenzel, C. (1986). An evaluation of institution-based respite care. *The Gerontologist, 26,* 77–82.

Schneider, L.S., Pollock, V. E., & Lyness, S. A. (1990). A metaanalysis of controlled trials of neuroleptic treatment in dementia. *Journal of American Geriatrics Society, 38,* 553–563.

Schulz, R., Visintainier, P., & Williamson, G. M. (1990). Psychiatric and physical morbidity effects of caregiving. *Journals of Gerontology: Psychological Sciences, 45,* P181–191.

Selye, H. (1976). *The stress of life* (Rev. ed.) (Preface and pp. 1–39). New York: McGraw Hill.

Semple, S.J. (1992). Conflict in Alzheimer's caregiving families: Its dimensions and consequences. *The Gerontologist, 32,* 648–655.

Sheehan, N. W., & Nuttall, P. (1988). Conflict, emotion, and personal strain among family caregivers. *Family Relations, 37,* 92–98.

Sieber, S. D. (1974). Toward a theory of role accumulation. *American Sociological Review, 39,* 567–578.

Skaff, M. M., Pearlin, L. I. (1992). Caregiving: Role engulfument and the loss of self. *The Gerontologist, 32* (5), 656–664.

Stephens, M. A. P., & Franks, M. M. (1995). Spillover between daughters' roles as caregiver and wife: Interference or enhancement? *Journals of Gerontology, 50B,* P9–P17.

Stephens, M. A. P., Franks, M. M., & Townsend, A. L. (1994). Stress and rewards in women's multiple roles: The case of women in the middle. *Psychology and Aging, 9,* 45–52.

Stephens, M. A. P., Norris, V. K., Kinney, J. M., Ritchie, S. W., & Grotz, R. C. (1988). Stressful situations in caregiving: Relations between caregiver coping and well-being. *Psychology and Aging, 3,* 208–209.

Stoller, E. P., & Pugliesi, K. L. (1989). Other roles of caregivers: Competing responsibilities or supportive resources. *Journals of Gerontology: Social Sciences, 44,* S231–S238.

Stone, R., Cafferata, G. L., & Sangl, J. (1987). Caregivers of the frail elderly: A national profile. *The Gerontologist, 27,* 616–626.

Strawbridge, W. J., & Wallhagen, M. I. (1991). Impact of family conflict on adult child caregivers. *The Gerontologist, 31,* 770–777.

Suitor, J. J., & Pillemer, K. (1992). Status transitions and marital satisfaction: The case of adult children caring for elderly parents suffering from dementia. *Journal of Social and Personal Relationships, 9,* 549–562.

Sundström, G. (1992). Care by families: An overview of trends. *Caring for Frail Elderly People, Social Policy Studies, 14.* Paris: OECD.

Tennstedt, S. L., Crawford, S., & McKinlay, J. B. (1993). Determining the pattern of community care: Is coresidence more important than caregiver relationship? *Journals of Gerontology: Social Sciences, 48,* S74–S83.

Tennstedt, S. L., McKinlay, J. B., & Sullivan, L. M. (1989). Informal care for frail elders: The role of secondary caregivers. *The Gerontologist, 29,* 677–683.

Teri, L. (1994). Behavioral treatment of depression in patients with dementia. *Alzheimer Disease and Associated Disorders, 8*(3), 66–74.

Thoits, P. A. (1983). Multiple Identities and psychological well-being: A reformulation and test of the social isolation hypothesis. *American Sociological Review, 48,* 174–187.

Thompson, E. H., Jr., Futterman, A. M., Callagher-Thompson, D., Rose, J. M., & Lovett, S. B. (1993). Social support and caregiver burden in family caregivers of frail elders. *Journals of Gerontology, 48,* S245–S254.

Toseland, R. W., Rossiter, C. M., Peak, T., & Smith, G. C. (1990). Comparative effectiveness of individual and group interventions to support family caregivers. *Social Work, 35,* 209–217.

Townsend, A. (1990). Nursing home care and family caregivers' stress. In M. A. P. Stephens, J. H. Crowther, S. E. Hobfall, & D. L. Tennenbaum (Eds.), *Stress and coping in later life families* (pp. 267–285). Washington, DC: Hemisphere.

Townsend, A. L., & Franks, M. M. (1995). Binding ties: Closeness and conflict in adult children's caregiving relationship. *Psychology and Aging, 10,* 343–351.

Townsend, A., Noelker, L., Deimling, G., & Bass, D. (1989). Longitudinal impact of interhousehold caregiving on adult children's mental health. *Psychology and Aging, 4,* 393–401.

Uchino, B. N., Kiecolt-Glaser, J. K., & Cacioppo, J. T. (1994). Construals of preillness relationship quality predict cardiovascular response in family caregivers of Alzheimer's disease victims. *Psychology and Aging, 9,* 113–120.

Verbrugge, L. M. (1983). Multiple roles and physical health of women and men. *Journal of Health and Social Behavior, 24,* 16–30.

Vitaliano, P. P., Young, H. M., Russo, J., Romano, J., & Magana-Amato, A. (1993). Does expressed emotion in spouses predict subsequent problems among care recipients with Alzheimer's disease? *Journals of Gerontology, 48,* P202–P209.

Walker, A. J., Martin, S. S. K., & Jones, L. L. (1992). The benefits and costs of caregiving and care receiving for daughters and mothers. *Journals of Gerontology, 47,* S130–S139.

Webster, P. S., & Herzog, A. R. (1995). Effects of parental divorce and memories of family problems on relationships between adult children and their parents. *Journals of Gerontology, 50B,* S24–S34.

Weihl, H. (1983). Three issues from the Israeli scene. *The Gerontologist, 23,* 576–578.

Weissert, W. G., Elston, J. M., Bolda, E. J., Zelman, W. N., Mutran, E., & Mangum, A. B. (1990). *Adult day care: Findings from a national survey.* Baltimore, MD: Johns Hopkins University Press.

White, L. (1992). The effect of parental divorce and remarriage on parental support for adult children. *Journal of Family Issues, 13,* 234–250.

Whitlatch, C. J., & Noelker, L. S. (in press). Caregiving and caring. In J. E. Birren (Ed.), *Encyclopedia of gerontology.* New York: Academic Press.

Whitlatch, C.J., Zarit, S.H., & von Eye, A. (1991). Efficacy of interventions with caregivers: A reanalysis. *The Gerontologist, 31,* 9–14.

Whitlatch, C. J., Zarit, S. H., Goodwin, P. E., & von Eye, A. (1995). Influence of the success of psychoeducational interventions on the course of family care. *Clinical Gerontologist, 16,* 17–30.

Williamson, G. M., & Schulz, R. (1993). Coping with specific stressors in Alzheimer's disease caregiving. *The Gerontologist, 33,* 747–755.

Worach-Kardas, H. (1983). The Polish family tradition. *The Gerontologist, 23,* 593–596.

Wright, L. K. (1993). *Alzheimer's disease and marriage: An intimate account.* Newbury Park, CA: Sage.

Wright, L., Clipp, E., & George, L. (1993). Health consequences of caregiver stress. *Medicine Exercise Nutrition and Health, 2,* 181–195.

Zarit, J. M., & Zarit, S. H. (in press). Til death do us part. In R. P. Halgin & S. K. Whitbourne (Eds.) *Partners in change: Growth through the therapeutic process.* New York: Oxford University Press.

Zarit, S.H. (1996). Clinical interventions for family caregiving. In S. H. Zarit & B. Knight (Eds.), *A guide to psychotherapy and aging: Clinical intervention in a life stage context.* Washington, DC: APA Books.

Zarit, S. H., & Eggebeen, D. J. (1995). Parent child relationships in adulthood and old age. In M. H. Bornstein (Ed.), *Handbook of parenting: Vol. 1. Children and parenting* (pp. 119–140). Mahwah, NJ: Lawrence Erlbaum.

Zarit, S. H., Johansson, B., & Berg, S. (1993). Functional

impairment and co-disability in the oldest old. *Journal of Aging and Health*, *5*, 291–305.

Zarit, S. H., Orr, N. K., & Zarit, J. M. (1985). *The hidden victims of Alzheimer's Disease: Families under stress*. New York: NYU Press.

Zarit, S. H., Stephens, M. A. P., Townsend, A. & Greene, R. (1996, November). Adult day care and the relief of caregiver strain. Paper presented at the annual meeting of the Gerontological Society of America, Washington, DC.

Zarit, S. H., Todd, P. A., & Zarit, J. M. (1986). Subjective burden of husbands and wives as caregivers: A longitudinal study. *The Gerontologist*, *26*, 260–266.

Zarit, S. H. & Whitlatch, C. J. (1992). Institutional placement: Phases of the transition. *The Gerontologist*, *32*, 665–672.

7.23
Rehabilitation in Old Age: Psychosocial Issues

CLEMENS TESCH-RÖMER
Ernst Moritz Arndt University, Greifswald, Germany
and
HANS-WERNER WAHL
German Center for Research on Aging at the University of Heidelberg, Germany

7.23.1 INTRODUCTION

Aging is associated with an increase in acute and chronic illness with serious consequences for daily living. To give the reader an idea of how prevalent these self-limiting conditions are in old age, the following empirical findings (Ebrahim, 1992; Kemp,1985) are used. The percentage of persons with arthritis increases from 1% for the less than 17 years old group to about 25% for the (noninstitutionalized) over 65 years old group. Heart conditions increase from 2.4% for the under 17 group to 23.4% for the over 65 group (these rates are significantly higher depending on the mode of data collection [self-reports versus medical expert rating; Jette, 1996). Visual and hearing disorders also increase dramatically with age. About one third of all persons 65 and older exhibits a significant hearing loss; about 8% suffer from severe age-related visual impairment. The prevalence of mental disorders also increases with age. The percentage of persons with major depression is about 11%; the percentage of elderly with at least some degree of dementia also hovers around 11%. Strokes, degenerative neurological disorders, pulmonary disorders, and most orthopedic disabilities increase with age at a similar rate. Also, there is convergent evidence that these prevalence rates increase dramatically from the young-old to the old-old and the oldest-old and are especially high in institutionalized settings (e.g., Jette, 1996; Suzman, Willis, & Manton, 1992; Schneekloth & Müller, 1995).

Whereas acute illnesses normally can be treated quite adequately in many old and very old persons, the burden of chronic illness (as well as the disabilities and functional losses in daily life that result from them) have become one of the most dramatic challenges for society, for gerontology in general, and for rehabilitation with elderly clients in particular. If our basic goal is to engender a "good" life into old age by fostering "active life expectancy" among the elderly (e.g., Crimmins, Hayward, & Saito, 1996), then rehabilitative work as the process of maximizing abilities after a disabling event (Kemp, 1996) gains crucial importance for the individual as well as for society.

Nevertheless, the burden imposed by chronic conditions, and the rehabilitative efforts to counteract them, deserve a highly differentiated analysis. Oversimplifying statements, whether positive or negative with respect to the power of rehabilitation to improve the lives of the elderly, are detrimental to research and can wreak havoc with the hopes and fears of the frail and chronically ill elderly and their families. On the one hand, the metamorphosis of gerontology from a decline and deficit view of old age toward a competence view that stresses the potentials and reserve capacities of old age has influenced significantly the field of geriatric rehabilitation. The body of empirical evidence underscores the success of rehabilitation in the elderly with respect to stroke, arthritis, cardiovascular disease, and falls (e.g., Andrews, 1987; Harris, O'Hara, & Harper, 1995; Kemp, 1985, 1996; Meier-Baumgartner, Nerenheim-Duscha, & Görres, 1992; Rubenstein et al., 1984; Schütz, 1993; Tallis, 1992). In addition, there is evidence that rehabilitation leads to better outcomes in the short and long run as compared to traditional medical treatment. On the other hand, convergent evidence from longitudinal and catamnestic studies show that the success of rehabilitation is tempered by everyday factors; further deterioration due to the underlying disease process, a lack of rehabilitation capacity in the homecare setting, poor ecological circumstances, or dependence-supporting behavior of the social environment (e.g., Horgas, Wahl, & Baltes, 1996; Meier-Baumgartner et al., 1992; Wahl & Baltes, 1993) can have a lasting, negative impact on the rehabilitation process.

With this in mind, it is accepted broadly in the academic field that rehabilitation with the elderly deserves additional research efforts in order to maximize its efficiency. For example, special problems that arise when treating the elderly must be considered, such as multimorbidity, concomitant cognitive impairments, reduced social networks, poor ecological conditions, longer time periods to regain certain functions, and lowered motivation ("I am too old; this is not worth the effort."). There is also general consensus within the professional field that rehabilitation truly deserves a multidisciplinary approach. The multiprofessional team should include high quality medical personnel, a psychiatrist, well-educated nursing staff, physical therapists, occupational therapists, speech pathologists, social workers, nutritionists, audiologists, and optometricians as well as experts in housing, design, and technical devices (Kemp, 1996; Saltz, 1995; Zeiss & Steffen, 1996). There is additional consent that rehabilitation of the elderly should take place in different settings such as the hospital, day-care center, home health care, and nursing home settings.

What is stressed in this chapter is that psychology as a research and applied field is essential to geriatric rehabilitation in all of these settings. The critical importance of addressing geropsychological and psychosocial issues in the field of geriatric rehabilitation is underscored by the two contrasting theoretical approaches briefly alluded to above. With respect to the competence view of rehabilitation in old age, the emergence and application of psychological intervention techniques such as behavioral or cognitive training programs has broadened significantly the scope of rehabilitation in different settings (in the nursing home setting in particular; e.g., Hussian & Davis, 1985; Wisocki, 1991). Also, there is general consensus that the differential success of rehabilitation programs has as much to do with underlying psychological and social issues (e.g., motivational issues, personality traits, sense of self-efficacy, ability to mobilize social support) as with the "objective" severity of the disease process. With respect to the limits and the fragility of rehabilitation success, the psychosocial perspective points to crucial aspects such as inadequate housing, certain neighborhood characteristics, and the attitudes and behaviors of significant others who may undermine the elderly's striving toward independent functioning (Baltes, 1996).

This chapter was written by two geropsychologists and thus presupposes that rehabilitation with the elderly can be effectively provided if a multidisciplinary and multiprofessional approach is applied. The task is to highlight the psychological and psychosocial perspective within geriatric rehabilitation. This is done in four sections: (i) general principles and geropsychological essentials of rehabilitation, (ii) psychosocial issues and strategies of rehabilitation with older adults (assessment issues, restoration of functional independence, cognitive retraining, psychotherapeutic intervention, motivation and compliance, role of social support, ecological aspects), (iii) psychosocial issues with respect to particular client groups (stroke, arthritis, the sensory impaired, demented patients), and (iv) final consideration of practical, research-related, and ethical problems of rehabilitation in old age.

7.23.2 GENERAL PRINCIPLES AND GEROPSYCHOLOGICAL ESSENTIALS OF REHABILITATION IN OLD AGE

7.23.2.1 General Principles

Rehabilitation is required whenever an impairment or a disability causes permanent, widespread disruption of the normal fit between person and environment. Central to understanding rehabilitation is the distinction between impairment, disability, and handicap (World Health Organization, 1980). Impairment is any loss or abnormality of psychological, physiological, or anatomical structure or function. Disability is any restriction, due to impairment, which limits the ability to perform an activity in the manner or within the range considered normal for a human being. Handicap is defined as a disadvantage resulting from an impairment or disability that limits or prevents the fulfillment of a role appropriate to a person's age, gender, social, and cultural circumstances. For example, a stroke might lead to pathological changes in the brain and quite often to unilateral paralysis (impairment). These stroke-induced impairments are responsible for deteriorations in walking, manual dexterity, memory, and speech performance (disability). These disabilities in turn lead to social consequences for the individual, preventing the person from participating in social roles and activities (handicap).

Rehabilitation can be regarded as a problem-solving and educational process aimed at reducing the disability and handicap experienced by someone as a result of disease, one that is always limited by the resources available (World Health Organization, 1980). Hence, rehabilitation is a set of procedures located between acute medical treatment and prevention. Of course, curable diseases should be treated medically, but whenever possible one should prevent disease instead of dealing with disabling and handicapping consequences. This statement is by no means trivial, as epidemiological data on stroke shows. Preventive measures are responsible for decreasing incidence rates for cardiovascular stroke (e.g., Svanborg, 1988; see also Fries, 1990). Nevertheless, rehabilitation is necessary in those cases where prevention or medical treatment are not effective. Hence, the focus of rehabilitative interventions is not the (underlying) disease but the functional level (e.g., Kemp, 1996). A medical diagnosis, that is knowledge about a certain impairment, does not necessarily imply knowledge about resulting disabilities and handicaps. Indeed, pronounced discrepancies in the emotional or functional outcomes between different patients suffering from "objectively" comparable diseases are more often the rule than the exception and require careful attention.

Rehabilitation is not only aimed at restoring the patients' rights, privileges, reputation, and/or proper condition, but also at realizing their potential, reablement, and resettlement (Ebrahim, 1992). However, rehabilitation with the elderly does not necessarily mean *restitutio ad integrum* (complete cure of disease, full elimination of handicap) but quite often *restitutio ad optimum* (improving functional capability and maximizing wellness). According to Williams (1984), rehabilitation in old age may be characterized as a set of techniques as well as a point of view or a philosophy. In accordance with this philosophy, the primary aim of rehabilitation is to restore an individual to their former functional status, or to maintain or maximize independent functioning (Lee & Itoh, 1990; Williams, 1994). Getting elderly clients to transfer themselves from the bed to a wheelchair may thus be a great rehabilitation success and have tremendous impact on the elderly persons' perception of life. At younger ages, the main goal of rehabilitation is the restoration of the individual's capacity to resume family and work roles. However, these are not necessarily the main goals of rehabilitation in old age. Rather, functional independence (self care and instrumental activities of daily living), the cultivation of leisure activities, and a sense of well-being, that is, improvement of life quality, are the main objectives of rehabilitation in old age (Andrews, 1991; Kemp, 1996; Mosqueda, 1996).

The general goals of geriatric rehabilitation are to control the underlying disease process, prevent secondary disabilities, restore functional abilities, facilitate the patient's adaptation, educate the patient regarding impairment, and modify or otherwise prepare the environment (Kemp, 1985; Saudan, 1990). The process of rehabilitation can be divided into five formal components (Ebrahim, 1992; Wade, 1992):

(i) *Assessment*. In addition to medical diagnosis, the identification, analysis, and measurement of problems in terms of disabilities and handicaps is an essential first step in the rehabilitation process.

(ii) *Planning*. This is extremely important in setting long-term, intermediate, and short-term goals. It is necessary to involve the patient as early and as intensively as possible in this planning procedure, since the acceptance of rehabilitation goals is important for motivation and compliance.

(iii) *Treatment*. Having identified the problems and formulated goals, the proper intervention should take place in order to reduce disability and minimize handicap. Treatment might consist of interventions aimed at the restoration of functional independence, cognitive retraining, psychotherapy or mobilization of social support.

(iv) *Care*. Although rehabilitation is aimed at restoring maximal functional capacity, very often care is necessary to support elderly persons and alleviate the consequences of disability.

(v) *Evaluation*. Great importance, although not a standard procedure in many rehabilitation settings, is the careful evaluation of the effectiveness of intervention which should consist of individual reassessment during or after the rehabilitation process (Görres, 1994).

Psychosocial and clinical-psychological issues play an important role in all of these components. Thus, rehabilitation should be based on a comprehensive psychological profile of the elderly client that includes neuropsychology evaluation as well as the assessment of personality, emotional-motivational functions and personal goals ((i) and (ii) above, assessment and planning). Individuals also need psychological support in order to cope with the existential crises normally following the onset of disability; treatment should focus on fostering behavioral, cognitive, and emotional changes, working on specific coping strategies, promoting self-esteem, improving family relations, and mobilizing other social network resources ((iii) and (iv) above; treatment and care). Finally, everyday life after rehabilitation should not only be seen in terms of functional gains but also in terms of life quality (subjective well-being, self-efficacy, and positive future expectations; (v) above; evaluation).

The goals of geriatric rehabilitation call for a thorough understanding of clinical psychology. Likewise, concepts from geropsychology and lifespan developmental psychology are fundamental to any rehabilitative endeavor. In the following pages, the theoretical foundations of geriatric rehabilitation are reviewed in some detail, before turning to psychosocial issues and strategies of rehabilitation with the elderly.

7.23.2.2 Geropsychological Essentials of Rehabilitation in Old Age

In practice, rehabilitation efforts will only be effective when essential concepts from gerontological and geropsychological research have been given due consideration. Because aging is a lifelong process, it is suggested that lifespan developmental psychology is crucial to gerontology and can contribute greatly to these conceptual essentials (e.g., Baltes, 1987; Lehr, 1993; 1996; Thomae, 1979).

First of all, the rehabilitation of the elderly should not be based on chronological age (or old age) per se but on aging. That is, the emphasis should lie on aging as a dynamic process which can be characterized, like any period of the lifespan, as the simultaneous occurrence of potentials and limits, gains and losses, continuity and change (Baltes, 1987; Thomae, 1979). A variety of studies within geropsychology and developmental psychology stresses the elderly person's potential for growth and development, contrasting starkly with a one-sided picture of mere decline (for overview, see Kruse, 1987; Lehr, 1996). Even when faced with severe competence losses, elderly persons are not reactive, helpless, or passive; instead, the majority of these elderly use a whole scope of coping strategies to deal actively and differentially with threats to their independence and life quality. Rehabilitation of the elderly should thus count on these coping capabilities to address severe illnesses or disabilities. Also, a major task of rehabilitation lies in the reactivation of the elderly person's potential to deal actively with their health threats, thereby regaining as much independent functioning in everyday life as possible. The strategy of selective optimization with compensation is a general adaptational tool to counteract detrimental health changes (e.g., Baltes & Baltes, 1990). From this point of view, rehabilitation in old age can be understood as the transmission of powerful compensation techniques and a mutual search for selective optimization opportunities (particularly in those cases in which the impairment and resulting disabilities can only be altered marginally). To conclude, rehabilitation in old age must base itself upon the insight that elderly persons possess certain fundamental physical and mental potentials (Kruse, 1992); agism must be scoured thoroughly from the rehabilitation effort.

Furthermore, the pronounced interindividual variability of the elderly must also be considered. Persuasive empirical indications from cognitive, personality, and social network research, show that heterogeneity is one of the defining criteria of the aged population (e.g., Nelson & Dannefer, 1992). The general implication for rehabilitation is that a highly individualized approach is necessary. In particular, there is reason to assume that the estimation of the rehabilitation potential deserves an individual point of view and can be significantly different even when the underlying disease (such as a certain type of stroke) is relatively similar between cases (Kruse, 1992). The mere fact that some individuals possess lifelong expertise in particular areas (whereas other individuals do not) may have tremendous implications for rehabilitation. The acknowledgment of variability also points to the need that rehabilitation efforts should not only focus on impairments and disabilities but also on remaining capacities and competencies.

Rehabilitative work must also view aging as an inherently biographical process (Lehr, 1996; Kruse, 1992; Thomae, 1996). Old age is a significant part of the individual biography and life course. Over the course of their lives, individuals develop particular attitudes and coping styles in dealing with everyday challenges and critical life events, such as the onset of severe health problems. Rehabilitation must not neglect these personal styles in dealing with illnesses; it may mean the difference between gaining a powerful tool to understand the idiosyncrasies of the elderly individual and jeopardizing the success of the rehabilitative effort. Individual development, biographical experiences, and evaluative standards also stress the importance of understanding the subjective interpretations assigned to competence losses in everyday life. It is commonplace in clinical work for subjective evaluations of illnesses, impairments, and disability to differ significantly from the ratings of physicians, clinical psychologists, and other professionals involved in the rehabilitation process. One consequence of these discrepancies can be that different goal attainment priorities between the elderly in rehabilitation and their professional surroundings emerge which may delay or even undermine rehabilitation success.

According to leading scholars in the field of lifespan developmental psychology (e.g., Baltes, 1987), aging must also be seen as a contextual phenomenon. One set of powerful factors is social influence. It is known from a body of classical work in gerontology that the course of aging is influenced by the way social networks have been arranged and maintained. Also that social contact means, on the one hand, mutual exchange, personal warmth, the opportunity to give and to receive, and in a sense even physical and cognitive training. On the other hand, social surroundings may hinder the elderly individual from using or exercising capabilities and may thus contribute to a decline in functioning. Rehabilitation should always consider the social embeddedness of aging processes, especially with regard to severe health problems. Thus, there is a need to integrate significant others in the rehabilitation process. These persons represent concrete links with the everyday world in which the elderly person will return; they may deserve training and education about how to interact with the elderly person after the rehabilitation program.

Aging is, however, also aging in place, that is, aging is also influenced by the physical environment (e.g., Lawton & Nahemow, 1973; Parmelee & Lawton, 1990; Saup, 1993; Wahl, 1992). Rehabilitation has to consider the simple fact that elderly faced with severe losses in competence do not normally age in clinical or institutional settings but in their own "world" at home. From this perspective, it is one of the challenges of rehabilitation to intervene as effectively as possible (which, in many cases, can only be done in a formal rehabilitation setting) but nevertheless as close to the everyday world of the elderly person as possible.

Finally, a very important construct in the rehabilitation of the aged stems from lifespan developmental psychology: plasticity (e.g., Baltes, 1987; Kruse, 1992). This term signifies that the course of aging is not predetermined or fixed, regardless of whether the process in question is one of "normal" aging or aging coupled with serious illnesses and disabilities. For example, cognitive training studies have underlined clearly the potential for significant gains which can sometimes exceed the level of untrained younger persons (Baltes, 1993; see also below). So-called control-enhancing interventions have proven their physical and psychological benefits even in frail elderly populations like nursing home residents (e.g., Rodin, 1986). Aging obviously is not a fixed and predetermined process but is subject to many different types of influences which may lead to differential outcomes. Rehabilitation may thus be regarded as one of the most powerful attempts to systematically influence aging organisms challenged by chronic disease processes.

In conclusion, the fact is emphasized that the fundamental principles and concepts of geriatric rehabilitation rest upon clinical as well as geropsychological insights. This should be kept in mind as some of the main psychosocial issues and strategies of rehabilitation in old age are discussed.

7.23.3 PSYCHOSOCIAL ISSUES AND STRATEGIES OF REHABILITATION IN OLD AGE

7.23.3.1 Assessment Issues

There is wide agreement that only comprehensive geriatric assessment (CGA) can serve as a basis for successful rehabilitative work with the elderly (e.g., Stuck, Siu, Wieland, Adams, & Rubenstein, 1992). Although not expressed explicitly in this widely used term, the assessment of psychological functioning is as a very important part of CGA. Furthermore, geropsychological knowledge and research can contribute to the shortcomings of CGA as it is commonly conducted in most rehabilitation settings. It should be mentioned that the aim of this section is not to give a complete overview of cognitive and neuropsychological assessment (which undoubtedly is also critical with respect to geriatric rehabilitation and its outcomes; see Chapter 7, this volume; see also Franzen & Martin, 1996; Rentz, 1991); instead, issues beyond the assessment of cognitive functioning will be discussed (cf. Lawton & Teresi, 1994). Comprehensive geriatric assessment has at least three major tasks: (i) to measure individual functional capacity, that is, losses as well as competencies at the beginning and during the course of the rehabilitation process; (ii) to contribute to the planning and prognosis of rehabilitation; and (iii) to serve as a tool for quality assurance and evaluation. To fulfill these tasks, CGA is basically aimed at the differential description of disease-related impairments to everyday life and functioning (see again the functional approach as one general principle of rehabilitation, above).

7.23.3.1.1 Activities of daily living and instrumental activities of daily living

One core issue of CGA is thus the estimation of decline and competence in activities of daily living (ADL) of varying complexity. In most research and practical work, basic ADL such as the capacity for eating, washing, or dressing are differentiated from instrumental activities of daily living (IADL), such as shopping, phone use, banking, or the intake of medications. A whole range of rather similar scales for the measurement of ADL and IADL can be found in the psychological literature. With respect to the basic ADL, the Barthel index has found wide use in geriatric rehabilitation (Mahoney & Barthel, 1965); prototypical IADL are represented in the widely applied Lawton and Brody scale (Lawton & Brody, 1969).

All of these scales are short and easy to apply. However, there are also problems: for one, the assessment of functional capacity is based mostly on face validity and still lacks theoretical foundation. It is thus strongly argued for closer links between the ADL/IADL literature (including their respective assessment devices in the clinical setting) and emerging theoretical and empirical research on everyday competence (e.g., Baltes, Maas, Wilms, & Borchelt, 1996; Willis, 1991, 1996). In particular, this latter work supports the notion that everyday competence depends heavily on personal and environmental variables that lie beyond chronic illness conditions such as cognitive performance and environmental barriers. One assessment implication of this insight is the need to "diagnose" the physical environment and always interpret a given degree of competence or impairment in everyday functioning (as assessed based on the common ADL/IADL approach) as the result of a transaction between personal capabilities and environmental circumstances. Furthermore, the existing everyday competence literature suggests that basic ADL and IADL are fundamentally different: the former are closely linked to basic physical capacity, whereas the latter depend heavily on motivation and socialization (e.g., preparing meals in elderly men). Second, functional capacity and thus the assessment of everyday performance should not only be focused on ADL and IADL; the capacity to solve everyday problems effectively (Willis, 1996) and to perform leisure activities in the social and nonsocial domain deserve to be assessed as well (e.g., Baltes et al., 1996) in order to gain a comprehensive picture of the everyday implications of chronic disablement.

7.23.3.1.2 Performance vs. reserve capacity

ADL/IADL scales can measure performance in functioning but not remaining reserve capacity, that is the individual's potential for further growth, which can be activated during the rehabilitation process. Although there is no *via regia* to approach this issue (which is a crucial one for planning the rehabilitation process), one important aspect in this regard is to consider the personality characteristics of the elderly client (see below).

Obviously, it would not make very much sense to expect that the reactivation of remaining reserve capacities always occurs under ideal personal and environmental conditions. Although it is always possible to alter personality (e.g., by psychotherapeutic intervention) or modify the social and physical surroundings, an adequate and realistic estimation of the current personal and living situation of the elderly client is indispensable. For example, anamnestic exploration should not only focus on the medical history but also on personal motivations, biographical key experiences with relevance for the coping with the current rehabilitation process, subjective evaluations of personal competencies, and coping styles (see the geropsychological essentials of rehabilitation described above). Another important area encompasses personality variables such as introversion—extraversion or anxiety. Both of these variables probably influence the rehabilitation process in different ways. For example, the personality characteristic of introversion versus extraversion may strongly influence the motivation to regain mastery over daily living tasks. Also, trait as well as state anxiety may undermine rehabilitation and transferral to the home situation if not taken seriously.

The results of all of these assessments can be crucial for the development of the final rehabilitation plan. Rehabilitation should always be done in close cooperation with the individual because the implementation of relevant goals and strategies depends heavily on the client's insight, motivation, and compliance. According to the contextuality of the aging process and the docility of the chronically ill organism to "pressing" environmental conditions (as stated quite early on in the so-called Environmental Docility Hypothesis, see Lawton & Simon, 1968), assessment should also include the description of the physical home environment (see, for example, Regnier & Pynoos, 1987). Also, the measurement of rehabilitation outcome should be regarded as more than mere ADL/IADL improvement. The basic aim of rehabilitation to contribute to life quality in general deserves the assessment of subjective well-being, depressivity, or of mood states as well (Kemp, 1996).

7.23.3.2 Restoration of Functional Independence

7.23.3.2.1 Functional independence as basic objective of geriatric rehabilitation

The restoration of functional independence can be regarded as one of the most important, though not the only, objective of geriatric rehabilitation. Independent functioning in daily life is highly valued within (Western) society; hence, the preservation or restoration of independence represents one of the most important life goals of most elderly. Basic ADL functions to be considered are self-care (such as eating, drinking, dressing, grooming, washing, and controlling urination and bowel movements) and mobility (getting in and out of bed, chair, or toilet, walking, and climbing stairs). For community dwelling elderly persons, being capable of performing instrumental activities of daily living is extremely important (doing household chores, shopping, cooking). There is also reason to assume that independent functioning in these daily living tasks is associated closely with related personal variables such as perceptions of control, self-efficacy, and competency; thus, personal autonomy can contribute much to good psychological adaptation in the course of aging.

Obviously, the majority of efforts within the multiprofessional team, such as physical or occupational therapy, is aimed toward improving functional capacity. It must once again be emphasized here that this goal does not necessarily entail the restoration of full independence. As Kemp (1996) has put it, to manage the step from "maximum assist" to "partial assist" can mean a dramatic gain for the elderly individual as well as their social environment. Most importantly, this "small" step can enable the individual to remain in a private household situation and to avoid relocation to a nursing home setting. Reliance upon functional criteria in rehabilitation is reliance upon personal variables, and the latter repeatedly have proven themselves superior to mere medical diagnoses in the prediction of important outcome variables (e.g., nursing home entry, daily life quality, life satisfaction, and even mortality; e.g., Kemp, 1996).

7.23.3.2.2 *Contributions from clinical geropsychology*

It would be shortsighted, however, to view the restoration of independence solely from a physical training perspective. Although bodily functions such as gross and fine mobility are important for performance of ADL and IADL (and should, thus, be trained by different means during geriatric rehabilitation), there is reason to assume that psychological factors are important as well. One factor is cognitive performance (e.g., Baltes et al., 1996; Willis, 1991); cognitive retraining can contribute significantly to the regaining of everyday competence. Also, since striving toward independence has much to do with the motivational and goal-directedness of each client, counseling and psychotherapeutic interventions can maximize the effects of medically-oriented treatments such as physical therapy and training in basic mobility (see respective sections below).

The restoration of functional independence in daily living tasks is also a prototypical case for the effectiveness of behavioral modification techniques based on social-learning principles, that is, it underscores the worth of a genuinely psychological intervention strategy. A whole body of research has demonstrated that such techniques (e.g., the use of different reinforcement procedures) can contribute significantly to the maintenance or restoration of functional independence in the elderly (e.g., Hasselkus, 1989; Smyer, Zarit, & Qualls, 1990; Wisocki, 1991). These approaches have particular rehabilitative value in institutionalized settings. Not long ago, the institutionalized elderly more or less led passive, sheltered lives under custodial care. In the 1990s, there is a basic consensus that institutions should be able to promote successful aging; they are not only expected to provide a secure and prosthetic environment, but also to stimulate autonomy (Baltes, Wahl, & Reichert, 1991). As was shown in a research program, the etiology and maintenance of dependence in institutions is related closely to the social environment, that is, the dependence-supportive behavior of staff and others in institutionalized settings. The systematic change of these interaction patterns by means of cognitive and behavioral training with staff led to a significant increase in the independent functioning of nursing home residents (e.g., Baltes & Wahl, 1996). Because a strong tendency has been found toward independence-supportive behavior within the home health setting (e.g., Baltes & Wahl, 1992), rehabilitative efforts based on cognitive and behavioral motivations should not be reserved solely for institutional settings.

Functional loss is thus not only a characteristic of the person but always a feature person–environment interchange. Naturally, this fact carries implications for rehabilitation. Disability may be reduced by increasing personal competence, changing situational demands, or employing effective compensation strategies (e.g., simplification or redesign of the task; see also Dixon & Bäckman, 1995). Due to practical constraints in terms of time, effort, or money, rehabilitation aimed toward the restoration of functional independence thus is forced frequently to make a decision of what is more promising, that is, to change the person, to change the environment, or to change the task performance itself. Assessment issues like the ones described above (i.e., information pertaining to the elderly client as well as their social and physical environment) is particularly helpful in selecting the best possible from these alternatives.

7.23.3.3 Cognitive Retraining

Cognitive capacity can be divided into two broad ability categories; fluid intelligence and crystallized intelligence (Baltes, 1984; Cattell, 1971; Horn & Hofer, 1992). Fluid intelligence, also called cognitive mechanics, encompasses the most basic cognitive processes and is measured mostly using memory tasks, problem-solving tasks, or perceptual speed tasks. Crystallized intelligence, or cognitive pragmatics, encompasses the experience and knowledge-related parts of cognitive capacity and is measured using knowledge or fluency tasks. Several studies have shown a decline in fluid intelligence already by middle age, while crystallized intelligence shows stability in adulthood and declines markedly only in old age (Salthouse, 1991; Schaie & Willis, 1993; Smith & Baltes, 1996). Such cognitive decline in old age seems characteristic of normal aging; it is not confined to elderly persons with a diagnosis of dementia (Reischies & Lindenberger, 1996), although it is more severe in such cases. Dementia is a syndrome due to brain disease in which there is impairment of multiple higher cortical functions, including memory, thinking, orientation, comprehension, learning capacity, and language (see also Chapter 10, this volume). The prevalence rates for dementia range from 3–7% for the population over 65 years, and increases dramatically with advancing age (Cooper, 1991a). Given cognitive decline in old age, and especially in the case of dementia, it is worth investigating whether (re)training might possibly help with these age- and/or disease-related losses.

7.23.3.3.1 Intelligence training

Experimental studies have demonstrated that cognitive interventions in old age are successful (Baltes & Lindenberger, 1988; Baltes,1993). In several studies, it could be shown that the cognitive performance of elderly people is modifiable (Baltes, Sowarka, & Kliegl, 1989; Blieszner, Willis, & Baltes, 1981; Willis, Blieszner, & Baltes, 1981). In these studies, the emphasis of training was on explaining and practicing rules for solving figural relations tasks and inductive reasoning problems. Even with few (5–10) training sessions, elderly participants increased their test scores in post-intervention assessments. Despite the gains achieved in cognitive training, it seems necessary to ensure the generalizability of these interventions (e.g., training in inductive reasoning, deductive reasoning, fluency, and memory techniques should help elderly people solve practical, everyday problems). Furthermore, the rehabilitative power of combining cognitive training with other intervention strategies (e.g., psychomotor training components, training in everyday problem solving) deserve consideration (see for instance Butler & Namerow, 1988, and their differentiation between cognitive retraining, aimed at improving cognitive "micro-processes," and skill acquisition training as a functional "macro-treatment" with greater rehabilitation impact; e.g., Oswald, Rupprecht, & Gunzelmann, 1998). Elderly persons at risk of dementia or even at low to moderate levels of dementia also can profit from cognitive training, although their training gains are much lower than those of healthy persons (Bäckman, Josephsson, Herlitz, Stigsdottir, & Viitanen, 1991; Baltes & Sowarka, 1995). Plasticity appears to be greatly reduced in dementia, even at the onset. Therefore, it has been argued that cognitive training might be a useful diagnostic tool for the early detection of dementia processes (e.g., the testing-the-limits approach; Baltes, Kühl, Gutzmann, & Sowarka, 1995).

7.23.3.3.2 Memory training

Decrease in memory capacity seems to be a marker of aging, at least in the subjective conceptions of elderly people (Abson & Rabbitt, 1988). More equivocal support for memory decline in old age has been reported (Fleischmann, 1989; Kausler, 1991). Nevertheless, memory training with older participants has been tested carefully. A wide variety of memory tasks (recognition, free recall, or pair-association learning) and memory strategies (including diverse mnemotechniques like verbal categorization, elaboration, visual imagery, and the method of loci; Fleischmann, 1982; Yesavage, Lapp, & Sheikh, 1989) have been examined. In the majority of these experiments, the effects of memory training in elderly people are positive. Interestingly, memory training which combines memory strategies with reattribution training, in order to reduce exaggerated achievement levels and change attribution patterns for success and failure, might help elderly people most (Lachman, Weaver, Bandura, Elliott, & Lewkowicz 1992; Weinert & Knopf, 1990). Memory training can be effective in mildly demented elderly persons as well (Ermini-Fünfschilling & Meier,1995). Still, the generalizability of memory training from laboratory settings to everyday memory functioning has yet to be proven (see also Camp, et al., 1993).

7.23.3.3.3 Reality orientation training

Persons suffering from dementia can profit greatly from training in time and space orientation (Kaschel, Zeiser-Kaschel, & Mayer, 1992). Dementia not only affects higher order problem solving but, in later stages, it also impedes basic functions like orienting in time (year, season, day of the month), space (rooms of apartment or institution), and contacting communication partners (staff members, family). Basic cognitive training encompasses orientation in time and space; also, reinforcement of the mechanics and pragmatics of intelligence may be included depending on the cognitive status of the rehabilitation client (e.g., Bäckman et al., 1991; Koh et al., 1994; Little, 1991; Rentz, 1991). Speech and communication therapy might also be very helpful in demented patients or patients suffering from stroke (Sarno, 1984; Jordan, Worral, Hickson, & Dodd, 1993). However, persons with dementia do not only profit from cognitive training in the strict sense of the word. A reactivating occupational therapy program can complement functional rehabilitation in long-term geriatric inpatients with slight to moderate dementia (Bach, Bach, Böhmer, Frühwald, & Grilc, 1995).

To summarize, it can be stated that although younger persons profit even more from cognitive interventions, intelligence and memory training are effective in the healthy elderly. Relatively smaller training effects have been demonstrated in the demented elderly, also. Despite the successes reported in such research, cognitive interventions which fit the everyday needs of elderly people are still the exception. Practical problem solving like reading (and understanding) public transportation schedules might be a good example (Schaie & Willis, 1986). It is also unclear whether cognitive interventions have substantial, long-term consequences. Especially in the case of dementia, however, such interventions might support the person and their caregivers in getting along with the ever-increasing complexity of everyday life.

7.23.3.4 Psychotherapeutic Intervention

Disability and handicap mean a more or less sudden decrease in the functional capacity of the elderly person; this may severely threaten mental balance and stability. Most threatening for elderly persons is the anticipation that living conditions must be changed dramatically in the near future (such as the relocation to an institutional setting) or that future life will only be possible at the cost of great dependency upon others. The psychological burden of losing one's own independence is compounded by the anticipation of becoming a burden to others, thereby negatively influencing the life course of loved ones. There is also broad evidence in the depression literature that severe physical chronic conditions are correlated significantly with depressive episodes (e.g., Schulz & Williamson, 1993; see also Gatz, Kasl-Godley, & Karel, 1996); in other words, besides functional impairments, the identity and self-esteem of the handicapped person are also threatened.

Geriatric rehabilitation seldom calls upon psychotherapy to play the role it should in addressing the psychological crisis experienced by the disabled elderly. Rehabilitation should, however, rise to meet the challenge of helping the elderly person to cope successfully with their disabilities and handicaps. To restate the argument: psychologists have more than only diagnostic tasks to fulfill in geriatric rehabilitation.

Because of the time limitations of normal rehabilitation efforts, individual and group psychotherapy based on a cognitive-behavioral philosophy seem particularly promising to deal with these problems, especially with depressive episodes (Hartke & Horowitz, 1991; Smyer, et al., 1990). However, treatment of depression is only one focus. There are further challenges having to do with the optimization of the rehabilitation success as well as with the maintenance of outcomes, particularly when transitioning from the hospital to the home situation. One task is to enhance motivation in certain clients, particularly in those who have started rehabilitation based on an externally induced motivation ("My wife suggested to try it."). Another approach with special importance for the maintenance of rehabilitation success in the "real world" employs coping skills training (see also Rodin, 1986). This powerful preventive tool serves to develop strategies and train the individual to deal with daily hassles, stress, and possible failure, all of which occur frequently after returning home.

Also, counseling with the goal of enhancing feelings of self-efficacy and competence (despite severe disabilities) may be an important task for clinical psychologists in geriatric rehabilitation. In some cases, psychological support with the goal of learning to accept irreversible losses is critical as well. Social competence training may be particularly helpful in those elderly living alone and running the risk of becoming still more isolated after the onset of chronic illnesses and the disabilities and handicaps they entail. Finally, counseling the relatives of the elderly clients (particularly those living with the client) may be crucial for the maintenance of rehabilitation success. If it is true, as research shows, that a dependence-supportive interaction pattern prevails in the private household setting (as well as in institutional settings), then the counseling and education of the persons in the elderly client's social sphere obviously becomes most important (Baltes & Wahl, 1992; Wahl & Baltes, 1993).

A point frequently not taken as seriously as it deserves should be mentioned at the end of this section, namely, rehabilitation with the mentally ill elderly (e.g., Häfner, 1986; see also Carstensen, Edelstein, & Dornbrand, 1996). The special rehabilitation needs of the mentally ill (e.g., those suffering from major depressive disorders or psychotic disturbances) are seldom acknowledged, even among professionals. Researchers and professionals in geriatric rehabilitation should be encouraged to give this subgroup of the chronically ill elderly the attention they rightfully deserve.

7.23.3.5 Considering Motivation and Compliance Issues

It is a truism to state that the motivation and compliance of the elderly person are necessary conditions for successful rehabilitation (King & Barrowclough, 1989; Ellul, Watkins, Ferguson, & Barer, 1992; Hartke, 1991; Trezona, 1991). The elderly person has to be convinced that participating in a rehabilitation program is worth the effort and cost. Hence, it is necessary to understand the personal attitudes and intentions of the person before starting the rehabilitation process (see, for example Wiesner & Tesch-Römer, 1996).

7.23.3.5.1 Motivation

Although the problem of motivating the elderly patient is often mentioned in the rehabilitation literature, rarely are specific measures for increasing motivation described. Quite often, elderly people are convinced that rehabilitation is not worthwhile, that improvement is impossible, that too much effort is required, or that the results of rehabilitation might threaten the current safe (albeit dependent) life situation. Improving motivation can be achieved through communication with the elderly person before and during rehabilitation, giving credence to individual goals, and simplifying steps needed to achieve rehabilitation objectives (Kemp, 1985). Specifically, changing pessimistic self-efficacy beliefs, strengthening self-esteem, increasing optimism, and exploring "possible selves" might be helpful in increasing motivation for rehabilitation (Guthrie & Harvey, 1994). Important aspects of the rehabilitation process that might enhance motivation are information (What should one know about the intervention?), choice (Which options are available?), goal-setting (What are long- and short-term goals?), attention to emotional needs (What does the disability/handicap mean to the person?), and dealing with social anxieties (What do other people think/expect?). Finally, it should be noted that lack of motivation could also be due to an endogenous depressive disorder. Similarly, motivational deficits can occur due to reactive depression following loss sustained in the initial illness or even a specific brain disease (like frontal lobe disorder, Vanderpool, 1984). In these cases, specific therapeutic interventions might be necessary.

7.23.3.5.2 Compliance

It is not enough that the person is motivated to start rehabilitation, they must also comply with the rehabilitative process, which can take weeks or months. Problems during the intervention process may result from low motivation, psychosocial crises, or cognitive decline (e.g., memory problems). Hence, elderly persons in rehabilitation should be helped to maintain a schedule if necessary. This can be achieved by keeping short-term goals clear and giving simple instructions for rehabilitation procedures. Moreover, motivation should be maintained by regularly encouraging and reinforcing the rehabilitation progress. Examples for the importance of compliance issues can be found in prosthetics use (Cameron & Quine, 1994), implementing safety features at home (El-Faizy & Reinsch, 1994), and continence training (Fonda, 1991).

7.23.3.5.3 Impact of the social network on motivation and compliance

The social network of the patient is very important in rehabilitation motivation and compliance. Motivation is not a personal characteristic, but a product of interpersonal interactions. Hence, motivation can be influenced significantly by rehabilitation staff, family members, and community services (Tucker, 1984). An example might be shaping the self-care behavior of elderly nursing home residents via social feedback from staff members (Baltes, Burgess, & Stewart, 1980; Baltes, Kindermann, & Reisenzein, 1986). It should be noted, however, that it is difficult for health professionals in institutional settings to rate rehabilitation motivation; rehabilitation decisions can be facilitated by describing specific behaviors, like mobility, self-care, independence, and socialization (King & Barrowclough, 1989).

Before beginning a rehabilitative intervention, it would seem useful to instill a sense of confidence in the elderly client, to persuade them that the long road ahead is not so very difficult and well worth the effort. Motivation is a complex product of the interaction between a person's values, the values held by significant others, history, talents and interests, personality, and treatment setting. As a rule of thumb, one should emphasize that if a derogatory, devalued label is applied to the person (either by the person or by the social network), rehabilitative efforts will fail; conversely, if the person is given positive feedback, the individual's motivation for rehabilitation will be enhanced.

7.23.3.6 The Role of Social Support

Social relations change with advancing age. The chance of living with a partner, especially for women, decreases, the size of the social network shrinks, and loneliness increases with advancing age (Wagner, Schütze, & Lang, 1996). Elderly people living in institutions are especially vulnerable to accumulated risk factors for social isolation and loneliness. Nevertheless, important aspects of the "social convoy" remain stable even in old age (Antonucci, 1985). Most elderly people have good relations and frequent contact with children and grandchildren, and elderly people at all ages name friends, acquaintances, or neighbors as parts of their social network. Moreover, elderly people are not solely receivers of social support; they also give support to members of their social network. At this point, one should distinguish between emotional and instrumental support. In rehabilitation, one might inquire regarding what role social support plays in the well-being of the disabled elderly, and how social support could be mobilized for the purpose of rehabilitation.

7.23.3.6.1 Effects of social support

There can be no doubt that social support, whether instrumental or emotional, helps the elderly individual cope with chronic illness and disabilities that remain even after the best rehabilitation efforts (e.g., Antonucci & Jackson, 1987; Silverstone, 1984). Several studies show that social support has positive effects upon a broad range of handicaps and in various rehabilitation settings. Chronic pain patients with supportive families tend to report less pain intensity, less reliance on medication, and greater activity levels than patients with non-supportive, disharmonic families (Jamison & Virts, 1990). In stroke patients, emotional support and moderate degrees of instrumental support are related to positive outcomes and recovery (Glass & Maddox, 1992). However, social support might be dysfunctional as well. Too much instrumental support might hinder the recovery of stroke patients. Hence, the positive and potentially negative sides of social support deserve consideration in this context. On the one hand, social partners should be integrated into the rehabilitation process as early as possible, since they are able to contribute significantly to the restoration and maintenance of functional independence of the elderly client. On the other hand, social interactions can also become detrimental to the elderly when social partners tend toward overcare (e.g., Baltes & Wahl, 1996), or care giving situations evoke an overflow of problematic psychodynamic elements (see Pearlin, Aneshensel, Mullan, & Whitlatch, 1996).

7.23.3.6.2 Mobilizing social support

Social relations (and the sources of social support) can be divided into informal and formal support givers (Silverstone, 1984). Among the informal support givers are spouses (especially wives), children (especially daughters), friends, and neighbors. The existence of a possible support giver does not necessarily mean that an elderly handicapped person receives help from network members. This is of some importance, because without some type of informal support, a return to the patient's home in the community might be very difficult. The burden (and the support) of the caregivers should also be acknowledged (see Chapter 22, this volume). The support offered by family (and friends) should be supplemented by formal support givers, such as primary health care, rehabilitation services, social workers, homemakers, meals-on-wheels, and so on. It should also be acknowledged that the (possibly short) acute phase of illness is usually followed by a recuperative phase and a (probably long) maintenance phase. Allocation of formal community services should depend on the needs and prospects of the care recipient and amount of resources available. Even in the case of psychiatric disorders, day-care, outpatient care, and community-based care can be implemented (Cooper, 1991b).

Hence, whenever possible, the global goal of rehabilitative efforts is to discharge elderly patients into the community, that is, back to their former, everyday living situation. Therefore, the mobilization of social support is important for helping the elderly person to live as independently as possible but with as much help from social partners at home as necessary. Living in the community and in one's own home means getting permanent and everyday support, even if this support takes the form of "small" gestures and signs from the neighborhood (Wagner, Schütze, & Lang, 1996).

7.23.3.7 Ecological Aspects of Rehabilitation

Although a "gestalt switch" from the elderly person to the environment took place in the 1960s and 1970s (see, for example, Lawton & Nahemow, 1973), gerontology in general and geriatric rehabilitation in particular is still very "person centered." From its inception, environmental gerontology persistently has considered the elderly person's surroundings as protective or risk factors for independent functioning. Of particular relevance here is the Environmental Docility Hypothesis, according to which the elderly suffering from competence losses and chronic conditions are particularly prone to environmental characteristics (e.g., Lawton, 1982; Lawton & Simon, 1968). A few simple statements can be emphasized. Independence in self-care always means independence in a certain bathroom environment (with certain supportive or constraining conditions). Independence in meal preparation always means independent meal preparation in a certain kitchen environment with specific features and equipment. Finally, independence in shopping always means independence within a certain neighborhood or meso-environment with supermarkets of varying proximity.

7.23.3.7.1 Person–environment fit as critical for rehabilitation

There is thus good reason to assume that discrepancies between the competence profile of the elderly person and the environment can undermine even the best person-centered rehabilitation effort (e.g., Lawton, 1982; Olbrich & Diegritz, 1995). This is true, for instance, with respect to the eastern part of Germany (the former German Democratic Republic), in which housing conditions are still significantly worse compared to those in the western part. As empirical analyses have revealed, discrepancies on measures of daily competence are at least in part caused by poor living environments within and outside the home (e.g., long distances to supermarkets and pharmacies) that are prevalent in the eastern regions of the country (Olbrich & Diegritz, 1995; Schneekloth & Potthoff, 1993).

Thus, rehabilitation should always be aimed at both training the elderly client to cope with environmental challenges and changing environmental features to suit their profile of deficits and competencies (e.g., Regnier & Pynoos, 1987; 1992; Parmelee & Lawton, 1990). Rehabilitation may thus be defined as the attempt to reduce all possible discrepancies between personal competence and environmental challenges by focusing on the person and their physical environment.

7.23.3.7.2 Considering objective and subjective environmental aspects within the everyday world

One should also note that the physical environments of the elderly are more than mere objective surroundings which vary in the amount of support they offer. Environments may also be viewed as materializations of personal biographies and as extensions of the personal self (Wahl & Oswald, in press); this concept is particularly relevant for the great number of elderly individuals who do not live for decades at the same location. Thus, alterations may indeed be helpful and necessary for the rehabilitation outcome from an objective perspective, but not from the elderly client's point of view. Geriatric practitioners should take these subjective evaluations seriously; the elderly individual's decision to refrain from modifying their home environment must be considered to be a valid choice, even though it might lower independence in daily functioning in the long run. Furthermore, elderly persons should not be seen as mere pawns of their environmental conditions. The creativity with which the elderly (particularly those suffering from chronic conditions) use their potential for compensation is very impressive; they demonstrate consistently a high degree of "proactivity" in adapting themselves to their living environments and vice versa (Lawton, 1989; see also Wahl & Oswald, in press).

The ecological approach to geriatric rehabilitation may be used to illustrate another basic issue. Environmental gerontology and psychology have always stressed the importance of remaining as close as possible to the everyday world of their subjects (see for example the concept of behavior setting proposed by Barker, 1968); likewise, rehabilitation efforts should also demonstrate a good measure of "ecological validity" (Wahl & Baltes, 1993). Rehabilitative work, particularly when it takes place in a hospital setting, should do its utmost remain close to the "life world" of the elderly individual; this is the most promising way to ensure the maintenance of rehabilitation outcomes in the home world.

7.23.3.7.3 New technologies and their rehabilitation potential

Finally the issue of old age and technology should be mentioned briefly, particularly so-called new technologies (e.g., Bouma & Graafmans, 1992; Charness & Bosman, 1990). What is emphasized here, is that there is no reason to assume that elderly persons are unable or unwilling to use new technologies. Instead, these devices could become major parts of the rehabilitative process in a variety of ways. For example, shopping via a home computer may be advantageous to the elderly person with significant impairment in mobility, and contribute greatly to self-efficacy and feelings of control. E-mail services or fax devices can facilitate the maintenance of social networks and social exchange, particularly when social isolation results from disablement.

7.23.4 PSYCHOSOCIAL REHABILITATION ISSUES WITH RESPECT TO PARTICULAR CLIENT GROUPS

Rehabilitation must change to suit different kinds of handicaps. With this in mind, four client groups, namely stroke patients, arthritis patients, the sensory impaired elderly, and demented elderly, are discussed in more detail in this subsection. Although it is clear that rehabilitation programs exist for other age-related handicaps as well (e.g., amputation, Marmann, 1994; falls and hip fracture, Campbell, 1992; Felsenthal & Stein, 1990), there are at least three reasons to concentrate on these four target groups. First, each of these illnesses represents a chronic condition that is highly prevalent in the population at large. Second, arthritis, sensory impairments, dementia, and to a lesser extent, stroke, do not receive the attention within geriatric rehabilitation which they deserve. Third, each patient group poses a significant, yet unique challenge to the rehabilitation professional.

7.23.4.1 Stroke Patients

Cerebrovascular diseases belong to the most prevalent diagnoses in old age (Steinhagen-Thiessen & Borchelt, 1996). Cerebral vascular accident (stroke) constitutes the third leading cause of death in the United States (following heart disease and cancer). About one third of stroke victims will die within the first three months after the stroke. Symptoms of stroke can be partial or complete paralysis, urinary incontinence, difficulties in swallowing, aphasia, and losses in memory and other cognitive functions (Wade, 1992). The functional consequences of stroke are often serious and concern overall physical ability (activities of daily living), walking, dexterity, and communication (Gibson & Caplan, 1984). Very often mood changes occur; many stroke victims develop depressive symptoms which might negatively influence the rehabilitation process (Goldberg, 1984). Early medical treatment of the stroke is extremely important, and it seems that specialized stroke units reduce morbidity and mortality among stroke victims (Langhorne, Williams, Gilchrist, & Howie, 1993). Once the clinical state has settled, one can expect a period of rapid recovery over the first 2–3 weeks, followed by slower but continuing improvement over the next five months (Wade & Langton-Hewer,1987). There is much debate whether functional improvement occurs after that, but some studies show that continued rehabilitative efforts might be helpful (Dam, et al., 1993). More information on pathophysiological changes can be found in geriatric textbooks (Abrams, Berkow, & Fletcher, 1990; Brocklehurst, Tallis, & Fillit, 1992; Evans & Williams, 1992; Pathy, 1991).

7.23.4.1.1 Critical issues of rehabilitation

Rehabilitation should start immediately after the onset of stroke. From the beginning, the patient should be mobilized and encouraged to be as independent as possible. Rehabilitation efforts should also be directed toward communication disorders, upper extremity function, and bowel and bladder care. Assessment is also crucial to stroke rehabilitation; detecting disabilities, discovering the relevant impairments, determining prognosis, planning the intervention process, and evaluating rehabilitation progress are the tasks of the interdisciplinary stroke rehabilitation team (Kruse, 1992, 1995; Rustemeyer, 1983). Physicians are responsible for medical diagnosis and treatment, although no effective medical therapy can ensure complete recovery from stroke. Hence, a variety of professions are involved in stroke rehabilitation. Physiotherapeutic exercises, such as those which improve range of motion, muscle strength, and endurance, are necessary for dealing with muscle spasticity and improving functional performance (Lee & Itoh, 1992). The Bobath method of treatment has been very influential in stroke rehabilitation, emphasizing the suppression of abnormal postures and movements before normal motor patterns are practiced (Bobath, 1971). Although physiotherapy should start early, even late physiotherapeutic intervention (12 months after stroke) can improve mobility (Wade, Collen, Robb, & Warlow, 1992). Occupational therapy is directed at training compensatory techniques for performing activities of daily living (Hasselkuss, 1989). Speech therapy is aimed at supporting stroke patients to overcome communication problems (Lehmann, 1992; Sarno, 1984; Vignolo, 1964).

Psychologists might carry out several important tasks in stroke rehabilitation. Changes concerning alterations in intellect, personality, and emotional behavior deserve attention in the diagnostic process as well as in psychotherapeutic interventions aimed at the elderly person or their social environment (Kruse, 1984). First, psychological and neuropsychological diagnostics are genuinely psychological tasks and highly relevant for assessing the specific problems of stroke patients (Lawton & Teresi, 1994). Since many patients suffer from depressive symptoms, psychological counseling might help the patient to cope with the losses resulting from the stroke and to recover from depressed mood. Clinical psychologists working with stroke patients need to plan realistic short-term goals, provide structure for working sessions, and carefully confront the patient with the denial of disability (Goldberg, 1984). Also group therapy with other stroke patients and family therapy, involving spouse and other family members, might be helpful.

Ideally, stroke patients should be able to return home after rehabilitation. It is necessary to plan carefully the discharge of the patient, involving family and community-based services as far as possible. If necessary, the patient's home should be altered to accommodate the needs of the stroke patient. For family members, caring for a relative suffering from stroke and its consequences is highly distressing; hence, community services should not only focus attention toward the neuropsychological aspects of stroke patients, but also toward the social functioning of caregivers who support them (Anderson, Linto, & Stewart-Wynne, 1995).

7.23.4.1.2 Effects of rehabilitation and challenges in the future

Since the treatment of stroke in older patients is the rule rather than the exception, research has been devoted to demonstrating the effectiveness of rehabilitation over spontaneous recovery. Meta-analyses show that stroke rehabilitation programs may improve the functional performance of stroke patients (Ottenbacher & Jennall, 1993). The extent of improvement appears to be related to the timely initiation of treatment, but not to the duration of intervention. Improvements are also associated with the patient's age, older patients taking longer to recover from stroke (Falconer, Naughton, Strasser, & Sinacore, 1994; Kalra, 1994). Regarding the institutional setting of stroke rehabilitation, it seems that early care in specialized stroke units might be most effective (Jørgensen et al., 1995; Kaste, Palomaki, & Sarna, 1995). In the further rehabilitation process, day hospitals may be more effective (and also economically advantageous) compared to conventional hospital management (Gladman, Forster, & Young, 1995; Hui, Lum, Woo, Or, & Kay, 1995).

The 1980s and 1990s have seen the establishment of special stroke units within hospitals. What is needed now are efforts for continuing rehabilitative efforts in the community, cooperation between professions, and better gerontological and geriatric education for professionals working in stroke rehabilitation. In particular, clinical psychologists working in geriatrics commonly report scarce academic preparation and training experiences and relate continuing education to higher satisfaction with geriatric work experiences (Lichtenberg & Rosenthal, 1994). The rehabilitation of a patient who has suffered a stroke is a challenge for the geriatric rehabilitation team and requires diagnostic, management, and counseling resources. Since so many psychomotor functions and psychosocial aspects are affected by a stroke, it can be taken as a general model for rehabilitation in old age. Although the medical treatment of risk factors for stroke (especially hypertension) has proven itself to be an effective prevention, stroke rehabilitation will continue to be an important part of geriatric medicine.

7.23.4.2 Arthritis Patients

The most common chronic condition in old age results from arthritis and rheumatism (US Department of Health and Human Services, 1992). Rheumatoid diseases are characterized by chronic inflammation of joints and soft tissues. Degenerative arthritis results from wearing out of joints (e.g., hip, knee) or from degeneration of bones (e.g., osteoporosis). Age at onset has an aggravating effect on disease expression in rheumatoid arthritis (Keitel, 1993). Symptoms of arthritic diseases are pain (like back pain or pain in the affected joints) and decreasing flexibility of the affected joints (e.g., hip, knee, foot, or fingers). Emotional consequences of arthritis can be increased depressive symptoms or dysphoria (Frank et al., 1992). Functional consequences of arthritic conditions are reduced mobility and losses in certain ADL functions (Badley & Tennant, 1993). Treatment of the several forms of rheumatoid and degenerative arthritis involves anti-inflammatory and analgesic drugs, although medical and physical treatment modalities are closely interrelated and should always be considered together (Baum, 1984). Hence, physical therapy and exercise programs are also extremely important. Sometimes surgery might be effective (like artificial hip joints). In some cases, dietary restrictions might be helpful (degenerative arthritis: weight loss; gout: restriction of calories and alcohol; osteoporosis: additional supply of calcium).

7.23.4.2.1 Physical therapy

In patients with degenerative joint disease, physical exercise programs should be used. Exercises to maintain muscle function are as important as exercises to strengthen specific muscle groups around the affected joint. In contrast, in elderly patients with arthritic conditions, it is necessary to control the underlying inflammatory disease before starting with exercise programs (Baum, 1984). Moreover, morning stiffness and afternoon fatigue make it necessary to schedule active therapy between the end of morning stiffness and the onset of fatigue. Exercise programs have been shown to be effective in increasing mobility, endurance, and functional status (Kovar et al., 1992). Also occupational therapy has positive effects on functional status (Helewa et al., 1991). Moreover, physiotherapy also seems to protect bone mass which may have implications for avoiding bone fractures in the long run (Shawe, Hesp, Gumpel, Sambrook, & Reeve, 1993).

7.23.4.2.2 Psychological interventions

Physical exercise programs not only improve physical health but can also improve mood and reduce anxiety and pain (Frobose & Schule, 1992). Hence, it is an important task for gerontopsychologists to strengthen the compliance of elderly arthritic patients with the therapeutic regimen and exercise programs. The perceived benefits of exercise programs can be an important determinant of exercise participation and compliance (Neuberger, Kasal, Smith, Hassanein, & DeViney, 1994). Moreover, certain sociodemographic characteristics (lower income, lower education, and higher chronological age) might lead to underuse of physical or occupational therapy provided by community services (Mayer-Oakes et al., 1992). The particular challenge for geropsychology with respect to arthritic patients lies in the chronic pain which may undermine life quality severely and permanently (Smith, Wallston, & Dwyer, 1995). The stress and coping literature in general, as well the intervention literature in particular, has not put enough emphasis on the question of what it means to age in the face of chronic and uncontrollable pain. Intervention may thus be aimed at direct alteration of the pain (e.g., by using biofeedback procedures) as well as supportive measures that enable the individual to live better with this chronic stressor (e.g., relaxation techniques, client-centered counseling). Controlled studies show that behavior-oriented interventions might influence knowledge about the disease and pain coping strategies, even if health status deteriorates because of the progressive nature of rheumatoid arthritis (Barry, Purser, Hazleman, McLean, & Hazleman, 1994; Kraaimaat, Brons, Geenen, & Bijlsma, 1995; Matussek, 1992; Simeoni, Bauman, Stenmark, & O'Brien, 1995). Since arthritic diseases affect mobility, the body self-image of an elderly person might be threatened. Clinical psychologists might help arthritic patients to cope with these losses (Jordan & Schmidt, 1988; Lehr, Kruse, & Kruse, 1992).

The musculoskeletal diseases account for the most frequent complaints among elderly persons. Since it is rarely possible to provide the patient with complete symptomatic relief, it is necessary to inform them about adequate health habits, concepts of preventive care, the value of physiotherapeutic and occupational exercises, and the gains to be achieved through behavioral and cognitive therapy.

7.23.4.3 Sensory Impaired Elderly

Losses in hearing and vision are very common in old age (Tesch-Römer & Wahl, 1996b). Hearing impairment undermines the elderly person's everyday communication, whereas losses in vision impede orientation within the physical environment. Aural rehabilitation with elderly suffering from hearing impairments includes technological devices like hearing aids and behavioral communication strategies (Kaplan, 1989; McCarthy & Sapp, 1993; Wahl & Tesch-Römer, 1996). Rehabilitation with the visually impaired elderly consists in orientation and mobility training, exercises in activities of daily living, and the use of magnifying optical devices (LaGrow & Blasch, 1992; Wahl & Oswald, 1996; Wahl & Tesch-Römer, 1996).

7.23.4.3.1 Hearing impairment

Hearing impairment is the second most prevalent chronic condition in old age; about 30% of those over 65 are so severely hearing-impaired that they would benefit from a hearing aid (Davis, 1989; US Department of Health and Human Services, 1992). Presbycusis (or hearing loss in old age) is a high-frequency symmetric hearing loss in old age beginning gradually around the fifth decade and leading progressively and irreversibly to moderate and severe losses of hearing capacity in higher ages (Corso, 1981; Fozard, 1990; Kline & Scialfa, 1996; Willott, 1991; Olsho, Harkins, & Lenhardt, 1985). Age effects for auditory and speech processing independent from hearing sensitivity have also been documented (Humes & Christopherson, 1991). Hearing loss in old age can have negative consequences in the areas of communication, social integration, well-being, and cognitive capacity (Marsiske, Delius, Lindenberger, Scherer, & Tesch-Römer, 1996; Rott, Wahl, & Tesch-Römer, 1996; Weinstein & Ventry, 1983).

There is no medical cure for presbycusis. The only way to help elderly hearing-impaired adults is through rehabilitation with hearing aids (Glass, 1986; Stephens & Goldstein, 1983). Hearing aids are small technical devices which amplify environmental sounds. Although there have been advances in hearing aid technology, hearing aids are problematic devices. Four problem areas in the use of hearing aids have been identified. Elderly hearing aid users complain of poor amplification, stigmatization, financial costs, and handling problems (e.g., inserting the hearing aid in the earmold or manipulating small levers; Franks & Beckmann, 1985; May, Upfold, & Battaglia, 1990). Nevertheless, the use of hearing aids reduces the subjective communication problems of elderly persons with hearing impairment (Tesch-Römer, 1997).

Elderly hearing-impaired patients should be supported in several ways (Tesch-Römer & Wahl, 1996a). Patients should be informed carefully about the functioning and handling of technical aids (in addition to hearing aids, a variety of listening devices exists; Kaplan, 1987). Since hearing with hearing aids is a new experience for the impaired person, they should adapt systematically to the hearing aid (e.g., use the hearing aid first in one-to-one communication and only later in group situations with background noise). Moreover, it could be useful to train the hearing impaired elderly in communication strategies and "hearing tactics," such as asking for well-articulated repetitions, occupying acoustically favorable positions, and lip reading (Vognsen, 1976).

7.23.4.3.2 Visual impairment

As is the case with respect to the elderly with hearing impairments, age-related low vision and its rehabilitation has only received due acknowledgment in the 1990s. The empirical work (Wahl, 1997; see also Wahl & Oswald, in press) has shown clearly that visual impairment has negative emotional and behavioral consequences. For example, significantly higher rates of clinically relevant depression and lower subjective well-being have been reported repeatedly (for overview, see Wahl, 1997; see also Horowitz, 1995). It should be mentioned here, however, that the negative impact on emotional adaptation does not substantially correlate with the objective loss in visual capacity. Regarding behavior, there can be no doubt that the visual loss has profound negative consequences with respect to daily living competence and independent functioning. Moreover, the visually impaired elderly are challenged by the fact that at least some of their preferred leisure activities (reading activities in particular) may become very difficult or even impossible without a good rehabilitation program. Finally, visual impairment is a prototypical environment-relevant loss in competence (Wahl, 1994). Thus, age-related loss in vision may be seen as a prototypical case for an ecological approach to geriatric rehabilitation.

The negative impact of significant (and irreversible) vision loss (e.g., caused by macular degeneration or diabetic retinopathia) makes a multidimensional rehabilitation approach necessary. The main goal of rehabilitation is the restoration of reading capability by the appropriate use of technical devices. A whole range of technical tools, from magnifying glasses to computer-based reading devices, exists (see, for example, Tesch-Römer & Wahl, 1996a). The challenge here is not the device itself but the implementation of these devices in the everyday world of the visually impaired elderly. Moreover, good training with a high degree of "ecological validity" is also needed. A second rehabilitation issue is training in orientation and mobility. The challenge with respect to these rehabilitation techniques lies in the fact that elderly persons often have concomitant impairments of a chronic nature, for example, coexisting hearing, motor, or cognitive impairments. A third issue is training in the domain of daily living tasks. In all of these rehabilitation efforts, training must take place within the elderly person's everyday world. Interventions in the environment of visually impaired elderly are frequently supportive and helpful. With respect to the social environment, it is very important to educate social partners to take the disabilities of their relatives and friends seriously while resisting the temptation to be overprotective. With respect to the physical environment, a whole range of alterations has been suggested (e.g., Hiatt, 1987) such as the enhancement of light conditions (without producing too much glare), the use of contrast and color, and the employment of technical innovations such as special telephones or talking appliances for the kitchen.

To conclude this section, the rehabilitative needs of sensory impaired persons have only been articulated in the 1990s. The aim of this section was thus not only to elaborate on the special needs of these groups of elderly (those with impairments in vision and hearing), but also to emphasize that the rehabilitation of these elderly must consist of more than the mere adoption of technical devices. Truly adequate interventions must implement the devices properly and facilitate the elderly person's adaptation to the new technology. And of course, rehabilitation must enable the individual to better cope with the psychosocial losses caused by the sensory impairment (e.g., Tesch-Römer & Nowak, 1995; Wahl & Oswald, 1996).

7.23.4.4 Demented elderly

Dementia is a very serious problem in the elderly, especially in the very old (see Chapter 10, this volume). In the most common form of dementia, Alzheimer's disease, aphasia, agnosia, and apraxia are present in various combinations as well as emotional and personality changes, memory disorders, slowness in rate of information processing, and the incapacity to fulfill daily living activities. It would therefore be reasonable to question the merit of rehabilitation efforts with the demented elderly. However, professionals as well as society as a whole, cannot neglect the burden and challenge of the tremendous and fast growing number of elderly suffering from dementia. Custodial care is obviously not the right answer. The responsibility for this problem should be shared by all and should address the challenge with those rehabilitative tools which promise at least some measure of success. In this context, it may not be wise to talk about "dementia" in general. There are different degrees of severity, and each patient exhibits a unique profiles of competencies; both of these factors crucially affect rehabilitation outcome.

Rehabilitation efforts undoubtedly should include reality orientation programs and training to cope, at least in part, with daily living challenges. Data suggest that rehabilitative work of this kind may be particularly promising when it starts in the early stages of the cognitive decline process. Intervention studies hint that further deterioration can be delayed by early cognitive training intervention (e.g., Oswald et al., 1988). Family members and other caregivers should be part of rehabilitative efforts, too (Pearlin et al., 1996; see also Chapter 22, this volume). Thus, the comprehensive care of the caregivers, as suggested in the literature on caregiver burden, may also be regarded as a very important part of the geriatric rehabilitation system. In a sense, it also serves important preventive purposes. As is known, being a caregiver for a demented individual heightens the risk of suffering from chronic physical or mental conditions in the long run. Finally, the treatment of dementia provides a prototypical example of how, given unchangeable person characteristics, the possibility of altering the physical environment always remains. This is particularly true in institutional settings, but also relevant in private home living. Some persuasive and empirically proven solutions for modifying and adjusting the environment have been suggested in the literature (e.g., Regnier & Pynoos, 1992).

7.23.5 PRACTICAL ISSUES, RESEARCH QUESTIONS, AND ETHICAL PROBLEMS

The last section of this chapter is concerned with some practical, research-oriented, and ethical problems associated with rehabilitation in old age. Practical problems concern the institutional organization of geriatric rehabilitation, the qualification of staff, and the assurance of rehabilitation quality. Research questions concern the effectiveness of interventions and the development and evaluation of innovative rehabilitation concepts. Finally, ethical problems deal for instance with the distribution of scarce resources within the health care system.

7.23.5.1 Practical Issues

Regarding the institutional organization of geriatric rehabilitation, it has been shown that specialized geriatric units or geriatric hospitals are more effective and more cost efficient than general medical wards (Görres, 1992b). An important problem for elderly patients after rehabilitation is returning home and maintaining independent living in the community. It could be helpful to view this problem from the perspective that individuals with disabilities are handicapped more by barriers in the environments than by their specific impairments (DeJong, Batavia, & McKnew, 1992) and that rehabilitative interventions should be realized in conjunction with community-based long-term care (Miller, 1991; see also Chapter 20, this volume). Another important practical problem is quality assurance (Görres, 1994; Meier-Baumgartner et al., 1992). Conceptions of rehabilitation programs might be very different from their practical implementation. Hence, it is necessary to control the quality of rehabilitative interventions. Three aspects of quality in medical care and rehabilitation can be distinguished (Donabedian, 1966): quality of structure, process quality, and outcome quality. Quality of structure concerns characteristics of the institution, the educational profile of staff, and quality of technical equipment. Process quality concerns characteristics of the rehabilitation process (diagnostics, development of rehabilitation goals, implementation of therapy and interventions, documentation of changes, and team communication). Outcome quality concerns the evaluation of changes stemming from rehabilitative efforts (reduced morbidity and mortality, increased functional independence, ability and motivation for independent living, patient satisfaction). Quality of rehabilitation structure and process are necessary conditions for outcome quality; but outcome quality certainly is what counts in evaluating rehabilitation services (Görres, 1992b).

7.23.5.2 Research Questions

For policy planning and program development, it seems necessary to gather epidemiological data on chronic diseases in old age. The lack of adequate epidemiological data might lead to underestimating the need for rehabilitation efforts. A second major research problem concerns the effectiveness of rehabilitation programs (Görres, Tschubar, & Meier-Baumgartner, 1991). Rehabilitation programs should be tested empirically regarding their effectiveness and efficiency by considering a psychosocial view of life quality as well as a cost-benefit ratio. Although it may be ethically questionable to evaluate rehabilitation programs involving experimental and control groups in pre/post-treatment designs, nevertheless controlled studies should be the standard procedure in rehabilitation research (Wottawa & Thierau, 1990). Finally, the development and evaluation of innovative rehabilitation programs is an important research task. It should be emphasized again that not only dramatic diseases (like stroke) should be the focus of future gerontological rehabilitation research. There are a variety of age-related diseases which urgently require rehabilitation (e.g., arthritis, vision problems and blindness, hearing loss).

7.23.5.3 Ethical Problems

There are several ethical issues concerning rehabilitation in old age (e.g., Spicker, Ingman, & Lawson, 1987). Thinking about rehabilitation implies reference to norms (What is the goal of rehabilitation?), making a decision between rehabilitation and care (When does rehabilitation promise progress in the individual?), and weighing individual and social benefits and costs (What are the gains of rehabilitation compared to the costs?). Considering rehabilitation goals, normative standards (e.g., independent living) could come in conflict with individual values (e.g., security and social contact). Hence, in developing rehabilitation goals, individual values should be considered carefully. Second, before an individual rehabilitation process is initiated, a decision has to be made regarding the rehabilitation potential of the particular individual; sometimes this decision concerns the alternatives rehabilitation vs. care. But even in geriatric, long-term care facilities, nursing does not necessarily have to fulfill a primarily custodial function; rather, it could also be performed according to a therapeutic model of rehabilitation (Burgio & Burgio, 1990). However, sometimes the general goal of rehabilitation has to be given up, and a decision to commit to long-term care be made. This decision might also involve considerations of costs and benefits (Brody, 1987; Hausman, 1987). There are individual costs connected with rehabilitation (e.g., time and effort), but these costs might be outweighed by the potential benefits of rehabilitation outcomes. Additionally, there are also material costs (e.g., financial support for rehabilitation programs). It should be emphasized, though, that rehabilitation is based on humanistic values. This basic ethical orientation stresses that the disabled elderly deserve, as much as anyone else, the opportunity to participate in all aspects of life (Kemp, 1985). Beyond humanistic arguments, however, one might add that current economic conditions make rehabilitation more efficient in the long run than long-term care.

Rehabilitation in old age is a promising field. Empirical research demonstrates the effectiveness of psychosocial interventions in a variety of chronic diseases. Moreover, rehabilitation in old age should not necessarily be dominated by the medical profession. Instead, clinical psychology should demonstrate its rich reservoir of intervention and therapeutic strategies, and clinical psychologists might more often lay hold of the leadership in interdisciplinary rehabilitation teams. Despite unsolved practical issues, open research questions, and difficult ethical problems, rehabilitation in old age is a gratifying field of expertise for clinical psychologists.

7.23.6 SUMMARY

In this chapter, general principles and geropsychological essentials of rehabilitation in old age are reviewed from a geropsychological perspective. Rehabilitation aims at reducing the disability and handicap experienced as a result of disease and impairment. Since aging is associated with increased chronic illness, the goal of rehabilitation in old age is not necessarily complete cure of disease but improving functional capability and maximizing wellness. An overview concerning psychosocial issues and strategies of rehabilitation in old is given, including comprehensive geriatric and psychosocial assessment, restoration of functional independence, cognitive and reality orientation training, therapeutic intervention, motivational and compliance problems, the role of social support, and the ecology of aging. Since different geriatric client groups have different rehabilitation needs, four highly prevalent and serious chronic conditions in old age are treated specifically, that is, stroke, arthritis, sensory impairment, and dementia. The chapter closes with perspectives for psychologists working in rehabilitative settings discussing practical issues, research questions, and ethical considerations.

7.23.7 REFERENCES

Abrams, W. B., Berkow, R., & Fletcher, A. J. (Eds.) (1990). *The Merck Manual of Geriatrics.* Rahway, NJ: Merck, Sharp, & Dohme Research Laboratories.

Abson, V., & Rabbitt, P. M. (1988). What do self-rating questionnaires tell us about changes in competence in old age? In M. M. Gruneberg, P. E. Morris, & R. N. Sykes (Eds.), *Practical aspects of memory: Current research and issues* (pp. 188–191). Chichester, UK: Wiley.

Anderson, C. S., Linto, J., & Stewart-Wynne, E. G. (1995). A population-based assessment of the impact and burden of caregiving for long-term stroke survivors. *Stroke, 26*, 843–849.

Andrews, K. (1987). *Rehabilitation of the older adult.* London: Edward Arnold.

Andrews, K. (1991). Rehabilitation of the elderly. In M. S. J. Pathy (Ed.), *Principles and practice of geriatric medicine* (pp. 1341–1365). Chichester, UK: Wiley.

Antonucci, T. C. (1985). Personal characteristics, social support, and social behavior. In R. H. Binstock & E. Shanas (Eds.), *Handbook of aging and the social sciences* (2nd ed., pp. 94–128). New York: Van Nostrand Reinhold.

Antonucci, T. C., & Jackson, J. S. (1987). Social support, interpersonal efficacy, and health: A life course perspective. In L. L. Carstensen & B. A. Edelstein (Eds.), *Handbook of clinical gerontology* (pp. 291–311). New York: Pergamon.

Bach, D., Bach, M., Böhmer, F., Frühwald, T., & Grilc, B. (1995). Reactivating occupational therapy: a method to improve cognitive performance in geriatric patients. *Age and Ageing, 24*, 222–226.

Bäckman, L., Josephsson, S., Herlitz, A., Stigsdotter, A., & Viitanen, M. (1991). The generalizability of training gains in dementia: Effects of an imagery-based mnemonic on face-name retention duration. *Psychology and Aging, 6*, 489–492.

Badley, E. M., & Tennant, A. (1993). Disablement associated with rheumatic disorders in a British population: problems with activities of daily living and level of support. *British Journal of Rheumatology, 32*, 601–608.

Baltes, M. M. (1996). *The many faces of dependency in old age.* Cambridge, UK: Cambridge University Press.

Baltes, M. M., Burgess, R. L., & Stewart, R. B. (1980). Independence and dependence in self-care behaviors in nursing home residents: An operant-observational study. *International Journal of Behavioral Development, 3*, 489–500.

Baltes, M. M., Kindermann, T., & Reisenzein, R. (1986). Die Beobachtung von unselbständigem und selbständigem Verhalten in einem deutschen Altenheim: Die soziale Umwelt als Einflußgröße [The observation of dependent and independent behavior in a German old age home: the social environment as an influencing factor]. *Zeitschrift für Gerontologie, 19*, 14–21.

Baltes, M. M., Kühl, K. P., Gutzmann, H., & Sowarka, D. (1995). Potential of cognitive plasticity as a diagnostic instrument: a cross-validation and extension. *Psychology and Aging, 10*, 167–172.

Baltes, M. M., Maas, I., Wilms, H.-U., & Borchelt, M. (1996). Alltagskompetenz im Alter: Theoretische Überlegungen und empirische Befunde [Everyday competence in old age: Theoretical issues and empirical findings]. In K. U. Mayer & P. B. Baltes (Eds.), *Die Berliner Altersstudie* [The Berlin Aging Study] (pp. 525–542). Berlin, Germany: Akademie Verlag.

Baltes, M. M., & Sowarka, D. (1995). Kognitive Intervention im Alter [Cognitive intervention in old age]. In R. Oerter & L. Montada (Eds.), *Entwicklungspsychologie* [Developmental psychology] (pp. 1116–1126). Weinheim, Germany: Psychologie Verlags Union

Baltes, M. M., & Wahl, H.-W. (1992). The dependency-support script in institutions: Generalization to community settings. *Psychology and Aging, 7*, 409–418.

Baltes, M. M., & Wahl, H.-W. (1996). Patterns of communication in old age: The Dependency-Support and Independence-Ignore Script. *Health Communication, 8*, 217–231.

Baltes, M. M., Wahl, H.-W., & Reichert, M. (1991). Successful aging in long-term care institutions. *Annual Review of Gerontology and Geriatrics, 11*, 311–338.

Baltes, P. B. (1984). Intelligenz im Alter [Intelligence in old age]. *Spektrum der Wissenschaft*, Mai 1984, 46–60.

Baltes, P. B. (1987). Theoretical propositions of life-span developmental psychology: On the dynamics between growth and decline. *Developmental Psychology, 23*, 611–626.

Baltes, P. B. (1993). The aging mind: Potential and limits. *The Gerontologist, 33*, 580–594.

Baltes, P. B., & Baltes, M. M. (1990). Psychological perspectives on successful aging: the model of selective optimization with compensation. In P. B. Baltes & M. M. Baltes (Eds.), *Successful aging. Perspectives from the behavioral sciences* (pp. 1–34). Cambridge, UK: Cambridge University Press.

Baltes, P. B. & Lindenberger, U. (1988). On the range of cognitive plasticity in old age as a function of experience: 15 years of intervention research. *Behavior Therapy, 19*, 283–300.

Baltes, P. B., Sowarka, D., & Kliegl, R. (1989). Cognitive training research on fluid intelligence in old age: What can older adults achieve by themselves? *Psychology and Aging, 4*, 217–221.

Barker, R. G. (1968). *Ecological psychology*. Stanford, CA: Stanford University Press.

Barry, M. A., Purser, J., Hazleman, R., McLean, A., & Hazleman, B. L. (1994). Effect of energy conservation and joint protection education in rheumatoid arthritis. *British Journal of Rheumatology*, *33*, 1171–1174.

Baum, J. (1984). Rehabilitation aspects of arthritis in the elderly. In T. F. Williams (Ed.), *Rehabilitation in the aging* (pp. 177–197). New York: Raven Press.

Blieszner, R., Willis, S. L., & Baltes, P. B. (1981). Training research in aging on the fluid ability of inductive reasoning. *Journal of Applied Developmental Psychology*, *2*, 247–265.

Bobath, B. (1971). *Adult hemiplegia: evaluation and treatment*. London: Heinemann.

Bouma, H., & Graafmans, J. A. M. (Eds.) (1992). *Gerontechnology*. Amsterdam: IOS Press.

Brocklehurst, J. C., Tallis, R. C., & Fillit, H. M. (Eds.). (1992). *Textbook of geriatric medicine and gerontology* (4th ed.). Edinburgh, UK: Churchill Livingstone.

Brody, B. (1987). Wholehearted and halfhearted care: national policies vs. individual choice. S. F. Spicker, S. R. Ingman, & I. R. Lawson (Eds.), *Ethical dimensions of geriatric care* (pp. 79–93). Dordrecht, The Netherlands: Reidel.

Burgio, L. D., & Burgio, K. L. (1990). Institutional staff training and management: A review of the literature and a model for geriatric, long-term-care facilities. *International Journal of Aging and Human Development*, *30*, 287–302.

Butler, R. W., & Namerow, N. S. (1988). Cognitive retraining in brain-injury rehabilitation: A critical review. *Journal of Neurologic Rehabilitation*, *2*, 97–101.

Cameron, I. D., & Quine, S. (1994). External hip protectors: Likely non-compliance among high risk elderly people living in the community. *Archives of Gerontology and Geriatrics*, *19*, 273–281.

Camp, C. J., Foss, J. W., Stevens, A. B., Reichard, C. C., McKitrick, L. A., & O'Hanlon, A. M. (1993). Memory training in normal and demented elderly populations: the E-I-E-I-O model. *Experimental Aging Research*, *19*, 277–290.

Campbell, A. J. (1992). Role of rehabilitation in fall recovery and prevention. *Reviews in Clinical Gerontology*, *2*, 53–65.

Carstensen, L. L., Edelstein, B. A. , & Dornbrand, L. (Eds.) (1996). *The practical handbook of clinical gerontology*. Thousand Oaks, CA: Sage.

Cattell, R. B. (1971). *Abilities: Their structure, growth, and action*. Boston: Houghton Mifflin.

Charness, N., & Bosman, E. A. (1990). Human factors and design for older adults. In J. E. Birren & K. W. Schaie (Eds.), *Handbook of the psychology of aging* (3rd ed., pp. 446–463). San Diego, CA: Academic Press.

Cooper, B. (1991a). The epidemiology of dementia. In R. Jacoby & C. Oppenheimer (Eds.), *Psychiatry in the elderly* (pp. 574–585). Oxford, UK: Oxford University Press.

Cooper, B. (1991b). Principles of service provision in old age psychiatry. In R. Jacoby & C. Oppenheimer (Eds.), *Psychiatry in the elderly* (pp. 274–300). Oxford, UK: Oxford University Press.

Corso, J. F. (1981). *Aging sensory systems and perception*. New York: Praeger.

Crimmins, E. M., Hayward, M. D., & Saito, Y (1996). Differentials in active life expectancy in the older population of the United States. *Journal of Gerontology: Social Sciences*, *51B*, S111–S120.

Dam, M., Tonin, P., Casson, S., Ermani, M., Pizzolato, G., Iaia, V., & Battistin, L. (1993). The effects of long-term rehabilitation therapy on poststroke hemiplegic patients. *Stroke*, *24*, 1186–1191.

Davis, A. C. (1989). The prevalence of hearing impairment and reported hearing disability among adults in Great Britain. *International Journal of Epidemiology*, *18*, 911–917.

DeJong, G., Batavia, A. I., & McKnew, L. B. (1992). The independent living model of personal assistance in national long-term-care policy. *Generations*, *16*, 89–95.

Dixon, R. A., & Bäckman, L. (Eds.) (1995).*Compensating for psychological deficits and declines. Managing losses and promoting gains*. Mahwah, NJ: Erlbaum.

Donabedian, A. (1966). Evaluating the quality of medical care. *Millbank Memorial Fund Quarterly*, *44*, 166–206.

Ebrahim, S. (1992). Rehabilitation. In J. C. Brocklehurst, R. C. Tallis, & H. M. Fillit (Eds.), *Textbook of geriatric medicine and gerontology* (4th ed., pp. 1038–1054). Edinburgh, UK: Churchill Livingstone.

El-Faizy, M., & Reinsch, S. (1994). Home safety intervention for the prevention of falls. *Physical and Occupational Therapy in Geriatrics*, *12*, 33–49.

Ellul, J., Watkins, C., Ferguson, N., & Barer, D. (1993). Increasing patient engagement in rehabilitation activities. *Clinical Rehabilitation*, *7*, 297–302.

Ermini-Fünfschilling, D., & Meier, D. (1995). Gedächtnistraining: Wichtiger Bestandteil der Milieutherapie bei seniler Demenz [Memory training: An important constituent of milieu therapy in senile dementia]. *Zeitschrift für Gerontologie und Geriatrie*, *28*, 190–194.

Evans, J. G., & Williams, T. F. (Eds.). (1992). *Oxford textbook of geriatric medicine*. Oxford, UK: Oxford University Press.

Falconer, J. A., Naughton, B. J., Strasser, D. C., & Sinacore, J. M. (1994). Stroke inpatient rehabilitation: A comparison across age groups. *Journal of the American Geriatrics Society*, *42*, 3–44.

Felsenthal, G., & Stein, B. D. (1990). Rehabilitation of dysmobility in the elderly: A case study of the patient with a hip fracture. In S. J. Brody & L. G. Pawlson (Eds.), *Aging and rehabilitation II: the state of the practice* (pp. 110–129). New York: Springer.

Fleischmann, U. M. (1982). Gedächtnistraining im höheren Lebensalter—Ansatzpunkte und Möglichkeiten [Memory training in old age—Foci and possibilities]. *Zeitschrift fr Gerontologie*, *15*, 53–62.

Fleischmann, U. M. (1989). *Gedächtnis und Alter. Multivariate Analysen zum Gedächtnis alter Menschen* [Memory and old age. Multivariate analyses of the memory of the elderly]. Bern, Switzerland: Huber.

Fonda, D. (1991). Management of the incontinent disabled patient. *Clinical Rehabilitation*, *5*, 331–336.

Fozard, J. L. (1990). Vision and hearing in aging. In J. E. Birren & K. W. Schaie (Eds.), *Handbook of the psychology of aging* (3rd ed., pp. 150–170). San Diego, CA: Academic Press.

Frank, R. G., Chaney, J. M., Clay, D. L., Shutty, M. S., Beck, N. C., Kay, D. R., Elliott, T. R., & Grambling, S. (1992). Dysphoria: a major symptom factor in persons with disability or chronic illness. *Psychiatry Research*, *43*, 231–241.

Franks, J. R., & Beckmann, N. J. (1985). Rejection of hearing aids: Attitudes of a geriatric sample. *Ear and Hearing*, *6*, 161–166.

Franzen, M. D. & Martin, R. C. (1996). Screening for neuropsychological impairment. In L. L. Carstensen, B. A. Edelstein, & L. Dornbrand (Eds.), *The practical handbook of clinical gerontology* (pp. 188–216). Thousand Oaks, CA: Sage.

Fries, J. F. (1990). Medical perspectives upon successful aging. In P. B. Baltes & M. M. Baltes (Eds.), *Successful aging. Perspectives from the behavioral sciences* (pp. 35-49). Cambridge, UK: Cambridge University Press.

Frobose, I., & Schule, K. (1992). Befindlichkeits- und Einstellungsänderungen beim Sport mit Rheumatikern [Mood and attitude change as a consequence of sports with rheumatic patients]. *Die Rehabilitation, 31*, 198–201.

Gatz, M., Kasl-Godley, J. E., & Karel, M. J. (1996). Aging and mental disorders. In J. E. Birren & K. W. Schaie (Eds.), *Handbook of the psychology of aging* (4th ed., pp. 365–382). San Diego, CA: Academic Press

Gibson, C. J. & Caplan, B. M. (1984). Rehabilitation of the patient with stroke. In T. F. Williams (Ed.), *Rehabilitation in the aging* (pp. 145–159). New York: Raven Press.

Gladman, J., Forster, A., & Young, J. (1995). Hospital- and home-based rehabilitation after discharge from hospital for stroke patients: analysis of two trials. *Age and Ageing, 24*, 49–53.

Glass, L. E. (1986). Rehabilitation for deaf and hearing-impaired elderly. In S. J. Brody & G. E. Ruff (Eds.), *Aging and rehabilitation* (pp. 218–237). New York: Springer.

Glass, T. A., & Maddox, G. L. (1992). The quality and quantity of social support: Stroke recovery as psychosocial transition. *Social Science and Medicine, 34*, 1249–1261.

Goldberg, R. (1984). Psychosocial aspects of stroke. In D. W. Krueger (Ed.), *Rehabilitation psychology* (pp. 293–300). Rockville, MD: Aspen.

Görres, S. (1992a). Stationäre Rehabilitation und Nachsorge älterer Menschen [Hospital rehabilitation and post-hospital care of the elderly]. In A. Mühlum & H. Oppl (Eds.). *Handbuch der Rehabilitation* [Handbook of rehabilitation] (pp. 401-423). Neuwied, Germany: Luchterhand.

Görres, S. (1992b). Qualitätssicherung in der Geriatrie [Quality assurance in geriatrics]. *Archiv für Wissenschaft und Praxis der Sozialen Arbeit, 23*, 90–111.

Görres, S. (1994). Qualitätssicherung in der Rehabilitation älterer Menschen [Quality assurance in the rehabilitation of the elderly]. *Die Rehabilitation, 33*, 64–68.

Görres, S., Tschubar, H., & Meier-Baumgartner, H.-P. (1991). Zur Bedeutung klinikinterner Erfolgskriterien in der geriatrischen Rehabilitation. Ergebnisse eines Nachsorgeprojekts zum Problem der Qualitätssicherung [On the importance of outcome criteria in geriatric rehabilitation: Findings from a post-hospital care project on the problem of quality assurance]. *Die Rehabilitation, 30*, 63–68.

Guthrie, S., & Harvey, A. (1994). Motivation and its influence on outcome in rehabilitation. *Reviews in Clinical Gerontology, 4*, 235–243.

Harris, R. E., O'Hara, P. A., & Harper, D. W. (1995). Functional status of geriatric rehabilitation patients: A one-year follow-up study. *Journal of the American Geriatrics Society, 43*, 51–55.

Hartke, R. J. (1991). The older adult's adjustment to the rehabilitation setting. In R. J. Hartke (Ed.), *Psychological aspects of geriatric rehabilitation* (pp. 73-96). Gaithersburg, MD: Aspen.

Hartke, R. J., & Horowitz, M. (1991). Psychotherapy with the older rehabilitation patient. In R. J. Hartke (Ed.). *Psychological aspects of geriatric rehabilitation* (pp. 229–248). Gaithersburg, MD: Aspen.

Hasselkus, B. R. (1989). Occupational and physical therapy in geriatric rehabilitation. *Physical and Occupational Therapy in Geriatrics, 7*, 3–20.

Hausman, D. M. (1987). Health care: efficiency and equity. In S. F. Spicker, S.R. Ingman, & I.R. Lawson (Eds.), *Ethical dimensions of geriatric care* (pp. 67–78). Dordrecht The Netherlands: Reidel.

Häfner, H. (1986). *Psychische Gesundheit im Alter* [Mental health in old age]. Stuttgart, Germany: Fischer.

Helewa, A., Goldsmith, C. H., Lee, P., Bombardier, C., Hanes, B., Smythe, H. A., & Tugwell, P. (1991). Effects of occupational therapy home service on patients with rheumatoid arthritis. *Lancet, 337*, 1453–1456.

Hiatt, L. G. (1987). Designing for the vision and hearing impairments of the elderly. In V. Regnier & J. Pynoos (Eds.), *Housing the aged* (pp. 341–371). New York: Elsevier.

Horgas, A., Wahl, H.-W., & Baltes, M. M. (1996). Dependency in late life. In L. L. Carstensen, B. A. Edelstein, & L. Dornbrand (Eds.), *The practical handbook of clinical gerontology*. Newbury Park, NJ: Sage.

Horn, J. L., & Hofer, S. M. (1992). Major abilities and development in the adult period. In R. J. Sternberg & C. A. Berg (Eds.), *Intellectual development* (pp. 44–99). New York: Cambridge University Press.

Hui, E., Lum, C. M., Woo, J., Or, K. H., & Kay, R. L. (1995). Outcomes of elderly stroke patients. Day hospital versus conventional medical management. *Stroke, 26*, 1616–1619.

Humes, L. E., & Christopherson, L. (1991). Speech identification difficulties of hearing-impaired elderly persons: The contributions of auditory processing deficits. *Journal of Speech and Hearing Research, 34*, 686–693.

Hussian, R. A. & Davis, R. L. (1985). *Responsive care.* Champain, IL: Research Press.

Jamison, R. N., & Virts, K. L. (1990). The influence of family support on chronic pain. *Behaviour Research and Therapy, 28*, 283-287.

Jette, A. M. (1996). Disability trends and transitions. In R. H. Binstock & L. K. George (Eds.), *Handbook of aging and the social sciences* (4th ed., pp. 94–116). San Diego, CA: Academic Press.

Jordan, F. M., Worral, L.E., Hickson, L. M., & Dodd, B. J. (1993). The evaluation of intervention programmes for communicatively impaired elderly people. *European Journal of Communication Disorders, 28*, 63–85.

Jordan, J., & Schmidt, M. (1988). Rehabilitationspsychologische Aspekte bei Erkrankungen des rheumatischen Formenkreises [Psychological aspects of rheumatic diseases relevant for rehabilitation]. In U. Koch, G. Lucius-Koene, & R. Stegie (Eds.), *Handbuch der Rehabilitationspsychologie* [Handbook of rehabilitation psychology] (pp. 455–478). Berlin, Germany: Springer.

Jørgensen, H. S., Nakayama, H., Raaschou, H. O., Larsen, K., Hubbe, P., & Olsen, T. S. (1995). The effect of a stroke unit: reductions in mortality, discharge rate to nursing home, length of hospital stay, and cost. A community-based study. *Stroke, 26*, 1178–1182.

Kalra, L. (1994). The influence of stroke unit rehabilitation on functional recovery from stroke. *Stroke, 25*, 821–825.

Kaplan, H. (1987). Assistive communication devices. In H. G. Mueller & V. C. Geoffrey (Eds.), *Communication disorders in aging: Assessment and management* (pp. 464–496). Washington, DC: Gallaudet University Press.

Kaplan, H. (1989). Communication problems of the hearing-impaired elderly: What can be done? *Pride Institute Journal of Long Term Health Care, 7*, 10–22.

Kaschel, R., Zaiser-Kaschel, H., & Mayer, K. (1992). Realitäts-Orientierungs-Training: Literaturüberblick und Implikationen für die neuropsychologische Gedächtnisrehabilitation [Reality orientation training: Literature review and implications for neuropsychological memory rehabilitation]. *Zeitschrift für Gerontopsychologie und -psychiatrie, 5*, 223–235.

Kaste, M., Palomaki, H., & Sarna, S. (1995). Where and how should elderly stroke patients be treated? A randomized trial. *Stroke, 26*, 249–253.

Kausler, D. H. (1991). *Experimental psychology, cognition, and human aging* (2nd ed.). New York: Springer.

Keitel, W. (1993). Verlauf der Rheumatoid-Arthritis bei Beginn im hheren Lebensalter [The course of rheumatoid arthritis beginning in advanced age]. *Zeitschrift für Rheumatologie, 52*, 138–141.

Kemp, B. (1985). Rehabilitation and the older adult. In J. E. Birren & K. W. Schaie (Eds.), *Handbook of the psychology of aging* (2nd ed., pp. 647–663). New York: Van Nostrand Reinhold.

Kemp, B. (1996). Rehabilitation. In J. E. Birren (Ed.), *Encyclopedia of Gerontology* (Vol 2, pp. 381–386). San Diego, CA: Academic Press.

King, P., & Barrowclough, C. (1989). Rating the motivation of elderly patients on a rehabilitation ward. *Clinical Rehabilitation, 3*, 289–291.

Kline, D. W., & Scialfa, C. T. (1996). Visual and auditory aging. In J. E. Birren & K. W. Schaie (Eds.), *Handbook of the psychology of aging* (4th ed., pp. 181–203). San Diego, CA: Academic Press.

Koh, K., Ray, R., Lee, J., Nair, A., Ho, T., & Ang, P.C. (1994). Dementia in elderly patients: can the 3R mental stimulation programme improve mental status? *Age and Ageing, 23*, 195–199.

Kovar, P. A., Allegrante, J. P., MacKenzie, C. R., Peterson, M. G., Gutin, B., & Charlson, M. E. (1992). Supervised fitness walking in patients with osteoarthritis of the knee. A randomized, controlled trial. *Annals of Internal Medicine, 116*, 529–534.

Kraaimaat, F. W., Brons, M. R. Geenen, R., & Bijlsma, J. W. (1995). The effect of cognitive behavior therapy in patients with rheumatoid arthritis. *Behavior Research and Therapy, 33*, 487–495.

Kruse, A. (1984). Der Schlaganfallpatient und seine Familie [The stroke patient and her/his family]. *Zeitschrift für Gerontologie, 17*, 359–366.

Kruse, A. (1987). Kompetenz bei chronischer Krankheit im Alter [Competence in chronic disease in the aged]. *Zeitschrift für Gerontologie, 20*, 355–366.

Kruse, A. (1992). Rehabilitation in der Gerontologie - theoretische Gundlagen und empirische Forschungsergebnisse [Rehabilitation in gerontology - theoretical base and empirical findings]. In A. Mühlum & H. Oppl (Eds.). *Handbuch der Rehabilitation* [Handbook of rehabilitation] (pp. 333–355). Neuwied, Germany: Luchterhand.

Kruse, A. (1995). Ergebnisse aus einer Längsschnittstudie zu Effekten der ambulanten Rehabilitation [Findings of a longitudinal study aimed at the outcome of home-based rehabilitation]. *Zeitschrift für Gerontologie und Geriatrie, 28*, 104–112.

Lachman, M. E., Weaver, S. L., Bandura, M., Elliott, E., & Lewkowicz., C. J. (1992). Improving memory and control beliefs through cognitive restructuring and self-generated strategies. *Journals of Gerontology: Psychological Sciences, 47*, P293–P299.

LaGrow, S. J., & Blasch, B. B. (1992). Orientation and mobility services for older persons. In A. Orr (Ed.), *Vision and aging: Crossroads for service delivery* (pp. 255–288). New York: American Foundation for the Blind.

Langhorne, P., Williams, B. O., Gilchrist, W., & Howie, K. (1993). Do stroke units save lives? *Lancet, 342*, 395–398.

Lawton, M. P. (1982). Competence, environmental press, and the adaption of older people. In M. P. Lawton, P. G. Windley, & T. O. Byerts (Eds.), *Aging and the environment. Theoretical approaches* (pp. 33–59). New York: Springer.

Lawton, M. P. (1989). Behavior-relevant ecological factors. In K.W. Schaie & C. Schooler (Eds.), *Social structure and aging: Psychological processes* (pp. 57–78). Hillsdale, NJ: Erlbaum.

Lawton, M. P. & Brody, E. M. (1969). Assessment of older people: Self-maintaining and instrumental activities of daily living. *The Gerontologist, 9*, 179–186.

Lawton, M. P., & Nahemow, L. (1973). Ecology and the aging process. In C. Eisdorfer & M. P. Lawton (Eds.), *Psychology of adult development and aging* (pp. 619–674). Washington, DC: American Psychological Association.

Lawton, M. P., & Simon, B. (1968). The ecology of social relationships in housing for the elderly. *The Gerontologist, 8*, 108–115.

Lawton, M. P., & Teresi, J. A. (Eds.). (1994). *Annual Review of Gerontology and Geriatrics. Focus on assessment techniques.* New York: Springer.

Lee, M. H. M., & Itoh, M. (1990). Rehabilitation. In W. B. Abrams, R. Berkow, & A. J. Fletcher (Eds.), *The Merck Manual of Geriatrics* (pp. 249–273). Rahway, NJ: Merck, Sharp, & Dohme Research Laboratories.

Lehmann, W. (1992). Diagnose und Therapie von geriatrischen Aphasiepatienten nach einem zerebrovaskulären Insult [Diagnosis and therapy of geriatric aphasic patients following cerobro-vascular stroke]. *Zeitschrift für Gerontologie, 25*, 271–277.

Lehr, U. (1993). Erkenntnisse psychologischer Grundlagenforschung für Prävention und Rehabilitation im Alter [Results of psychological basic research relevant for prevention and rehabilitation in old age]. In A. Niederfranke (Ed.), *Fragen geriatrischer Rehabilitation* [Questions of geriatric rehabilitation]. (pp. 39–46). Stuttgart, Germany: Kohlhammer.

Lehr, U. (1996). Psychologie des Alterns [Psychology of aging] (8th ed.). Heidelberg, Germany: Quelle & Meyer.

Lehr, U., Kruse, A., & Kruse, M. (1992). Rheumatische Erkrankungen im höheren Lebensalter - Psychologische Aspekte [Rheumatic diseases in advanced age - psychological aspects]. *Zeitschrift für Rheumatologie, 51*, 290–294.

Lichtenberg, P. A., & Rosenthal, M. (1994). Characteristics of geriatric rehabilitation programs: A survey of practitioners. *Rehabilitation Psychology, 39*, 277–281.

Little, A. (1991). Psychological treatments. In R. Jacoby & C. Oppenheimer (Eds.), *Psychiatry in the elderly* (pp. 400–415). Oxford, UK: Oxford University Press.

Mahoney, F. I., & Barthel, D. W. (1965). Functional evaluation: The Barthel Index. *Maryland Medical Journal, 14*, 61–65.

Marmann, C. (1994). Der geriatrisch Amputierte nach Entlassung aus erfolgreicher Rehabilitation [The geriatric amputee after discharge from successful rehabilitation]. *Die Rehabilitation, 33*, 69–75.

Marsiske, M., Delius, J., Lindenberger, U., Scherer, H., & Tesch-Römer, C. (1996). Sensorische Systeme im Alter [Sensory systems in old age]. In K. U. Mayer & P. B. Baltes (Eds.). *Die Berliner Altersstudie* [The Berlin Aging Study] (pp. 379–403). Berlin, Germany: Akademie Verlag.

Mattussek, S. (1992). Die "cP-Schule Hannover": Entwicklung eines Curriculums und Durchführung einer kontrollierten Studie zur Schulung von Patienten mit einer chronischen Polyarthritis [The "Hannover Chronic Polyarthritis School": Development of a curriculum and conductance of a controlled study of education of patients with chronic arthritis]. *Zeitschrift für Rheumatologie, 51*, Suppl. 1: 41–50.

May, A. E., Upfold, L. J., & Battaglia, J. A. (1990). The advantages and disadvantages of ITC, ITE and BTE hearing aids: Diary and interview reports from elderly users. *British Journal of Audiology, 24*, 301–309.

Mayer-Oakes, S. A., Hoenig, H., Atchison, K. A., Lubben, J.E., De-Jong, F., & Schweitzer, S. O. (1992). Patient-related predictors of rehabilitation use for community-dwelling older Americans. *Journal of the American Geriatrics Society, 40*, 336–342.

McCarthy, P. A., & Sapp, J. V. (1993). Rehabilitative considerations with the geriatric population. In J. G. Alpiner & P. A. McCarthy (Eds.), *Rehabilitative audiology: Children and adults* (2nd ed., pp. 331–373). Baltimore: Williams & Wilkins.

Meier-Baumgartner, H.-P., Nerenheim-Duscha, I., & Görres, S. (1992). *Die Effektivität von Rehabilitation* bei älteren Menschen unter besonderer Bercksichtigung psychosozialer Komponenten bei ambulanter, teilstationärer und stationärer Betreuung [Outcome of rehabilitation with the elderly]. Stuttgart, Germany: Kohlhammer.

Miller, J. A. (1991). *Community-based long-term care:*

Innovative models. Newbury Park, NJ: Sage.
Mosqueda, L. (1996). Geriatric rehabilitation. In L. L. Carstensen, B. A. Edelstein, & L. Dornbrand (Eds.), *The practical handbook of clinical gerontology* (pp. 468–480). Thousand Oaks, CA: Sage.
Nelson, E. A., & Dannefer, D. (1992). Aged heterogeneity: Fact or fiction? the fate of diversity in gerontological research. *The Gerontologist*, *32*, 17–23.
Neuberger, G. B., Kasal, S., Smith, K. V., Hassanein, R., & DeViney, S. (1994). Determinants of exercise and aerobic fitness in outpatients with arthritis. *Nursing Research*, *43*, 11–17.
Olbrich, E., & Diegritz, U. (1995). Das Zusammenwirken von Person- und Umweltfaktoren im Alltag: Eine kritische Diskussion von Aktivitäten des täglichen Lebens und instrumentellen Aktivitäten des täglichen Lebens [On the interaction of person and environment in everyday life: A critical discussion of activities of daily living and instrumental activities of daily living]. *Zeitschrift für Gerontopsychologie und -psychiatrie*, *8*, 199–212.
Olsho, L. W., Harkins, S. W., & Lenhardt, M. L. (1985). Aging and the auditory system. In J. E. Birren & K. W. Schaie (Eds.), *Handbook of the psychology of aging* (2nd ed., pp. 332–377). New York: Van Nostrand Reinhold.
Oswald, W. D., Rupprecht, R., & Gunzelmann, T. (1998). Effekte eines einjährigen Gedächtnis-, Kompetenz- und psychomotorischen Trainings auf die Leistungsfähigkeit im höheren Lebensalter [Effects of a one-year memory, competence and psychomotor training on performance in old age]. In A. Kruse (Ed.), *Jahrbuch der Medizinischen Psychologie. Psychosoziale Gerontologie, Band II: Intervention* [Yearbook of Medical Psychology. Psychosocial gerontology, Vol II: Intervention] (pp. 94–107). Göttingen, Germany: Hogrefe.
Ottenbacher, K. J., & Jannell, S. (1993). The results of clinical trials in stroke rehabilitation research. *Archives of Neurology*, *50*, 37–44.
Parmelee, P. A., & Lawton, M. P. (1990). The design of special environments for the aged. In J. E. Birren & K. W. Schaie (Eds.), *Handbook of the psychology of aging* (3rd ed., pp. 464–488). San Diego, CA: Academic Press.
Pathy, M. S. J. (Ed.). (1991). *Principles and practice of geriatric medicine* (2nd ed.). Chichester, UK: Wiley.
Pearlin, L. I., Aneshensel, C. S., Mullan, J. T., & Whitlatch, C. J. (1996). Caregiving and its social support. In R. H. Binstock & L. K. George (Eds.), *Handbook of aging and the social sciences* (4th ed., pp. 283–302). San Diego, CA: Academic Press.
Regnier, V., & Pynoos, J. (Eds.) (1987). *Housing the aged: Design directives and policy considerations*. New York: Elsevier.
Regnier, V., & Pynoos, J. (1992). Environmental intervention for cognitively impaired older persons. In J. E. Birren, R. B. Sloane, & G. D. Cohen (Eds.), *Handbook of mental health and aging* (2nd ed., pp. 763–792). San Diego, CA: Academic Press.
Reischies, F. M., & Lindenberger, U. (1996). Grenzen und Potentiale kognitiver Leistungsfähigkeit im Alter [Limits and potentials of cognitive performance in old age]. In K. U. Mayer & P. B. Baltes (Eds.), *Die Berliner Altersstudie* [The Berlin Aging Study] (pp. 351–377). Berlin, Germany: Akademie Verlag.
Rentz, D. M. (1991). The assessment of rehabilitation potential: Cognitive factors. In R. J. Hartke (Ed.), *Psychological aspects of geriatric rehabilitation* (pp. 97–114). Gaithersburg, MD: Aspen.
Rodin, J. (1986). Aging and health: Effects of the sense of control. *Science*, *233*, 1271–1276.
Rott, C., Wahl, H.-W., & Tesch-Römer, C. (1996). Zur Bedeutung von Seh- und Hörveränderungen für den Alternsprozess [On the meaning of visual and hearing impairment or the aging process]. In C. Tesch-Römer & H.-W. Wahl (Eds.), *Seh- und Höreinbussen älterer Menschen: Herausforderungen in Medizin, Psychologie und Rehabilitation* [Visual and hearing impairment in old age: Challenges within medicine, psychology, and rehabilitation] (pp. 89–106). Darmstadt, Germany: Steinkopff.
Rubenstein, L. Z., Josephson, K. R., Wieland, D., English, P. A., Sayre, J. A., & Kane, R. L. (1984). Effectiveness of a geriatric evaluation unit. *New UK Journal of Medicine*, *311*, 1664–1670.
Rustemeyer, J. (1983). Rehabilitative Massnahmen [Rehabilitation strategies]. In D. Platt (Ed.), *Handbuch der Gerontologie. Band 1: Innere Medizin* [Handbook of gerontology, Vol. 1, Internal Medicine] (pp. 13–32). Stuttgart, Germany: Fischer.
Salthouse, T. A. (1991). *Theoretical perspectives on cognitive aging*. Hillsdale, NJ: Erlbaum.
Saltz, C. C. (1995). Rehabilitation. In G. L. Maddox (Ed.), *The encyclopedia of aging* (2nd ed., pp. 798–799). New York: Springer.
Sarno, M. T. (1984). Communication disorders in the elderly. In T.F. Williams (Ed.), *Rehabilitation in the aging* (pp. 161–176). New York: Raven Press.
Saudan, Y. (1990). Prinzipien der funktionellen Rehabilitation im Alter [Principles of functional rehabilitation in old age]. In F. Martin & J.-P. Junod (Eds.), *Lehrbuch der Geriatrie* [Textbook of geriatrics] (pp. 696–707). Bern, Switzerland: Huber.
Saup, W. (1993). *Alter und Umwelt. Eine Einführung in die Ökologische Gerontologie*. [Aging and environment. An introduction to environmental gerontology]. Stuttgart, Germany: Kohlhammer.
Schaie, K. W., & Willis, S. L. (1986). Can decline in adult intellectual functioning be reversed? *Developmental Psychology*, *22*, 223–232.
Schaie, K. W., & Willis, S. L. (1993). Age difference patterns of psychometric intelligence in adulthood: Generalizability within and across ability domains. *Psychology and Aging*, *8*, 44–55.
Schneekloth, U., & Müller, U. (1995). *Hilfe- und Pflegebedürftige in Heimen. Endbericht zur Repräsentativerhebung im Rahmen des Forschungsprojekts "Möglichkeiten und Grenzen selbständiger Lebensführung in Einrichtungen."* [Persons with basic care needs in institutions. Research report]. München, Germany: Infratest Sozialforschung und Infratest Epidemiologie und Gesundheitsforschung.
Schneekloth, U., & Potthoff, P. (1993). *Hilfe- und Pflegebedürftige in privaten Haushalten. Bericht zur Repräsentativerhebung im Forschungsprojekt "Möglichkeiten und Grenzen selbständiger Lebensführung."* [Persons with basic care needs in private households. Research Report]. München, Germany: Infratest Sozialforschung und Infratest Epidemiologie und Gesundheitsforschung.
Schulz, R., & Williamson, G. M. (1993). Psychosocial and behavioral dimensions of physical frailty. *The Journals of Gerontology*, *48* (Special Issue), 39–43.
Schütz, R. M. (1993). Geriatrische Rehabilitation—eine Standortbestimmung [Geriatric rehabilitation—A point of view]. In A. Niederfranke (Ed.), *Fragen geriatrischer Rehabilitation* [Questions of geriatric rehabilitation] (pp. 16–20). Stuttgart, Germany: Kohlhammer.
Shawe, D., Hesp, R., Gumpel, J. M., Sambrook, P. N., & Reeve, J. (1993). Physical activity as a determinant of bone conservation in the radial diaphysis in rheumatoid arthritis. *Annals of Rheumatic Diseases*, *52*, 579–581.
Silverstone, B. (1984). Social aspects of rehabilitation. In T. F. Williams (Ed.), *Rehabilitation in the aging* (pp. 59–79). New York: Raven Press.
Simeoni, E., Bauman, A., Stenmark, J., & O'Brien, J. (1995). Evaluation of a community arthritis program in

Australia: Dissemination of a developed program. *Arthritis Care Research, 8*, 102–107.
Smith, C. A., Wallston, K. A., & Dwyer, K. A. (1995). On babies and bathwater: disease impact and negative affectivity in the self-reports of persons with rheumatoid arthritis. *Health Psychology, 14*, 64–73.
Smith, J., & Baltes, P. B. (1996). Altern aus psychologischer Perspektive: Trends und Profile im hohen Alter [Aging from a psychological point of view: Trends and profile in the oldest old]. In K.U. Mayer & P.B. Baltes (Eds.), *Die Berliner Altersstudie* [The Berlin Aging Study] (pp. 221–250). Berlin, Germany: Akademie Verlag.
Smyer, M. A., Zarit, S. H. & Qualls, S. H. (1990). Psychological intervention with the aging individual. In J. E. Birren & K. W. Schaie (Eds.), *Handbook of the psychology of aging* (3rd ed., pp. 375–403). San Diego, CA: Academic Press.
Spicker, S. F., Ingman, S.R., & Lawson, I.R. (Eds.) (1987). *Ethical dimensions of geriatric care; Value conflicts for the 21st century.* Dordrecht, The Netherlands: Reidel.
Steinhagen-Thiessen, E., & Borchelt, M. (1996). Morbidität, Medikation und Funktionalität im Alter [Morbidity, medication, and functionality in old age]. In K. U. Mayer & P. B. Baltes (Eds.), *Die Berliner Altersstudie* [The Berlin Aging Study] (pp. 151–183). Berlin, Germany: Akademie Verlag.
Stephens, S. D. G., & Goldstein, D. P. (1983). Auditory rehabilitation for the elderly. In R. Hinchcliffe (Ed.), *Hearing and balance in the elderly* (pp.174–200). Edinburgh, UK: Churchill Livingstone.
Stuck, A. E., Siu, A. L., Wieland, G. D., Adams, J., & Rubenstein, L. Z. (1993). Comprehensive geriatric assessment: A meta-analysis of controlled trials. *Lancet, 342*, 1032–1036.
Suzman, R. M., Willis, D. P., & Manton, K. G. (Eds.) (1992). *The oldest old.* New York: Oxford University Press.
Svanborg, A. (1988). The health of the elderly population: Results from longitudinal studies with age-cohort comparisons. In D. Evered & J. Whelan (Eds.), *Research and the ageing population* (pp. 3–16). Chichester, UK: Wiley.
Tallis, R. (1992). Rehabilitation of the elderly in the 21st century. The F. E. Williams Lecture 1992. *Journal of the Royal College of Physicians of London, 26*, 413–422.
Tesch-Römer, C. (1997). Psychological effects of hearing aid use in older adults. *Journal of Gerontology. Psychological Sciences, 52B*, P127–P138.
Tesch-Römer, C., & Nowak, M. (1995). Bewältigung von Hör- und Verständnisproblemen bei Schwerhörigkeit [Coping with hearing and communication problems in aural impairment]. *Zeitschrift für Klinische Psychologie, 24*, 35–45.
Tesch-Römer, C., & Wahl, H.-W. (Eds.) (1996a). *Seh- und Höreinbussen älterer Menschen: Herausforderungen in Medizin, Psychologie und Rehabilitation* [Visual and hearing impairment in old age: Challenges within medicine, psychology, and rehabilitation]. Darmstadt, Germany: Steinkopff.
Tesch-Römer, C., & Wahl, H.-W. (1996b). Was es bedeutet, (nicht) hören und sehen zu können [What it means (not) to be able to hear or see]. In C. Tesch-Römer & H.-W. Wahl (Eds.), Seh- und Höreinbussen älterer Menschen: Herausforderungen in Medizin, Psychologie und Rehabilitation [Visual and hearing impairment in old age: Challenges within medicine, psychology, and rehabilitation] (pp. 1–12). Darmstadt, Germany: Steinkopff.
Thomae, H. (1979). The concept of development and life span developmental psychology. In P. B. Baltes & O. G. Brim (Eds.), *Life span developmental psychology* (Vol. 2, S282–S312). New York: Academic Press.
Thomae, H. (1996). *Das Individuum und seine Welt: Eine Persönlichkeitstheorie* [The individual and her/his world] (2nd ed.). Göttingen, Germany: Hogrefe Verlag.
Trezona, R.R., Jr. (1991). The assessment of rehabilitation potential: Emotional factors. In R. J. Hartke (Ed.), *Psychological aspects of geriatric rehabilitation* (pp. 115–134). Gaithersburg, MD: Aspen Publishers.
Tucker, S.J. (1984). Patient staff interaction with the spinal cord patient. In D.W. Krueger (Ed.), *Rehabilitation psychology* (pp. 257–266). Rockvill, MD: Aspen.
US Department of Health and Human Services (1992). *Vital and health statistics: Current estimates from the National Health Interview, 1991. Series 10: Data from the National Health Survey, No. 184.* Hyattsville, MD: National Center for Health Statistics.
Vanderpool, J. P. (1984). Stressful patient relationships and the difficult patient. In D. W. Krueger (Ed.), *Rehabilitation psychology* (pp. 167–181). Rockvill, MD: Aspen.
Vignolo, L. A. (1964). Evolution of aphasia and language rehabilitation. *Cortex, 1*, 344–367.
Vognsen, S. (Ed.) (1976). *Hearing tactics: How hearing impaired persons may solve their hearing problems in their daily life.* Copenhagen, Denmark: State Hearing Centre.
Wade, D. T. (1992). Stroke rehabilitation. In J. G. Evans & T. F. Williams (Eds.), *Oxford textbook of geriatric medicine* (pp. 321–328). Oxford, UK: Oxford University Press.
Wade, D. T., Collen, F. M., Robb, G. F., & Warlow, C. P. (1992). Physiotherapy intervention late after stroke and mobility. *British Medical Journal, 304*, 609–613.
Wade, D. T., & Langton-Hewer, R. (1987). Functional abilities after stroke: measurement, natural history, and prognosis. *Journal of Neurology, Neurosurgery, and Psychiatry, 50*, 177–182.
Wagner, M., Schütze, Y., & Lang, F. (1996). Soziale Beziehungen alter Menschen [Social relations of the elderly]. In K. U. Mayer & P.B. Baltes (Eds.), *Die Berliner Altersstudie* [The Berlin Aging Study] (pp. 301–319). Berlin, Germany: Akademie Verlag.
Wahl, H.-W. (1992). Ökologische Perspektiven in der Gerontopsychologie: Ein Blick in die vergangenen drei Jahrzehnte und in die Zukunft [Ecological perspectives in geropsychology: Viewing three decades backwards and into the future]. *Psychologische Rundschau, 43*, 232–248.
Wahl, H.-W. (1994). Visual impairment in later life: A challenge for environmental gerontology. *Aging and Vision News, 6*, 1–2.
Wahl, H.-W. (1997). *Ältere Menschen mit Sehbeeinträchtigung: Eine empirische Untersuchung zur Person-Umwelt-Transaktion.* [Age-related visual impairment: An empirical study of person-environment transaction]. Frankfurt, Germany: Peter Lang.
Wahl, H.-W., & Baltes, M. M. (1993). Ökopsychologische Aspekte geriatrischer Rehabilitation [Ecological aspects of geriatric rehabilitation]. In A. Niederfranke (Ed.), *Fragen geriatrischer Rehabilitation* [Questions of geriatric rehabilitation]. (pp. 63–69). Stuttgart, Germany: Kohlhammer.
Wahl, H.-W., & Oswald, F. (1996). Schwere Seheinbussen im Alter aus psychologischer Sicht: Belastung und Bewältigungsmöglichkeiten [Severe visual impairment in old age from a psychological point of view: Stress and coping potential].. In C. Tesch-Römer & H.-W. Wahl (Eds.), *Seh- und Höreinbussen älterer Menschen: Herausforderungen in Medizin, Psychologie und Rehabilitation* [Visual and hearing impairment in old age: Challenges within medicine, psychology, and rehabilitation] (pp. 127–148). Darmstadt, Germany: Steinkopff.
Wahl, H.-W., & Oswald, F. (in press). The person/environment perspective of visual impairment. In B. Silverstone, M. A. Lang, B. Rosenthal, & E. Faye (Eds.), *The Lighthouse handbook on vision and rehabilitation.* New York: Oxford University Press.

Wahl, H.-W., & Tesch-Römer, C. (1996). Über die Technik hinaus - Psychosoziale Aspekte der Rehabilitation bei Hör- und Seheinbussen im Alter [Beyond technique - Psychosocial aspects of rehabilitation of hearing and vision loss in old age]. In C. Tesch-Römer & H.-W. Wahl (Eds.), *Seh- und Höreinbussen älterer Menschen: Herausforderungen in Medizin, Psychologie und Rehabilitation* [Visual and hearing impairment in old age: Challenges within medicine, psychology, and rehabilitation] (pp. 203–231). Darmstadt, Germany: Steinkopff.

Weinert, F. E., & Knopf, M. (1990). Gedächtnistraining im höheren Erwachsenenalter - Lassen sich Gedächtnisleistungen verbessern, während sich das Gedächtnis verschlechtert? [Memory training in old age - Improvement of memory performance and memory impairment at the same time?] In R. Schmitz-Scherzer, A. Kruse, & E. Olbrich (Eds.), *Altern - Ein lebenslanger Prozess der sozialen Interaktion* [Aging - A lifespan process of social interaction] (pp. 91–102). Darmstadt, Germany: Steinkopff.

Weinstein, B. E., & Ventry, I. M. (1983). Audiometric correlates of the Hearing Handicap Inventory for the Elderly. *Journal of Speech and Hearing Disorders, 48*, 379–384.

Wiesner, M., & Tesch-Römer, C. (1996). Hörgerätebenutzung im Alter: Der Zusammenhang zwischen Intention und Verhalten [Use of an hearing aid in old age—The link between intention and behavior]. *Zeitschrift für Gerontologie, 26*, 273–279.

Williams, T. F. (Ed.) (1984a). *Rehabilitation in the aging*. New York: Raven Press.

Williams, T. F. (1994). Rehabilitation in old age. In R.P. Abeles, H.C. Gift, & M.G. Ory (Eds.), *Aging and quality of life* (pp. 121–132). New York: Springer.

Willis, S. (1991). Cognition and everyday competence. *Annual Review of Gerontology and Geriatrics, 11*, 80–109.

Willis, S. L. (1996). Everyday problem solving. In J. E. Birren & K. W. Schaie (Eds.), *Handbook of the psychology of aging* (4th ed., pp. 287–307). San Diego, CA: Academic Press.

Willis, S. L., Blieszner, R., & Baltes, P. B. (1981). Intellectual training research in aging: Modification of performance on the fluid ability of figural relations. *Journal of Educational Psychology, 73*, 41–50.

Willott, J.F. (1991). *Aging and the auditory system: Anatomy, physiology, and psychophysics.* San Diego, CA: Singular Publishers.

Wisocki, P. A. (Ed.) (1991). *Handbook of clinical behavior therapy with the elderly client.* New York: Plenum.

World Health Organisation. (1980). *International classification of impairments, disabilities and handicaps.* Geneva, Switzerland: World Health Organization.

Wottawa, H., & Thierau, H. (1990). *Lehrbuch Evaluation* [Textbook evaluation]. Bern, Switzerland: Huber.

Yesavage, J. A., Lapp, D., & Sheikh, J. L. (1989). Mnemonics as modified for use by the elderly. In L.W. Poon, D.C. Rubin, & B.A. Wilson (Eds.), *Everyday cognition in adulthood and late life* (pp. 598–611). Cambridge, UK: Cambridge University Press.

Zeiss, A. M., & Steffen, A. M. (1996). Interdisciplinary health care teams: The basic unit of geriatric care. In L. L. Carstensen, B. A. Edelstein, & L. Dornbrand (Eds.), *The practical handbook of clinical gerontology* (pp. 423–450). Thousand Oaks, CA: Sage.

7.24
Interdisciplinary Health Care Teams in Geriatrics: An International Model

ANTONETTE M. ZEISS,
VA Palo Alto Health Care System, CA, USA
and
ANN M. STEFFEN
University of Missouri at St. Louis, MO, USA

7.24.1 INTRODUCTION

As a mental health practitioner, you often receive referrals for the evaluation and treatment of patients who attend a variety of specialty clinics at your medical center. Your most recent referral is to assess and treat Sam P., a 76 year-old man exhibiting symptoms of depression. The Medical Resident treating Sam's cardiovascular disease and arthritis in the hospital's Geriatric clinic had become alarmed and made the referral after Sam began to cry and then refused to answer questions during his most recent medical appointment.

Your clinical decisions regarding the assessment and treatment of Sam P. will be influenced by your model of depression and how it is treated in older adults. Sam's response to treatment, however, will also depend upon your ability to work effectively with professionals from a variety of disciplines who are involved in his care. What difference in your work would there be if you were an official member of the interdisciplinary geriatric clinic team, as opposed to operating separately as a referral service? Few of us have received formal training in the advantages and tasks involved in working in interdisciplinary team settings. This chapter is designed to introduce both the conceptual and practical issues that are a part of interdisciplinary team work.

7.24.2 WHY TEAMS?

Geriatric patients are characterized by two pervasive qualities: their problems are complex and chronic (Binstock & George, 1990; Birren & Schaie, 1990; Dornbrand, Hoole, & Pickard, 1992; Schneider & Rowe, 1990). Problem complexity has many dimensions, including the following: patients may have multiple problems, each exacerbating the others; problems may present differently in geriatric patients than in younger patients; geriatric patients are likely to present inconsistent information about their health concerns; current problems are influenced in complex ways by a lengthy history of medical and/or psychosocial problems; and patients bring complex attitudes towards health care based on their past involvement with other health care providers (Hickey & Rakowski, 1981). Chronic health problems, such as cardiovascular complaints, arthritis, or pulmonary decline, are more typical of older individuals than younger ones (Federal Council on Aging, 1981). While older patients can, of course, also present with acute problems, the typical health care visit is more likely to be prompted by chronic concerns among elders (Woolf, Kamerow, Lawrence, Medalie, & Estes, 1990; Zawadski & Eng, 1988).

Older patients are also more heterogeneous than younger patients. While age typically brings decline, as measured by average capacity, on many biological functions (e.g., visual acuity, cardiac efficiency, speed of male erection, lung capacity), age is also typically characterized by increased variability (Fries & Crapo, 1981). Looking within a group of older adults, the range of capacities will be highly variable for any function, with some individuals displaying better function than the average younger person, whereas others display severe decline. There is also variability within individuals, with some functions remaining at high levels and others showing decline of varying degrees.

Because of these issues, the model of patient care which is the best fit for the management of such patients (i.e., those with chronic, complex problems which present in diverse ways and where stereotyped expectations about patients are inappropriate) is the interdisciplinary team model. This chapter will review basic aspects of interdisciplinary team theory, the natural history of team development, skills necessary for interdisciplinary teamwork, strategies for interdisciplinary team treatment planning, and models of effective interdisciplinary teams.

There has been a growing international awareness of the role of interdisciplinary care in a variety of settings. In Europe, concerns about the care of cancer patients led the Council of Europe in 1987 to create a Select Committee of experts to consider coordination of care for patients. The Committee recommended "the provision of joint professional education as a means of improving teamwork in cancer care ..." (Jones, 1992). The European Health Committee has funded a review of interdisciplinary training of health care staff in member states, and the World Health Organization has supported the development of a network for interprofessional education, based in Linkoping, Sweden (Goble, 1994). In the USA, a network of geriatric education centers (GECs) has been created to provide didactic and clinical training to a wide range of health professionals. These GECs are sponsored by the Bureau of Health Professions of the US Health Resources and Services Administration. Also in the US, the Interdisciplinary Team Training Program (ITTP) is funded by the Division of Veterans Affairs in 12 medical centers to promote direct service and training in a variety of inpatient and outpatient settings.

7.24.3 INTERDISCIPLINARY TEAM THEORY

To say that a group of health care providers is a "team" says very little, as there are many different kinds of teams, organized in different ways to perform different functions. A group that is a team shares a common workplace and set of patients, but teams differ among themselves in their membership composition, commitment to common goals, degree of collaboration in accomplishing team-related tasks, handling of leadership, and the kind of attention paid to team processes. While these factors theoretically could be combined in a large number of ways, in practice the five kinds of teams shown in Table 1 are commonly identified (Takamura; 1985; Takamura, Bermost, & Stringfellow, 1979). Interdisciplinary teams will be described in some detail, along with briefer descriptions of the other kinds of health care team organization.

7.24.3.1 Types of Teams

Unidisciplinary teams (from the Latin "uni," or one) are made up of many providers from a single background, such as a group of public health nurses providing home care. All team members share the same professional skills and training, speak a common language of health care, and function in the same role within the group.

Intradisciplinary teams (from the Latin "intra," or within) are also composed of professionals from one discipline, but include team members from different levels of training and skills within the discipline. For example, a geriatric mental health outpatient clinic team might be composed of a Licensed Psychologist, a postintern, prelicensing psychological assistant, a psychological technician, and two psychology practicum students.

The term *Multidisciplinary team* is often used as if it were synonymous with *interdisciplinary team*, but the two are actually different in very important ways. A multidisciplinary team (from the Latin "multi," or many) is composed of members from more than one discipline, so that the team can offer a greater breadth of services to patients. However, in a multidisciplinary team, each discipline does its own assessment, generates its own treatment plan, implements the plan, evaluates progress, and refines the plan based on their own evaluation (see Figure 1). Team members share information with each other, typically at meetings attended by all team members. There is no attempt to generate or implement a common plan, although members may choose to utilize information obtained in the meeting to revise their own goals or intervention strategies. Multidisciplinary teams are hierarchically organized, that is, there is a designated program "Chief," who is usually the highest ranking professional (commonly an MD). The designated leader is responsible for overseeing the program, leading meetings, resolving conflicts, allocating case load, and so on. Other team members feel responsible only for the clinical work of their discipline, and need not share a sense of responsibility for program function and team effectiveness.

Interdisciplinary teams (from the Latin "inter," or among) also are composed of members from more than one discipline, making a breadth of resources available to patients. Interdisciplinary teams work much more collaboratively, however, as shown in Figure 2. Individual team members do their own assessment, but generally have worked out overall assessment strategies so that patients are not asked redundant questions or submitted to

Table 1 Types of health care teams.

Type of team	*Defining characteristics*
Unidisciplinary team	Members from a single discipline; all members have the same role
Intradisciplinary team	Members from a single discipline, but at different levels of training; roles and responsibilities assigned by training level
Multidisciplinary team	Members from different disciplines; team members have independent roles and meet to share information
Interdisciplinary team	Members from different disciplines; team members have interdependent, collaborative roles and meet to plan treatment and evaluate response
Transdisciplinary team	Members from different disciplines, but team members largely have similar roles and responsibilities

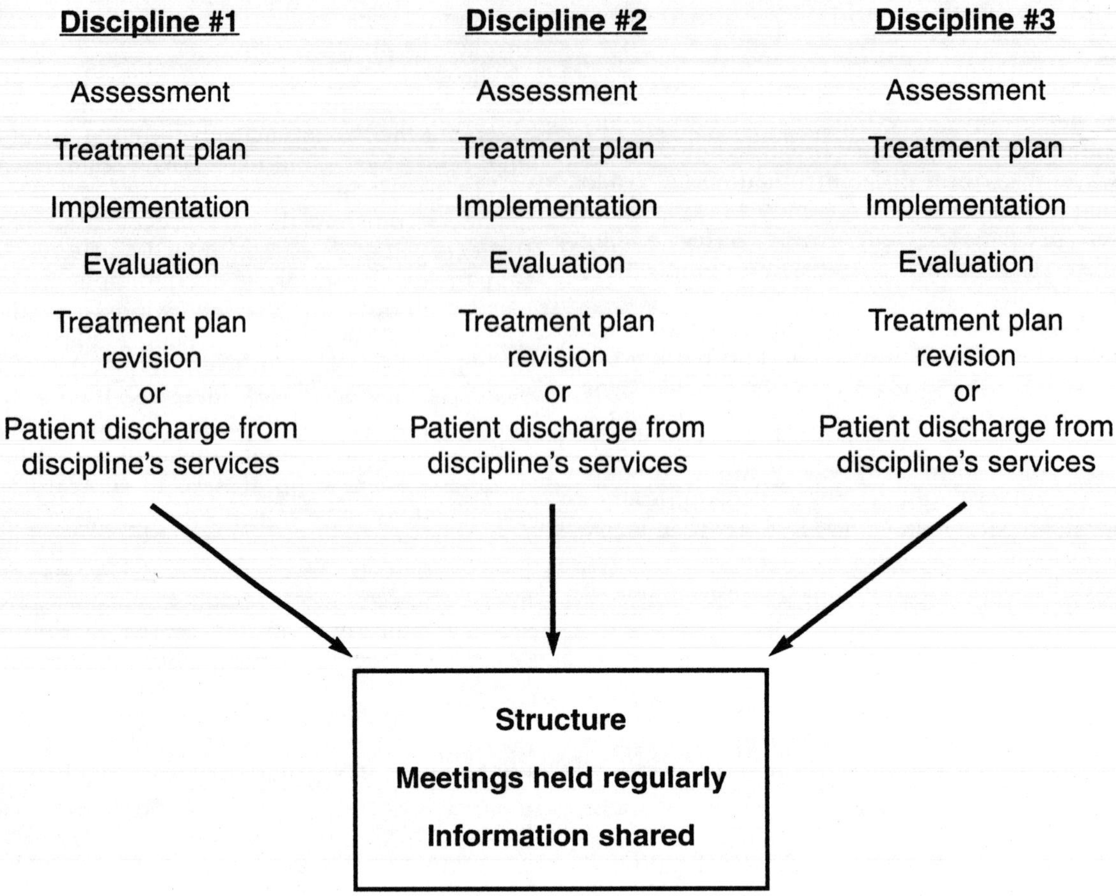

Figure 1 Organization of multidisciplinary team care.

repeated tests. Assessment information is shared with the team as a whole to generate an overall conceptualization of the relationships among biological, psychological, and social aspects of the case (the "biopsychosocial" model). This model is used to generate shared team goals for overall outcomes and to delineate how different disciplines will work together to create desired outcomes. Team members then can implement interventions, either individually or collaboratively as necessary, and evaluate progress. Those evaluations become new assessment data, which are brought back to the team to revise the team's goals and/or strategies for reaching them. This process is repeated as often as necessary until goals are achieved and the patient can either be discharged or a maintenance plan can be put in place.

In an interdisciplinary team, the group as a whole takes responsibility for program effectiveness and team function. Leadership functions are shared among members, with the expectation that everyone must be equally committed to both the clinical content of the program and the process in which team members work together. All team members are assumed to be colleagues, and there is no hierarchical team organization. One member may be designated team "coordinator," but this is understood to be an administrative role and does not imply that the team member has higher status, a stronger say in resolving conflict, or the ability to make unilateral decisions. Because interdisciplinary teamwork requires so much collaboration and consensus decision-making, team members must have a high degree of interpersonal skill. The team must make a commitment to spending time developing effective working strategies and to attending consistently to the process of working together as well as to the quality of the outcomes of their work. Communication skills, role development, leadership skills, conflict resolution skills, and skills for comprehensive conceptualization of cases are necessary for all team members.

This approach has also been labeled "interprofessional care," especially in Europe. A new journal which is rapidly becoming a primary source of articles on interdisciplinary care is titled the *Journal of Interprofessional Care*. Interdisciplinary and interprofessional seem to be interchangeable terms; there do not seem to

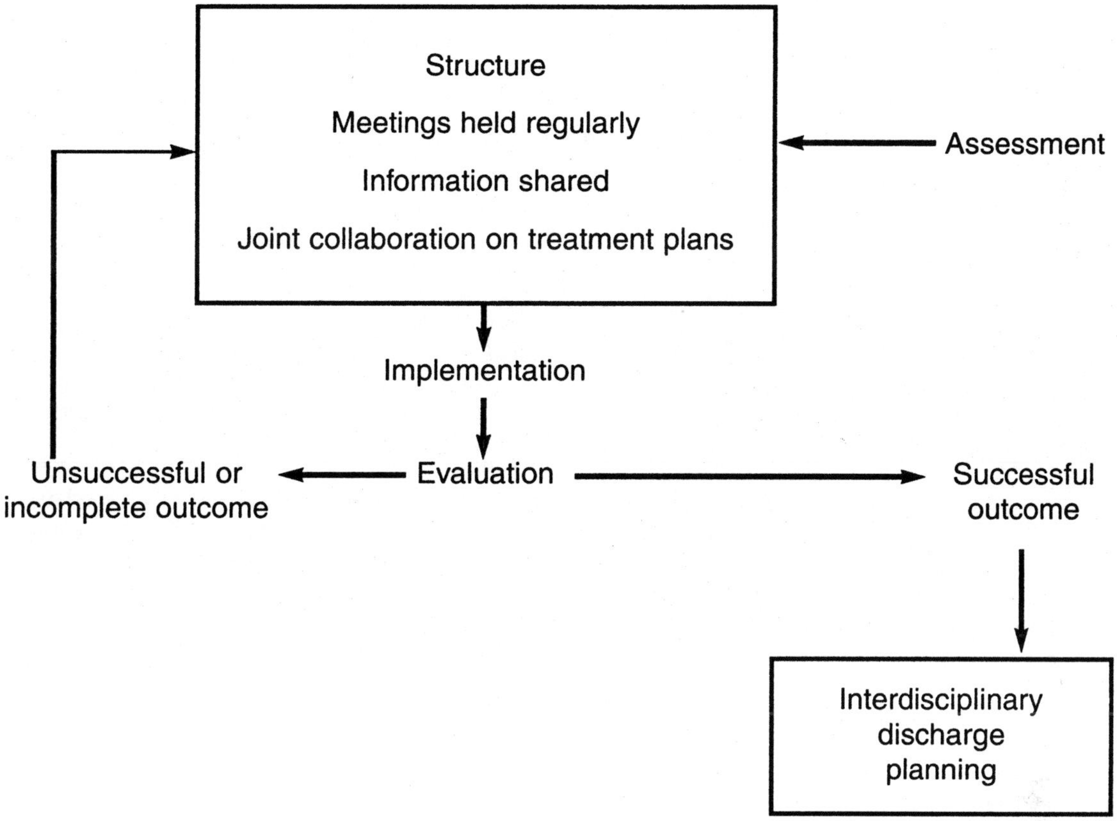

Figure 2 Organization of interdisciplinary team care.

be important conceptual distinctions between them.

In *transdisciplinary teams* (from the Latin "trans," or beyond), disciplinary lines are blurred, and team members share role functions to a high degree. For example, nurses, psychologists, social workers, and occupational therapists in an adult day health care program might all drive the van to bring in patients, run groups, see individual cases for supportive counseling, supervise lunchtime interactions, work with patients on increasing physical and cognitive activity, and so on. This model does not have wide application in geriatric settings, since patients generally need the special skills of each discipline, obtained through extensive specialized training, not just generic skills that many disciplines might share.

7.24.3.2 Advantages of Interdisciplinary Teams

The major reason to adopt a particular model of health care is that it provides the most cost-effective results. In cost-effectiveness analyses, effectiveness should be considered first: for example, does the approach reduce symptoms, increase quality of life, promote health, and prevent future illness? If more than one approach is effective, then it is meaningful to ask what the relative costs of each approach are and to select the program that provides the greatest effectiveness for the least cost. Well-functioning interdisciplinary teams provide cost-effective care by increasing the effectiveness of outcomes, thereby decreasing costs for continued treatment (e.g., Hendriksen, Lund, & Stromgard, 1984). There are four usual ways in which this occurs. First, interdisciplinary teams reduce duplication of services, compared to multidisciplinary teams, because team members plan carefully how to allocate resources and to cover necessary tasks. This may involve the collaboration of more than one discipline but precludes duplication. For example, on a multidisciplinary team both the social worker and the psychologist might begin individual psychotherapy for depression with a patient; this would not happen on an interdisciplinary team. Second, a related cost-saving impact is that problems do not fall through the cracks when care is organized by an interdisciplinary team. It is not uncommon on units staffed by multidisciplinary teams for discharge to be planned and then delayed repeatedly as the staff discover that not all the necessary work has been done; for example, the home care coverage is arranged before the physical therapist has become aware of the need to see the patient, and then home care plans have to be rearranged. A third advantage is that interdisciplinary teams can generate more creative interventions, since the ideas and knowledge of a group can be brought to bear and team members can stimulate each other's ideas. Finally, interdisciplinary teams can reduce institutional costs, because they increase staff morale and reduce staff turnover (Lichtenberg, Strzepek, & Zeiss, 1990; Sbordone & Sherman, 1983). As a result, more continuous care can be provided and the cost of recruiting and training replacement staff is reduced.

While there is a need for more research to examine each of the elements of this argument in favor of the cost-effectiveness of teams, the evidence available does support the interdisciplinary team approach. For example, Zeiss & Okarma (1985) compared interdisciplinary team approaches to multidisciplinary care in an outpatient rheumatology clinic setting. Interdisciplinary team approaches were shown to improve patient outcomes on measures of quality of life (such as life satisfaction, self-rated pain, and depression) and measures of health care utilization (e.g., inpatient stays, the most costly care delivery modality). Another study in Sweden compared the outcomes of two groups of female outpatients with rheumatoid arthritis; one group had interdisciplinary care and the other standard care by a rheumatologist. While there were no significant differences in joint function or disease activity, overall health improved significantly over one year only in the interdisciplinary group (Ahlmen, Sullivan, & Bjelle, 1988). Other research showing the effectiveness and/or cost-effectiveness of interdisciplinary teams is reviewed in Lichtenberg (1994) and West and Poulton (1997).

Concern is sometimes expressed that interdisciplinary teams may be too costly, because of the number of disciplines involved. However, interdisciplinary teams have no specific complement of personnel; it is not necessary that every team have a physician, nurse, psychologist, social worker, pharmacist, occupational therapist, and so on. Teams need to include members of those professions who are essential to provide effective care for the identified patient population. Thus, a well-designed interdisciplinary team involves no more personnel than would normally staff a clinic or inpatient unit for that population. The staff are simply organized differently than they would be if the unit had some other type of team (or no team framework at all).

7.24.3.3 Disadvantages of Interdisciplinary Teams (and Ways to Deal With Them)

Even though interdisciplinary teams can be effective, they are not necessarily the treatment of choice in all care settings. Settings where patients have simple, routine problems would probably benefit more from some other form of care, since in-depth discussion of each case is unnecessary if everyone is going to receive essentially the same straightforward intervention. A clinic offering acute care to generally healthy adults, for example, is best staffed by nurses working with physicians; adding staff and meetings for the majority of the presenting concerns would serve no useful purpose. If a 40-year-old woman comes down with bronchitis, adding collaborative care from a social worker, pharmacist, psychologist, and other disciplines to a routine medical visit is unlikely to be cost-effective or satisfying to either the patient or the providers. It is rare, however, that elderly individuals have straightforward problems or benefit from routinized care. If an 80-year-old woman comes down with bronchitis, it may be essential to know that she is caregiver for a demented husband, what other medications she is taking, what her immune status is, and other issues pertinent to her physical and emotional well-being. Social work, pharmacy, psychology, psychiatry, and/or other team members may be essential in planning not only acute treatment for her bronchitis but also backup care for her demented husband.

The other potential drawback of interdisciplinary teams is that they are not organized to provide rapid response in crisis situations; they are organized to provide care for chronic, complex problems. If a patient calls with an acute problem on Tuesday morning, and the next team meeting is not scheduled until the following Monday afternoon, there must be a way for individual team members, or a smaller set of team members, to make emergency decisions. Interdisciplinary teams can handle this by allocating such authority to team members, with the understanding that the issues will be raised at the next team meeting so that the implications of the crisis can be factored into the team's overall plan and the treatment responsibilities of other team members.

7.24.4 NATURAL HISTORY OF TEAM DEVELOPMENT

Groups do not immediately become well-functioning interdisciplinary teams by deciding to make a commitment to that model of care. Much learning and development within the team must occur, over a period of time which lasts at least several months and sometimes longer. The term "team building" is sometimes used to describe activities during this period, but it is a particularly inappropriate term, because of the implications of the word "building," which could imply that a solid structure, impervious to change, is being built. In fact, good teams learn to change continually and to respond fluidly to new demands, new patients, new staff, new health care policies, and so on, through a coordinated, collaborative process. Thus, the term "team development" is preferable, since it implies an ongoing, fluid process.

7.24.4.1 Processes of Team Development

The sequence of experiences that groups go through in the process of developing cohesion and a high level of function has been described by many authors (e.g., Center for Interdisciplinary Education in Allied Health, 1980; Gersick, 1989; Scholtes, 1988), but most influentially by Tuckman (1965). He identified four processes which usually occur in sequence in the process of team development. He labeled these four processes Forming, Storming, Norming, and Performing; they will be described in more detail. It is important to note that these are processes, not stages. If these four processes are seen as four stages that all teams must go through, the opportunity to understand each team's unique pattern can be obscured. In addition, since these are fluid processes, it is not helpful to think of the team as being in only one stage at any given time. For example, a team may be still Storming with regard to some issues while it has already progressed to Performing in other areas. Furthermore, teams can change by leaping forward or falling back in response to personnel changes, the development of new treatment options, stresses or positive events in team members' lives, or a variety of other events. Nonetheless, these processes can be examined to help in conceptualizing the changes and skills necessary for effective team functioning without falling into a rigid stage theory framework.

7.24.4.1.1 Forming

Teams may be formed when programs develop, expand, or are consolidated. A new team must deal with a number of issues, including which staff are part of the team; which patients will be served; what resources are available, such as hospital beds or outpatient visit rooms; how the team treatment planning process will be organized; and so on. Early in the life of the team, these decisions about content matters take priority, and little attention is paid to the process of working together. Team members typically feel a bit awkward with each other, and are willing to develop team relationships but unsure of what that involves. Team members may have concerns about trust, wondering whether it is all right, for example, to express disagreement or concern about how the group is working together.

7.24.4.1.2 Storming

As the team continues to work together, process issues become unavoidable. It becomes clear that team members do not always agree about content issues, for example, how the team treatment planning should be set up. Differences in personal style may need to be faced: one person may handle concerns directly in ways that others see as too brusque, or a team member may try so hard to be tactful that no one can tell what he or she is saying. Team members may make different assumptions about basic working structure, for example, some may assume that starting the meeting at 10 a.m. means 10 on the dot, whereas others assume it means any time before 10.15 a.m. More substantive issues may arise, for example, different beliefs about whether the first-level intervention for depression should be antidepressant medication or psychotherapy. The group will have to learn to voice disagreement in a way that communicates a desire to stay engaged and work out the issues fairly in a collaborative process. If it cannot, the group will likely disband or fall back to multidisciplinary functioning, where individuals can make autonomous decisions without the need for collaboration and consensus.

7.24.4.1.3 Norming

If the group can work on areas of disagreement constructively, a working strategy will evolve. This strategy can be thought of as "ground rules" or norms which describe the way the group will work together and resolve conflict. Norms can be very specific (e.g., "starting at 10 a.m. means any time before 10.05 a.m.") or more general (e.g., "When team members disagree we will engage in a complex process to show our respect and trust for each other and remind each other that good people can disagree; then we will start to work on the substance of the issue"). If the norms developed are reasonable and effective, the group will set aside time to check on its progress (often referred to as "process time") and to continue clarifying its norms. In addition, content decisions will be made and acted on, and the group will begin to feel cohesive.

If the norms are ineffective, the group will feel stuck and rising frustration will throw the group back into Storming. For example, if the team develops a norm that polite agreement will be voiced on most occasions when disagreement occurs, team meetings may seem peaceful at first, but team members who disagree privately are likely to implement their own ideas rather than the ideas ostensibly agreed on in the meeting. This leads to hard feelings and the belief that meetings waste time; the group will have to learn to express disagreement openly and honestly before effective norms can be established that really resolve issues from the Storming process.

7.24.4.1.4 Performing

Over time, the group will develop a high level of effectiveness, called "performing," in which the team becomes expert at using its process to make decisions and get work done. Ground rules will rarely need to be explicitly stated; the group might seem to be on automatic pilot, especially to outsiders who see a seamless performance with deceptively little effort being needed to make complex decisions. The group will feel cohesive and morale will be high.

7.24.4.1.5 Team evolution

Unfortunately, maintaining function in Performing mode consistently over time is unlikely and not a realistic team goal. Key staff members leave; a needed new discipline is added to the team; the program is moved to a different building; or trainees rotate through at four-month intervals. The group must be able to change accordingly, and it is likely that the team must go back through the four processes of team development before settling into Performing mode again. The new team and its resources and responsibilities must be examined in a Forming phase. Old norms may no longer work (e.g., if the team member whose role it was to draw out quieter team members has left), so there will be a Storming process as the implications of change for the day-to-day life of the team become clear. The team will develop new norms, which maintain as much of what worked before as possible, but which also enthusiastically embrace the different skills and personal style of any new team members. If continual change is a reality, for example, if new trainees appear at frequent intervals, the team will develop metanorms for how to allow trainees to have some impact on the group, without constantly having to redefine the group from scratch.

7.24.4.2 Dilemmas of Team Work

One helpful way to think about the processes groups need to go through to become performing teams is summarized in Table 2. Groups must learn to deal effectively with three inevitable challenges: interdependence, complexity, and disagreement.

The first issue the team faces is interdependence; by definition, an interdisciplinary team seeks to share responsibility for patients by working collaboratively. Early in the life of the team, this usually leads to turf battles, as each team member realizes that his or her skills overlap, often substantially, with the skills of other team members. In well-functioning teams, this will be a source of camaraderie and confidence, but early in the team's development, members can fight over who "should" be doing various activities. For example, teams might argue about whether social work or psychology "should" do family therapy, or whether pharmacy or nursing "should" do home visits to check patients' medicine cabinets and prevent mistakes in the home drug regimen. In the Storming process, these issues will be highlighted in order to develop team-specific agreements (norms) about how such tasks will be distributed and/or shared. The section on team role maps below (7.24.5.3) gives more detail on this process.

The second issue is complexity. By definition, interdisciplinary teams are established to deal with complexity, and case discussions, to be useful, must increase the complexity of the

Table 2 Dilemmas of teamwork.

Theme	*Problem*	*Opportunity*	*Work to be done*
Interdependence	Turf battles	Collaboration	Knowledge of and respect for diversity and shared abilities
Complexity	Endless assessment	Comprehensive care	Conceptualization, key issues, language of function
Disagreement	Destructive conflict	Integration of multiple perspectives	Communication skills

whole group's understanding of the interrelationships of each patient's biological, functional, social, and psychological problems. On a well-functioning team, this leads to a breadth of understanding that allows effective comprehensive care. Early in the life of the team, it can lead to information overload and frustration that cases are discussed seemingly without end. In the Storming process, the team must develop strategies for integrating information and capturing the team's complex understanding of the patient in a written format that facilitates treatment planning and implementation. Section 7.24.6 provides some examples of formats teams can use for developing treatment plans that capture complexity and promote collaborative intervention.

The third issue is disagreement. Interdisciplinary teams rely on healthy conflict, in which the different perspectives and knowledge of team members can be presented. It is illusory to believe that these different perspectives will always be complementary; sometimes they are in direct contradiction. For example, the patient may have told one team member that he is sleeping better since starting a behavioral sleep hygiene program, but told another team member that his sleep problems are unchanged. Teams that are having problems are likely to treat these differences as issues in which one team member is right and the other is wrong, leading to conflict destructive to team cohesion and effective patient care. However, in a functioning team, the team members will recognize that there is direct conflict and see it as an opportunity to learn something more about the patient and themselves. The patient may be trying to manipulate one team member to obtain pain medications. Or the patient may be more demented than the team realized and generating unreliable answers to questions. It is also possible that different team members have different interview styles that elicit different information from the patient, or team members may attend selectively to different kinds of information patients present. The important point to remember is that the ability to consider multiple possibilities and integrate multiple perspectives in handling conflict is the hallmark of a highly functioning team. A detailed analysis of strategies for learning to handle conflict effectively are beyond the scope of this chapter, but important sources giving such analysis are presented in Section 7.24.8.

Thus, interdisciplinary teams must develop the capacity not only to deal with the patient issues that the program was originally designed to treat, but also to deal with the interpersonal world of collaborative care. Skills that are necessary for all team members include knowledge and respect for other team members' abilities, the capacity to conceptualize cases holistically, the expertise to develop written team treatment plans which capture the clinical conceptualization, communication skills, leadership skills, conflict resolution skills, and the capability to anticipate and respond to change.

7.24.5 DEVELOPMENT OF INTERDISCIPLINARY TEAM SKILLS

7.24.5.1 Formal Educational Settings

Since the mid-1980s there has been an increase in university-based gerontology programs. However, these programs may not result in the development of skills needed for working in interdisciplinary environments. Clark (1993) argues that the basic departmental structure of universities can create problems for maintaining a truly interdisciplinary perspective. Interdisciplinary principles and practice cannot be taught in a classroom with didactic methods over a short period of time. Instead, interdisciplinary experiences must be integrated into the program at a variety of points, so that students can master the conceptual frameworks and acknowledge the differing value orientations of different disciplines. In discussing interdisciplinary education embedded in specific university departments, Mitchell (1993) states that exposure to clinical settings is essential for beginning health care students if they are to change their traditional orientation and embrace an interdisciplinary perspective of patient care. For example, only 9% of first-year physiotherapy students acknowledged the importance of being able to communicate with other health professionals (Mitchell, 1993); it appears that these students had already developed specific beliefs about therapeutic practice.

Clark's (1993) guidelines for interdisciplinary education involved the following recommendations for educators who need to: (i) clarify the educational objectives of interdisciplinary programs, (ii) attend to team process issues by including a substantial experiential component, (iii) develop educational methods and materials for communicating across disciplines, (iv) focus on obtaining high-level institutional support for interdisciplinary programs, and (v) recognize that interdisciplinary education represents a true educational revolution.

7.24.5.2 On-the-job Training

The majority of professionals are exposed to interdisciplinary team concepts for the first time when at work. Most interdisciplinary health care teams are not formed with the intent to be time limited, and teams have the additional challenge of continuously changing group membership. Because of these factors, team skills need to be taught on an ongoing basis to individuals with very different beginning skill levels. Drinka (1994) points out that it is often the task of ongoing members to teach new members how to collaborate and assume leadership within the team. This process may be difficult at times, since developing a collaborative set involves integrative problem-solving skills in professionals who may be used to working independently. All team members must feel empowered to participate in conflict resolution. While individual members will have varying degrees of formal power, informal power is also important, particularly for new team members. Informal power can be gained through organizational skills, developing increased knowledge about the other disciplines, demonstrating commitment to the team's mission, and increased tenure (Drinka, 1994). Teams can facilitate this process through inservices and retreats that foster both an increased knowledge of other disciplines and a sense of ownership of the team's mission. Individual members may also protect the rights of new members by drawing them into discussions, for example, by asking their opinion before soliciting the view of established team members. Team members also need to feel comfortable enough with the team to disagree in order to avoid poor decision-making (Heinemann, Farrell, & Schmitt, 1994). In addition to team retreats that provide opportunities for informal social activities, team members can practice brain-storming exercises and rotate the role of "devil's advocate," thus formalizing the importance of alternative views (Heinemann et al., 1994).

7.24.5.3 Role Definition on Interdisciplinary Teams

One of the activities which helps a team progress is the development of a shared understanding of the roles of each team member. An example of such a role map is shown in Figure 3; this role map is adapted from one generated for a hospital-based home care team (HBHC). This Department of Veterans Affairs program serves home-bound older patients and their caregivers; all team members drive to each patient's home to assess needs and provide services. Team members shown in the figure are a physician, four nurse practitioners, a social worker, an occupational therapist, a pharmacist, and a psychologist. Each discipline is represented by an oval, and each oval overlaps with others. Within each discipline's oval are listed the components of their role. In the part of the oval that does not overlap with other ovals appear clinical responsibilities assumed only by that discipline. In areas where two circles overlap, clinical responsibilities appear which either discipline might perform or which the two team members might perform as co-therapists. For example, either psychology or medicine might do cognitive screening.

There are also areas where three, or even more, ovals overlap. In those intersections appear tasks which several team members might perform, for example, nursing, medicine, or pharmacy might all educate patients about the effects and side effects of medications. Figure 3 has been simplified for clarity and does not include all the roles of any of the disciplines, but a more complex version could be generated that did demonstrate the complete range of tasks performed.

Generating and/or examining such a diagram provides several kinds of information. First, it can delineate all the clinical services which patients could receive from this team. Second, it clarifies for each discipline what they offer to the team and what the team will expect them to provide. Third, it clarifies areas which, on a well-functioning team, will be opportunities for conjoint efforts or, in a poorly-functioning team, will be sources of conflict that can be termed "turf battles." If pharmacy and nursing each want to hold the unique right in this setting to educate the patient about medications, for example, the two disciplines are likely to be in conflict about this issue. If each sees the other as a collaborative resource instead, team work (and patient care) will be enhanced. Fourth, Figure 3 suggests which disciplines may have the most difficulty speaking each other's language. The roles of pharmacy and psychology, for example, overlap very little in this setting. In a well-functioning team, members will see these as complementary functions and take pride in being able to provide a range of services well beyond the purview of any discipline. In a poorly functioning team, members will complain about the time taken to discuss issues outside their own scope of practice and compete for time to discuss the issues most closely connected to their own role.

To generate a role map which captures the realities of a specific program and the disciplines on its team takes some time, but is usually well worth the effort. Each team member needs to specify his/her role and present it for team discussion; often this results in adding tasks to the list which the team member did not specify but recognized when mentioned by other team

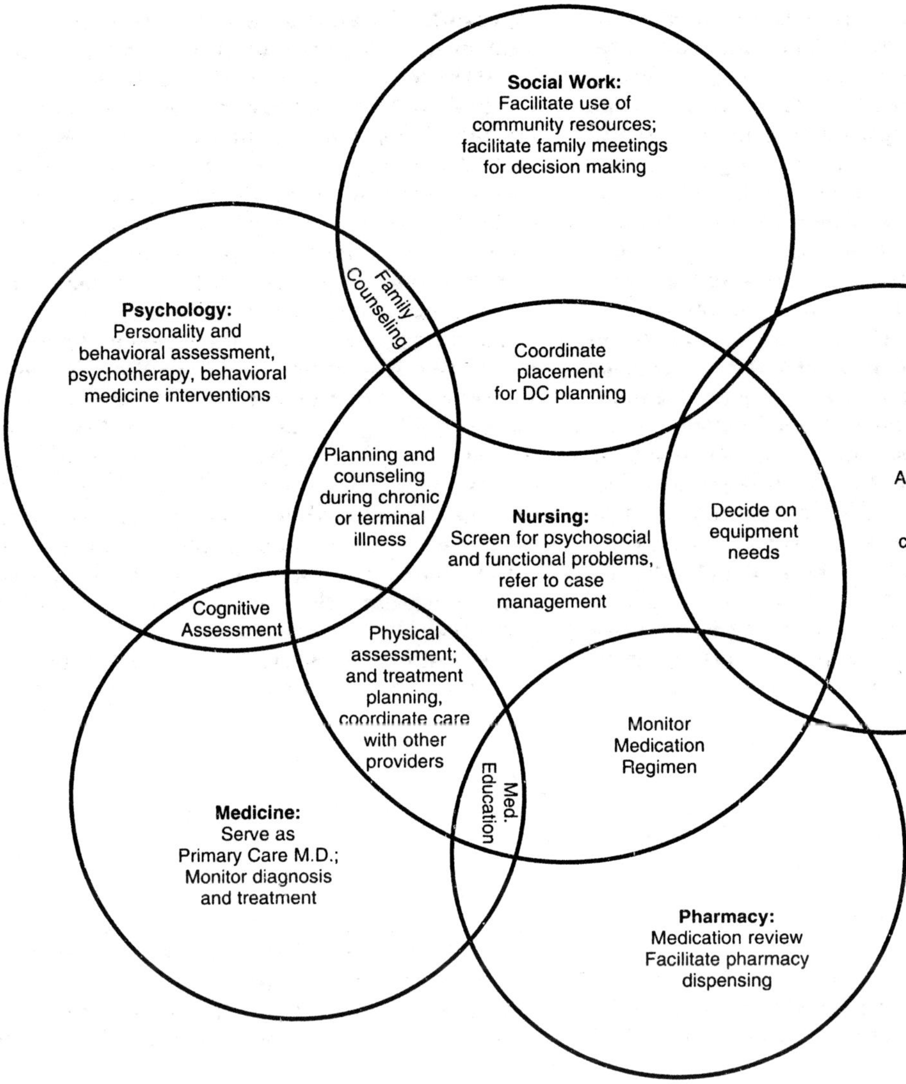

Figure 3 Geriatric interdisciplinary team role map.

members. This also begins to highlight the areas of overlap, as team members recognize some of their own tasks on colleagues' lists. After all disciplines have presented their roles, someone on the team, or a small group, needs to organize the lists to capture graphically areas of overlap and areas of unique function. This document can then become a tool to help in shaping norms and to help in the process of socializing new team members and reaching or returning to the Performing level of team process.

7.24.6 INTERDISCIPLINARY TEAM TREATMENT PLANNING

Interdisciplinary teams generate treatment plans through two interlocking processes. First, the team must be able to conceptualize patients broadly, incorporating all the relevant information and the relationships between different problems. Thus, the team must go beyond simply listing patient concerns on a problem list, to look at the relationships among problems. For example, a patient's depression may be triggered by loss of independence in activities of daily living (ADL) and the depression may be the primary reason (because of the patient's apathy and hopelessness) for medication nonadherence. Psychology or psychiatry could list depression on the problem list; occupational therapy could list difficulties with ADL; pharmacy could list medication nonadherence. But the efforts of each discipline to deal with these problems will be enriched if the linkages among problems are understood.

This type of conceptualization will be demonstrated in more detail in the case study in Section 7.24.7.

Second, the team must have a structured format for guiding and capturing on paper the treatment planning process. That structure should, at minimum, specify which problems will be treated, what the goals of treatment are, what treatment strategies will be used, and which team members will be involved. It is helpful to indicate which team members will be involved by name as well as discipline, to emphasize accountability. The plan may indicate time frames, specifying which interventions should begin immediately, which will be implemented after progress is made on initial problems, and the expected time frame to accomplish the goals. The plan could also include space to update status of progress generally, such as noting if the treatment goals are accomplished

The plan should be available to all team members to guide their activities in implementing their own roles, and it should be available at team meetings to guide discussion. To ensure continuous availability, teams can circulate copies to all members or keep charts in an easily accessible place. To guide team discussions, plans can be shown using overhead transparencies, or circulated at the meeting, or a team member can review highlights of the plan before case discussion.

7.24.7 INTERDISCIPLINARY TEAM CONCEPTS IN ACTION: TEAM RESPONSE TO A GERIATRIC PATIENT WITH MULTIPLE MEDICAL PROBLEMS AND DEPRESSION (SAM P.)

In order to further clarify the use of the team treatment planning process, we return now to the case which opened the chapter, Sam P., a man referred to a mental health practitioner for the assessment and treatment of depression. Let's look at this case in more detail to see how an interdisciplinary perspective influences his treatment. This case also offers the opportunity to contrast how an interdisciplinary team would approach the planning and treatment processes differently from a multidisciplinary team.

Sam P. is a man in his mid-70s of Italian-American background. He has been married to his wife, Pauline, for 40 years: they have been in the same two-storey home for their entire marriage and enjoy gardening, visiting with family and friends, and participating in some church activities. For the last 15 years, Sam has had progressively greater trouble with day-to-day function as a result of his medical problems. His arthritis results in joint pain, especially in his hands, knees, and hips. This joint pain also negatively affects his sexual function. Sam's cardiovascular disease results in impaired blood flow, especially to his legs, to the extent that he gets cramping pain in his legs after walking as little as half a block. Impaired blood flow also has impaired Sam's ability to get and keep an erection. Taken together, these problems have affected almost every aspect of Sam's life. He has trouble getting up and downstairs in his home, he cannot do the gardening he enjoys, he has trouble joining family and friends on outings, and he and his wife have stopped any form of physical intimacy because of his frustration with his sexual function problems.

Sam is taking various medications for his medical problems and comes to the geriatric clinic every three months on average. At the clinic, the medical residents rotate every four months; Sam feels frustrated when he has to retell information to a new doctor. He sometimes gets disgusted and angry with clinic staff, and forgets the questions he has about his medications. On several occasions, Sam has lost track of his medication schedule, became overmedicated, and developed severe nausea, diarrhea, and cognitive confusion. At other times, he has failed to take medication for days at a time, resulting in increased pain and decreased energy.

Sam says that he sometimes feels depressed and useless. He and his wife used to baby-sit their infant granddaughter, but Sam can no longer keep up with a toddler and gets rattled by too much noise and activity. Sam used to enjoy activities in his neighborhood, such as pot-lucks and reading groups, but has stopped going because of his physical problems. His major independent forms of recreation before his decline were driving his friends on outings and attending Elks Club meetings; he has also stopped trying to do these things. He reports that he is often "blue" and tearful, and describes a poor appetite and waking early, about 4 a.m., several days a week.

During the 40 years of their marriage, Sam and Pauline enjoyed physical intimacy and Sam describes feeling sad and frustrated that he "can't perform." Besides problems with erections, Sam often feels tired and is afraid that having intercourse would put too much physical stress on his joints. Sam also admits to feeling self-conscious about the way he looks and has a hard time believing that his wife still finds him sexually attractive.

You can see from this case description that a competent professional in any one discipline cannot address the many issues involved in Sam's physical and mental health. Like many older adults, his treatment should involve the cooperation of a number of disciplines, including nursing, social work, medicine, psychiatry, pharmacy, occupational therapy, and psychology. The psychologist involved in the case would probably conduct a careful mood assessment, then contact the psychiatry consult service to determine if Sam's medication regimen is commonly associated with depression. Several key issues likely to be related to Sam's negative mood would be examined: decreased participation in activities that are both meaningful and pleasurable for him; beliefs that he is no longer useful to others; and disruption of his marital intimacy, both physically and emotionally, as a result of his sexual dysfunction. The psychologist may consider some neuropsychological assessment to evaluate Sam's short-term memory, given that he has forgotten to take some doses of medication in the past and taken too much medicine at other times. There are additional areas that could be targeted for change, such as his frustration and communication difficulties with clinic staff. Psychiatry and psychology may discuss together the usefulness of prescribing antidepressant medications.

The other disciplines involved in his care would have their own concerns and areas of interest. The geriatric medical resident assigned to Sam would continue to evaluate choice of medications with the goals of reducing pain and minimizing joint damage, and maximizing cardiac function and circulation. The nursing staff may want to further educate Sam and his family about his medical diagnoses and the reasons for daily fluctuations in pain and function. Occupational therapy might work with Sam on selecting assistive devices to aid him in difficult tasks (e.g., buttons, zippers, jar lids), create hand splints to protect his hands from further arthritic damage, and plan ways for him to continue important daily activities (e.g., design a table-top garden for which he does not have to kneel). The social worker involved in the case would be aware that Sam and Pauline's two-storey house is a problem because of Sam's swollen knees and peripheral neuropathy, and would discuss housing and long-term plans with them. Sam's episodes of overdosing on medications would be concerning to the pharmacist, who may consider ways to reduce the likelihood of this re-occurring.

So far, it may appear that each professional could execute her or his own treatment plans without the input of the other disciplines (i.e., as a multidisciplinary team). Upon closer inspection, the evaluation and treatment goals in each area overlap in a way that creates the potential for conflict as well as cooperation. For example, the psychologist's suggestions for increasing pleasant activities may appear to directly contradict what Sam has been told by the occupational therapist and the geriatric medical resident. In addition, the psychologist and social worker might be convinced that his medication overdose and seeming confusion during appointments are related to complex issues such as anxiety about his illness, some recent decline in short-term memory that should be monitored, his response to the staffing patterns of the clinic, and a lack of support from his family. This may contradict the pharmacist's approach that the main issue is regulating medication regimens and providing more education about the purpose of each medication. From a different perspective, the medical resident may believe that too much time is spent in team meetings discussing Sam's emotional and psychosocial reactions to his illness. After all, the severity of his symptoms would decline significantly if he would just carefully follow his medication regimen and not engage in strenuous physical activity. These conflicts might be traced to several aspects of the team setting: poor patterns of communication during and outside of team meetings, a decision-making process that minimizes opportunities for discussion or dissent, and a lack of understanding and respect for each discipline's norms and perspectives for patient care.

In contrast to how a multidisciplinary team would approach the patient, the interdisciplinary team in this case would spend more time and attention coordinating Sam's evaluation and care. Through regularly scheduled opportunities for education during team meetings, the interdisciplinary team members would develop a greater understanding of the competencies and perspectives of the other disciplines. This would result in the team's enhanced ability to identify shared treatment goals and the specific needs for collaboration necessitated by each patient.

What team response could be expected in Sam's case? The following section describes an interdisciplinary effort focused on several interwoven goals and strategies. From the information provided in the case description plus some additional assessments, a treatment plan was developed. An important issue that became clear during interdisciplinary discussion was that Sam's care had been fragmented and spread across several specialty clinics, rather than being consolidated in a primary care setting and coordinated. Sam's loss of mobility was a particular focus. He had been seen by orthopedics, who planned hip replacement surgery with the expectation that he would be able to return to most of his prior activities after surgery. However, when seen by cardiology, he was told that hip replacement surgery was unnecessary and that he would be more mobile if his cramping pain (known as claudication) was treated with a medication to improve cardiovascular performance. Sam tried that medication, but stopped using it because of side effects, especially headaches. When he stopped using it, he did not go back to cardiology to try another medication, nor did he go back to orthopedics, because of his pain, difficulty getting to the doctor for appointments, and his general discouragement and depression. Thus, his treatment plan was based on the idea that his care needed to be coordinated, not fragmented, and that regaining mobility would be key to resolving many of the other issues that Sam presented. The three interwoven issues that were targeted as initial goals thus became: (i) decrease depression; (ii) reduce joint pain; and (iii) improve cardiovascular performance. It was expected that improvements in these three areas would result in improved function across a variety of activities, including increased mobility, return to valued social and recreational activities, and improved sexual function with his wife. These functional changes were also considered important aspects of the treatment plan, and are woven into it. The frst two elements of the treatment plan are shown in more detail in Table 3. This also shows how the goals for the first two problems are related to specific intervention strategies, the disciplines working together to provide services, and the time frame for completing each intervention. The reader will also notice from Table 3 that the suggested interventions were linked closely to a jointly developed conceptualization of each problem.

After targeting Sam's main problems and agreeing on etiological models for each, the team identified goals that could be linked to time-specific interventions facilitated by team members. The first, central issue was addressing Sam's discouragement about treatment and alienation from health care providers. A plan was developed to provide Sam with more personalized and consistent care by establishing a stable staff person on the interdisciplinary team as his primary contact person. This staff member (the social worker in this case) could help him use his medical appointments more effectively and efficiently and provide support and encouragement to pursue more vigorous treatment of his medical problems. This intervention also improved the team's overall knowledge of Sam's medical and psychosocial status. The team believed that improving Sam's involvement with care and motivation to participate fully in care were crucial in meeting the second goal of reducing joint pain in his hips by rescheduling hip replacement surgery. In turn, reducing that joint pain was essential to work on increasing mobility.

The team viewed Sam's depression as heavily influenced by his progressively decreasing involvement in pleasurable activities due to chronic pain and decreased mobility. The team encouraged Sam to participate in brief psychotherapy with the team psychologist, with the further expectation that the psychologist and Sam would work with the occupational therapist on selecting activities and environments that would match his interests and degree of physical disability. As his physical situation improved, with surgery and medication, the level of activity could increase, but they could also develop strategies for increased pleasure, satisfaction, and sense of competence even before the surgery. This could help combat his discouragement and passive withdrawal from treatment, just as the closer relationship with the team did. Antidepressant medications were not recommended by the psychiatrist because of the strong situational components tied to his recent depression (i.e., decreased involvement in pleasant activities, chronic pain) and Sam's difficulty in managing his other medications.

Sam was initially surprised at the team's feedback that his feelings of depression were important and could be treated. He had expected someone in the clinic to tell him to "not be so emotional and just deal with it." After talking to the psychologist about the team's view of his depression, Sam attended four individual sessions with the psychologist and learned to identify the activities that were most closely linked with feelings of happiness and satisfaction. Sam and the therapists carefully planned ways to retain the daily activities most meaningful to him and to adapt activities, like gardening, that he had believed must be given up. He reported that, while still feeling sad at times, he was less tearful and more energetic. In addition, his appetite and sleep schedule returned to a more normal basis.

The team also arranged an appointment for Sam and his wife to meet with the geriatric medical resident and the psychologist. During this visit, Sam and Pauline were able to discuss their concerns about the impact of Sam's pain and physical functioning on sexual activity. They agreed to try different body positions and touching that resulted in less pressure on his affected joints. Sam also began to use a warm bath and pain medication just prior to making love and reported that this was helpful. After Sam's hip replacement surgery and improved function with cardiovascular treatment, the therapists helped Sam and his wife work out additional positions and timing for sexual activity and to continue communicating clearly

Table 3 Treatment plan for Sam P.

Problem area	*Treatment goal*	*Intervention*	*Disciplines involved*	*Timeframe*
(1) Depression (linked to discouragement about treatment, reduced pleasant activities, and loss of marital and sexual intimacy)	(1) Increase	(1) Offer following therapies:	(1)	(1)
	(i) Understanding of and confidence in treatment providers and potential treatment outcomes	(i) Consolidate care in geriatrics clinic; appoint a long-term staff member to meet with client every visit to assist in clarifying issues and questions for the medical resident; preclinic discussion of case with resident to ensure knowledge of treatment plan and consistent follow-up	(i) Social worker as long term staff contact; entire team involved	(i) Ongoing
	(ii) Pleasant activities	(ii) Brief psychotherapy using OT as consultant on adapting activities	(ii) Psychology and	(ii) 4 months
	(iii) Level of physical intimacy	(iii) Joint appointments with patient and wife for problem-solving re. sexual activity	(iii) Medicine and psychology	(iii) 6 months
(2) Joint pain, particularly in hips, knees, and hands (believed by the team to be primarily a result of osteoarthritis, exacerbated by lack of joint protection activities)	2(i) Decrease pain	2(i)(a) Reschedule hip surgery, with close communication between geriatrics clinic and orthopedics	2(i)(a) Medicine	2(i)(a) 1 month
		(i)(b) Increase consistent use of pain medication through education and increasing motivation	(i)(b) Pharmacy and psychology	(i)(b) 2 months
		(i)(c) Use hand splints to reduce pain and prevent deformity	(i)(c) OT	(i)(c) 2 months
	(ii) Prevent further problems	(ii) Patient and family education about arthritis self-management	(ii) Nursing and psychology	(ii) 3 months
	(iii) Reduce stress on joints in day to day life	(iii) Assist patient and wife make long range plans about housing if still needed after hip surgery; adapt gardening and daily tasks using joint protection techniques and assistive devices	(iii) Social work and OT	(iii) 6 months, if needed

OT, occupational therapy.

about their expectations and occasional problems.

Sam was able to keep better track of his medications through the suggestions and encouragement of the pharmacist and the nurse, especially after his depression began to resolve with treatment. They helped him understand the differences between different medications in his regimen and set up a procedure for organizing his weekly medication regimen. There were no further instances of taking too much medication, and Sam was better able to report to the geriatric resident on whether different medications were having their intended impact.

Ultimately, Sam did have hip replacement surgery, which resulted in a significant improvement in his pain and mobility. During his postsurgery recovery, the work on depression and maintaining a strong team relationship continued, resulting in a rapid recovery and reestablishment of a wide spectrum of activities, including a return to more social contact. After the surgery, Sam was able to stay in his two-storey house, so the social work intervention which was considered was not, in the end, necessary.

7.24.8 RESOURCES AND TRAINING MATERIALS

While the case of Sam P. demonstrated an interdisciplinary team at work in a hospital setting, this type of case formulation and treatment is important when working with older adults in a variety of mental and physical health care settings. This chapter has introduced the concepts and practice of interdisciplinary teamwork, with the expectation that more resources and experience will be needed for those wanting to apply this information to their own work groups. This section discusses additional written materials and training guides that may be useful.

The disciplines of industrial/organizational psychology, social psychology, and business management have traditionally devoted the most attention to studying group behavior, decision-making, and conflict resolution. However, a separate literature on interdisciplinary team functioning in health care settings has also developed. Some basic early work is covered in an annotated bibliography (Czirr & Rappaport, 1984). Early work will be mentioned, but the chapter will emphasize more recent publications and training approaches. While it is beyond the scope of this chapter to review these literatures in depth, the following section outlines several articles and books that provide a context for understanding interdisciplinary team issues.

7.24.8.1 Outcomes and Descriptions of Interdisciplinary Teams

The literature on team functioning in geriatrics is dominated by articles describing and evaluating interdisciplinary programs (e.g., Rubenstein et al., 1984; Zimmer, Eggert, & Schiverton, 1990) and discussing barriers to effective team functioning (e.g., Saltz, 1992; Chafetz, West, & Ebbs, 1988). Qualls and Czirr (1988) discuss how models for professional functioning differ across disciplines and influence team participation and collaboration. Goldstein (1989) looks at team functioning from the perspective of physicians and offers practical advice for developing team approaches in geriatric health care settings. Drinka and Streim (1994) provide case examples of teams functioning ineffectively and suggest intervention strategies to help teams escape from "health care purgatory." In his book *A Guide to Psychological Practice in Geriatric Long-term Care*, Lichtenberg (1994) does an excellent job advocating for an interdisciplinary approach in long-term care settings. The chapter on creating effective interdisciplinary teams is particularly useful for those needing more information on models for training nursing assistants, organizational interventions in long-term care settings, and specific examples of team-development approaches (including the Department of Veterans Affairs' Interdisciplinary Team Training Program). Lichtenberg also reviews the empirical literature on the relationship between team functioning and patient outcome, noting studies such as the work by Feiger and Schmitt (1979) that demonstrate a relationship between collegiality in interdisciplinary health teams and improved physical, social, and emotional functioning in patients.

7.24.8.2 Team Training Guides

There are a variety of "hands-on" training manuals for those interested in practical advice and examples of team development exercises. Some of these guides target work groups in business, while others are specific to health care settings. Several are particularly helpful. While not specific to health care environments, *The Team-Building Sourcebook* (Phillips & Elledge, 1989) is a comprehensive resource for practicing team consultants and others who are involved in team development. This guide discusses the steps of the team development process and provides numerous examples and activities to be used in addressing the specific needs of a given team. A strength of this resource text is the inclusion of agendas and workshop suggestions for a variety of tasks, giving specific amounts of time for team development activities. For example, the implementation section of the source book outlines the possible contents of team development workshops lasting from four hours to two days. Eleven modules are presented with step-by-step instructions for conducting team development sessions, complete with handouts and materials to be used in flip charts.

The Team Handbook: How to Use Teams to Improve Quality (Scholtes, 1988) is another excellent team-training guide. Although it was also developed with business consulting in mind, the handbook is relevant for health-care professionals. This work discusses quality improvement concepts, then shows how productive meetings and cooperative work groups are important components of increasing team efficacy. Scholtes addresses common problems in team settings (e.g., dominating or reluctant participants, feuding team members) and makes specific recommendations on how to work through these difficulties. The handbook also includes an entire chapter of team development activities and exercises, from handling introductions to helping team members make observations about group processes.

A Guide to Team Development was developed by an interdisciplinary team (Center for Interdisciplinary Education in Allied Health, 1980) at The University of Kentucky's Center for Interdisciplinary Education in Allied Health. This field manual was designed for faculties who train students in team development. It identifies tasks and exercises focused on organizing team meetings, goal setting, decision-making, generating an open and creative environment for team problem-solving, and evaluating the team process.

An assessment tool for evaluating interdisciplinary training efforts is The Interdisciplinary Education Perception Scale (IEPS) (Luecht, Madsen, Taugher, & Petterson, 1990). The IEPS is an attitude inventory that assesses perceptions of professionals, and has four factors: beliefs about competence and autonomy; perceived need for cooperation; perceptions of actual cooperation among different disciplines; and understanding others' values.

The Centre for the Advancement of Interprofessional Postgraduate Education has identified interprofessional training initiatives throughout the United Kingdom (CAIPE, 1989). The University of Newcastle Health Care Research Unit also developed a report that suggested practical steps for increasing collaboration among health care professionals. More broadly in Europe, an organization, the European Network for Development of Multiprofessional Education in Health Sciences (EMPE), has been developed to promote interprofessional education (Goble, 1994). This organization offers expert resources and opportunities for meeting to share educational plans, implementation strategies, and data. Resources for promoting interprofessional collaboration have also been developed in Finland (Lamska, Hietanen, & Lamsa, 1994) and Romania (Stephenson & McCreery, 1994).

7.24.8.3 Communication Training

There are occasions when a group has already accomplished many of the tasks needed to function as an interdisciplinary team, yet team members have difficulty resolving conflict or communicating clearly. Two books are recommended that specifically address conflict resolution and communication skills. Gottman, Notarius, Gonso, and Markman's *A Couple's Guide to Communication* (1976) is a classic in the psychotherapy and counseling literature for very good reasons. Although it targets communication difficulties in married couples, this work provides the rationale and description of exercises that can improve communication in a variety of contexts and settings. The first five chapters in the book, covering skills such as listening, validation, constructively expressing grievances, negotiating agreements, and handling hidden agendas, are especially helpful. A highly recommended book by Fisher, Ury, and Patton (1991), *Getting to YES: Negotiating Agreement Without Giving In*, is based on work done by the Harvard Negotiation Project. *Getting to YES* addresses both the conceptual orientation and practical implications of principled negotiation, a method of negotiation that can be used in a wide variety of circumstances. In principled negotiation (also called negotiation on the merits), negotiators are encouraged to separate the people from the problem, focus on interests instead of positions, generate a variety of alternatives before making decisions, and base results on some objective standard. These authors also discuss handling several common dilemmas in negotiations, including negotiating with someone who is more powerful and working with others who continue to rely on positional bargaining or unprincipled tactics.

7.24.8.4 Factors that Influence Team Functioning

Interdisciplinary teams are based on nonhierarchical interactions, but team members come from a larger social structure that often emphasizes rank and status. Work has been done in areas such as the behavior of low-ranking group members, and cultural and gender differences, as they influence the decision-making strategies of groups. Lichtenberg, Strzepek, and Zeiss (1990) discuss factors that limit the participation of psychiatric aides in treatment teams. They use a particular program, the Veterans Administration's Interdisciplinary Team Training in Geriatrics Program (ITTG; now known as the Interdisciplinary Team Training Program or ITTP), as an example of how to bring about change.

Mechanic (1962) discussed the attributes of the social structure of an organization that led to greater power and influence by lower ranking group members. When these concepts are applied to team members from traditionally lower-ranked disciplines (i.e., recreational therapists, nursing assistants, clerks), Mechanic's work has implications for team interventions. For example, teams can increase opportunities for these staff to interact and have access to other professionals, which will increase their influence in teams and improve the quality of team decisions. The team can also develop ways to recognize explicitly that individuals from low-ranking disciplines often have important expert knowledge that is not readily available to others in the team.

On a related topic, Kirchmeyer and Cohen (1992) discuss the concept of constructive conflict and then demonstrate empirically how specific behaviors in multicultural groups may increase the participation of ethnic minorities. This approach is described in more detail by Tjosvold (1991), who presents some actions that can be taken by designated group leaders to encourage the active involvement of all team members. Kelley and Streeter (1992) review issues and research on gender in organizations, covering such wide topics as trends in work patterns and perceived gender differences in performance and job attitudes.

7.24.9 HELPING WITH INTERDISCIPLINARY TEAM DEVELOPMENT

It should be clear that all interdisciplinary teams, no matter how motivated and talented the members, will have difficulty from time to time. The material presented thus far is intended to provide a theoretical background for how teams function, an example of good interdisciplinary team treatment planning, and information on resources where more can be learned about team functioning and essential skills for teamwork. It is also helpful to consider how to try to have a positive impact as a team member or how to help with program development.

First, there is a need to respect a fundamental tenet of interdisciplinary team development: by definition, no single person can make a group become an interdisciplinary team. Even with enthusiasm about interdisciplinary team ideas and a desire to see them put into action, no single person can make this occur, even if he or she has the institutional power to define program goals and organizational structure. Interdisciplinary teams ultimately depend on and are the embodiment of a powerful principle: people support what they help create. A group can only become an interdisciplinary team if the group members decide themselves that they want to take on the responsibilities of shared leadership and interdependent functioning. An individual's role can be one of bringing the concept to the table and trying to generate shared enthusiasm for it, but it cannot be mandated from above. If the group must function in a way mandated by authority, it is, by definition, not an interdisciplinary team.

If the group embraces the interdisciplinary concept, an individual can help create experiences that will move the group forward. It is usually essential early in the life of the team to generate a vision statement that articulates team members' understanding of program goals, including what patients are to be served, what resources are available to serve them, and the expected impact of the program. This can help the team negotiate the Storming process by providing a grounding in a commonly held set of values.

When the team has a shared sense of purpose, other training experiences largely mirror the organization of this chapter. Team members need to learn about interdisciplinary concepts and to confirm their commitment to shared responsibility for the success of the team. They need to recognize how much there is to know, for example, about each others' professions, about sharing leadership, and about communication skills and conflict resolution. The group optimally will decide together on strategies for appropriate additional training. Team members can train each other, or it may be necessary to bring in a team consultant. It will be especially important to bring in a consultant if the team cannot handle successfully the Storming process, either because the group avoids all conflict or because conflict escalates uncontrollably. There are systems level factors that encourage team members to ignore conflict. For example, factors such as low staff-to-patient ratios, lack of proximate office space that would allow informal staff contact, and few direct incentives for team process meetings

(Drinka, 1994) all point to the benefits of having a consultant assist in the process of team development.

In the training process, it is particularly helpful to find a balance between content and process. During process time, team members can share personal reactions to the tensions and pleasures of interdisciplinary work and discuss experiences with communication styles in the group. During content training, it is very helpful to have the group develop its own unique role map. This also provides an opportunity for each discipline to educate the others about its skills, training experiences, licensure status, and model of health care. The group can also look at different approaches to team treatment planning and choose one that best fits the team's mission and style of working.

Any team member can suggest such strategies and contribute to implementing the group's decisions. If the group does not develop effectively, or one individual seems to make all the suggestions or guide all the training experiences, bringing in a team consultant would be a good idea. The more one person tries to carry a reluctant team, the less interdisciplinary it will be, and the more that person will become the *de facto* leader of a multidisciplinary team. In such cases, the most helpful thing to be done is to relinquish power in order to encourage other team members to join in the process of assessing the team's problems and generating solutions.

7.24.10 SUMMARY

Interdisciplinary teams are a particularly appropriate way to organize health care for geriatric patients, who typically have complex, chronic problems. The interdisciplinary team provides care in which several disciplines coordinate assessment and treatment, so that problems can be dealt with consistently and comprehensively. Interdisciplinary teams are characterized by a nonhierarchical organization, in which responsibility for the effective functioning of the team is shared by all team members. This requires that team members be excellent representatives of and advocates for their disciplines. It also requires that team members have training in team theory, leadership skills, and communication skills, including conflict resolution skills. Interdisciplinary teams go through a process of development. Newly formed teams work out goals and basic models of function; this process usually highlights areas of disagreement among team members in strategies of care and/or personal interaction styles. As groups work out these disagreements, they develop shared norms which define the team's working strategies. With experience, most interdisciplinary teams reach a high level of function and deliver cost-effective care while supporting staff morale.

Interdisciplinary teams come about through the efforts of health care providers who are committed to the idea that patients will be best served when their care is coordinated and provided by team members who challenge, learn from, and rely on each other. Interdisciplinary teams depend on the wise and creative integration of diverse viewpoints. Sometimes those are complementary, but sometimes they are conflicting. The team must learn to value diversity, remain cohesive when viewpoints conflict, and negotiate agreement to which all team members are committed.

7.24.11 REFERENCES

Ahlmen, M., Sullivan, M., & Bjelle, A. (1988). Team versus non-team outpatient care in rheumatoid arthritis. *Arthritis and Rheumatism, 31*, 471–479.

Binstock, R. H., & George, L. K. (1990). *Handbook of aging and the social sciences*. San Diego, CA: Academic Press.

Birren, J. E., & Schaie, K. W. (1990). *Handbook of the psychology of aging*. San Diego, CA: Academic Press.

Center for Interdisciplinary Education in Allied Health (1980). *A guide to team development*. Lexington, KY: College of Allied Health Professions, University of Kentucky.

Centre for the Advancement of Interprofessional Post-graduate Education (CAIPE) (1989). A report of a national survey on interprofessional education in primary health care.

Chafetz, P., West, H., Ebbs, E. (1987). Overcoming obstacles to cooperation in interdisciplinary long term care teams. *Journal of Gerontological Social Work, 11*, 131–140.

Clark P. (1993). A typology of interdisciplinary education in gerontology and geriatrics: Are we really doing what we say we are? *Journal of Interprofessional Care, 7*, 217–227.

Czirr, R., & Rappaport, M. (1984). Toolkit for teams: Annotated bibliography on Interdisciplinary Health Teams. *Clinical Gerontologist, 2*, 47–54.

Dornbrand, L., Hoole, A. J., & Pickard, C. G. (1992). *Manual of clinical problems in adult ambulatory care*. Boston, MA: Little, Brown.

Drinka, T. J. K. (1994). Interdisciplinary geriatric teams: Approaches to conflict as indicators of potential to model teamwork. *Educational Gerontology, 20*, 87–103.

Drinka, T. J. K., & Streim, J. E. (1994). Case studies from purgatory: Maladaptive behavior within geriatric health care teams. *The Gerontologist, 34*, 541–547.

Federal Council on Aging, United States Department of Health and Human Services (1981). The need for long term care: Information and issues. *DHHS Publication (OHDS) 81-20704*. Washington, DC: United States Government Printing Office.

Feiger, S. M., & Schmitt, M. H. (1979) Collegiality in interdisciplinary health teams: Its measurement and its effects. *Social Science Medicine, 13*, 217–229.

Fisher, R., Ury, W., & Patton, B. (1991). *Getting to YES: Negotiating agreement without giving in*. New York: Penguin.

Fries, J. F., & Crapo, L. M. (1981). *Vitality and aging: Implications of the rectangular curve.* San Francisco: Freeman.

Gersick, C. J. (1989). Marking time: Predictable transitions in task groups. *Academyof Management Journal, 32,* 274–309.

Goble, R. (1994). Multiprofessional education: European Network for Development of Multiprofessional Education in Health Sciences (EMPE). *Journal of Interprofessional Care, 8,* 85–92.

Goldstein, M. (1989). Physicians and teams. In R. J. Ham (Ed.) *Geriatric medicine annual* (pp. 256–275), Oradell, NJ: Medical Economics Books.

Gottman, J., Notarius, C., Gonso, J., & Markman, H. (1976). *A couple's guide to communication.* Champaign, IL: Research Press.

Heinemann, G. D., Farrell, M. P., & Schmitt, M. H. (1994). Groupthink theory and research: Implications for decision making in geriatric health care teams. *Educational Gerontology, 20,* 71–85.

Hendriksen, C., Lund, E., & Stromgard, E. (1984). Consequences of assessment and intervention among elderly people: A three year randomised controlled trial. *British Medical Journal, 289,* 1522–1524.

Hickey, T., & Rakowski, W. (1981). Consistency in patients' health and treatment expectations at a Geriatric Clinic. *Journal of the American Geriatrics Society, 29,* 278–284.

Jones, R. V. H. (1992). Teamwork in primary care: How much do we know about it? *Journal of Interprofessional Care, 6,* 25–2 9.

Kelley, K., & Streeter, D. (1992). The roles of gender in organizations. In K. Kelley (Ed.), *Issues, Theory, and Research in Industrial/Organizational Psychology* (pp. 285–337). Oxford, UK: Elsevier.

Kirchmeyer, C., & Cohen, A. (1992). Multicultural groups: Their performance and reactions with constructive conflict. *Group & Organization Management, 17,* 153–170.

Lamska, A., Hietanen, I., & Lamsa, J. (1994). Education for holistic care: A pilot programme in Finland. *Journal of Interprofessional Care, 8,* 31–43.

Lichtenberg, P. (1994). *A guide to psychological practice in geriatric long-term care.* New York: Haworth Press.

Lichtenberg, P., Strzepek, D., & Zeiss, A. (1990). Bringing psychiatric aides into the treatment team: An application of the Veterans Administration's ITTG model. *Gerontology and Geriatrics Education, 10,* 63–73.

Luecht, R. M., Madsen, M. K., Taugher, M. P., & Petterson, B. J. (1990). Assessing professional perceptions: Design and validation of an interdisciplinary education perception scale. *Journal of Allied Health, 19,* 181–191.

Mechanic, D. (1962). Sources of power of lower participants in complex organizations. *Administrative Science Quarterly, 7,* 349–364.

Mitchell, M. (1993). Models of therapeutic practice amongst first year students: A problem for educators in the health professions? *Journal of Interprofessional Care, 7,* 247–252.

Phillips, S., & Elledge, R. (1989). *The Team-Building Sourcebook.* San Diego, CA: University Associates.

Qualls, S., & Czirr, R. (1988). Geriatric health teams: Classifying models of professional and team functioning. *The Gerontologist, 28,* 372–376.

Rubenstein, L., Wieland, D., English, P., Josephson, K., Sayre, J., & Abrass, I. (1984). The Sepulveda VA Geriatric Evaluation Unit: Data on four-year outcomes and predictors of improved patient outcomes. *Journal of the American Geriatrics Society, 32,* 503–512.

Saltz, C. (1992). The interdisciplinary team in geriatric rehabilitation. Special Issue: Geriatric Social Work Education. *Journal of Gerontological Social Work, 18,* 133–142.

Sbordone, R. J., & Sherman, L. T. (1983). The Psychologist as a consultant in a nursing home: Effect on staff morale and turnover. *Professional Psychology: Research and Practice, 14,* 240–250.

Schneider, E. L., & Rowe, J. W. (1990). *Handbook of the biology of aging.* San Diego, CA: Academic Press.

Scholtes, P. R. (1988). *The Team Handbook: How to Use Teams to Improve Quality.* Madison, WI: Joiner Associates.

Stephenson, P., & McCreery, R. (1994). Two heads are better than one: Interprofessional collaboration for capacity building in health systems research in Romania. *Journal of Interprofessional Care, 8,* 57–61.

Takamura, J. (1985). Introduction—Health teams. In L. J. Campbell & S. Vivell (Eds.), *Interdisciplinaryteam training for primary care in geriatrics: An educational model forprogram development and evaluation* (pp. II.64—II.67). Washington, DC: United States Government Printing Office.

Takamura, J., Bermost, L., & Stringfellow, L. (1979). *Health team development team.* University of Hawaii, HI: John A. Burns School of Medicine.

Tjosvold, D. (1991). *The conflict-positive organization: Stimulate diversity and create unity.* Reading, MA: Addison-Wesley.

Tuckman, B. W. (1965). Developmental sequence in small groups. *Psychological Bulletin, 64,* 384–399.

West, M. A. & Poulton, B. C. (1997). A failure of function: Teamwork in primary health care. *Journal of Interprofessional Care, 11,* 205–216.

Woolf, S. H., Kamerow, D. B., Lawrence, R. S., Medalie, J. H., & Estes, E. H. (1990). The periodic health examination of older adults: The recommendations of the US Preventive Services Task Force. *Journal of the American Geriatrics Society, 38,* 817–823.

Zawadski, R. T., & Eng, C. (1988). Case management in capitated long-term care. *Health Care Financing Review,* Annual Suppl., 75–81.

Zeiss, A. M., & Okarma, T. (1985). Effects of interdisciplinary health care teams on elderly arthritic patients: A randomized prospective trial of alternative team models. *Proceedings of the Sixth Annual Conferenceon Interdisciplinary Health Team Care.* (pp. 21–35). Hartford, CN: University of Connecticut School of Allied Health Professions, Nursing, Pharmacy, & Medicine.

Zimmer, J., Eggert, G., & Schiverton, P. (1990). Individual versus team case management in optimizing community care for chronically ill patients with dementia. *Journal of Aging and Health, 2,* 357–372.

Subject Index

Every effort has been made to index as comprehensively as possible, and to standardize the terms used in the index in line with the following standards:

Thesaurus of Psychological Index Terms, APA, Eighth Edition, for the selection of psychological terms.

Thesaurus of ERIC Descriptors, ERIC, Twelfth Edition, for the selection of education terms not covered by the above.

EMTREE Thesaurus for the selection of medical terms not covered by the above.

IUPAC Recommendations for the nomenclature of chemical terms, with trivial names being employed where normal usage dictates.

In general, the index follows the recommendations laid down in BS ISO 999:1996.

In view of the diverse nature of the terminology employed by the different authors, the reader is advised to search for related entries under the appropriate headings.

The index entries are presented in word-by-word alphabetical sequence. Chemical terms are filed under substituent prefixes, where appropriate, rather than under the parent compound name; this is in line with the presentation given in the *Thesaurus of Psychological Index Terms*.

The index is arranged in set-out style, with a maximum of three levels of heading. Location references refer to page number; major coverage of a subject is indicated by bold, elided page numbers; for example,

professional licensing, oral examinations **1234–55**
  and public accountability 266

See cross-references direct the user to the preferred term; for example, character *see* personality

See also cross-references provide the user with guideposts to terms of related interest, from the broader term to the narrower term, and appear at the end of the main heading to which they refer; for example

credentialing
  see also professional certification; professional licensing; recredentialing